This book is dedicated to my daughters, Terri Spence, Lorrie Shives, and Debbie Moore; to my grandchildren, Jeffray, Jennifer, and Zachary; and to the memory of my parents, Pete and Christine Rebraca.

Tamera L. Althoff, MSN, RN
Associate Professor
North Dakota State College of Science
Wahpeton, North Dakota

Kathleen C. Banks, MSN
Assistant Professor AD Nursing
Kent State University, East Liverpool Campus
East Liverpool, Ohio

Catherine Batscha, MSN
Clinical Instructor
University of Illinois, Chicago College of Nursing
Chicago, Illinois

Terry Broda, BSN, RN, CDDN
Nursing Instructor
John Abbott College
Montreal, Québec, Canada

Denise Doliveira, MSN, RN
Assistant Professor
Community College of Allegheny County, Boyce Campus
Monroeville, Pennsylvania

Florencetta Hayes Gibson, PhD, APRN, LMFT
Director, Associate Professor, School of Nursing
University of Louisiana at Monroe
Monroe, Louisiana

Jessica Greni, MSN, RN
ADN Director/Faculty
Howard College
Big Spring, Texas

Leslie E. Guthrie, MS, BSN, RN, CLC, NRP
Assistant Professor of Nursing
Bacone College
Muskogee, Oklahoma

Pamela Gwin, BSN, RN,C
Director, Vocational Nursing Program
Brazosport College
Lake Jackson, Texas

Jane S. Hopson, MSN, RN
Coordinator, Practical Nursing Program
Northeast Alabama Community College
Rainsville, Alabama

Leanna Huscher, MSN, RN
Associate Professor
Kansas Wesleyan University
Salina, Kansas

Linda Kisker, MSN, BSN, RN
Professor of Nursing
Kansas City Kansas Community College
Kansas City, Kansas

Kathryn Kornegay, PhD, RN, CARN-AP
Professor of Nursing
Southeast Missouri State University
Cape Girardeau, Missouri

Dimitra Loukissa, PhD, RN
Assistant Professor
Rush University
Chicago, Illinois

Tamar Jones Lucas, MSN, BSN, RN, BC
Associate Degree Nursing Instructor
Itawamba Community College
Fulton, Mississippi

Jane S. Mahoney, DSN, APRN, BC
Assistant Professor
University of Texas Health Science Center at Houston
Houston, Texas

Sherri Melrose, PhD, RN
Assistant Professor
Centre for Nursing and Health Studies, Athabasca University
Calgary, Alberta, Canada

Norma Ponzoni, PhD (c), RN
Nursing Professor
John Abbott College
Ste Anne de Bellevue, Québec, Canada

iv

Since its inception, the goal has been to produce a textbook that addresses the current concepts used in psychiatric–mental health nursing to foster competency in practicing nurses and other mental health professionals. Several nursing journals were reviewed to obtain information relevant to the content included in this text: *ADVANCE for Nurses, ADVANCE for Nurse Practitioners, American Journal for Nurse Practitioners, American Journal of Nursing, Clinical Advisor: A Forum for Nurse Practitioners,* and the *Journal of Psychosocial and Mental Health Nursing.* Additional journals utilized were *Clinical Psychiatry News, Current Psychiatry,* and *Neuropsychiatry News.* Information regarding psychotropic medication was obtained from several sources including current editions of the *Nurse Practitioners' Prescribing Reference.* Several Internet resources, including the World Health Organization and Centers for Disease Control and Prevention, were utilized to obtain relevant information and current statistics related to various psychiatric–mental health disorders.

Comments by reviewers helped this author to identify specific content that should be included in this seventh edition of *Basic Concepts of Psychiatric-Mental Health Nursing.* Consideration was given to the limited amount of time and various clinical settings in which nurse educators are able to present psychiatric–mental health nursing content. Reviewers recommended:

- Retaining the following threads throughout the text: psychobiological and developmental theories related to specific disorders; economic, spiritual, and religious factors affecting mental health; cultural and ethnic diversity; loss and grief; the nurse's role in clinical psychopharmacology; management of pain and sleep disturbances; client empowerment; and the utilization of behavior therapy as a nursing intervention when appropriate

- Expanding content regarding historical perspectives of the various psychiatric–mental health disorders
- Adding content about forensic nursing practice, the psychiatric–mental health nurse's role in disaster intervention, and the identification and treatment of the impaired nurse
- Expanding content about spirituality, schizophrenia, substance-related disorders, and disorders of childhood and adolescence
- Adding current information regarding psychiatric research that focuses on genetic, biologic, and psychosocial theories
- Discussing current technological advances used in the delivery of care
- Reorganizing the lengthy chapter on psychopharmacology
- Adding current content on clinical psychopharmacology in the disorder chapters, including the practice of "off-label prescribing," the identification of target symptoms for specific drugs, the assessment and treatment of metabolic syndrome, and the importance of recognizing FDA black box warnings as they relate to nursing interventions
- Retaining information related to nursing specialties such as legal, holistic, parish, and addictions nursing
- Retaining content regarding clients who are seriously and persistently mentally ill, including the homeless and incarcerated
- Retaining, and expanding when indicated, pedagogic content such as key terms, learning objectives, nursing research, NCLEX-style multiple-choice questions, critical thinking questions, and Internet resources

As noted in the 6th edition, understanding the neuropathology or pathophysiology of a psychiatric–mental health disorder presents a challenge to student nurses as they enter a new phase of nursing education. Clinical psychopharmacology, which includes a working knowledge of the pharmacodynamics and pharmacokinetics of psychoactive drugs and the potential for drug–drug interactions, is an integral part of psychiatric–mental health nursing care. Furthermore, students must be given the opportunity to feel competent using crisis and disaster intervention techniques because both have become topics affecting the mental health of all age groups.

The availability of settings for student nurse clinical experiences continues to be limited due to changes in Medicaid and Medicare reimbursement, limited insurance coverage for both outpatient and inpatient psychiatric care, and the decentralization of settings where mental health care is provided (eg, private practice, community mental health centers, mobile mental health units, and school systems). For example, insurance carriers require health care providers to obtain precertification prior to an initial consult for clients with mental health concerns. This precertification process often delays or may deny treatment. If precertification is obtained, the insurance carriers then require the health care providers to complete a treatment plan stating the number of estimated visits the client will require, what type of treatment will be initiated, and where the treatment will occur. Finally, the out-of-pocket expenses or co-payments imposed on clients may affect their decision to continue or discontinue treatment. As a result of these changes and limitations in the delivery of psychiatric–mental health care, student nurses are now challenged to apply the basic concepts of psychiatric–mental health nursing in diverse settings.

Text Organization

The text is organized into seven units. An in-depth review of chapter content and a detailed literature search were conducted to provide the student with the most current information available. Suggestions by reviewers were considered and added to enhance content.

Unit I, **Psychiatric–Mental Health Nursing,** includes three chapters. Chapter 1 focuses on the development of self-awareness and addresses student issues and concerns regarding psychiatric clinical experiences. Chapter 2 discusses the history and trends of psychiatric–mental health nursing from 1773 to present. It describes basic concepts such as mental health and mental illness, factors affecting mental

health maintenance, misconceptions about mental illness, different levels of communication used by clients and health care providers, the use of defense mechanisms, and the ANA standards of practice. The current state of psychiatric nursing, including career opportunities and the expanded role of the nurse, is addressed. Chapter 3 addresses the development of psychiatric–mental health nursing theory and its application to practice.

Unit II, **Special Issues Related to Psychiatric–Mental Health Nursing**, consists of five chapters. Chapter 4 discusses spiritual, cultural, and ethnic issues psychiatric–mental health nurses face as they provide care to various diverse clients in the clinical setting. Nursing implications derived from research on ethnopharmacology are also addressed. Chapter 5 discusses the major ethical and legal issues that occur in psychiatric–mental health nursing.

Chapter 6, a new chapter, focuses on the history of forensic nursing, the scope and standards of forensic nursing practice, the forensic nurse's code of ethics, and forensic nursing education. Chapter 7 provides information to familiarize the student with the concepts of loss, grief, and end-of-life care as they are experienced by individuals, families, or their significant others. Chapter 8 discusses the continuum of care available to clients as they progress from the most restrictive clinical setting (inpatient) to the least restrictive clinical setting in which they may reside.

Unit III, **Components of the Nurse–Client Relationship**, includes four chapters. Chapters 9 and 10 discuss the application of the six steps of the nursing process and the use of the *Diagnostic and Statistical Manual of Mental Disorders, Fourth Edition, Text Revision (DSM-IV-TR)* in the psychiatric setting. Chapters 11 and 12 address therapeutic communication and relationships and the therapeutic milieu.

Unit IV, **Interactive Therapies**, consists of three chapters. They describe the different therapeutic approaches used by psychiatric–mental health nurses to meet the needs of clients and their families and significant others. The approaches include Crisis and Disaster Intervention (Chapter 13), Individual Psychotherapy (Chapter 14), and Family, Couple, and Group Therapy (Chapter 15).

Unit V, **Special Treatment Modalities**, includes three chapters. Chapter 16 addresses the science of psychopharmacology and the rationale for the use of various psychoactive agents, including the newest agents available at the time of publication. Generic and trade names, as well as daily dose ranges of various agents, are listed. Chapter 17, Somatic Therapies, discusses the history of ECT, its indications for use in the psychiatric clinical setting, contraindications, adverse effects, advances in the technique, and nursing interventions. A discussion of recent advances in somatic therapies (e.g., VNS, TMS, and MST) is also included. Chapter 18 describes the concept of holistic nursing and discusses the common complementary and alternative (CAM) therapies classified by the National Institute of Health that are used in the treatment of insomnia, pain, stress and anxiety, depression, and cognitive decline.

Unit VI, **Clients With Psychiatric Disorders,** contains 10 chapters (Chapters 19 through 28). The chapter order has been reorganized to introduce the more common psychiatric disorders first, focusing on:

- Anxiety disorders
- Somatoform and dissociative disorders
- Mood disorders
- Schizophrenia and schizophrenic-like disorders
- Eating disorders
- Personality development and personality disorders
- Substance-related disorders
- Sexuality and sexual disorders
- Cognitive disorders
- Delusional and shared psychotic disorders

Each chapter describes the historical perspective of a disorder, if applicable; discusses the etiology of specific disorders, including the discussion of specific theories if appropriate; presents the clinical symptoms and diagnostic characteristics of each disorder incorporating the *DSM-IV-TR* criteria when applicable; focuses on the application of the nursing process; and explains the continuum of care. Most of these chapters contain a drug summary table listing the generic name and trade name of the more common drugs used, the daily dosage range, adverse effects, and nursing implications. Specific target symptoms of certain drugs are listed if the drug is used for stabilization of more than one symptom or is used in off-label prescribing.

Unit VII, **Special Populations,** includes seven chapters (Chapters 29 through 35) that address the needs of clients who exhibit clinical symptoms of:

- Disorders of infancy, childhood, and adolescence
- Ineffective coping with the psychosocial aspects of aging
- Suicidal ideation or behavior or who request physician-assisted suicide
- Dual diagnosis
- Abuse and violence
- Ineffective coping associated with AIDS
- Serious and persistent mental illness

Pedagogic Features

Reviewers recommended that several pedagogic features introduced in the sixth edition be retained in this edition's text. Revisions in each of the features were made when appropriate to reflect changes in or expansion of content. Pedagogic features include:

- Learning objectives at the beginning of each chapter
- Key terms at the beginning of each chapter linked to the expanded glossary
- Self-awareness prompts
- Clinical examples of clients with specific psychiatric–mental health disorders
- Boxes to highlight features such as med alerts, assessment or screening tools, subtypes of a specific disorder, and nursing interventions
- Recurring boxes that address supporting evidence for practice
- Drug summary tables in clinical disorder chapters that include generic/trade name, dosage range, adverse effects, and nursing interventions
- Recurring boxes summarizing the major clinical symptoms and diagnostic characteristics associated with specific psychiatric mental health disorders incorporating the *DSM-IV-TR* criteria
- Recurring boxes highlighting examples of North American Nursing Diagnosis Association (NANDA) nursing diagnoses for specific disorders
- Recurring boxes providing examples of client outcomes for specific disorders
- Key concepts summarized at the end of each chapter

New and Expanded Features and Content

The seventh edition now provides:

- Examples of unique pilot or outreach intervention programs such as In Shape (Chapter 12), Project SMART (Chapter 20), community- and school-based interventions (Chapter 29), and Signs of Suicide Prevention Programs (Chapter 31)

- Examples of current research and surveys pertaining to specific psychiatric mental health disorders including schizophrenia, eating disorders, substance abuse, dementia, and autism
- Expanded content in Chapter 2 describing events during the 21st century that have influenced history and trends in psychiatric–mental health nursing
- New content in Chapter 4 addressing spiritual, cultural, and ethnic issues
- New content in Chapter 5 focusing on ethical and legal issues such as advance psychiatric directives
- One new chapter, Chapter 6, describing forensic nursing practice
- New content in Chapter 7 describing the use of a legal document, 5 Wishes, that enables a dying client to plan his or her end-of-life care
- New and expanded content in Chapter 9 regarding the assessment of supporters or caregivers of clients, cultural assessment of diverse client populations, and assessment of clients exhibiting impaired communication and thought process
- New content in Chapter 10 regarding the concept of evidence-based nursing practice
- New content in Chapter 11 discussing therapeutic interaction with difficult clients who exhibit angry, manipulative, suspicious, demanding, uncooperative, or escalating behavior
- Expanded content in Chapter 12 focusing on interventions related to personal and sleep hygiene, pain management, restraint and seclusion standards for protective care, and therapeutic lifestyle change counseling
- New content in Chapter 13 discussing disaster intervention
- New content in Chapter 14 focusing on nursing diagnosis for individuals, including children and adolescents, participating in individual psychotherapy
- Expanded content in Chapter 15 including the addition of couple therapy
- Expanded content in Chapter 16 describing the science of psychopharmacology
- New and expanded content in Chapter 17 describing the history of ECT, recent advances in somatic therapies, and nursing diagnoses related to clients utilizing somatic therapies
- New and expanded content in Chapter 18 describing practice recommendations by the White House

Commission on Complementary and Alternative Medicine Policy and the establishment of safety classifications of medical herbs by the American Herb Products Association

- New and expanded content in Chapter 20 related to somatoform and dissociative disorders
- New and expanded content in Chapter 21 including an historical perspective of mood disorder, biologic theories related to mood disorder, clinical symptoms and characteristics of mood disorder with postpartum onset, and pain management of clients with a mood disorder
- New and expanded content in Chapter 22 including history of schizophrenia, clinical symptoms of metabolic syndrome, Phase I of the Clinical Antipsychotic Trials Intervention Effectiveness (CATIE) in Schizophrenia, and application of the nursing process
- New and expanded content in Chapter 23 focusing on the history of eating disorders, research, and application of the nursing process
- Expanded content in Chapter 24 regarding individuals at risk for the development of personality disorders, clinical symptoms and diagnostic characteristics, and application of the nursing process
- New content in Chapter 25 including the history of substance use and abuse, prescription drug abuse, Internet addiction, Stages of Change Model, detoxification, and the impaired nurse
- New and expanded content in Chapter 26 discussing sexual aggression in adolescents, new diagnostic labels regarding women's sexual problems, medical management of clients with sexual disorders, and treatment of children with sexually abusive behavioral problems
- New and expanded content in Chapter 27 addressing the history of dementia, dementia with Lewy bodies, behavioral intervention techniques and programs, medication management of clients with cognitive disorders, and research related to cognitive disorders
- New content in Chapter 28 describing the history of delusional and shared psychotic disorders
- New and expanded content in Chapter 29 including history of child and adolescent psychiatry, recent research regarding autism, clinical symptoms of ADHD in adults, attachment theory, child and adolescent psychosis, and community- and school-based interventions

- New and expanded content in Chapter 30 focusing on the history of geriatric psychiatry; assessment of elderly clients, with specific content addressing the treatment of Native American, African American, Hispanic, and Asian American elderly clients; pain management; and stabilization of sleep–rest activity
- New and expanded content in Chapter 31 including new theories, assessment tools for adolescents, suicide prevention programs, and empowerment of survivors of suicide
- Expanded content in Chapter 32 focusing on the application of the nursing process during the treatment of clients with dual diagnosis
- New and expanded content in Chapter 33 discussing child abduction, groups at risk for domestic or intimate partner violence, etiology of youth violence, and hate crimes
- New and expanded content in Chapter 34 related to the history and etiology of HIV/AIDS
- Expanded content in Chapter 35 related to special populations of the homeless, hate crimes against the homeless, and the application of the nursing process including assessment, medication management and education, continuum of care, and empowerment of clients with SPMI
- Updated selected references and suggested readings

Ancillary Package

An Instructor's Resource CD-ROM is available to faculty adopting this text and a back-of-book CD-ROM is available for students. There is also a companion website at thePoint*. **The Instructor's Resource CD-ROM** includes:

- PowerPoint lectures intended to provide significant lecture, classroom, and/or online teaching support.
- Testbank containing approximately 350 multiple-choice NCLEX-style question
- Answers to the NCLEX-style questions found at the end of each chapter
- An Image Bank
- Answers to the movie viewing guides

Student Resource CD-ROM

A back-of-book CD-ROM is an invaluable learning tool that provides an NCLEX alternate format tutorial, clinical simulations, and movie viewing guides, as indicated by the M●VIE viewing GUIDES icon in the text. Also included are a Glossary, updated Internet Resources, and a Spanish-English Audio Glossary.

---

*thePoint is a trademark of WKHealth

ACKNOWLEDGMENTS

Since the inception of the first edition of this textbook began in the early 1980s, the emergence of the biopsychosocial model or paradigm of psychiatric–mental health nursing has challenged authors such as myself to reevaluate the format in which psychiatric–mental health nursing content should be presented. The seventh edition of this textbook would not have materialized without the guidance and support of the staff at Lippincott Williams and Wilkins. I would like to express my sincere appreciation to the following individuals who were readily accessible throughout this project: Margaret Belcher Zuccarini, Senior Acquisitions Editor; Helen Kogut, Senior Managing Editor; Michelle Clarke, Managing Editor; and Debra Schiff, Senior Production Editor.

Recognition is also given to the individuals who reviewed the 6th edition of this text and the proposed manuscript of the 7th edition. Their candid comments and constructive criticism regarding the use of this text in the academic or clinical setting by nursing students were considered during the revision process.

Contents

Psychiatric–Mental Health Nursing

CHAPTER 1 / SELF-AWARENESS

*It takes so much more skill to understand the human mind
and emotions than it does to give a shot.* —FUNDERBURK, 2001

AFTER STUDYING THIS CHAPTER, YOU SHOULD BE ABLE TO:

1. Describe at least two personality traits in yourself that could affect your ability to interact with clients in the clinical setting.
2. Articulate how self-awareness can be an effective tool in the clinical setting.
3. Determine whether your personal issues and concerns about your psychiatric nursing clinical experience have been resolved.

Emotionally stable
Extrovert
Facilitate
Introspection
Introvert
Judgmental
Open-minded
Personality traits
Prejudice
Self-awareness
Stereotyped

Student nurses have described psychiatric–mental health nursing as a challenging experience that provides an opportunity for personal and professional growth. Working with clients who exhibit wide-ranging clinical symptoms of different psychiatric–mental health disorders can elicit a variety of emotional or behavioral responses. Psychiatric clients are often **stereotyped** or categorized by the public as being poor, violent, confused, or unable to care for themselves. Consider these questions as you prepare for your psychiatric–mental health nursing experience:

- Do you have any fears?
- Do you feel nervous knowing that you will be interacting with clients in a psychiatric–mental health clinical setting?
- Do you feel adequately prepared to provide interventions for clients with clinical symptoms of a mental illness?
- Do you have any concerns that have not been answered by your instructor or peers?
- Do you have any **prejudice** or feelings of intolerance about persons who are hospitalized in psychiatric–mental health facilities?

In 1957, a paper entitled "Facilitating Student Learning Through the Teacher's Use of Self" was presented at the curriculum conference of the National League for Nursing (NLN). The paper's author, Catherine Norris, stated that one of the greatest contributions a teacher can make is to help students discover who they are, what they can do, and where they want to go. She also noted that students need someone to listen to them, someone to be concerned about how they feel, and someone to help them obtain satisfaction during their nursing experience (Norris, 1957).

This chapter addresses some of the common issues and concerns you may have as you prepare for this unique experience and addresses the concept of self-awareness.

Frequently Asked Questions by Student Nurses

Psychiatric–mental health nursing clinical rotations may occur in many different settings. Although each setting provides a unique experience, students frequently ask the same basic questions. These questions are addressed in the following sections.

Will the Client Know That I Am a Student Nurse?

Many clients are very aware of the persons responsible for providing care. Thus, they also are aware of the arrival of new persons, such as student nurses, on the unit. The unit staff or clinician is responsible for informing clients about the purpose of the clinical rotation and explaining that the student nurses will be present for a specific time period. Clients who are cognitively impaired, who are withdrawn, or who have difficulty communicating for various reasons also may be assigned to your care to **facilitate** or further enhance or expand your learning experience.

How Do I Introduce Myself?

You have probably become accustomed to wearing a name tag that displays your given name and title (eg, M. Jones, Student Nurse). Additionally, you typically wear some type of uniform that identifies you as a professional student nurse.

In the past, when psychiatric clinical experience occurred in the state hospital setting, student nurses introduced themselves by only their first name because they did not want to provide the clients with any personal information. Today, because clients may have a medical diagnosis in addition to their psychiatric diagnosis, clients may be seen in a variety of clinical settings, such as an outpatient clinic, different units in the general hospital, the emergency room psychiatric triage unit, the practitioner's office, a long-term care facility, or the local community mental health center. Members of the staff in the psychiatric hospital may wear name tags that display a first name only. In other settings, the staff members may wear name tags that state a given name and title (eg, J. Smith, RN). Any identification, such as a name tag worn, and what is presented depends on your educational institution's policy. In any event, informing the client that you are a student nurse is appropriate. (Refer to Chapter 11 for a more thorough discussion of communication skills and the establishment of a therapeutic relationship with a client.)

What Do I Wear?

Street clothes are generally worn in the clinical setting unless uniforms including "scrubs" and laboratory coats are required in areas where both medical and psychiatric–mental health nursing care are provided.

The student nurse may feel uncomfortable at first because he or she has lost the "props" (uniform and stethoscope) that assist in establishing one's identity and ability to communicate with clients. The school of nursing generally provides the student with a list of what is considered to be appropriate attire.

What if I Say the Wrong Thing?

Utilize the communication skills you have developed in previous clinical rotations. Do not be afraid that you might say the wrong thing. If you are sincere and honest, show respect for the client, and display a caring attitude, the staff and clients will give you their trust.

Will I Be Left Alone With a Client?

Your instructor and the unit staff or a clinician will determine which clients are appropriate for an assignment and whether you may be left alone with the client. They will provide you with information about the plan of care, including nursing interventions.

What if the Client Becomes Violent?

A potential for violence exists in any health care setting. However, studies have shown that the risk is greater in psychiatric–mental health care facilities. Nursing staff and clinicians are experienced in assessing the client's potential for violence and have developed specific procedures to follow when a client becomes disruptive or violent. Familiarize yourself with these procedures. Then if a client becomes disruptive or exhibits the potential for violence, notify your instructor and a member of the nursing staff immediately and be ready to follow the staff member's instructions.

Recommendations by Student Nurses

Student nurses made the following recommendations during postclinical conferences when they were asked to evaluate their personal psychiatric nursing clinical experiences:

- Avoid making assumptions about any client's medical or psychiatric history.

- Don't hesitate to approach your clinical supervisor or a staff member with questions about your assigned client's needs or plan of care.
- Feel free to discuss with your instructor any feelings that you have about your clinical rotation or your assigned client.
- Take time to adjust to a slower pace.
- Don't become frustrated with a client who refuses to speak to you.
- Be patient with a client who requires repeated prompting to complete a task.
- Recognize that listening, observing, and self-awareness are important tools that you possess when providing care.

Self-Awareness

Self-awareness refers to the ability to recognize the nature of one's own behavior, attitude, and emotions. It can be an effective tool when interacting with clients who are exhibiting anxiety (Chapter 19), depression (Chapter 21), confusion (Chapter 27), or psychosis (Chapter 22). Have you ever reflected on your **personality traits** or distinguishing characteristics of your personality?

In general, most individuals display extrovert or introvert behavior. An **extrovert** is an outgoing person who relates more easily to people and things in the environment, likes to take charge of situations, and has little difficulty socializing. An **introvert** is a quiet individual who relates better to the inner world of ideas, thoughts, and feelings; prefers to be a follower; and usually lets others initiate and direct interactions. Both of these personality traits can be effective in the clinical setting depending upon the needs of individual clients.

Are you an open-minded individual or do you display a judgmental attitude? Individuals who display an **open-minded** attitude do not make decisions until they are aware of all the facts pertaining to a certain situation. Persons who display **judgmental** attitudes are often inflexible and run the risk of neglecting the perception of others, possibly arriving at an opinion based on their own values without enough facts or enough regard for what other people may feel or think. The student nurse needs to be aware of these traits so that they do not interfere with one's ability to develop a therapeutic relationship with clients.

Most individuals are considered to be **emotionally stable**. That is, they are able to interact with others without displaying undue anger, fear, frustration, or other inappropriate behavior. Nurses need emotional

SELF-AWARENESS PROMPT

This exercise contains several responses a person may exhibit during interactions with other individuals. Check those responses that best describe your behavior and reflect on how such reactions could affect your interactions with clients, peers, or your instructors. When interacting with others, I:

- ☐ Feel uncomfortable offering constructive criticism
- ☐ Hesitate to disagree
- ☐ Evade topics that are uncomfortable
- ☐ Have difficulty responding to negative comments
- ☐ Am embarrassed when given a compliment
- ☐ Enjoy giving directions or explaining a task
- ☐ Am a good listener but will also initiate conversation
- ☐ Accept criticism as a learning experience
- ☐ Avoid making judgemental statements
- ☐ Am cordial and display respect

stability to cope with human suffering, emergencies, and other stresses. They should be caring, sympathetic, responsible, and detail oriented. They must also be able to direct or supervise others, correctly assess a client's biopsychosocial status, and determine when a referral or consultation is required. These qualities are often developed over time, as one matures and engages in interactions with clients and others during clinical experiences. Clients in the psychiatric–mental health clinical setting should receive emotional support as part of their plan of care.

The following Self-awareness Exercise has been designed to help you identify personality traits that you may possess. Consider the examples found in the Self-awareness Prompt. These examples were given to stimulate your **introspection** or self-reflection prior to clinical experience in the psychiatric setting. The examples also should help you to understand attitudes and behaviors displayed by clients. After you resolve basic issues and concerns about this clinical experience, self-confidence in your ability to interact with clients in a variety of settings will grow.

Throughout this text, Self-Awareness Prompts are presented to encourage you to examine attitudes and feelings toward clients exhibiting various clinical symptoms. Critical Thinking Questions and Multiple Choice Questions are also included at the end of each

chapter to enhance your personal and professional growth.

KEY CONCEPTS

◆ Psychiatric–mental health nursing is a challenging experience that provides an opportunity for personal and professional growth.

◆ As student nurses prepare for their psychiatric nursing clinical rotation, they often ask the same basic questions, such as: Will the client know that I am a student nurse?; How do I introduce myself?; What do I wear?; What if I say something wrong?; Will I be left alone with a client?; and What if the client becomes violent?

◆ Practicing self-awareness is an effective way to prepare for interactions with various clients in the psychiatric setting.

For additional study materials, please refer to the Student Resource CD-ROM located in the back of this textbook.

CHAPTER WORKSHEET

CRITICAL THINKING QUESTIONS

1. Reflect back on the first time you were told that part of your nursing experience included a psychiatric nursing clinical rotation. Where were you? Who told you? What was your initial reaction? How did you feel? How did you resolve your feelings?
2. Identify your personality traits. Are you more comfortable performing tasks or relating to people? Are you flexible, or do you prefer an orderly routine? Are you an introvert or extrovert?
3. Discuss how each of the personality traits identified in the previous question could affect your ability to interact with clients in the psychiatric–mental health clinical setting.

REFLECTION

Review the chapter opening quote by Funderburk. Explain its significance to psychiatric–mental health nursing and your role as a student nurse.

NCLEX-STYLE QUESTIONS

1. You are told to wear street clothes and a name tag when providing care for your assigned client at the local community mental health center. Which of the following items of clothing do you think would be most appropriate for a female student to wear in the clinical setting?
   a. Shorts, T-shirt, and tennis shoes
   b. Blue jeans, a shirt, and cowboy boots
   c. Mini-skirt, a sleeveless blouse or shirt, and sandals
   d. Slacks, a sweater, and loafers

2. Your first assignment in the psychiatric–mental health clinical setting is to provide care for a female client who appears sad and verbalizes hopelessness to the staff. You are uncertain how to approach the client. Which of the following actions would be the most effective?
   a. Ask a peer to introduce you to the client.
   b. Wait for the client to approach you to avoid bothering the client.
   c. Ask a staff member what approach is usually effective with the client.
   d. Discuss your feelings with your instructor before approaching the client.

3. One of your peers states that your assigned client looks like a "drug addict." Which of the following best describes your peer?
   a. Introvert
   b. Judgmental attitude
   c. Extrovert
   d. Prejudice

4. You overhear two of your friends talking about mental illness. They agree that mentally ill persons are not capable of living alone or working. Your friends are exhibiting which of the following?
   a. Stereotyping
   b. Prejudice
   c. Introspection
   d. Censorship

5. When assuming the role of a student nurse in the psychiatric–mental health setting, which behavior would be least effective in helping to achieve personal and professional growth?

   a. Completing a task for a client instead of repeatedly prompting him to finish it
   b. Taking time to adjust to a slower pace
   c. Avoiding frustration when a client refuses to interact
   d. Using listening and observing skills throughout the client's care

6. As part of your preparation for your psychiatric–mental health rotation, you and your classmates participate in self-awareness exercises. Which of the following statements would indicate that you and your classmates have developed some self-awareness? Select all that apply.
   a. "I'm basically a quiet, thinking kind of person."
   b. "My lack of spontaneity can be a problem sometimes."
   c. "I usually don't take things at face value."
   d. "My personality is just fine."
   e. "People being inflexible frustrates me."
   f. "I usually try to stay on schedule."

Selected References

Funderburk, A. (2001, Sept/Oct). Through the eyes of a student. *American Psychiatric Nursing Association News, 13*(5).

Norris, C. (1957). Facilitating student learning through the teacher's use of self. Paper presented at Conference of the National League of Nursing. In S. Smoyak & S. Rouslin (Eds.), *Collection of classics in psychiatric nursing literature* (pp. 50–56). Thorofare, NJ: Charles B. Slack.

Suggested Readings

Chapman, R., & Orb, A. (2001). Coping strategies in clinical practice: The nursing students' lived experience. *Contemporary Nurse, 11*(1), 95.

Dunham, K. S. (2004). *How to survive and maybe even love nursing school: A guide for students by students* (2nd ed.). Philadelphia: F.A. Davis.

English, D., & Macontel, E. D. (2001). A handbook for student nurses to guide clinical experiences in the school setting. *Journal of School Nursing, 17*(4), 213–217.

Grenade, E., & MacDonald, E. (1995). Risk of physical assaults among student nurses. *Occupational Medicine, 45*(5), 256–258.

Spouse, J. (2002). *Professional learning in nursing.* Malden, MA: Blackwell Publishing.

Stockhausen, L. J. (2005). Learning to become a nurse: Students' reflections on their clinical experiences. *Australian Journal of Advanced Nursing, 22*(3), 8–14.

CHAPTER 2 / HISTORY AND TRENDS
IN PSYCHIATRIC–MENTAL
HEALTH NURSING

The twenty years in this era (1915–1935) brought an awakening of interest in raising standards of care in psychiatric work, a growing realization of the role of nurses and the nursing profession in the needed improvements, and gradual inclusion in basic nursing curricula of the dominant psychiatric concepts available at this time. —PEPLAU, 1956

LEARNING OBJECTIVES

AFTER STUDYING THIS CHAPTER, YOU SHOULD BE ABLE TO:

1. Distinguish between mental health and mental illness.
2. Identify factors that influence the development of mental health.
3. Evaluate the levels of communication used when a person interacts with others.
4. Define *ego defense mechanism*.
5. Identify examples of defense mechanisms, including the purpose that each serves.
6. Analyze the role of a significant other or support person in maintaining mental health.
7. Define *psychiatric-mental health nursing*.
8. Differentiate Peplau's five phases in the emergence of psychiatric nursing from 1773 through 1936.
9. Interpret the educational objectives of psychiatric nursing during the early 20th century as described by the National League for Nursing (NLN).
10. Describe the purpose of the Scope and Standards of Psychiatric-Mental Health Nursing Practice.
11. Articulate the current state of psychiatric–mental health nursing.

KEY TERMS

Burnout
Ego defense
    mechanisms
Forensic nursing
Mental disorder
Mental health
Mental illness
Nursing informatics
Parish nursing
Privileging process
Psychiatric–mental
    health nursing
Self-actualization
Significant others
Standards of practice
Telehealth

Psychiatric–mental health nursing involves the diagnosis and treatment of human responses to actual or potential mental health problems. It is a specialized area of nursing practice that uses theories of human behavior as its scientific framework and requires the purposeful use of self as its art of expression. It is concerned with promoting optimum health for society. Comprehensive services focus on prevention of mental illness, health maintenance, management of and referral for mental and physical health problems, diagnosis and treatment of mental disorders, and rehabilitation (Haber & Billings, 1993).

According to the American Nurses Association's *A Statement on Psychiatric–Mental Health Clinical Nursing Practice* (1994, p. 7), psychiatric nurses must be able to make rapid comprehensive assessments; use effective problem-solving skills in making complex clinical decisions; act autonomously as well as collaboratively with other professionals; be sensitive to issues such as ethical dilemmas, cultural diversity, and access to psychiatric care for underserved populations; be comfortable working in decentralized settings; and be sophisticated about the costs and benefits of providing care within fiscal constraints.

This chapter serves two major purposes: to introduce the concepts of mental health and mental illness and to describe the historical development of the role of the psychiatric–mental health nurse.

Concept of Mental Health

Although there is no universal definition of mental health, people in the helping professions seem to agree that **mental health** is a positive state in which one is responsible, displays self-awareness, is self-directive, is reasonably worry free, and can cope with usual daily tensions. Such individuals function well in society, are accepted within a group, and are generally satisfied with their lives. Other definitions refer to the ability to solve problems; fulfill one's capacity for love and work; cope with crises without assistance beyond the support of family or friends; and maintain a state of well-being by enjoying life, setting goals and realistic limits, and becoming independent, interdependent, or dependent as the need arises without permanently losing one's independence.

Cultural beliefs influence how mental health and mental illness are determined. For instance, acceptable behavior in one cultural group may or may not be tolerated in another group (Johnson, 1997). See Chapter 4 for detailed information about cultural and ethnic issues.

Factors Influencing Mental Health

Three factors influence the development of mental health: inherited characteristics, nurturing during childhood, and life circumstances.

Inherited Characteristics

Some theorists believe that no one is completely normal and that the ability to maintain a mentally healthy outlook on life is due, in part, to one's genes (Kennedy, Pato, Bauer, Carvalho, & Pato, 1999; Kolb, 1977). Similarly, genetic defects resulting in innate differences in sensitivity and temperament that prompt various responses to the environment may predispose a person to cognitive disability, schizophrenia, or bipolar disorder. Genetic theories are discussed in specific chapters of this book when applicable.

Nurturing During Childhood

Nurturing during childhood refers to the interaction between the family and child, which also affects the development of mental health. Positive nurturing begins with bonding at childbirth and includes development of the feelings of love, security, and acceptance. The child experiences positive interactions with parents and siblings. Negative nurturing includes circumstances such as maternal deprivation, parental rejection, sibling rivalry, and early communication failures. Individuals who are exposed to poor nurturing may develop poor self-esteem or poor communication skills. They may also display socially unacceptable behavior as they seek to meet their basic needs.

Life Circumstances

Life circumstances can influence one's mental health from birth. Individuals who experience positive circumstances are generally emotionally secure and successful in school and are able to establish healthy interpersonal relationships. Negative circumstances such as poverty, poor physical health, unemployment,

SUPPORTING EVIDENCE FOR PRACTICE 2.1
The Relationship Between Environment and Mental Health

PROBLEM UNDER INVESTIGATION / The effects of housing quality on mental health and the ability to function

SUMMARY OF RESEARCH / Researchers collected pre- and postmove data on 31 low-income women with children living in metropolitan areas of Michigan to evaluate the effect of environment on their mental health postmove. The women were moving their families to better-quality housing through participation in Habitat for Humanity. Environmental indicators included structural quality, privacy, indoor climactic conditions, cleanliness, clutter, child resources, and neighborhood quality. The Demoralization Index of the Psychiatric Epidemiology Research Instrument (PERI), a standardized symptoms check list for nonclinical populations, was used to measure psychological distress. The women's PERI scores improved postmove. These findings provided strong evidence that mental health is related to housing quality and an improvement in housing quality can benefit mental health.

SUPPORT FOR PRACTICE / Health care providers have recognized that a relationship between environment and mental health exists, but little scientific research exists to prove how individuals are affected by their surroundings. Nursing research is needed to examine the correlations and relationships that exist between individuals and their surroundings.

SOURCE: Diffendal, J. (2003). Better homes, gardens . . . . and mental health? ADVANCE for Nurse Practitioners. [Online]. Retrieved January 30, 2003, from http://www.advancefornp.com/npfeature2.html

abuse, neglect, and unresolved childhood loss generally precipitate feelings of hopelessness, helplessness, or worthlessness. These negative responses place a person at risk for depression, substance abuse, or other mental health disorders. Supporting Evidence for Practice 2-1 provides information about the possible impact of the environment on mental health.

Characteristics of Mental Health

Abraham Maslow (1970), an eminent psychologist and writer, identified a "hierarchy of needs" to describe an individual's motivation to experience **self-actualization**, or mental health. To achieve self-actualization, a person must progress through five levels (Fig. 2-1). Also, an individual may reverse progression through these levels depending on various circumstances.

According to Maslow, mentally healthy people who achieve self-actualization are able to:

- have positive self-concepts and relate well to people and their environment.
- form close relationships with others.
- make decisions pertaining to reality rather than fantasy.
- be optimistic and appreciate and enjoy life.

FIGURE 2.1   Maslow's hierarchy of needs.

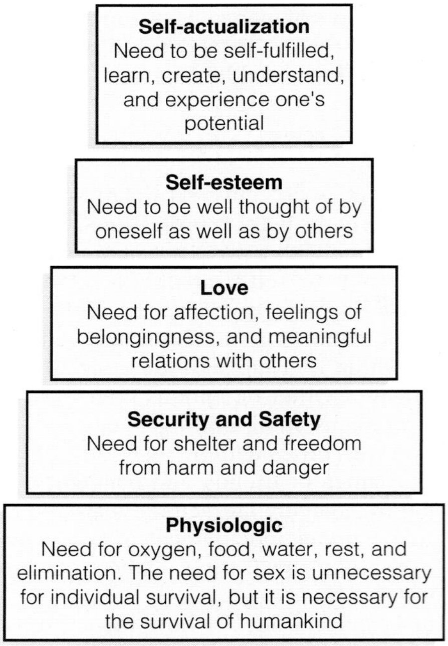

Self-actualization
Need to be self-fulfilled, learn, create, understand, and experience one's potential

Self-esteem
Need to be well thought of by oneself as well as by others

Love
Need for affection, feelings of belongingness, and meaningful relations with others

Security and Safety
Need for shelter and freedom from harm and danger

Physiologic
Need for oxygen, food, water, rest, and elimination. The need for sex is unnecessary for individual survival, but it is necessary for the survival of humankind

- be independent or autonomous in thought and action, relying on personal standards of behavior and values.
- be creative, using a variety of approaches as they perform tasks or solve problems.

In addition, self-actualized individuals display behavior that is consistent as they appreciate and respect the rights of others. They also display a willingness to listen and learn from others, and show reverence for the uniqueness of and difference in others.

Factors Affecting Mental Health Maintenance

Factors that influence the ability to achieve and maintain mental health include engaging in interpersonal communication and resorting to the use of ego defense mechanisms (Powell, 1995). The presence of significant others, or support people, also plays a role in maintaining mental health.

Interpersonal Communication

A relationship is only as good as the intent of the interaction that occurs during interpersonal communications between two or more individuals. Powell (1995) discusses five levels of communication that affect an individual's personal growth and maturity during interpersonal encounters: cliché conversation; reporting facts; revealing ideas and judgments; spontaneous, here-and-now emotions; and open, honest communication. The levels range from 5 to 1, with level 5 indicating superficial communication in which no emotions are shared. Level 1 reflects open communication in which two individuals share their emotions. Box 2-1 briefly summarizes these five levels of communication. Interpersonal communication is discussed at length in Chapter 11.

Ego Defense Mechanisms

Ego defense mechanisms, also referred to as *defense mechanisms,* are considered protective barriers used to manage instinct and affect in stressful situations (Freud, 1946). They may be used to resolve a mental conflict, to reduce anxiety or fear, to protect one's self-esteem, or to protect one's sense of security. Depending upon their use, they can be therapeutic or pathologic, because all defense mechanisms include a distortion of reality, some degree of self-deception, and

---

BOX 2.1 FIVE LEVELS OF COMMUNICATION

Level 5: Cliché Conversation: No sharing of oneself occurs during this interaction. Statements such as "How are you doing?" and "Talk to you later" are superficial. No personal growth can occur at this level.

Level 4: Reporting of Facts: Communicating at this level reveals very little about oneself and minimal or no interaction is expected from others. No personal interaction occurs at this level.

Level 3: Revelation of Ideas and Judgments: Such communication occurs under strict censorship by the speaker, who is watching the listener's response for an indication of acceptance or approval. If the speaker is unable to read the reactions of the listener, the speaker may revert to safer topics rather than face disapproval or rejection.

Level 2: Spontaneous, Here-and-Now Emotions: Revealing one's feelings or emotions takes courage because one faces the possibility of rejection by the listener. Powell (1995) states that if one reveals the contents of the mind and heart, one may fear that such emotional honesty will not be tolerated by another. As a result, the speaker may resort to dishonesty and superficial conversation.

Level 1: Open, Honest Communication: When this type of communication occurs, two people share emotions. Open communication may not occur until people relate to each other over a period of time, getting to know and trust each other.

---

what appears to be irrational behavior. Such mechanisms are supposedly in action by 10 years of age. Table 2-1 provides brief explanations and examples of commonly used defense mechanisms.

Significant Others or Support People

Although mental health can be maintained by engaging in positive interpersonal communication and using ego defense mechanisms, people may also reach out to individuals or groups for support during periods of increased stress or anxiety. Such people are referred to as **significant others** or *support people.* For instance, labor and delivery is generally considered

Review the levels of communication in Box 2.1. Which levels do you use during most interactions? Do the levels differ as you interact with friends, coworkers, families, or clients? If the answer is yes, explain why you think the levels differ.

to be a normal healthy biologic process; however, many women desire the presence or encouragement of a support person, one who assists the woman in coping with the stress and anxiety that may occur during the labor and delivery process as well as during the postpartum recovery period.

Harry Stack Sullivan, an eminent psychiatrist, states that people mistakenly believe that they can solve their own problems and maintain control of their lives

TABLE 2.1 ▮ Definition and Examples of Commonly Used Ego Defense Mechanisms

EGO DEFENSE MECHANISMS	DEFINITION	EXAMPLE
Compensation	Unconscious use of a specific behavior to make up for a real or imagined inability or deficiency, thus maintaining self-respect or self-esteem	Unattractive man selects expensive, stylish clothes to draw attention to himself.
Conversion	Unconscious expression of a mental conflict as a physical symptom to relieve tension or anxiety	Woman experiences blindness after witnessing a robbery.
Denial	Unconscious refusal to face thoughts, feelings, wishes, needs, or reality factors that are intolerable	Woman denies that her marriage is failing by telling her estranged husband that all couples go through marital slumps and "things will be better tomorrow."
Displacement	Unconscious shifting of feelings such as hostility or anxiety from one idea, person, or object to another	Teen-aged son slams door when told he can't attend a concert.
Dissociation	Separation and detachment of a strong, emotionally charged conflict from one's consciousness	Male victim of car-jacking exhibits symptoms of traumatic amnesia the next day.
Identification	Unconscious attempt to identify with personality traits or actions of another to preserve one's self-esteem or to reach a specific goal	Teenager dresses, walks, and talks like his favorite basketball player.
Introjection	Unconscious application of the philosophy, ideas, customs, and attitudes of another person to one's self	Psychiatric client who claimed to be Moses grew a beard and long hair, wore a blanket and sandals, and read his Bible daily.
Projection	Unconscious assignment of unacceptable thoughts or characteristics of self to others	Man who was late for work blames wife for not setting the alarm clock.
Rationalization	Unconscious justification of one's ideas, actions, or feelings to maintain self-respect, prevent feelings of guilt, or obtain social approval	Student states he didn't make the golf team because he was sick.
Reaction-formation	Unconscious demonstration of the opposite behavior, attitude, or feeling of what one would normally show in a given situation	Man who dislikes his mother-in-law is very polite and courteous toward her.

(Continued)

TABLE 2.1 Definition and Examples of Commonly Used Ego Defense Mechanisms *(Continued)*

EGO DEFENSE MECHANISMS	DEFINITION	EXAMPLE
Regression	Retreat to past developmental stages to meet basic needs	Woman acts like a teenager on her first date with a fellow employee.
Restitution	Negation of a previous consciously intolerable action or experience	Man sends flowers to fiancée after embarrassing her at a cocktail party.
Sublimation	Unconscious rechanneling of intolerable or socially unacceptable impulses or behaviors into activities that are personally or socially acceptable	College student with hostile feelings joins the debate team.
Substitution	Unconscious replacement of unacceptable impulses, attitudes, needs, or emotions with those that are more acceptable	A student nurse decides to be a teacher because he or she is unable to master clinical competencies.
Suppression	Voluntary rejection of unacceptable thoughts or feelings from conscious awareness	Student who failed a test states she isn't ready to talk about her grade.
Symbolization	Use of external objects to become an outward representation of an internal idea, attitude, or feeling	An engagement ring symbolizes love and a commitment to another person.

without assistance from anyone or anything (Evans, 1997). Sullivan believed that those who attempt to solve problems by themselves may become consumed by their problems and suffer some type of mental disorder or illness. Mental health, in part, is determined by relationships between those who either love or refuse to love one another. Support people or significant others can be anyone with whom the person feels comfortable, trusts, and respects. A support person can act as a sounding board, simply listening while one vents various feelings or emotions, or he or she may interact as the need arises. Box 2-2 provides examples of situations in which a support person might be used.

Personal Strategies for Mental Health Maintenance

Burnout, also referred to as *compassionate fatigue*, may occur when one provides care for others at work and home but loses the ability to take care of ones self. Cell phones, e-mail, fax machines, pagers, and the use of computers have increased personal stress because people feel like they are working "24/7" (24 hours a day, 7 days a week). Such technology even has an impact on vacations because individuals take their "portable offices" with them. When the individual can no longer cope with the stress, compulsive behaviors such as

drug abuse or gambling may become distractions from the reality of burnout. As the burnout progresses, serious health problems or mental illness may occur (DeBarth, 2005).

BOX 2.2 EXAMPLES OF SITUATIONS INVOLVING THE USE OF A SUPPORT PERSON

- A female employee contemplating a legal separation from her husband discusses marital problems with a co-worker.
- A male client diagnosed with cancer asks to see his minister to discuss his concerns about his family and his future.
- A young mother hospitalized for emergency surgery arranges for her sister to provide care for her young children.
- A teenager whose parents are contemplating divorce explores feelings of guilt, anger, and resentment with her school counselor.
- A paraplegic who lives alone requires someone to be on-call 24 hours a day.

Many individuals have sought alternate ways to reduce stress and enhance their well-being while balancing the responsibilities between work and time spent at home. Stress-management programs are one way to combat the increasing demands on individuals both professionally and personally. Box 2-3 lists examples of additional personal strategies people use to reduce stress and enhance well-being.

Concept of Mental Illness

Like diabetes or cerebral palsy, mental illness is no one's fault. It can be caused by chemical imbalances in the brain, transfer of drugs across the placental barrier, or by organic changes within the brain. Additionally, if a person is unsuccessful in dealing with environmental stresses because of faulty inherited characteristics, poor nurturing during childhood, or negative life circumstances, mental illness may develop. The American Psychiatric Association defines **mental illness** or **mental disorder** as an illness or syndrome with psychological or behavioral manifestations and/or impairment in functioning as a result of a social, psychological, genetic, physical/chemical, or biologic disturbance. The disorder is not limited to relations between the person and society. The illness is characterized by symptoms and/or impairment in functioning (Shahrokh & Hales, 2003).

BOX 2.3 PERSONAL STRATEGIES FOR REDUCING STRESS AND ENHANCING WELL-BEING

- Aerobic exercise
- Aromatherapy
- Martial arts
- Massage
- Meditation
- Progressive relaxation techniques
- Self-hypnosis
- Walking
- Yoga

Other definitions refer to mental illness as a disorder causing people to display abnormal behavior more consistently than most people; a psychopathology exhibiting frequent irresponsibility, the inability to cope, frequently being at odds with society, and an inaccurate perception of reality; and the absolute absence or constant presence of a specific behavior that has a socially acceptable range of occurrences. Table 2-2 compares characteristics of mental health and mental illness.

Misconceptions About Mental Illness

Altrocchi (1980) lists several misconceptions about abnormal behavior and mental illness.

Summarized, they are as follows:

1. *Abnormal behavior is different or odd, and easily recognized.* We are all irrational at times and behave in an unusual or different manner. Such behavior may occur in a variety of environments and still may go unnoticed by others.
2. *Abnormal behavior can be predicted and evaluated.* Newspaper articles and television newscasts prove otherwise. Family members have verbalized complete surprise when confronted about acts of abuse or violence committed by loved ones, often describing the suspect as nice, quiet, friendly, or pleasant.
3. *Internal forces are responsible for abnormal behavior.* Although internal forces may cause abnormal behavior, other factors (eg, people, culture, and environment) can influence one's behavior.
4. *People who exhibit abnormal behavior are dangerous.* According to statistics provided by the National Institute of Mental Health (2004), more than 40 million Americans have a psychiatric diagnosis at any given time. Approximately 60% to 65% of those individuals who are hospitalized for psychiatric treatment are discharged and live with their families.
5. *Maladaptive behavior is always inherited.* Heredity plays a part in the development of some types of abnormal behavior; however, learning also influences behavior. Children learn early in life how to satisfy their needs. They, as well as adults, may observe specific behaviors used by others to meet their needs. As a result, they may imitate behavior that they believe to be acceptable to others.

TABLE 2.2 Characteristics of Mental Health and Mental Illness

MENTAL HEALTH	MENTAL ILLNESS
Accepts self and others	Feels inadequate
	Has poor self-concept
Is able to cope with or tolerate stress	Is unable to cope
Can return to normal functioning if temporarily disturbed	Exhibits maladaptive behavior
Is able to form close and lasting relationships	Is unable to establish a meaningful relationship
Uses sound judgment to make decisions	Displays poor judgment
Accepts responsibility for actions	Is irresponsible or unable to accept responsibility for actions
Is optimistic	Is pessimistic
Recognizes limitations (abilities and deficiencies)	Does not recognize limitations (abilities and deficiencies)
Can function effectively and independently	Exhibits dependency needs because of feelings of inadequacy
Is able to distinguish imagined circumstances from reality	Is unable to perceive reality
Is able to develop potential and talents to fullest extent	Does not recognize potential and talents because of poor self-concept
Is able to solve problems	Avoids problems rather than coping with them or attempting to solve them
Can delay gratification	Desires or demands immediate gratification
Mental health reflects a person's approach to life by communicating emotions, giving and receiving, working alone as well as with others, accepting authority, displaying a sense of humor, and coping successfully with emotional conflict.	Mental illness reflects a person's inability to cope with stress, resulting in disruption, disorganization, inappropriate reactions, unacceptable behavior, and the inability to respond according to the person's expectations and the demands of society.

6. *Mental illness is incurable.* Much progress has occurred in the diagnosis and treatment of mental illness. Early detection and treatment may alleviate symptoms and allow the person to function normally in society. People with chronic mental disorders may receive maintenance doses of medication, attend various therapies, or care for themselves with minimal supervision. As a result of deinstitutionalization and the implementation of managed care, clients are empowered to function as independently as possible. Community resources are used to provide education for the client and family. Ongoing supervision and support are available to minimize recidivism.

Diagnosis of a Mental Illness

Diagnosis of a client's mental illness is achieved through examination and analysis of data. This diagno-

sis is an integral part of the theory and practice of nursing. Chapters 9 and 10 address the nursing process and its application to clients with mental health issues. The *Diagnostic and Statistical Manual of Mental Disorders (4th Edition, Text Revision; DSM-IV-TR)* published by the American Psychiatric Association and used by many different disciplines, is included in the discussion of nursing diagnosis in Chapter 10. Unit 6, Clients With Psychiatric Disorders, and Unit 7, Special Populations, discuss the clinical symptoms and methods used to diagnose the presence of a specific mental illness.

Historical Development of Psychiatric–Mental Health Nursing

A review of the social changes occurring before 1773 is necessary to understand the emergence of psychiatric–mental health nursing. The origins of most of psychiatry's concepts begin with prehistoric times, when primitive people believed spirits possessed the body and had to be driven out to effect a cure. Before the 5th century BC, the Greeks, Romans, and Arabs believed that emotional disorders were an organic dysfunction of the brain.

Hippocrates (460-375 BC) described a variety of personalities, or temperaments, and proposed that mental illness was a disturbance of four body fluids, or "humors." Aristotle (382-322 BC) concluded that the mind was associated with the heart, whereas Galen (130-200 AD), a Greek physician, stated that emotional or mental disorders were associated with the brain. Treatment approaches during this time-frame included the use of sedation, good nutrition, good physical hygiene, music, and recreational activities such as riding, walking, and listening to the sounds of a waterfall. Fresh air, sunshine, and pure water were thought to promote healing for the mentally ill.

Middle Ages to 1773

During the Middle Ages, humane treatment of mentally ill people suffered a setback as mentally ill individuals were excluded from society and confined in asylums or institutions. Various theories pertaining to demonic possession also were advanced. Specifically, persons who displayed abnormal behavior were considered lunatics, witches, or demons possessed by evil spirits. Superstition, mysticism, magic, and witchcraft prevailed as patients were locked in asylums, flogged, starved, tortured, or subjected to bloodletting. Beheading, hanging, and burning at the stake were common occurrences. Exorcism was practiced in some monasteries.

During this same period, physicians described symptoms of depression, paranoia, delusions, hysteria, and nightmares. Persons displaying such symptoms were thought to be incompetent and potentially dangerous. The first mental hospital, Bethlehem Royal Hospital, opened in England in 1403. Pronounced "Bedlam," the name came to symbolize the inhumane treatment of persons who were put on public display for twopence a look. Harmless inmates sought charity on the streets. In 1724, a Puritan clergyman by the name of Cotton Mather (1663-1728) broke with superstition by discounting the fact that mental illness was the result of demonic possession and witchcraft, explaining that mental illnesses were the result of physical changes within the body (Mental Wellness.com, 2003).

1773 to 1956

In contrast, the 18th century is regarded as an era of reason and observation. In 1843, there were approximately 24 hospitals available for the treatment of mental illness. Clifford Beers (1876-1943) wrote an account of his experience as a mental patient, *The Mind That Found Itself*, vividly describing the norm of institutional care. He later founded the National Committee for Mental Hygiene, predecessor to the National Mental Health Association (NMHA). Emil Kraepelin first described Alzheimer's disease in 1910, and in the 1920s Harry Stack Sullivan established a ward for clients with the diagnosis of schizophrenia, demonstrating the positive impact of a therapeutic milieu that allowed clients to return to the community. The first human frontal lobotomy was performed in 1936, and electrotherapy was established in the 1940s. Fountain House, a psychiatric rehabilitation center for mentally ill clients was established in New York City in 1947 (Mental Wellness.com, 2003).

According to Peplau (1956), the historical development of psychiatric nursing also began in 1773. Peplau identified five eras, or phases, in the establishment of psychiatric nursing, both as an aspect of all nursing and as a specialty in nursing. Table 2-3 summarizes these eras.

Phenothiazines and other major tranquilizers were introduced in the United States between 1952 and the 1960s to treat the major symptoms of psychoses, enabling clients to be more responsive to therapeutic care. During this time, open-door policies were implemented in large mental institutions, allowing clients to leave the units or wards while under supervision.

Other Developments Since the 1950s

In 1963, the Community Mental Health Act authorized funding for the establishment of community health centers to provide the following services to the public: emergency mental health care, such as crisis centers and telephone hotlines; patient care or hospitalization, such as daycare centers and therapeutic communities; aftercare, including halfway houses and foster homes; and consultation services, as provided in counseling centers. This act promoted the specialization of psychiatric nursing services as the provision of care shifted to the community. Nurse practitioners or clinical specialists could provide direct care to psychiatric clients in a variety of settings. In 1970, the deinstitutionalization of

TABLE 2.3 Development of Psychiatric–Mental Health Nursing

Phase 1: The Emergence of Psychiatric–Mental Health Nursing (1773–1881)	• Special institutions for individuals with psychiatric disorders were built. • Benjamin Rush wrote the first American textbook on psychiatry. • Attendants were hired to socialize with patients. • Philippe Pinel classified clients according to their observable behaviors. • Schools of nursing were established in Boston and Philadelphia by 1872. • Dorothea Lynde Dix devoted time to improving conditions for the mentally ill.
Phase 2: Development of the Work Role of the Psychiatric Nurse (1882–1914)	• Training schools for nurses in the psychiatric setting were established at McLean Hospital in Belmont, Massachusetts, and at Buffalo State Hospital in New York (1882). • Trained nurses were employed in state mental hospitals (1890). • First undergraduate psychiatric nursing program was established. • National Society for Mental Hygiene was founded in 1909. • Large state mental hospitals were built in rural areas.
Phase 3: Development of Undergraduate Psychiatric Nursing Education (1915–1935)	• Linda Richards, the first graduate nurse in the United States, suggested that mentally ill clients receive the same quality care as physically ill clients. • Student nurses received clinical experience in state mental hospitals. • Textbooks focusing on psychiatric nursing practice were written. • Educational objectives for undergraduate psychiatric nursing education were discussed at National League for Nursing conventions. • Harriet Bailey wrote the first psychiatric nursing textbook, Nursing Mental Diseases. • Insulin shock therapy, electroconvulsive therapy, and prefrontal lobotomy were introduced in the psychiatric clinical setting. • The National Committee for Mental Hygiene was established.
Phase 4: Development of Graduate Psychiatric Nursing Education (1936–1945)	• Clinical experiences in psychiatric hospitals were standardized by 1937. • Approximately half of all nursing schools provided psychiatric nursing courses; however, participation in psychiatric courses did not become a requirement for nursing licensure until 1955. • The National League of Nursing Education developed curriculum guidelines for psychiatric nursing graduate education. By 1943, three university-sponsored graduate programs existed.
Phase 5: Development of Consultation and Research in Psychiatric Nursing Practice (1946–1956)	• The Mental Health Act of 1946 provided funding of graduate nursing programs to prepare psychiatric clinical nurses. • Yearly grants were given to the National League for Nursing to evaluate psychiatric programs. • Nurses who served with the armed forces were able to secure an education through the GI Bill. • The National League of Nursing Education formed a committee in 1956 to review and revise a proposed guide for the development of an advanced clinical course in psychiatric nursing. The Brown Report, a product of the committee's meeting, stressed that interest in the field of psychiatry should be stimulated to facilitate research focusing on the prevention and cure of mental illness.

clients from state mental hospitals to community living was considered a positive move; however, insufficient federal funding resulted in an increase in the number of homeless mentally ill people.

Recent events include the President's New Freedom Commission on Mental Health (2002), an executive order by President George W. Bush to promote increased access to educational and employment opportunities for people with mental health disabilities. A final report, dated March 5, 2003, urges federal, state, and local governments to develop a recovery-oriented mental health system that embraces the values of self-determination, empowering relationships, meaningful roles in society, and elimination of stigma and discrimination. The NMHA issued a policy position statement urging mental health associations, mental health service provider organizations, and other advocates to promote peer support as a unique

SELF-AWARENESS PROMPT

Reflect on the history and trends that have occurred in psychiatric nursing. What trends have been implemented into your nursing curriculum? How do you think they will affect the development of your psychiatric nursing skills?

and essential element of recovery-oriented mental health systems (NMHA, 2005).

In October 2002, the National Alliance for the Mentally Ill (NAMI) initiated the Campaign for the Mind of America, a multiyear effort to promote investment in recovery and to prevent the abandonment of another generation of Americans with mental illness to neglect and hopelessness. NAMI is also working with other advocacy groups in psychiatry to advance the conversation on mental illness (NAMI, 2002; Norton, 2004).

The Paul Wellston Mental Health Equitable Treatment Act of 2003 states that it is illegal to discriminate between mental health and physical health insurance coverage unless there are comparable limi-

tations imposed on medical and surgical insurance benefits (Norton, 2004). As of July 2005, the Act was still under debate in the Senate.

As mentioned herein, during the 20th century, psychiatric nursing began to evolve as a clinical specialty. Nurses were previously involved as managers and coordinators of activities as they provided therapeutic care based on the medical model. With advanced study and clinical practice experienced in a master's program in psychiatric nursing, clinical specialists and nurse practitioners gained expert knowledge in the care and prevention of psychiatric disorders. Table 2-4 lists historical events influencing psychiatric nursing from 1856 to the present. Box 2-4 provides examples of research on biologic aspects of mental illness during the period known as the Decade of the Brain (1990–2000).

Standards of Psychiatric–Mental Health Nursing Practice

Standards of practice are authoritative statements used by the nursing profession to describe the responsibilities for which nurses are accountable. They pro-

---

BOX 2.4 RESULTS OF RESEARCH ON BIOLOGIC ASPECTS OF MENTAL ILLNESS

- Molecular targets have been identified in the treatment of bipolar disorder.
- Panic attacks appear to induce a long-lasting rise in LDL and total cholesterol in men, placing them at increased risk of cardiovascular disease.
- High-dose electroconvulsive therapy on the right brain maximizes therapy efficacy while minimizing adverse effects on memory.
- Schizophrenia may be caused by a virus, autoimmune phenomena or frontal lobe dysfunction.
- Approximately 60% of chronic alcoholics may experience cerebral atrophy, cortical shrinkage, and ventricular dilatation in the frontal lobe. Electroencephalograms are poorly synchronized.
- Increased episodes of depression and mania cause changes in brain structure and function, which lead to treatment-resistant depression.
- Alcoholics can be delineated into type A or B subgroups based on the disease's etiologic elements, onset and course, presenting symptoms, and drinking pattern.

- A combination of electroconvulsive therapy and lithium may achieve rapid control of an acute manic episode.
- Prozac may significantly improve the clinical symptoms of bulimia.
- Endozepine-1, a newly described brain chemical is likened to endogenous diazepam (Valium).
- Untreated hypothyroidism may play an unheralded role in treatment resistance and in the development of rapid cycling in bipolar patients.
- Clozaril has proven to be a safe, effective drug for psychotic clients with a history of neuroleptic malignant syndrome.
- Desyrel and Eldepryl have proved effective in the management of behavioral symptoms of Alzheimer's disease.
- Serotonin reuptake inhibitors such as Prozac augment previously ineffective tricyclic therapy in the treatment of depression.

Other examples are included in the text.

TABLE 2.4 Events Influencing Psychiatric–Mental Health Nursing

The following is a chronologic listing of some important events influencing psychiatric nursing:

1856–1929	Emil Kraepelin differentiated manic-depression psychosis from schizophrenia and stated that schizophrenia was incurable.
1856–1939	Sigmund Freud introduced psychoanalytic theory and therapy. He explained human behavior in psychological terms and proved that behavior can be changed in certain situations.
1857–1939	Eugene Bleuler described the psychotic disorder of schizophrenia (formerly referred to as *dementia "praecox"*).
1870–1937	Alfred Adler focused on the area of psychosomatic medicine, referring to organ inferiority as the causative factor.
1875–1961	Carl Jung described the human psyche as consisting of a social mask (persona), hidden personal characteristics (shadow), feminine identification in men (anima), masculine identification in women (animus), and the innermost center of the personality (self).
1940–1945	World War II veterans received financial support and vocational rehabilitation for psychiatric and physical disabilities.
1946–1971	Care of mentally ill persons was brought into the mainstream of health care. World Federation for Mental Health provided funds for research and education.
1947	Helen Render wrote *Nurse–Patient Relationships in Psychiatry.*
1949	The National Institute of Mental Health was established to (1) provide grants-in-aid; (2) fund training programs and demonstration projects; and (3) provide support for research.
1952	Hildegard E. Peplau wrote *Interpersonal Relations in Nursing,* a text that provided the basis for the development of therapeutic roles in nurse–client relationships. This book was of paramount importance in the development of psychiatric nursing as a profession.
1955	The Joint Commission on Mental Illness and Health was developed to study and evaluate needs and resources.
1961	The World Psychiatric Association examined the social consequences of mental illness.
1963–1979	The Economic Opportunity Act stressed improvement of social environments to prevent the development of mental illness. The Mental Retardation Facilities and Community Mental Health Centers Construction Act provided federal funds to help state and local agencies decentralize mental health care; provided community services and facilities to treat substance abusers; and proposed that community mental health programs include special programs to treat children and the elderly. Fifty graduate psychiatric nursing programs were established in the United States. Private psychiatric hospitals, as well as psychiatric units in general hospitals, were established. Insurance companies provided coverage for psychiatric care. Deinstitutionalization and community living for mentally ill patients was emphasized, focusing on teaching them activities of daily living and self-care. Canadian and American nurses laid groundwork for formation of North American Nursing Diagnosis Association.
1980s	Mental Health Systems Act (1980), designed to strengthen existing community efforts and to develop new initiatives, was never implemented due to 1981 legislation. Omnibus Budget Reconciliation Act (1981) drastically curtailed federal funding for health care services. Emphasis placed on American Nurses Association (ANA) specialty certification exam.
1990s	Insurance companies made drastic cuts in coverage for psychiatric care. Formation of National Alliance for the Mentally Ill (NAMI). Greater emphasis placed on the biologic aspects of mental illness and on advances in neuropharmacology. This era is referred to as the "Decade of the Brain."
2001	New Freedom Initiative to promote increased access to educational and employment opportunities for people with disabilities signed by President George W. Bush.
2002	New Freedom Commission on Mental Health introduced to transform mental health care in America
2002	NAMI initiated Campaign for the Mind of America
2003	Paul Wellston Mental Health Equitable Treatment Act introduced in Senate

vide direction for professional nursing practice and a framework for the evaluation of practice. They also define the nursing profession's accountability to the public and the client outcomes for which nurses are responsible.

In 1967, the American Nurses Association (ANA) published the *Statement on Psychiatric and Mental Health Nursing Practice.* A revision followed in 1976. Belief that the scope of practice is linked to practice standards resulted in the publication of *Standards of Psychiatric and Mental Health Nursing Practice* in 1982. Broader general standards of nursing practice are delineated in the *Standards of Clinical Nursing Practice* (ANA, 1991).

In May 1999, a workgroup convened to review and revise, if necessary, the *A Statement on Psychiatric-Mental Health Clinical Nursing Practice and Standards of Psychiatric-Mental Health Clinical Nursing Practice* published in 1994. The current revision, *Scope and Standards of Psychiatric-Mental Health*

Nursing Practice (ANA, 2000), is divided into two sections, Standards of Care and Standards of Professional Performance, as described in Boxes 2-5 and 2-6.

Psychiatric–Mental Health Nursing Today

"The nursing shortage has struck just about everywhere in the United States and there's no relief in sight—but its effects vary by region and specialty...it's clear that experienced nurses are in short supply in all areas of nursing, particularly specialty areas" (Valentino, 2002, p. 24).

Many registered nurses have left nursing for better opportunities and higher-paying jobs. In 2002, there were nearly a half million licensed nurses not employed in nursing. The Bureau of Labor Statistics predicts that more than 1 million new nurses will be needed by the year 2010. This predicted need is based

---

BOX 2.5 STANDARDS OF CARE

Standard I. Assessment: The psychiatric-mental health nurse collects client health data.

Standard II. Diagnosis: The psychiatric-mental health nurse analyzes the assessment data in determining diagnoses.

Standard III. Outcome Identification: The psychiatric-mental health nurse identifies expected outcomes individualized to the client.

Standard IV. Planning: The psychiatric-mental health nurse develops a plan of care that is negotiated among the client, nurse, family, and health care team and prescribes evidence-based interventions to attain expected outcomes.

Standard V. Implementation: The psychiatric-mental health nurse implements the interventions identified in the plan of care.

Standard Va. Counseling: The psychiatric-mental health nurse uses counseling interventions to assist clients in improving or regaining their previous coping abilities, fostering mental health, and preventing mental illness and disability.

Standard Vb. Milieu Therapy: The psychiatric-mental health nurse provides, structures, and maintains a therapeutic environment in collaboration with the client and other health care providers.

Standard Vc. Promotion of Self-Care Activities: The psychiatric-mental health nurse structures interventions around the client's activities of daily living to foster self-care and mental and physical well-being.

Standard Vd. Psychobiologic Interventions: The psychiatric-mental health nurse uses knowledge of psychobiologic interventions and applies clinical skills to restore the client's health and prevent future disability.

Standard Ve. Health Teaching: The psychiatric-mental health nurse, through health teaching, assists clients in achieving satisfying, productive, and healthy patterns of living.

Standard Vf. Case Management: The psychiatric-mental health nurse provides case management to coordinate comprehensive health services and ensure continuity of care.

Standard Vg. Health Promotion and Health Maintenance: The psychiatric-mental health nurse employs strategies and interventions to promote and maintain mental health and prevent mental illness.

Advanced Practice Intervention Vh–Vj: The following interventions (Vh-Vj) may be performed only by the APRN-PMH.

Standard Vh. Psychotherapy: The APRN-PMH uses individual, group, and family psychotherapy and other therapeutic treatments to assist client in preventing mental illness and disability, treating mental health disorders, and improving mental health status and functional abilities.

Standard Vi. Prescriptive Authority and Treatment: The APRN-PMH uses prescriptive authority procedures and treatments, in accordance with state and federal laws and regulations, to treat symptoms of psychiatric illness and improve functional health status.

Standard Vj. Consultation: The APRN-PMH provides consultation to enhance the abilities of other clinicians to provide services for clients and effect change in the system.

Standard VI. Evaluation: The psychiatric–mental health nurse evaluates the client's progress in attaining expected outcomes.

APRN-PMH, advanced practice registered nurse-psychiatric mental health.

Reprinted with permission from American Nurses Association (2000). *Scope and standards of psychiatric-mental health nursing practice.* Washington, DC: American Nurses Publishing.

on several factors. Nurses are retiring or leaving the profession for several reasons, such as low wages for physically demanding work, mandatory overtime, burnout, job dissatisfaction, increased nurse-to-client ratios, and work-related injuries. Salaries, when adjusted for inflation, have remained the same since 1992, whereas malpractice suits involving client safety issues have increased. The lack of part-time shifts or flex time, variations in health delivery systems, reimbursement by Medicare and Medicaid, and local customs and culture have also altered the need for nurses (Stokowski, 2004; Valentino, 2002).

Education

A paradigm shift is taking place in education, moving from the traditional classroom to the presentation of knowledge via distance education, multimedia cen-

---

BOX 2.6 **STANDARDS OF PROFESSIONAL PERFORMANCE**

Standard I. Quality of Care: The psychiatric–mental health nurse systematically evaluates the quality of care and effectiveness of psychiatric–mental health nursing practice.

Standard II. Performance Appraisal: The psychiatric–mental health nurse evaluates one's own psychiatric–mental health nursing practice in relation to professional practice standards and relevant statutes and regulations.

Standard III. Education: The psychiatric–mental health nurse acquires and maintains current knowledge in nursing practice.

Standard IV. Collegiality: The psychiatric–mental health nurse interacts with and contributes to the professional development of peers, health care clinicians and others as colleagues

Standard V. Ethics: The psychiatric–mental health nurse's assessments, actions, and recommendations on behalf of clients are determined and implemented in an ethical manner.

Standard VI. Collaboration: The psychiatric–mental health nurse collaborates with the client, significant others, and health care providers in giving care.

Standard VII. Research: The psychiatric–mental health nurse contributes to nursing and mental health through the use of research methods and findings.

Standard VIII. Resource Utilization: The psychiatric–mental health nurse considers factors related to safety, effectiveness, and cost in planning and delivering client care.

Reprinted with permission from American Nurses Association (2000). *Scope and standards of psychiatric-mental health nursing practice.* Washington, DC: American Nurses Publishing.

ters, and cyberspace. The beginning nurse needs to have basic competencies related to computer literacy and **nursing informatics,** a specialty that integrates nursing science, computer science, and information science to manage and communicate data, information, and knowledge in nursing practice (Reavis & Brykczynski, 2002; Newbold, 2001).

Schools of nursing offer a variety of programs to prepare students for the practice of psychiatric-mental health nursing.

Licensed Practical or Vocational Nursing Programs

Licensed practical or vocational nursing schools generally address the topics of human behavior or mental health and mental illness, and may integrate mental health concepts into courses such as pediatrics, obstetrics, and the aging process. Psychiatric nursing clinical experience usually is not offered in 1-year programs, although state board examinations do include questions pertaining to basic mental health concepts. If a licensed practical or vocational nurse elects to continue training to become a registered nurse, psychiatric nursing experience must be obtained in either an associate's or baccalaureate degree nursing program.

Associate's Degree Nursing Programs

Associate's degree programs may offer a 5- to 10-week course in psychiatric nursing with or without clinical rotation in psychiatric–mental health settings. Some schools integrate psychiatric nursing concepts throughout the 2-year program, after core courses in developmental or abnormal psychology. Psychiatric nursing experience may occur in a medical–psychiatric unit, private psychiatric hospital, state psychiatric facility, or community mental health setting. Alternate sites used for clinical experience may include shelters for the homeless, public school systems, penal institutions, and triage units in the general hospital setting. Emphasis is on nursing intervention under the direction of a more experienced registered nurse.

Baccalaureate Degree Nursing Programs

Baccalaureate degree programs usually provide more time for psychiatric nursing and clinical experiences. Emphasis is placed on theoretical foundations, the assessment process, mathematical statistics, group dynamics, client and family education, and the nurse's role in preventive care.

Master's Degree Nursing Programs

Graduate schools offering a master's degree in psychiatric or mental health nursing usually require a certain number of credit hours related to core courses, clinical experience, research, electives, and a practicum. The graduate student may elect to become a clinical nurse specialist or a nurse practitioner, depending on the courses available.

Continuing Education

The Board of Nursing of each state has established continuing education guidelines that must be completed prior to license renewal. Nurses may also apply for certification of competency in psychiatric nursing by organizations such as the ANA. Certification is available for various levels of psychiatric nursing, such as generalist, clinical specialist, and nurse practitioner. Review courses are available prior to taking the test. See Box 2-7 for examples of certification organizations.

Career Opportunities

Currently, the field of psychiatric–mental health nursing offers a variety of opportunities for specialization.

BOX 2.7 CERTIFICATION ORGANIZATIONS

Examples of certification organizations include but are not limited to the following:

American Academy of Nurse Practitioners: www. aanp.org

American Holistic Nurses Certification Corporation: www.ahna.org

American Nurses Credentialing Center: www.nursing world.org/ancc/certification/certs.html

National Board of Certification of Hospice and Palliative Nurses: www.nbchpn.org/

Psychiatric Nurse Certification: www.calapna.org/ certf.htm

TABLE 2.5 Use of Psychiatric–Mental Health Nursing Skills in Career Opportunities

CAREER OPPORTUNITIES	USE OF PSYCHIATRIC–MENTAL HEALTH NURSING SKILLS
Obstetric nursing	Helping the mother in labor and support person cope with anxiety or stress during labor and delivery
	Providing support to bereaved parents in the event of fetal demise, inevitable abortion, or the birth of an infant with congenital anomalies
	Providing support to a mother considering whether to keep her child or give the child up for adoption
Forensic nursing	Providing services to incarcerated clients
	Acting as a consultant to medical and legal agencies
	Serving as an expert witness in court
	Providing support for victims of violent crime
Oncologic nursing	Helping cancer patients or other terminally ill individuals on oncology units work through the grieving process
	Providing support groups for families of terminally ill patients
Industrial (occupational health) nursing	Implementing or participating in industrial substance abuse programs for employees and their families
	Providing crisis intervention during an industrial accident or the acute onset of a physical or mental illness (eg, heart attack or anxiety attack)
	Teaching stress management
Public health nursing	Assessing the person both physically and psychologically (eg, the newly diagnosed diabetic client may develop a low self-concept, or the recovering stroke client may exhibit symptoms of depression due to a slow recovery)
Office nursing	Assisting the client by explaining somatic or emotional concerns during the assessment process
	Providing support with the problem-solving process when people call the office and the physician is unavailable
	Acting as a community resource person
Emergency room nursing	Providing crisis intervention as the need arises (eg, during natural disasters, accidents, or unexpected illnesses causing increased anxiety, stress, or immobilization)

Examples include nurse liaison in the general hospital, therapist in private practice, consultant, educator, expert witness in legal issues, employee assistance counselor, mental health provider in long-term care facilities, and work in association with a mobile psychiatric triage unit. A new model of family practice has been proposed in which the client is center stage and a multidisciplinary team is the source of care. This model is expected to provide a variety of services for clients to manage and prevent acute injuries, illnesses, and chronic diseases, as well as rehabilitation and supportive care (Hoppel, 2004). According to the American Psychiatric Association and the American Academy of Family Physicians, 42% of clients diagnosed with depression and 47% diagnosed with general anxiety disorder were first diagnosed by a primary care clinician. Additionally, more than 40% of antidepressants are prescribed by primary care clinicians and nearly one third of undiagnosed, asymptomatic adults say they would first turn to their primary care physician for help with a mental health issue (Worcester, 2004). Such a model of care provides an excellent career opportunity for the psychiatric-mental health nurse.

In addition, psychiatric–mental health nursing experience as a student provides a valuable foundation for career opportunities after graduation. Table 2-5 lists such positions and gives examples of how psychiatric-mental health nursing experience can be an asset to them.

Expanded Role of the Nurse

The role of nurses continues to expand. For example, the American Board of Managed Care Nursing (ABMCN), formed in 1998, promotes excellence and professionalism in managed care nursing (see Chapter 8) by recognizing individuals who, through voluntary certification, demonstrate an acquired knowledge and expertise in managed health care. The managed care nurse's role is to advocate for all clients enrolled in managed health care plans, to administer benefits within the confines of the managed care plan, and to provide customer service during all of the nurse's encounters with members of the managed care plan. Managed care nurses develop and implement wellness and prevention programs and disease management programs. The nurse's role in managed care moves along the continuum from direct client care to administrator (ABMCN, 2004).

Another area of expansion is parish nursing, which developed in the early 1980s in the Midwest. **Parish nursing** is a program that promotes health and wellness of body, mind, and spirit using the community health nursing model as its framework. The church congregation is the client. The parish nurse is a member of the church congregation, spiritually mature, and is a licensed registered nurse with a desire to serve the members and friends of his or her congregation. Much of the nurse's time is spent helping to improve quality of life and wellness in a faith-based setting (Dryden, 2004).

The International Parish Nurse Resource Center of St. Louis, Missouri endorses a standard curriculum for parish nurses. It assists the participant to:

- explore theoretical and practical knowledge that is necessary to develop and implement an outcome-oriented, faith-based nursing practice.
- differentiate among body, mind, and spiritual dimensions of clients
- assess spiritual needs of clients
- recognize the various components of the parish nursing role
- understand various theological concepts from Christian, Jewish, and Eastern religions that affect individual healing and wellness
- discover the various components of a health ministry as they relate to community health and wellness (Florida Nurse, 2004).

Although parish nurses are volunteers, some are paid by grants, the hospital, or the congregation. In 1998, the ANA recognized parish nursing as a specialty focusing on disease prevention and health promotion (Hamlin, 2000).

Additionally, nurses have recently become subject to the **privileging process** that physicians have enjoyed for years. Nurses provide comprehensive services, including health promotion, disease prevention, acute and chronic illness management, and management of psychiatric disorders for hospitalized clients and those admitted to subacute and long-term care facilities.

The role of nurses is also expanding in the area of **telehealth,** or telephone nursing. It is an effective method to teach clients and consumers about health care and disease management. As technology becomes cheaper and more reliable, and demand for this convenient delivery method grows, experts predict more dramatic changes in the delivery of health care in the 21st century after legislative, technical, and practice barriers are overcome. Confidentiality issues, imperfect software, faulty equipment, and reimbursement issues present challenges.

Finally, **forensic nursing** is expected to become one of the fastest growing nursing specialties of the 21st century. Forensic nursing focuses on advocacy for and ministration to offenders and victims of violent crime and the families of both. Refer to Chapter 6, Forensic Nursing Practice, for additional information about forensic nursing.

Perhaps the greatest challenge to nursing lies in the future, as we identify and develop clinical provider performance measures that are relevant to the care we provide and the people we serve.

KEY CONCEPTS

◆ Mental health is a positive state in which one functions well in society, is accepted within a group, and is generally satisfied with life.

◆ Open and honest communication fosters personal growth and maturity.

◆ Ego defense mechanisms are protective barriers used to manage instinct and affect in stressful situations.

◆ Significant others or support people enable clients to maintain mental health by allowing them to vent thoughts or emotions during times of increased anxiety or stress.

◆ Mental illness is characterized by psychological or behavioral manifestations and/or impairment in functioning due to a social, psychological, genetic, physical/chemical, or biologic disturbance.

◆ Humane treatment of mental illness suffered a setback in the Middle Ages.

◆ The emergence of psychiatric nursing began in the 18th century.

◆ Humane treatment of mentally ill people improved during the 19th century.

◆ Training schools for nurses in the psychiatric setting were started in 1882, with nurses being employed in state mental hospitals by 1890.

◆ Literature written by psychiatric nurses described philosophy of practice, the role of the nurse in a psychiatric facility, and psychiatric nursing curriculum.

◆ Undergraduate psychiatric nursing education was developed between 1915 and 1935; graduate education in psychiatric nursing evolved between 1936 and 1945.

◆ Standards of practice for psychiatric nursing were published in 1982.

◆ During the 20th century, practice sites have changed and career opportunities have expanded as nurse practitioners have been credentialed and allowed to participate in the privileging process.

◆ Forensic nursing has been described as one of the fastest-growing nursing specialties of the 21st century.

For additional study materials, please refer to the Student Resource CD-ROM located in the back of this textbook.

 ## CHAPTER WORKSHEET

CRITICAL THINKING QUESTIONS

1. You have been asked to make a presentation to a local women's club whose members are especially interested in maintaining their mental health as they age. Outline a 20-minute presentation that includes basic information on mental health, misconceptions about mental illness, and maintenance of mental health.
2. During the Middle Ages, persons who displayed abnormal behavior were often treated inhumanely. Today, many mentally ill persons end up on the streets of our cities. Analyze how society handles persons with mental illness and compare the social, political, and economic issues that affect care for this segment of the population.
3. The American Nurses Association issued *Standards of Psychiatric–Mental Health Nursing Practice* in 1982. Explain why standards of practice are necessary and delineate the nurse's responsibility for these standards.

REFLECTION

Review the quote at the beginning of the chapter. According to Peplau (1956), several trends occurred in psychiatric–mental health nursing between 1915 and 1935. Explain the impact of these trends on the delivery of care to clients during the 21st century.

NCLEX-STYLE QUESTIONS

1. Which of the following statements about causation of mental illness would the nurse identify as incorrect?
   a. Life circumstances can influence one's mental health from birth.
   b. The inability to deal with environmental stresses can result in mental illness.
   c. Mental health is influenced by relationships between persons who either love or refuse to love one another.
   d. Inherited characteristics exert minimal to no influence on one's mental health.

2. Which of the following would the nurse expect as the *least* likely reason for using defense mechanisms?
   a. Improved insight
   b. Protection of self-esteem
   c. Reduced anxiety
   d. Resolution of a mental conflict

3. A client talks to the nurse about safe, neutral topics, without revealing feelings or emotions. The nurse determines that the client's motivation for remaining on this superficial level of communication is most likely which of the following?

a. Fear of rejection by the nurse
b. Lack of awareness of feelings
c. Poor communication ability
d. Poor emotional maturity

4. The following events are associated with influencing psychiatric–mental health nursing. Place the events in the proper chronological order, beginning from the earliest to the most recent.
a. Formation of the National Alliance for the Mentally Ill (NAMI)
b. Introduction of the psychoanalytic theory and therapy
c. Establishment of the National Institute of Mental Health
d. Curtailment of federal funding for health care services
e. Publication of Peplau's *Interpersonal Relations in Nursing*

5. Which of the following nursing functions is different in current psychiatric–mental health nursing practice when compared with practice from 1915 to 1935?
a. Careful client assessment
b. Concerns about the effect of environmental conditions
c. Focus on understanding the causes of mental illness
d. Use of nursing diagnosis

6. The certified nurse practitioner of psychiatric nursing performs which of the following functions not performed by the psychiatric nurse generalist?
a. Case management and health promotion
b. Counseling and establishment of nursing diagnosis
c. Health teaching and milieu therapy
d. Psychotherapy and prescribing medications

Selected References

Altrocchi, J. (1980). *Abnormal behavior.* New York: Harcourt Brace Jovanovich.

American Board of Managed Care Nursing. (2004). *Managed care nursing.* Retrieved January 30, 2004, from http://www. abmcn.org

American Nurses Association. (1991). *Standards of clinical nursing practice.* Kansas City: Author.

American Nurses Association. (1994). *A statement on psychiatric-mental health clinical nursing practice and standards of psychiatric-mental health clinical nursing practice.* Washington, DC: American Nurses Publishing.

American Nurses Association. (2000). *Scope and standards of psychiatric-mental health nursing practice.* Washington, DC: American Nurses Publishing.

DeBarth, K. (2005). Compassion fatigue: Burnout in the health professions. *Clinician News, 9*(6), 16–17.

Dryden, P. (2004). Heaven sent—Parish nurses are making a difference. *Medscape Nurses 6*(1). Retrieved May 13, 2004, from http://www.medscape.com/viewarticle/474866

Evans, F. Barton. (1997). *Harry Stack Sullivan: The interpersonal theory of psychiatry.* New York: Routledge.

Florida Nurse. (2004). The International Parish Nurse Endorsed Standard Curriculum for Parish Nurses. September 2004, p. 18.

Freud, A. (1946). *The ego and the mechanisms of defense.* New York: International Universities Press.

Haber, J., & Billings, C. (1993). Primary mental health care: A vision for the future of psychiatric-mental health nursing. *American Nurses Association Council Perspectives, 2*(2), 1.

Hamlin, L. (2000). Parish nursing: Ties faith and healing. *Vital Signs, 10*(23), 6–7.

Hoppel, A. M. (2004). The future of family medicine. *Clinician News, 8*(8), 1, 26–28.

Johnson, B. S. (1997). *Psychiatric-mental health nursing: Adaptation and growth* (4th ed.). Philadelphia: Lippincott-Raven Publishers.

Kennedy, J. L., Pato, J., Bauer, A., Carvalho, C., & Pato, O. (1999). Genetics of schizophrenia. Current findings and issues. *CNS Spectrum, 4*(5), 17–21.

Kolb, L. C. (1977). *Modern clinical psychiatry.* Philadelphia: W. B. Saunders.

Maslow, A. (1970). *Motivation and personality* (2nd ed.). New York: Harper & Row.

Mental Wellness.com. (2003). History of mental illness. Retrieved August 14, 2006, from http://www.mental wellness.com

National Alliance for the Mentally Ill. (2002). Campaign for the mind of America. Retrieved July 10, 2005, from http://www. nami.org

National Institute of Mental Health. (2004). Myths about mental illness. Retrieved January 30, 2004, from http://www.nimh. nih.gov/

National Mental Health Association. (2005). NMHA policy positions: The role of peer support services in the creation of recovery-oriented mental health systems. Retrieved July 10, 2005, from http://www.nmha.org/ position/peersupport. cfm

Newbold, S. K. (2001). A new definition for nursing informatics. *ADVANCE for Nurses, 2*(17), 13–14.

Norton, P. G. W. (2004). Advocacy groups joining forces in psychiatry. *Clinical Psychiatry News, 32*(4), 108.

Peplau, H. E. (1956). Historical development of psychiatric nursing: A preliminary statement of some facts and trends. In S. Smoyak & S. Rouslin (Eds.), *Collection of classics in psychiatric nursing literature* (1982, pp. 10–46). Thorofare, NJ: Charles B. Slack.

Powell, J. (1995). *Why am I afraid to tell you who I am?* Grand Rapids, MI: Zondervan.

President's New Freedom Commission on Mental Health: Executive Order. (2002, May 3). Federal Register, *67*(86).

Reavis, C. W., & Brykczynski, K. A. (2002). The high-tech classroom. *ADVANCE for Nurse Practitioners, 10*(3), 67–74.

Shahrokh, N., & Hales, R. E. (Eds.). (2003). *American psychiatric glossary* (8th ed.). Washington, DC: American Psychiatric Press, Inc.

Stowkowski, L. (2004). Trends in nursing: 2004 and beyond. *Topics in Advanced Practice Nursing eJournal, 4*(1). Retrieved January 1, 2005, from http://www.medscape.com

Valentino, L. M. (2002). Future employment trends in nursing. *American Journal of Nursing, 2002, Career Guide*, 24–28.

Worcester, S. (2004). Teamwork closes mental health gap. *Clinical Psychiatry News, 32*(11), 1, 7.

Suggested Readings

American Nurses Association. (1982). *Standards of psychiatric and mental health nursing practice.* Kansas City: Author.

Canadian Nurses Association. (1998). *Canadian standards of psychiatric and mental health nursing practice* (2nd ed.). Ottawa, ON: Standards Committee of the Canadian Federation of Mental Health Nurses.

In brief: More than one million new nurses needed by 2010. (2002, January/February). *The American Nurse.* Washington, DC: American Nurses Publishing.

Molea, J. (2004). The dangers of stress. *Vital Signs, 14*(1), 6–7, 30.

Smoyak, S., & Rouslin, S. (Eds.). (1982). *A collection of classics in psychiatric nursing literature.* Thoroughfare, NJ: Charles B. Slack.

Studzinski, S. R. (2002). Patient education trends: The main tool is cyberspace. *ADVANCE for Nurse Practitioners, 10*(10), 89–90.

Taylor, R. (1998). Forensic nursing: Standards for a new specialty. *American Journal of Nursing, 98*(2), 73.

Willing, J. (2003). Digital evolution. *ADVANCE for Nurses, 4*(3), 17–19.

CHAPTER 3 / DEVELOPMENT OF PSYCHIATRIC–MENTAL HEALTH NURSING THEORY

By unfolding the development of our theoretical past, we gain insights that improve our understanding of our current progress, and we are empowered to achieve our disciplinary goals. By looking at our theoretical present, we see shadows of our past as well as visions of our future. Reconstructing our theoretical heritage is a process that involves reconstructing our present reality. —MELEIS, 2005

LEARNING OBJECTIVES

AFTER STUDYING THIS CHAPTER, YOU SHOULD BE ABLE TO:

1. Define *conceptual framework*.
2. Explain the purpose of theory.
3. Describe three types of theory used in psychiatric nursing.
4. Analyze the theories of Hildegard Peplau, Dorothea Orem, Sister Callista Roy, Martha Rogers, and Rosemarie Parse.
5. Articulate how nursing theory is applied to practice.
6. Interpret the phrase *eclectic approach*.

KEY TERMS

Behavioral Nursing theory
Cognator
Conceptual framework
Eclectic approach
Interaction-oriented approach
Interpersonal theory
Needs-oriented approach
Outcome-oriented approach
Regulator
Systems-oriented theory
Theory
Theory of Adaptation
Theory of Human Becoming

Before the 1950s, the medical model dominated psychiatric–mental health nursing practice. Physicians and psychiatrists assessed, diagnosed, and planned care for individuals with psychiatric disorders. Nurse practitioners were taught and supervised mainly by physicians and psychiatrists who incorporated the theories of individuals such as Freud, Sullivan, Skinner, Bowen, or Erikson into their practice. However, during this same period, nursing leaders began to emerge to provide impetus for the development of psychiatric nursing as an independent discipline (Fitzpatrick, Whall, Johnston, & Floyd, 1982). Table 3-1 describes how various theoretical frameworks of other disciplines influenced the development of psychiatric nursing theory. Specific theoretical models of personality development are discussed in Chapter 24.

Terminology such as conceptual models or frameworks and theories have been used freely and interchangeably to refer to any conceptualization of nursing reality. The interchangeable use of these terms has presented a problem to the pure semanticists in the field of nursing. For example, although it is a paper written to describe her view of nursing, Florence Nightingale's *Notes on Nursing: What It Is, and What It Is Not* (1859), is considered to be nursing's first environmental theory (Gropper, 1990).

Conceptual frameworks (a group of concepts linked together to describe a specific viewpoint) were developed by theorists such as Hildegard Peplau in 1952, Virginia Henderson in 1955, Martha Rogers in 1970, Imogene King in 1971, Dorothea Orem in 1971, and Sister Callista Roy in 1971. These frameworks provided a foundation and strategy for theory development by introducing orderliness into the research process and providing ideas for statements of theoretical hypotheses (ie, predicted relationships among variables under investigation). Hypotheses lead to empirical studies that seek to confirm or discredit predictions. Theoretical hypotheses eventually lead to the development of theories, which are abstract generalizations that present systematic explanations about the relationships among variables.

Early theorists focused on interpersonal relationships between client and nurse, behavioral responses to stress and the environment, and approaches to self-

TABLE 3.1 Theoretical Frameworks Influencing the Development of Psychiatric Nursing Theory

THEORIST	THEORY	IMPACT ON NURSING THEORY
Sigmund Freud	Psychoanalytic theory	Nurses began to focus on human behavior, early stages of sexual development, and use of maladaptive defense mechanisms.
Harry Stack Sullivan	Interpersonal theory	Nurses recognized that humans are social beings who develop interpersonal relationships that could result in stress or anxiety, the use of maladaptive behaviors, or alteration of the development of one's personality.
B.F. Skinner	Behavior theory	Nurses recognized that interventions could be used to bring about changes in thoughts, feelings, and observed behavior.
Murray Bowen	Family Systems theory	Nurses developed an understanding of individual and family behaviors and their relationship to each other.
Eric Erikson	Developmental theory	Nurses recognized that personality development begins at birth and continues across the lifespan until death.

Adapted from Boyd (2004), Johnson (1997), Meleis (2005), and Videbeck (2004).

care deficit. The phrase **systems-oriented theory** also evolved at this time. For example, in systems-oriented theory the individual is considered part of the family system. Stress in one part of the system (eg, family) affects other parts of the system. Changes in family structure contribute to changes in the behavior of individuals.

Since the 1970s, nursing theories based on caring, cultural care diversity and universality, modeling and role modeling, energy fields, and human becoming have emerged. Table 3-2 provides a chronology of nursing theorists and theories.

This chapter highlights the major theories and nursing theorists and describes the application of nursing theory to psychiatric–mental health nursing practice.

Theory

Theory is considered a branch of science dealing with conceptual principles that describe, explain, and predict a class of phenomena. Meleis (2005) defines theory as an organized, coherent, and systematic artic-

ulation of a set of statements related to significant questions in a discipline that is communicated in a meaningful whole. It is a symbolic depiction of aspects of reality that are discovered or invented to describe, explain, predict, or prescribe responses, events, situations, conditions, or relationships.

Theories can be tested, challenged, modified, or replaced, or they can become obsolete. For example, Rosemarie Parse's theory of human becoming was initially called the *Man-Living-Health Theory* when it was first published in 1981. Parse synthesized her theory from works by European philosophers and the American theorist Martha Rogers. The name was officially changed to the *Theory of Human Becoming* in 1992 to remove the word "man" from its title.

Nursing Theories

Johnson (1997) noted that theory is necessary for the further development of nursing as a profession. Several nurse theorists, such as Hildegard Peplau, Dorothea Orem, Sister Callista Roy, and Rosemarie Parse, have focused on concepts specifically related to

---

TABLE 3.2 Chronology of Nursing Theorists and Theories

YEAR	THEORIST	THEORY
1859	Florence Nightingale	Environmental theory
1952	Hildegard Peplau	Interpersonal theory
1955	Virginia Henderson	Needs theory
1960	Faye Abdellah	Patient-centered theory
1961	Josephine Patterson and Loretta Zderad	Interaction theory
1961	Ida Orlando	Interaction theory
1964	Ernestine Weidenbach	Interaction theory
1964	Joyce Travelbee	Interaction theory
1966	Myra Levine	Conservation theory
1970	Martha Rogers	Unitary Human Being theory
1971	Imogene King	Systems theory Updated
1971	Dorothea Orem	Self-care Deficit theory Updated
1971	Sister Callista Roy	Adaptation theory
1972	Betty Neuman	Systems theory
1973	Madeleine Leininger	Cultural Care Diversity theory
1978	Joyce Fitzpatrick	Rhythm theory
1979	Jean Watson	Human Caring theory
1981	Rosemarie Parse	Human Becoming theory
1983	Helen Erickson, Evelyn Tomlin, and Mary Ann Swain	Modeling and Role Modeling theory

psychiatric nursing. Other theorists are discussed in the text where relevant.

Peplau's Interpersonal Theory

Hildegard Peplau was responsible in part for the emergence of theory-based psychiatric nursing practice. She believed that the nurse serves as therapist, counselor, socializing agent, manager, technical nurse, mother surrogate, and teacher. Her **Interpersonal theory** incorporates communication and relationship concepts from Harry Stack Sullivan's Interpersonal theory. Her theory focuses primarily on the nurse–client relationship in which problem-solving skills are developed. Four phases occur during this interactive process: orientation, identification, exploitation, and resolution (Meleis, 2005; also available at http://www.sandiego.edu/academics/nursing/theory/).

Analysis of this theory (Johnson, 1997) reveals that it is effective in long-term care, home health, and psychiatric settings where time allows for the development of a nurse–client relationship and, hopefully, a resolution to promote health. However, the theory's effectiveness is limited in short-term, acute care nursing settings, where hospitalizations last for only a few hours or a few days. It is also ineffective when the client is considered to be a group of individuals, a family, or a community.

Orem's Behavioral Nursing Theory

Orem's **Behavioral Nursing theory** focuses on self-care deficit. It proposes that the recipients of nursing care are persons who are incapable of continuous self-care or independent care because of health-related or health-derived limitations (Johnson, 1997; McFarland &Thomas, 1991; also available at: http://www.sandiego.edu/academics/nursing/theory/).

Human beings are described as integrated wholes functioning biologically, symbolically, and socially. Because of an individual's self-care deficits, a nurse, family member, or friend may educate or consult with the individual to improve the deficit. This theory is used in the psychiatric setting, where individuals may neglect self-care needs such as eating, drinking, rest, personal hygiene, and safety because of their underlying disorder.

Roy's Theory of Adaptation

Roy's **theory of Adaptation,** modeled from a behavioral theory, states that human beings use coping mechanisms to adapt to both internal and external stimuli. Two major internal coping mechanisms are the regulator and the cognator. The **regulator** mechanism refers to an individual's physiologic response to stress, whereas the **cognator** mechanism pertains to perceptual, social, and information-processing functions. Coping behavior occurs in four adaptive modes: physiologic, self-concept, role function, and interdependence. Individuals sustain health through the integration of the four modes of adaptation. This theory is used in the psychiatric setting as the nurse assesses client behavior and stimuli and develops a plan of care to assist the client in adaptation in the four modes—contributing to health, quality of life, and dying with dignity. (Johnson, 1997; McFarland & Thomas, 1991; also available at: http://www2.bc.edu/~royca/).

Parse's Theory of Human Becoming

Parse's **theory of Human Becoming** presents an alternative to both the conventional biomedical approach and the bio-psycho-social-spiritual approach of most other theories of nursing. Parse first published this theory in 1981. Parse's Human Becoming theory posits quality of life from each person's own perspective as the goal of nursing practice. In other words, the role of the nurse is to guide the client or simply be with him or her to bear witness to the client's experiences. Three themes are noted: meaning, rhythmicity, and transcendence.

The first theme, meaning, refers to clients' coparticipating in creating what is real for them through self-expression in living their values in a chosen way rather than according to the expectation of others. The second theme, rhythmicity, explains that in living moment to moment, one determines whether to show or not to show aspects of oneself as opportunities and limitations emerge in moving with and apart from others. The third theme, transcendence, explains that moving beyond the "now" moment is forging a unique personal path for oneself in the midst of ambiguity and continuous change.

Parse's theory is considered by some advanced practitioners to be an excellent framework for community psychiatric nursing in which the nurse focuses on the client's experiences, not problems; bears witness to the client's experiences; respects the individual's capacity for self-knowing; and assists the client in co-creating a valuable space for the client to voice the lived experience of health (Parse, 2003; also available at http://www.Sandiego.edu/academics/nursing/theory). Humanly lived experiences such as loss and grief are believed to respond well to interventions based on Parse's theory. Clients with mood disorders and psychotic disorders also have benefited from interventions promoting independence and empowerment.

Application to Practice

Meleis (2005) discusses the application of nursing theory to psychiatric nursing practice. Using nursing theory, nurses focus on various aspects of care depending on identified needs or presenting problems of psychiatric clients. Several approaches may be used: needs oriented; interaction oriented; outcome oriented; and eclectic.

Needs-Oriented Approach

With a **needs-oriented approach**, nurses are actively doing and functioning. They problem-solve, perform physiologic and psychosocial activities for the client, supplement knowledge, and may become temporary self-care agents for clients with self-care deficits.

Interaction-Oriented Approach

The **interaction-oriented approach** is used by nurses who rely on interactions and include themselves in the sphere of other actions. They view themselves as a therapeutic tool and evaluate their actions according to the client's response. They counsel, guide, and teach clients, helping them to find meaning in their situations. They appear to be process oriented.

Outcome-Oriented Approach

The **outcome-oriented approach** is used by nurses who are viewed as goal setters. They are referred to as controllers, conservators, and healers without touch. They focus on maintaining and promoting energy and harmony with the environment. They do not view themselves as therapeutic agents, because they focus on enhancing the development of health environments.

Eclectic Approach

The **eclectic approach** is an individualized style that incorporates the client's own resources as a unique person with the most suitable theoretical model. Therapists may specialize in one particular conceptual framework or combine aspects of different ones. The therapist realizes there is no one way to deal with all of life's stresses or problems of living and is open to new ideas and approaches as the need arises.

Agreement Among Nursing Theorists

Although nursing theorists differ in their beliefs and concepts, they do agree on some points (Meleis, 2005). The following are some of the statements of agreement that guide student nurses as they enter the area of psychiatric nursing:

- Nursing theories offer a beginning articulation of what nursing is and what roles nurses play.
- Nursing theories provide descriptions of how to help clients become comfortable, how to deliver treatment with the least damage, and how to enhance high-level wellness.
- Nursing theories offer a beginning common language and a beginning agreement about who the nursing care recipients are.
- Nurses should not view the recipients only through biologic glasses or psychological glasses, but rather through holistic glasses. Clients are more than the sum total of their psychological, sociological, cultural, or biologic parts.
- Recipients of care respond to events in a holistic way.
- Recipients have needs, and nursing assists them in meeting those needs.

Nurses provide care for clients who are in constant interaction with their environment. They may have unmet needs, may be unable to care for themselves, or may be unable to adapt to the environment as a result of interruptions or potential interruptions in health. The role of nurses is to provide therapeutic care so that clients are able to adapt to the environment and meet identified needs related to self-care ability, health, and well-being.

KEY CONCEPTS

◆ In the past, psychiatric nursing practice was dominated by the medical model.

◆ Although Florence Nightingale's publication of *Notes on Nursing. What It Is, and What It Is Not* (1859), was written to express her views on nursing, it is considered to be nursing's first environmental theory.

◆ Conceptual frameworks of nursing care were first developed in the 1950s by Peplau and Henderson. These frameworks paved the way for research and the development of nursing theories.

◆ Early psychiatric nursing theories focused on interpersonal relationships (Peplau), behavioral responses to stress and the environment (Roy), and self-care deficit (Orem).

◆ Nursing theories have since emerged based on caring, cultural care diversity and universality, modeling and role modeling, energy fields, and human becoming.

◆ Theory has been defined as a science that deals with conceptual principles that describe, explain, and predict a class of phenomena. A theory is an organized, coherent, and systematic articulation of a set of statements related to significant questions in a discipline that are communicated in a meaningful whole. Theory is necessary for the further development of nursing as a profession.

◆ In the psychiatric setting, the nurse may use needs-oriented, interaction-oriented, outcome-oriented, and eclectic approaches to care. The role of nurses is to provide therapeutic care to promote adaptation to the environment and to meet identified needs related to self-care ability, health, and well-being.

For additional study materials, please refer to the Student Resource CD-ROM located in the back of this textbook.

CHAPTER WORKSHEET

CRITICAL THINKING QUESTIONS

1. A 50-year-old client with a history of chronic depression tells the nurse that he feels he is a failure because he has lost his job due to company layoffs. Describe how the nursing care of this client differs using the theoretical approach of Peplau as compared with Roy's theoretical approach.
2. Using Parse's theory of nursing, explain how the nurse assists a client who has been a victim of abuse to focus on becoming a survivor.
3. Summarize the positive and negative points of each of the theories discussed in the chapter. Select one of the theories and discuss how it could be used in a recently encountered client situation.

REFLECTION

Reflect on the development of psychiatric nursing and nursing theories by Peplau, Roy, and Parse. Do they remain appropriate, or should modifications be considered to meet the multifaceted needs of clients in the 21st century?

NCLEX-STYLE QUESTIONS

1. All nursing theorists agree that nursing theories provide which of the following? Select all that apply.
   a. An expansive description of what nursing is
   b. A description of how to promote high-level wellness
   c. The view of the recipient as a biologic being
   d. A beginning description of nurses' roles
   e. A highly developed common language

2. Nursing theorists concur in viewing humans as beings who are primarily which of the following?
   a. Biologic
   b. Holistic
   c. Psychological
   d. Sociological

3. The psychiatric nurse is providing care for a newly admitted client who is homeless and has not been able to bathe or change clothes for 2 weeks. Which of the following theorists would the nurse apply, using a needs approach to guide the nursing interventions for this client situation?
   a. Leininger
   b. Orem
   c. Peplau
   d. Roy

4. The nurse refers a client with a nursing diagnosis of "Dysfunctional Grieving related to the death of a spouse" to a grief support group. The nurse's recommendation emphasizes coping mechanisms in adaptation, illustrating which of the following nursing theories?
   a. Levine
   b. Henderson
   c. Peplau
   d. Roy

5. The nurse uses concepts of several theoretical approaches in the practice of psychiatric nursing. This practice can be said to be which of the following?
   a. Eclectic
   b. Limited in scope
   c. Interaction oriented
   d. Research based

6. The psychiatric nurse focuses on the use of self as a therapeutic tool and evaluates nursing actions according to client response. Which of the following best describes this nurse's practice?
   a. Interaction oriented
   b. Eclectic
   c. Needs oriented
   d. Outcome oriented

Selected References

Boyd, M. A. (2004). *Psychiatric nursing: Contemporary practice* (3rd ed.). Philadelphia: Lippincott Williams & Wilkins.

Fitzpatrick, J., Whall, A., Johnston, R., & Floyd, J. (1982). *Nursing models and their psychiatric-mental health application.* Bowie, MD: Robert J. Brady.

Gropper, E. I. (1990). Florence Nightingale: Nursing's first environmental theorist. *Nursing Forum, 25*(3), 30–33.

Johnson, B. S. (1997). *Psychiatric-mental health nursing: Adaptation and growth* (4th ed.). Philadelphia: Lippincott-Raven.

McFarland, G. K., & Thomas, M. D. (1991). *Psychiatric-mental health nursing: Application of the nursing process.* Philadelphia: J. B. Lippincott.

Meleis, A. I. (2005). *Theoretical nursing: Development and progress* (3rd ed.). Philadelphia: Lippincott Williams & Wilkins.

Nightingale, F. (1859). *Notes on nursing: What it is, and what it is not.* London: Harrison.

Parse, R. R. (2003). *Community: A human becoming experience.* Boston: Jones and Bartlett.

Videbeck, S. L. (2004). *Psychiatric-mental health nursing* (2nd ed.). Philadelphia: Lippincott Williams & Wilkins.

Suggested Readings

DeChasnay, M. (2004). *Caring for the vulnerable: Perspectives in nursing theory, practice, and research.* Boston: Jones & Bartlett.

Marriner-Tomey, A. & Aligood, M. R. (2002). *Nursing theorists and their work.* St. Louis, MO: C. V. Mosby.

McKenna, H. (1997). *Nursing models and theories.* London: Rutledge.

Powers, B. A. & Knapp, T. K. (1995). *Dictionary of nursing theory and research.* Thousand Oaks, CA: Sage Publications.

Redic, L. (2000). Nursing theory, research vital to practice. *ADVANCE for Nurse Practitioners, 8*(5), 16.

Sitzman, K. (2004). *Understanding the work of nurse theorists: A creative beginning.* Boston: Jones & Bartlett.

Taylor, E. J. (2001). *Spiritual care: Nursing theory, research, & practice.* St. Paul, MN: Prentice Hall.

Watson, J. (1999). *Nursing human science and human care* (2nd ed.). New York: National League for Nursing.

CHAPTER 4 / SPIRITUAL, CULTURAL, AND ETHNIC ISSUES

*Health Care Organizations should ensure that patients/consumers receive effective, understand-
able and respectful care that is provided in a manner compatible with their cultural health
beliefs and practices and preferred languages.* —OFFICE OF MINORITY HEALTH (2000)

LEARNING OBJECTIVES

AFTER STUDYING THIS CHAPTER, YOU SHOULD BE ABLE TO:

1. Articulate the importance of understanding the meaning of the following terminology when providing care for culturally diverse clients: *religion, spirituality*, and *spiritual distress.*
2. Discuss the relationships among culture, ethnicity, and human behavior.
3. Identify how ethnocentrism and stereotyping can affect nursing care.
4. Differentiate the three modes of culturally congruent care according to Leininger.
5. Discuss the use of mental health services by ethnic groups.
6. Explain how the different perceptions of mental health by providers and clients can affect the use of mental health services.
7. Compare and contrast different cultural beliefs about mental illness.
8. Discuss nursing implications derived from research on ethnopharmacology.
9. Summarize how the nurse uses knowledge about spirituality and culture when caring for clients from various ethnic groups.

KEY TERMS

Acculturation
Culture
Culture-bound syndrome
Cultural care accommodation/negotiation
Cultural care preservation/maintenance
Cultural care repatterning/restructuring
Ethnic group
Ethnicity
Ethnocentrism
Ethnopharmacology
Religion
Spiritual distress
Spirituality
Stereotyping
Subculture
Yin-yang

Psychiatric–mental health nursing provides client care that maintains mental health, prevents potential problems, and treats human response to actual problems of mental illness. Although Abraham Maslow's theory states that all human behavior is motivated by basic human needs, the expression of these needs depends on the complex relationships among biology, psychology, and culture (Maslow, 1987). Psychiatric nursing considers how the relationships among these factors affect the client with a mental illness. With the increased cultural diversity in the United States, the nurse encounters clients with spiritual beliefs, customs, and lifestyles different from her or his own. Therefore, it is essential to incorporate knowledge about clients' spiritual needs as well as their cultural diversity into psychiatric–mental health nursing care.

This chapter focuses on how spirituality, culture, ethnicity, and the process of **acculturation** (the ways in which individuals and cultural groups adapt and change over time) affect individual and family behavior, including the implications for psychiatric nursing practice.

Spirituality

Spirituality can be understood within a wide range of contexts. It has been defined as that aspect of every human being, rooted in our unique createdness that is on a sacred journey of completeness, sometimes seeking to connect with and trust in the divine being (Vink, 2003). The concept of spirituality also refers to a person's belief in a "power," not necessarily a Creator, apart from his or her own existence. Spirituality is not confined to architectural designs such as churches, synagogues, or temples.

The terms *spirituality* and *religion* are often used interchangeably, but for many they have different meanings. Spirituality, which goes beyond religion and religious affiliation, is a personal quality that strives for inspiration, reverence, awe, meaning, and purpose in life. **Religion** is an organized system of beliefs and practices that focus on a higher power that governs the universe. It has been described as a specific manifestation of one's spiritual drive to create meaning in the world and to develop a relationship with God. Although many clients consider themselves both spiritual and religious, some clients may consider themselves spiritual, but not religious. Conversely, other clients may consider themselves religious, but not spiritual.

Spirituality and religious beliefs can affect a client's recovery rate and attitude toward treatment. They can be a source of strength as the client deals with stress, or they may contribute to conflicts. Carpenito-Moyet (2006) defines **spiritual distress** as the state in which an individual or group experiences, or is at risk of experiencing, a disturbance in the belief or value system that provides strength, hope, and meaning to life. The distress may be related to challenges to the belief system, separation from spiritual ties, or personal or environmental conflict.

Andrews and Boyle (2003) discuss several reasons why nurses fail to provide spiritual care to culturally diverse clients. They state that the nurse may:

- view religious and spiritual needs as a private matter between the client and his or her Creator
- deny the existence of spiritual needs or feel uncomfortable about one's own religious beliefs
- lack knowledge about the religious beliefs or spirituality of others
- mistake spiritual needs for psychosocial needs
- believe that the spiritual needs of clients are the responsibility of a family or pastor

The goal of spiritual nursing care is to promote the client's physical, emotional, and spiritual health. The nurse who provides spiritual interventions recognizes that the balance of physical, psychosocial, and spiritual well-being is essential to overall good health (Andrews & Boyle, 2003).

Cultural perceptions regarding mental illness as a spiritual concern are addressed later in this chapter. Spiritual assessment and interventions as part of the nursing process are addressed in detail in Chapter 12, The Therapeutic Milieu.

Culture and Nursing

Culture is a broad term referring to a set of shared beliefs, values, behavioral norms, and practices that are common to a group of people sharing a common identity and language. The United States has more than 100 cultural groups, whose members have thousands of beliefs and practices related to what is considered appropriate behavior in conducting one's life, maintaining health, and preventing and treating illness. For example, providing care for an elderly parent with a chronic illness can require significant lifestyle changes and self-sacrifice for the care-giving son or daughter. Cultural background can affect willingness to sacrifice individual needs to fulfill familial obligations. For example, the Vietnamese culture values family and community over individual needs, whereas European American middle-class culture emphasizes fulfilling individual needs. Thus, one's cultural background can shape decision-making and behavior in this situation.

Much of an individual's behavior and way of thinking is automatic and originates from childhood learning. Learning about acceptable and expected behavior in one's culture occurs from earliest childhood through socialization. Children acculturate more quickly than adults because they are exposed to other cultures through schooling. They also learn cultural characteristics as they associate with others. The family has the first and most profound influence on the development of traditional values and practices. However, the community, school, church, government, and media also play significant roles. For example, loss and grief are painful for all individuals, yet how we express and process this experience depends almost completely on culture (DiCicco-Bloom, 2000).

A **subculture** is a smaller group that exists within a larger culture. Members of a subculture may share commonalities, such as age, gender, race, ethnicity, socioeconomic status, religious and spiritual beliefs, sexual orientation, occupation, and even health status. Therefore, an individual is influenced both by the larger cultural group (ie, society) and by membership in multiple subcultures. The client and the nurse thus can be members of quite different subcultures, as well as share membership in other particular subcultures. In psychiatric–mental health nursing, the nurse must be sensitive to factors affecting the client and to the influences on his or her own behavior.

Introspection and self-analysis regarding one's own cultural background and membership in particular subcultures is important. Cultural sensitivity requires the nurse to develop awareness of his or her attitudes, beliefs, and values (DiCicco-Bloom, 2000). Values and beliefs that are not examined and analyzed can influence the nurse's judgment about clients, thereby

SELF-AWARENESS PROMPT

Select a client assigned to your care. How is the client's cultural background different from yours? Do any of your values conflict with the client's beliefs and values? What are your expectations of this client? Explain your answers.

affecting the nurse–client relationship. For example, the nurse, as a member of a helping profession (a distinct subculture) relying on principles of good communication, places value on maintaining eye contact when talking with a client. If the client happens to be a member of a Native American culture, however, avoidance of eye contact is considered a sign of respect. Therefore, the nurse may misinterpret this behavior as a sign that the client is not interested in communicating with the nurse.

Ethnicity, or **ethnic group,** refers to people in a larger social system whose members have common ancestral, racial, physical, or national characteristics, and who share cultural symbols such as language, lifestyles, and religion (Andrews & Boyle, 2003). For example, hundreds of different Native American and Alaskan tribes and many different Asian and Pacific Island ethnic groups exist. There are also different ethnic groups of African Americans, including individuals from Africa, the Caribbean, and other parts of the world. Other examples of ethnic groups include people who share membership in American culture, but trace their ethnic identity to Western and Eastern Europe. Thus, ethnicity differs from culture in that ethnic identity is often defined by specific geographic origins as well as other unique characteristics that differ from the larger cultural group.

The tendency to believe that one's own way of thinking, believing, and behaving is superior to that of others is called **ethnocentrism.** Hunt (2001) presents an example of an ethnocentric response by a nurse as follows: "Ms. Wang is noncompliant with her treatment. She won't take her real medicine and only takes the teas given her by the community herbalist." The belief that only prescribed medication is useful or helpful to the client leads the nurse to conclude that the client is noncompliant. A nurse who respects another's belief system would discuss with this client the reasons she does not want to take the prescribed medication.

Judgments or generalizations about members of a particular ethnic group or a subculture different from one's own can lead to the problem of **stereotyping,** or assuming that all members of a particular group are alike. Although information about different ethnic groups can be valuable to the nurse, this information represents generalizations about behavior. No assumptions can be made about an individual client unless the generalization is tested with the individual (DiCicco-Bloom, 2000). To avoid stereotyping, the nurse must remember that each individual is unique and has a unique cultural heritage that differs not only from other ethnic groups but also from others within one's own group. Therefore, the use of the word "some" is important when referring to a particular subculture or ethnic group.

Culturally Congruent Nursing Care

Nursing is no stranger to the issue of cultural diversity. Our society is becoming a kaleidoscope of racial and ethnic groups, behaviors, values, world perspectives, social customs, and attitudes. The professed gold standard is to guarantee culturally relevant care in a multicultural society where cross-cultural communication and cultural sensitivity are the norm, and care is provided by culturally competent nurses who were educated in programs with a culturally diverse student body and faculty. These programs place students in rural sites or culturally diverse, underserved areas for clinical experiences. Multicultural medical and psychiatric issues are incorporated into the curriculum. If nurses are to deliver culturally diverse care effectively, they need to reflect upon their values and beliefs, seek direction from their professional organizations, and

SELF-AWARENESS PROMPT

Think of an example of when you first encountered a client from an ethnic or age subculture different than yours. What were your attitudes or expectations about this client? How did the client differ from what you expected?

modify their own behavior (Gooden, Porter, Gonzalez, & Mims, 2001).

Madeline Leininger, a nurse with a background in cultural anthropology, developed a theory of nursing based on the concept of culturally congruent care (Leininger, 1991). Leininger's model uses worldview, social structure, language, ethnohistory, environmental context, and generic (folk) and professional systems to provide a comprehensive and holistic view of influences on culture care and well-being (Andrews & Boyle, 2003). According to Leininger, the nurse who plans and implements care for clients from diverse ethnic groups will do so using one of three culturally congruent nursing care modes. These modes are:

- Cultural care preservation/maintenance
- Cultural care accommodation/negotiation
- Cultural care repatterning/restructuring

In **cultural care preservation/maintenance,** the nurse assists the client in maintaining health practices that are derived from membership in a certain ethnic group. For example, a client with a Chinese background may want foods that are considered "hot" to counteract an illness that is considered "cold." The nurse helps the client select and obtain foods congruent with these beliefs.

In **cultural care accommodation/negotiation,** the nurse adapts nursing care to accommodate the client's beliefs or negotiate aspects of care that would require the client to change certain practices. For example, a Native American client may wish to have a tribal healer visit him in the hospital and perform a healing ceremony. The nurse accommodates this wish and negotiates with the client about incorporating the rituals of the tribal healer into his medical treatment. If rituals and other spiritually focused activities are important to the client, clinicians must respect and work with, not against, this philosophy.

In **cultural care repatterning/restructuring,** the nurse educates the client to change practices that are not conducive to health. Lefever and Davidhizar (1991) describe how members of a particular Eskimo ethnic group believe that wrapping red yarn around the head can cure pain in the head. The nurse repatterns or teaches a client from this culture that if head pain persists, the continued wrapping of red yarn may delay needed treatment.

Regardless of the model of culturally competent nursing care used, the nurse demonstrates sensitivity and respect for the individual client's beliefs, norms, values, and health practices. The use of assessment and communication skills and nursing implementations that enhance and support cultural perspectives of the client are the means to deliver this care.

Population Groups

The federal government divides the U.S. population into several broad cultural groups, also referred to as *pan-ethnic groups*. These groups are referred to in research studies and statistics, and therefore are important for the nurse to understand. The categories and population percentages are as follows: Hispanic, 12.55%; non-Hispanic white, 69.13%; non-Hispanic black, 12.06%; non-Hispanic American Indian and Eskimo, 0.74%; non-Hispanic Asian, 3.6%; non-Hispanic Hawaiian or Pacific Islander, 0.13%; non-Hispanic other, 0.17%; and two or more races, 1.64% (Social Science Data Analysis Network [SSDAN], 2004). In the United States, white Americans are referred to as the majority population, and the other groups are called *ethnic minorities*. In 2005, the Hispanic population was considered to be the largest of the pan-ethnic minority groups, and by 2025, their number is expected to double.

Note that these broad divisions ignore the unique characteristics of and differences among people in these groups. For example, the category of "white" fails to make any distinction among people who trace their ethnic origin from the various countries of Western and Eastern Europe. Think of three persons tracing their origin from England, Poland, and Russia. All three persons would be classified as white, although they do not completely share language, customs, beliefs, or ethnic identity. The category of "Asian/Pacific Islander" includes people from more than 60 different countries (Andrews & Boyle, 2003). The Hispanic category is composed of diverse ethnic groups, including people from Mexico, Cuba, Puerto Rico, Spain, and Central and South America (Munet-Vilaro, Folkman, & Gregorich, 1999). In discussing the issue of racial–ethnic blending, Ferrante states that 1 of every 24 children in the United States is classified as a race different from one or both of the parents due to adoption, biracial, or multiracial status (2001). Andrews and Boyle (2003), in their discussion of pan-ethnic groups, point out that the nurse should ask the client, "With what cultural group or groups do you identify?" This question allows the client to establish his or her own ethnicity and helps the nurse to avoid making assumptions about ethnicity.

Use of Mental Health Services by Ethnic Groups

In the United States, members of diverse ethnic groups do not use mental health care to the same extent as members of the dominant European American middle class. According to the U.S. Surgeon General's report on mental health, an important reason for the underuse of mental health services by members of diverse ethnic groups is that language, values, and belief systems may be quite different in the providers as compared with these clients (U.S. Department of Health and Human Services [DHHS], 1999). The socioeconomic status of diverse ethnic groups, specifically that people in these groups are more likely to be affected by poverty and lack of health insurance, must also be considered (U.S. DHHS, 1999).

Nature of the Mental Health System

The U.S. mental health system was not designed to respond to the cultural and linguistic needs of diverse ethnic populations. In a historical review of U.S. psychiatric treatment, Moffic and Kinzie (1996) point out that treatment originally consisted of generic psychiatry (ie, assuming that humans the world over are no different and will react to given stressors in the same manner). The recognition that beliefs, values, family expectations, and other ingredients combine uniquely in various ethnic groups has been slow. Further, the values and beliefs of mental health care providers often differ from those of clients from diverse ethnic groups. The system itself, and most mental health providers, has a European American middle-class orientation, perhaps with biases, misconceptions, and stereotypes regarding other cultures (U.S. DHHS, 1999).

Nursing also tends to have the same values as the European American middle-class culture. DiCicco-Bloom (2000) reports that in 1996, nearly 90% of nurses reported themselves as white non-Hispanic, as compared with 72% of the U.S. population. The differences between providers' and clients' values, beliefs, health practices, and language contribute to the difficulties in delivering services to people from diverse ethnic groups.

Emphasis being placed on the individual, versus on the relationship between the individual and society, illustrates how values of the provider and the client may clash. European American middle-class culture is primarily individualistic, emphasizing freedom of choice and personal responsibility. The dominant set of values is oriented toward individuals, who are viewed as accountable for decision-making, self-care, and many other self-oriented tasks. Privacy rights and personal freedom are based on the value of individualism. In many ethnic groups, however, individualism is not a primary value. Instead, these groups are *sociocentric,* emphasizing the mandatory responsibility of the individual to the family and larger society. For example, Hispanic, Asian, and African traditions typically paint a more social picture of life, emphasizing balance and cooperation over individualistic concerns (Mitchell, 2004). Consequently, psychiatric treatment's emphasis on client self-responsibility is congruent with European American middle-class values, but not necessarily with the values of other ethnic groups. This essential difference in values can help account for the underuse of mental health services by ethnic groups, as well as the fact that when care is utilized, it is not perceived as helpful.

Guarnaccia (1998) provides an example of the effect of differences regarding individual and personal responsibility. A middle-aged Hispanic mother of a 25-year-old son with schizophrenia asked for advice from her support group, which consisted primarily of white members, about how to handle her son's refusal to take his medication. Their advice was to not allow her son to live at home unless he agrees to take medication. If the support group were more culturally aware, they would have understood that interdependence is valued in Hispanic families, and the mother would not consider turning her son out of her home. Thus, the support group was not helpful to this woman's situation.

Socioeconomic Status of Ethnic Groups

The Surgeon General's 1999 report stated that many racial and ethnic groups have limited financial resources (U.S. DHHS, 1999). There is an association between lower socioeconomic status (in terms of income, education, and occupation) and mental illness; however, no one is certain whether one influences the other. Certainly, substandard housing, unemployment or underemployment, poor nutrition, lack of preventive care, and limited access to medical care create severe stressors for affected families. Statistics from the 1990 U.S. census indicate that 23.4% of all foreign-born residents, including children and youth, who entered the United States between 1980 and 1990 are at or below the poverty level, as compared with 9.5% of the U.S.-born population (U.S. Bureau of the Census, 1993). This lack of finances can block needed psychiatric care from too many people, regardless of whether they have health insurance with inadequate mental health benefits, or are one of the 44 million Americans who lack any insurance (U.S. DHHS, 1999). More recent statistics indicate the following percentages of uninsured ethnic groups: white, 14.2%; African American, 21.2%; Asian and Pacific Islander, 20.8%; and Hispanic, 33.4% (U.S. Bureau of the Census, 1999). Thus, it is evident that many people from diverse ethnic groups lack adequate health insurance, are affected by poverty, or both.

Poor living conditions and lack of financial resources contribute to life stressors, thus affecting the need for psychiatric–mental health services. Although the need for services may be increased, help may not be accessible because of lack of finances. Even when available, services may not be used because of the substantial cultural differences between the providers and the users of these services.

Psychiatric–mental health care, like other health care, tends to occur as crisis intervention for those individuals without income sufficient to meet basic needs. The nurse working in the community or in a hospital emergency department encounters many clients who, because they are unable to pay for wellness care or early intervention, seek treatment only for severe illness. This is also true of psychiatric–mental health care. The psychiatric–mental health nurse encounters clients with multiple, complex problems related to the effects of poverty, whose insurance plans do not pay for psychiatric care or who are without family resources for payment.

Cultural Perceptions: Mental Illness as a Spiritual Concern

Some ethnic groups believe that mental illness is related to spiritual issues. For example, some Asian cultures interpret mental illness as a supernatural event caused by an offense to deities or spirits. The remedy

CLINICAL EXAMPLE 4.1

CULTURALLY COMPETENT CARE FOR THE CLIENT WITH SCHIZOPHRENIA

RS, a woman with an Hispanic background, was admitted to an inpatient psychiatric unit for treatment of schizophrenia. Her family brought her to the mental health center because she had been refusing to wash or change her clothes and would not sleep more than 3 hours at a time—she felt she had to remain on guard in the house in case something bad happened. When admitted, RS had multiple religious objects in her purse and carried a Bible everywhere she went. She claimed to have been visited by God and was on a special mission to save the world. Her family reported that she had always been very religious but had never talked like this before. They also told the nurse that the Bible she carried was a family Bible and was very important to her. The initial nursing plan of care involved asking RS to leave the purse and Bible in her room and encouraging her to participate with other clients in the milieu activities. She refused to leave her purse or Bible in her room and would not participate in any of the activities. The psychiatric treatment plan involved individual and group psychotherapy as well as medication with neuroleptics or antipsychotics to reduce delusional thinking. The primary nurse assigned to RS recognized that these spiritual objects were very important to her security and sense of well-being. Therefore, the nurse negotiated with the client that she would be able to keep her purse and Bible if she agreed to participate in the milieu activities and accept the medication and therapies. RS was agreeable to this plan.

involves appeasing or demonstrating respect for the spirits offended. The client with this belief may first seek help from spiritual advisors, such as Buddhist monks or other religious leaders (Vandiver & Keopraseuth, 1998). The nurse recognizes this and assists such clients to incorporate their spiritual beliefs into psychiatric care. The nurse encourages the client to maintain contact with his or her spiritual advisor while receiving psychiatric services. This is an example of Leininger's cultural care preservation/maintenance.

For some African American ethnic groups, especially those tracing their origin to Haiti, mental illness may be viewed as the result of a "hex" or "spell" put on the affected person. The removal of the hex involves the use of voodoo, plant roots, or both (working of roots) to prepare potions to bring about good or evil (Griffith & Baker, 1993). The nurse's respect for this belief, while encouraging acceptance of psychiatric care, is an example of Leininger's cultural care accommodation/negotiation.

Many members of Hispanic cultures rely heavily on the Roman Catholic Church. The client from this culture who is being treated by psychotherapy or medication may wish to integrate spiritual rituals into the prescribed plan of care (Bechtel, Davidhizer, & Tiller, 1998). Clinical Example 4-1: Culturally Competent Care for the Client With Schizophrenia illustrates how cultural care accommodation/negotiation can be used to assist a client with mental illness to accept psychiatric care.

Cultural Perceptions: Mental Illness as Imbalance or Disharmony in Nature

In some Native American cultures, mental illness is seen as a sign of imbalance with the rest of the natural world. This concept of balance in Native American culture can be compared with the idea of homeostasis in Western medicine; however, the Native American concept is broader in scope and includes the natural world as well as the human body (Thompson, Walker, & Silk-Walker, 1993). A similar concept of balance or harmony is expressed in Chinese culture. In this culture, the state of health exists when there is a finely balanced and rhythmic working of the body, an adjustment of the body by its physical environment, and harmonious relationships between bodily functions and emotions (Gaw, 1993). In such a concept of health, "chi" is an all-pervasive force that flows unrestricted through the body. Blockages in this system cause pain and disease (Mitchell, 2004). The chi force is believed to be regulated by **yin-yang.** Yin represents female, cold, and darkness; yang represents male, hot, and light (Andrews & Boyle, 2003).

Yamamoto, Silva, Justice, Chang, and Leong (1993) provide an interesting example of the nursing implications of these beliefs. A young Laotian client with major depression refused to take the antidepressant medication nortriptyline (Pamelor) because it was in a yellow and orange capsule. She believed too much heat in her body caused her illness, and therefore the treatment prescribed should be a "cold" color. She accepted another antidepressant that was blue in color. The nurse providing culturally congruent care is sensitive to the client's belief system regarding both mental illness and its acceptable treatment.

Cultural Expressions of Mental Illness and Nursing Implications

The expression of symptoms of mental illness and how they are perceived varies widely among cultures. Currently, the prevalence of mental disorders among ethnic groups in the United States is inadequately understood (U.S. DHHS, 1999). Major psychiatric disorders occur in every society and primary symptoms are similar across cultures. However, the secondary features of these disorders can be strongly influenced by culture (Kavanagh, 2003). In many ethnic groups, there is no distinction among physical, mental, and spiritual illness. Therefore, an individual suffering from severe environmental stressors or emotional distress might express this distress as a physical problem. For example, the experience of depression in the Taiwan Chinese culture usually takes the form of somatic illness. Complaints such as insomnia, anorexia, and weight loss thus may be an expression of depressive illness. Epidemiologic studies have confirmed that African Americans also have relatively high rates of somatization (U.S. DHHS, 1999).

The *Diagnostic and Statistical Manual of Mental Disorders (4th Edition, Text Revision; DSM-IV-TR)* recognizes that specific cultures may express mental distress differently from the European American middle-class majority culture. The term **culture-bound syndrome** denotes recurrent locality-specific patterns of aberrant behavior and troubling experience that are prominent in folk belief and practice (American Psychiatric Association, 2000; Sadock & Sadock, 2003). These syndromes appear to fall outside conventional Western psychiatric diagnostic categories. Table 4-1 lists examples of culture-bound syndromes. (The *DSM-IV-TR* provides a list of culture-bound syndromes from around the world.) The nurse must be aware that individuals from diverse ethnic groups might describe troubling experiences in terms of physical problems or specific culture-bound syndromes.

Psychiatric Nursing of Ethnic Groups
Ethnopharmacologic Considerations

Ethnopharmacology is the study of how ethnicity affects drug metabolism. It has special relevance to psychiatric nursing care in the aftermath of the Decade of the Brain (1990–2000) and the explosion of knowledge regarding psychotropic medications. The nurse needs to know that ethnic differences affect the efficacy of psychoactive medications and the incidence of adverse effects.

Research has demonstrated that the biotransformation or metabolism of psychoactive medications depends on biologic, cultural, and environmental factors (Mohr, 1998). The biologic or genetic basis for the differences in response to psychotropic drugs among different ethnic groups is related to the hepatic cytochrome P450 microsomal enzyme system (Lin, 1996). A specific P450 isozyme, the CYP2D6 enzyme, is responsible for metabolizing most antidepressant drugs, tricyclic antidepressants, and selective serotonin reuptake inhibitors (Mohr, 1998). Individuals who possess strong enzyme activity are known as "extensive metabolizers," whereas those with slower rates of enzyme activity are "poor metabolizers" (Mohr, 1998). People who are poor metabolizers are more likely to have adverse effects at doses of medication lower than recommended for a particular drug. For example, research related to the rate of CYP2D6 enzyme activity found that more than one third of the East Asian population is considered "poor metabolizers" (Smith & Mendoza, 1996). In contrast, only 1% to 2% of whites are "poor metabolizers." Thirty-three percent of African Americans have been found to be slower than whites in metabolizing psychotropic medications (Lin, Poland, Wan, Smith, & Lessner, 1996). This decreased metabolism can lead to an increased incidence of adverse effects, especially extrapyramidal symptoms, when standard doses of psychotropic drugs are used in clients from the ethnic groups described earlier.

Asian and African American clients may also require lower doses of lithium because each of these groups has been found to have a lower concentration of a particular plasma protein known to bind lithium. When lithium is in the form of nonbound lithium, it crosses the blood–brain barrier more readily to reach the central nervous system (Mohr, 1998). Mohr (1998) also cites an interesting study of lithium therapy in which Chinese clients did not complain about polyuria and

TABLE 4.1 Culture-Bound Syndromes

SYNDROME	ASSOCIATED CULTURE(S)	DESCRIPTION OF SYMPTOMS
Amok	Malaysia, Laos, Philippines, Polynesia	Dissociative episode followed by outburst of violent behavior directed at people or objects
Ataque de nervios	Latin-American and Latin-Mediterranean groups	Uncontrollable shouting, crying, trembling, and verbal or physical aggression. Occurs frequently as direct result of stressful family event
Bilis and colera	Latin-American and Latin-Mediterranean groups	Acute nervous tension, headache, trembling, screaming, stomach disturbance, and even loss of consciousness. Cause is thought to be strong anger or rage
Boufée delirante	West Africa and Haiti	Sudden outburst of agitated and aggressive behavior, confusion, and psychomotor excitement
Brain fag	West Africa	Difficulty concentrating, remembering, and thinking. Associated with challenge of schooling
Nervios	Latin America	General state of vulnerability to stressful life experiences. Wide range of symptoms of emotional distress
Dhat	India	Severe anxiety and hypochondriacal concerns
Falling-out or blacking out	Southern U.S. and Caribbean groups	Sudden collapse; may occur without warning, but sometimes preceded by feelings of dizziness. Person claims inability to see and may feel powerless to move.
Ghost sickness	American Indian tribes	Preoccupation with death and the deceased. Bad dreams, weakness, feelings of danger, anxiety, and hallucinations may occur.
Hwa-byung (wool-hwa-byung), "anger syndrome"	Korea	Insomnia, fatigue, panic, fear of impending death, indigestion, and anorexia
Pibloktog	Eskimo cultures	Abrupt dissociative episode accompanied by extreme excitement
Rootwork	African American, European American, and Caribbean groups	Illness ascribed to hexing, witchcraft, sorcery, or evil influence of another person
Shenjing shuairo (neurasthenia)	China	Physical and mental fatigue, dizziness, headaches, sleep disturbance, and memory loss
Susto, "fright" or "soul loss"	Latin American, Mexican, Central, and South American cultures	Illness attributed to frightening event that causes the soul to leave the body and results in unhappiness and sickness

Reprinted with permission from the *Diagnostic and Statistical Manual of Mental Disorders, 4th Edition, Text Revision*. Copyright 2000, American Psychiatric Association.

polydipsia because in Chinese tradition, water consumption and excretion were positive effects, ridding the body of toxins and aiding digestion. In this example, the nurse can focus client teaching on the risk of lithium toxicity with excessive diuresis and encourage reporting of this adverse effect.

Table 4-2 provides selected cultural implications of drugs used in the treatment of clients with psychiatric disorders.

Nursing Implications

Psychiatric–mental health nurses need to be aware of the increased incidence of adverse effects in both Asian and African American ethnic groups, with a focus on continued data collection related to dosage and the incidence of adverse effects. The nurse plays a key role in communicating and collaborating with the physician in evaluating the effects of psychotropic medica-

TABLE 4.2   Selected Cultural Implications of Psychotropic Agents

DRUG	CLINICAL FINDING
Antianxiety drugs diazepan (Valium) alprazolam (Xanax)	Some clients of Asian descent metabolize these drugs more slowly than do whites and require smaller doses.
Antidepressants	Asians and Hispanics may respond better to lower doses than do whites; nature of variation unclear.
Antipsychotics haloperidol (Haldol)	Blacks and whites appear to exhibit the same degree of adverse effects; Chinese clients require lower doses.
Antimanics lithium	Japanese clients may require lower doses than do whites.

Reprinted with permission: Kudzma, E.C. (1999). Culturally competent drug administrations. *American Journal of Nursing, 99*(B), 46–51.

tions on the client, including the effect of drug dosage. The nurse also teaches the client and family about measures to counteract adverse effects and the importance of reporting any adverse effects experienced.

Nonbiologic factors, such as nutrition and diet, also influence the action and adverse effects of psychotropic medications. For example, herbal and homeopathic remedies taken by clients can alter responses to medications. Ginseng can either inhibit or accelerate metabolism, possibly affecting both drug absorption and elimination (Kudzma, 1999). The nurse asks assessment questions related to the use of herbal and homeopathic remedies and communicates this information to the physician in collaborating in the treatment plan. (See Chapter 18, Complementary and Alternative Medical Therapy, for a discussion of herbal remedies.)

Role of Family

Families play an important role in providing support for individuals with psychiatric problems. However, the definition of what constitutes a family differs by ethnic group, as do the roles assumed by different family members. In some ethnic groups, the family may include the nuclear family, the extended family, and community members. Often, members of diverse ethnic groups will not seek psychiatric treatment until supports provided by family and community have been exhausted.

A study by Guarnaccia (1998) reports that African American and Hispanic ethnic groups tend to have large social support networks, and seek advice from these networks more frequently than from psychiatric professionals. When a client does enter the psychiatric treatment system, family members often expect to be involved in the care.

Asian American ethnic groups tend to emphasize family obligations, filial piety, and respect for one's parents and siblings. Typically there is a wide family network of grandparents, uncles, aunts, cousins, and godparents (Vandiver & Keopraseuth, 1998). Guilt and shame may be used as social sanctions to control behavior. Therefore, those with a mental illness may be viewed as bringing shame on the family.

The length of time that the family has lived in the United States is also important to consider in psychiatric care. Moffic and Kinzie (1996) discuss that the longer refugees live in the United States, the more pressing family and generational problems become. As younger members of the family embrace the new culture and older family members continue to cling to the culture they left behind, conflict may develop.

Nursing Implications

The nurse needs to be sensitive to issues affecting the psychiatric needs of both the client and the family. As part of the initial assessment, encourage the client to identify those people considered family members. Family members who accompany the client and expect to be part of the treatment planning are included in any teaching done by the nurse. A psychoeducational approach, in which the nurse educates the family about the illness and offers supportive understanding of the family experience, may help in this situation.

Role of Healers

Most ethnic cultures have traditional healers who speak the client's native tongue, usually make house calls, and may cost significantly less than Western medical–psychiatric care (Andrews & Boyle, 2003). Culturally diverse clients with a mental health problem, comorbid medical illness, or terminal illness will often seek the services of these healers because the client and family can least afford conflicts, emotional trauma, and the stress of having the nurse or clinician not understand their cultural values. Table 4-3 provides examples of healers and their scope of practice.

Nursing Implications

Several cultural variables, such as the client's views on illness causation, experience with the health care sys-

tem, religious beliefs, goals for care, and views about death if the client is terminally ill, need consideration and exploration. (Chapter 7 discusses loss, grief, and end-of-life care.) In many societies, it is considered an act of rudeness to tell a client that he or she is going to die. The nurse asks each client or the family decision-maker about the use of a healer during assessment procedures. If a healer is used or desired, the nurse is responsible for including this in the client's multidisciplinary treatment plan (Klessig, 1998).

Role of Translators

Communication is vital to the delivery of all health care services, including psychiatric–mental health services. Clients who are non–English speaking or who have difficulty with English require a translator or interpreter. Language interpretation is an art that is best practiced by trained professionals. In an ideal situation, the translator has knowledge of the client's particular ethnic group and an appropriate mental health professional background. If a translator with these

TABLE 4.3 Healers and Their Scope of Practice	
CULTURE	**SCOPE OF PRACTICE**
Hispanic	
Curandero	Treats almost all of the traditional illnesses. Some may not treat illness caused by witchcraft for fear of being accused of possessing evil powers
Espiritualista or spiritualist	Emphasizes prevention of illness or bewitchment through use of medals, prayers, amulets
Black (African American)	
Spiritualist	Assists with financial, personal, spiritual, or physical problems
Voodoo priest or priestess or Hougan	Knowledgeable about properties of herbs; interprets signs and omens. Able to cure illness caused by voodoo
Chinese	
Herbalist	Knowledgeable in diagnosis of illness and herbal remedies
Acupuncturist	Diagnoses and treats yin-yang disorders by inserting needles into meridians, pathways through which life energy flows
Native American	
Shaman	Uses incantations, prayers, and herbs to cure a wide range of physical, psychological, and spiritual illnesses
Crystal gazer, hand trembler (Navajo)	Diviner diagnostician who can identify the cause of a problem, either by using crystals or placing a hand over sick person

Andrews, M., & Boyle, J.S. (2003). *Transcultural concepts in nursing care* (4th ed.). Philadelphia: Lippincott Williams & Wilkins. Adapted with permission.

qualifications is unavailable, then someone from the client's culture is used. Privacy and confidentiality issues may affect the selection of a translator. The use of a family member is controversial. A family member may leave out information that the family member believes the client would not like to hear. A child is not an appropriate family member to use as a translator (Kanigel, 1999).

Nursing Implications

If a translator is used, the nurse still speaks directly to the client and uses eye contact that is congruent with the client's culture. Interrupting the client and the translator or using medical jargon or slang is avoided. Asking the client's permission to discuss emotionally charged questions is important.

THE NURSING PROCESS

ASSESSMENT

Cultural nursing assessment, or *culturologic nursing assessment*, has been described as a systematic appraisal or examination of individuals, groups, and communities as to their cultural beliefs, values, and practices to determine nursing needs and intervention practices within the cultural context of the individuals being evaluated (Andrews & Boyle, 2003).

Cultural assessment of a mentally ill client can be part of the initial data collection for a nursing history. The first essential question to ask is, "With what culture or ethnic group(s) do you identify?" Many clients from multiracial or ethnic backgrounds identify with the group that was most influential in their early family life.

Andrews and Boyle (2003) present a comprehensive transcultural nursing assessment guide that focuses on communication, cultural affiliations, cultural restrictions and sanctions, developmental considerations, educational background, health-related beliefs and practices, kinship and social networks, nutrition, spirituality and/or religious affiliation, and values orientation. The nurse may conclude this assessment by asking the client, "Is there anything else that I need to know that will help me to provide care for you?"

Cultural assessment information related to the composition and frequency of contact with the family or social network, including the nature of these relationships, aids in identifying support persons to be included in the plan of care. Information about religious and spiritual practices and the use of healers helps the client maintain practices that are congruent with his or her ethnic group. The explanation by the client and family as to the cause of the illness and beliefs about treatment provide relevant data with which to ensure culturally relevant treatment. The client's use of any alternative therapies, including herbal or other dietary substances or remedies, can affect prescribed psychotropic medications. Box 4-1 illustrates sample cultural assessment questions.

NURSING DIAGNOSES AND OUTCOME IDENTIFICATION

Data related to spiritual, cultural, and ethnic issues are collected and analyzed along with other client data. Determining the nursing diagnoses appropriate for the client is contingent on the specific problems or needs identified from the collected data. Analysis of data helps to determine how nursing care can preserve or maintain practices that are important to the client. The nurse analyzes spiritual, cultural, or ethnic issues that

---

BOX 4.1 BRIEF CULTURAL ASSESSMENT GUIDE FOR A CLIENT WITH A MENTAL ILLNESS

- With what culture or ethnic group(s) do you identify?
- Who are the members of your family and where do they live?
- Do you have any special cultural or spiritual beliefs or practices that should be considered in planning your treatment?
- Is there someone in your culture who practices healing? Have you used their services?
- What is your explanation of your illness?
- What do you believe will be important for your treatment for you to get better?
- Do you take any special herbal remedies or receive any other kinds of treatments?
- What is your usual daily diet? Do you have special dietary practices or beliefs that should be considered in planning your treatment?

may present problems in accepting nursing care to plan for negotiation, repatterning, or restructuring.

In general, data related to spiritual, cultural, and ethnic issues are used in the etiology section of the nursing diagnosis. The nurse determines client outcomes that are relevant to the diagnosis and realistic for the client's unique situation. Table 4-4 lists some sample nursing diagnoses and statements of outcome.

IMPLEMENTATION

Nursing interventions are selected to enable the client to accomplish the stated outcome. Interventions specific to spiritual, cultural, and ethnic considerations include those that enable the nurse to establish a trusting relationship; to communicate with the ethnically diverse client, including the family or social network in the care plan; and to incorporate the spiritual and cultural beliefs of the client and family in treatment.

Establishing a Trusting Relationship

The nurse's attitude of wanting to learn about the client's ethnicity demonstrates respect and acceptance of ethnically diverse clients. Other measures to establish a trusting relationship include asking the client how he or she wishes to be addressed, respecting the client's version of acceptable eye contact, and allowing the client to choose seating for comfortable personal space.

Communicating With Client and Family

The initial nursing intervention is establishing the client's fluency in the English language during the assessment interview. If the client requires a translator, the nurse collaborates with the treatment team to obtain an appropriate person. The nurse carefully avoids using slang, jargon, and complex sentences with clients who have minimal understanding of the English language. Nonthreatening communication strategies are best because members of some ethnic groups are intimidated by direct questions. A supportive and empathetic—rather than confrontational—approach is used. For example, rather than ask a series of direct questions, the nurse encourages clients to tell their story in their own words. Careful listening enables the nurse to gather necessary assessment data. Sufficient time is allotted for clients to clarify and express feelings about their situation.

The nurse also includes the family in discussions about treatment where appropriate. For example, the nurse asks, "What would you like to see happen as a result of treatment?" This question helps establish client and family expectations about the treatment process. The nurse also ensures that the family is part of any teaching related to the client's illness. If the client's family includes a large social network, the members of this group are also included in discussions about treatment.

TABLE 4.4 Nursing Diagnoses and Statements of Outcome for Clients From Diverse Cultures	
DIAGNOSIS	**OUTCOME**
Ineffective Coping related to feelings of guilt and shame secondary to cultural beliefs about mental illness	The client will verbalize relief from feelings of guilt and shame.
Spiritual Distress related to cultural beliefs about the nature of mental illness	The client will seek spiritual guidance that is congruent with cultural beliefs.
Impaired Verbal Communication related to difficulty speaking and understanding the English language	The client will use the services of a translator to communicate with health care providers.
Ineffective Role Performance related to inability to fulfill culturally expected positions secondary to symptoms of mental illness	The client will return to usual role in family and/or work group.
Noncompliance related to nonacceptance of psychiatric treatment secondary to cultural beliefs	The client will reconcile cultural beliefs with recommended treatment approach.

A client from a different culture verbalizes spiritual distress during the assessment and requests that his spiritual advisor be notified of his admission to the hospital. Which culturally congruent nursing care mode developed by Leininger would be appropriate? How comfortable would you be utilizing this mode? Explain your answer.

Incorporating Cultural Beliefs

The nurse is not expected to be an expert about each and every culture group; however, the nurse can ask the clients to share cultural norms as they understand them. The nurse's knowledge about the client's culture is used in selecting culturally congruent actions. For example, the nurse learns that a client from a Native American ethnic group believes that his depression is caused by failing to properly honor his ancestors. The remedy involves a special ceremony conducted by a tribal shaman. The nurse communicates this to the treatment team and facilitates the shaman's ceremony in the psychiatric inpatient unit. The nurse supports the client and family in their beliefs regarding the use of healers and facilitates their use in treatment. The use of brief therapy and self-help groups can be particularly effective for clients and families from diverse ethnic groups, and the nurse assists in the referral for these groups.

EVALUATION

As part of the evaluation process, the nurse determines whether the nursing care provided enabled the client to accomplish the stated outcomes. Nursing care is also evaluated to ensure that respect and understanding of the ethnically diverse client and family have been demonstrated. The use of appropriate nursing interventions, including communication strategies congruent with the client's spirituality and culture, is also evaluated. Client and family expression of satisfaction with nursing care is important and is the final measure of the success of incorporating spiritual and cultural considerations in the nursing process. Nursing Plan of Care 4-1 provides an example of the nursing process for a client from a diverse ethnic group.

NURSING PLAN OF CARE 4.1

THE CLIENT FROM A DIFFERENT CULTURE

Mai, a 22-year-old Chinese female, was brought to the college health office by her roommate, who was concerned because Mai had stopped going to class, slept only 2 hours per night, and complained of headaches and stomach pains. The roommate stated that this behavior began after Mai received a D grade on an important paper. Mai verbalized to the college health nurse that she wanted to kill herself. After psychiatric evaluation, Mai was then admitted into the psychiatric inpatient unit, accompanied by her aunt. Nursing admission assessment reveals that client's appearance is neat and clean, she maintains minimal eye contact, and she speaks softly in brief responses to any questions. She tells the nurse that she believes she is ill because of an imbalance of too much yin and requests yang foods and beverages.

DSM–IV–TR DIAGNOSIS: Major depressive disorder, moderate, without psychotic features

ASSESSMENT: Personal strengths: Alert, oriented to person, place, and time; supportive roommate; self-care ability intact; previous good adjustment to role as college student; recognition of illness along with explanation about illness that is congruent with her culture

Weaknesses: Suicidal thoughts; current inability to function in usual role; sleep disturbance and physical complaints

NURSING DIAGNOSIS: Risk for Self-Directed Violence related to thoughts of suicide secondary to receiving a poor grade

OUTCOME: Within 72 hours, the client will state that she wants to live.

Planning/Implementation	Rationale
Implement suicide precautions, respecting client's version of acceptable eye contact and personal space requirements	Individuals at high risk for suicide need constant supervision and limitation of opportunities to harm self
Encourage client to discuss recent stressful events in her life	Client needs to identify and express the feelings that underlie the suicidal behavior or thoughts
Contact family members (after obtaining client's permission) and encourage visits	Increasing client's support system may help decrease future suicidal behavior
Administer ordered antidepressant medication, teaching client about action and side effects	Chemical control can help the client regain self-control while exploring feelings and problems

NURSING DIAGNOSIS: Ineffective Coping related to receiving a poor grade and as evidenced by various physical complaints and client's belief that imbalance of yin-yang has occurred

OUTCOME: Within 72 hours, the client will verbalize decreased complaints of physical symptoms and improved sleep.

Planning/Implementation	Rationale
Respect client's beliefs about meaning of symptoms	Showing respect demonstrates interest and caring
Ask client about specific foods and beverages that would be acceptable dietary practices and yang remedies	Involving the client in her plan of care demonstrates respect of her cultural beliefs and can help to increase a sense of responsibility and control
Maintain sleep chart to document actual sleep patterns	Clients with clinical symptoms of depression often experience insomnia due to erratic sleep patterns, daytime napping, or underlying anxiety
Teach client relaxation techniques, encouraging use when experiencing headache or stomach pain	Relaxation techniques are used to reduce stress and minimize somatic symptoms

EVALUATION: Client's aunt and cousin participated in family conference and were helpful in facilitating client's adopting more realistic view of poor grade received. Client verbalized wish to live and was able to sleep 6 hours each night. Foods that were acceptable were provided by dietary department. Discharge plans included referral to the college counselor for follow-up treatment along with recommendation to continue antidepressant medication.

KEY CONCEPTS

◆ Spirituality is an aspect of every human being that refers to a person's belief in a higher power apart from one's own existence. It is a personal quality that strives for inspiration, reverence, awe, meaning, and purpose in life. Spirituality is not confined to architectural designs.

◆ Although the terms *spirituality* and *religion* are often used interchangeably, they have different meanings. Religion is an organized system of beliefs and practices that focus on a higher power that governs the universe. A client may consider himself or herself to be both spiritual and religious, spiritual but not religious, or religious but not spiritual.

◆ Culture is a broad term referring to a set of shared beliefs, values, behavioral norms, and practices that are common to a group of people sharing a common identity and language. A subculture is a smaller group that exists within a larger society. Members of a subculture may share commonalities such as age, gender, race, ethnicity, socioeconomic status, religious or spiritual beliefs, sexual orientation, occupation, and even health status.

◆ An individual is influenced by membership in her or his culture as well as by membership in multiple subcultures. The client and the nurse can share or differ in membership in both culture and subculture. When cultural membership differs between nurse and client, there is a need for increased knowledge and sensitivity regarding the impact of these differences on nursing care.

◆ The nurse is responsible for identifying, understanding, and providing care to clients from diverse ethnic groups. Ethnocentrism, or the tendency to believe that one's own way of thinking, believing, and behaving is superior to that of others, is counteracted by the nurse's use of self-analysis.

◆ The nurse provides culturally congruent nursing care so that the client's cultural perspective is preserved or maintained and negotiates with the client when changing the client's practices is necessary for health.

◆ Many diverse ethnic groups in the United States do not use the services of the mental health system because of factors such as differences in language, values, and beliefs between providers and clients.

◆ Many people from diverse ethnic groups in the United States have limited financial resources and experience increased incidence of mental health problems associated with lower socioeconomic status. The need for mental health services is increased; however, statistics indicate that people from these groups do not take advantage of services.

◆ Many people from diverse ethnic groups believe that mental health problems are related to spiritual issues or are evidence of an imbalance in the natural order of the human body or nature. Culturally congruent nursing care respects these views and accommodates the client's and family's beliefs.

◆ Specific cultures may express mental distress in unique ways that are known as culture-bound syndromes.

◆ Ethnicity influences the metabolism of drugs and can influence effects, adverse effects, and recommended dosage. The nurse applies knowledge of ethnopharmacology when administering medications to individuals from diverse ethnic groups.

◆ The nurse considers the role of the family, social network, and ethnic healers in planning care for the client with a mental illness.

◆ Communication with people who do not speak English is facilitated by the use of translators.

◆ The nurse assesses membership in a cultural or ethnic group, composition of the family, religious and spiritual practices, cultural beliefs about cause of mental illness, and practices that are considered helpful in treating the client with a mental illness.

◆ Implementation of nursing interventions for clients from diverse ethnic groups includes measures that are helpful in establishing trust, communicating with client and family, and incorporating cultural beliefs.

For additional study materials, please refer to the Student Resource CD-ROM located in the back of this textbook.

CHAPTER WORKSHEET

CRITICAL THINKING QUESTIONS

1. With what culture or ethnic group do you identify? Interview your parents, grandparents, and other relatives regarding beliefs about mental illness, including causation and treatment.
2. What influence, if any, do you anticipate that this knowledge will have on your ability to provide care for culturally diverse clients in the psychiatric clinical setting?
3. Research a particular ethnic culture common in your community. Determine members' beliefs about health, illness, and practices that are considered health enhancing, especially in relation to mental health. Has your nursing education addressed these issues? If not, what changes can be made to incorporate this information into your psychiatric nursing clinical experience?

REFLECTION

Reread the quote at the beginning of the chapter and then research the plan of care of a culturally diverse client. Do the nursing interventions facilitate effective transcultural mental health care? If not, what changes can be made to implement culture-specific care?

NCLEX-STYLE QUESTIONS

1. The nurse interviews a client who expresses the cultural belief that mental illness is caused by offending one's ancestors. When planning care for this client, which of the following has priority?
   a. Questioning the validity of the belief
   b. Expecting poor response to psychiatric treatment
   c. Respecting this belief
   d. Seeking assistance of family members

2. The client from Korea who is admitted to the inpatient psychiatric unit has difficulty speaking English. Which of the following interventions would be best?
   a. Communicating with gestures and pictures
   b. Evaluating client's understanding of written English
   c. Planning to assign the client to a private room
   d. Using the services of a translator

3. A Hispanic client requests that a *curandero* visit the psychiatric unit to perform a healing ceremony. The nurse facilitates this visit by advocating for the client in the treatment team meeting. According to Madeline Leininger's model, the nurse is demonstrating:
   a. Accommodation/negotiation
   b. Preservation/maintenance
   c. Repatterning/restructuring
   d. Supporting/providing

4. The nurse prepares to administer an antianxiety medication to an adult client who is Asian American. The nurse anticipates which of the following about the dosage of this medication?
   a. Equal to the usual adult dose
   b. Higher than the usual adult dose
   c. Lower than the usual adult dose
   d. Spaced evenly around the clock

5. The nurse uses which of the following when determining problem areas for the client with a mental illness who is from the Philippines?
   a. Yes–no direct questioning
   b. Indirect questioning
   c. Confrontational strategies
   d. Family-provided information

6. A client of Native Indian descent is found to have the culture-bound syndrome of ghost sickness. Which of the following would the nurse expect to assess? Select as many as apply.
   a. Uncontrollable crying and shouting
   b. Preoccupation with death and the deceased
   c. Indigestion and anorexia
   d. Bad dreams and hallucinations
   e. Feelings of anxiety and danger
   f. Sudden outburst of agitation and aggression

Selected References

American Psychiatric Association. (2000). *Diagnostic and statistical manual of mental disorders* (4th ed., text revision). Washington, DC: Author.

Andrews, M., & Boyle, J. S. (2003). *Transcultural concepts in nursing care* (4th ed.). Philadelphia: Lippincott Williams & Wilkins.

Bechtel, G. A., Davidhizer, R., & Tiller, C. (1998). Patterns of mental health care among Mexican Americans. *Journal of Psychosocial Nursing and Mental Health Services, 36*(11), 20–27.

Carpenito-Moyet, L. J. (2006). *Handbook of nursing diagnosis* (11th ed.). Philadelphia: Lippincott Williams & Wilkins.

DiCicco-Bloom, B. (2000). Practical approaches to developing cultural competency. *Home Health Care Management and Practice, 12*(2), 30–39.

Ferrante, J. (2001). Cross cultural psychiatry. *American Journal of Psychiatry, 158*(1), 155–156.

Gaw, A. C. (1993). Psychiatric care of Chinese Americans. In A. Gaw (Ed.), *Culture, ethnicity and mental illness* (pp. 245–279). Washington, DC: American Psychiatric Press.

Gooden, M. B., Porter, C. P., Gonzalez, R. I., & Mims, B. L. (2001). Rethinking the relationship between nursing and diversity. *American Journal of Nursing, 101*(1), 63–65.

Griffith, E., & Baker, F. M. (1993). Psychiatric care of African Americans. In A. Gaw (Ed.), *Culture, ethnicity and mental illness* (pp. 147–168). Washington, DC: American Psychiatric Press.

Guarnaccia, P. (1998). Multicultural experiences of family caregiving: A study of African American, European American and Hispanic American families. In H. Lefley (Ed.), *Families coping with mental illness: The cultural context* (pp. 45–61). San Francisco: Jossey-Bass.

Hunt, R. (2001). *Introduction to community-based nursing.* Philadelphia: Lippincott Williams & Wilkins.

Kanigel, R. (1999, September). Integrative medicine: Bridging the culture gap. *Hippocrates, 19*–21.

Kavanagh, K. (2003). Transcultural perspectives in mental health. In M. Andrews & J. S. Boyle (Eds.), *Transcultural concepts in nursing care* (4th ed., pp. 272–314). Philadelphia: Lippincott Williams & Wilkins.

Klessig, J. (1998). Death and culture: The multicultural challenge. *Annals of Long-Term Care, 6*(9), 285–290.

Kudzma, E. C. (1999). Culturally competent drug administrations. *American Journal of Nursing, 99*(8), 46–51.

Lefever, D., & Davidhizar, R. E. (1991). American Eskimos. In J. N. Giger & R. E. Davidhizar (Eds.), *Transcultural nursing* (pp. 261–292). St. Louis, MO: Mosby–Year Book.

Leininger, M. (1991). *Culture care diversity and universality: A theory of nursing.* New York: National League for Nursing Press.

Lin, K. M. (1996). Psychopharmacology in cross-cultural psychiatry. *Mount Sinai Journal of Medicine, 63,* 283–284.

Lin, K. M., Poland, R. E., Wan, Y., Smith, M. W., & Lessner, I. M. (1996). The evolving science of pharmacogenetics: Clinical and ethnic perspectives. *Psychopharmacology Bulletin, 32,* 205–217.

Maslow, A. H. (1987). *Motivation and personality* (3rd ed.). New York: Harper and Brothers.

Mitchell, H. B. (2004). *Roots of wisdom* (4th ed.). Belmont, CA: Wadsworth.

Moffic, H. S., & Kinzie, D. (1996). The history and future of cross-cultural psychiatric services. *Community Mental Health Journal, 32*(6), 581–592.

Mohr, W. K. (1998). Cross-ethnic variations in care of psychiatric patients: A review of contributing factors and practice considerations. *Journal of Psychosocial Nursing and Mental Health Services, 36*(5), 16–21.

Munet-Vilaro, F., Folkman, S., & Gregorich, S. (1999). Depressive symptomatology in three Latino groups. *Western Journal of Nursing Research, 21*(2), 209–224.

Office of Minority Health. (2000). Assuring cultural competence in health care: Recommendations for national standards and an outcomes-focused research agenda. Action: Final. *Federal Register, 63*(247), 80865–80879.

Sadock, B. J., & Sadock, V. A. (2003). *Kaplan & Sadock's synopsis of psychiatry: Behavioral sciences/clinical psychiatry* (9th ed.). Philadelphia: Lippincott Williams & Wilkins.

Smith, M. W., & Mendoza, R. P. (1996). Ethnicity and pharmacogenetics. *Mount Sinai Journal of Medicine, 63,* 285–290.

Social Science Data Analysis Network (SSDAN). (2004). *Analysis of Census 2000.* Retrieved January 30, 2004, from http://www.censusscope.org/us/chart_race.html

Thompson, J. W., Walker, R. D., & Silk-Walker, P. (1993). Psychiatric care of American Indians and Alaska Natives. In A. Gaw (Ed.), *Culture, ethnicity, and mental illness* (pp. 189–234). Washington, DC: American Psychiatric Press.

United States Bureau of the Census. (1993, July). *The foreign-born population in the United States, 1990 census of the population.* Washington, DC: United States Department of Commerce.

United States Bureau of the Census. (1999, March). *The uninsured.* Washington, DC: United States Department of Commerce.

United States Department of Health and Human Services. (1999). *Mental health: A report of the Surgeon General.* Washington, DC: Department of Health and Human Services, Substance Abuse and Mental Health Services Administration, Center for Mental Health Services, National Institutes of Health, National Institute of Mental Health.

Vandiver, V. L., & Keopraseuth, K. O. (1998). Family wisdom and clinical support: Culturally relevant strategies for working with Indochinese families who care for a relative with mental illness. In H. Lefley (Ed.), *Families coping with mental illness: The cultural context* (pp. 75–88). San Francisco: Jossey-Bass.

Vink, C. (2003). *Towards a definition of spirituality.* [Slide presentation.] Retrieved March 8, 2005, from http://www.cappe.org/presentations/presentation2003_files/outline.htm

Yamamoto, J., Silva, J. A., Justice, L. R., Chang, C. Y., & Leong, G. B. (1993). Cross-cultural psychotherapy. In A. Gaw (Ed.), *Culture, ethnicity and mental illness* (pp. 104–114). Washington, DC: American University Press.

Suggested Readings

Brown, D. (2000, September 29). Nation's uninsured down marginally. *Citizen's Voice, 23*(19), 12.

Mendyka, B. (2000). Exploring culture in nursing: A theory-driven practice. *Holistic Nursing Practice, 15*(10), 32–41.

O'Reilly, M. L. (2004). Feature Article: Spirituality and mental health clients. *Journal of Psychosocial Nursing and Mental Health Services, 42* (7).

Prunell, L., & Paulinka, B. (2003). *Transcultural health care: A culturally competent approach.* Philadelphia: F. A. Davis.

Simons, R. C. (2001). Introduction to culture-bound syndromes. *Psychiatric Times, 18*(11), 63–64.

Solomon, P. (1998). The cultural context of interventions for family members with a seriously ill relative. In H. Lefley (Ed.), *Families coping with mental illness: The cultural context* (pp. 5–15). San Francisco: Jossey-Bass.

CHAPTER **5** / ETHICAL AND LEGAL ISSUES

Nurses, therapists, and other health care workers are expected to make informed and effective patient care decisions quickly by utilizing rational problem solving skills. —ROSS, 2001

LEARNING OBJECTIVES

1. Construct the six-step model of ethical nursing care designed by Chally and Loriz.
2. Articulate why nurses must become knowledgeable about genetics and the issues surrounding this topic.
3. Recognize five forms of nursing malpractice.
4. Discuss implications for psychiatric care related to the Tarasoff ruling of duty to warn.
5. Compare the criteria for voluntary and involuntary admission to a psychiatric facility.
6. Interpret the concept of *competency.*
7. Compare the legal rights of adults and minors admitted to psychiatric facilities.
8. Discuss the impact of the Omnibus Reconciliation Act (OBRA) on the placement of clients with psychiatric disorders in long-term care facilities.
9. Distinguish the legal phrases *diminished capacity, not guilty by reason of insanity*, and *guilty but mentally ill*.
10. Explain forensic psychiatry and the role of the forensic nurse.

KEY TERMS

Assault
Autonomy
Battery
Beneficence
Bill of Rights for
   Registered Nurses
Civil commitment
Client confidentiality
Client privacy
Code of Ethics for
   Nurses
Defamation
Diminished capacity
Doctrine of Charitable
   Immunity
Ethics
Failure of duty to warn
False imprisonment
Fidelity
Forensic psychiatry
Genetic testing
Guilty but mentally
   ill
Incompetent
Informed consent
Intentional tort

Involuntary admission	Not guilty by reason of insanity	Slander
Libel	Nurse Practice Act	Tarasoff decision
Malpractice	Omnibus Reconciliation Act	Veracity
Miranda warning	Paternalism	Voluntariness hearing
Negligence	Risk management	Writ of habeas corpus

Historically, the care of those deemed mentally ill included questionable practices and involved the loss of individual rights. Ethical and legal issues concerning nurse–client relationships were identified and subsequently addressed by the nursing profession. For example, nursing as a profession is influenced in each state by legislative acts referred to as **Nurse Practice Acts.**

In the early 1900s, all states had accepted the **Doctrine of Charitable Immunity,** or the Good Samaritan Act. Initially, this doctrine originally provided immunity from prosecution for hospitals, churches, and schools. If a client was harmed by the negligence of another, the doctrine prevented the client from suing to recover damage. In 1959, California became the first state to enact Good Samaritan legislation. Since that time, all states have implemented similar legislation to protect health care providers who render assistance at the scene of an emergency without threat of a legal action (Morrison & Bagalio, 2004).

The concept of health care **risk management,** a systematic approach to the prevention of financial loss, evolved in the mid-1970s to decrease liability exposures, integrate risk reduction strategies, and ultimately create a risk-free environment (Miranda, Saliba, Cerimele, et al., 2004). Preventive law in medicine was addressed and standards of psychiatric-mental health clinical nursing practice were developed.

The everyday practice of psychiatric-mental health nursing is full of values-laden decisions requiring the use of critical thinking skills. Such decisions demand a knowledge of the law, particularly the rights of clients, their legal status, and the prescribed quality of their care. This chapter discusses the major ethical and legal issues that occur in psychiatric-mental health nursing.

Ethics in Nursing

Ethics has been defined as a branch of philosophy that refers to the study of values or values-laden decisions that conform to moral standards of a group or a profession (Kelly, 1998). In 1950, the American Nurses Association (ANA) developed a *Code of Ethics for Nurses* to use when faced with ethical challenges. Specifically, the ANA identified four primary principles to guide ethical decisions. Governing the relationship between nurse and client, these principles include the client's right to **autonomy** (making decisions for oneself), the client's right to **beneficence** (doing good by the nurse), the client's right to justice or fair treatment, and the client's right to **veracity** (honesty and truth by the nurse) regarding the client's condition and treatment. The ethical principle of **fidelity** is closely related to veracity. It implies that the nurse is faithful to duties, obligations, and promises when providing care for the client (ANA, 1985).

In 1994, the ANA Center for Ethics and Human Rights conducted a survey to identify ethical dilemmas most frequently encountered by nurses on a daily or weekly basis. Respondents noted the most common dilemmas to be cost-containment issues that jeopardize client welfare; end-of-life care; informed consent; incompetent, unethical, or illegal practices of colleagues; and access to care. As a result of this survey, a task force was formed to thoroughly revise the 1985 code of ethics (Chally & Loriz, 1998; Daly, 1999). The revised code (ANA, 2001b) is described in Box 5-1.

BOX 5.1   CODE OF ETHICS FOR NURSES—PROVISIONS

1. The nurse, in all professional relationships, practices with compassion and respect for the inherent dignity, worth, and uniqueness of every individual, unrestricted by considerations of social or economic status, personal attributes, or the nature of health problems.
2. The nurse's primary commitment is to the patient, whether an individual, family, group, or community.
3. The nurse promotes, advocates for, and strives to protect the health, safety, and rights of the patient.
4. The nurse is responsible and accountable for individual nursing practice and determines the appropriate delegation of tasks consistent with the nurse's obligation to provide optimum patient care.
5. The nurse owes the same duties to self as to others, including the responsibility to preserve integrity and safety, to maintain competence, and to continue personal and professional growth.
6. The nurse participates in establishing, maintaining, and improving health care environments and conditions of employment conducive to the provision of quality health care and consistent with the values of the profession through individual and collective action.
7. The nurse participates in the advancement of the profession through contributions to practice, education, administration, and knowledge development.
8. The nurse collaborates with other health professionals and the public in promoting community, national, and international efforts to meet health needs.
9. The profession of nursing, as represented by associations and their members, is responsible for articulating nursing values, for maintaining the integrity of the profession and its practice, and for shaping social policy.

Voted on and accepted by the American Nurses Association House of Delegates on June 30, 2001.

The *Code of Ethics for Nurses* is available for sale from American Nurses Publishing at (800) 637-0323 or www.nursesbooks.org.

Reprinted with permission from American Nurses Association. (©2001). *Code of Ethics for Nurses with Interpretive Statements.* Washington, DC: American Nurses Publishing, American Nurses Association.

"This new code will serve the profession even more efficiently because it clearly explains the mission of nursing in society and how nurses partner with the public with regard to health promotion, patient recovery, and illness prevention" (White, 2001, p. 73). The code is also expected to better serve nurses involved in legal challenges.

Model of Ethical Nursing Care

Commonly, nurses think that they know what is best for their clients, often imposing their own methods for care and treatment decisions. This behavior, referred to as **paternalism,** may occur in the psychiatric clinical setting where clients exhibit clinical symptoms of confusion, depression, or anxiety or when clients are unable to communicate their needs because of communication disorders or mental retardation. The nurse may fail to recognize an ethical dilemma as a result of lack of training in ethics or lack of available resources to describe ethical issues (Box 5-2 lists examples of nursing resources on ethics). The nurse may also fail to act or intervene when an ethical dilemma is identified. Failure to act can violate the *Code of Ethics for Nurses With Interpretive Statements* (ANA, 1985). This action could constitute a breach of standard of care and violate a state's Nurse Practice Act. The nurse may be subject to liability if the breach of care results in any harm or injury to the client.

Chally and Loriz (1998) developed a six-step ethical decision-making model for nurses to use when confronted with ethical dilemmas or moral problems that involve two or more mutually exclusive, morally correct courses of action. During the implementation of this model, the nurse must respect the individuality of all clients, protect clients from harm, treat all clients equally, and evaluate the result of full disclosure regarding treatment. The following is an example of the application of the six steps of Chally and Loriz's model during an ethical dilemma:

BOX 5.2 EXAMPLES OF NURSING RESOURCES ON ETHICS

Books: Chambliss, D. F. (1996). *Beyond caring: Hospitals, nurses, and the social organization of ethics.* Chicago: University of Chicago Press.

Continuing education courses: LearnWell.org at http://www.learnwell.org/ provides courses in ethics with instant online processing and certification 24/7.

Ethic rounds or discussions: Hospital-based committees discuss ethical situations.

Journals: *Nursing Ethics: An International Journal for Healthcare Professionals*

  Journal of Bioethics

  Journal of Nursing Law

Online resources: International Centre for Nursing Ethics lists seminars, issues of *Nursing Ethics Journal,* and assists student nurses with research in ethics.

ANA Center for Ethics and Human Rights: Addresses complex ethical and human rights issues.

Staff development programs: Hospital-based nursing education programs are given to comply with various credentialling boards such as the joint Commission for Accreditation of Health Care Organizations (JCAHO).

---

1. *Clarify the ethical dilemma.* A client exhibits clinical symptoms of major depression and verbalizes suicidal thoughts but refuses to take antidepressant medication. The nurse evaluates whose problem it is, who should make the decision regarding the use of antidepressant medication, who is affected by the decision, and what ethical principles are related to the problem.

2. *Gather additional data,* including any legal issues related to the ethical dilemma. The nurse considers the following situations. Does the client have a suicide plan? Is anyone else aware of the client's depression, or does the client wish to keep the information confidential? Who would be responsible if the client did commit suicide?

3. *Identify options* to determine what alternate, acceptable solutions are available. For example, does the client have a significant other or support group? Is the client agreeable to a suicide contract? Should the client be admitted to an inpatient psychiatric program? What options does the client propose?

4. *Make a decision* to determine which option is the most acceptable and therapeutic. Discuss this decision with the client, considering risks and benefits.

5. *Act* or carry out the decision. Collaboration with others may be necessary.

6. *Evaluate* the impact of the decision regarding what went right or what went wrong.

Ethics in Pain Management

Concentration on pain management—considered the fifth vital sign—and comfort measures should be an ethical responsibility of all clinician–client relationships. Psychiatric–mental health nurses provide care for clients who verbalize symptoms of pain, especially those clients who present with a comorbid medical condition, terminal illness, or clinical symptoms of a somatoform disorder (see discussion in Chapter 20). Individuals with a history of substance abuse, especially narcotics, may also present with complaints of pain. The nurse may find it difficult to determine whether such clients are indeed experiencing pain or are attempting to obtain their addictive drugs of choice.

In 1995, the *Journal of the American Medical Association* published a study in which 4,300 terminally ill clients were followed up on until their deaths. According to the data, 50% of the clients' physicians claimed that they had no indication of the clients' end-of-life wishes. In the same study, 2,300 terminally ill clients were assigned a registered nurse who intervened weekly with each client, the client's physician, and the client's family. Again, 50% of the physicians claimed that they were unaware of their clients' wishes regarding pain management and end-of-life care. More than 50% of the family members stated that their loved ones suffered moderate to severe pain in the last 3 days of life (Dunegan, 2000; issues related to end-of-life care are addressed in Chapter 7).

Although rating tools to assess pain intensity and guidelines for pain management are available, some nurses still have difficulty participating in the pain management of their assigned clients. In the past, nurses were overly cautious because most available pain medication was highly addictive. Nurses were faced with ethical dilemmas, that is, administering pain medication but not wanting to promote substance abuse by clients. Now, more than 30 states have established clinician guidelines for pain management. The federal and state licensing boards meet regularly with representatives from the Drug Enforcement Agency (DEA) to review the actions of clinicians who prescribe pain medication. In addition, the federal government has mandated that any hospital receiving federal funding must make pain management a priority. Pain must be rated and relieved, with the effectiveness evaluated for every client. Clinicians who refuse to address the pain and suffering of clients may be sanctioned. Box 5-3 lists examples of situations in the psychiatric setting that may pose ethical dilemmas associated with pain management.

BOX 5.3 EXAMPLES OF ETHICAL DILEMMAS ASSOCIATED WITH PAIN MANAGEMENT

- A 23-year-old male client with a suspected history of substance abuse (narcotics) is hospitalized with a back injury. He requests a "stronger pain pill" because he feels that the prescribed muscle relaxant and nonsteroidal anti-inflammatory agent are not effective.
- A 31-year-old woman, married and the mother of two small children, with a history of fibromyalgia was admitted to the emergency department for treatment of what she describes as an accidental overdose of pain pills. She asks for a prescription of Xanax, an antianxiety agent that she has taken in the past, to help her deal with insomnia secondary to pain because pain medication "never helps."
- A 67-year-old retired car salesman is admitted to the nursing home for rehabilitation after hip surgery. He tells you that pain medication is ineffective but that a "shot or two of whiskey" helps him to relax at night and fall asleep. His wife reveals to you in private that she thinks her husband fell because he drinks too much but that she doesn't know what to do about it.

Ethics in Genetic Testing and Clinical Research

Nurses in every specialty care for clients and/or families who have or are at risk for the development of various genetic disorders, such as Huntington's disease, cystic fibrosis, or muscular dystrophy, and common diseases such as heart disease and diabetes that are caused by altered genes. A genetic marker also has been identified for eating disorders. Research scientists continue to search for genetic markers related to various psychiatric disorders. Research also focuses on the development of second- and third-generation psychotropic medications with fewer adverse effects to alleviate clinical symptoms of psychiatric disorders.

Nurses must become knowledgeable about genetics and the issues surrounding this topic. **Genetic testing,** the laboratory analysis of cells for gene products (eg, proteins, enzymes, metabolites) or DNA analysis (eg, chromosomal analysis), promises early identification of diseases and cure. Genetic testing also is making advances in prenatal predictive testing. Genetic testing may allow providers to discover a person's genetic predisposition to a given disease; to predict the onset, extent, and severity of the disease; and to determine treatment options. Caring for clients who undergo genetic testing presents ethical dilemmas because it tests our knowledge as well as our conscience. A potential for coercion exists, for example, when grown children urge parents to undergo genetic testing for a disease known to determine their own risk (Sanders, 2001b; Silberstein, 2003; Spahis, 2002).

Genetics or biotechnology is not unique to the 21st century. Gregor Mendel, a botanist, is considered to be the founder of genetics in 1865. The X and Y chromosomes were identified in 1905. In 1941, the term *genetic engineering* was coined. In 1982, insulin was genetically engineered; in 1989, a gene for cystic fibrosis was found. Since then, a series of events occurred that led President George W. Bush to announce the funding of embryonic stem-cell research on August 9, 2001 (Sanders, 2001b).

Nurses can participate in clinical research, including research associated with psychiatric–mental health. Karigan (2001) identifies three ethical dilemmas that the nurse may confront during participation in clinical research if he or she is not familiar with research protocol. The first ethical dilemma addresses the issue of **informed consent** (the client's right of self-decision). Violations of the ethical principles of informed consent are committed when there is no consent; when a consenting client is not fully informed of the details of the research study, including expected outcomes, benefits, or risks; or when the client is not continually informed of study changes or results.

A second ethical dilemma may involve documentation of research protocols. Nurses need to know the outline of the protocol and how to locate specific information related to it. The protocol outline should be kept in a designated location, readily available so that nurses can refer to any guidelines that pertain to their roles. If the nurse is unable to locate the protocol and is given an order to administer an investigational drug or provide a specific treatment, the nurse may refuse the physician's order until consultation with appropriate resources—such as a pharmacist—occurs.

The third ethical dilemma may involve the client's right to full disclosure about the research study or trial. If the client makes any statements that indicate misunderstanding or lack of understanding about research protocol, or if the client indicates perceived coercion by others, the nurse is responsible for alerting the program research investigator of such statements.

Legal Issues in Nursing

The role of the nurse in this highly technical profession has undergone a significant change; duties have expanded and responsibility has increased. Consequently, nurses, now more than ever, are subject to the scrutiny of federal and state regulations as well as the legal system. Indeed, the legal profession has demonstrated a vested interest in the welfare of clients by advertising their services on television, on the Internet, in newspapers, and in various publications. Referring to death cases, doctor or hospital malpractice, nursing home neglect, misdiagnosis, and accidents, one such advertisement on the back page of a telephone directory reads as follows:

> *Medical Malpractice: Representing Accident Victims for Over 25 Years.*
> *Free consultation at home or in the hospital. No fee or costs if no recovery.*
> *Call 24 hours a day, 7 days a week.*

As a response to a nursing staff survey regarding nursing recidivism in early 2001, the ANA issued the **Bill of Rights for Registered Nurses** to aid nurses in improving the workplace and to ensure their ability to provide safe, quality client care. It states that nurses have the right to a safe environment, to practice in a manner that ensures the provision of safe care through adherence to professional standards and ethical practice, and to advocate freely on behalf of themselves and their clients (ANA, 2001a; Box 5-4).

Malpractice

Conduct that falls below the standard of care established by law for the protection of others and involves an unreasonable risk of harm to a client is referred to as **negligence. Malpractice** is a type of negligence that applies only to professionals, such as licensed nurses (Schipske, 2002). Nursing malpractice law is generally based on fault. Before a nurse can be held legally liable, it must be shown that the nurse's conduct fell below the professional standard of other professionals with the same education and training. The following four elements must be present to constitute nursing malpractice (Schipske, 2002):

1. Failure to act in an acceptable way
2. Failure to conform to the required standard of care
3. Approximate cause, which requires that there be a reasonably close connection between the defendant's conduct and the resultant injury (ie, the performance of the health care provider caused the injury)
4. The occurrence of actual damage

Cases of malpractice involving nurses have risen over the years. Croke (2003) lists several factors that contributed to the increase in the number of malpractice cases against nurses: (1) delegation of duties to unlicensed assistive personnel; (2) early discharge of clients without proper referral for outpatient care; (3) increased workloads in the clinical setting; (4) advances in technology that require nurses to have technological skills; (5) increased autonomy and responsibility in the exercise of advanced nursing skills; (6) better-informed consumers capable of recognizing insufficient or inappropriate care; and (7) the expanded legal definitions of liability that holds all professionals to a higher standard of accountability. Eskreis (1998) identifies seven common "legal pitfalls": client falls; failure to follow physician orders or established protocols; medication errors; improper use of equipment; failure to remove foreign objects; failure to provide sufficient monitoring; and failure to commu-

BOX 5.4 THE AMERICAN NURSES ASSOCIATION'S BILL OF RIGHTS FOR REGISTERED NURSES

Registered nurses promote and restore health, prevent illness, and protect the people entrusted to their care. They work to alleviate the suffering experienced by individuals, families, groups, and communities. In so doing, nurses provide services that maintain respect for human dignity and embrace the uniqueness of each patient and the nature of his or her health problems, without restriction in regard to social or economic status. To maximize the contributions nurses make to society, it is necessary to protect the dignity and autonomy of nurses in the workplace. To that end, the following rights must be afforded.

1. Nurses have the right to practice in a manner that fulfills their obligations to society and to those who receive nursing care.
2. Nurses have the right to practice in environments that allow them to act in accordance with profes-

sional standards and legally authorized scopes of practice.
3. Nurses have the right to a work environment that supports and facilitates ethical practice, in accordance with the *Code of Ethics for Nurses* and its interpretive statements.
4. Nurses have the right to freely and openly advocate for themselves and their patients, without fear of retribution.
5. Nurses have the right to fair compensation for their work, consistent with their knowledge, experience, and professional responsibilities.
6. Nurses have the right to a work environment that is safe for themselves and their patients.
7. Nurses have the right to negotiate the conditions of their employment, either as individuals or collectively, in all practice settings.

Disclaimer: The American Nurses Association (ANA) is a national professional association. ANA policies reflect the thinking of the nursing profession on various issues and should be reviewed in conjunction with state association policies and state board of nursing policies and practices. State law, rules, and regulations govern the practice of nursing. The ANA's *Bill of Rights for Registered Nurses* contains policy statements and does not necessarily reflect rights embodied in state and federal law. ANA policies may be used by the state to interpret or provide guidance on the profession's position on nursing.

Adopted by the ANA Board of Directors: June 26, 2001

Reprinted with permission from American Nurses Association. (©2001). *Bill of Rights for Registered Nurses.* Washington, DC: American Nurses Publishing, American Nurses Association.

nicate. Any or all of these incidents could occur in the psychiatric clinical setting. In an effort to reduce malpractice suits, many states have mandated the completion of continuing education programs related to health care safety issues prior to license renewal.

The Joint Commission on Accreditation of Healthcare Organizations (JCAHO), a national organization whose mission is to improve the quality of care provided at health care institutions in the United States, hold institutions accountable for ensuring a safe environment for clients, and grant accreditation, has defined what constitutes a potential malpractice "sentinel event" (2002). Such an event may result in an unanticipated death or major loss of function not related to the natural course of the client's illness or underlying condition. Examples of "sentinel events" that could occur in the psychiatric clinical setting include suicide or rape.

Other forms of malpractice include intentional torts such as assault and battery, defamation, and false imprisonment. **Intentional torts** refer to willful or wanton conduct to do a wrongful act with disregard of the interests of others. **Assault** is an act that puts another person in apprehension of being touched or of bodily harm without consent. **Battery** is unlawful touching of another without consent. For example, during the involuntarily admission of a client to a psychiatric–mental health facility (ie, has not signed the voluntary admission form or consent for treatment), emergency orders are necessary to provide any type of nursing intervention. Touching the client, administering medication, or completing a physical examination could result in a malpractice suit based on a complaint of assault and battery.

Defamation involves injury to a person's reputation or character through oral (**slander**) or written

(libel) communications to a third party. For example, if a physician tells the administration of a hospital that a nurse is unfit to care for clients in a psychiatric-mental health facility, the nurse could sue the physician for defamation, possibly being rewarded with a financial judgment.

Finally, **false imprisonment** is the intentional and unjustifiable detention of a person against his or her will. Detention can occur with the use of physical restraint, barriers, or threats of harm. For example, suppose a client with alcohol abuse voluntarily admits himself to a substance abuse treatment center. He attempts to leave and is forcibly restrained. The client could sue for false imprisonment and be awarded a financial judgment.

In the psychiatric-mental health clinical setting, knowledge of the law and of the bill of rights for psychiatric-mental health clients (discussed later in this chapter) in addition to the provision of quality care greatly reduces the risk of malpractice litigation. Legal issues could arise in various practice settings involving situations such as child abuse, breach of confidentiality, failure to provide for informed consent, family violence, mental retardation, prenatal substance abuse, rape, sexual assault, spouse or significant-other abuse, and suicide. Box 5-5 lists potential legal issues the psychiatric-mental health nurse could face.

Breaches of Client Confidentiality and Privacy

Breaches of client confidentiality and privacy are two forms of malpractice that have become increasingly common because of the widespread use of computers or personal digital assistants (PDAs), e-mail, fax machines, copy machines, pagers, and cell phones to share client information with other health care professionals (Badzek & Gross, 1999). **Client confidentiality** refers to the nondisclosure of private information related by one individual to another, such as from client to nurse. **Client privacy** is defined as the right to be left alone and free from intrusion or control by the public or, in this situation, health care providers. Only health care workers taking care of a client are able to review the client's medical records. Sharing information with anyone else requires the client's informed consent. As of April 14, 2003, health care providers are required to implement systems to ensure compliance with privacy provisions that evolved from the Health Insurance Portability and Accountability Act (HIPAA) of 1996 (Box 5-6). Under

| BOX 5.5 | POTENTIAL LEGAL ISSUES IN PSYCHIATRIC–MENTAL HEALTH NURSING* |

Abandonment: Premature termination of a professional relationship with a client or withdrawal of services without adequate notification, leaving the client unattended when health care is still needed

Diversion of narcotics: Writing or calling in fraudulant prescriptions for narcotics or diverting controlled substances from a health care facility

Falsification of medical records: Entering information into a client's medical record that is known to be inaccurate

Impairment: Professional misconduct due to chemical, mental, or physical impairment

Negligence: Failure to act, or conduct that falls below the accepted standard of care established by law, resulting in an injury or loss to the client

Unprofessional practice: Departure from, or failure to conform to, minimum standards of nursing practice

*The issues of assault, battery, defamation of character, false imprisonment, and nursing malpractice are discussed in detail within the text.

the new regulations, mental health records, other than psychotherapy notes, are considered protected health information that can be disclosed only for payment, treatment, and "health-care operations." Generally speaking, psychotherapy records cannot be released without the authorization of the client (Starr, 2004).

Because of the stigma attached to psychiatric-mental health care, and clauses regarding preexisting conditions or limited coverage listed in insurance policies, clients are taking various measures to protect their privacy. They may withhold or provide inadequate information to the health care professional, pay out of pocket for covered services, change providers frequently, or avoid seeking care. Such practices can compromise the quality of care an individual receives. A dilemma occurs when the health care provider attempts to obtain additional information from a previous provider or when a referral is made to secure a second opinion regarding the client's medical condition.

BOX 5.6 | HIPAA PRIVACY PROVISIONS RULE

- Patient records are secure, not readily available to those who do not need them to carry out treatment, payment, or health care operations activities.
- Employees have access to only the minimum patient information that is necessary to do their job.
- Disclosure is made only to individuals who need to know the information to treat the patient, conduct the practice's operations, or obtain payment for services.
- Patients are aware of their rights under the Privacy Rule.
- A patient's written authorization is obtained before disclosing the patient's information for any purpose other than treatment, payment, or practice/facility operations.

Patients' rights include setting boundaries on the use and release of health records; requesting and obtaining audits of how a health care provider used or disclosed the patient's information in the last 6 years; examining their own records; obtaining copies and requesting correction of their own records; requesting to receive confidential communications at alternate locations or by alternate means; and filing complaints about a suspected violation of privacy, which may trigger an investigation.

Every practice will be expected to have relevant authorization forms, policies, procedures, security safeguards, training, and a privacy officer, and to notify patients of their right to privacy.

Sources: Standards for Privacy of Individually Identifiable Health Information, "Final Rule" printed in the *Federal Register* on December 28, 2000, pp. 82462–82829. The rules are codified as 45 Code of Federal Regulations Parts 160 and 164; and Public Law 104-191.

In 1995, the ANA House of Delegates approved a policy titled *Privacy and Confidentiality Related to Access to Electronic Data.* This policy provides nurses with guidelines to ensure privacy and confidentiality related to medical records. In 1998, a policy titled *Core Principles of Telehealth* was also endorsed by the ANA Board of Directors to regulate telecommunication technologies used to provide long-distance care, education, and client data. Detailed information related to these policies can be obtained by contacting American Nurses Publishing at (800) 637-0323 (*Core Principles of Telehealth* is Publication No. 9901TH).

Failure of Duty to Warn

Failure of duty to warn is another form of malpractice the psychiatric–mental health nurse faces. In 1976, the California Supreme Court refocused psychiatric tort law in the landmark case of *Tarasoff v. Regents of the University of California.* In this case, a male client informed his psychologist that he intended to kill a young woman. The psychologist informed the police, who, in turn, interviewed the man. Neither the police nor the psychologist warned the woman of the threat to her life. The client subsequently murdered the woman, and her parents brought a successful suit against the psychologist and the Regents of the University of California for failure of duty to warn. This duty to warn takes precedence over the duty to protect a client's confidentiality. According to Tarasoff, the protective privilege ends where public peril begins (Felthous, 1989; Perlin, 1999).

The **Tarasoff decision** reshaped the configuration of mental health practice and altered the relationship between clinicians and public authorities (Perlin, 1999). Application of Tarasoff may be emphasized in cases involving sexual abuse in which the third party is a pedophile; cases in which violent or self-destructive behavior is identified by the clinician; and cases in which the defendant is not a mental health professional but rather a friend, significant other, or family member who is aware of the potential for danger but neglects to warn the potential victim.

Bill of Rights for Psychiatric–Mental Health Clients

Psychiatric clients who voluntarily seek help retain civil rights during hospitalization. Conversely, those who are committed involuntarily lose the right to leave the hospital during treatment unless the attending clinician writes an order for a leave of absence or discharge from the facility. The following is a summary of rights for all clients undergoing hospitalization or outpatient treatment, or receiving emergency care. These rights are adapted from the Mental Health Systems Act of 1980 and the Protection and Advocacy Bill for Mentally Ill Individuals Act of 1986. They include the rights to:

1. receive treatment, including (a) treatment in a humane psychological and physical environment; (b) adequate treatment in a least-restrictive environment; (c) a current, written, individualized treatment plan; and (d) informed consent concerning one's condition, progress, explanations of procedures, risks involved, alternative treatments, consequences of alternative treatments, and any other information that may help the client to make an intelligent, informed choice.
2. refuse treatment, unless such action endangers others, or withdraw from treatment if risks outweigh benefits.
3. have a probable-cause hearing within 3 court days of admission to secure a speedy recovery from involuntary detention if found sane in a court of law (**writ of habeas corpus**).
4. maintain client privacy and confidentiality: Information, records, and correspondence may be disclosed only with the client's written consent. The exception occurs when the public becomes endangered; the client is transferred to another facility; the client's attorney, law enforcement officers, or a court requests information; the client participates in research; or insurance companies require information to complete insurance claims.
5. communicate freely with others by letter, telephone, or visits, unless such activities are specifically restricted in one's treatment plan.
6. have personal privileges: (a) wearing one's own clothing; (b) maintaining personal appear-

ance to individual taste; and (c) receiving the basic necessities of life.
7. maintain one's civil rights, including the right to (a) be legally represented; (b) be employed; (c) hold public office; (d) vote; (e) execute a will; (f) drive; (g) marry; (h) divorce; or (i) enter into a contract.
8. engage in religious freedom and education.
9. maintain respect, dignity, and personal identity.
10. maintain personal safety and assert grievances.
11. be transferred and receive continuity of care.
12. access own records.
13. obtain an explanation of cost of services.
14. obtain aftercare: Individuals discharged from mental health facilities have the right to adequate housing and aftercare planned by professional staff.

Discontinuation of treatment without providing alternatives to care constitutes abandonment by the mental health professional.

Advance Psychiatric Directives

The 1990 Patient Self-Determination Act gave clients with the diagnosis of psychiatric disorders the right to formulate legal documents known as advance psychiatric directives (APDs; similar to advance directives for end-of-life care) to indicate what treatments they would accept or refuse. APDs are created when a mental health professional certifies that the client has mental capacity (ie, is of sound mind to make decisions) to formulate the document. The purpose of APDs is to inform a doctor, institution, or judge what types of confinement and treatment the client wants and does not want. It also appoints a friend or family member as agent to make mental health decisions if the client is incapable of doing so. Furthermore, APDs promote autonomy and empowerment; enhance communication between the client, family, and members of the treatment team; protect the client from inappropriate, unwanted, or possible harmful treatment; protect the client from unnecessary involuntary hospitalizations; and may shorten length of hospitalization. Currently, 29 states allow APDs within statutes of living wills and/or durable power of attorney for health care, and 17 states have statutes to support them (Lachman, 2006). Additional information regarding APDs can be obtained from the Bazelon Center for Mental Health Law (http://www.bazelon.org/issues/advancedirectives/index.htm).

Psychiatric Hospitalization

Psychiatric hospitalization can be traumatic or supportive, depending on the situation, attitude of family and friends, response of staff, and the manner in which the admission occurs. Admission to a psychiatric facility can occur as an emergency or as a scheduled admission and can be classified as voluntary or involuntary.

The type of admission depends on the client's mental status and his or her presenting clinical symptoms. Is the client legally competent to make decisions and consent to treatment, or does the client demonstrate significant personality deterioration and resultant defects in business and social judgment? Competent clients who admit themselves voluntarily have the right to refuse any treatment prescribed and may initiate their own discharge at any time. The attending physician may write the order as a routine discharge, or as against medical advice (AMA) if the physician feels that the client should remain in the facility but does not wish to invoke the involuntary admission procedure.

If clients pose a threat to themselves or others, they may be admitted and detained for at least 72 hours by an **involuntary admission.** For example, in most states, a physician, licensed clinical psychologist, master's-prepared psychiatric nurse, or master's-prepared licensed clinical social worker may initiate an involuntary admission. The form for involuntary admission usually states that the following conditions exist:

- There is reason to believe said person is mentally ill and (a) has refused voluntary examination after conscientious explanation and disclosure of the purpose of the examination or (b) is unable to determine for herself or himself whether examination is necessary.
- Either (a) without care or treatment, said person is likely to suffer from neglect or refuse to care for self, or (b) there is substantial likelihood that in the near future said person will inflict serious bodily harm on self or another person.

During these 72 hours, the client still retains the right to make decisions regarding care, including the decision to refuse treatment or prescribed medication. Some hospitals have established a 72-hour emergency treatment policy that identifies specific interventions for clients who refuse to sign the voluntary admission form and are at risk of hurting themselves or others.

If within 72 hours the client's condition does not improve and the client does not sign the voluntary admission forms authorizing treatment and continued stay in the facility, first and second opinions by two psychiatrists are completed and a court hearing is set. On the basis of information presented at the hearing, the client may be court-ordered to remain in the facility for a specified period (**civil commitment**) or may be released from the facility.

If individuals admitted to a psychiatric facility are judged to be (adjudicated) **incompetent** to make decisions (ie, incapable of giving informed consent), the court will appoint a guardian to make decisions for them. Guardianship may continue after they are released from the facility or transferred to a long-term care psychiatric institution.

Individuals may decide to elope from a facility. If they were admitted under a voluntary status, they can be brought back to the facility only if they again voluntarily agree. If they refuse to return, the physician must discharge them or initiate civil commitment procedures. If a client elopes after an involuntary admission, the police are notified. Then if the client is located, he or she is returned to a crisis center or the mental health facility from which the elopement occurred.

Hospitalization of Minors

State laws regarding the age and legal rights of minors vary. Such rights include the right to purchase cigarettes or alcoholic beverages, obtain an abortion, or obtain medical treatment without consent. In the past, parents or guardians made decisions regarding admission to psychiatric facilities and commitment for treatment. Now, in most states, a minor—considered anyone under 18 years of age who has not been court-ordered to receive treatment—has a right to a **voluntariness hearing** at the time of admission to a facility. During a private interview, an objective professional, such as the registered nurse, asks the minor if he or she has voluntarily agreed to obtain psychiatric care or if coercion has occurred. The U.S. Supreme Court has stated that such a neutral fact finder has the authority to refuse admission of a minor if a parent has erred in the decision to have the minor institutionalized or to seek treatment for psychiatric care.

In most states, minors under the age of 18 years but at least 14 years of age have the opportunity to petition the court for full rights as an adult if factors make it inappropriate for the minor's parents to retain control over the minor (eg, the minor is married or on active duty with the armed forces). A minor who becomes emancipated is granted adult rights and has the privilege of consenting to medical, dental, and psychiatric care without parental consent, knowledge, or liability (Harbet, 2003).

Long-Term Care Facilities

As of August 1, 1988, new regulations regarding the admission of clients with psychiatric disorders to long-term care facilities (nursing homes) were established. These regulations, based on the **Omnibus Reconciliation Act** (OBRA) of 1987, state that a long-term care facility must not admit, on or after January 1, 1989, any new resident needing active treatment for mental illness or mental retardation. A screening document called the Preadmission Screening and Annual Resident Review (PASARR) determines whether the client needs active psychiatric treatment.

If a client already resides in a long-term care facility and requires psychiatric treatment, the proper course of action may be unclear. Should the client be discharged, transferred to a psychiatric facility, or treated within the facility? This confusion also impedes discharge planning for clients admitted to psychiatric treatment facilities. Some long-term care facilities are willing to admit psychiatric clients if they are stabilized and in the care of a psychiatrist or psychiatric nurse practitioner.

Forensic Psychiatry

The involvement of mental health professionals in the operations of the legal system has been the subject of debate and discussion. The issue of criminal responsibility involves questions of moral judgments and related legal and public policy issues rather than medical, psychiatric, or psychological judgments. However, mental health professionals are called on to provide assistance and consultation about a wide range of civil, criminal, and administrative proceedings (Curran, McGarry, & Shah, 1986). For example, a judge may order a client to undergo a psychiatric evaluation before trial or may request the appearance of an expert witness to provide data related to a criminal lawsuit.

The U.S. judicial system has guarded the right of an accused person to receive a fair, impartial criminal trial by determining whether the individual is competent to stand trial. Various pleas may be introduced. The plea of **diminished capacity** is used to assert that

because of mental impairment, such as mental retardation, the defendant could not form the specific mental state required for a particular offense, such as first-degree murder. The defendant is typically found guilty of a lesser offense such as manslaughter. The plea of **not guilty by reason of insanity** is entered in the presence of a mental disease, such as delusional disorder, at the time of the commission of an alleged criminal act. **Guilty but mentally ill** is a third plea that may be used by individuals who exhibit clinical symptoms of a *DSM-IV-TR* psychiatric disorder such as pyromania, substance abuse, or sexual offenses. The criminal act occurred because of the client's illness, but the client is responsible for his or her behavior (eg, an individual who is a substance abuser robs a store to obtain money to purchase drugs).

Evaluation of an individual's competency and mental condition at the time of an alleged crime constitutes the specialized area of mental health referred to as **forensic psychiatry.** If a defendant is found competent to stand trial, criminal trial and related proceedings will continue. If a defendant is found mentally incompetent, a judicial decision about treatment or habilitation must be made. Elements of mental competency to stand trial are summarized in Box 5-7.

If it is determined that a defendant could benefit from psychiatric treatment, commitment to an appropriate facility is the most common disposition. Law-related mental health service programs are provided in many different settings, such as centralized state institutions with security units, community and regional forensic mental health programs, court clinics, state and local correctional institutions, and community corrections programs.

Reevaluation for mental incompetency occurs periodically, generally every 6 months, so that courts can review an individual's treatment progress and rule on restoration of competency. A person's commitment may be extended if it appears that competency can be restored in the foreseeable future, or it may be terminated if pretrial competency does not appear attainable (Curran, McGarry, & Shah, 1986).

Role of the Forensic Nurse

Nurses may play a role in forensic psychiatry. The role of the forensic nurse varies according to legal status of the client, treatment setting, and ANA Standards for Practice in the Correctional Setting. The forensic nurse may function as a staff nurse in an emergency room or correctional setting, a nurse scientist, a nurse investi-

The client:

- has mental capabilities to appreciate his or her presence in relation to time, place, and things.
- has elementary processes enabling him or her to comprehend that he or she is in a court of justice, charged with a criminal offense.
- comprehends that there is a judge on the bench.
- comprehends that a prosecutor will try to convict him or her of a criminal charge.
- comprehends that he or she has a lawyer who will undertake to defend him or her against the charge.
- comprehends that he or she will be expected to tell his or her lawyer the circumstances, to the best of his or her mental ability, and the facts surrounding him or her at the time and place of the alleged law violation.
- comprehends that there is or will be a jury present to pass upon evidence adduced as to his or her guilt or innocence of such charges.
- has memory sufficient to relate those things in his or her own personal manner.

SELF-AWARENESS PROMPT

A young male client with the history of mental illness has been brought to the emergency room by the police for a psychiatric evaluation. During the initial assessment, he tells you that he was "manhandled" by the police and that he is being held against his will. What are his rights as an individual receiving emergency care? What course of action should you take?

gator, an expert witness, or an independent consulting nurse specialist. The roles of health educator, client advocate, and counselor are also fulfilled. (This role is discussed more fully in Chapter 6, Forensic Nursing Practice.)

Whatever his or her function, the nurse must be familiar with the law and legal provisions related to the area in which care is rendered. An ethical dilemma could occur because the duty to the legal system (not the client) could conflict with the issue of confidentiality. Informing the client of the limits of confidentiality is similar to the **Miranda warning,** in which a person who is arrested is informed of his or her legal rights. In other words, the client is aware, before the onset of care, that the nurse may be legally required to repeat anything the client has discussed in a confidential manner. Security standards must be maintained at all times.

The forensic nurse must adhere to principles of honesty, strive for objectivity, and maintain professional skills, interest, and empathy. Clients may present as seriously mentally ill individuals manifesting psychoses.

They may exhibit severe psychiatric disturbances such as personality disorders, violent or suicidal behavior, alcoholism, or substance abuse. Special populations may include minorities, the elderly, women, and clients with HIV or AIDS.

Because of the changing nature of the legal system, forensic nurses need continual updates of information. Johnson (1997, p. 782) states, "continuing education and professional development efforts are necessary to provide nurses with ongoing, specific and relevant information and are critical to the promotion and advancement of forensic psychiatric nursing as a specialty practice." Conversely, if the forensic practitioner does not feel well informed or supported, the practitioner may retreat from the institutional scene in haste, frustration, or anger.

The Forensic Nurse as a Legal Nurse Consultant and an Expert Witness

The legal nurse consultant (LNC) is a specialty field within the scope of forensic nursing. LNCs play an invaluable role in advocating patient rights and safety. According to the American Association of Legal Nurse Consultants (AALNC), the LNC evaluates, analyzes, and renders informed opinions on the delivery of health care, including professional conduct, documentation in medical records, and medication errors, and the resulting outcomes (Sanders, 2001a). For example, an LNC may serve as a consultant for a law firm that specializes in malpractice claims, testify as an expert witness in court, or review and respond to issues included in affidavits.

The task of the forensic nurse serving as an expert witness is to combine empathy with a willingness to translate complex, scientific, and psychiatric findings into clear and pertinent meaning. Factors that determine expert witness status include level of education, clinical training, licensure, specialty board certification, experience, and reputation. Scholarship, or the participation in workshops and the publication of articles in leading journals, adds to one's reputation as an expert witness (Curran, McGarry, & Shah, 1986).

In today's medical–legal environment, the expert witness also must be familiar with courtroom procedures, the subtleties of expert testimony, and the limitations of his or her own potential liability. An expert witness may serve as a consultant about the quality of care provided in a malpractice claim (eg, Were the standards of care met?), may conduct evaluations of hospital policies and procedures, or may provide testimony in court. For example, a client may be seeking a financial judgment because a practitioner prescribed the wrong medication for treatment. The expert witness may be asked to provide information about whether the nursing care associated with the administration of the medication reflected adherence to the standards of nursing care.

KEY CONCEPTS

◆   The practice of psychiatric nursing involves ethical decisions regarding such issues as when to hospitalize a client involuntarily, when to use pain-medication management on a substance abuse unit, and when genetic testing would be of benefit to a client. A code of ethics has been developed by the ANA to guide nurses to employ certain principles when faced with such ethical challenges.

◆   Psychiatric nursing demands knowledge of the law as it pertains to client rights, client legal status, and the quality of care rendered. The ANA developed a Bill of Rights for Registered Nurses identifying the rights needed to provide high-quality client care in a safe work environment.

◆   Nurses are subject to malpractice liability, such as for medication errors, improper use of equipment, and failure to follow physician orders or established protocols. Intentional torts such as assault and battery, defamation, and false imprisonment are also classified as forms of professional malpractice.

◆   The use of technology such as e-mail and fax machines has contributed to breaches of client confidentiality and privacy.

◆   The landmark Supreme Court case *Tarasoff v. Regents of the University of California* has reshaped the configuration of psychiatric practice and altered the relationship between clinicians and public authorities. The duty to warn takes precedence over the duty to protect confidentiality.

◆   The civil rights of psychiatric clients are protected by law. Clients who are involuntarily committed to treatment (civil commitment) lose the right to liberty. State laws govern the legal rights of minors admitted to a psychiatric facility.

◆   The judicial system has guarded the right of accused persons to receive a fair, impartial criminal trial by determining competency to stand trial. Pleas that may be entered include diminished capacity, not guilty by reason of insanity, or guilty but mentally ill.

◆   The role of the forensic nurse is challenging because the nurse must be familiar with the law and legal provisions for clients in the clinical setting. Ethical dilemmas may occur because the nurse's primary responsibility is to the legal system, not the client.

For additional study materials, please refer to the Student Resource CD-ROM located in the back of this textbook.

 CHAPTER WORKSHEET

CRITICAL THINKING QUESTIONS

1. You are working the evening shift in a psychiatric facility when you are asked to admit a new client. As you begin your assessment, the client informs you he has been brought there against his will and does not intend to stay. You notice that neither the voluntary admission form nor the consent for treatment has been signed. You excuse yourself and inform the charge nurse of your findings. Ignoring your concerns, she says, "Don't worry, get him admitted and then I'll talk to him." What do you do?

2. While working in a long-term care facility, you begin to admit a new client. She informs you that she is under the care of a psychiatrist, but states, "Don't worry, my hallucinations are mostly controlled." Keeping in mind the Omnibus Reconciliation Act of 1987, explore the actions that you must take.

3. For several days you have been caring for a 15-year-old girl who was admitted for episodes described by her parents as "outbursts of rage." She confides in you that her parents forced her to come to the hospital and she feels like a prisoner. What do you need to consider before taking action?

REFLECTION

Review the quote presented at the beginning of the chapter and then imagine the following: You are providing care for a client undergoing a clinical research drug study. The client informs you that she suspects that she is pregnant but has not seen a doctor to confirm the pregnancy. What informed and effective care decisions do you need to make before taking action?

NCLEX-STYLE QUESTIONS

1. When faced with an ethical dilemma that involves two mutually exclusive yet morally correct courses of action, the nurse takes specific steps to arrive at a decision. Place the following steps in the order that the nurse would do to arrive at an ethical decision.
   a. Gather additional data about the dilemma
   b. Make a decision
   c. Clarify the problem and those involved
   d. Carry out the decision
   e. Identify options
   f. Evaluate the decision's impact

2. A client has signed the consent for electroconvulsive therapy (ECT) treatments scheduled to begin in the morning. The client tells the nurse, "I really don't know why I need this procedure, but everybody has been telling me that it is the best thing." The basis for the ethical dilemma facing the nurse in this situation most likely involves which of the following?
   a. Determining whether client has given informed consent
   b. Identifying whether client and family disagree on treatment
   c. Deciding whether client is expressing anxiety about treatment
   d. Judging whether treatment team is following ethical principles

3. The nurse fails to assess a client in physical restraints according to the frequency stipulated in the hospital's policy. The nurse's behavior could legally constitute which of the following?
   a. False imprisonment
   b. Breach of client privacy
   c. Defamation
   d. Negligence

4. Which of the following represents inappropriate maintenance of client confidentiality by the psychiatric nurse?
   a. Discussing client's current problems and past history in treatment team meeting
   b. Explaining to client's visitor that it is inappropriate to discuss client's care
   c. Sending copy of client records to referring agency without client's written consent
   d. Telling a coworker that it is inappropriate to discuss client's problems in the cafeteria

5. Which of the following represents appropriate criteria for the involuntary admission of a client into a psychiatric facility?
   a. Client who is competent but refuses admission
   b. Client who has threatened suicide
   c. Client who has a long history of mental illness
   d. Client whose family has requested admission

6. A client on a day pass from a psychiatric inpatient unit runs a red light while driving and is involved in an accident resulting in the death of another. The client's lawyer subpoenas the nurse to testify at the trial that the client was delusional when released for the day pass. The nurse understands that the lawyer is attempting to establish the legal defense of which of the following?
   a. Diminished capacity
   b. Guilty but mentally ill
   c. Not guilty by reason of insanity
   d. Special circumstances of responsibility

Selected References

American Nurses Association. (1985). *Code of ethics for nurses with interpretive statements.* Washington, DC: Author.

American Nurses Association. (2001a). *Bill of rights for registered nurses.* Washington, DC: Author.

American Nurses Association. (2001b). *Code of ethics for nurses with interpretive statements* (revised). Washington, DC: Author.

Badzek, L., & Gross, L. (1999). Confidentiality and privacy. *American Journal of Nursing, 99*(6), 52–54.

Chally, P. S., & Loriz, L. (1998). Ethics in the trenches: Decision making in practice. *American Journal of Nursing, 98*(6), 17–20.

Croke, E. M. (2003). Nurses, negligence, and malpractice. *American Journal of Nursing, 103*(9), 54–64.

Curran, W. J., McGarry, A. L., & Shah, S. A. (1986). *Forensic psychiatry and psychology.* Philadelphia: F. A. Davis.

Daly, B. J. (1999). Ethics: Why a new code? *American Journal of Nursing, 99*(6), 64.

Dunegan, L. J. (2000). The ethics of pain management. *Annals of Long-Term Care, 8*(11), 23–26.

Eskreis, T. R. (1998). Seven common legal pitfalls in nursing. *American Journal of Nursing, 98*(4), 34–40.

Felthous, A. (1989). *The psychotherapist's duty to warn or protect.* Springfield, IL: Thomas.

Harbet, S. C. (2003). *Emancipated minors.* Retrieved April 3, 2003, from http://chhd.csun.edu/shelia/436/lecture0405. html

Johnson, B. S. (1997). *Psychiatric-mental health nursing: Adaptation and growth* (4th ed.). Philadelphia: Lippincott-Raven Publishers.

Joint Commission on Accreditation of Healthcare Organizations. (2002). JCAHO–Sentinel events and alerts. Retrieved July 23, 2005, from http://www.jointcommission.org/Sentinel Events/SentinelEventAlert.

Karigan, M. (2001). Ethics in clinical research. *American Journal of Nursing, 101*(9), 26–31.

Kelly, K. V. (1998). The ethic of humility and the ethics of psychiatry. *Psychiatric Times, 15*(6), 49–51.

Lachman, V. D. (2006). Psychiatric advance directives. *ADVANCE for Nurses, 7*(3), 3–17.

Miranda, F., Saliba, G., Cerimele, R., Lowery, K., & Riegel-Gross, K. (2004). Risk management. *ADVANCE for Nurses, 5*(24), 13–14.

Morrison, H., & Bagalio, S. (2004). Being a good Samaritan. *ADVANCE for Nurses, 5*(21), 15–16.

Perlin, M. L. (1999). Tarasoff at the millennium: New directions, new defendants, new dangers, new dilemmas. *Psychiatric Times, 16*(11), 20–21.

Ross, B. A. (2001). Critical thinking. Part 1: The eight elements of reasoning. *Vital Signs, 11*(1), 21–24.

Sanders, C. (2001a). Forensic nursing part two: Legal nurse consultants and sexual assault nurse examiners. *Vital Signs, 11*(13), 13–18.

Sanders, C. (2001b). Genetic testing—What health care professionals need to know. *Vital Signs, 11*(22), 13–16.

Schipske, G. (2002). The difference between negligence and malpractice. *ADVANCE for Nurse Practitioners, 10*(5), 26.

Silberstein, N. (2003). Genetic technology training. *ADVANCE for Nurses, 4*(23), 25–26.

Spahis, J. (2002). Human genetics: Constructing a family pedigree. *American Journal of Nursing, 101*(7), 44–50.

Starr, D. S. (2004). Mental health confidentiality. *Clinical Advisor, 7*(3), 93.

White, G. (2001). The code of ethics for nurses. *American Journal of Nursing, 101*(10), 73–75.

Suggested Readings

American Hospital Association. (1974). *A patient's bill of rights.* Chicago: Author.

American Nurses Association. (1994). *Standards of psychiatric-mental health clinical nursing practice.* Washington, DC: Author.

Buppert, C. (2003). HIPAA patient privacy. *American Journal for Nurse Practitioners, 7*(1), 17–22.

Calabro, M. D., & Tukosi, B. (2003). Participative ethical decision-making: A model for primary care. *ADVANCE for Nurse Practitioners, 11*(6), 83.

Cook, A. F., Haas, H., Guttmannova, K., & Joyner, J. C. (2004). An error by any other name. *American Journal of Nursing, 104*(6), 32–44.

Grady, P. A., & Collins, F. S. (2003). Genetics and nursing science: Realizing the potential. *Nursing Research, 52*(2), Editorial Page.

Horner, S. D. (2004). Ethics and genetics. *Clinical Nurse Specialist, 18*(5), 228–236.

Hughes, R. G. (2004). First, do no harm: Avoiding near misses. *American Journal of Nursing, 104*(5), 81–84.

Mental Health Systems Act, Pub. L. No. 96–398, Title V, § 501.94, Stat. 1598 (October 7, 1980).

Nehring, W. M., & Lashley, F. R. (2004). Calculated safety. *ADVANCE for Nurses, 5*(18), 30–31.

Starr, D. S. (2002). Decision on a duty to warn. *Clinical Advisor, 5*(7), 96–100.

Starr, D. S. (2004). The duties of informed consent. *Clinical Advisor, 7*(4), 83.

CHAPTER 6 / FORENSIC NURSING PRACTICE

Forensic nursing is the cutting edge issue in education, practice and research as we prepare for issues in health care in the 21st century. —INTERNATIONAL ASSOCIATION OF FORENSIC NURSES, 2005D

LEARNING OBJECTIVES

AFTER STUDYING THIS CHAPTER, YOU SHOULD BE ABLE TO:

1. Articulate the history of forensic nursing practice.
2. Discuss the purpose of the International Association of Forensic Nurses (IAFN).
3. Analyze the scope of forensic nursing practice.
4. Interpret the *Forensic Nurse's Code of Ethics.*
5. Distinguish three different educational programs available to nurses who desire to become forensic nurses.
6. Explain the rationale for Standard III of the forensic nurse's *Standards of Professional Performance*.
7. Compare and contrast four practice areas of forensic nursing.

KEY TERMS

e-practice
Forensic Nurse's Code of Ethics
Forensic nursing education
Forensic nursing practice
Genomic health care
International Association of Forensic Nurses (IAFN)
Pharmacogenomics
Scope of forensic nursing practice
Sexual assault nurse examiner (SANE)
Standards of Care
Standards of Forensic Nursing Practice
Standards of Professional Performance

Introduction to Forensic Nursing Practice

Forensic nursing practice is one of the fastest growing nursing specialties of the 21st century. Increased reports by the news media of violent acts are a constant reminder of the violence that is occurring in our society. Acts of violence affect our relationships, homes, schools, workplaces, and communities.

Before the recognition of forensic nursing as a specialty by the American Nurses Association (ANA) in 1995, forensic nursing was a respected practice in the scientific investigation of death. It has been a significant resource in the field of forensic psychiatry as nurses worked with victims of violence and perpetrators in primary care, in the emergency room, and in psychiatric and correctional institutional settings. Forensic nurses provide a vital link in the multidisciplinary treatment of victims, perpetrators, survivors, or individuals falsely accused of abuse and violence (ANA & IAFN, 1999). This chapter focuses on the history of forensic nursing, the scope and standards of forensic nursing practice, the forensic nurse's code of ethics, and forensic nursing education.

History of Forensic Nursing Practice

The emergence of modern forensic nursing began with the establishment of the **sexual assault nurse examiner (SANE)** programs in the mid-1970s in Minnesota, Tennessee, and Texas. SANEs are trained to collect forensic evidence from sexual assault survivors. Their role as a member of the Sexual Assault Response Team is discussed in Chapter 33, Clients Experiencing Abuse and Violence.

The formal recognition of forensic nursing was accomplished at the Annual Meeting of the American Academy of Forensic Sciences in Anaheim, California, in February 1991. In that same year, the ANA published a position statement on violence as a nursing practice issue.

During the summer of 1992, several SANEs met to discuss the formation of the **International Association of Forensic Nurses (IAFN)**, a diverse body of nurses who apply concepts and strategies to provide intervention to victims of crime or perpetra-

tors of criminal acts (IAFN, 2005b). Their mission focuses on the development, promotion and dissemination of information about the science of forensic nursing as well as the establishment and improvement of standards of practice (IAFN, 2005c). Three years later, the *Scope and Standards of Nursing Practice in Correctional Facilities* was published (ANA, 1995). When the IAFN requested that the ANA recognize forensic nursing as a specialty, the ANA responded to this request and jointly created the *Scope and Standards of Forensic Nursing Practice* with the IAFN in 1997.

Each year, the IAFN holds a Scientific Assembly at which experts present topics on the latest advances in the field of forensic science and nursing. Papers are accepted for poster presentation at the meeting. Associate members of the IAFN include physicians, criminologists, law enforcement officials, paramedic/emergency technicians, and other interested professionals. The organization also provides a quarterly publication, *On the Edge* (IAFN, 2005b).

Scope of Forensic Nursing Practice

Forensic nursing practice is a unique practice of the expansive role of registered nurses and is independent and collaborative in nature. It has been recognized as a significant resource in forensic psychiatric practice and in the treatment of incarcerated clients. The victim can be the client, the family, the significant other, the alleged perpetrator, or the public in general. The **scope of forensic nursing practice** encompasses three areas (ANA & IAFN, 1999; IAFN, 2005d):

- Application of the nursing-related sciences, including biopsychosocial education, to public or legal proceedings
- Application of the forensic aspects of health care in scientific investigation
- Treatment of trauma or death victims and perpetrators (or alleged perpetrators) of abuse, violence, criminal activity, and traumatic accidents

The forensic nurse provides direct services to nursing, medical, and/or law-related agencies, as well as consultation and expert testimony in areas related to questioned investigative processes, adequacy of services delivered, and specialized diagnoses of specific conditions as related to forensic nursing and/or pathology (ANA & IAFN, 1999; IAFN, 2005d). Sharing responsibility with the legal system to augment resources available to victims and perpetrators of trauma or violence represents a holistic approach to legal issues for clients in clinical and community-based facilities (Muscari, 2004).

Unique Characteristics of Forensic Nursing

The scope of forensic nursing is considered to be multidimensional and possesses unique characteristics because it is compelled to provide direction to health care providers, educators, attorneys, researchers, and administrators, as well as other health professionals, legislators, and the public in general. Examples of unique characteristics listed under the forensic nurse's scope of nursing practice appear in Box 6-1.

Standards of Forensic Nursing Practice

The *Standards of Forensic Nursing Practice* consists of *Standards of Care* and *Standards of Professional Performance*. Forensic nursing *Standards of*

BOX 6.1   EXAMPLES OF FORENSIC NURSING SCOPE OF PRACTICE

- Identifying injuries and deaths with forensic implications
- Collecting evidential material required by law enforcement or medical examiners
- The scientific investigation of death
- Provisions of care in uncontrolled or unpredictable environments and providing continuity of care from the emergency department to the court of law
- Providing expert witness testimony
- Interacting with grieving families
- Thoroughly reviewing and analyzing medical records

Source: ANA & IAFN. (1999, February, 3rd reprint). *Scope and standards of forensic nursing practice* (pp. 4–5). Washington, DC: American Nurses Publishing.

Care describes a competent level of forensic nursing practice as demonstrated by the nursing process. It also delineates services that are provided to all clients of forensic nurses or practitioners including the provision of culturally and ethnically applicable services, maintaining a safe environment, and planning for continuity of care and services.

Standards of Professional Performance describes a competent level of behavior by the forensic nurse, including activities related to quality of services, performance appraisal, education, collegiality, ethics, collaboration, research, and resource utilization (ANA & IAFN, 1999).

Forensic nurses should be self-directed and purposeful in seeking necessary knowledge and skills to enhance their career goals. Membership in nursing organizations, certification in a specialty or advanced practice area, and further academic education are also considered to be desirable activities to enhance the forensic nurse's professionalism (ANA & IAFN, 1999).

The Forensic Nurse's Code of Ethics

Adherence to the *Forensic Nurse's Code of Ethics* is a condition of initial and continued membership set forth by the IAFN. A brief description of the responsibilities and obligations of the forensic nurse as stated in the Code of Ethics is listed in Box 6-2.

Forensic Nursing Education

The forensic nurse is prepared through a synthesis of education and experience in nursing, forensic science, and law enforcement. This specialized education develops a clinician qualified to respond to the challenge health care faces in the protection of the legal, civil, and human rights of victims and perpetrators of violent crimes (ANA & IAFN, 1999).

SELF-AWARENESS PROMPT

The ANA *Code of Ethics for Nurses*—Provisions is listed in Chapter 5, Ethical and Legal Issues. Compare and contrast it with the *Forensic Nurse's Code of Ethics*. How do these two codes differ? Explain your answer.

Standard III of the *Standards of Professional Performance* addresses **forensic nursing education.** The Standard states that the forensic nurse acquires and maintains current knowledge in forensic nursing practice and integrates that learning into daily practice. To achieve this standard, the forensic nurse:

- Participates in ongoing activities related to clinical knowledge and professional issues
- Seeks experience to maintain competence
- Seeks knowledge and skills appropriate to the practice setting (ANA & IAFN, 1999).

Forensic nursing education can be obtained through colleges and universities that offer online courses, distance learning, or on-campus education. A registered nurse who is interested in forensic nursing has the option of participating in continuing education courses, certification programs, and undergraduate or graduate programs.

Forensic nursing curriculum courses include interviewing skills; documentation; collection of forensic evidence; and criminal, procedural, and constitutional law. Courses in forensic law and forensic science are also available (Burgess, Berger, & Boersma, 2004; Doerfler, 2004; Grady & Collins, 2003; Horner, 2004). Box 6-3 lists examples of colleges or universities that provide forensic nursing education.

Practice Areas

Forensic nurses practice within various settings whenever and wherever a medical–legal interest and forensic issues interact. This practice can occur in the primary care setting; the emergency room department; community or private hospital setting; clinics; legal arenas; businesses; educational, industrial, and correctional institutes; or other health care environments (ANA & IAFN, 1999).

BOX 6.2 FORENSIC NURSING RESPONSIBILITIES AND OBLIGATIONS

- *Responsibility to the public and the environment.* Forensic nurses are actively concerned with the health and welfare of the community at large and have a professional responsibility to serve the public welfare, especially disadvantaged citizens, and to further the cause of science and justice. They should understand and anticipate the environmental consequences of their work or the work of other communities and be prepared to stand up and oppose environmental problems or degradation.
- *Obligation to science.* Forensic nurses should seek to advance nursing and forensic science, understand the limits of their knowledge, and respect the truth. Their scientific contributions should be thorough, accurate, and unbiased in design, operationalization, and presentation.
- *Care of the profession.* Forensic nurses should remain current in their profession, share ideas, keep accurate and complete records, maintain integrity, and understand that conflicts of interest and scientific misconduct, such as fabrication, falsification of truth, slander, libel, and plagiarism are incompatible with and a violation of this Code of Ethics.
- *Dedication to colleagues.* As employers, forensic nurses should promote and protect the legitimate interest of their employees, perform work honestly and competently, fulfill obligations, and safeguard proprietary information. They should treat subordinates and associates with respect and regard the tutelage of students as a trust conferred by society to promote the student's learning and professional development.
- *Fidelity to clients.* Clients should be served faithfully and incorruptibly, with respect to confidentiality. They should be advised honestly and charged fairly.

Source: IAFN. (2005a). Code of Ethics. Retrieved February 15, 2005, from http://www.forensic.nurse.org/about/code.html

Special Roles of the Forensic Nurse

The nurse may desire to specialize as a child abuse nurse examiner, forensic nurse examiner (FNE), forensic clinical nurse specialist or advanced practice forensic nurse, SANE, sexual assault forensic examiner

BOX 6.3 EXAMPLES OF FORENSIC NURSING EDUCATION PROGRAMS

Duquesne University, Pittsburgh, PA: www.nursing.duq.edu
- MSN in Forensic Nursing
- Post-Master's Certificate in Forensic Nursing

Johns Hopkins University School of Nursing, Baltimore, MD: www.son.jhmi.edu
- MSN with Forensic Clinical Nurse Specialization

Kaplan University, Davenport, IA: www.kaplan.edu/hcp/programs
- Forensic Nursing Certification
- Online Forensic Nursing Courses
- Post-RN Forensic Nurse Certification

Monmouth University, West Long Branch, NJ: www.monmouth.edu/academica/schools/graduate/programs
- MSN with Forensic Nursing courses
- Graduate Certificate in Forensic Nursing

Quinnipiac University, Hamden, CT: www.quinnipiac.edu/x1338.xml
- Forensic Clinical Nurse Specialist

University of Pennsylvania, Philadelphia, PA: www.nursing.upenn.edu
- MSN with Forensic Nursing courses

CLINICAL EXAMPLE 6.1

INVESTIGATION OF VIOLENT BEHAVIOR

On Saturday, February 26, 2005, the Wichita, Kansas, police announced the capture of the "BTK killer" (bind-torture-kill) who had murdered at least 10 people over the last three decades. He had taunted detectives with poems, word puzzles, and boastful letters, and reached out to police several times. On one occasion, he called 911 to direct authorities to his most recent victim. In March 2004, he sent a letter claiming credit for an unsolved strangling in 1986. Before his capture, he sent a word-search puzzle to a local TV station, wrote a letter to police, and left packages containing various clues (eg, his autobiography, the driver's license and jewelry of his victims) in public areas in Wichita. The suspect was described as married, the father of two adult children, and an animal-control officer who also had the responsibility for citing residents who violated municipal codes. He also served as president of his church council and a Cub Scout leader.

Functions of the Forensic Nurse
The functions of the forensic nurse during the investigation of this case could include:
1. Collection of evidential material required by law enforcement or medical examiners
2. Scientific investigation of the death of known victims
3. Crisis intervention for family or friends of the victims
4. Interaction with grieving families or friends of the victims
5. Provision of expert witness testimony regarding the client's violent behavior

Source: Huffstutter, P. J., & Simon, S. (2005, February 7). We have BTK Killer, Kansas police say. *Orlando Sentinel,* p. A1, A25; and ANA & IAFN. (1999). *Scope and standards of forensic nursing practice* (pp. 3–4). Washington, DC: American Nurses Publishing.

(SAFE), sexual assault response team nurse (SART), nurse death examiner, or nurse coroner. Clinical Example 6-1 depicts details of violent behavior in which the forensic nurse could utilize his or her expertise.

Specialty roles will continue to develop as health care providers focus on issues of genetic therapy, **genomic health care** (a highly individualized plan of care that utilizes information related to phenotype responses and gene functions), **pharmacogenomics** (prescribing drugs based on the client's complete DNA structure), **e-practice** (use of electronic technology in the delivery of health care), and euthanasia. Box 6-4 lists specific practice areas of forensic nurses. Information regarding the role of the forensic nurse as a legal nurse consultant and expert witness is found in Chapter 5, Ethical and Legal Issues. The role of the forensic nurse is also included in chapters that discuss sexual disorders, suicidal clients, and incarcerated clients.

BOX 6.4 PRACTICE AREAS OF FORENSIC NURSES

- Forensic nursing sexual assault examiners
- Forensic nursing educators/consultants
- Nurse coroners
- Death investigators
- Legal nurse consultants
- Nurse attorneys
- Correctional nurses
- Clinical nursing specialists in trauma, transplant, and critical care nursing
- Forensic pediatric nurses
- Forensic gerontology nurses
- Forensic psychiatric nurses

KEY CONCEPTS

◆ Forensic nursing practice is considered to be one of the fastest growing nursing specialties of the 21st century. Sexual assault nurse examiners (SANEs) were trained in the mid-1970s to collect forensic evidence from sexual assault survivors; the formal recognition of forensic nursing occurred in 1991; the International Association of Forensic Nurses (IAFN) was formed during the summer of 1992; the American Nurses Association (ANA) published the *Scope and Standards of Nursing Practice in Correctional Facilities* in 1995; and finally, in 1997, at the request of the IAFN, the ANA collaborated with IAFN and created the *Scope and Standards of Forensic Nursing Practice.*

◆ The scope of forensic nursing practice, as defined by ANA and IAFN, encompasses three areas:

   • Application of the nursing-related sciences, including biopsychosocial education to public or legal proceedings
   • Application of the forensic aspects of health care in scientific investigation
   • Treatment of trauma or death victims and perpetrators (or alleged perpetrators) of abuse, violence, criminal activity, and traumatic accidents

◆ Forensic nursing is a unique, multidimensional discipline that provides direction to health care providers, educators, attorneys, researchers, and administrators, as well as other health professionals, legislators, and the public in general.

◆ The *Standards of Forensic Nursing Practice* consist of *Standards of Care* and *Standards of Professional Performance.* The *Standards of Care* describes a competent level of forensic nursing practice and delineates services provided to all clients of forensic nurses or practitioners. The *Standards of Professional Performance* describes a competent level of behavior in the forensic nurse's role.

◆ The *Forensic Nurse's Code of Ethics* addresses the nurse's responsibility to the public and the environment, obligation to science, care of the profession, dedication to colleagues, and fidelity to clients.

◆ Forensic nursing education can be obtained through colleges and universities that offer a variety of programs online, by distance learning, or on-campus. These programs may focus on continuing education, certification, or undergraduate or graduate studies that specialize in the field of forensic nursing.

◆ According to Standard III of the *Standards of Professional Performance,* forensic nurses are expected to acquire and maintain current knowledge in forensic nursing practice and to integrate the learning into daily practice.

◆ Forensic nurses practice in settings whenever and wherever a medical–legal interest and forensic issues interact, such as in the primary care setting, hospital, clinics, legal arenas, businesses, and the like.

For additional study materials, please refer to the Student Resource CD-ROM located in the back of this textbook.

CHAPTER WORKSHEET

CRITICAL THINKING QUESTIONS

1. Review the *Forensic Nurse's Code of Ethics* with a peer. Analyze the first code, *Responsibility to the public and the environment.* Discuss what activities a forensic nurse could perform to serve the public welfare, especially disadvantaged citizens. Cite examples of environmental problems or degradation that the forensic nurse might oppose.

2. Reflect on your observation and assessment skills. In what way would you be able to assist a forensic nurse in the collection of data on a client who complained of being physically abused during hospitalization? Cite examples of evidential material that would be collected.

3. Visit the Web site of at least three of the forensic nursing programs listed in Box 6.3. Do any of the programs offer a forensic nursing specialty that is of interest to you? If so, what additional educational preparation would you need to pursue this specialty?

REFLECTION

Reflect on the quote at the beginning of the chapter about forensic nursing. Articulate your understanding of this statement. Do you think forensic nurses should be able to function as a nurse coroner or death investigator? Explain the rationale for your answer.

NCLEX-STYLE QUESTIONS

1. The forensic nurse is incorporating information about a client's phenotype and gene function in the client's plan of care. The nurse is involved with
   a. genomic health care.
   b. e-practice.
   c. pharmacogenomics.
   d. euthanasia.

2. Which of the following is *least* descriptive of forensic nursing practice?
   a. Wide-ranging client population serviced
   b. Independent yet collaborative practice role
   c. Responsibilities independent of the legal system
   d. Collection of necessary evidence

3. Which of the following actions would violate the *Forensic Nurse's Code of Ethics*?
   a. Seeking clarification of confusing information
   b. Manipulating research data to meet the situation
   c. Treating associate providers with respect
   d. Maintaining client confidentiality

4. When describing the specific activities related to forensic nursing, which of the following would the nurse be *least* likely to include?
   a. Reviewing the medical record of a victim of assault and battery
   b. Testifying as an expert witness in a criminal court proceeding
   c. Providing emotional support to a victim of intimate partner violence
   d. Providing direct care to a hospitalized patient who was injured in an automobile accident.

5. According to the *Standards of Professional Performance*, the forensic nurse must demonstrate competent behavior by engaging in which of the following?
   a. Provision of cultural services
   b. Performance appraisal
   c. Maintenance of a safe environment
   d. Planning for continuity of care

6. Forensic nursing is considered one of the fastest growing nursing specialties in the 21st century. Place the following events in the development of forensic nursing in the proper sequence from earliest to most recent.
   a. Formal recognition of forensic nursing practice
   b. Publication of *Scope and Standards of Nursing Practice in Correctional Facilities*
   c. Establishment of sexual assault nurse examiner (SANE) programs
   d. Formation of the International Association of Forensic Nurses (IAFN)
   e. Creation of the *Scope and Standards of Forensic Nursing Practice*

Selected References

American Nurses Association. (1995). *Scope and standards of nurse practitioners in correctional facilities*. Washington, DC: American Nurses Publishing.

American Nurses Association & International Association of Forensic Nurses. (1999, February, 3rd reprint). *Scope and standards of forensic nursing practice*. Washington, DC: American Nurses Publishing.

Burgess, A. W., Berger, A. D., & Boersma, R. B. (2004). Forensic nursing. *American Journal of Nursing, 104*(3), 58–64.

Doerfler, R. E. (2004). Embracing the E-Revolution: How technology can maximize your practice. *ADVANCE for Nurse Practitioners, 12*(6), 35–42.

Grady, P.A., & Collins, F.S. (2003, March/April). Genetics and nursing science: Realizing the potential. *Nursing Research, 52*(2), 69.

Horner, S. D. (2004). Ethics and genetics. *Clinical Nurse Specialist, 18*(5), 228–231.

Huffstutter, P. J., & Simon, S. (2005, February 7). We have BTK killer, Kansas police say. *Orlando Sentinel,* pp. A1, A25.

International Association of Forensic Nurses. (2005a). Code of Ethics. Retrieved August 16, 2006, from http://www. forensicnurse.org/membership/membershipEthics.cfm

International Association of Forensic Nurses. (2005b). History. Retrieved February 15, 2005, from http://www. forensicnurse.org/about/history.html

International Association of Forensic Nurses. (2005c). Mission. Retrieved February 15, 2005, from http://www. forensicnurse.org/about/mission.html

International Association of Forensic Nurses. (2005d). What is forensic nursing? Retrieved February 15, 2005, from http://www.forensicnurse.org/about/default.html

Muscari, M. E. (2004). Forensic techniques. Retrieved September 11, 2004, from http://nursing.advance-web.com/common/ Editorial/Editorial.aspx?CC=40302

Suggested Readings

American Association of Colleges of Nursing. (2002). Violence as a public health problem. Retrieved March 10, 2004, from http://www.aacn.nche.edu/Publications/positions/ violence.htm

Courson, S. (2003 update). The investigative specialty of forensic nursing. *Pennsylvania State Nurses Association Career Center.* Retrieved August 16, 2006, from http://www. panurses.org

International Association of Forensic Nurses. (2003a). Council report of the IAFN. *On the Edge, 9*(4), 24.

International Association of Forensic Nurses. (2003b). Nurses. SANE-A certification exam. *On the Edge 9*(1), 13–14.

Keefe, S. (2006). Forensic nursing. A valuable resource for sexual assaults, death scenes and other health consequences of violence. *ADVANCE for Nurses, 7*(5), 33–34.

McKoy, Y. D. (2005). Forensic nursing: A challenge for nursing education. *Forensic Nurse.* Retrieved February 26, 2005, from http://www.forensicnursemag.com

Standing Bear, Z. G. (1999, May). Crime scene responders: The imperative sequential steps. *Critical Care Nursing Quarterly, 22*(1), 75–89.

U. S. Department of Justice. (2003). Advancing justice through DNA technology. Retrieved November 13, 2003, from http://www.usdoj.gov/ag/dnapolicy book_cov.htm

CHAPTER 7 / LOSS, GRIEF, AND END-OF-LIFE CARE

In this sad world of ours, sorrow comes to all... It comes with bittersweet agony... [Perfect] relief is not possible, except with time. You cannot now realize that you will ever feel better... And yet this is a mistake. You are sure to be happy again. To know this, which is certainly true, will make you feel less miserable now. —ABRAHAM LINCOLN

LEARNING OBJECTIVES

AFTER STUDYING THIS CHAPTER, YOU SHOULD BE ABLE TO:

1. Discuss the concepts of *loss, grief,* and *end-of-life care.*
2. Describe at least three types of losses that an individual can experience.
3. Explain the grief process.
4. Differentiate between *normal* and *unresolved* or *dysfunctional grief.*
5. Define *advance care planning.*
6. Articulate the needs of dying persons and their survivors.
7. State the rationale for The Dying Person's Bill of Rights.
8. Compare the perceptions of death by children during various growth stages.

KEY TERMS

Advance care planning
Advance directive
Anticipatory grief
Bereavement
Durable health care power of attorney
Dying declaration exception to hearsay
The Dying Person's Bill of Rights
Dysfunctional grief
End-of-life care
Grief
Grief process
Health care directive
Health care proxy
Hospice care
Living will
Loss
Mourning
Palliative care
Patient Self-Determination Act
Suffering
Unresolved grief

Peorole are complex, biopsychosocial beings.
When they become ill, undergo diagnosis for altered
health states, experience a loss, or progress into the
end stage of life, their responses are the result of the
complex interaction of biopsychosocial changes that
occur. Because we live in a culture marked by dramatically different responses to the experiences of loss
and grief, nurses often feel inadequate in planning
interventions to facilitate grief management and the
healing process.

This chapter provides information to familiarize the
student with the concepts of loss, grief, and end-of-life
care as they are experienced by individuals, families,
and/or their significant others.

Loss

Loss is one of the most important issues experienced
during one's lifetime. The concept of **loss** can be
defined in several ways. The following definitions have
been selected to familiarize the student with the concept of loss

- Change in status of a significant object
- Any change in an individual's situation that reduces
  the probability of achieving implicit or explicit goals
- An actual or potential situation in which a valued
  object, person, or other aspect is inaccessible or
  changed so that it is no longer perceived as valuable
- A condition whereby an individual experiences
  deprivation of, or complete lack of, something that
  was previously present

Everyone has experienced some type of major loss
at one time or another. Clients with psychiatric disorders, such as depression or anxiety, commonly
describe the loss of a spouse, relative, friend, job, pet,
home, or personal item.

Types of Loss

A loss may occur *suddenly* (eg, death of a child due to
an auto accident) or *gradually* (eg, loss of a leg due to
the progression of peripheral vascular disease). It may
be *predictable* or occur *unexpectedly*. Loss has been
referred to as *actual* (the loss has occurred or is occurring), *perceived* (the loss is recognized only by the
client and usually involves an ideal or fantasy), *antici-*

patory (the client is aware that a loss will occur),
temporary, or *permanent*. For example, a 65-year-old
married woman with the history of end-stage renal
disease is told by her physician that she has approximately 12 months to live. She may experience several
losses that affect not only her, but also her husband
and family members, as her illness gradually progresses. The losses may include a predictable decline
in her physical condition, a perceived alteration in her
relationship with her husband and family, and a permanent role change within the family unit as she
anticipates the progression of her illness and actual
loss of life. Whether the loss is traumatic or temperate
to the client and her family depends on their past
experience with loss; the value the family members
place on the loss of their mother/wife; and the cultural, psychosocial, economic, and family supports that
are available to each of them. Box 7-1 describes losses
identified by student nurses during their clinical experiences.

Grief

Grief, mourning, and bereavement are closely related to
loss, and sometimes the terms are used interchangeably. **Grief** is a normal, appropriate emotional response
to an external and consciously recognized loss. It is usually time-limited and subsides gradually. Staudacher
(2000) refers to grief as a stranger who has come to
stay in both the heart and mind. **Anticipatory grief**
refers to the reactions that occur when an individual,
family, significant other, or friends are expecting a loss
or death to occur. It includes all of the thinking, feeling,
cultural, and social reactions that occur regarding a loss
or death. Anticipatory grief allows the individual and
others to get used to the reality of the loss or death and
to complete unfinished business (eg, saying "good-bye,"
"I love you"). **Mourning** is a term used to describe an
individual's outward expression of grief regarding the
loss of a love object or person. The individual experiences emotional detachment from the object or person, eventually allowing the individual to find other
interests and enjoyments. Some individuals experience
a process of grief known as **bereavement** (eg, feelings
of sadness, insomnia, poor appetite, deprivation, and
desolation).

BOX 7.1 EXAMPLES OF LOSSES IDENTIFIED BY STUDENT NURSES

- Loss of spouse, friend, and companion. The client was a 67-year-old woman admitted to the psychiatric hospital for treatment of depression after the death of her husband. During a group discussion that focused on losses, the client stated that she had been married for 47 years and had never been alone. She described her deceased husband as her best friend and constant companion. The client told the student and group that she felt better after expressing her feelings about her losses.
- Loss of body image and social role as the result of a below-the-knee amputation. The client was a 19-year-old girl who was involved in a motorcycle accident. She had shared her feelings with the student nurse about her "new" body image and dating after hospitalization.
- Loss of a loved one owing to fetal demise or intrauterine death. The student nurse had been assigned to a young woman, who was in her twenty-eighth week of pregnancy and delivered a preterm newborn who died immediately after birth. The following day, the client expressed a sincere thanks to the student nurse for supporting her during such a difficult time in her life.
- Loss of physiologic function, social role, and independence because of kidney failure. A 49-year-old woman was admitted to the hospital for improper functioning of a shunt in her left forearm. She was depressed and asked that no visitors be permitted in her private room. She shared feelings of loneliness, helplessness, and hopelessness with the student nurse as she described the impact of kidney failure and frequent dialysis treatment on her lifestyle. Once an outgoing, independent person, she was housebound because of her physical condition and "resented what her kidneys were doing to her."

Grief Theory

Grief theory proposes that grief occurs as a process. The **grief process** is all-consuming, having a physical, social, spiritual, and psychological impact on an individual that may impair daily functioning. Feelings vary in intensity, tasks do not necessarily follow a particular pattern, and the time spent in the grieving process varies considerably, from weeks to years (Schultz & Videbeck, 2002).

Several authors have described grief as a process that includes various stages, characteristic feelings, experiences, and tasks. Staudacher (2000) states there are three major stages of grief: shock, disorganization, and reorganization. Westberg (2004) describes ten stages of grief work, beginning with the stage of shock and progressing through the stages of expressing emotion, depression and loneliness, physical symptoms of distress, panic, guilt feelings, anger and resentment, resistance, hope, and concluding with the stage of affirming reality. Kübler-Ross (1969) identifies five stages of the grieving process: denial, anger, bargaining, depression, and acceptance; however, progression through these stages does not necessarily occur in any specific order. Her basic premise has evolved as a result of her work with dying persons. The creation of hospices, palliative care, and programs on pain management has been attributed to the work of Kübler-Ross. The care of the dying is in the forefront of medicine and the voices of the dying are increasingly recognized (Munoz, 2004). Box 7-2 discusses Kübler-Ross's five stages of the grief process.

Unresolved or Dysfunctional Grief

Unresolved or **dysfunctional grief** could occur if the individual is unable to work through the grief process after a reasonable time. The cause of dysfunctional grief is usually an actual or perceived loss of someone or something of great value to a person. Clinical features or characteristics include expressions of distress or denial of the loss; changes in eating and sleeping habits; mood disturbances, such as anger, hos-

SELF-AWARENESS PROMPT

Identify at least one loss that you or a member of your family has experienced. Was it an actual, perceived, or anticipated loss? How did you and/or members of your family respond to the loss? What type of support, if any, was offered to help you with the grief process? Was it sufficient to meet the needs of yourself and/or members of your family?

(Chapter 21), or psychosis (Chapter 22). Kishiyama (2004) lists practical tips for clients' experiencing grief. Paraphrased, they include:

- Allowing oneself to experience feelings of pain, anger, etc.
- Sharing personal feelings with others
- Talking out loud to one's loved one to release feelings
- Maintaining or resuming a daily schedule or routine to avoid feeling overwhelmed
- Avoiding the use of alcoholic beverages to avoid feeling more depressed
- Sleeping, eating, and exercising regularly
- Delaying the making of any major decisions immediately after the loss
- Asking for help to deal with a loss to avoid unresolved or dysfunctional grief

End-of-Life Care

The following statement was retrieved from the Aging with Dignity organization's Web site (http://www.agingwithdignity.org):

> Something is terribly wrong: The majority of Americans want to die at home surrounded by family and friends, but most end up dying in the hospital or nursing home, cared for by strangers. Half of these Americans die in pain that could have been treated. Sick people have come to fear losing their dignity or burdening their families more than they fear death. And this is all happening in a country that is meant to prize the rights of individuals and champion respect for personal wishes.

End-of-life care refers to the nursing care given during the final weeks of life when death is imminent. The American culture is marked by dramatically different responses to the experience of death. On one hand, death is denied or compartmentalized with the use of medical technology that prolongs the dying process and isolates the dying person from loved ones. On the other hand, death is embraced as a frantic escape from apparently meaningless suffering through means such as physician-assisted suicide. Both require compassionate responses rooted in good medical practice and personal religious beliefs.

The **Patient Self-Determination Act** (PSDA), passed in 1990, states that every competent individual

---

BOX 7.2 FIVE STAGES OF GRIEF IDENTIFIED BY KÜBLER-ROSS

- *Denial:* During this stage, the person displays a disbelief in the prognosis of inevitable death. This stage serves as a temporary escape from reality. Fewer than 1% of all dying clients remain in this stage. Typical responses include: "No, it can't be true," "It isn't possible," and "No, not me." Denial usually subsides when the client realizes that someone will help him or her to express feelings while facing reality.
- *Anger:* "Why me?" "Why now?" and "It's not fair!" are a few of the comments commonly expressed during this stage. The client may appear difficult, demanding, and ungrateful during this stage.
- *Bargaining:* Statements such as "If I promise to take my medication, will I get better?" or "If I get better, I'll never miss church again" are examples of attempts at bargaining to prolong one's life. The dying client acknowledges his or her fate but is not quite ready to die at this time. The client is ready to take care of unfinished business, such as writing a will, deeding a house over to a spouse or child, or making funeral arrangements as he or she begins to anticipate various losses, including death.
- *Depression:* This stage is also a very difficult period for the family and physician because they feel helpless watching the depressed client mourn present and future losses. "The dying patient is about to lose not just one loved person but everyone he has ever loved and everything that has been meaningful to him" (Kübler-Ross, 1971, p. 58).
- *Acceptance:* At this stage the client has achieved an inner and outer peace due to a personal victory over fear: "I'm ready to die. I have said all the good-byes and have completed unfinished business." During this stage, the client may want only one or two significant people to sit quietly by the client's side, touching and comforting him or her.

---

tility, or crying; and alterations in activity levels, including libido (sex drive). The person experiencing dysfunctional grief idealizes the lost person or object, relives past experiences, loses the ability to concentrate, and is unable to work purposefully because of developmental regression. The grieving person may exhibit symptoms of anxiety (Chapter 19), depression

has the right to make decisions about his or her health care and is encouraged to make known in **advance directives** (ADs; legal documents specifying care) end-of-life preferences, in case the individual is unable to speak on his or her own behalf (Allen, 2002; Robinson & Kennedy-Schwartz, 2001). Advance directives evolved as new technologies to sustain life were being developed and a perception existed that physicians hadn't developed good judgment on how to use this new power. The belief was that if illness or injury prevented a client from making decisions about one's health care, the best alternative would be to follow instructions issued by the client before the onset of the illness or injury, when the individual could still think about the choice (Silverman, 2004).

Advance Care Planning

Advance care planning is a thoughtful, facilitated discussion that encompasses a lifetime of values, beliefs, and goals for the client and family. Advance care planning often involves completion of an AD. The two most common forms of advance directives are the **living will** or the **health care directive** and the **durable health care power of attorney** or **health care proxy** (Allen, 2002; Norlander, 2001).

The living will is a document filled out by the client with specific instructions addressing issues of cardiopulmonary resuscitation (CPR); life support systems such as the use of a ventilator or intubation; tube feedings or artificial nutrition and hydration; and emergency measures such as surgery, blood transfusion, or antibiotics to treat end-stage diseases. Living wills give some guidance, but a document called Five Wishes enables all caretakers to know and understand the desires of a dying client. Each wish gives a specific desire regarding end-of-life care (Box 7-3).

A durable health care power of attorney permits an individual to name a health care decision-maker or surrogate to make medical decisions in the event that the individual is unable to make these decisions or give informed consent. If a health care power of attorney or surrogate has not been named, the law allows a health care proxy to be appointed to act on behalf of the client (eg, an individual has a stroke and is unable to communicate his wishes). Examples of health care proxies include spouses, guardians, or parents.

A unique form of advance directive, the **dying declaration exception to hearsay** allows statements referred to as "death bed declarations" to be honored by the medical and nursing staff. For example, a client,

---

BOX 7.3 FIVE WISHES

Each of the following wishes makes a specific desire for the client. Five Wishes meets the legal requirements in several states. Summarized, the wishes are:

Wish 1: State the name of the person you want to make health care decisions about medical tests, treatments or surgery, or admission to a hospital, hospice or nursing home when you can't make the decisions yourself.

Wish 2: Describe the kind of medical treatment you want or don't want. Choices are listed for clinical situations such as a coma, near-death situation, permanent and severe brain damage without recovery, or any other condition under which the client does not wish to be kept alive.

Wish 3: State how comfortable you want to be. Several choices are given regarding activities of daily living, pain management, and relaxation techniques or interventions.

Wish 4: Describe how you want people to treat you. This wish addresses the spiritual needs of the client during the dying process, such as having someone present at bedside, having prayers said at a vigil or in church, having visits from a chaplain or one's spiritual advisor, and expressing the desire whether to die at home or in the hospital.

Wish 5: Explain what you would like your loved ones to know. This wish addresses how the client wants to be remembered and gives him or her the opportunity to relay funeral and memorial wishes.

Sources: Gilbert, S. (2004). Living 'til the end. Using the Five Wishes to prepare for the end of life. *ADVANCE for Nurses, 5*(5), 27; and Aging With Dignity: http://www.agingwithdignity.org.

---

who is aware that death is imminent and has not completed a living will, may inform the nursing staff that he wants all medication, including intravenous (IV) therapy, to be discontinued. Such a request can be honored if documented (Scanlon, 2003).

Ethnic Considerations and Cultural Sensitivity

Our health care system is based on a scientific, biomedical model of disease. Many other cultures have a more spiritual or nature-based view (Norlander, 2001). Nurses need to acknowledge that their view of end-of-life care might be quite different from views held by clients and their families or significant others. Ethnicity and race significantly influence end-of-life decisions and treatments. Cultural competence demands that nurses view clients through their own eyes and the eyes of the client and family. Many culturally diverse clients and families have had negative experiences with health care providers as a result of the lack of attention to cultural needs, or they have experienced additional stressors such as limited financial resources and health coverage. Such influences could have profound effects upon establishing trust with a client when planning end-of-life care (Mazanec & Tyler, 2003).

Andrews and Boyle (2003) discuss stages of grief and bereavement observed in culturally diverse clients such as Native Americans, Buddhists, Mexican Americans, Puerto Ricans, and Eurasians. The magnitude of stress and its meaning to such individuals varies significantly cross-culturally. Contemporary grieving practices of various cultural groups demonstrate a wide range of expression of emotion related to personal losses. Hindering or interfering with the practices that the culturally diverse client and family find meaningful can disrupt the grieving process and precipitate physical or psychological symptoms that may lead to serious physical illness or even death.

Palliative Care and Hospice Care

The terms *palliative care* and *hospice care* are associated with end-of-life care. According to the World Health Organization (WHO), **palliative care** is the active total care of clients whose disease is not responsive to curative treatment. The Institute of Medicine (IOM) emphasizes that palliative care seeks to prevent, relieve, reduce, or soothe the symptoms of disease or disorder without effecting a cure.

On April 30, 2004, the National Consensus Project for Quality Palliative Care released the first national Clinical Practice Guidelines for Quality Palliative Care. They focus on coordination and delivery of care; spiritual, cultural, ethical, and legal aspects of palliative care; and care when the client's death is imminent (Foley, 2004). Nursing outcomes focus primarily on promoting quality of life while emphasizing the relief of pain, suffering, and symptom management; and assisting clients and families to reach personal goals, reconcile conflicts, and derive meaning from their

experiences at end of life. Palliative care can and should exist outside of hospice programs because not all clients who receive palliative care are near the end of life. Palliative care may be provided in the early stages of a chronic disease or terminal illness (Ferrell & Coyle, 2002; Norlander, 2001; Puntillo, 2001).

Hospice care refers to a program that supports the client and family through the dying process and the surviving family members through the process of bereavement. It is based on a biopsychosocial model rather than a disease model of care. The essential philosophy of hospice care is the focus on comfort, dignity, and personal growth at life's end. This encompasses biomedical, psychosocial, and spiritual aspects of the dying experience, emphasizing quality of life and healing or strengthening interpersonal relationships rather than prolonging the dying process at any and all cost. Hospice care also supports the well-being of those in caregiving roles and provides bereavement care for survivors (Medscape, 2004).

Hospice care can be traced back to early Western Civilization when shelter and rest was provided for weary or sick travelers on long journeys. In the 1970s, a group of clergy, health care workers, and other individuals felt that individuals were being deprived of the natural dying process and were being robbed of dignity. Out of these concerns, the first hospice was established in 1974 in New Haven, Connecticut, and the natural process of dying was returned to the home. Although most clients are cared for in the home or in a nursing home, they can receive hospice care in a variety of settings (Hospice of the Plains, Inc, 2005).

Typically, to qualify for hospice care, Medicare or other insurance companies require that the individual be terminally ill, have a medical prognosis with a life expectancy of 6 months or less if the illness runs its normal course (eg, end-stage chronic obstructive pulmonary disease or cancer), and no longer wishes to pursue aggressive treatment options (Klimkiewicz, 2001).

Both palliative care and hospice care address issues related to the manifestations of suffering, including physical and emotional responses, pain, and the act of dying. The American Nurses Credentialing Center (ANCC) and the National Board for Certification of Hospice and Palliative Nurses (NBCHPN) offer certification opportunities for nurses in home health and hospice care. Both agencies have partnered to create an advanced practice palliative care nursing certification.

Manifestations of Suffering

Suffering has been described as a process or state of severe distress associated with injury or events that threaten the composure, integrity, and fulfillment of our intentions. Manifestations of suffering may be behavioral (eg, withdrawal or avoidance of contact with family or caregiver), emotional (eg, anger or depression), physical (eg, impaired sleep or fatigue), or spiritual (eg, a sense of alienation or emptiness) (Norlander, 2001; Rushton, 2001).

Norlander (2001) lists the several key concepts of suffering that should be considered when assessing a client. Summarized, they state:

- Suffering involves physical, psychosocial, and spiritual aspects.
- Suffering should be assessed routinely when providing care.
- Not all suffering requires intervention.
- Many interventions for suffering can be implemented by nurses.
- Members of the multidisciplinary treatment team can often perform interventions.

After the nurse has identified the source of the client's suffering, a holistic plan of care can be implemented based on the client's needs. Interventions may vary according to the type of distress the client is experiencing. (Chapters 9 and 10 address the nursing process.) Box 7-4 lists common responses associated with suffering at the end of life.

Pain

"The role of the nurse in pain management cannot be overemphasized. As skilled clinicians, we need to be competent in assessing pain and understanding the principles of pain management. As advocates, we need to work with physicians and other health team members to develop the most effective care plan for the patient. As guides, we need to work with the patient and family to find the highest level of comfort" (Norlander, 2001, p. 20).

The Agency for Health Care Policy and Research (AHCPR; 1994, p. 12) defined pain as "an unpleasant sensory and emotional experience associated with actual or potential tissue damage or described in terms of such damage." Box 7-5 lists the ABCDE mnemonic of pain assessment and management as stated by AHCPR.

In 1996, the WHO (1996) developed an *Analgesic Ladder* that outlines the principles of analgesic selection and titration as well as the use of adjunctive drug therapy to ease pain or to counteract adverse effects in the treatment of clients with cancer. For example,

---

BOX 7.4   COMMON RESPONSES ASSOCIATED WITH SUFFERING AT END OF LIFE

- **Behavioral:** Avoidance, controlling, distancing
- **Emotional:** Anger, anxiety, depression, emotional outbursts, frustration, guilt, sarcasm, emotional withdrawal from family or friends
- **Physical:** Fatigue, fluctuation in vital signs, impaired sleep, impaired mental processes such as confusion or delirium, persistent physical symptoms such as pain, weight gain or loss
- **Spiritual:** Verbalization of a sense of hopelessness, emptiness, or meaninglessness

Adapted from: Kearney, M. (1996). *Mortally wounded.* New York: Simon & Schuster; and Norlander, L. (2001). *To comfort always: A nurse's guide to end of life care.* Washington, DC: American Nurses Publishing.

BOX 7.5   ABCDE MNEMONIC OF PAIN MANAGEMENT

A: Ask about the client's pain regularly and assess the pain systematically.

B: Believe the client, family, and/or significant other in their reports of pain and what relieves it.

C: Choose pain-control options that are appropriate for the client, family, or significant other. Consider the setting in which the client is receiving care.

D: Deliver nursing interventions in a timely, logical, and coordinated fashion.

E: Empower the client, family, and/or significant other. Enable client to control his or her course to the greatest extent possible.

Source: Agency for Health Care Policy and Research. (1994). *Management of cancer pain, clinical practice guideline number 6.* Rockville, MD: Department of Health and Human Services, p. 24.

control of mild pain may be achieved with the use of a non-narcotic analgesic. As the severity of pain increases, a narcotic analgesic would be administered. In the case of severe or persistent pain, a combination of medications such as an opioid and non-narcotic analgesic or opioid and salicylate would be used. Additional medication may be added to relieve adverse effects secondary to the use of pain medication or to relieve clinical symptoms of anxiety or depression.

In 1991, the American Nurses Association issued a position statement regarding the promotion of comfort and relief of pain in dying clients. It maintained that efforts to relieve pain and other symptoms in dying patients are the obligations of the nurse and may require increasing titration of medication to achieve adequate symptom control. Although such aggressive measures may interfere with maintaining life and may hasten death, these nursing interventions are considered to be ethically justified. The Joint Commission on Accreditation of Healthcare Organizations (JCAHO) recently issued pain treatment standards mandating pain assessment in all hospitalized clients, including those in the psychiatric setting. These guidelines have helped to alleviate the fear prevalent among health care professionals that the use of analgesic or sedative medications will promote tolerance or addiction to pain medication, hasten death, or be viewed as an act of euthanasia.

The Act of Dying

"A recently published study found that persons who are terminally ill are able to discuss death, dying, and bereavement with their caregivers with minimal stress" (Fink, 2005, p. 10). Although death is inevitable, clients do have a choice regarding the medical procedures, drugs, and nutritional or respiratory support that they can receive during the final stage of life, referred to as the *act of dying.* Supporting Evidence for Practice 7-1 highlights a study on end-of-life ethical concerns. Bad deaths, those accompanied by unnecessary and severe suffering, are often the result of the clinician's failure to follow recommended end-of-life guidelines for the care of dying clients. Few clinicians outside of hospice and palliative care programs have the skills necessary to manage the dying process (LaDuke, 2001). Early recognition of impending death and the recognition of a client's life choices can lead to a good death.

Fink (2005) identifies critical psychosocial and psychiatric issues to be addressed as the client accepts the reality of death. They include the following: existential and spiritual concerns, making amends with family and friends, preparing advance directives, leaving legacies and memories for children, planning custody arrangements for dependent children, differentiating grief from depression and treating each appropriately, mate-

---

SUPPORTING EVIDENCE FOR PRACTICE 7.1

Providing Interventions for End-of-Life Ethical Concerns of Clients in the Psychiatric–Mental Health Clinical Setting

PROBLEM UNDER INVESTIGATION / Elders discuss ethical concerns related to aging and end-of-life issues

SUMMARY OF RESEARCH / Eighteen elders between the ages of 70 years and 92 years of age, ten of their children, and two of their grandchildren were interviewed by a nurse researcher to explore end-of-life ethical concerns and how they and their family members responded to the concerns. Ethical concerns included issues such as personal health and caregiver burden; maintaining spirituality; ethnic identity; worry about the health of a loved one; concern about the loved one's death; and facing death. Researchers concluded that most elders wanted to avoid pain and dis-

comfort, to avoid being a burden on their families, and to achieve a natural, peaceful death. Family members described the importance of positive interpersonal family relationships and the need to assist elders in resolving conflicts.

SUPPORT FOR PRACTICE / Planning of nursing interventions for ethical concerns and unresolved conflicts of elders and their family members should focus on the promotion of healthy and positive choices for quality-of-life and end-of-life decision-making.

SOURCE: Cameron, M.D. (2002). Older persons' ethical problems involving their health. Nursing Ethics, 9, 537–556.

TABLE 7.1 ⬛ Needs of Dying Persons and Survivors

DYING PERSON'S NEEDS	SURVIVOR'S NEEDS
Vent anger and frustration	Provide a quality of life for the dying person while preparing for a life without that loved one
Share the knowledge that the end is near	Be available to offer comfort and care even though the survivor feels like running away to escape the pain of death
Ensure the well-being of loved ones who will be left behind, because the person resents the fact that life will go on without him or her	Hope that the loved one will somehow live in spite of obvious deterioration and inability to function. At this time, the survivor may pray for the peace of death.
Vent feelings or irritation at omissions or neglect, although the person feels guilty over the pain this causes	Vent feelings or irritation and guilt over the dying person's demands and increased dependency needs
Remain as independent as possible, fearing he or she will become unlovable	Live and appreciate each day as one plans for a future without the loved one
Be normal and natural at a time when nothing appears to be normal or natural. The dying client generally experiences the fears of pain, loss of control, and dying alone. The client has a need to maintain security, self-confidence, and dignity.	Reassure the dying person that the survivor will "continue in his or her footsteps" by holding the family together, raising the children, or managing the business, while knowing that such talk about the future is painful to the dying client

---

rial stress, sexual concerns, loss of physical function, and dealing with psychiatric symptoms and syndromes such as depression and anxiety (p. 10).

The act of dying is a very personal matter, and end-of-life care such as hospice offers a final respite and a time for acceptance and peace for both the client and the client's family or significant other (Klimkiewicz, 2001).

Holst (1984) created a list of needs experienced by dying persons and their survivors while they face conflicts and dilemmas during this critical time in their lives. These needs are summarized in Table 7-1.

Families and clients may grieve many losses before the disease finally takes life. Optimism, spontaneity, holidays, long-range planning, dreams, retirement, and grandparenthood are just a few of the many losses experienced as a client and his or her family live with a terminal illness (Holst, 1984).

In 1975, **The Dying Person's Bill of Rights** was developed (Box 7-6). Every nursing unit should have this bill of rights posted in a readily accessible area to remind members of the health care team about their responsibilities for providing holistic health care. If the nurse feels uncomfortable in planning care to meet

these rights or needs, a team conference should be held to enlist suggestions or help from other members of the team.

In 1997, there was a strong recommendation by the IOM that health care professionals commit to improving care for dying clients, especially symptom management. Since that time, many agencies within the U. S. Department of Health and Human Services are involved with research initiatives to improve end-of-life care. The funded studies include a wide range of populations and modalities. Clients with life-limiting conditions can benefit from research developments as understanding of the unique aspects of end-of-life care improves (Knebel, 2002).

Spiritual Needs

One of the most important, but difficult, areas to assess when a client is dying is the realm of spirituality (Norlander, 2001). Although hospice and most palliative care programs address the spiritual issues of dying clients and their families and/or significant others, not all clients receive palliative or hospice care. Becoming

---

BOX 7.6 **THE DYING PERSON'S BILL OF RIGHTS***

I have the right to:

Be treated as a living human being until I die.

Maintain a sense of hopefulness, however changing its focus may be.

Be cared for by those who can maintain a sense of hopefulness, however changing this might be.

Express my feelings and emotions about my approaching death in my own way.

Participate in decisions concerning my care.

Expect continuing medical and nursing attention even though "cure" goals must be changed to "comfort" goals.

Not die alone.

Be free from pain.

Have my questions answered honestly.

Not be deceived.

Have help from and for my family in accepting my death.

Die in peace and with dignity.

Retain my individuality and not be judged for my decisions, which may be contrary to beliefs of others.

Discuss and enlarge my religious and/or spiritual experiences, whatever these may mean to others.

Expect that the sanctity of the human body will be respected after death.

Be cared for by caring, sensitive, knowledgeable people who will attempt to understand my needs and will be able to gain some satisfaction in helping me face my death.

---

*The Dying Person's Bill of Rights was created at a workshop on "The Terminally Ill Patient and the Helping Person" in Lansing, Michigan, sponsored by the Southwestern Michigan Inservice Education Council and conducted by Amelia J. Barbus, Associate Professor of Nursing at Wayne State University in Detroit, Michigan. From the *American Journal of Nursing,* January, 1975, p. 99.

---

familiar with the attitudes and requirements of various religious groups is crucial to addressing the spiritual needs of clients, families, and/or significant others.

Clients may not verbalize their desire or need for spiritual support. Pumphrey (1977) discusses how clients search for an understanding listener and spiritual support by sending out feelers or making remarks such as "I haven't gone to church much lately" or "My pastor is so busy, I hate to bother him while I'm in the hospital." Norlander (2001) cites helpful questions the nurse may ask during the assessment of the dying client's spiritual needs. Nursing interventions begin with listening and acknowledging the client's spirituality. Ideally, the nurse should be able to respond to each client's spiritual needs as naturally as he or she responds to the client's physical needs. If addressing various spiritual concerns is uncomfortable, the nurse can suggest that the client talk to the hospital chaplain, the client's own clergy, members of his or her congregation, or other clients with similar religious beliefs. If none of these options seems appropriate, the nurse can provide quiet time for private meditation or prayer (Cohen & Koenig, 2002).

Culture also can influence a client's spiritual needs. Andrews and Hanson (2003) as well as Norlander (2001) discuss the assessment of spiritual needs in culturally diverse clients who are actively dying. Four areas to be explored include the environment, behavior, verbalization, and interpersonal relationships. For example, are religious objects visible? Does the client or family wear clothing that has religious significance? Is a trained interpreter available? Are written resources available for the client or family in their own language? Is space available to accommodate extended families? Have nonrestrictive visiting hours been instituted? Has the family or client requested important rituals such as a traditional healing ceremony? Are special dietary requests made? Such observations enable the nurse to address spiritual needs of the client, family, and/or significant other.

Children and Death

Although children's growth varies both physically and emotionally, books that discuss children and the impact of dying outline general growth stages, citing the needs and understanding of children in each phase of development.

Preschool children between the ages of 3 and 5 years have a fear of separation from their parents and are unable to think of death as a final separation. They perceive death as a temporary trip to heaven or some other place in which the person still functions actively by eating, sleeping, and so forth. If a child displays guilt feelings because the child "wished something awful would happen when angry at mommy or daddy," he or she needs to be told that wishes do not kill. Conversely, the well-adjusted child who appears to be brave and displays little emotion while appearing to accept a parent's death should be seen by a professional counselor to ensure that no psychological problem is developing.

Children between the ages of 5 and 6 years see death as a reversible process that others experience, whereas children from 6 to 9 years of age begin to accept death as a final state. Death is conceptualized as a destructive force, a frightening figure, a bogey monster, or an angel of death who comes during the night "to get bad people." Children of this age believe they will not die if they avoid the death figure.

By the age of 10 years, some children begin to realize that death is an inevitable state that all human beings experience because of an internal process. They also believe that the body of a dead person slowly rots until only bones remain as insects infest the coffin and prey on the body. The child may verbalize words such as *afterlife, cremation, rebirth,* and *reunion* at this age.

Adolescents are able to intellectualize their awareness of death, although they usually repress any feelings about their own death. Adolescents often hide the fact that they are mourning. They are inexperienced in coping with a stressor and may not shed tears or voice their emotions regarding their loss.

Children and adolescents are capable of feeling the great loss of a loved person one moment and yet becoming fully absorbed in something funny the next. Adults need to be aware of this capability so that they do not misinterpret such behavior as disrespect or lack of love for the deceased person. In addition, as a child matures and his or her concept of death changes, the child may have to mourn a loss more than once. For example, a child may lose a parent while at the age where he or she believes that death is not permanent; thus, the child believes that he or she will see the parent again. However, after the

SELF-AWARENESS PROMPT

Reflect on your personal ethnic and cultural background. How do you and your family view end-of-life care? Do you feel comfortable providing end-of-life care for clients whose cultural beliefs and practices may differ from yours? If not, what could you do to improve your comfort level?

child matures, he or she may mourn the loss again and in a new way.

Various studies have been performed to evaluate children and their responses to death. Christ (2001) reports the findings of a qualitative intervention study regarding the understanding of death by 157 children ages 3 to 17 years and their ability to mourn the death of a parent from cancer. According to Christ, most children and adolescents can adapt effectively to the death of a parent and even learn and grow from the experience; however, they cannot do it alone. The findings of the study and developmental conceptions of death, behavioral responses, and interventions are summarized in Table 7-2.

KEY CONCEPTS

◆ Loss has been described as a condition whereby an individual experiences deprivation of, or complete lack of, something that was previously present, such as a job, pet, home, personal item, or loved one. The individual may experience an actual loss, perceive that a loss has occurred, or anticipate that a loss will occur.

◆ Grief is a normal, appropriate emotional response to an external and consciously recognized loss. Anticipatory grief gives an individual, family, significant other, or friends an opportunity to adjust to the reality of an expected loss or death and to complete unfinished business such as saying "good-bye" or "I love you." Failure to work through the grief process could result in unresolved or dysfunctional grief.

◆ "End of life" refers to the final weeks of life when death is imminent. The Patient Self-Determination Act of 1990 states that every competent individual has the right to make decisions about his or her health

TABLE 7.2 Research Results: Mourning the Death of a Parent From Cancer

AGE GROUP	DEVELOPMENTAL CONCEPTIONS, RESPONSES, AND INTERVENTIONS
Ages 3–5 years	Children did not understand that death was permanent and irreversible. Mourning was nonspecific and included behaviors such as irritability, toileting regression, nightmares, and somatic symptoms. Play bereavement groups helped to improve communication and to decrease clinical symptoms.
Ages 6–8 years	Children had difficulty understanding the circumstances that led to the death of a parent. They focused on themselves as the cause when something bad happened. Mourning behaviors included joyful reminiscences of the parent, with sporadic crying and sadness. Children believed the parent was in a place such as heaven and were convinced that the deceased parent could see them and still care for them. Play bereavement groups, contact with peers with similar losses, reminiscences of parent, and rituals such as visiting the parent's gravesite were considered to be therapeutic.
Ages 9–11 years	Behaviors included spending time with peers and looking for ways to be helpful with caretaking functions. Mourning included compartmentalization of their emotions, and intellectualization of their feelings by writing reports about cancer and treatment options. Children responded favorably to encouragement of appropriate reminiscences of the deceased parent and structural family rituals.
Ages 12–14 years	Behaviors included marked egocentrism (concern about self) and fluctuating emotional responses and needs. Mourning occurred in private areas such as their bedrooms; however, they did talk about dreams and speaking with the deceased parent. Limit-setting and formal family reminiscence experiences enabled the children to express feelings that they avoided in informal discussions.
Ages 15–17 years	Behaviors included the presence of anticipatory grief during the parent's terminal illness. The teenagers acknowledged that their family's future would be changed. Mourning symptoms for most of the teenagers were similar to those of adults but shorter in duration. Clinical symptoms included lack of interest, sleeping problems, and inability to concentrate. Sharing of grief experiences with their peers who had lost their parents to death or divorce appeared to be beneficial. The teens were encouraged to maintain independent functioning.

Source: Christ, G. H. (2001). Facilitating mourning following parental death. *Psychiatric Times, 18*(9), 39–45.

care. This includes the use of advance directives such as the living will and durable health care power of attorney. These documents address the issues of CPR, life support, artificial nutrition and hydration, and emergency measures to treat end-stage diseases.

◆ Acknowledging that our view of end-of-life care might differ from views held by our clients and their families or significant others is important. Lack of knowledge regarding the ethnicity, culture, and race of a client could have a profound effect on establishing trust with a client when planning end-of-life care.

◆ Palliative care seeks to prevent, relieve, reduce, or soothe the symptoms of disease or disorder without effecting a cure. Palliative care may be provided in the early stages of a chronic disease or terminal illness. Hospice care supports the client and family during the dying process (medical prognosis of 6 months or less) and the surviving family members through the process of bereavement. Both palliative care and hospice care address issues related to the manifestations of suffering including physical and emotional responses, pain, and the act of dying.

◆ Not all clients receive palliative or hospice care. Nurses need to familiarize themselves with the attitudes and requirements of various religious groups so that they can address the spiritual needs of their clients, families, and/or significant others.

◆ The concept of death changes as children undergo various developmental stages. Preschool children fear separation from their parents and are unable to think of death as a final separation. Five- and 6-year-olds see death as a reversible process, whereas 6- to 9-year-olds begin to accept death as a final state. By the age of 10 years, some children begin to realize that death is an inevitable state. Adolescents are able to intellectualize their awareness of death, although they usually repress any feelings about their own death.

For additional study materials, please refer to the Student Resource CD-ROM located in the back of this textbook.

CHAPTER WORKSHEET

CRITICAL THINKING QUESTIONS

1. Your best friend hasn't been herself lately; in fact, you are becoming increasingly worried about her. It has been 18 months since her father died of lung cancer. She is smoking more, missing class, and reacting angrily when questioned. You feel her grief is dysfunctional at this point. How might you help her?
2. Mrs. Kessler, a 78-year-old widow, has been under your care for several days. She has openly spoken about her wishes for a dignified death, with "none of that mechanical stuff." You have just overheard her son and doctor planning additional surgery for her without her involvement in the decision. What action should you take and why?

REFLECTION

A new neighbor tells you that his wife of 30 years was killed in an automobile accident 3 months ago, and he is having difficulty adjusting to living alone. Reflect on the chapter opening quote by Abraham Lincoln. How would you interpret the meaning of this quote? What significance does it have in relation to the neighbor's disclosure about the loss of his wife?

NCLEX-STYLE QUESTIONS

1. When assessing a client experiencing dysfunctional grief, which of the following would the nurse expect to assess? Select all that apply.
   a. Changes in libido
   b. Acknowledgement of the loss
   c. Diminished ability to concentrate
   d. Expressions of hostility
   e. Reliving of past experiences

2. A 27-year-old male client who recently lost his wife due to terminal cancer relates that he and his wife discussed her end-of-life wishes including her burial service. The client states that he is now unable to sleep; has a poor appetite; and feels sad even when in the company of their two children, ages 5 and 7 years. Which of the following responses to the death of his wife is the client experiencing?
   a. Mourning
   b. Anger
   c. Acceptance
   d. Bereavement

3. A woman diagnosed with terminal breast cancer discusses with her husband her wishes for end-of-life care, including her funeral. Which type of loss is this couple experiencing?
   a. Perceived loss
   b. Anticipatory loss
   c. Temporary loss
   d. Sudden loss

4. A client whose husband died last month of a sudden cardiac arrest tells you that her 4-year-old child asks, "When is Daddy coming home?" When explaining to the mother about the child's concept of death, which of the following would you include?
   a. Death is an irreversible process.
   b. Death is a final state.
   c. Death is a destructive force.
   d. Death is a temporary separation.

5. Palliative care differs from hospice care because palliative care
   a. may be provided in the early stages of a chronic disease.
   b. requires that a client is a Medicare recipient.
   c. does not provide care for hospitalized clients.
   d. does not provide spiritual support for family members.

6. Several health care agencies have addressed the issue of pain management for terminally ill clients. In 1991, which of the following issued a position statement regarding the promotion of comfort and relief of pain in dying clients?
   a. The Agency for Health Care Policy and Research
   b. The Joint Commission on Accreditation of Healthcare Organizations
   c. The American Nurses Association
   d. The World Health Organization

Selected References

Agency for Health Care Policy and Research. (1994). *Management of cancer pain. Clinical practice guideline number 9*. Rockville, MD: Department of Health and Human Services. AHCPR Publication No. 94–0592.

Aging With Dignity.org. (n.d.). Aging with dignity. Retrieved August 17, 2006, from http://www.agingwithdignity.org

Allen, R. (2002). The challenges of advance directives. *Vital Signs, 12*(7), 12–13.

Andrews, M. M., & Boyle, J. S. (2003). *Transcultural concepts in nursing care* (4th ed.). Philadelphia: Lippincott Williams & Wilkins.

Andrews, M. M., & Hanson, P. A. (2003). Religion, culture, and nursing. In M. M. Andrews & J. S. Boyle (Eds.), *Transcultural concepts in nursing care* (4th ed.). Philadelphia: Lippincott Williams & Wilkins.

Cameron, M. D. (2002). Older persons' ethical problems involving their health. *Nursing Ethics, 9*, 537–556.

Christ, G. H. (2001). Facilitating mourning following parental death. *Psychiatric Times, 18*(9), 39–45.

Cohen, A. B., & Koenig, H. G. (2002). Spirituality in palliative care. *Geriatric Times, 3*(6), 25.

Ferrell, B. R., & Coyle, N. (2002) An overview of palliative nursing care. *American Journal of Nursing, 102*(5), 26–31.

Fink, P. J. (2005). Helping the terminally ill. *Clinical Psychiatry News, 33*(20), 10.

Foley, S. (2004). National Consensus Project releases palliative care guidelines. *American Journal of Nursing, 104*(11), 45.

Gilbert, S. (2004). Living 'til the end. Using the Five Wishes to prepare for the end of life. *ADVANCE for Nurses, 5*(5), 27.

Holst, L. (1984, April 6). To love is to grieve. *The Lutheran Standard*.

Hospice of the Plains, Inc. (2005). The history of hospice. Retrieved July 26, 2005, from http://www.plains.net/~hospice/history.html

Kearney, M. (1996). *Mortally wounded*. New York: Simon & Schuster.

Kishiyama, K. (2004). Tips for grieving. *Neuropsychiatry Reviews, 5*(6), 19.

Klimkiewicz, I. (2001). Dealing with death and dying. *ADVANCE for Nurses, 2*(24), 31–32.

Knebel, A. R. (2002). Research initiatives to improve end-of-life care. *Geriatric Times, 3*(6), 23–25.

Kübler-Ross, E. (1969). *On death and dying*. New York: Macmillan.

Kübler-Ross, E. (1971). What is it like to be dying? *American Journal of Nursing*.

LaDuke, S. (2001). Terminal dyspnea & palliative care. *American Journal of Nursing, 101*(11), 26–31.

Mazanec, P., & Tyler, M. K. (2003). Cultural considerations in end-of-life-care. *American Journal of Nursing, 103*(3), 50–60.

Medscape from WebMD. (2004). What is hospice? Retrieved September 30, 2004, from http://www.medscape.com/viewarticle/487401

Munoz, R. A. (2004). On death and dying. *Clinical Psychiatry News, 32*(11), 66.

Norlander, L. (2001). *To comfort always: A nurse's guide to end of life care*. Washington, DC: American Nurses Publishing.

Pumphrey, J. (1977, December). Recognizing your patient's spiritual needs. *Nursing 1977*.

Puntillo, K. (2001). Symptom management at end of life: The importance of nursing. *The American Nurse*, (May/June), 19.

Robinson, E. M., & Kennedy-Schwartz, J. (2001). Ethical issues: Caring for incompetent patients and their surrogates. *American Journal of Nursing, 101*(7), 75–76.

Rushton, C. H. (2001). Caregiver suffering is a dimension of end-of-life care. *The American Nurse*, (November/December), 9–10.

Scanlon, C. (2003). Ethical concerns in end-of-life care. *American Journal of Nursing, 103*(1), 48–56.

Schultz, J. M., & Videbeck, S. L. (2002). *Lippincott's manual of psychiatric nursing care plans* (6th ed.). Philadelphia: Lippincott Williams & Wilkins.

Silverman, J. (2004). Advance directives may undermine good care. *Clinical Psychiatry News, 32*(6), 92.

Staudacher, C. (2000). *Beyond grief: A guide for recovering from the death of a loved one*. New York: Barnes & Noble, Inc.

Westberg, G. (2004). *Good grief*. Philadelphia: Augsburg Fortress Press.

World Health Organization. (1996). *Cancer pain relief and palliative care. Report of a WHO expert committee* (pp. 1–75). Geneva, Switzerland: Author.

Suggested Readings

Cappelli, L. (2003). Suffering: A holistic model of assessment. *Oncology Issues 18*(5), 31.

Franklin, D. (2005): After a stillbirth, the needs of grieving parents can vary. *Clinical Psychiatry News, 33*(2), 76.

Henderson, M. (2004). Nuts and bolts of advance care planning. *American Journal for Nurse Practitioners, 8*(9), 41–52.

Jennings, J. (2005). *Living with grief: Ethical dilemmas at the end of life.* Totowa, NJ: Biblio Distribution.

Lefkof, J., & Glazer, G. (2002). Grief after miscarriage. *ADVANCE for Nurse Practitioners, 10*(10), 79–82.

Meleski, D. (2002). Families with chronically ill children. *American Journal of Nursing, 102*(5), 47–53.

Matzo, M. L. (2004). Palliative Care: Prognostication and the chronically ill. *American Journal of Nursing, 104*(9), 40–50.

Norton, S. A., Tilden, V. P., Tolle, S. W., Nelson, C. A., & Talamantes Eggman, S. (2003). Life support withdrawal: Communication and conflict. *American Journal of Critical Care, 12*(6), 548–555.

Paice, J. (2002). Managing psychological conditions in palliative care. *American Journal of Nursing, 102*(11), 36–44.

Panke, J. T. (2002). Difficulties in managing pain at the end of life. *American Journal of Nursing, 102*(7), 26–34.

Pitorak, E. F. (2003). Care at the time of death. *American Journal of Nursing, 103*(7), 42–52.

Stevens, S. (2005). The dark days of grief. *ADVANCE for Nurse Practitioners, 13*(3), 31–33.

Many patients leave the hospital with ongoing medical (or mental health) needs, and they need a health care continuum that works...treating the whole person from wellness to illness to recovery, within the community. —GREEN & LYDON, 1998

LEARNING OBJECTIVES

AFTER STUDYING THIS CHAPTER, YOU SHOULD BE ABLE TO:

1. Explain the meaning of the phrases *continuum of care* and *managed care.*
2. Differentiate the roles of the utilization review nurse, quality assurance nurse, and discharge planner.
3. Identify the implications of managed care for both psychiatric clients and nurses.
4. Construct the continuum of care available to a client with the diagnosis of major depression.
5. Articulate how the components of community-based health care compare with those of community mental health.
6. Identify the types of community mental health services that are available to psychiatric clients.
7. Analyze the role of the community mental health nurse.

KEY TERMS

Case management
Community-based health care
Community mental health
Community Mental Health Centers Act
Continuum of care
Cybertherapy
Deinstitutionalization
Discharge planner
Managed care
National Mental Health Act
Nurse case manager
Programs for Assertive Community Treatment (PACT)
Pre-admission Screening and Annual Resident Review (PASARR)
Prospective payment system (PPS)
Quality assurance nurse
Subacute care unit
Utilization review nurse

ommunities provide different types of treatment programs and services for clients with illnesses, including psychiatric–mental health disorders. A complete range of programs and services that treats the whole person from wellness to illness to recovery within the community is called the **continuum of care** (Green & Lydon, 1998). However, not every community has every type of service or program on the continuum.

The continuum of care is designed to meet the biopsychosocial needs of a client at any given time. The delivery of such services has been referred to as **community-based health care**. Hunt (1998) defined the following essential components of community-based care: enhancement of client self-care abilities; preventive care; planning care within the context of the client's family, culture, and community; and collaboration among a diverse team of professionals (Fig. 8-1). *Community mental health* (discussed later in this chapter) is an example of one aspect of this integrated system that uses a variety of settings and disciplines to provide comprehensive, holistic health care.

This chapter focuses on the continuum of care available to clients as they progress from the most restrictive clinical setting (inpatient) to the least restrictive clinical setting in which they may reside. Trends affecting delivery of care, such as case management, managed care, prospective payment system, and the Mental Health Parity Act, are addressed (Box 8-1). The concept

and history of community mental health is also described extensively.

Inpatient Care

Acute care facilities including psychiatric hospitals and subacute units are considered to be the most restrictive clinical settings in which mental health services are available. Although long-term care facilities provide 24-hour inpatient care, outpatient mental health services may be an option if a client is medically stable and able to be transported to a community center for psychiatric services.

Acute Care Facilities

The continuum of care begins in the acute care facility. Examples of different acute care facilities in which psychiatric care may originate include the medical–psychiatric unit of a hospital, transitional-care hospital,

FIGURE 8.1 Continuum of care. Client being seen for follow-up in an outpatient mental health clinic.

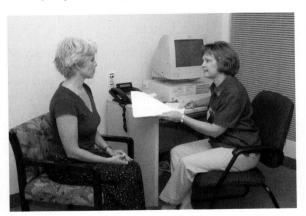

BOX 8.1 **TRENDS AFFECTING DELIVERY OF CARE**

Case Management: The method used to achieve managed care by coordinating services required to meet the needs of a client. Nurses are used in this role.

Managed Care: A system, financed by insurance companies, that controls the balance between cost and quality of care (cost containment). Health care providers are reimbursed for criteria-driven services received by consumers. Examples include health maintenance organizations (HMOs) and preferred provider organizations (PPOs).

Prospective Payment System: A per diem payment system, mandated by the Balanced Budget Act of 1997, that covers all costs (routine, ancillary, and capital) related to services where Medicare Part A is the payer. For additional information, visit the Health Care Financing Administration's website at *www.hcfa.gov.*

The Mental Health Parity Act: Effective January 1, 1998, it requires equal insurance coverage for mental illness in business health plans.

freestanding psychiatric hospital, community-based psychiatric hospital, or forensic hospital.

As a result of the tremendous pressure being exerted on health care to control costs, the average length of client stay in a psychiatric hospital has been dramatically shortened from the standard of the last decade. In the past, it was not unusual for a client to remain hospitalized for several weeks or months until clinical symptoms were considered to be stabilized.

Because hospitalization length of stay has been limited, most clients undergo crisis stabilization and then are transitioned or discharged to a less restrictive environment. To ease the transition, **case management** is used. The **nurse case manager** coordinates the continuum of care and determines the providers of care for a particular condition—such as depression—during the transition process. The nurse case manager may assume three different roles: utilization review nurse/manager, quality assurance nurse/manager, and discharge nurse/planner. In today's health care climate, the **utilization review nurse** is responsible for monitoring a client's care to ensure that it is appropriate and given in a timely manner. Utilization review nurses working for insurance companies or health care maintenance organizations determine whether a client's clinical symptoms meet the appropriate psychiatric or medical necessity criteria or clinical guidelines, as developed by the company and organization. If admission criteria for psychiatric hospitalization are met, a specific amount of time, such as 3 or 5 days, is approved or certified by the insurance provider. If the client requires additional time, the attending clinician must request re-certification. The **quality assurance nurse** is accountable for the overall quality of care being delivered and often serves as a member of the risk management team, investigating any legal issues that may develop during the client's hospitalization. The nurse who serves as a **discharge planner** coordinates all the facets of a client's admission and discharge. The discharge planner reviews the client's current response to treatment, past medical history, and assesses what family or friend support is available once the client is ready to be discharged. This concept is referred to as **managed care** (Shay, 2005).

The per diem **prospective payment system (PPS)** by Medicare is also a form of managed care. It governs payment for treatment by setting forth specific criteria. The per diem rate covers all costs related to services provided and is based on client need and resources used. For psychiatric treatment, this system applies in general hospitals, subacute or transitional care units, long-term care facilities, or psychiatric facilities where Medicare Part A is the payer. (Part B applies to outpatient treatment or consultant services.) Consequently, the case manager's position is a mix of clinical and financial responsibilities that are intended to reduce costs and improve outcomes (Joers, 2001; Patterson, 2002). Case management is also utilized to prevent hospitalization. For example, specially trained individuals coordinate or provide psychiatric, financial, legal, and medical services to help a child, adolescent, or adult client live successfully at home and in the community.

As clients transition to less restrictive clinical settings, nurses are challenged to assess the client's psychiatric and medical needs accurately while developing a therapeutic plan of care, all within a short period of time. Limited time also is available for client and family education. The plan of care must be reviewed by the multidisciplinary treatment team to ensure comprehensive care in the context of environmental, psychosocial, medical, financial, and functional issues after discharge (Green & Lydon, 1998). Where the client goes after leaving the psychiatric hospital depends on the care needed, available social support systems, and his or her insurance coverage. For instance, the client's freedom to select a clinician or therapist may be limited because the insurance company or health care maintenance organization establishes working relationships and contracts with preferred providers.

The continuum of care may continue in subacute care units, transitional care units, assisted-living or skilled nursing facilities, or adult day care, or may be part of home health care, as depicted in Figure 8-2 (Tellis-Nayak, 1998).

Subacute Care Units

Hospitalized clients with psychiatric problems may be transferred to **subacute care units**, which are generally located in long-term care facilities. These units provide time-limited, goal-oriented care for clients who do not meet the criteria for continued hospitalization. For example, a client with the diagnosis of bipolar disorder who is recovering from open reduction and internal fixation of a fractured hip requires rehabilitation prior to weight bearing. Both medical and psychiatric needs can be met in the subacute care unit. Such units have also been referred to as *postacute care units* or "rehab units."

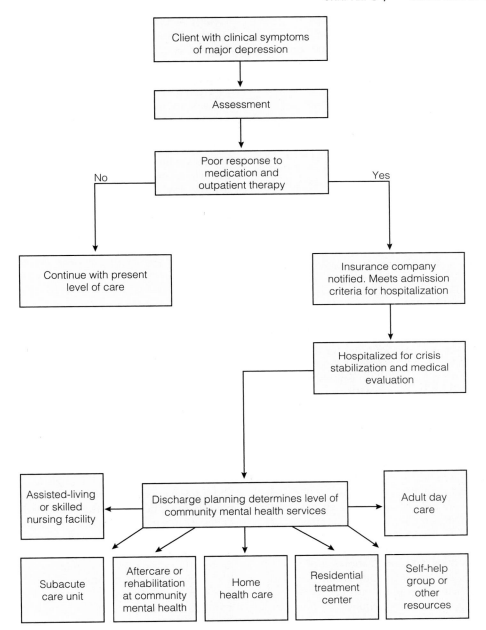

FIGURE 8.2   Continuum of care decision tree.

Clinical nurse specialists, nurse practitioners, or psychiatric liaison nurses have been used in the subacute setting to ensure continuum of care while medical needs are addressed and to assist with discharge planning. Length of stay and services provided are generally dictated by criteria developed by insurance providers or Medicare.

Nurses may be confronted with culture shock as they apply subacute care skills to clients. Endless paperwork, such as long assessment forms and documentation necessary to comply with various guidelines, rules, and regulations, can result in frustration. The psychosocial needs of clients may go unnoticed or unmet if task-oriented procedures take precedence.

Long-Term Care Facilities

Over the last decade, the long-term care environment has changed rapidly due to the establishment of subacute and rehabilitation units within long-term care (LTC) facilities. The average client can be admitted to the LTC facility for short-term rehabilitation, behavioral problems, some chronic care issues, or respite care. Today, most clients go home for services that were once provided in LTC facilities. As a result, the clients that are admitted to LTC facilities have more complex conditions or multiple problems. The prevalence of admitted clients with a dual medical and psychiatric disorder has increased as a result of these changes. Frequently seen comorbid psychiatric diagnoses include dementia, delirium, organic anxiety disorder, mood disorder, and adjustment disorder.

Clients with psychosocial needs may be admitted from a general hospital or from home, or they may be transferred from another LTC facility. Direct admissions may also occur from psychiatric hospitals or community mental health centers (CMHCs) after clinical symptoms are stabilized and continuum of care is necessary. For example, a 45-year-old female client with multiple sclerosis is admitted to a psychiatric facility to stabilize clinical symptoms of schizophrenia, paranoid type. The Department of Children and Family Services requests protective services after psychiatric care because of inadequate living conditions in her home. Discharge plans include placement in an LTC facility until alternate living conditions can be arranged.

Federal legislation and evolving regulations shape the delivery of services. The Nursing Home Reform Act of the Omnibus Budget Reconciliation Act of 1987 set forth guidelines regarding the admission of persons who have psychiatric disorders into LTC facilities. All nursing home applicants are required to be given a preadmission screening test, referred to as Level 1 **Pre-Admission Screening and Annual Resident Review (PASARR)**, to determine the presence or absence of a serious mental illness. If a client does meet the criteria for a serious mental illness (excluding dementia or organic brain disorders), state mental health authorities must provide mental health services or arrange for these services to be provided in the LTC

facility. Mental health services may be provided in nursing home facilities by clinicians who have a contractual agreement with the facility, unless the disorder requires specialized services such as substance abuse counseling, electroshock therapy, or intense individual or group psychotherapy (Kaplan, 2001).

In response to these guidelines, psychiatric and psychological services are now provided in most LTC facilities. Nurse practitioners working in collaboration with physicians or psychiatrists are reimbursed for services, which may include consultation or diagnostic interview, follow-up visits to monitor response to medication, brief individual psychotherapy, full individual psychotherapy, group psychotherapy, family psychotherapy, and consultation with family and the medical staff. The clients most in need of admission into LTC facilities often are those who also have the greatest need for psychiatric services. For example, clients may exhibit anxiety or depression resulting from relocation or loss, delirium caused by adverse effects of medication or a medical problem (eg, a urinary tract infection), or behavioral disturbances as a result of an alteration in mental status. The attending clinician often requests a psychiatric consultation or evaluation to determine the cause of the change in mental status, mood, or behavior.

Community Mental Health

Community mental health can best be described as a movement, an ideology, or a perspective that promotes early comprehensive mental health treatment in the community, accessible to all, including children and adolescents. It derives its values, beliefs, knowledge and practices from the behavioral and social sciences (Panzetta, 1985). According to the Surgeon General and community-based mental health studies, fewer than one half of children and youth meeting the diagnostic criteria for emotional or behavioral problems have received community mental health care; therefore, multiple levels of intervention are central to a public health approach to mental health services (Imperio, 2001).

Mental health services provided in the community may include emergency psychiatric care and crisis intervention, partial hospitalization and day-treatment programs, case management, community-based residential treatment programs, aftercare and rehabilitation, consultation and support, and psychiatric home care. The primary goal of community mental health is to deliver comprehensive care by a professional multidisciplinary team using innovative treatment approaches. Miller (1981) describes five major ideological beliefs influencing community mental health:

1. Involvement and concern with the total community population
2. Emphasis on primary prevention
3. Orientation toward social treatment goals
4. Comprehensive continuity of care
5. Belief that community mental health should involve total citizen participation in need determination, policy establishment, service delivery, and evaluation of programs

Historical Development of Community Mental Health

The community mental health movement, often considered to be the third revolution in psychiatry (after the mental hygiene movement in 1908 and the development of psychopharmacology in the 1950s), gained prominence in the early 1960s. Before this time, psychiatric treatment had occurred primarily in psychiatric institutions or psychiatric hospitals. Three very early community programs included a farm program established in New Hampshire in 1855, a cottage plan in Illinois in 1877, and community boarding homes for clients who were discharged from state psychiatric hospitals in Massachusetts in 1885. Although successful, these initial efforts were limited until after World War II, when social, economic, and political factors were favorable to stimulate the community mental health movement.

In 1946, the **National Mental Health Act** provided funding for states to develop mental health programs outside of state psychiatric hospitals. This act also provided funding for the establishment of the National Institute of Mental Health (NIMH) in 1949. Early in 1952, an international committee from the World Health Organization (WHO) defined the components of community mental health as outpatient treatment, rehabilitation, and partial hospitalization. Later in the decade, state- and federally funded programs mandated the broadening of services to include 24-hour emergency walk-in services, community clinics for state hospital clients, traveling mental health clinics, community vocational rehabilitation programs, halfway houses, and night and weekend hospitals.

In October 1963, U.S. President John F. Kennedy, who supported the improvement of mental health care, approved major legislation significantly strengthening community mental health. This legislation, the **Community Mental Health Centers Act,** authorized the nationwide development of CMHCs to be established outside of hospitals in the least restrictive setting in the community. It was believed that these centers would provide more effective and comprehensive mental health treatment than the often remote, state-run hospitals that previously served as the primary setting for psychiatric client care.

In conjunction with these congressional mandates, states began the massive process of **deinstitutionalization,** moving chronically mentally ill clients from the state psychiatric hospitals back to their homes or to community-supervised facilities. This movement, a controversial and much-debated social policy, occurred within the framework of the major and comprehensive social reforms of the 1960s. The federally funded CMHCs were also mandated to provide comprehensive services for this new population, some of whom had been in institutions for as long as 25 years.

The positive and negative effects of deinstitutionalization continue to have a significant influence in the field of community mental health. Unfortunately, state and federal governments have not provided a financial budget necessary to meet the needs of seriously ill psychiatric clients.

As noted in Chapter 2, on April 29, 2002, the New Freedom Commission on Mental Health was formed as a result of an executive order by President George W. Bush. This commission has been charged with studying the mental health system in the United States. Section 4 of the Executive Order states that "the Commission shall focus on community-level models of care that efficiently coordinate the multiple health and human service providers and public and private payers involved in mental health treatment and delivery of services" (Bush, 2002). The goal of the Commission is to recommend improvements to the U.S. mental health service system both for adults with serious mental illness and for children with severe emotional disorders. Several creative community programs have been identified and are listed in Table 8-1.

Concepts of Community Mental Health

Panzetta (1985) has documented eight fundamental concepts that he believes are the foundation for community mental health:

TABLE 8.1 █ Examples of Creative Community-Based Mental Health Programs

TYPE OF PROGRAM	DESCRIPTION OF PROGRAM	GOAL OF PROGRAM
Nurse–Family Partnership	Located in 270 communities in 23 states; nurses visit high-risk pregnant women	Teach positive parenting and coping skills
School–based mental health	Located in Dallas, Texas; formed by a school principal and physician; nurses and counselors visit students	Identify mental health problems of students Tailor classroom activities to meet specific needs
IMPACT (Improving Mood & Providing Access to Collaborative Treatment)	Located in California; consists of a mental health professional and medical team	Identify depression in older adults
Care for the homeless	Located in California	Identify the homeless Provide safe housing Engage them in care
Suicide prevention	Located in the U.S. Air Force	Encourages personnel to seek help for emotional pain and trauma Provides education and training regarding stress management

SOURCE: Hoppel, A.M. (2003). Mental health system failing Americans, government report says. *Clinician News, 7*(2), 7–8.

1. A multidisciplinary team, consisting of psychiatrist, psychologist, social workers, nurses, and mental health counselors
2. Prevention of mental illness
3. Early detection and treatment
4. Comprehensive, multifaceted treatment program
5. Continuity of care
6. Group and family therapy
7. Environmental and social support and intervention
8. Community participation, support, and control

In their well-documented description of overall community health services, Solomon and Davis (1985) discuss the belief that community mental health should be based on identified needs of deinstitutionalized individuals with specific psychiatric disorders such as schizophrenia, bipolar disorder, or major depression. The results of their comprehensive survey indicate that more than 85% of the population of discharged psychiatric clients had a need for community mental health services. Crosby (1987) wrote that community-focused mental health services were based on the premise that confined institutional living did not assist the resident with a psychiatric illness to acquire the skills to reintegrate into community life.

He claimed that community treatment could provide the wide range of needed services, would ensure more support from family and friends, and could strengthen the psychiatric client's need for independence and self-care. Crosby further promoted the theory that all community mental health should be based on the concepts of structure, support, and conceptual awareness for adaptation to societal norms and expectations.

The fundamental concepts and beliefs expressed in the 1980s about the need for community mental health services still hold true today. Unfortunately, an adequate financial budget from state and federal governments to develop community mental health services to meet these needs remains lacking. The hope is that the results of the New Freedom Commission on Mental Health will inspire government officials to revisit this issue.

Types of Community Mental Health Services

Psychiatric Emergency Care

The Community Mental Health Centers Act of 1963 mandated that communities make the necessary provisions for psychiatric emergency care. It was believed that accessible emergency services were needed to provide crisis intervention, to prevent unnecessary hospitalizations, and to attempt to decrease chronicity of and dependence on institutional care. At that same time, providing these critical support services placed additional pressure on communities because of the increased population of chronically mentally ill clients residing outside institutions. Jails were often inappropriate, psychiatrists were either overburdened or uncooperative, and mental health centers operated only during regular business hours.

Community mental health administrators and clinicians responded either by establishing an emergency clinic at the local mental health center or by contracting with a general hospital in the same community to provide emergency care on a 24-hour-per-day basis. Since that time, other methods of providing psychiatric emergency care have included the use of mobile crisis units and crisis residence units. Crisis residence units provide short-term (usually fewer than 15 days) crisis intervention and treatment. Clients receive 24-hour-per-day supervision.

Because of the psychiatric client's increasing reliance on these emergency services in the last decade, hospitals have assumed a key role in providing and managing crisis intervention and psychiatric emergency care. Nurius (1983–1984) notes that hospitals often functioned as the "revolving door" between clients and the mental health services network, focusing on crisis stabilization services. The research that Nurius and others have conducted indicates that the people who use community-based emergency services most commonly tend to be young, unemployed veterans of the mental health system and either chronically mentally ill or chronic substance abusers.

The psychiatric emergency room is often located in a separate room or a specially allocated section of the hospital emergency department. The triage staff may include members of several psychiatric disciplines: psychiatric nurses, social workers, mental health counselors, and marriage and family therapists. The primary focus is on crisis stabilization through the therapeutic interview and immediate mobilization of available community- and client-centered resources and support systems. A nurse practitioner or clinical nurse specialist may supervise the triage area. The nurse may have a collaborative agreement with a consulting psychiatrist to prescribe necessary psychotropic medication or to support admission to a psychiatric inpatient unit. The staff who provide these critical services must be knowledgeable and skillful in the areas of psychi-

atric assessment, including the administration of a complete mental status examination; application of crisis intervention theories; individual and family counseling; and use of resources in the specific community that can provide emergency housing, financial aid, and medical and psychiatric hospitalization.

Day-Treatment Programs

Day-treatment programs are also known as *day hospital* or *partial hospitalization programs*. The first day-treatment program in North America was established in Montreal, Canada, shortly after the end of World War II. Day-treatment programs are usually located in or near the CMHC or in an inpatient treatment facility such as a psychiatric hospital. The programs usually provide treatment for 30 to 90 days, operating for 6 to 8 hours per day, 5 days a week. Most of these programs can accommodate up to 25 persons. These persons are not dysfunctional enough to require psychiatric hospitalization, but need more structured and intensive treatment than traditional outpatient services alone can provide. These programs generally provide all the treatment services of a psychiatric hospital, but the clients are able to go home each evening.

Day-treatment programs are usually supervised by a psychiatrist and staffed by psychologists, social workers, psychiatric nurses, family therapists, activity therapists, and mental health counselors. Multidisciplinary assessments usually include a physical examination; a complete psychiatric evaluation; psychological, educational, and nursing assessments; a substance abuse assessment; and a psychosocial history. A treatment plan, which is usually formulated within 10 days of admission to the program, is reviewed weekly by the multidisciplinary treatment team. Examples of day-treatment program interventions are listed in Box 8-2.

Research shows that day-treatment programs have been successful, as evidenced by the increase in the number of programs in communities. Clients participating in day-treatment programs have fewer hospitalizations, a decrease in psychiatric symptoms, more successful work experiences, and better overall social functioning in the community (National Alliance for the Mentally Ill [NAMI], 1999).

Residential Treatment Programs

Clients with a diagnosis of chronic schizophrenia, a severe affective disorder, borderline personality disorder, and mental retardation are viewed as individuals

---

BOX 8.2 EXAMPLES OF DAY-TREATMENT PROGRAM INTERVENTIONS

- Family therapy—multifamily groups
- Client and family education
- Individual therapy
- Group therapy
- Therapeutic education or vocational training
- Drug and alcohol education
- Recreational therapy
- Expressive therapies (eg, art, movement, psychodrama)

BOX 8.3 EXAMPLES OF RESIDENTIAL TREATMENT PROGRAMS

- *Group homes:* Halfway houses, therapeutic community homes
- *Personal care homes:* Boarding homes, congregate care facilities, social rehabilitation residential programs
- *Foster homes:* Domiciliary care, group foster homes, transitional care facilities
- *Satellite housing:* Apartment clusters, transitional residences, independent living with aftercare support
- *Independent living:* Lodgings, single-room occupancy with therapeutic support

---

who benefit from participation in residential treatment programs. The goals of these programs are to improve self-esteem and social skills, promote independence, prevent isolation, and decrease hospitalization. In many communities, residential placements are a key element in the services provided by CMHC advisory boards. Indeed, residential placements have become one of the leading areas of program expansion in the care of the psychiatric client. Numerous clients now are able to leave an LTC facility or psychiatric hospital for another structured living situation. Historically, the first community program of this type, called Tueritian House, was established in New York City shortly after World War II. Today there are thousands of innovative residential treatment programs throughout the United States. Examples of such programs are included in Box 8-3.

Each type of residential treatment program offers different support services. The services provided include shelter, food, housekeeping, personal care and supervision, health care, individual or group counseling, vocational training or employment, and leisure and socialization opportunities. Staffing for these residential programs ranges from professional psychiatric staff present at all times in the facility to provide support and supervision, to staff only on call for crisis intervention and stabilization. Continued research into these programs has led many community mental health experts to conclude that they are a successful means of therapeutic support and intervention and are particularly effective with the chronically mentally ill client.

Children or adolescents may benefit from placement in therapeutic group homes or community residence programs. This setting usually includes six to ten children or adolescents per home. The home may be linked with a day-treatment program or specialized educational program. Family support services such as parent training or a parent support group may also be offered.

Psychiatric Home Care

With the increased emphasis on community mental health in the 1960s, programs were established to treat the psychiatric client at home with a visiting nurse providing care. An early project in Louisville, Kentucky, had clients with acute schizophrenia living at home with their families. A public health nurse or a nurse from the local Visiting Nurses Association visited these clients at least weekly. The nurse's role was to conduct a psychiatric assessment, dispense medication, and provide individual and family counseling. In addition, a psychiatrist evaluated the home client every few months.

During the 1970s, psychiatric home care programs declined as the focus increasingly centered on day-treatment and residential treatment programs. However, in the late 1980s, the concept of psychiatric home care was revitalized as community resources became scarcer. Pelletier (1988) writes that psychiatric home care can fill the gap in the mental health continuum of care by providing nursing resources as adjunctive to outpatient treatment.

The advantages of home care are well known and include cost-effectiveness, client satisfaction, and decreased disruption of relationships with family and friends. Home care also presents a significant opportunity for psychiatric nurses to promote client independence in the home environment by assessing functional abilities or self-care tasks and incidental abilities such as medication management, housekeeping, and managing finances (Sanders, 2001).

The age of clients receiving psychiatric home care can vary. Any individual who has had a chronic psychiatric illness for at least 2 years may apply for Medicare or Medicaid health care coverage. Therefore, clients may be children, adolescents, adults, or elderly persons.

Independent psychiatric nurse practitioners who have contracts with insurance companies or who are providers for Medicare and Medicaid can provide psychiatric services in the home environment. Medicare and Medicaid have made provisions to use a billing code that indicates a house call was made.

The Health Care Financing Administration (HCFA) has established the following criteria for the provision of psychiatric home care services:

1. A psychiatrist must certify that the client is homebound.
2. The client must have a *Diagnostic and Statistical Manual of Mental Disorders, 4th Edition, Text Revision* (*DSM-IV-TR*) psychiatric diagnosis that is acute or an acute exacerbation of a chronic illness.
3. The client must require the specialized knowledge, skills, and abilities of a psychiatric registered nurse.

Richie and Lusky (1987) define the major features of psychiatric home care as the provision of comprehensive care, ongoing interdisciplinary collaboration, and accountability to client and community. They have identified three major client populations that use this community service. The first group is the elderly who do not have a history of chronic mental illness, but who are experiencing acute psychological and developmental problems. A common client in this group is an elderly person who lives alone and is experiencing increasing physical limitations that cause severe isolation and major depression. The second population is the chronically mentally ill who require long-term medication and ongoing supportive counseling. Such clients are often diagnosed with schizophrenia, bipolar illness, depression, or a schizoaffective disorder. The third population consists of clients in need of crisis intervention and short-term psychotherapy.

Aftercare and Rehabilitation

When clients are discharged from a psychiatric hospital, CMHCs provide support and rehabilitation for the client. Many of these clients require only minimal support, with weekly or biweekly individual or family therapy and medication evaluation. Most of these clients, however, represent the chronically mentally ill population. They experience repeat hospitalizations and require diverse support functions from the treatment team at the CMHC. Therapeutic services provided by most CMHCs are highlighted in Box 8-4.

One of the most effective and novel approaches community mental health care providers use is the **Programs for Assertive Community Treatment (PACT),** also referred to as ACT. PACT is a service-delivery model that provides comprehensive, locally based treatment to clients with serious and persistent mental illnesses. Unlike other community-based programs, PACT is not a case-management program that connects individuals to mental health, housing, or rehabilitation agencies or services. It provides highly individualized services directly to consumers. The key features include treatment of the psychiatric disorder (eg, psychopharmacology, individual supportive therapy, mobile crisis intervention), rehabilitation (eg, behaviorally oriented skill teaching, supported employment, support for resuming education), and support services (eg, legal and advocacy services, financial support, transportation). This approach has been described as a hospital without walls. The goal of this integrated program is to help clients with schizophrenia and related disorders, such as depression or substance abuse, stay out of psychiatric hospitals and live independently. Available 24 hours a day, 7 days a week, the program provides professional staff to meet clients where they live and provide at-home support at whatever level is needed to solve any problem. PACT has significantly reduced hospital admissions and improved both functioning and quality of life for those it serves (NAMI, 2005).

Other community programs have developed and been successful. Warner-Robbins (2003) describes a community program in Oceanside, California, that helps incarcerated women transition from prison to society. Welcome Home Ministries began in 1996 as a result of the need to provide aftercare to released incarcerated clients who spoke of deprivation, poverty, emotional and physical abuse, drug addiction, and repeated incarceration. Volunteers visit clients in prison. Clients also are provided with transportation to

---

BOX 8.4 THERAPEUTIC SERVICES PROVIDED BY COMMUNITY MENTAL HEALTH CENTERS (CMHCs)

- *Medication:* Psychotropic medication is generally regarded as essential in the treatment of chronically ill clients. The individual often continues this medication regimen after the acute symptoms have subsided and he or she returns to the community. The CMHC psychiatrist or nurse practitioner is responsible for conducting a full medication assessment and for supervising a safe and strategic medication care plan.
- *Individual and family therapy:* In the last several years, many significant developments have occurred in community-based family therapy with the psychiatric client. Family interventions focus on altering the emotional climate within the family and reducing stress. Significant emphasis is placed on educating the family about the client's illness and teaching more effective communication and problem-solving skills.
- *Crisis intervention:* The psychiatric client in the community is vulnerable to stress and often lacks the self-care skills to cope with unexpected stressful situations. CMHCs usually assume responsibility for 24-hour crisis intervention by contracting with hospital emergency rooms or by establishing their own hotline or psychiatric emergency room.

- *Social skills training:* Many CMHC clients lack social skills and experience much difficulty in maintaining good interpersonal relationships. In response to this need, many centers have established social skills training programs that use role-playing and individual and group therapy to teach interpersonal skills.
- *Medical care:* Clients recently discharged from a psychiatric hospital may suffer from a significant physical illness. Poor physical health is one of the most important factors affecting the recovery of psychiatric clients in the community. A comprehensive treatment program at a CMHC should include a means of obtaining medical services for clients through contracting or referral. Laboratory service is also provided to monitor drug levels, liver profiles, electrolytes, and so forth.
- *Vocational training:* Many clients also experience difficulty in finding a suitable job. CMHCs offer programs that focus on honing job skills, improving interview techniques, writing résumés, filling out applications, and job searching. To be fully effective, these vocational rehabilitative programs should continue after the CMHC client obtains a job, because he or she will need continued skills training, support, and stress management.

---

a preferred destination when released from jail, and are given the opportunity to attend monthly meetings to support and encourage one another.

Role of the Community Mental Health Nurse

Nurses play a major role in the provision of quality services to the psychiatric client in the community. Psychiatric nurses, along with other health care professionals, participated in the movement of the 1960s to deinstitutionalize and move significant numbers of hospitalized patients back to the community. Nurses assumed positions in the newly established CMHCs and provided the necessary aftercare services. These early community projects encouraging the use of nurses were based on the belief that psychiatric nurses would provide optimal transition from the hospital to the community.

In the 1970s and 1980s, the role of the community mental health nurse expanded as nurses assumed key leadership positions in all community programs, including day treatment, residential homes, community mental health prevention programs, and psychiatric home care programs. Today, the psychiatric nurse practicing in the community provides counseling, support, and coordination of care and health teaching. The role is comprehensive and challenging and requires adaptability and flexibility. A nurse clinician with an advanced degree may function as a nurse therapist employing individual, group, and family therapy. Prescriptive privileges may be allowed, depending on the state's department of professional regulation. Many insurance companies, as well as government-funded Medicare and Medicaid programs, approve reimbursement for psychiatric nursing services provided in the home, in LTC facilities, or in community-based mental health settings.

To emphasize the need for a clear theoretical framework for the practice of community mental health nursing, Dr. Jeanne Miller (1981) described two areas of concern to community mental health nurses. The first concern was the attempt by nurses to improve the quality of direct client care through means such as primary nursing, psychiatric home care, and case management. At the same time, community mental health nurses were becoming more concerned about societal and community conditions that could contribute to health problems and to the needs of persons with mental illness. Miller further stated that community mental health nurses should continue to broaden their role to include a more holistic approach in the assessment, planning, and implementation of community services. Being prepared to respond to the increasingly complex challenge of providing optimal mental health care by going beyond the traditional roles of psychiatric nursing also was important. Miller encouraged these specialized nurses to go beyond providing therapy and education, to include interventions that reduce vulnerability to mental illness and enhance strengths in the individual and the community.

The Continuum of Care in the 21st Century

As a result of the increase in computer accessibility, a health care revolution is occurring on the World Wide Web (Leipsic, 1999; Sherer, 1999). In the past, psychiatric Internet resources were limited to library holdings and journal abstracts. However, clinicians are now able to obtain practice updates, the most current journal summaries and publications, and continuing education credits online. Individuals are using the Internet to enhance their understanding of diseases and treatment.

Mental health care providers and consumers are venturing into more direct therapeutic resources on the Internet. Web sites provide resources similar to self-help groups. For example, http://masteringstress.com is a Web site that guides clients through a series of branching statements toward resolving stress-related problems (Sherer, 1999). Chat rooms provide the client with the opportunity to access support groups online. Educational resources are readily accessible and can generally be downloaded at no charge. Medication information and adverse-effect profiles (patient monographs) are available for client education.

SELF-AWARENESS PROMPT

Concern has been raised regarding the use of the Internet as a resource for clients with psychiatric–mental health issues. Do you believe that some clients would benefit from this practice? If so, state two examples of the types of resources that you feel would be helpful to a client. If not, explain why Internet resources would not be beneficial.

A debate within the psychiatric community is expected regarding the use of the Internet as a practice extender, or **cybertherapy.** Concern has been voiced that clients could develop a false sense that their psychiatric condition is improving. The real beneficiaries of the Internet may be persons who do not qualify for therapeutic intervention but are motivated for treatment.

The continuum of care also extends into the primary care practice. Primary care practitioners and medical specialists often are expected to provide follow-up care to clients who received limited psychiatric care because of limited insurance coverage. Approximately 25% of all clients in the primary care setting have a diagnosis of mood disorder and are treated by the primary care clinician. Frequent complaints by clients in the primary care setting also include anxiety, chronic pain, insomnia, and phobias. The presence of mental health practitioners on site in the primary care setting has resulted in improved recognition and treatment of psychiatric disorders (Weiner, 1999).

In the primary care practice, the nurse practitioner can provide consultation, diagnostic evaluation, psychotherapy, and evaluation and management of psychotropic medication in the medical setting. The client receives comprehensive health care in a nonthreatening environment.

KEY CONCEPTS

◆ Trends such as case management, managed care, and prospective payment systems have affected the delivery of health care, including psychiatric–mental health care, to children, adolescents, and adult clients during the last decade.

◆ Nurses are challenged to accurately assess a client's psychosocial and medical needs in a limited amount of time during transitions between levels of care.

◆ Care provided by community mental health services is based on the client's psychiatric and medical needs, available social support systems, and availability of reimbursement for care.

◆ The admission of psychiatric clients to long-term care facilities is regulated by the Nursing Home Reform Act of the Omnibus Budget Reconciliation Act of 1987.

◆ The components of community-based health care also apply to community mental health services. These components include enhancement of client self-care abilities; preventive care; planning care in the context of the client's family, culture, and community; and collaboration among a diverse team of professionals.

◆ The role of the community mental health nurse today is comprehensive and challenging, requiring adaptability and flexibility. Various levels of care are provided, depending on the nurse's education and qualifications. The nurse is challenged to include interventions that reduce vulnerability to mental illness and enhance strengths in the individual and the community.

◆ The use of the Internet has been referred to as a practice extender, because both clinicians and consumers of health care use online knowledge to enhance their understanding of diseases and treatment.

For additional study materials, please refer to the Student Resource CD-ROM located in the back of this textbook.

CHAPTER WORKSHEET

CRITICAL THINKING QUESTIONS

1. Interview a local community mental health nurse about the system in which she or he works. How does that system reflect Panzetta's eight fundamental concepts for community mental health?
2. Visit a group home or personal care home in a local community. What support services,

staffing, and therapeutic interventions are available? What are the strengths and weaknesses of this type of program? After assimilating this information, discuss how a group home might be accepted in the neighborhood where you live.
3. Visit the Web site of a mental health support group on the Internet. What information is available? How would the nurse be able to use this information to benefit his or her client?

REFLECTION

Review the quote at the beginning of the chapter. Interview a client in your present clinical practice setting. Assess the client's medical and mental health needs. What health care service(s) should be used to ensure an effective continuum of care for the client? Are such services available in the community? If not, what alternative interventions could be employed?

NCLEX-STYLE QUESTIONS

1. Which of the following terms best refers to a nurse who is employed by a health care maintenance organization and determines if a client's symptoms meet the appropriate psychiatric or medical necessity criteria?
   a. Case manager
   b. Utilization reviewer
   c. Primary nurse
   d. Community mental health nurse

2. Which of the following reflects most accurately the direct impact of managed care on psychiatric nursing care planning?
   a. Assessing and planning for client care must occur in a short period of time.
   b. Family members need to be involved in planning care.
   c. Clients require follow-up or provision for continuum of care.
   d. All treatment team members should be involved with planning.

3. The nurse manager in an LTC unit is talking with the family of a newly admitted client with a diagnosis of schizophrenia, paranoid type.

The daughter voices concern that her father's behavior seems worse since his admission. Which of the following is the best action the nurse can take?

a. Explain that psychotropic medications can be adapted according to behavior.
b. Initiate treatment-team review of the client's behavior since admission.
c. Speak to the nursing assistants about the client's current behavior.
d. Refer client's daughter to the physician in charge of her father's care.

4. A client with chronic schizophrenia is to be discharged from the psychiatric facility to a group home. The nurse interprets this type of care as indicative of which of the following?

a. Crisis intervention
b. Partial hospitalization program
c. Residential treatment program
d. Psychiatric home care

5. The nurse working in a community mental health center is asked to speak to a parent–teacher group at an elementary school regarding discipline issues. This is an example of which of the following functions of community mental health centers?

a. Concern with total community populations
b. Emphasis on primary prevention
c. Provision of continuity of care
d. Social and environmental interventions

6. When preparing a teaching plan for the family of a client who will be receiving psychiatric home care, which of the following would the nurse incorporate into the teaching plan? Select all that apply.

a. This type of care, although effective, can be costly
b. There is less disruption in the client's relationship with family
c. The client's level of independence is fostered
d. Clients typically receive less satisfaction from this type of care
e. The client can engage in all types of recreational community activities

Selected References

Bush, G. W. (2002). President's New Freedom Commission on Mental Health. Retrieved January 31, 2005, from http://www.mentalhealthcommission.gov/reports/Finalreport/toc_exec.html

Crosby, R. (1987). Community care of the chronically mentally ill. *Journal of Psychosocial Nursing and Mental Health Services,* (1).

Green, K., & Lydon, S. (1998). The continuum of patient care. *American Journal of Nursing, 98*(10), 16bbb–16ddd.

Hoppel, A. M. (2003). Mental health system failing Americans, government report says. *Clinician News, 7*(2), 7–8.

Hunt, R. (1998). Community-based nursing. *American Journal of Nursing, 98*(10), 44–47.

Imperio, W. A. (2001). Surgeon General confronts gaps in mental health care. *Clinical Psychiatry, 29*(2), 1, 10–11.

Joers, D. M. (2001). Case management: Ripe for technology. *ADVANCE for Nurses, 2*(19), 27–28.

Kaplan, A. (2001). Ensuring appropriate treatment for patients. *Psychiatric Times, 18*(9), 1, 5–7.

Leipsic, J. (1999). The Internet as practice extender. *Psychiatric Times, 16*(11), 62–63.

Miller, J. (1981). Theoretical basis for the practice of community mental health nursing. *Issues in Mental Health Nursing,* (3).

National Alliance for the Mentally Ill. (1999). Schizophrenia fact sheet. Retrieved July 5, 2002, from http://www.nami.org

National Alliance for the Mentally Ill. (2005). PACT; Program of Assertive Community Treatment. Retrieved August 1, 2005, from http://www.nami.org

Nurius, P. (1983–1984). Emergency psychiatric services: A study of changing utilization patterns and issues. *International Journal of Psychiatry in Medicine, 13.*

Panzetta, A. (1985). Whatever happened to community mental health? Portents for corporate medicine. *Hospital and Community Psychiatry,* (11).

Patterson, T. S. (2002). Nurse life care planner. *ADVANCE for Nurses, 3*(12), 15–16.

Pelletier, L. (1988). Psychiatric home care. *Journal of Psychosocial Nursing and Mental Health Services,* (3).

Richie, F., & Lusky, K. (1987, Fall). Psychiatric home health nursing: A new role in community mental health. *Community Mental Health Journal.*

Sanders, C. (2001). Functional independence in home care. *Vital Signs, 11*(18), 17–20.

Shay, B. (2005). *Case management.* Retrieved July 29, 2005, from http://medi-smart.com/profile7.htm

Sherer, R. A. (1999). Access to mental health resources: A revolution on the Internet. *Supplement to Psychiatric Times, 16*(12) 6.

Solomon, P., & Davis, J. (1985, Spring). Meeting community service needs of discharged psychiatric patients. *Psychiatric Quarterly.*

Tellis-Nayak, M. (1998). The postacute continuum of care: Understanding your patient's options. *American Journal of Nursing, 98*(8), 44–49.

Warner-Robbins, C. (2003). *Welcome Home Ministries.* Retrieved August 16, 2006, from http://www.welcome homeministries.com/CarmenArticle.htm

Weiner, J. S. (1999, November 11-14). *How to integrate mental health clinics into primary care practice.* Presentation delivered at the 12th Annual United States Psychiatric & Mental Health Congress Conference, Atlanta, GA.

Suggested Readings

American Board of Managed Care Nursing. (2005). *What is the American Board of Managed Care Nursing?* Retrieved July 29, 2005, from http://www.abmcn.org/right_pageframe.htm

Bull, M. J., Luo, D., & Maruyamar, G. M. (2000). Measuring continuity of elder's posthospital care. *Journal of Nursing Management, 8*(8), 41-60.

Cooney, J. P., Landers, G. M., Etchason, J., & Williams, J. (2001). Rough passages for long-term care: The churning effect. *Long-Term Care Interface, 2*(1), 38-44.

Emanuel, M., & Tugrul, K. (Eds.). (2004). Treatment team: Optimizing clinical outcomes in community mental health. *Treatment Team Today, 1*(1), 5-9.

MacReady, N. (2005). Partial hospitalization benefits phobia and anxiety patients. *Clinical Psychiatry News, 33*(2) 23.

Renick, O., & Ransom, S. (2001). The search for Eden: An alternative path for nursing homes. *Long-Term Care Interface, 2*(1), 45-48.

Webster, J., & Cowart, P. (1998). Innovative practice: Care for your chronically ill patients beyond the hospital walls. *American Journal of Nursing, 98*(9), 16aaa-16bbb.

Components of the Nurse–Client Relationship

CHAPTER 9 / ASSESSMENT OF PSYCHIATRIC–MENTAL HEALTH CLIENTS

The first step in the nursing process, the assessment of the client, is crucial. Assess the client in a holistic way, integrating any relevant information about the client's life, behavior, and feelings. The focus of care, beginning with the initial assessment, is toward the client's optimum level of health and independence from the hospital. —SCHULTZ & VIDEBECK, 2005

LEARNING OBJECTIVES

AFTER STUDYING THIS CHAPTER, YOU SHOULD BE ABLE TO:

1. Define the nursing process.
2. Articulate the purpose of a comprehensive nursing assessment.
3. Differentiate the purpose of a focused and a screening assessment.
4. Explain the significance of cultural competence during the assessment process.
5. Recognize how disturbances in communication exhibited by a client can impair the assessment process.
6. Describe the importance of differentiating among the six types of delusions during the assessment process.
7. Interpret the five types of hallucinations identified in psychiatric disorders.
8. Recognize the differences between obsessions and compulsions.
9. Determine levels of orientation and consciousness during the assessment process.
10. Reflect on how information obtained during the assessment process is transmitted to members of the health care team.
11. Formulate the criteria for documentation of assessment data.

KEY TERMS

Acute insomnia
Affect
Blocking
Circumstantiality
Clang association
Compulsions
Delusions
Depersonalization
Echolalia
Flight of ideas
Hallucinations
Illusion
Insight
Insomnia
Looseness of association

Memory	Neurovegetative changes	Secondary insomnia
Mood	Obsessions	Tangentiality
Mutism	Perseveration	Verbigeration
Neologism	Primary insomnia	Word salad

The nursing process is a six-step problem-solving approach to nursing that also serves as an organizational framework for the practice of nursing (Fig. 9-1). It sets the practice of nursing in motion and serves as a monitor of quality nursing care. Nurses in all specialties practice the first step, assessment. This chapter focuses specifically on the assessment of clients with psychiatric disorders, including those clients who may have a coexisting medical diagnosis.

Client Assessment

The assessment phase of the nursing process includes the collection of data about a person (child, adolescent, adult, or older adult client), family, or group by the methods of observing, examining, and interviewing. The type of assessment that occurs depends on the client's needs, presenting symptoms, and clinical setting. For example, an adolescent client who attempts suicide may be assessed in the emergency room, or an older adult may be assessed in a nursing home to rule out the presence of major depression secondary to a cerebral vascular accident.

Two types of data are collected: objective and subjective. *Objective data* include information to determine the client's physical alterations, limits, and assets (Nettina, 2001). Objective data are tangible and measurable data collected during a physical examination by inspection, palpation, percussion, and auscultation. Objective data can also include observable client behavior such as crying or talking out loud when no one else is in the room. Laboratory results and vital signs also are examples of objective data. *Subjective data* are obtained as the client, family members, or significant others provide information spontaneously during direct questioning or during the health history. It can also include any statements made by the client,

for example, "I hate my life and I want to die." Subjective data also are collected during the review of past medical and psychiatric records. This type of data collection involves interpretation of information by the nurse.

Types of Assessment

Three kinds of assessment exist: comprehensive, focused, and screening assessments. A *comprehensive assessment* includes data related to the client's biologic, psychological, cultural, spiritual, and social needs. This type of assessment is generally completed in collaboration with other health care professionals such as a physician, psychologist, neurologist, and social worker. A physical examination is performed to rule out any physiologic causes of disorders such as anxiety, depression, or dementia. For example, more than 30% of clients with dermatologic diseases have reported the presence of depressive and anxiety disorders. Neuroimaging has been included as part of a comprehensive assessment to avoid misdiagnosis or a serious delay in the diagnosis of some psychiatric disorders. It has been used to confirm psychiatric diagnoses in clients who exhibited auditory hallucinations, symptoms of bipolar disorder, behavioral symptoms of acute onset dementia, and atypical headache symptoms (Johnson, 2005; Novick, 2004; Romano, 2004; Wright, 2005). Many psychiatric facilities require a comprehensive assessment, including medical clearance, before or within 24 hours of admission to avoid medical emergencies in the psychiatric setting.

A *focused assessment* includes the collection of specific data regarding a particular problem as determined by the client, a family member, or a crisis situation. For example, in the event of a suicide attempt, the nurse would assess the client's mood, affect, and

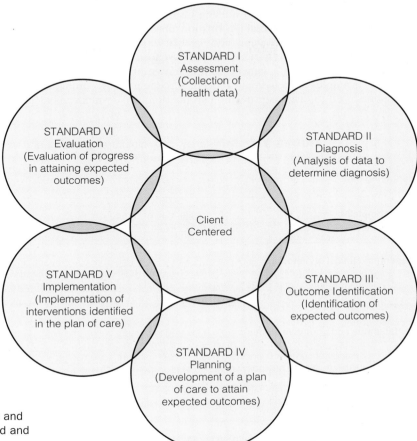

FIGURE 9.1 Standards of care and the nursing process: an integrated and client-centered framework.

behavior. Data regarding the attempted suicide and any previous attempts of self-destructive behavior would also be collected (see Chapter 31).

A *screening assessment* includes the use of assessment or rating scales to evaluate data regarding a specific problem or behavior. Although a client's history may remain stable, his or her mental status or behavior can change from day to day or hour to hour. The psychiatric mental status examination is one type of screening assessment that can be used in a variety of locations such as the emergency room, the physician's office, or an outpatient clinic. This assessment provides a description of the client's appearance, speech, mood, thinking, perceptions, sensorium, insight, and judgment (Sadock & Sadock, 2003). Other examples of screening assessments or rating scales used to evaluate data regarding a

particular problem or behavior include the Folstein Mini Mental State Examination, Brief Psychiatric Rating Scale (BPRS), Dementia Rating Scale, Drug Attitude Inventory (DAI-10), Impulsivity Scale, or the Hamilton Rating Scale for Depression (HRSD).

Although rating scales provide useful symptom frequency and severity data, client reliability and credibility are reasonable concerns. However, the rating scales can provide objective information about clients in a variety of situations and help confirm the diagnosis of a psychiatric disorder (Menaster, 2004). For example, a screening assessment using the Abnormal Involuntary Movement Scale could be utilized to evaluate the frequency and severity of a client's movement disorder during administration of neuroleptic medication to stabilize clinical symptoms of schizophrenia.

During any assessment, the psychiatric–mental health nurse uses a psychosocial nursing history and assessment tool to obtain factual information, observe client appearance and behavior, and evaluate the client's mental or cognitive status. A sample psychosocial nursing history and assessment form is shown in Figure 9-2. Examples of assessment tools or screening instruments used to diagnose specific psychiatric disorders are discussed in the appropriate chapters of Units VI and VII.

Cultural Competence During Assessment

According to the 2000 census, more than 6.8 million Americans identified themselves as multiracial such as

FIGURE 9.2 Sample psychosocial nursing history and assessment form.

Identifying data: AJ is a 38-year-old recently widowed white female referred by Dr. S for a psychiatric evaluation.

Chief complaint: Inability to sleep, loss of appetite, decreased concentration, and lack of motivation since the death of her husband last month. "My doctor tells me that I am depressed."

Presenting clinical symptoms: Client presents with a flat affect, poor eye contact, and unkempt appearance. Speech is monotonous and difficult to hear. Exhibits blocking. Gait is slow and deliberate upon entering the room. Slouched posture is noted when seated. Responds to questions but does not initiate conversation. Denies any alteration in thought process such as delusions or hallucinations. Denies any self-destructive thoughts or plans.

Mental status and cognitive abilities: Alert. Oriented to person, place, and time. Recent and remote memory are intact although blocking does occur at times. Object recall is delayed but correct. Admits to decreased attention span and concentration since the death of her husband. Judgment is appropriate. Insight is limited. She is unable to identify any positive coping skills or personal strengths.

Previous psychiatric history: None. There is no family history of psychiatric illness.

Medical history including any medication taken: No known allergies. The results of the last complete physical examination, including laboratory test results and ECG, were within normal limits. She presently takes no medication and has not required any in the past except for over-the-counter medication for pain or cold. Both parents and two younger siblings are alive and well. There is no history of major illness, surgeries, or hospitalizations.

Psychosocial history: AJ is a college graduate with a degree in accounting. She works part time. She has two children, a son 8 years of age and a daughter who is 6 years old. AJ is Protestant and is active in her religious community. Until the death of her husband, she played duplicate bridge and golfed with him twice a month. She is a nonsmoker, drinks socially, and has never taken illicit drugs. She has a good relationship with her parents and two siblings, who have been supportive during the illness and recent death of her husband.

Identified strengths:
No physical problems
Judgment, memory, and orientation intact
Supportive family
College graduate
Active in religious community

white/other, white/Native American, white/Asian, white/black, Asian/other, black/other, and three or more races. Cultural competence experts realize that nurses cannot learn the customs, languages, and specific beliefs of every client they see. But the psychiatric–mental health nurse must possess sensitivity, knowledge, and skills to provide care to culturally diverse groups of clients to avoid labeling persons as noncompliant, resistant to care, or abnormal. For example, the act of suicide is accepted in some cultures as a means to escape identifiable stressors such as marital discord, illness, criticism from others, and loneliness (Andrews & Boyle, 2003).

Several client cultural assessment approaches, identified by Mackey-Padilla (2005) and Kanigel (1999), can be used during the assessment and treatment of diverse client populations. These approaches are:

1. Assess and clarify the client's cultural values, beliefs, and norms.
2. Assess the client's degree of cultural assimilation/acculturation.
3. Assess the client's perspective regarding feelings and symptoms. Questions would include "What do you call your illness?," "What do you think causes it?," and "How have you treated it?"
4. Elicit the client's expectations and ask what the client feels is important for the health care provider to know about the client's biopsychosocial needs. Negotiate treatment. Explain what assessment tools may be used. Ask the client whether there is a need to clarify any information as the assessment process occurs.
5. Learn how to work with interpreters. Using a family member as an interpreter is contraindicated because a family member may omit data or give erroneous information. (According to the recent Health Insurance Portability and Accountability Act [HIPAA] privacy rules policy, the client must give permission to include a family member or an interpreter in the interview; otherwise a breach of client confidentiality could occur.)
6. When using an interpreter, talk to the client rather than the interpreter. Observe the client's eyes and face for nonverbal reactions.
7. Seek collaboration with bilingual community resources, such as a social worker, for assistance in meeting biopsychosocial needs of clients who have difficulty communicating in a second language.

Talking openly and communicating with the client can provide valuable information about compliance and behavior. Acknowledging that differences do exist is the most important thing that the psychiatric-mental health nurse can do. Refer to Chapter 4 for more detailed information about cultural competence of the psychiatric–mental health nurse.

Collection of Data

Many data are collected by the psychiatric–mental health nurse during a comprehensive assessment, which may take place in a variety of settings such as the primary care setting, general hospital, or psychiatric clinical setting. Specific questions or guidelines are at times included in the assessment to alert the nurse to information that could be overlooked or misinterpreted. Clients are often reluctant to discuss their mental or emotional problems because of the stigma that mental illness has historically carried. They may not have the self-awareness to realize that their emotional symptoms may play a role in their physical and general well-being.

Appearance

General appearance includes physical characteristics, apparent age, peculiarity of dress, cleanliness, and use of cosmetics. A client's general appearance, including facial expressions, is a manner of nonverbal communication in which emotions, feelings, and moods are related. For example, people who are depressed often neglect their personal appearance, appear disheveled, and wear drab-looking clothes that are generally dark in color, reflecting a depressed mood. The facial expression may appear sad, worried, tense, frightened, or distraught. Clients with mania may dress in bizarre or overly colorful outfits, wear heavy layers of cosmetics, and don several pieces of jewelry.

Affect, or Emotional State

Affect is defined as an individual's present emotional responsiveness. It is the observable manifestation of one's emotions or feelings inferred from facial expressions (eg, anger, sadness, or happiness). For example, when complemented by his teacher a child smiles. He is expressing an affective or emotional response to the complement. (The terms *affect* and *emotion* are commonly used interchangeably.) **Mood** is a descriptive term that refers to the presence of pervasive and sustained emotions or feelings described by a person (Sadock & Sadock, 2003; Shahrokh & Hales, 2003). For example, a woman who cries frequently and says she misses her deceased husband who died last month, is exhibiting a depressed mood. The relationship between one's affect and mood is of particular significance. The term *congruent* is used to describe consistency between a person's affect and mood (eg, "The client's affect is congruent with his mood."). Conversely, affect can be widely divergent or incongruent from what one says or does. For example, a client may appear happy in the presence of family members but, when alone, abuses alcohol in an attempt to alleviate a depressed mood. *Apathy* is a term that may be used to describe an individual's display of lack of emotion, interest, or concern.

A lead question such as "What are you feeling?" may elicit such responses as "nervous," "angry," "frustrated," "depressed," or "confused." Ask the person to describe the nervousness, anger, frustration, depression, or confusion. Is the person's emotional response constant or does it fluctuate during the assessment? When performing the interview, always record a verbatim reply to questions concerning the client's mood and note whether an intense emotional response accompanies the discussion of specific topics. Affective responses may be appropriate, inappropriate, labile, blunted, restricted or constricted, or flat. An emotional response out of proportion to a situation is considered inappropriate. The lack of an affective response to a very emotional event may also be considered inappropriate, such as no display of emotion when discussing a close relative's death or when discussing another traumatic event. Box 9-1 describes the various affective responses.

Under ordinary circumstances, a person's affect varies according to the situation or subject under discussion. The person with emotional conflict may have a persistent emotional reaction based on this conflict. As the examiner or observer, identify the abnormal emotional reaction and explore its depth, intensity, and persistence. Such an inquiry could prevent a person who is depressed from attempting suicide.

Behavior, Attitude, and Coping Patterns

Asking about suicidal risk, violent behavior, or substance abuse during client assessments is embarrass-

---

BOX 9.1   TYPES OF AFFECTIVE RESPONSES

Blunted affect: Severe reduction or limitation in the intensity of a one's affective responses to a situation

Flat affect: Absence or near absence of any signs of affective responses, such as an immobile face and monotonous tone of voice when conversing with others

Inappropriate affect: Discordance or lack of harmony between one's voice and movements with one's speech or verbalized thoughts

Labile affect: Abnormal fluctuation or variability of one's expressions, such as repeated, rapid, or abrupt shifts

Restricted or constricted affect: A reduction in one's expressive range and intensity of affective responses

---

ing for many nurses. Such embarrassment may result in the nurse's judging a client or making assumptions about the client (Blair, 2005). To avoid such mistakes when assessing clients' behavior and attitude, consider the following factors:

- Do they exhibit strange, threatening, suicidal, self-injurious, or violent behavior? Aggressive behavior may be displayed verbally or physically against self, objects, or other people. Are they making an effort to control their emotions?
- Is there evidence of any unusual mannerisms or motor activity, such as grimacing, tremors, tics, impaired gait, psychomotor retardation, or agitation? Do they pace excessively?
- Do they appear friendly, embarrassed, evasive, fearful, resentful, angry, negativistic, or impulsive? Their attitude toward the interviewer or other helping persons can facilitate or impair the assessment process.
- Is behavior overactive or underactive? Is it purposeful, disorganized, or stereotyped? Are reactions fairly consistent?

If clients are in contact with reality and able to respond to such a question, ask them how they normally cope with a serious problem or with high levels of stress. Responses to this question enable the nurse to assess clients' present ability to cope and their judgment. Is there a support system in place? Are clients using medication, alcohol, or illicit drugs to cope? Their behavior may be the result of inadequate coping patterns or lack of a support system.

Clients experiencing paranoia or suspicion may isolate themselves, appear evasive during a conversation, and demonstrate a negativistic attitude toward the nursing staff. Such activity is an attempt to protect oneself by maintaining control of a stressful environment.

Communication and Social Skills

"The manner in which the client talks enables us to appreciate difficulties with his thought processes. It is desirable to obtain a verbatim sample of the stream of speech to illustrate psychopathologic disturbances" (Small, 1980, p. 8).

The client may hesitate to communicate with a complete stranger on the first meeting unless the nurse is able to display empathy for the client's distress and establish trust with the client. Consider the following factors while assessing clients' ability to communicate and interact socially:

- Do they speak coherently? Does the flow of speech seem natural and logical, or is it illogical, vague, and loosely organized? Do they enunciate clearly?
- Is the rate of speech slow, retarded, or rapid? Do they fail to speak at all? Do they respond only when questioned?
- Do clients whisper or speak softly, or do they speak loudly or shout?
- Is there a delay in answers or responses, or do clients break off their conversation in the middle of a sentence and refuse to talk further?
- Do they repeat certain words and phrases over and over?
- Do they make up new words that have no meaning to other people?
- Is their language obscene?
- Does their conversation jump from one topic to another?
- Do they stutter, lisp, or regress in their speech?
- Do they exhibit any unusual personality traits or characteristics that may interfere with their ability to socialize with others or adapt to hospitalization? For example, do they associate freely with others, or

do they consider themselves "loners"? Do they appear aggressive or domineering during the interview? Do they feel that people like them or reject them? How do they spend their personal time?
- With what cultural group or groups do they identify?

A review of data collection enables the nurse to integrate specific purposeful communication techniques during interactions with the client. These techniques are chosen to meet the needs of the client and may be modified based on their effectiveness during the nurse–client interaction (Schultz & Videbeck, 2005).

Impaired Communication

During assessment, clients may demonstrate impaired communication. The following terminology defined by Shahrokh and Hales (2003) and Sadock and Sadock (2003) is commonly used to describe this impaired communication: blocking, circumstantiality, clang association, echolalia, flight of ideas, looseness of association, mutism, neologism, perseveration, tangentiality, verbigeration, and word salad.

Blocking.   **Blocking** refers to a sudden stoppage in the spontaneous flow or stream of thinking or speaking for no apparent external or environmental reason. Blocking may be due to preoccupation, delusional thoughts, or hallucinations. For example, while talking to the nurse, a client states, "My favorite restaurant is Chi-Chi's. I like it because the atmosphere is so nice and the food is..." Blocking is most often found in clients with schizophrenia experiencing auditory hallucinations.

Circumstantiality.   With **circumstantiality,** the person gives much unnecessary detail that delays meeting a goal or stating a point. For example, when asked to state her occupation, a client may give a very detailed description of the type of work she did. This impairment is commonly found in clients with mania and those with some cognitive impairment disorders, such as the early stage of dementia or mild delirium. Individuals who use substances may also exhibit this pattern of speech.

Clang Association.   **Clang association** is a type of thinking in which the sound of a word (eg, punning or rhyming), substitutes for logic during communication. For example, a client who was asked, "Would you like to go for a walk?" responded, "Talk helps a lot." Individuals with a thought disorder such as schizophrenia or atypical psychosis exhibit clang association.

Echolalia.   **Echolalia** is the parrot-like repetition of overheard words or phrases. Individuals with a developmental disorder, neurologic disorder, or schizophrenia may exhibit echolalia in a mocking or mumbling manner or with staccato intonation.

Flight of Ideas.   **Flight of ideas** is characterized by overproductivity of talk and verbal skipping from one idea to another. Although talk is continuous, the ideas are fragmentary. Connections between segments of speech often are determined by chance associations; for example, "I like the color blue. Do you ever feel blue? Feelings can change from day to day. The days are getting longer." It is most commonly observed in clients with mania.

Looseness of Association.   **Looseness of association,** synonymous with the term *derailment,* is a disturbance of thinking shown by speech in which ideas shift from one unrelated, or minimally unrelated subject to another. The individual speaks in complete sentences, but the relationship between sentences does not make sense; for example, "Mary went swimming. I like turkey." Clients with impaired thought disorders such as schizophrenia, delusional disorder, or dementia exhibit looseness of association.

Mutism.   **Mutism** refers to the refusal to speak even though the person may give indications of being aware of the environment. Mutism may occur due to conscious or unconscious reasons and is observed in clients with catatonic schizophrenic disorders, profound depressive disorders, and stupors of organic or psychogenic origin.

Neologism.   **Neologism** describes the use of a new word or combination of several words coined or invented by a person and not readily understood by others; for example, "His phenologs are in the dryer." This impairment is found in clients with certain schizophrenic disorders.

Perseveration.   With **perseveration,** the person emits the same verbal response (eg, "When do we eat?" or "I have to go to the bathroom") to various questions. Perseveration is also defined as repetitive motor response to various stimuli. This impairment is found in clients experiencing some cognitive impairment disorders and clients experiencing catatonia.

Tangentiality.   **Tangentiality** occurs when a person responds to a question with a reply that is appropriate to the general topic but does not specifically answer the question. For example, a client is asked if she has a good appetite. She responds that she usually eats when she is hungry. Clients experiencing thought disorders such as schizophrenia or dementia exhibit tangentiality.

Verbigeration.   **Verbigeration** describes the meaningless repetition of specific words or phrases (for example, "bad dog"). It is observed in clients with certain psychotic reactions or clients with cognitive impairment disorders.

Word Salad.   **Word salad** is a disturbance in form of thought. The client's speech contains a mixture of words and phrases that lack comprehensive meaning or logical coherence. Clients with the diagnosis of dementia or schizophrenia exhibit word salad.

Content of Thought

In the psychiatric–mental health clinical setting, variations in thought content frequently are noted. These variations may include delusions, hallucinations, depersonalization, obsessions, and compulsions. Alterations in thought process can be related to a mood disorder (eg, depression) or to an organic condition (eg, dementia).

Delusions

Delusions are fixed false beliefs not true to fact and not ordinarily accepted by other members of the person's culture. They cannot be corrected by an appeal to the reason of the person experiencing them. Delusions occur in clients with various types of psychotic disorders, such as cognitive impairment disorder and schizophrenic disorder, and in clients with some affective disorders. Sadock and Sadock (2003) list 13 types of delusions. Table 9-1 describes the more frequently reported types of delusions.

Hallucinations and Illusions

Hallucinations are sensory perceptions that occur in the absence of an actual external stimulus. They may be auditory, visual, olfactory, gustatory, or tactile in nature (Table 9-2). *Command hallucinations* are false

TABLE 9.1 Types of Delusions Frequently Reported

DELUSION	DESCRIPTION
Delusion of reference or persecution	The client believes that he or she is the object of environmental attention or is being singled out for harassment. "The police are watching my every move. They're out to get me."
Delusion of alien control	The client believes his or her feelings, thoughts, impulses, or actions are controlled by an external source. "A spaceman sends me messages by TV and tells me what to do."
Nihilistic delusion	The client denies reality or existence of self, part of self, or some external object. "I have no head."
Delusion of poverty	The client is convinced that he or she is, or will be, bereft of all material possessions.
Delusion of grandeur	A client experiences exaggerated ideas of her or his importance or identity. "I am Napoleon!" or "I am Jesus!"
Somatic delusion	The client entertains false beliefs pertaining to body image or body function. The client actually believes that she or he has cancer, leprosy, or some other terminal illness.

perceptions of orders that a person may feel obligated to obey or unable to resist. Hallucinations occur in clients with substance-related disorders, schizophrenia, and manic disorders. **Illusion** is a term used to describe the misperception of a real external stimulus such as noise or shadows. For example, a client with the diagnosis of dementia may misinterpret the sound of rustling leaves to be the sound of voices. It is not unusual for clients to experience illusions during the withdrawal from alcohol or other substances.

Depersonalization

Depersonalization refers to a feeling of unreality or strangeness concerning self, the environment, or both. For example, clients have described out-of-body sensa-

TABLE 9.2 Types of Hallucinations

HALLUCINATION	EXAMPLE
Auditory hallucination	AS tells you that he hears voices frequently while he sits quietly in his lounge chair. He states, "The voices tell me when to eat, dress, and go to bed each night!"
Visual hallucination	Ninety-year-old EK describes seeing spiders and snakes on the ceiling of his room late one evening as you make rounds.
Olfactory hallucination	AJ, a 65-year-old psychotic client, states that she smells "rotten garbage" in her bedroom, although there is no evidence of any foul-smelling material.
Gustatory (taste) hallucination	MY, a young client with delirium, complains of a constant taste of salt water in her mouth.
Tactile hallucination	NX, a middle-aged woman undergoing symptoms of alcohol withdrawal and delirium tremens, complains of feeling "worms crawling all over [her] body."

tions in which they view themselves from a few feet overhead. These people may feel they are "going crazy." Causes of depersonalization include prolonged stress and psychological fatigue, as well as substance abuse. Clients with schizophrenia, bipolar disorders, and depersonalization disorders have described this feeling.

Obsessions

Obsessions are insistent thoughts, recognized as arising from the self. The client usually regards the obsessions as absurd and relatively meaningless. However, they persist despite his or her endeavors to be rid of them. Persons who experience obsessions generally describe them as "thoughts I can't get rid of" or by saying, "I can't stop thinking of things... they keep going on in my mind over and over again." Obsessions are typically seen in clients with anxiety (eg, obsessive-compulsive disorder).

Compulsions

Compulsions are insistent, repetitive, intrusive, and unwanted urges to perform an act contrary to one's ordinary wishes or standards. For example, a client expresses the repetitive urge to gamble although his wife has threatened to divorce him if he does not stop playing poker. If the person does not engage in the repetitive act, he or she usually experiences feelings of tension and anxiety. Compulsions are frequently seen in clients with anxiety, obsessive–compulsive disorder, or personality, body dysmorphic, eating, or autism spectrum disorders.

Orientation

During the assessment, clients are asked questions about their ability to grasp the significance of their environment, an existing situation, or the clearness of conscious processes. In other words, are they oriented to person, place, and time? Do they know who they are, where they are, or what the date is? Levels of orientation and consciousness are subdivided as follows: confusion, clouding of consciousness, stupor, delirium, and coma (Table 9-3).

Memory

Memory is the ability to recall past experiences. Typically, memory is categorized as recent and long-term memory. *Recent memory* is the ability to recall events in the immediate past and for up to 2 weeks previously. *Long-term memory* is the ability to recall remote past experiences such as the date and place of birth, names of schools attended, occupational history, and chronologic data relating to previous illnesses. Loss of recent memory may be seen in clients with dementia, delirium, or depression. Long-term memory loss usually is a result of a physiologic disorder resulting in brain dysfunction.

Memory defects may result from lack of attention, difficulty with retention, difficulty with recall, or any combination of these factors. Three disorders of memory include:

- Hyperamnesia, or an abnormally pronounced memory

TABLE 9.3 Levels of Orientation and Consciousness

LEVEL	DESCRIPTION
Confusion	Disorientation to person, place, or time, characterized by bewilderment and complexity
Clouding of consciousness	Disturbance in perception or thought that is slight to moderate in degree, usually due to physical or chemical factors producing functional impairment of the cerebrum
Stupor	A state in which the client does not react to or is unaware of his or her surroundings. The client may be motionless and mute, but conscious
Delirium	Confusion accompanied by altered or fluctuating consciousness. Disturbance in emotion, thought, and perception is moderate to severe. Usually associated with infections, toxic states, head trauma, and so forth
Coma	Loss of consciousness

- Amnesia, or loss of memory
- Paramnesia, or falsification of memory

Intellectual Ability

Intellectual ability is an indication of a person's ability to use facts comprehensively. During an assessment, a client may be asked general information such as the names of the last three presidents. He or she may also be asked to calculate simple mathematical problems and correctly estimate and form opinions concerning objective matters. For example, the person may be asked a question such as, "What would you do if you found a wallet in front of your house?" The nurse evaluates reasoning ability and judgment by the response given. Abstract and concrete thinking abilities are evaluated by asking the client to explain the meaning of proverbs such as "an eye for an eye and a tooth for a tooth."

Insight Regarding Illness or Condition

Insight is defined as self-understanding, or the extent of one's understanding about the origin, nature, and mechanisms of one's attitudes and behavior. Does the client consider himself or herself ill? Does the client understand what is happening? Is the illness threatening to the client? Clients' insights into their illnesses or conditions range from poor to good, depending on the degree of psychopathology present. Insightful clients are able to identify strengths and weaknesses that may affect their response to treatment.

Spirituality

"Spiritual assessment should, at a minimum, determine the patient's denomination, beliefs, and what spiritual practices are important to the patient" (Joint Commission for the Accreditation of Healthcare Organizations, 2005).

Spirituality involves the client's beliefs, values, and religious culture. Obtaining a spiritual history enables nurses to identify significant spiritual practices that may influence care. For example, a hospitalized client exhibiting spiritual anxiety verbalizes a need to connect with his or her own spiritual support system before consenting to treatment. Questions asked in a matter-of-fact fashion can focus on the religious background of the client, parents, spouse, or significant other; the client's current religious affiliation or important spiritual beliefs; whether the client is currently active in a religious community; whether religious beliefs serve as a coping mechanism; and to what extent religious or spiritual issues are pertinent to the client's current situation (Larson, Larson, & Puchalski, 2000). A sample spiritual needs assessment is shown in Figure 9-3.

Sexuality

"Sexuality depends on four interrelated psychosexual factors: sexual identity, gender identity, sexual orientation, and sexual behavior" (Sadock & Sadock, 2003, p. 692).

Sexuality may be a factor having an impact on, effecting, or contributing to psychiatric illness with a client for a number of reasons. For example, a client may be impotent, may have lost a sexual partner, or may have been a victim of sexual abuse or a hate crime. An interviewer should be careful about using non–gender-specific terms when asking about significant others: use "partner" instead of assuming a heterosexual relationship as clients may be hesitant in revealing their sexual history/orientation if they feel they will be judged on their responses. The following questions may be helpful in initiating a discussion on the topic of sexuality:

- Does the client express any concerns about sexual or gender identity, activity, or function?
- When did these concerns begin?
- Does the client prefer a male or female clinician to discuss these concerns?

The age and sex of the clinician may affect the responses given. For example, a 50-year-old male client may feel uncomfortable discussing issues related to sexuality with a nurse who appears to be the same age as his daughter. A female client with the clinical symptoms of depression may be reluctant to discuss sexual abuse with a male nurse. Obtaining a sexual history is discussed in detail in Chapter 26, Sexuality and Sexual Disorders.

Neurovegetative Changes

Neurovegetative changes involve changes in psychophysiologic functions such as sleep patterns, eating patterns, energy levels, sexual functioning, or bowel functioning. Persons with depression (see

Name: _____

Age: _____

Marital status: _____

Religious affiliation: _____

Name of local clergy contact: _____

Address of clergy: _____

_____

_____

Phone number of clergy: _____

Receptive to visits by parish, clergy, or laypersons: ☐ Yes ☐ No

Name and address of congregation: _____

_____

_____

Should congregation be notified: ☐ Yes ☐ No

Advance directives in place: ☐ Yes ☐ No

Spiritual life review including description of higher power and coping skills: _____

_____

_____

_____

Request for spiritual interventions:

☐ Inspirational matter or music
☐ Prayer or meditation
☐ Sacraments or anointing
☐ Scriptural ministry
☐ Last Rites

FIGURE 9.3 Spiritual needs assessment form.

Chapter 21) usually complain of insomnia or hypersomnia, loss of appetite or increased appetite, loss of energy, decreased libido, and constipation, all signs of neurovegetative changes. Persons who are diagnosed as psychotic may neglect their nutritional intake, appear fatigued, sleep excessively, and ignore elimination habits (sometimes to the point of developing a fecal impaction).

During the collection of data, specific questions are asked about the client's appetite and eating pattern, energy level and ability to perform activities of daily living, sexual functioning (discussed earlier), bowel functioning or elimination patterns, and sleep pattern. Because sleep disturbances also can occur as a primary medical or psychiatric symptom, sleep pattern is addressed in the next section in more detail.

Sleep Pattern

Asking clients about their sleep patterns and any problems is an often-neglected but extremely important area to investigate. It has been estimated that as many as one third of clients seen in the primary care setting may experience occasional difficulties in sleeping, and 10% of those persons may have chronic sleep problems (Brown, 1999). A simple yet valuable question to ask clients is, "Do you have difficulty sleeping at night or staying awake during the day?"

It is important that the nurse understand that sleep patterns change throughout the life cycle. Newborns sleep many short periods of sleep for a total of approximately 16 to 20 hours of sleep per day. As children get older, sleep becomes more organized and extended during the night. Adolescents require 9 to 10 hours of sleep; most adults need approximately 7 to 9 hours of sleep; and the elderly tend to have a pattern of early rising and early sleep, interspersed with a nap, totaling approximately 6 hours per day (Redeker & Nadolski, 2004).

Insomnia, difficulty initiating or maintaining sleep, is a symptom with many different causes. It is 1.3 times more common in women than in men, and 1.5 times more common in the elderly than in persons younger than 65 years of age. The Sleep in America Poll, conducted in 2003 by the National Sleep Foundation (NSF, 2003), reported that 48% of adults experienced one or more symptoms of insomnia at least a few nights per week. It often occurs in clients with psychiatric–mental health disorders. Therefore, nurses must question the client about any sleep pattern disturbance to plan appropriate measures. See Supporting Evidence for Practice 9-1.

SUPPORTING EVIDENCE FOR PRACTICE 9.1

Nursing Assessment and Interventions for Clients in the Psychiatric–Mental Health Setting Who Experience Insomnia

PROBLEM UNDER INVESTIGATION / Identification and treatment of primary insomnia versus insomnia related to mental disorders

SUMMARY OF RESEARCH / Subjects included 216 clients between the ages of 14 and 89 years in five clinical sites. Sleep specialists evaluated each client. Results indicated that poor sleep hygiene and negative conditioning (eg, frustration related to sleeplessness and disproportionate concern about the inability to sleep) contributed to a diagnosis of primary insomnia. The presence of a psychiatric disorder (eg, anxiety disorder, psychotic disorder, adjustment disorder, and personality disorder) contributed more to the diagnosis of insomnia related to a mental disorder. However, psychiatric disorders (eg, mood disorder, personality disorder, and anxiety disorder) were also identified as contributing to a diagnosis of primary insomnia in 77% of the cases. Researchers concluded that behavioral treatment aimed at improving sleep hygiene habits and reducing negative conditioning behaviors, combined with pharmacotherapy, may be beneficial for clients with insomnia.

SUPPORT FOR PRACTICE / Nursing-oriented interventions to combat insomnia in the psychiatric–mental health clinical setting generally focus on nonpharmacologic approaches such as changes in daily and prebedtime routines. For example, a client with the diagnosis of depression may avoid daytime naps, eliminate stimulants such as caffeine, and avoid the use of alcohol after dinner, but go to bed early in the evening to avoid stress. However, going to bed earlier may not help, and the client may awaken earlier in the morning and complain of fatigue throughout the day.

Encouraging the client to keep a journal of daily activities and a sleep log will assist the nurse in evaluating the effectiveness of sleep hygiene changes and the need for medication to induce sleep due to primary insomnia or insomnia related to a mental disorder.

SOURCE: Nowell, P. D., et al. (1997, Oct.) Clinical factors contributing to the differential diagnosis of primary insomnia and insomnia related to mental disorders. American Journal of Psychiatry 154(10), 1412-1426.

Acute or **primary insomnia** refers to the inability to initiate or maintain sleep or nonrestorative sleep for at least 1 month. It is often caused by emotional discomfort such as chronic stress, hyperarousal, poor sleep hygiene (drinking coffee just prior to sleep), environmental noise, or jet lag. It is not caused by the direct physiologic effects of a substance or a general medical condition. **Secondary insomnia** is the inability to initiate or maintain sleep or nonrestorative sleep due to a psychiatric disorder such as depression, anxiety, or schizophrenia; general medical or neurologic disorders; pain; or substance abuse (Brown, 1999). The Epworth Sleepiness Scale is a simple questionnaire to assess clients who suffer from excessive daytime sleepiness. The client rates the chances that he or she would doze off or fall asleep during eight different routine daytime situations (eg, sitting and reading, watching television, or sitting and talking to someone). A total score of 10 or more suggests that the client may need further evaluation for an underlying sleep disorder. To obtain free copies of the Epworth Sleepiness Scale, call 866-373-2287. Chapter 12 contains additional information regarding the treatment of insomnia. See Box 9-2 for a list of common sleep disorders.

Medical Issues

Clients with medical problems commonly present with clinical symptoms of a comorbid psychiatric–mental health disorder. In the past, psychiatric nurses were trained to assess clients for emotional and behavioral changes in the psychiatric–mental health clinical setting, whereas other members of the multidisciplinary treatment team attended to medical issues. However, collaboration and communication among psychiatric nurses, primary care doctors, and other clinicians are becoming increasingly critical. Comorbid depression with various major medical illnesses such as cardiovascular disease, stroke, or Parkinson's disease can impede medical treatment and increase mortality if the depression is not identified and treated (Ellen, 2001).

Pain

Pain, a major yet largely avoidable health problem, is considered a multidimensional experience that potentially affects the individual physically, emotionally, spiritually, and socially. Pain may be associated with a general medical condition (eg, cancer), psychological factors (eg, pain not accounted for by a medical or

---

| BOX 9.2 | COMMON SLEEP DISORDERS |

Insomnia: Difficulty initiating or maintaining sleep

Jet lag: Sleepiness and alertness that occur at an inappropriate time of day relative to local time, occurring after repeated travel across more than one time zone

Narcolepsy: Overwhelming sleepiness in which the individual experiences irresistible attacks of refreshing sleep, cataplexy (loss of muscle tone), and/or hallucinations or sleep paralysis at the beginning or end of sleep episodes

Nightmare disorder: Repeated awakenings from the major sleep period or naps with detailed recall of extended and extremely frightening dreams, usually involving threats to survival, security, or self-esteem

Restless legs syndrome: Characterized by insomnia associated with crawling sensations of the lower extremities; frequently associated with medical conditions such as arthritis or pregnancy

Sleep apnea: A breathing-related sleep disorder due to disrupted ventilation or airway obstruction in which the individual may experience a lack of airflow. The normal sleeping pattern is completely disrupted several times throughout the night

Sleep terror disorder: Recurrent episodes of abrupt awakening from sleep usually accompanied by a panicky scream, intense fear, tachycardia, rapid breathing, and diaphoresis. The individual is unresponsive to efforts of others to provide comfort and there is no detailed dream recall

---

neurological condition), or it may be associated with both psychological factors and a general medical condition (eg, associated with functional impairment and emotional distress). The Joint Commission on Accreditation of Healthcare Organizations (JCAHO) has developed standards that create new expectations for the assessment and management of pain in accredited hospitals and other health care settings, including behavioral health facilities. Clinicians are now expected to assess, record, and treat pain as routinely as they would the other four vital signs.

Initially, pain is assessed using a pain-intensity rating scale appropriate to the client's age and ability to communicate. This baseline pain assessment is used for comparison with all future assessments.

Self-report of pain is the most reliable and valid pain assessment tool. If the client is unable to communicate, data are obtained by observing behavior, obtaining proxy reports from family or significant others, or by the documentation of physiological parameters (Dempsey, 2001).

Physiological Responses to Medication

Psychiatric–mental health nurses are also expected to be knowledgeable about the potential for adverse effects of various medications that could precipitate a change in a client's emotions, behavior, or mental status. For example, a client diagnosed with Parkinson's disease and comorbid depression is placed on carbidopa (Sinemet) by his attending physician. Over the last 3 months, he has been seen twice a month by the psychiatric–mental health nurse for supportive therapy to discuss his adjustment to the changes in his physical condition and his relationship with his family. During a visit to the mental health clinic, the client complains that he has not felt right since he began taking the carbidopa. He reports that he has difficulty concentrating, has strange and bizarre dreams, and states that his eyes are "playing tricks" on him. The psychiatric–mental health nurse recognizes that the potential adverse effects of his current drug therapy with carbidopa include central nervous system disturbances such as confusion, disorientation, or visual hallucinations. After reassessing the client to rule out the clinical symptoms of major depression, the nurse educates the client about the potential adverse effects of carbidopa and advises the client to contact his family doctor to discuss his physiological response to the medication.

Psychiatric–mental health nurses also must obtain accurate information from clients about any medications that they are taking, whether by prescription or over the counter, to prevent the possibility of any drug–drug interactions or accidental overdose if the use of psychotropic medication is indicated. Chapter 16 presents a detailed discussion of the pharmacokinetics and pharmacodynamics of drug therapy.

Supporters or Caregivers Assessment

Informal supporters or caregivers (eg, spouse, parents, significant other) of clients with the diagnosis of a psychiatric disorder may be prone to depression, anxiety, grief, fatigue, changes in social relationships, or other issues. Such a role has been recognized as an activity with perceived benefits and burdens. Originally designed for use in long-term care, the Caregiver Strain Index is a tool that can be used in any clinical setting to identify individual supporters or caregivers of any age or families with potential caregiving concerns. This 13-question tool measures strain related to care provision and focuses on the following domains: employment, financial, physical, social, and time. It effectively identifies individuals who may benefit from more in-depth assessment and follow-up. Additional information regarding this tool can be obtained at http://www.hartfordign.org (Sullivan, 2004). Recognizing the importance of including supporters or caregivers in the client's plan of care, this text includes content such as transcultural considerations and client/family education when appropriate.

Documentation of Assessment Data

Assessment information is documented on the nursing admission–history form used by the specific psychiatric or mental health facility. The multidisciplinary team planning client treatment reviews this information, in conjunction with history and physical examination information, summary of social history, and summary of psychological testing. Nurses can provide invaluable information if they follow the criteria of good documentation. Such information is significant to the members of the interdisciplinary team, who use the data in planning treatment and disposition of clients. Thorough documentation shows client progress, lack of progress, or evidence of regression. The details of the client's conduct, appearance, and attitude are significant. Increased skill in observation and collection of data results in more concise and precise documentation.

Documentation is also important in research because it provides an accurate record of the client's symptoms, behavior, treatment, and reactions. Moreover, documentation is recognized by legal authorities, who frequently use the information for testimony in court.

Documentation should adhere to specific criteria. Documentation should be:

- *Objective:* The nurse documents what the client says and does so by stating facts and quoting the client's conversation.

- *Descriptive:* The nurse describes the client's appearance, behavior, and conversation as seen and heard. Subjective statements such as 'patient was depressed' should not be included, as they are subject to the interpretation of the interviewer. A more appropriate way to document this would be, "Patient stated, 'I feel depressed.'"
- *Complete:* All examinations, treatments, medications, therapies, nursing interventions, and the client's reaction to each should be on the client's chart. Samples of the client's writing or drawing should be included.
- *Legible:* Documentation should be written legibly, using acceptable abbreviations only, and no erasures. Correct grammar and spelling are important, and complete sentences should be used.
- *Dated:* The day and time of each entry must be noted. For example, "MS was quiet and withdrawn all day today, 2/17; however, later in the evening at 9:15 PM, she began pacing the corridor and wringing her hands." The nurse needs to state the time at which the client's behavior changed, as well as describe any pertinent situations that might be identified as the cause of this behavioral change.
- *Logical:* Documentation should be presented in logical sequence.
- *Signed:* The form should be signed by the person making the entry.

Examples of Documentation

Nurses use various forms of documentation, including SOAP (subjective data, objective data, assessment, and plan of care) and DAP (objective and subjective data, assessment, and plan of care). Nursing documentation should reflect the effectiveness of treatment plans. Multidisciplinary progress notes have become more prevalent because they depict a chronologic picture of the client's response to therapeutic interventions implemented by various disciplines. Social workers, activity therapists, and occupational therapists often combine their progress notes with those written by the nursing staff in SAP and DAP form. An example of DAP documentation by members of the multidisciplinary team is presented in Box 9-3. Problems identified in the plan of care and addressed in documentation are entered in the column labeled "Problem Number." Both objective and subjective data are included at "data" (D). A summary of the client assessment is listed at "A" and the plan of care at "P."

KEY CONCEPTS

◆   The nursing process is a six-step problem-solving approach to nursing that also serves as an organizational framework for the practice of nursing.

◆   The nurse collects both objective and subjective data during the assessment. Objective data are collected by inspection, palpation, percussion, and auscultation. Subjective data are obtained through questioning, interviewing, or reviewing past medical records.

◆   The nurse determines which of the three types of assessment (comprehensive, focused, or screening) to use based on the client's needs, presenting symptoms, and clinical setting.

◆   The assessment of culturally diverse clients can be challenging to the nurse and requires an understanding of the client's perspective regarding his or her illness.

◆   During an assessment, the nurse explores the client's ability to function biologically, behaviorally, cognitively, culturally, psychologically, and spiritually.

◆   Informal supporters or caregivers (eg, spouse, parents, significant other) of clients may be prone to depression, anxiety, grief, fatigue, changes in social relationships, or other issues and may benefit from an assessment such as the Caregiver Strain Index.

◆   Following the criteria for documentation of assessment data provides pertinent information to be used during the development of a client's plan of care.

For additional study materials, please refer to the Student Resource CD-ROM located in the back of this textbook.

BOX 9.3 EXAMPLE OF DAP NURSING PROGRESS NOTES

DATE AND TIME	PROBLEM NUMBER	NAME AND TITLE	MULTIDISCIPLINARY TREATMENT TEAM PROGRESS NOTES
2/7/00 9:00 AM	#1	J Smith, ARNP	D: RK was eating breakfast at 8:00 AM when she began to perspire profusely and stated, "I don't know what's wrong with me, but I feel jittery inside. I feel like something terrible is going to happen." When asked to describe her feelings, RK replied, "I can't. I just have an awful feeling inside." Affect blunted. Pallor noted. Tearful during interaction. Minimal eye contact. Voice tremulous.
			P = 120, R = 28, BP = 130/80. No signs of acute physical distress noted at this time.
			A: Expressing fear of the unknown and inability to maintain control of her emotions. Recognizes she is experiencing symptoms of anxiety but is unable to use effective coping skills.
			P: Encourage verbalization of feelings when able to interact/ communicate needs.
			Explore presence of positive coping skills.
			Administer prescribed antianxiety agent.
			Monitor response to medication.
2/7/00 2:00 PM	#1	M Smith, LCSW	D: RK attended group therapy from 1:00 PM to 2:00 PM
			A: Informed members of group of incident that occured at 9 AM today. Appeared calm. Good eye contact. Did not express fears.
			P: Focus on present coping skills. Encourage attendance and participation in group therapy on M-W-F.

Note: Problem #1 refers to the nursing diagnosis, Ineffective Individual Coping.

CHAPTER WORKSHEET

CRITICAL THINKING QUESTIONS

1. While in the clinical setting, observe the general appearance (physical characteristics, facial expressions, apparent age, dress, hygiene, and use of cosmetics) of several clients. Record your assessments and then compare with the assessments written in the clients' charts.

2. As you assess Mr. Chan, you notice that he stops his answers in mid-sentence and also uses words that are unfamiliar to you. How would you continue your assessment to determine whether he is blocking and using neologisms, or if there is a cultural or language barrier?

3. To assess how a client normally copes with a problem, it can be helpful to provide a scenario, ask the client to identify and talk through the problem, and then listen to the client's problem-solving methods. (Such scenarios must be applicable to the individual client.) What kind of scenario might you provide to a 16-year-old

male, a 45-year-old worker who recently became unemployed, and a 76-year-old widow?

REFLECTION

Review the quote at the beginning of the chapter, and then complete an assessment of a client in your clinical practice setting. What information did you obtain? How was that information crucial to the client's care?

NCLEX-STYLE QUESTIONS

1. Which of the following questions would be most appropriate to use during the psychiatric admission assessment to obtain data about the client's affect?
   a. "What are you feeling?"
   b. "Are you happy or sad?"
   c. "You look upset; are you?"
   d. "What brought you to the hospital?"

2. The nurse asks a client with a diagnosis of bipolar disorder where he lived during the past year. The client replies, "Yes, I wanted to paint the living room blue but then decided on white. Of course there were nail holes in the wall, so I had to patch them before I could paint. Do you know how many different shades of white there are?" The nurse interprets the client's response as an example of which of the following?
   a. Blocking
   b. Circumstantiality
   c. Perseveration
   d. Neologism

3. The nurse expects a client exhibiting flight of ideas to do which of the following?
   a. Make sudden stops in the flow of conversation
   b. Coin new words or combinations of several words
   c. Provide excessive detail that delays starting a point
   d. Talk excessively while frequently shifting from one idea to another

4. A client tells the nurse that his body is made of wood and is quite heavy. The nurse interprets this as which of the following?

   a. Compulsion
   b. Hallucination
   c. Depersonalization
   d. Obsession

5. Which finding would lead the nurse to suspect that a female client has insight into the mental disorder she is experiencing?
   a. Demonstration of self-understanding related to the origin of behavior
   b. Verbalization of acceptance of her mental illness
   c. Placement of responsibility for problems on dysfunctional family
   d. Suggestion that problems are related to bad nerves

6. Which of the following would the nurse assess as indicative of neurovegetative changes? Select all that apply.
   a. Amnesia
   b. Flat affect
   c. Insomnia
   d. Constipation
   e. Perseveration
   f. Loss of appetite

Selected References

Andrews, M. M., & Boyle, J. S. (2003). *Transcultural concepts in nursing care* (4th ed.). Philadelphia: Lippincott Williams & Wilkins.

Blair, B. H. N. (2005). Assessing for risky behavior. *ADVANCE for Nurses, 6*(3), 27–28.

Brown, D. B. (1999). Managing sleep disorders: Solutions in primary care. *Clinician Reviews, 9*(10), 51–64.

Dempsey, S. K. (2001). Pain assessment. *ADVANCE for Nurses, 2*(2), 11–12.

Ellen, E. F. (2001). Treating the patient as a whole person. *Psychiatric Times, 18*(6), 1, 6, 10, 12–13.

Joint Commission for the Accreditation of Healthcare Organizations. (2005). Standards clarification on spiritual assessment. Retrieved March 8, 2005, from http://www.jcaho.org

Johnson, K. (2005). Imaging may lead to test for bipolar. *Clinical Psychiatry News, 33*(1), 1, 6.

Kanigel, R. (1999). Integrative medicine: Bridging the culture gap. *Hippocrates, 9*, 19–21.

Larson, D. B., Larson, S. S., & Puchalski, C. M. (2000). The once-forgotten factor in psychiatry, Part 1: Residency training addresses religious and spiritual issues. *Psychiatric Times, 17*(1), 18–23.

Mackey-Padilla, J. (2005). National standards on culturally and linguistically appropriate services in health care. Final report, March, 2001. Retrieved January 31, 2005, from http://www.medscape.com/viewarticle/497283_print

Menaster, M. (2004). Psychometrics: A valuable tool. *Clinical Psychiatry News, 32*(4), 12–13.

Nettina, S. M. (2001). Nursing practice and the nursing process. In S. M. Nettina (Ed.), *The Lippincott manual of nursing practice* (6th ed., pp. 2–6). Philadelphia: Lippincott Williams & Wilkins.

National Sleep Foundation. (2003). 2003 Sleep in America poll. Retrieved August 2, 2005, from http://www.sleepfoundation.org

Novick, L. (2004). Psychiatric comorbidity tied to skin diseases underestimated. *Clinical Psychiatry News, 32*(4), 92.

Nowell, P. D., Buysse, D. J., Reynolds, C. F., III, Hauri, P. J., Roth, T., Stepanski, E. J., et al. (1997, October). Clinical factors contributing to the differential diagnosis of primary insomnia and insomnia related to mental disorders. *American Journal of Psychiatry, 154*(10), 1412–1426.

Redeker, N. S., & Nadolski, N. (2004). Treating insomnia in primary care. *American Journal for Nurse Practitioners, 8*(3), 61–68.

Romano, C. J. (2004). Do you see what I hear? Imaging auditory hallucinations. *Neuropsychiatry Review, 5*(6), 1, 12, 20.

Sadock, B. J., & Sadock, V. A. (2003). *Kaplan & Sadock's synopsis of psychiatry, behavioral sciences/clinical psychiatry* (9th ed.). Philadelphia: Lippincott Williams & Wilkins.

Schultz, J. M., & Videbeck, S. L. (2005). *Lippincott's manual of psychiatric nursing care plans* (7th ed.). Philadelphia: Lippincott Williams & Wilkins.

Shahrokh, N., & Hales, R. E. (Eds.). (2003). *American psychiatric glossary* (8th ed.). Washington, DC: American Psychiatric Press, Inc.

Small, S. M. (1980). *Outline for psychiatric examination.* East Hanover, NJ: Sandoz Pharmaceuticals.

Sullivan, M. T. (2004). Caregiver strain index. *Dermatological Nursing, 16*(4), 385–386.

Wright, W. (2005, April). Practitioners on the front line: Assessing patients for migraine. *Supplement to the Clinical Advisor,* 1–8.

Suggested Readings

Allen, R. P., & Hening, W. A. (2005). Diagnosis and treatment of restless legs syndrome. *Clinician Reviews, 15*(3), 57–68.

Bradberry, C. (2001). Pain—the fifth vital sign. *Vital Signs, 11*(1), 10.

Buckley, T. (2002). Reflex sympathetic dystrophy. *ADVANCE for Nurses, 3*(8), 27–28.

Carpenito, L. J. (2006). *Handbook of nursing diagnosis* (11th ed.). Philadelphia: Lippincott Williams & Wilkins.

Giuliano, V. (2004, April). The forgotten role of diagnostic imaging with regard to mental health. *Central Florida M.D. News, 6*(4), 10.

Haskins, B. (2000). Serving and assessing deaf patients: Implications for psychiatry. *Psychiatric Times, 17*(12), 29–32.

Khouzam, H. R., Gill, T., & Tan, D. (2005). When 'agitation' spells a medical problem. *Current Psychiatry, 4*(2), 87–88.

Kubose, S. (2000). Not enough time for the mini-mental state exam? Try the micro-mental. *Neuro Psychiatry, 1*(6), 17.

Kwentus, J. A. (2000). Sleep problems. *Clinical Geriatrics, 8*(9), 64–72.

McCaffery, M. (2001). Using the 0-to-10 pain rating scale. *American Journal of Nursing, 101*(10), 81–82.

McCaffery, M., & Pasero, C. (2001). Assessment and treatment of patients with mental illness. Implementing the JCAHO pain management standards. *American Journal of Nursing, 101*(7), 69–70.

Morgan, C. D., & Bober, J. F. (2005). Psychological testing: Use do-it-yourself tools or refer? *Current Psychiatry, 4*(6), 56–66.

Penny, J. T. (2000). I didn't sleep a wink last night: Sleep disorders. *ADVANCE for Nurses, 10*(23), 17–22.

Stansberry, T. T. (2001). Narcolepsy: Unveiling a mystery. *American Journal of Nursing, 101*(8), 50–53.

Warner, P. H., Rowe, T., & Whipple, B. (1999). Shedding light on the sexual history. *American Journal of Nursing, 99*(6), 34–41.

Zunkel, G. M. (2005). Insomnia: Overview of assessment and treatment strategies. *Clinician Reviews, 15*(7), 38–44.

CHAPTER 10 / NURSING DIAGNOSIS, OUTCOME IDENTIFICATION, PLANNING, IMPLEMENTATION, AND EVALUATION

Making accurate nursing diagnoses takes knowledge and practice. If the nurse uses a systematic approach to nursing diagnosis validation, then accuracy will increase. The process of making nursing diagnoses is difficult because nurses are attempting to diagnose human responses. Humans are unique, complex, and ever-changing; thus, attempts to classify these responses have been difficult. —CARPENITO-MOYET, 2006

LEARNING OBJECTIVES

AFTER STUDYING THIS CHAPTER, YOU SHOULD BE ABLE TO:

1. Articulate the purpose of using a nursing diagnosis in the psychiatric–mental health setting.
2. Distinguish among the four types of nursing diagnoses.
3. State the use of the phrase *possible nursing diagnosis*.
4. State the rationale for using the *Diagnostic and Statistical Manual of Mental Disorders, 4th Edition, Text Revision (DSM-IV-TR)* in the psychiatric–mental health setting.
5. Discuss the rationale for using outcome identification as part of the nursing process.
6. Compare and contrast the use of the following when developing a plan of care: clinical pathways, concept mapping, critical pathways, and evidence-based nursing practice.
7. Construct a plan of care in the psychiatric setting.
8. Interpret the nurse's role when implementing nursing interventions.
9. Explain the rationale for the evaluation phase of the nursing process.

KEY TERMS

Actual nursing diagnosis
Clinical pathways
Concept mapping
Critical pathways
Cues
Decision trees
DSM-IV-TR
Evidence-based nursing practice
Expected outcomes
Inferences
Nursing diagnosis
Risk nursing diagnosis
Standardized nursing plans of care
Syndrome nursing diagnosis
Wellness nursing diagnosis

As stated in Chapter 9, the nursing process consists of six steps and uses a problem-solving approach. The first step, assessment, has already been covered in detail. This chapter focuses on the remaining five steps:

1. Nursing diagnosis
2. Outcome identification
3. Planning (formulation of a nursing plan of care)
4. Implementation of nursing actions or interventions
5. Evaluation of the client's response to interventions

The nursing process has been referred to as an ongoing, systematic series of actions, interactions, and transactions.

Nursing Diagnosis

The **nursing diagnosis** is a statement of an existing problem or a potential health problem that a nurse is both competent and licensed to treat. The North American Nursing Diagnosis Association (NANDA) defines a nursing diagnosis as a clinical judgment about individual, family, or community responses to actual or potential health problems or life processes. A nursing diagnosis provides the basis for selecting nursing interventions to achieve outcomes for which the nurse is accountable.

The psychiatric–mental health nurse analyzes the assessment data before determining which nursing diagnosis would be most appropriate. Analysis of the data involves differentiating cues from inferences, assuring validity, and determining how much data are needed. **Cues** are facts collected during the assessment process, whereas **inferences** are judgments that the nurse makes about cues. The inferences that nurses make are only as valid as the data used (Carpenito-Moyet, 2006).

Data, when valid, can be assumed to be factual and true. Validation of data may occur by rechecking data collected, asking someone to analyze the data, comparing subjective and objective data, or asking the client to verify the data. To determine if a sufficient number of valid cues are present to confirm a nursing diagnosis, the nurse should consult a list of defining characteristics for the diagnosis suspected (Carpenito-Moyet, 2006).

Nursing diagnoses are not to be written in terms of cues, inferences, goals, client needs, or nursing needs. Caution is advised regarding making legally inadvisable or judgmental statements as part of the nursing diagnosis. Finally, nursing diagnostic statements should not be stated or written to encourage negative responses by health care providers, the client, or the family.

Carpenito-Moyet (2006) classifies nursing diagnoses into actual, risk, wellness, and syndrome diagnoses (Table 10-1). An **actual nursing diagnosis** is based on the nurse's clinical judgment on review of validated data. A **risk nursing diagnosis** is based on the nurse's clinical judgment of the client's degree of vulnerability to the development of a specific problem. A **wellness nursing diagnosis** focuses on clinical judgment about an individual, group, or community transitioning from a specific level to a higher level of wellness. A **syndrome nursing diagnosis** refers to a cluster of actual or high-risk diagnoses that are predicted to be present because of a certain event or situation.

The nurse may elect to use the phrase *possible nursing diagnosis* (eg, Possible Activity Intolerance related to obesity, Possible Loneliness related to hospitalization, Possible Noncompliance related to illiteracy) when a suspected problem requires additional data to confirm a diagnosis; however, it is not a type of diagnosis.

Diagnostic Systems

The NANDA diagnostic system was originally organized around nine human response patterns (exchanging, communicating, relating, valuing, choosing, moving, perceiving, knowing, and feeling). In 2000, NANDA approved a new Taxonomy II, which addresses several domains (health promotion, nutrition, elimination, activity/rest, perception/cognition, self-perception, role relationships, sexuality, coping/stress tolerance, life principles, comfort, and growth/development) and 167 nursing diagnoses (NANDA, 2006). The psychiatric–mental health nursing (PMHN) diagnostic system is organized around eight human response processes (activity, cognition, ecological, emotional, interpersonal, perception, physiologic, and valuation). The psychiatric nursing community has agreed to use the existing NANDA classifications until further integration of the two models occurs (Boyd, 2002). Indeed, the American Nurses Association (ANA) Task Force continues to work on the development of a single

TABLE 10.1   Classifications of Nursing Diagnoses

CLASSIFICATION	EXAMPLES
Actual Nursing Diagnoses	Acute Pain related to surgery as evidenced by. . . Anxiety related to chemotherapy as evidenced by. . . Sleep Deprivation related to acute pain as evidenced by. . .
Risk Nursing Diagnoses	Risk for Impaired Parenting related to divorce Risk for Suicide related to depression Risk for Post-Trauma Syndrome related to auto accident
Wellness Nursing Diagnoses	Readiness for Enhanced Community Coping related to identified support groups and role responsibilities Readiness for Enhanced Spiritual Well-Being related to inner peace and identified purpose to one's life Readiness for Enhanced Family Coping related to common identified goals and open communication
Syndrome Nursing Diagnoses	Impaired Environmental Interpretation Syndrome related to disorientation and confusion Rape-Trauma Syndrome related to sexual assault as evidenced by. . . Relocation Stress Syndrome related to high degree of environmental change secondary to frequent moves

classification system that will incorporate psychiatric nursing diagnoses. Box 10-1 lists nursing diagnoses commonly seen in the psychiatric–mental health clinical setting.

The following are two examples of NANDA nursing diagnoses identified by student nurses who assessed clients in the medical–psychiatric clinical setting:

1. A 52-year-old male was diagnosed with acute heart failure and metabolic acidosis. This man's chief complaint was shortness of breath. History revealed two heart attacks, chronic constipation, and kyphosis. After completion of a psychosocial assessment, the student nurse analyzed the data, which included observations of clinical symptoms of anxiety and verification of the client's statements. The student nurse validated the data with the clinical instructor and consulted a list of defining characteristics for the diagnoses suspected. The student nurse then noted the following nursing diagnoses pertaining to psychosocial needs of the client:
   - Anxiety, moderate level, related to physical condition and hospitalization as evidenced by tremulous voice, increased verbalization with pressured speech, tremors of hands when speaking, and diaphoresis

   - Ineffective Coping related to separation from family and home, change in physical status, and limited mobility
   - Disturbed Sleep Pattern related to anxiety secondary to physical illness as evidenced by the inability to fall asleep
   - Ineffective Sexuality Patterns related to fear and anxiety about sexual functioning secondary to physical illness

2. A 45-year-old female with chronic heart failure and lymphoma was admitted for chemotherapy. Chief complaints included shortness of breath, rapid weight loss, and fatigue. The student collected data regarding the client's emotional response to her medical condition and her ability to cope with the diagnosis of a terminal condition. The student nurse then validated the psychosocial data with the head nurse and asked the client to verify her statements made during the assessment. After the defining characteristics for the nursing diagnoses were confirmed, the following nursing diagnoses were made:
   - Anticipatory Grieving related to terminal condition as evidenced by denial, anger, and the statement "I don't have long to live"
   - Situational Low Self-Esteem due to alterations

BOX 10.1 EXAMPLES OF NURSING DIAGNOSES IN PSYCHIATRIC–MENTAL HEALTH NURSING

- Acute Confusion
- Anticipatory Grieving
- Anxiety
- Bathing/Hygiene Self-Care Deficit
- Decisional Conflict
- Deficient Diversional Activity
- Deficient Knowledge
- Delayed Growth and Development
- Disturbed Body Image
- Disturbed Sleep Pattern
- Dressing/Grooming Self-Care Deficit
- Dysfunctional Grieving
- Fear
- Feeding Self-Care Deficit
- Hopelessness
- Imbalanced Nutrition: Less Than Body Requirements
- Impaired Adjustment
- Impaired Memory
- Impaired Parenting
- Impaired Social Interaction
- Impaired Verbal Communication
- Ineffective Coping
- Ineffective Health Maintenance
- Ineffective Role Performance
- Ineffective Sexuality Patterns
- Interrupted Family Processes
- Noncompliance
- Post-Trauma Syndrome
- Powerlessness
- Relocation Stress Syndrome
- Risk for Injury
- Risk for Loneliness
- Risk for Other-Directed Violence
- Risk for Self-Directed Violence
- Social Isolation
- Spiritual Distress
- Toileting Self-Care Deficit

- Anxiety, acute, related to illness, hospitalization, and separation from spouse as evidenced by increased restlessness, rapid pulse, and increased questioning about illness

Diagnostic and Statistical Manual of Mental Disorders, 4th Edition, Text Revision (DSM-IV-TR)

As discussed in Chapter 2, Standard II of the Standards of Care states that the psychiatric–mental health nurse "analyzes the assessment data in determining nursing diagnoses" (ANA, 2000). Clinical nurse specialists, nurse practitioners, psychiatrists, psychologists, and licensed clinical social workers are often responsible for making a psychiatric diagnosis when a psychiatric problem exists. To ensure consistency and commonality of language, the American Psychiatric Association (APA) has published a multiaxial system of psychiatric disorder classification, the *Diagnostic and Statistical Manual of Mental Disorders, 4th Edition, Text Revision* (**DSM-IV-TR**). This classification is the accepted standard for identifying psychiatric disorders. Insurance companies require a diagnosis using the *DSM-IV-TR* for reimbursement. There are five axes in the classification system, as described briefly in Box 10-2.

The *DSM-IV-TR* is used by clinicians and researchers of many different disciplines in various settings. It also is used to identify and communicate accurate public health statistics (such as the prevalence of a specific psychiatric disorder in the general population including specific culture, age, and gender-related statistics).

Just as the ANA and PMHN association have formed a task force to develop a single nursing classification system, the APA has worked closely with the World Health Organization (WHO), developers of the International

SELF-AWARENESS PROMPT

Making accurate nursing diagnoses takes knowledge and practice. Do you have difficulty differentiating one diagnosis (eg, Disturbed Sleep Pattern) from another (eg, Activity Intolerance)? What resources do you use? Do they present a systematic approach to the organization of data and formulation of a nursing diagnosis?

of body image as evidenced by negative statements about self
- Defensive Coping demonstrated by the increased use of suppression, projection, dissociation, and denial

---

BOX 10.2 *DSM-IV-TR* MULTIAXIAL SYSTEM

Axis I: Clinical Disorders and Other Conditions That May Be a Focus of Clinical Attention

Examples: 293.0: Delirium Due to a General Medical Condition, 300.02: Generalized Anxiety Disorder Schizophrenia, 295.30: Paranoid Type, V15.81: Noncompliance with Treatment, V65.2: Malingering, 313.82: Identity Problem

Axis II: Personality Disorders and Mental Retardation

Examples: 301.83: Borderline Personality Disorder, 301.0: Paranoid Personality Disorder, 317: Mild Mental Retardation, 318.2: Profound Mental Retardation

Axis III: General Medical Conditions (with ICD-9-CM codes)

Examples: 850.9 (ICD-9-CM code): Concussion, 333.1: Medication-Induced Postural Tremor, 428.0 (ICD-9-CM code): Congestive Heart Failure

Axis IV: Psychosocial and Environmental Problems

This axis is for reporting psychosocial and environmental problems that may affect the diagnosis, treatment, and prognosis of mental disorders. The problems are grouped into the following categories: primary support group, social environment, educational, occupational, housing, economic, access to health care services, interaction with the legal system/crime, and other

psychosocial and environmental problems. Examples include a negative life event, an environmental difficulty or deficiency, inadequate social support, or interpersonal stress.

Axis V: Global Assessment of Functioning (GAF)

This axis is for reporting the clinician's judgment of the individual's overall level of functioning. It is useful in planning interventions and measuring outcomes. The clinician is to consider the client's psychological, social, and occupational functioning on a hypothetical continuum of mental health–illness. Impairment in functioning due to physical or environmental limitations is not to be considered. Following are two examples of the continuum coding scale of 0 to 100:

91–100: Superior functioning in a wide range of activities, life's problems never seem to get out of hand, is sought out by others because of his or her many positive qualities. No symptoms. The client's functioning score should be rated between 91 and 100.

41–50: Serious symptoms (eg, suicidal ideation, severe obsessional rituals, frequent shoplifting) or any serious impairment in social, occupational, or school functioning (eg, no friends, unable to keep a job). The client's functioning score should be rated between 41 and 50.

With permission from The American Psychiatric Association. (2000). *Diagnostic and statistical manual of mental disorders* (4th ed., text revision). Washington, DC.

Statistical Classification of Diseases and Related Health Problems (ICD-9-CM and ICD-10), to ensure that both systems are compatible and correspond more closely. For example, ICD codes are used for selected medical conditions and medication-induced disorders included in Axis III (General Medical Conditions) of the *DSM-IV-TR* multiaxial system.

Decision Trees for Differential Diagnoses

The *DSM-IV-TR* presents structured **decision trees** to help the clinician understand the organization and hierarchical structure of the *DSM-IV-TR* classification. Each decision tree guides the clinician through a series of questions to rule in or rule out various disor-

ders. Answers to these questions help the clinician determine whether or not various disorders can be ruled out. However, these questions are not meant to replace actual diagnostic criteria. Rather, they are to assist in the decision-making process. A decision tree has been developed for each of the following categories: disorders due to a general medical condition, substance-induced disorders, psychotic disorders, mood disorders, anxiety disorders, and somatoform disorders.

Outcome Identification

Expected outcomes are measurable client-oriented goals that are realistic in relation to the client's present and potential capabilities. When possible, the nurse, client, significant others, and multidisciplinary team members work together to formulate these outcomes. Also, because the formulation of outcomes involves the client, the nurse and multidisciplinary team members must understand the problems identified by the client and the outcomes the client hopes to achieve. Expected outcomes serve as a record of change in the client's health status (ANA, 2000).

Expected outcomes can be difficult to formulate. Clients with psychiatric–mental health disorders may engage in power struggles or focus on issues seemingly unrelated to identified needs or existing problems. Haas, Sanyer, and White (2001) identify several types of client behavior that could impede the formulation of expected outcomes and affect the nursing plan of care. They include noncompliance, manipulation, demonstration of lack of trust, verbalization of multiple complaints, and increased dependency on caregivers.

Outcomes or measurable client-oriented goals are both short term and long term. They should be clearly stated by the nurse and should describe the expected end result of care. Outcomes are the consequences of a treatment or an intervention.

The outcome statement should be directly related to the nursing diagnosis. For example, an appropriate outcome statement for the nursing diagnosis of Defensive Coping would be: "The client will verbalize the reality of his or her current illness, identifying specific fears and concerns."

Planning

Once the various biopsychosocial needs of the client are identified, the next phase of the nursing process occurs. This phase involves developing a plan of care to guide therapeutic intervention and achieve expected outcomes (Fig. 10-1). The use of resources, alternatives/options, referrals, groups and consultations may be included in the plan of care to assist in treatment and recovery (Dixon, 2003).

Plan of Care

The plan of care, or nursing care plan, is individualized and identifies priorities of care and proposed effective interventions. It includes client education to achieve the stated outcomes. Stating the rationale for the planning and implementation of each nursing intervention is an effective way to help students understand the development of the plan of care. The responsibilities

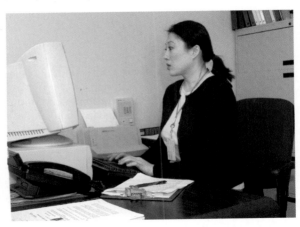

FIGURE 10.1 Nurse developing a plan of care using relevant client data.

of the psychiatric–mental health nurse, client, and multidisciplinary team members are indicated. Team members are allowed access to the plan of care when it is documented, modifying and updating the plan as necessary (ANA, 2000).

A key element of the plan of care is priority setting. Priority setting considers the urgency or seriousness of the problem or need and its impact on the client. Is there a threat to the client's life, dignity, or integrity? Are there problems or needs that negatively affect the client? Do problems exist that affect normal growth and development? Maslow's hierarchy of needs, discussed in Chapter 2, is commonly used as the guide for problem-solving during the formulation of a plan of care. For instance, because of their urgency, physiologic needs such as the stabilization of a comorbid medical condition, as well as the need for safety and security, take precedence over self-esteem and self-actualization needs.

Ideally, while goal setting, the nurse and client mutually discuss and state expected outcomes based on the nursing diagnosis. If the client is actively psychotic and unable to participate in the development of the plan of care, the mental health team formulates a plan for the client.

Remember the following general principles when writing plans of care:

- Individualize or personalize the plan of care according to the nursing diagnosis or problem list. Ask yourself, "If a person who knew nothing about the client read the plan, what would this person learn about the client's needs?"

- Use simple, understandable language to communicate information about the client's care.
- Be specific when stating nursing interventions. State the rationale for each intervention.
- Prioritize nursing care (eg, list nursing interventions for risk for injury or risk of self-harm before those for bathing/hygiene self-care deficit)
- State expected outcomes for each nursing diagnosis. If appropriate, consider both short- and long-term goals.
- Indicate the responsible party or discipline (eg, nursing, activity therapy) for each nursing intervention.

Standardized nursing plans of care are often used in the clinical setting for specific nursing diagnoses such as Anxiety and Fear. These plans summarize current nursing practices and interventions for particular clients according to medical or nursing diagnoses. Expected outcomes are defined (Boyd, 2002). **Concept mapping,** one alternative to the nursing plan of care, offers a method to represent assessment data visually and enhances critical thinking. It enables the nurse to synthesize assessment data, develop comprehensive plans of care focusing on multiple problems, and effectively apply nursing care (Schuster, 2002). **Clinical pathways** map the sequence of the standards of care that are necessary to achieve desired outcomes for a specific disorder or condition (eg, pneumonia) within a particular period of time. **Critical pathways** are plans of care that contain interdisciplinary practice guidelines (eg, for bipolar disorder) with predetermined standards of care (Critical and Clinical Pathways, 2003).

Although clinical and critical pathways were developed to treat medical and surgical disorders or conditions, they are used to plan care for clients with comorbid medical and psychiatric diagnoses. Daily flow charts are used to track a client's clinical symptoms, nursing diagnoses, nursing interventions, and expected outcomes. Other members of the multidisciplinary treatment team can also track their interventions.

Managed care companies use standardized nursing plans of care and clinical pathways to balance quality of care and cost containment. Their intent is to avoid or limit what is perceived to be unnecessary treatment, such as the use of trade-name drugs instead of generic drugs, the request for repetitive laboratory work, and the use of various therapies when the prognosis of the client's illness is limited or poor.

Implementation

During implementation, the nurse uses various skills to put the plan of care into action. Standard V of the Standards of Care describes interventions planned by the psychiatric–mental health nurse. These interventions are categorized based on the nurse's level of education and certification. **Evidence-based nursing practice** is a term used to describe the process by which nurses make clinical decisions (eg, choose nursing interventions) using the best available research evidence, their clinical expertise, and client preferences. Several nursing journals provide evidence-based nursing research data, including *Applied Nursing Research, Clinical Nursing Research, Nursing Research, Evidence Based Nursing,* and *Annual Review of Nursing Research* (University of Minnesota, 2005). The following is a list of interventions used by all nurses in the psychiatric–mental health clinical setting:

- Counseling interventions to help the client improve or regain coping abilities
- Maintenance of a therapeutic environment or milieu
- Structured interventions to foster self-care and mental and physical well-being
- Psychological and biologic interventions to restore the client's health and prevent future disability
- Health education
- Case management
- Interventions to promote mental health and prevent mental illness

The advanced practice psychiatric–mental health nurse provides additional interventions. These include:

- Individual, group, family, and child therapy
- Pharmacologic agent prescription
- Consultation to enhance the abilities of other clinicians to provide services for clients and effect change in the system.

During this stage of the nursing process, the nurse implements care based on nursing theory (see Chapter 3). The psychiatric–mental health nurse commonly faces numerous challenges in delivering care for clients in the psychiatric–mental health setting. Significant changes can occur in a client's mood, affect, behavior, or cognition, often unexpectedly. Additionally, because of the client's condition and psychiatric diagnosis, vigilance is needed to establish trust with the client, promote the client's strengths, and set mutual goals with the client to promote wellness.

Evaluation

The evaluation phase of the nursing process focuses on the client's status, progress toward goal achievement, and ongoing reevaluation of the care plan. Four possible outcomes may occur: (1) the client may respond favorably or as expected to nursing interventions; (2) short-term outcomes (goals) may be met but long-term goals may remain unmet; (3) the client may be unable to meet or achieve any outcomes (goals); or (4) new problems or needs may be identified, requiring the nurse to modify or revise the plan of care. All members of the multidisciplinary treatment team, as well as the client,

should be encouraged to provide feedback regarding the effectiveness of the plan of care. As a result of the evaluation process, the care plan is maintained, modified, or totally revised. A brief sample care plan for a client with the *DSM-IV-TR* diagnosis of Insomnia is shown in Nursing Plan of Care 10-1.

NURSING PLAN OF CARE 10.1

THE CLIENT WITH INSOMNIA RELATED TO DEPRESSED MOOD

Jim, a 58-year-old white male, was seen by the nurse practitioner 2 weeks after the death of his wife. They had been married 30 years and never had any children. Jim's sister and brother-in-law suggested that he tell his primary clinician that he was having difficulty adjusting to the death of his wife. During the visit, Jim confided in the nurse that he had not been sleeping well. His affect was blunted as he stated that he thought he would be the first to die. He informed the nurse that he did not want to take any medication for insomnia or depression but that he was willing to try alternative measures to sleep better at night.

ASSESSMENT: Personal strengths: Employed; college graduate; motivated for treatment; good support system; insightful

Weaknesses: None identified

NURSING DIAGNOSIS: Disturbed Sleep Pattern related to depression as evidenced by difficulty remaining asleep and statement by client that he is not sleeping well

OUTCOME: By the next visit client will report that the time spent in sleeping has improved by 1 to 2 hours.

(Continued on following page)

Planning/Implementation	Rationale
Explore client's present sleep habits	Clients who are depressed may sleep during the day-time and require less sleep at night
Assist the client to determine the desired amount of sleep each night including time to retire and time to rise	Establishing a routine sleep pattern promotes sleep hygiene and deters erratic sleep habits
Provide client with educational material regarding positive behaviors to promote sleep, such as relaxation techniques, reading, warm bath, and so forth	The client has the opportunity to try various techniques to facilitate an effective sleep pattern
Provide client with a sleep diary and ask the client to return in 7 days to evaluate his progress	Keeping a sleep diary allows the client to identify any behaviors or stressors that may interfere with his sleep pattern

EVALUATION: Client kept a sleep diary for 7 days. When he returned in 1 week for a follow-up visit, he stated that he was able to sleep 5 to 6 hours each night. He also stated that he was able to discuss his feelings with his sister and brother-in-law and had decided to attend grief counseling at their church.

KEY CONCEPTS

◆   The nursing diagnosis is a clinical judgment based on analysis of valid data. It provides the basis for selecting appropriate nursing interventions.

◆   Actual, risk, and wellness nursing diagnoses are based on the clinical judgment of the nurse. A syndrome nursing diagnosis is used in reference to a cluster of diagnoses that are predicted to be present because of a certain event or situation. Although the phrase *possible nursing diagnosis* is used when a diagnosis cannot be confirmed, it is not a type of nursing diagnosis.

◆   The NANDA approved a new Taxonomy II in the year 2000. It addresses several domains and includes 167 nursing diagnoses. The psychiatric–mental health nursing diagnostic system is organized around eight human responses. The psychiatric–mental health nursing community has agreed to use the existing NANDA classifications until further integration of the two models occurs.

◆   Clinical nurse specialists, nurse practitioners, psychiatrists, psychologists, and licensed clinical social workers use the *DSM-IV-TR* to make a psychiatric diagnosis when a psychiatric problem exists.

◆   Outcomes are measurable client-oriented goals that are the expected consequences of a treatment or intervention.

◆   The plan of care must be individualized to meet the identified needs of the client, his/her family and/or significant other. The needs are prioritized according to urgency or seriousness of identified problems.

◆   Plans of care may be standardized to achieve desired outcomes for medical, surgical, or psychiatric disorders. Concept mapping enables the nurse to synthesize assessment data, develop comprehensive plans of care focusing on multiple problems, and effectively apply nursing care. Clinical pathways map the sequence of the standards of care necessary to achieve desired outcomes for a specific disorder or condition within a particular period of time. Critical pathways contain interdisciplinary practice guidelines with predetermined standards of care.

◆   Implementation of the nursing plan of care is guided by nursing theory. Delivery of care can be challenging in the psychiatric clinical setting. The nurse may utilize evidence-based nursing practice to determine which nursing interventions would be the most effective for a specific nursing diagnosis.

◆   Four possible outcomes of a plan of care may be identified during the evaluation process. Depending on these outcomes, the plan of care may be maintained, modified, or totally revised.

For additional study materials, please refer to the Student Resource CD-ROM located in the back of this textbook.

CHAPTER WORKSHEET

CRITICAL THINKING QUESTIONS

1. Identify your own level of need attainment according to Maslow's hierarchy of needs. Develop a care plan for yourself, being sure to include short- and long-term goals to promote your growth and development.

2. Every time you take a report from Susan Fowler, RN, you find that her care plans are incomplete and the nursing actions do not seem appropriate for the clients as you assess them. What actions can you take to help the clients, Susan, and yourself?

3. Using a clinical case with which you are familiar, prepare a 10-minute presentation that will help the members of a multidisciplinary treatment team to see the nursing process in action.

4. Develop a plan of care for the client described in the following paragraph, focusing on the client's emotional or psychosocial needs:

> A 50-year-old man complains of chronic low back pain from degenerative disk disease and other somatic symptoms. He alleges that he is disabled and cannot work or pursue his hobbies because of his back pain. This person was divorced approximately 6 years ago at age 44, and described the divorce in great detail during his initial assessment. He refers to himself as a failure, stating, "I never could do anything well enough to please my father and then my marriage ended in divorce. Things never did go right for me. I don't have any friends." He states that he has difficulty falling asleep at night, has lost 18 pounds in the last year, and "does not feel like" eating. He has no social or civic involvements and alleges financial problems because he is receiving only Social Security disability benefits of $637.00 per month. During the interview, his voice became tremulous as he discussed his divorce. He rubbed the arm of the chair incessantly, chain-smoked four cigarettes, and complained of headaches, dizziness, restlessness in his legs, and back pain.

REFLECTION

The chapter opening quote states that making accurate nursing diagnoses takes knowledge and practice. As you developed the plan of care for the client listed in Question 4 of the Critical Thinking Questions, did you have any difficulty arriving at a nursing diagnosis or diagnoses? How did you validate data? How did you classify your nursing diagnoses (eg, actual, risk, wellness, or syndrome diagnosis)?

NCLEX-STYLE QUESTIONS

1. Assessment of a client reveals a long history of alcohol use. The client tells the nurse in the inpatient alcohol treatment unit, "I really don't have a problem with drinking because I drink only on weekends." Which of the following nursing diagnoses would most likely be the priority?
   a. Ineffective Denial
   b. Situational Low Self-Esteem
   c. Acute Confusion
   d. Risk for Injury

2. Which of the following outcomes is most appropriate for the client with a nursing diagnosis of Social Isolation related to inability to trust as evidenced by withdrawal from others?
   a. The client will ask the nurse for permission to be excused from activities.
   b. The client will identify positive qualities in self and others.
   c. The client will state that his or her level of trust in others is improved.
   d. The client will spend time with peers and staff members in unit activities.

3. The multidisciplinary treatment team is developing a plan of care for a client who has been living on the streets for several years. The client has delusions and frequently responds to auditory hallucinations. Which of the following client needs would be the priority?
   a. Self-esteem
   b. Love and belonging
   c. Self-actualization
   d. Physical safety

4. The nurse reviews the psychiatric history of a client with the *DSM-IV-TR* diagnosis of Borderline Personality Disorder. This diagnosis is coded on which of the following diagnostic axes?
   a. Axis I
   b. Axis II
   c. Axis III
   d. Axis IV

5. A client tells the nurse, "I never could do anything well enough to please my mother, and my wife never thought I'd amount to anything before she divorced me." Which of the following would be the priority nursing diagnosis for this client?
   a. Disturbed Thought Processes
   b. Disturbed Body Image
   c. Anxiety
   d. Chronic Low Self-Esteem

6. After presenting a class about nursing interventions applicable to all nurses in psychiatric–mental health clinical settings, which of the following, if stated by the group, would indicate to the presenter that the teaching was successful? Select all that apply.
   a. Counseling to improve client abilities
   b. Maintaining a therapeutic milieu
   c. Prescribing antipsychotic medications
   d. Providing group therapy
   e. Performing health education

Selected References

American Nurses Association. (2000). *Scope and standards of psychiatric–mental health nursing practice*. Washington, DC: American Nurses Publishing.

American Psychiatric Association. (2000). *Diagnostic and statistical manual of mental disorders* (4th ed., text revision). Washington, DC: Author.

Boyd, M. A. (2002). *Psychiatric nursing: Contemporary practice* (2nd ed.). Philadelphia: Lippincott Williams & Wilkins.

Carpenito-Moyet, L. J. (2006). *Handbook of nursing diagnosis* (11th ed.). Philadelphia: Lippincott Williams & Wilkins.

Critical and Clinical Pathways. (2003). Retrieved April 10, 2003, from http://www.nlm.nih.gov/archive/20040829/pubs/cbm/critpath.html

Dixon, M. (2003). Assessing psychosocial needs of psychiatric patients and their families. *Vital Signs, 12*(1), 8.

Haas, L. J., Sanyer, O. M., & White, G. L. (2001). Caring for the frustrating patient. *Clinician, 11*(10), 75–78.

North American Nursing Diagnosis Association. (2006). *Nursing diagnoses: Definitions and classification, 2005-2006.* Philadelphia: Author

Schuster, P. M. (2002). *Concept mapping.* Philadelphia: F. A. Davis.

University of Minnesota. (2005). Evidence based nursing. Retrieved August 12, 2005 from http://evidence.ahc.umn.edu/ebn.htm

Suggested Readings

Duke University School of Nursing. (2005). NANDA. Retrieved August 14, 2005, from http://www.duke.edu/~goodw010/vocab/NANDA.html

Koch, J., & Alverson, E. (2001). Case study in clinical decision-making. *American Journal for Nurse Practitioners, 5*(4), 42–52.

Meszaros, L. (2004). Focus on mental health. Fine-tuning the role of the PCP. *Central Florida M. D. News, 6*(4), 11–13.

Nettina, S. M. (Ed.). (2004). *The Lippincott manual of nursing practice* (8th ed.). Philadelphia: Lippincott Williams & Wilkins.

Schultz, J. M., & Videbeck, S. L. (2004). *Lippincott's manual of psychiatric nursing care plans* (7th ed.). Philadelphia: Lippincott Williams & Wilkins.

University of New Mexico College of Nursing. (2005). Concept map: Developing and implementing concept maps. Retrieved August 12, 2005, from http://hsc.unm.edu/consg/conct/concept%20map.shtml

Verispan. (2005). Vital signs. *Clinical Psychiatry News, 33*(6), 1.

CHAPTER 11 / THERAPEUTIC COMMUNICATION AND RELATIONSHIPS

Listen

When I ask you to listen to me and you start giving advice, you have not done what I asked.

When I ask you to listen to me and you begin to tell me why I shouldn't feel that way, you are trampling on my feelings.

When I ask you to listen to me and you feel you have to do something to solve my problem, you have failed me, strange as that may seem.

Listen! All I asked was that you listen, not talk or do—just hear me.

And I can do for myself; I'm not helpless. Maybe discouraged and faltering, but not helpless.

When you do something for me that I can and need to do for myself, you contribute to my fear and weakness.

But, when you accept as a simple fact that I do feel what I feel, no matter how irrational, then I can quit trying to convince you and can get about the business of understanding what's behind this irrational feeling.

And when that's clear, the answers are obvious and I don't need advice.

So, please listen and just hear me. And, if you want to talk, wait a minute for your turn; and I'll listen for you. —ANONYMOUS

LEARNING OBJECTIVES

AFTER STUDYING THIS CHAPTER, YOU SHOULD BE ABLE TO:

1. Explain the process of communication.
2. Distinguish the factors that influence communication.
3. Describe the importance of assessing nonverbal communication.
4. Articulate the relationship between comfort zones and effective communication skills.
5. Identify factors that contribute to ineffective communication.
6. Compare and contrast social and therapeutic communication.
7. Formulate a list of therapeutic communication techniques.
8. Demonstrate an understanding of the importance of confidentiality in the clinical setting.
9. Develop a sample process recording in the clinical setting.
10. Construct a list of the essential conditions for a therapeutic relationship as described by Carl Rogers.
11. Describe the six subroles of the psychiatric–mental health nurse identified by Hildegard Peplau.

KEY TERMS

Comfort zones
Communication
Countertransference
Nonverbal communication
Parataxic distortion
Process recording
Professional boundaries
Social communication
Therapeutic communication
Therapeutic relationship
Transference

12. Explain the phases of a therapeutic one-to-one relationship.
13. Articulate a list of potential boundary violations that may occur during a therapeutic relationship.

Verbal communication
Zones of distance
  awareness

elationships between psychiatric–mental health nurses and clients are established through communication and interaction. Communication between two human beings can be difficult and challenging. When we communicate, we share significant feelings with those to whom we are relating. If the interaction facilitates growth, development, maturity, improved functioning, or improved coping, it is considered therapeutic (Rogers, 1961). This chapter discusses the psychiatric–mental health nurse's ability to establish a therapeutic relationship with the client using a biopsychosocial approach.

Communication

Communication refers to the giving and receiving of information involving three elements: the sender, the message, and the receiver. The sender prepares or creates a message when a need occurs and sends the message to a receiver or listener, who then decodes it. The receiver may then return a message or feedback to the initiator of the message.

Factors Influencing Communication

Communication is a learned process influenced by a person's attitude, sociocultural or ethnic background, past experiences, knowledge of subject matter, and ability to relate to others. Interpersonal perceptions also affect our ability to communicate because they influence the initiation and response of communication. Such perception occurs through the senses of sight, sound, touch, and smell. Environmental factors that influence communication include time, place, the number of people present, and the noise level (Fig. 11-1).

Attitude

Attitudes are developed in various ways. They may be the result of interaction with the environment; assimilation of others' attitudes; life experiences; intellectual processes; or a traumatic experience. Attitudes can be described as accepting, caring, prejudiced, judgmental, and open or closed minded. An individual with a negative or closed-minded attitude may respond with, "It won't work" or "It's no use trying." Conversely, the individual with a positive or open-minded attitude may state, "Why not try it? We have nothing to lose."

Sociocultural or Ethnic Background

Various cultures and ethnic groups display different communication patterns. For example, some people of French or Italian heritage often are gregarious and talkative, willing to share thoughts and feelings. Some people from Southeast Asian countries such as Thailand or Laos, who often are quiet and reserved, may appear stoic and reluctant to discuss personal feelings with persons outside their families. However, with our "cultural melting pot" society, variations do exist, so generalizations should not be made.

Past Experiences

Previous positive or negative experiences influence one's ability to communicate. For example, teenagers who have been criticized by parents whenever attempting to express any feelings may develop a disturbed self-concept and feel that their opinions are not worthwhile. As a result, they may avoid interacting with others, become indecisive when asked to give an opinion, or agree with others to avoid what they perceive to be criticism or confrontation. Persons with a developmental disability or children may often try to give the expected "correct" response to get approval

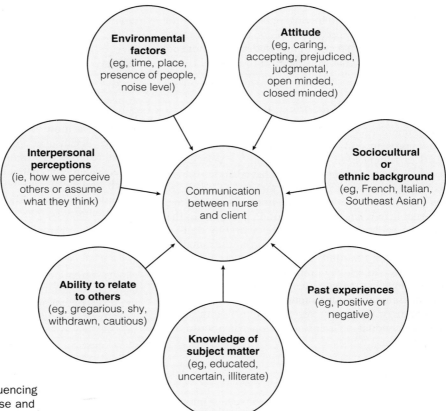

FIGURE 11.1 Factors influencing communication between nurse and client.

from the interviewer, although the answers may in fact not be true or representative of the actual situation.

Knowledge of Subject Matter

A person who is well educated or knowledgeable about certain topics may communicate with others at a high level of understanding. The receiver of the message may be unable to comprehend the message, or consider the sender to be a "know-it-all expert." As a result of this misperception, the receiver, not wanting to appear ignorant, may neglect to ask questions or even nod in agreement and may not receive the correct information.

Ability to Relate to Others

Some people are "natural-born talkers" who claim to have "never met a stranger." Others may possess an intuitive trait that enables them to say the right thing at the right time and relate well to people. "I feel so comfortable talking with her," "She's so easy to relate to," and "I could talk to him for hours" are just a few comments made about people who have the ability to relate well with others. Such an ability can also be a learned process, the result of practicing effective communicative skills over time.

Interpersonal Perceptions

Interpersonal perceptions are mental processes by which intellectual, sensory, and emotional data are organized logically or meaningfully. Satir (1995) warns of looking without seeing, listening without hearing, touching without feeling, moving without awareness, and speaking without meaning. In other words, inattentiveness, disinterest, or lack of use of one's senses during communication can result in distorted perceptions of others. The following passage reinforces the importance of perception: "I know that you believe you understand what you think I said, but I'm not sure you realize that what you heard is not what I said" (Lore, 1981).

Environmental Factors

Environmental factors such as time, place, number of people present, and noise level can influence communication. Timing is important during a conversation. Consider the child who has misbehaved and is told by his mother, "Just wait until your father gets home." By the time the father does arrive home, the child may not be able to relate to him regarding the incident that occurred earlier. Some people prefer to "buy time" to handle a situation involving a personal confrontation. They want time to think things over or "cool off."

The place in which communication occurs, as well as the number of people present and noise level, has a definite influence on interactions. A subway, crowded restaurant, or grocery store would not be a desirable place to conduct a disclosing, serious, or philosophic conversation.

Types of Communication

Communication is the process of conveying information verbally, through the use of words, and nonverbally, through gestures or behaviors that accompany words. Nonverbal communication also can occur in the absence of spoken words.

Verbal Communication

An individual uses **verbal communication** to convey content such as ideas, thoughts, or concepts to one or more listeners. Five levels of interpersonal, verbal communication were discussed in Chapter 2. Open, honest communication occurs in therapeutic relationships when the content of verbal communication is congruent with the speaker's nonverbal behavior (that is, when words match gestures and behaviors). To effectively use verbal communication, one must use the spoken word as a communication tool while being mindful of its potential to affect outcomes. Verbal communication allows us to present ourselves to each other, using words to convey the most com-

plex dimensions of ourselves—aspects that are not obvious from appearance or action (Frazier, 2001).

Nonverbal Communication

As presented in Chapter 9, clients may reveal their emotions, feelings, and mood through their general appearance or their behavior, termed **nonverbal communication.** Nonverbal communication is said to reflect a more accurate description of one's true feelings because people have less control over nonverbal reactions. Vocal cues, gestures, physical appearance, distance or spatial territory, position or posture, touch, and facial expressions are nonverbal communication techniques used in the psychiatric–mental health clinical setting.

Vocal Cues.   Pausing or hesitating while conversing, talking in a tense or flat tone, or speaking tremulously are vocal cues that can agree with or contradict a client's verbal message. Speaking softly may indicate a concern for another, whereas speaking loudly may be the result of feelings of anger or hostility. For example, a person who is admitted to the hospital for emergency surgery may speak softly but tremulously, stating, "I'm okay. I just want to get better and go home as soon as possible." The nonverbal cues should indicate to the nurse that the client is not okay and the client's feelings need to be explored.

Gestures.   Pointing, finger tapping, winking, hand clapping, eyebrow raising, palm rubbing, hand wringing, and beard stroking are examples of nonverbal gestures that communicate various thoughts and feelings. They may betray feelings of insecurity, anxiety, apprehension, power, enthusiasm, eagerness, or genuine interest.

Physical Appearance.   People who are depressed may pay little attention to their appearance. They may appear unkempt and unconsciously don dark-colored clothing, reflecting their depressed feelings. Persons who are confused or disoriented may forget to put on items of clothing, put them on inside out, or dress inappropriately. Weight gain or weight loss also may be a form of nonverbal communication. People who exhibit either may be experiencing a low self-concept or feelings of anxiety, depression, or loneliness. The client with mania may dress in brightly colored clothes with several items of jewelry and excessive make-up. People with a positive self-concept may communicate such a feeling by appearing neat, clean, and well dressed.

BOX 11.1 FOUR ZONES OF DISTANCE AWARENESS OR SPATIAL TERRITORY

Intimate zone: Body contact such as touching, hugging, and wrestling

Personal zone: 1½ to 4 feet; "arm's length"; some body contact such as holding hands; therapeutic communication occurs in this zone

Social zone: 1 to 12 feet; formal business; social discourse

Public zone: 12 to 25 feet: no physical contact; minimal eye contact; people remain strangers

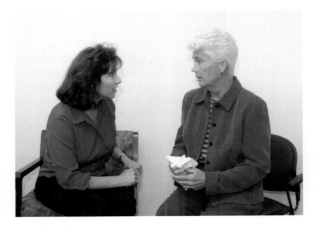

FIGURE 11.2 Nurse communicating at eye level with a client.

Distance or Spatial Territory. Adult, middle-class Americans commonly use four **zones of distance awareness** (Hall, 1990). These four zones include the intimate, personal, social, and public zones (Box 11-1). Actions that involve touching another body, such as lovemaking and wrestling, occur in the intimate zone. The personal zone refers to an arm's length distance of approximately 1½ to 4 feet. Physical contact, such as hand holding, still can occur in this zone. This is the zone in which therapeutic communication occurs. The social zone, in which formal business and social discourse occurs, occupies a space of 4 to 12 feet. The public zone, in which no physical contact and little eye contact occurs, ranges from 12 to 25 feet. People who maintain communication in this zone remain strangers.

Position or Posture. The position one assumes can designate authority, cowardice, boredom, or indifference. For example, a nurse standing at the foot of a client's bed with arms folded across chest gives the impression that the nurse is in charge of any interaction that may occur. A nurse slumped in a chair, doodling on a pad, gives the appearance of boredom. Conversely, a nurse sitting in a chair, leaning forward slightly, and maintaining eye contact with a client gives the impression that the nurse is interested in what the client says or does (Fig. 11-2).

Touch. Reactions to touch depend on age, sex, cultural background, interpretation of the gesture, and appropriateness of the touch. The nurse should always exercise caution when touching people. For example, hand shaking, hugging, holding hands, and kissing typically denote positive feelings for another person. The client with depression or who is grieving may respond to touch as a gesture of concern, whereas the client who is sexually promiscuous may consider touching an invitation to sexual advances. A child suffering from abuse may recoil from the nurse's attempt to comfort, whereas a person who is dying may be comforted by the presence of a nurse sitting by the bedside silently holding his or her hand. A psychotic client may misinterpret touch as a threat or an attack and may react accordingly.

Facial Expression. A blank stare, startled expression, sneer, grimace, and broad smile are examples of facial expressions denoting one's innermost feelings. For example, the client with depression seldom smiles. Clients experiencing dementia often present with apprehensive expressions because of confusion and disorientation. Clients experiencing pain may grimace if they do not receive pain medication or other interventions to reduce their pain.

Social and Therapeutic Communication

Two types of communication—social and therapeutic—may occur when the nurse works with clients or families who seek help for physical or emotional needs. **Social communication** occurs daily as the nurse greets the client and passes the time of day with what is referred to as "small talk." Comments such as "Good morning. It's a beautiful day out," "How are your children?" and "Have you heard any good jokes lately?" are examples of socializing. During a **therapeutic communication,** the nurse helps or encourages the client to communicate perceptions, fears, anxieties, frustrations, expectations, and increased dependency needs. "You look upset. Would you like to share your feelings with someone?" "I'll sit with you until the pain medication takes effect," and "No, it's true that I don't know what it is like to lose a husband, but I would think it would be one of the most painful experiences one might have," are just a few examples of therapeutic communication with clients.

Table 11-1 compares social and therapeutic communication as discussed by Purtilo and Haddad (2002). Purtilo also recommends the following approaches and techniques for nurses participating in a therapeutic interaction:

- Translate any technical information into layperson's terms.
- Clarify and restate any instructions or information given. Clients usually do not ask doctors or nurses to repeat themselves.

- Display a caring attitude.
- Exercise effective listening.
- Do not overload the listener with information.

Additional therapeutic communication techniques, and examples of how a nurse might use them in conversation with a client, are provided in Table 11-2.

Confidentiality During Communication

Client confidentiality is important during nurse–client communication because, as discussed in Chapter 5, the client has a right to privacy. All information concerning the client is considered personal property and is not to be discussed with other clients or outside the hospital setting. When discussing a client (eg, during preclinical or postclinical conference), the client's name and any descriptive information that might identify him or her should not be mentioned. Nurses may find it necessary to reassure a client that confidentiality will be maintained except when the information may be harmful to the client or others and except when the client threatens self-harm. One way to convey this is simply to state, "Only information that will be helpful in assisting you toward recovery will be provided to others on the staff." The nurse has an obligation to share such information with the nursing staff

---

TABLE 11.1   Social Versus Therapeutic Communication

SOCIAL	THERAPEUTIC
Social communication may be referred to as doing a favor for another person, such as lending someone money, taking food to a housebound elderly couple, or giving advice to a young girl who has just broken her engagement.	Therapeutic communication promotes the functional use of one's latent inner resources. Encouraging verbalization of feelings after the death of one's child or exploring ways to cope with increased stress are examples of therapeutic helping.
A personal or intimate relationship occurs.	A personal, but not intimate, relationship occurs.
The identification of needs may not occur.	Needs are identified by the client with the help of the nurse if necessary.
Personal goals may or may not be discussed.	Personal goals are set by the client.
Constructive or destructive dependency may occur.	Constructive dependency, interdependency, and independence, are promoted.
A variety of resources may be used during socialization.	Specialized professional skills are used while employing nursing interventions.

SOURCE: Adapted from Purtilo & Haddad, A.M. (2002). *Health professionals and patient interaction* (2nd ed.). Philadelphia: W.B. Saunders.

TABLE 11.2 Therapeutic Communication Techniques

TECHNIQUES	EXAMPLES
Using silence	
Accepting	Yes. That must have been difficult for you.
Giving recognition or acknowledging	I noticed that you've made your bed.
Offering self	I'll walk with you.
Giving broad openings or asking open-ended questions	Is there something you'd like to do?
Offering general leads or door-openers	Go on. You were saying...
Placing the event in time or in sequence	When did your nervousness begin?
Making observations	I notice that you're trembling. You appear to be angry.
Encouraging description of perceptions	What does the voice seem to be saying? How do you feel when you take your medication?
Encouraging comparison	Has this ever happened before? What does this resemble?
Restating	*Client:* I can't sleep. I stay awake all night. *Nurse:* You can't sleep at night.
Reflecting	*Client:* I think I should take my medication. *Nurse:* You think you should take your medication?
Focusing on specifics	This topic seems worth discussing in more depth. Give me an example of what you mean.
Exploring	Tell me more about your job. Would you describe your responsibilities?
Giving information or informing	His name is... I'm going with you to the beauty shop.
Seeking clarification or clarifying	I'm not sure that I understand what you are trying to say. Please give me more information.
Presenting reality or confronting	I see no elephant in the room. This is a hospital, not a hotel.
Voicing doubt	I find that hard to believe. Did it happen just as you said?
Encouraging evaluation or evaluating	Describe how you feel about taking your medication. Does participating in group therapy enable you to discuss your feelings?
Attempting to translate into feelings or verbalizing the implied	*Client:* I'm empty. *Nurse:* Are you suggesting that you feel useless?
Suggesting collaboration	Perhaps you and your doctor can discuss your home visits and discover what produces your anxiety.
Summarizing	During the past hour we talked about your plans for the future. They include...
Encouraging formulation of a plan of action	If this situation occurs again, what options would you have?
Asking direct questions	How does your wife feel about your hospitalization?

or with the client's doctor. Also, family members should be told that permission must be obtained from clients 18 years of age and older before the attending physician, social worker, or other members of the health care team can discuss the client's progress with them. If the client is younger than 18 years of age, the consent of the legal guardian is required before information can be released.

Effective Therapeutic Communication

To become more effective therapeutic communicators, nurses sometimes must stretch beyond their comfort zones when interacting with clients. **Comfort zones** encompass the way we dress and what we can and cannot do, and have a direct effect on the way we deal with people (Powell, 1995). For example, the communication comfort zone of a student nurse may be limited to interacting with peers or instructors in the classroom or in postclinical conference. Interacting with a mentally ill client on a psychiatric unit might require the student to stretch beyond his or her comfort zone. Box 11-2 provides some guidelines for establishing broader comfort zones for effective therapeutic communication.

Ineffective Therapeutic Communication

Despite the nurse's attempt to use effective therapeutic communication skills, problems or stalls may occur. Unrealistic expectations of the client or nurse, or the

---

BOX 11.2 GUIDELINES FOR ESTABLISHING BROADER COMFORT ZONES FOR EFFECTIVE THERAPEUTIC COMMUNICATION

- **Know yourself:** What motivates your interest in helping others? Identify your emotional needs so that they do not interfere with the ability to relate to others. Be aware of any mood swings that you may exhibit. Clients are sensitive to the emotions and reactions of helping persons. One student stated that at the beginning of a therapeutic interaction, "Mr. Williams asked me what was wrong today. I tried not to show that I had a headache. He said I wasn't my usual cheery self. I'm surprised he realized I wasn't feeling up to par."
- **Be honest with your feelings:** Do not wear a mask to protect yourself or avoid contact with others. Your body language, gestures, and tone of voice can reveal your true feelings or reactions to client behavior. Your nonverbal communication may contradict your spoken words if you are not honest with the client. For example, nurses working with cancer clients often find it difficult relating to terminally ill persons. They may avoid contact as much as possible, so that their emotions are not revealed to the clients when they are asked questions such as, "Will I be getting better?" "Is it cancer?" or "Am I going to die?" It is okay to cry with a terminally ill client who is emotionally upset or depressed.
- **Be secure in your ability to relate to people:** Do not allow the behavior of others to threaten or intimidate you. Remember that all behavior has meaning. Ask yourself, "What is the client trying to communicate?"
- **Be sensitive to the needs of others:** Listen attentively by maintaining eye contact, focusing your attention on the speaker, and assuming a personal

distance of $1\frac{1}{2}$ to 4 feet. Use tact and diplomacy while conversing with others.
- **Be consistent:** To encourage the development of client trust, be consistent in what you say and do.
- **Recognize symptoms of anxiety:** Knowing anxiety when it appears in yourself and those with whom you relate is important. Anxiety impairs communication if the person is unable to concentrate or express feelings (see Chapters 19 and 20 for more information).
- **Watch your nonverbal reactions:** Be aware of your body language because it emphasizes and modifies verbal messages. Use gestures cautiously to emphasize meanings, reactions, or emotions.
- **Use words carefully:** When relating to others, try to use the following words cautiously: I, you, they, it, but, yes, no, always, never, should, and ought. Satir (1995) refers to these words as "powerful words" that may be used thoughtlessly, appear to be accusations, be easily misunderstood, cause confusion or ambivalence, or imply stupidity.
- **Recognize differences:** The fact that people may have cultural, personality, or age differences or have conflicting loyalties can impair communication.
- **Recognize and evaluate your own actions and responses:** When you converse with someone, are you open or closed minded, cooperative or uncooperative, supportive or nonsupportive? Are you available when needed, or do you tend to put someone on hold if you are busy? Instead of cutting a conversation short in the middle of a self-disclosing interaction, refer the client to someone who can be supportive regarding the issue at hand.

maladaptive use of defense mechanisms by the client, can affect the communication process. Other causes of ineffective therapeutic communication include the following:

- *Failure to listen:* Some individuals are doers rather than listeners, focusing on task-oriented nursing instead of therapeutic communication. Also, the client may not hear the message sent, for example because of stress, anxiety, fear, denial, or anger.
- *Conflicting verbal and nonverbal messages:* Ambivalence on the part of the sender may confuse the receiver, who senses conflicting signals that cause doubts about the helping person's interest in him or her.
- *A judgmental attitude:* Someone who displays prejudice or a judgmental attitude when relating to others may never really get to know the person. A sensitive person may pick up on judgmental attitudes and refuse to relate to others, thinking that all people are judgmental.
- *Misunderstanding because of multiple meanings of English words:* The sender should select words that are not confusing in meaning. Consider the word "therapy." It may mean treatment of a disease, rehabilitation, or counseling. The sender needs to specify what meaning he or she intends.
- *False reassurance:* Clichés such as "Everything will be okay" or "Don't worry, the doctor will make you well" are examples of false reassurance. No one can predict or guarantee the outcome of a situation. There are too many variables, such as a person who desires to maintain a sick role, nonsupportive families, or an illness that is irreversible (eg, cancer or multiple sclerosis). Clients who receive false reassurance quickly learn not to trust people if they do not respond to treatment as predicted.
- *Giving of advice:* Giving of advice may facilitate dependency and may also cause the client to feel inadequate because she or he is not given the opportunity to make choices pertaining to personal care. Feelings of dependency and inadequacy may then impair therapeutic communication if the client receives no positive feedback during nurse–client interactions. Encouraging problem-solving and decision-making by the client is more constructive.
- *Disagreement with or criticism of a person who is seeking support:* Belittling a client may result in the development of a low self-concept because the client believes his or her thoughts and feelings are unimportant. Such negative feedback can interfere

with the client's ability to cope with stressors. Any hope of establishing a therapeutic relationship is lost if this occurs. The person may feel unsupported and may not risk divulging further information about himself/herself, for fear of more ridicule.

- *The inability to receive information because of a preoccupied or impaired thought process:* The receiver may be prepared to hear a message different from the one sent. Someone who is preoccupied with thoughts is not as receptive to messages as a person with a clear mind. Impaired thought processes, such as delusions or hallucinations, also interfere with communication. A person who hears voices saying that she or he is being poisoned may not be receptive to a nurse's request to take medication.
- *Changing of the subject if one becomes uncomfortable with the topic being discussed:* For example, during a physical examination, a young female client confides in the nurse that she is unable to have oral sex with her husband. The nurse feels uncomfortable with the topic of oral sex and tells the client that she wants to take her vital signs before her laboratory work is drawn, thus cutting off communication.

The One-to-One Nurse–Client Therapeutic Relationship

A **therapeutic relationship** is a planned and goal-directed communication process between a nurse and a client for the purpose of providing care to the client and the client's family or significant others. An understanding of the factors influencing communication, realization of the importance of nonverbal communication, development of effective communication skills, recognition of the causes of ineffective communication, and ability to participate in a therapeutic communication process provide the foundation for developing a therapeutic relationship with a client.

During the therapeutic relationship, clients might distort their perceptions of others. Therefore, they may relate to the nurse not on the basis of the nurse's realistic attributes, but wholly or chiefly on the basis of interpersonal relationships with important figures (such as parent, sibling, employer) in the client's life. For example, a client exhibits the same attitudes and behaviors toward a male nurse that she originally displayed toward her estranged husband before their separation. This behavior is referred to as **transference** or **parataxic distortion** (Yalom, 1995). **Countertransference** occurs when the nurse responds unrealistically to the client's behavior or interaction. Both can interfere with the development of a therapeutic relationship.

Conditions Essential for a Therapeutic Relationship

According to Rogers (1961), eight conditions are essential for a therapeutic relationship to occur. They include the following:

- *Empathy:* Empathy is the nurse's ability to zero in on the feelings of another person or to "walk in another's shoes."
- *Respect:* The nurse considers the client to be deserving of high regard.
- *Genuineness:* The nurse is sincere, honest, and authentic when interacting with the client.
- *Self-disclosure:* The nurse shares appropriate attitudes, feelings, and beliefs and serves as a role model to the client (but does not force her opinions on the client).
- *Concreteness and specificity:* The nurse identifies the client's feelings by skillful listening and maintains a realistic, not theoretical, response to clinical symptoms.
- *Confrontation:* The nurse uses an accepting, gentle manner after having established a good rapport with the client. The use of confrontation is limited to situations where the nurse–client relationship is well established and can tolerate this strong method, which may otherwise be considered threatening by the client.

- *Immediacy of relationship:* The nurse shares spontaneous feelings when he or she believes the client will benefit from such a discussion.
- *Client self-exploration:* The nurse encourages the client to learn positive adaptive or coping skills.

Boundaries of Therapeutic Relationships

The foundation of a nurse–client therapeutic relationship is based on trust and respect for the dignity and worth of the client. **Professional boundaries** are limits that protect the space between the professional nurse's power and the client's vulnerability in a therapeutic relationship. They separate therapeutic behavior of the registered nurse from any behavior that, well intentioned or not, could diminish the benefit of care to clients, families, significant others, or communities. Furthermore, professional boundaries provide security, order, and safe connections based on client need. (Peterson, 1992; Waite, 2004). A relationship becomes unacceptable, and a boundary violation occurs, with infringement on a client's therapeutic needs or basic rights. The nurse is responsible for maintaining professional boundaries; to act as a client advocate; and to intervene, when appropriate, to prevent or stop boundary violations (Nurses Board of South Australia, 2002). Examples of professional boundary violations are included in Box 11-3.

BOX 11.3 EXAMPLES OF PROFESSIONAL BOUNDARY VIOLATIONS

- Keeping secrets with a client
- Spending free time with a client
- Sharing personal, intimate information with a client
- Discussing work concerns with a client
- Displaying favoritism toward one client at the expense of others
- Socializing with a client during an ongoing therapeutic relationship
- Allowing a client to perform personal tasks for nursing personnel
- Giving personalized gifts to a client
- Receiving personalized gifts from a client or his or her family member or significant other

Roles of the Psychiatric–Mental Health Nurse in a Therapeutic Relationship

According to psychiatrist Harry Stack Sullivan (1968), all personal growth, personal damage, and regression, as well as personal healing, are a result of our relationships with others. Peplau (1952) incorporated Sullivan's concepts of interpersonal relationships into her interpersonal theory, part of which describes the subroles of the psychiatric nurse. The six subroles of the psychiatric nurse during a therapeutic relationship are as follows:

- Nurse-teacher: The nurse-teacher educates clients about specific illnesses and medication prescribed to promote stabilization of their condition.
- Mother surrogate: The nurturing needs of clients who are unable to carry out simple tasks are met by the subrole of the mother surrogate.
- Technical nurse: The technical nurse usually completes vital signs checks, medical or surgical treatment procedures, administration of medication, and physical assessment.
- Nurse-manager: The nurse-manager is responsible for creating a therapeutic environment in which clients feel safe and accepted.
- Socializing agent: Social skills, such as interacting with others in a group setting, are promoted by the nurse who acts as a socializing agent.
- Counselor or nurse-therapist: The counselor or nurse-therapist uses therapeutic skills to help clients identify and deal with stressors or problems that have resulted in dysfunctional coping.

The nurse can assume any of these roles at various times during the nurse-client relationship.

Phases of a Therapeutic Relationship

As part of her interpersonal theory, Peplau (1952) described the phases, also referred to as stages, of one-to-one nurse-client therapeutic relationships established in psychiatric-mental health nursing, applicable for use in both inpatient and outpatient settings. Such relationships can be divided into three phases: initiating or orienting, working, and terminating. Each phase is associated with specific therapeutic tasks or goals to be accomplished.

Initiating or Orienting Phase

The first step of the therapeutic relationship is called the *initiating* or *orienting phase.* During this phase, the nurse sets the stage for a one-to-one relationship by becoming acquainted with the client. The nurse also begins the assessment process. The nurse and client may experience anxiety with this first meeting. When initiating the relationship, a comment such as "Sometimes it's hard to talk to a stranger" may be an effective starting point for a discussion.

Communication styles of the nurse and client are explored to facilitate rapport and open communication as the client begins to share feelings and conflicts. The client must feel accepted as she or he begins to develop trust with the nurse. This feeling of acceptance and trust should set the pace of the relationship. The client is a unique person who is ill and may be experiencing feelings of loneliness, fear, anger, disgust, despair, or rejection. As a client, the person seeks comfort and help in handling stressors. In doing so, the client accepts another's assistance in problem-solving or goal-setting. Therapeutic tasks accomplished by the psychiatric-mental health nurse during the initiating phase include:

1. Building trust and rapport by demonstrating acceptance
2. Establishing a therapeutic environment, ensuring safety and privacy
3. Establishing a mode of communication acceptable to both client and nurse
4. Initiating a therapeutic contract by establishing a time, place, and duration for each meeting, as well as the length of time the relationship will be in effect
5. Assessing the client's needs, coping strategies, defense mechanisms, strengths and weaknesses

Working Phase

The second phase of the therapeutic relationship is known as the *working* (or *middle*) *phase*. The client begins to relax, trusts the nurse, and is able to discuss mutually agreed-on goals with the nurse as the assessment process continues and a plan of care develops. Perceptions of reality, coping mechanisms, and support systems are identified at this time. Alternate behaviors and techniques are explored to replace those that are maladaptive. The nurse and client discuss the meaning behind such behavior, as well as any reactions by the nurse such as fear, intimidation, embarrassment, or anger. During the working phase, the client focuses on unpleasant, painful aspects of life while the nurse provides support. Therapeutic tasks accomplished by the psychiatric–mental health nurse during the working phase include:

1. Exploring client's perception of reality and providing constructive feedback
2. Helping client develop positive coping behaviors
3. Identifying available support systems
4. Promoting a positive self-concept by focusing on what the client can do and not what the client cannot do
5. Encouraging verbalization of feelings
6. Promoting client independence by teaching new skills
7. Developing a plan of action with realistic goals
8. Implementing the plan of action
9. Evaluating the results of the plan of action

Terminating Phase

The final step of the therapeutic relationship is the *terminating phase*. The nurse terminates the relationship when the mutually agreed-on goals are reached, the client is transferred or discharged, or the nurse has finished the clinical rotation. The nurse discusses the termination phase with the client, encourages the client to identify the progress that the client has made, and explores the necessity of any referrals that may be of benefit to the client. As separation occurs, clients commonly exhibit regressive behavior, demonstrate hostility, or experience sadness. The client may attempt to prolong the relationship as clinical symptoms of separation anxiety are experienced. However, termination needs to occur if a therapeutic relationship is to be a complete process. Preparation for termination actually begins during the initiating phase. Mutually accepted goals resulting in the termination of a therapeutic relationship include the client's ability to:

1. Provide self-care and maintain his or her environment
2. Demonstrate independence and work interdependently with others
3. Cope positively when experiencing feelings such as anxiety, anger, or hostility
4. Demonstrate emotional stability
5. Identify the progress the client has made

Utilizing Therapeutic Interactions With Difficult Clients

Dealing with clients who are angry, manipulative, suspicious, demanding, uncooperative, or who display escalating behavior is a part of the job that all nurses must endure at one time or another. McCabe-Maucher (2005), a nurse and licensed psychotherapist, discusses several useful communication strategies that the student can use when interacting with clients who display difficult behaviors during an interaction. Summarized, they state that the nurse:

1. Shouldn't take the client's words personally. The client is probably not angry with the nurse but rather reacting to a stressful situation.
2. Should validate the client's emotions. Acknowledging the client's feelings can have a calming effect on his or her tirade.
3. Speak slowly in a soft, low voice. Humans tend to mirror one another's behavior.
4. Maintain a safe physical distance from the client. Advancing forward in the direction of the client may be viewed as provocative and can instigate unpredictable behavior.
5. Ask simple questions such as, "How can I help you?" Such an approach may diffuse a tense situation.
6. Appear confident and speak in a firm yet amicable tone to maintain control of the situation. Don't hesitate to ask for assistance from other personnel.
7. Be familiar with the facility's emergency plan and do not hesitate to employ it if the situation warrants serious action.

Graber and Mitcham (2002) interviewed several nurses in a study, Spirituality in the Lives of Compassionate Clinicians Working in Hospitals, funded by the Fetzer Institute. One aim of the study, considered to be the most important one, was to determine how the most caring and compassionate nurses and other clinicians communicated with hospitalized clients, including difficult patients. Graber and Mitcham concluded that nurses who were sensitive to the needs of the clients, displayed confidence and empathy, and demonstrated a high degree of emotional intelligence were able to interact therapeutically with the clients. Therapeutic interactions and interventions for clients who exhibit difficult behavior are addressed in several of the disorder chapters.

Process Recording

A **process recording** is a tool used in various formats to analyze nurse–client communication. The tool, which focuses on verbal and nonverbal communication, is used to teach communication skills to student nurses in the clinical setting. Student–client role-play situations are one method used to familiarize students with the process recording. Interview guidelines may be given explaining how to intervene with a client who gets up and leaves during an interview; what to do if another client interrupts the interaction; what to do if a client asks the student to keep a secret; and why a student should not write the interactions verbatim during the interview. The process recording format displayed in Box 11-4 has been used successfully in an associate's degree program; Box 11-5 contains an example of a process recording by a second-year associate's degree student during her clinical rotation on a medical floor in a general hospital. Although the client in this scenario was diagnosed as having acute low

---

BOX 11.4 PROCESS RECORDING FORMAT

Client's initials:

Age:

Nursing diagnosis:

Goal of interaction: State your goal.

Description of environment: Give a visual description of the setting in which the conversation took place, including noise level and odors.

Appearance of the client: Give a description of the client's physical appearance.

Verbal communication: State the communication verbatim, including what the client states and your responses. List in sequential order and identify therapeutic and nontherapeutic techniques used during the conversation. Identify any defense mechanisms used by the client.

Nonverbal communication: Include your thoughts and feelings, as well as any facial expressions, gestures, position changes, or changes in eye contact, voice quality, and voice tone by the client or yourself.

Evaluation of interaction: Discuss whether the goal was met. What changes would you make, if any, after evaluating this interaction?

---

back pain, the staff had observed symptoms of anxiety and suggested that the student and client would both benefit from the assignment.

BOX 11.5 EXAMPLE OF PROCESS RECORDING

Client's initials: JW

Age: 33

Nursing diagnosis: Anxiety related to hospitalization, limited mobility, and pain

Goal of interaction: To explore coping skills to reduce anxiety

Description of environment: A private room at the end of the corridor with no offensive odors or disturbing noises. The room was rather bare, with no evidence of get-well cards, pictures, or plants. The lights were turned off and the curtains were drawn

Appearance of client: The client was dressed in a hospital gown and was found lying with his back to the door as I entered the room.

(Continued on following page)

BOX 11.5	EXAMPLE OF PROCESS RECORDING *(Continued)*	

STUDENT	CLIENT	INTERPRETATION
"Good morning. My name is.... I will be your nurse for this morning." (Smiling; speaking softly; gazing directly at JW while walking to the side of the bed.) a. Giving recognition b. Giving information c. Offering self	"Oh. How long will you be here?" (Turns over in bed and briefly gazes at me with a blank facial expression; speaks in a low voice.)	Client doesn't want to be bothered. Client may be in pain. Client is uncertain about my capabilities.
"I'll be here until 1:30. I understand you are having back pain. Could you describe the pain to me?" a. Giving information b. Encouraging description of perception	"It started as I moved a chair in my living room." (Maintains eye contact and grimaces as he moves.)	Client appears to have difficulty with mobility. Client may not wish to interact at this time.
"Tell me about the pain." (Maintaining eye contact while sitting in chair beside his bed.) a. Exploring b. Active listening	"It's a sharp, stabbing pain that occurs whenever I move from side to side or try to get up and walk." (Facial expression is more relaxed with less grimacing.)	Client is responding to individual attention.
	"It also bothers me when I have a lot on my mind, like problems at home."	Client is beginning to disclose his feelings.
	"I've never had a back injury."	
	"My doctor told me I should see a counselor because it could be due to my nerves."	
"How do you feel about your doctor's recommendation?" (Maintaining eye contact; sitting.) a. Encouraging description of perceptions	"I guess he knows what he is doing." (Breaks eye contact; fingers sheets nervously.)	Client is becoming uncomfortable with the conversation.
"Perhaps you and the counseler can discover the cause of your back pain? Then you'll be able to prevent future hospitalizations." a. Suggesting collaboration	"I hope so. I can't afford to miss any more work." (Became more relaxed. Eye contact improved.)	Client appears to be relieved that he will be able to discuss his feelings with a counselor and possibly avoid hospitalization in the future.

Evaluation: JW is willing to undergo counseling at the suggestion of his family doctor to identify the cause of recurrent back pain. I feel that this interaction was effective because it showed JW that I cared about him as a person and displayed an active interest in his physical condition.

KEY CONCEPTS

◆ Communication is a learned process influenced by a variety of factors.

◆ Nonverbal communication reflects a more accurate description of emotions, feelings, and mood because people have less control over nonverbal reactions.

◆ Individual comfort zones directly affect the way people relate to others, possibly limiting one's ability to be an effective communicator.

◆ Communication is described as social or therapeutic depending on what occurs between the client and nurse. Therapeutic communication promotes the functional use of one's latent inner resources, whereas social communication occurs on a superficial level.

◆ Ineffective therapeutic communication or stalls can occur as a result of several factors including, but not limited to, unrealistic expectations of the client and nurse, the presence of impaired cognition, or the maladaptive use of defense mechanisms.

◆ Information concerning a client is considered to be the personal property of the client and is to be kept confidential, unless the client threatens self-harm or the information presented by the client poses a threat to the safety of the client or others.

◆ The psychiatric–mental health nurse is responsible for maintaining professional boundaries with the client during a therapeutic relationship and for intervening, when appropriate, to prevent or to stop actual boundary violations.

◆ Peplau described six subroles assumed by the psychiatric–mental health nurse during a therapeutic relationship, depending on the needs of the client: teacher, mother surrogate, technical nurse, manager, socializing agent, and counselor or nurse–therapist.

◆ Three phases of a therapeutic relationship were identified by Peplau: the initiating or orienting phase, during which the nurse assesses the client and initiates a relationship; the working phase, during which trust develops as the assessment process continues and a plan of care is developed; and the terminating phase that occurs when mutually agreed-on goals are reached or termination is necessary for other reasons.

◆ The process recording is used in the clinical setting as a teaching tool. Nonverbal and verbal communication, defense mechanisms, and therapeutic techniques are documented by the student nurse, who, with the instructor, analyzes the nurse–client interaction.

For additional study materials, please refer to the Student Resource CD-ROM located in the back of this textbook.

 ## CHAPTER WORKSHEET

CRITICAL THINKING QUESTIONS

1. Imagine that you enter a client's room and find her crying quietly. She looks up and tells you that her doctor has just announced that she needs surgery. Construct an imaginary conversation in which you encourage her to explore her fears, anxieties, and feelings, using Purtilo's and Rogers' essentials of therapeutic communication.

2. Discuss with other nurses the three phases of the one-to-one nurse–client relationship described by Peplau. Ask them to share experiences with clients in which they have and have not been able to accomplish the appropriate goals of each phase. Analyze these therapeutic interactions and reflect on strategies for improving them.

3. After studying your own use of therapeutic techniques, you realize that you are reluctant to give information and ask direct questions. How would you go about improving your use of these techniques?

REFLECTION

Reflect on the quote at the beginning of the chapter. Do any of the statements apply to you? If so, which ones? What actions can you take to improve your listening skills?

NCLEX-STYLE QUESTIONS

1. The nurse pays close attention to the client's nonverbal communication based on an understanding of which of the following?

    a. Clients have a tendency to tell the nurse what is expected.

b. Nonverbal communication may more accurately reflect the client's feelings than his or her verbal communication does.

c. Nonverbal communication provides the nurse with complete assessment.

d. Verbal communication may be misinterpreted.

2. The nurse tells a client who expresses concern about the ability to solve her problems, "I'm sure you'll do the right thing." Which of the following provides the best analysis of the nurse's response to the client?

   a. The response allows the client to move toward independence.

   b. Such a response gives the nurse more time to think about the situation.

   c. The response provides the client with support and encouragement.

   d. This type of response represents an example of false reassurance.

3. The client states, "I'm not sure what to do. What do you think would be best?" The nurse refrains from giving advice for which of the following reasons?

   a. Advice may be more appropriate if it comes from the physician.

   b. The client is only testing the nurse's ability as a helping person.

   c. The nurse may not be aware of the client's options.

   d. It is more useful to encourage client problem-solving.

4. During the initial phase of the nurse–client relationship, which of the following should occur?

   a. Encouraging verbalization of feelings

   b. Establishing therapeutic contract

   c. Exploring alternate behaviors

   d. Evaluating plan of action

5. The nurse works with a group of clients in a partial hospitalization program on behaviors appropriate for a job interview. According to Peplau, the nurse is functioning in which of the following roles?

   a. Counselor

   b. Socializing agent

   c. Surrogate parent

   d. Teacher

6. When reviewing a student's process recording, the instructor evaluates the interaction for the use of therapeutic techniques. Which of the following statements reflects the use of therapeutic communication techniques? Select all that apply.

   a. "You really should stop smoking all the time."

   b. "I notice that you are trembling."

   c. "You seem to be angry right now."

   d. "Don't worry, the doctors know what to do."

   e. "If you're Superman, go ahead and fly away."

   f. "Would you describe how you take your medications?"

Selected References

Frazier, L. (2001). Getting your word's worth: The spoken word as a health intervention. *ADVANCE for Nurse Practitioners, 9*(5), 73–77.

Graber, D. R., & Mitcham, M. (2002). Caring and communication. *ADVANCE for Nurses, 3*(23), 19–20.

Hall, E. (1990). *The hidden dimension.* New York: Doubleday.

Lore, A. (1981). *Effective therapeutic communication.* Bowie, MD: Robert J. Brady.

McCabe-Maucher, A. (2005). Managing angry patients. *ADVANCE Online Editions for Nurses.* Retrieved January 7, 2005, from http://nursing.advanceweb.com/common/Editorial

Nurses Board of South Australia. (2002). Standard for therapeutic relationships and professional boundaries. Retrieved August 1, 2005, from http://www.nursesboard.sa.gov.au/word/standards_ther_rel_prof_boundaries.doc

Peplau, H. (1952). *Interpersonal relations in nursing.* New York: Putnam.

Peterson, M. (1992). *At personal risk: Boundary violations in professional-client relationships.* New York: W. W. Norton and Company.

Powell, J. (1995). *Will the real me please stand up? 25 guidelines for good communication,* Allen, TX: Resources for Christian Living.

Purtilo, R., & Haddad, A. M. (2002). *Health professionals/patient interaction* (2nd ed.). Philadelphia: W. B. Saunders.

Rogers, C. (1961). *On becoming a person.* Boston: Houghton Mifflin.

Satir, V. (1995). *Making contact.* Berkeley, CA: Celestial Arts.

Sullivan, H. S. (1968). *The interpersonal theory of psychiatry.* New York: W. W. Norton & Co.

Yalom, I. D. (1995). *The theory and practice of group psychotherapy.* New York: Basic Books.

Waite, R. (2004). Maintaining boundaries. *ADVANCE for Nurses, 5*(14), 25–26.

Suggested Readings

Baker, S. K. (2001). Difficult people. *ADVANCE for Nurses, 2*(9), 25-26.

Carpenito-Moyet, L. J. (2006). *Handbook of nursing diagnosis* (11th ed.). Philadelphia: Lippincott Williams & Wilkins.

College of Registered Nurses of Manitoba. (2002). Professional boundaries for therapeutic relationships. Retrieved August 1, 2005, from http://www.crnm.mb.ca/boundary.htm

Cox, R. P. (1998). IPRs revisited: Using process recordings to develop nursing students' critical thinking skills. *Journal of Nursing Education, 37*(1), 37-41.

Forchuk, C., Westwell, J., McMartin, W., Bamki-Azzapardi, W., Kosterewa, D., & Hux, M. (2000). The developing nurse-client relationship. *Journal of American Psychiatric Nurses Association, 6*(1), 3-10.

Peternelj-Taylor, C. (2002). Professional boundaries. A matter of therapeutic integrity. *Journal of Psychosocial Nursing Mental Health Services, 40*(4), 22-29.

*The **therapeutic milieu** is an environment that is structured and maintained as an ideal, dynamic setting in which to work with clients. This milieu includes safe physical surroundings, all treatment team members, and other clients.* —SCHULTZ & VIDEBECK, 2005

LEARNING OBJECTIVES

AFTER STUDYING THIS CHAPTER, YOU SHOULD BE ABLE TO:

1. Define *milieu therapy*.
2. Articulate the standards for a therapeutic milieu or environment as set forth by Joint Commission on Accreditation of Healthcare Organizations (JCAHO).
3. Identify participants in the therapeutic milieu or environment.
4. Discuss the role of the psychiatric–mental health nurse in the therapeutic milieu or environment.
5. Describe the components of the therapeutic milieu or environment.
6. Formulate a list of educational strategies to promote client education.
7. Explain the importance of providing interventions to meet a client's spiritual needs.
8. Develop a list of nursing interventions to promote an optimal balance of rest and activity.
9. Articulate the rationale for pain management in the therapeutic milieu or environment.
10. Explain the rationale for the use of seclusion and restraints.
11. Describe examples of behavior therapy techniques.
12. Identify clients who would benefit from participation in occupational, educational, art, music, or recreational therapy.

KEY TERMS

Activities of daily living
Assertiveness training
Aversion therapy
Behavior therapy
Cognitive behavior therapy
Flooding
Implosive therapy
Limit-setting
Milieu therapy
Pavlov's Theory of Conditioning
Protective nursing care
Skinner's Theory of Operant Conditioning
Sleep pattern disturbance
Systematic desensitization
Therapeutic lifestyle change counseling (TLC)
Therapeutic milieu
Ward Atmosphere Scale (WAS)

Milieu therapy refers to socioenvironmental therapy in which the attitudes and behavior of the staff in a treatment service and the activities prescribed for the client are determined by the client's emotional and interpersonal needs (Shahrokh & Hales, 2003). The environment in which the treatment service is delivered is referred to as the therapeutic milieu. It is structured to control, stabilize, and improve problematic emotions and behavior and enables the client to use problem-solving skills to cope with self, others, and environmental stressors. Milieu therapy promotes personal growth and client interactions. The focus is on social relationships as well as occupational and recreational activities. Deinstitutionalization, the use of psychotropic agents, respect for client rights, creation of the multidisciplinary treatment team, and the use of therapeutic groups have contributed to the development of a therapeutic milieu or environment for individuals with psychiatric–mental health disorders.

This chapter describes the development of the therapeutic milieu, including the criteria for establishing it. It also highlights the components involved including the participants and specific interventions used in a therapeutic milieu. Finally, the chapter discusses the need for evaluating the therapeutic milieu to determine its effectiveness for psychiatric–mental health disorders.

Development of the Therapeutic Milieu

As noted in the opening quote for this chapter, therapeutic milieu refers to an environment that is structured to provide clients with the opportunity to interact with staff and other clients. It developed as a result of Henry Stack Sullivan's belief that interactions among clients are beneficial because clients have the opportunity to practice interpersonal relationship skills, provide feedback to peers about behavior, and work together to develop problem-solving skills (Sullivan, 1968).

A therapeutic milieu can exist in a variety of settings. Clients with psychiatric–mental health disorders may be treated in the hospital, the community, at home, or in private practice of a counselor or therapist.

The term *therapeutic milieu* has often been used interchangeably with *therapeutic environment*. It has also been used to describe contemporary treatment settings in which the biopsychosocial needs of individuals such as the terminally or chronically ill, victims of abuse, children with medical problems, and elderly clients are met. Examples include hospice programs, safe houses, Ronald McDonald Houses, halfway houses, geriatric residential treatment centers, and respite programs. Each of these programs provide individualized milieu therapy for clients and their families and/or significant others.

Regardless of the therapeutic milieu setting, certain criteria must be met to help clients develop a sense of self-esteem and personal worth, feel secure, establish trust, improve their ability to relate to others, and return to the community. The Joint Commission on Accreditation of Healthcare Organizations (JCAHO) has set forth a comprehensive list of standards as a guide in the development of a therapeutic milieu. These standards serve as criteria for JCAHO accreditation surveys. These standards are reflected in the criteria listed in Box 12-1.

Components of a Therapeutic Milieu

Today, as noted earlier in the text, inpatient stays are often limited to crisis stabilization unless a client has a diagnosis of serious and persistent mental illness (Chapter 35) and do not allow clients time to develop meaningful relationships. As a result of this change in the health care environment and health care delivery system, psychiatric nursing is moving toward noninstitutional care with an emphasis on outpatient functions and small treatment units. The components of a therapeutic milieu that were originally provided in psychiatric institutions have been incorporated into community mental health settings (Chapter 8). This movement has resulted in nurses working collaboratively and cooperatively with clients, clients' families, each other, and other health care providers in order to provide safe, competent, ethical care that will benefit clients. Collaboration is also needed to ensure the client's need for accessible, affordable health care is met.

BOX 12.1 CRITERIA FOR ESTABLISHING A THERAPEUTIC MILIEU

The therapeutic milieu should:

- be purposeful and planned to provide safety from physical danger and emotional trauma. It should have furniture to facilitate a homelike atmosphere. Provisions for privacy and physical needs are necessary.
- promote interaction and communication among clients and personnel and provide safety from emotional trauma.
- provide a testing ground for new patterns of behavior while clients take responsibility for their actions. Behavioral expectations—including the existing rules, regulations, and policies—should be explained to clients.
- provide for consistent limit-setting. This criterion reflects aspects of a democratic society. All clients are treated as equally as possible with respect to restrictions, rules, and policies.
- encourage participation in group activities and free-

flowing communication in which clients are free to express themselves in a socially acceptable manner.
- provide for client respect and dignity. Adult–adult interactions should prevail when appropriate, promoting equal status among the parties involved, exchange of interpersonal information, and avoidance of any "power plays." Clients should be encouraged to use personal resources to resolve problems or conflicts.
- convey an attitude of overall acceptance and optimism. Conflict among staff members must be handled and resolved in some manner to maintain a therapeutic milieu. Clients are perceptive of such reactions and may feel that they are the cause of conflicts among personnel.
- allow for continual assessment and evaluation of clients' progress, with modifications in treatment and nursing interventions as needed.

Participants in the Therapeutic Milieu

Members of several disciplines collaborate in the promotion of a therapeutic milieu. Referred to as the *psychiatric multidisciplinary treatment team,* members include psychiatric–mental health nurses; psychiatric nurse assistants or technicians; psychiatrists; clinical psychologists; psychiatric social workers; occupational, educational, art, musical, psychodrama, recreational, play, pet, and speech therapists; chaplains; dietitians; and auxiliary personnel. Table 12-1 presents a summary of these roles. The psychiatric–mental health nurse assumes responsibility for the management and coordination of activities in the milieu. Due to budgetary constraints, the occupational therapist or the recreational therapist often may serve as the music and art therapist, especially in smaller, privately owned, or community-based hospitals.

The multidisciplinary treatment team participates in regularly scheduled meetings to allow team members to discuss the client's progress and to review the client's individualized plan of care. Clients and their family members, significant others, and support persons are invited to participate in these meetings (Fig. 12-1). Treatment methods have evolved from passive, isolated ones to methods that emphasize interaction

and cooperation. Clients and their families or significant others who attend the meetings are able to participate in planning and problem-solving. Their input is encouraged as clients develop positive coping skills and are empowered to demonstrate accountability and responsibility in interdependent relationships.

Interventions Used in the Therapeutic Milieu

Various interventions can be used in the therapeutic milieu in either the inpatient or outpatient setting. Interventions that meet the basic needs of the client in the psychiatric–mental health setting are addressed here. Interactive therapies such as crisis intervention, individual and group therapy, and family therapy, as well as special treatment modalities such as psychopharmacology, electroconvulsive therapy, and alternative therapies, are discussed in Chapters 13 through 18 of this text.

Client Education

Client education, also referred to as *sharing information,* promotes self-care and independence, prevents complications, and reduces recidivism and hospital readmissions. As Gallagher and Zeind (1998, p.16aaa)

TABLE 12.1 Multidisciplinary Treatment Team

DISCIPLINE	DESCRIPTION
Psychiatric nurse	A registered nurse specializing in psychiatric nursing by employing theories of human behavior and the therapeutic use of self. Gives holistic nursing care by assessing the client's mental, psychological, and social status. Provides a safe environment, works with clients dealing with everyday problems, provides leadership, and assumes the role of client advocate. Nurses with master's degree, clinical specialty, or certification in psychiatric–mental health nursing; conducts individual, family, or group therapy. In certain states, the nurse practitioner is granted prescriptive privileges.
Psychiatric nurse assistant or technician	High school graduate who receives in-service education pertaining to the job description. Assists the mental health team in maintaining a therapeutic environment, providing care, and supervising client activities.
Psychiatrist	Licensed physician with at least 3 years of residency training in psychiatry, including 2 years of clinical psychiatric practice. Conducts therapy sessions and serves as leader of the multidisciplinary treatment team. Prescribes medication and somatic treatment. Specializes in the diagnosis, treatment, and prevention of mental and emotional disorders.
Clinical psychologist	Person with doctoral degree in clinical psychology, who is licensed by state law and a psychology internship (supervised work experience). Provides a wide range of services, from diagnostic testing, interpretation, evaluation, and consultation to research. May treat clients individually or in a group therapy setting.
Psychiatric social worker	College graduate with a baccalaureate, master's, or doctoral degree. Uses community resources and adaptive capacities of individuals and groups to facilitate positive interactions with the environment. Conducts the intake interview; family assessment; individual, family, and group therapy; discharge planning; and community referrals.
Occupational therapist	College graduate with a baccalaureate or master's degree in occupational therapy. Uses creative techniques and purposeful activities, as well as therapeutic relationship, to alter the course of an illness. Assists with discharge planning and rehabilitation, focusing on vocational skills and activities of daily living to raise self-esteem and promote independence.
Educational therapist	College graduate who specializes in educational therapy. Determines effective instructional methods, assessing the person's capabilities and selecting specialized programs to promote these capabilities. May include remedial classes, special education for "maladjusted" children, or continuing education for hospitalized students with emotional or behavioral problems (eg, anorexia nervosa, depression, or substance abuse).
Art therapist	College graduate with a master's degree and specialized training in art therapy. Encourages spontaneous creative artwork to express feelings of emotional conflicts. Assists the client in analyzing expressive work. Uses basic child psychiatry to diagnose and treat emotional or behavioral problems. Attention is paid to the use of colors as well as symbolic or real-life figures and settings.
Musical therapist	College graduate with a master's degree and training in music therapy. Focuses on the expression of self through music such as singing, dancing, playing an instrument, or composing songs and writing lyrics. Music therapy promotes improvement in memory, attention span, and concentration and provides an opportunity for one to take pride in one's achievement.
Psychodrama therapist	College graduate with advanced degree and training in group therapy. This therapy is also referred to as role-playing therapy. People are encouraged to act out their emotional problems through dramatization and role playing. This type of therapy is excellent for children, adolescents, and people with marital or family problems. The therapist helps the people to explore past, present, and potential experiences through role play and assists group members in developing spontaneity and successful interactional tools. The audience may participate by making comments about and interpretations of the people acting.

(Continued on the following page)

TABLE 12.1 Multidisciplinary Treatment Team (Continued)

DISCIPLINE	DESCRIPTION
Recreational or activity therapist	College graduate with a baccalaureate or master's degree and training in recreational or activity therapy. Focuses on remotivation of clients by directing their attention outside themselves to relieve preoccupation with personal thoughts, feelings, and attitudes. Clients learn to cope with stress through activity. Activities are planned to meet specific needs and encourage the development of leisure-time activities or hobbies. Recreational therapy is especially useful with those people who have difficulty relating to others (eg, the regressed, withdrawn, or immobilized person). Examples of recreational activities include group bowling, picnics, sing-alongs, and bingo.
Play therapist	A psychiatrist, licensed psychologist, psychiatric nurse, psychiatric social worker, or other person trained in counseling. A play therapist observes the behavior, affect, and conversation of a child who plays in a protected environment with minimal distractions, using games or toys provided by the therapist. The therapist tries to gain insight into the child's thoughts, feelings, or fantasies and helps the child to understand and work through emotional conflicts.
Pet therapist	Also referred to as an animal-assisted therapist. A trained practitioner with experience with animal behavior. Provides animal-assisted visitation and animal-assisted therapy. Uses certified therapy animals to visit clients and families at the bedside or in a common waiting area. Provides therapy on a one-to-one basis. The goals of animal-assisted therapy include the reduction of stress; improvement in emotional well-being, self-concept, and social interaction; and behavior modification.
Speech therapist	College graduate with a master's degree and training in speech therapy. Speech therapists assess and treat disturbed children or people who have developmental language disorders involving nonverbal comprehension, verbal comprehension, and verbal expression. Failure to develop language may occur as a result of deafness, severe mental disability, gross sensory deprivation, institutionalization (eg, an orphanage), or an abnormality of the central nervous system. The speech therapist may work with a neurologist or otologist in such cases.
Chaplain	College graduate with theological or seminary education. Identifies the spiritual needs of the client and support persons and provides spiritual comfort as needed. If appropriately trained, a chaplain may act as a counselor. The chaplain may attend the intake interview and staff meetings to provide input about the client as well as to plan holistic health care.
Dietitian or clinical nutritionist	Person with graduate-level education in the field of nutrition. The dietitian serves as a resource person to the multidisciplinary treatment team as well as a nutritional counselor for clients with eating disorders, such as anorexia nervosa, bulimia, pica, and rumination.
Auxiliary personnel	Volunteers, housekeepers, or clerical help who come in contact with clients. Such persons receive in-service training on how to deal with psychiatric emergencies as well as how to interact therapeutically with clients.

assert, "Today's patients want to be well-informed consumers of health care." The nurse is often challenged in the role of teacher or educator by barriers such as lack of educational resources, limited time spent with the client, the client's lack of education to comprehend information, language or cultural differences between the client and nurse, and the client's physical or emotional disabilities (Katz, 1997).

According to the 1992 National Adult Literacy Survey conducted by the Department of Education's National Center for Education Statistics, approximately 40 million adults in the United States can't understand written materials because of limited or low literacy. Older adults and members of inner-city minority groups are twice as likely to have poor reading abilities compared with the general population. However, despite these statistics, written patient education materials provided by health care facilities continue to be a primary source of information for many clients. Therefore, educational material should contain famil-

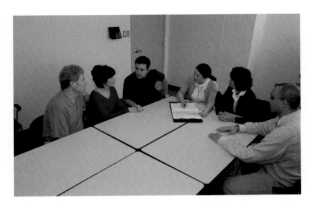

FIGURE 12.1 Multidisciplinary team meeting.

iar words and short sentences, and define any essential medical or psychiatric terminology in simple language (Winslow, 2001). The nurse should also consider the client's cultural and ethnic identity when developing educational material.

Before initiating client education, the nurse assesses what the client already knows and what his or her knowledge deficits are. The nurse also assesses whether the client is accessible and amenable to teaching before initiating a learning/teaching/information session. If the patient is not ready or open at the time, then the nurse is wasting his or her time.

The following is a list of educational strategies the nurse can use to promote client education after the client is ready to learn or to share information.

- Prioritize the client's needs and focus on everyday issues (eg, safety vs. nutritional needs).
- Present specific information (eg, "Let's discuss what you should do when you experience what you describe as panic attacks.").
- Use simple language and avoid speaking in a monotone.
- Utilize different educational approaches depending on the client's ability to relate to the written word, video or audio presentations, or ability to use the Internet.
- Involve the client's family members and support persons in the educational process.
- Educate and reinforce information while providing care.

Client educational group sessions are also an important intervention for clients who are typically admitted to a psychiatric facility to stabilize their symptoms until they are cleared for outpatient treatment. Nurses can address issues such as medication management, drug and alcohol abuse, stress, diet and exercise, and smoking (Sherman, 2003). Topics such as anger management, interventions for hallucinations or delusions, and the benefits of attending rehabilitation meetings are also included in client education. (Nursing interventions including client education regarding these various topics are discussed in the various disorder chapters in Units VI and VII.)

Sherman (2003) describes a unique group approach to client education, the News Hour. Clients are encouraged to talk about whatever interests them within a certain timeframe or allotted time period. Each client takes a turn, and this allows for exchange and sharing of thoughts. The purpose of this therapeutic intervention is to help clients improve their social skills, focus on others, and realize that they can effect change themselves if they stay informed.

Spiritual Interventions

Criteria for establishing a therapeutic milieu state that the staff should convey an overall acceptance of clients. According to the American Nurses Association's (ANA) *Code of Ethics for Nurses—Provisions* (2001), nurses must ensure human dignity for all clients regardless of differences in religion or spiritual beliefs. Because the nurse provides care for clients of different cultural and ethnic backgrounds, issues related to spirituality may be overlooked or misunderstood. As noted in Chapter 4, it is imperative that the nurse understands the concept of spirituality and the client's religious affiliation.

The psychiatric–mental health nurse plays a key role in planning interventions to meet the spiritual needs of a client. The client's initial assessment should include spiritual values and the client's existing religious support system (see Chapter 9 for a sample spiritual needs assessment). Various tools may be used to assess the client's spirituality. Sumner (1998) identifies additional instruments used to measure spiritual perspective; these include Reed's Spiritual Perspective Scale, Ellison's Spiritual Well-Being Scale, and Elkin's Spiritual Orientation Inventory. However, the nurse may encounter barriers related to specific spiritual beliefs of clients when providing appropriate care. These barriers may include the following:

- Disease is a divine punishment or test of faith.
- Modern science is the result of "false teachings."
- Drugs or medication are not an acceptable intervention.

- Psychiatric–mental health nursing does not respect certain restrictions (eg, dietary, clothing, activities).
- The nurse does not understand the client's spiritual or religious beliefs.

When barriers are encountered, the psychiatric–mental health nurse has the option of enlisting the help of members of the multidisciplinary treatment team, members of the client's family, or the client's spiritual advisor to determine appropriate interventions.

Some religious groups condemn modern scientific practice, whereas others support medicine in general. Therefore, the psychiatric–mental health nurse needs to be familiar with the attitudes and requirements of different religious groups. After the nurse has established a therapeutic relationship with a client, the nurse should inform the multidisciplinary treatment team of the client's spiritual and religious needs. As a plan of care is developed, the help of other personnel identified by the client may be elicited to provide spiritual support. Spiritual support interventions may include communicating acceptance of and respect for the client's spiritual beliefs and practices, providing privacy and quiet as needed for ritual or devotional practices, praying or meditating with the client, instilling hope, and collaborating with the client's spiritual counselor (Carpenito-Moyet, 2006; Kearns, 2002; Sumner, 1998).

Personal and Sleep Hygiene Management

Some clients cannot manage self-care activities such as personal hygiene or may report sleep disturbances because of clinical symptoms or as a result of adverse effects of medication therapy.

Assessments of the client's general appearance and sleep pattern were discussed in Chapter 9. NANDA-approved nursing diagnoses relating to these issues and commonly used in the psychiatric setting include Self-Care Deficit (Feeding Self-Care Deficit, Bathing/Hygiene Self-Care Deficit, Dressing/Grooming Self-Care Deficit, Toileting Self-Care Deficit), Disturbed Sleep Pattern, and Sleep Deprivation.

Nurses use the phrase **activities of daily living** (ADL) to describe the client's ability to provide self-care; that is, feed, bathe, dress, and toilet himself or herself. Factors such as regression, excessive ritualistic behavior, acute confusion or cognitive deficits, pain, decreased motivation, fatigue, psychosis, anxiety, or depression may alter the client's ability to perform self-care, contributing to self-care deficit. For example,

an individual with depression may neglect personal hygiene, dress in a slovenly manner, and exhibit a poor appetite. Nursing interventions would focus on promoting participation in bathing, dressing, and eating; encouraging independence; praising involvement; and exploring the client's feelings about the need for assistance. The presence of perceptual, visual, hearing, cognitive, or physical deficits determines the interventions the nursing staff uses; however, the nurse should avoid increasing the client's dependency by doing for the client what he or she has demonstrated the ability to do independently (Carpenito-Moyet, 2006).

Clients in psychiatric–mental health settings frequently describe **sleep pattern disturbances.** Clients with depression may complain of the inability to stay asleep, or may complain of sleeping too much. Clients experiencing anxiety generally complain of the inability to fall asleep. Individuals with confusion, delirium, or dementia may exhibit a reversal in their sleep pattern (ie, sleep during the day and wander at night). Clients experiencing psychotic symptoms may describe dreams or nightmares and express the fear of falling asleep because of hallucinations or delusions. Individuals with a terminal illness have been known to exhibit insomnia due to an expressed fear of dying in their sleep. Children may exhibit sleep disturbances related to fear, enuresis, reluctance to retire, or desire to sleep with parents (Carpenito-Moyet, 2006).

Drugs may interfere with sleep and wakefulness in a variety of ways. Drugs may decrease the rapid eye movement (REM) sleep interval causing sleep deprivation; alter sleep and wakefulness because of central nervous system adverse affects; cause insomnia; produce fatigue; or produce daytime fatigue and sleepiness (Munro, 2002).

A sleep diary can be a useful tool in determining a client's sleep pattern. Figure 12-2 depicts a 2-week sleep diary commonly used to determine a client's current sleep efficiency. Various nursing interventions are helpful in promoting an optimal balance of rest and activity. A treatment-selection decision tree to promote sleep hygiene is shown in Figure 12-3.

Interventions are aimed at client education, behavioral change, and self-efficacy, allowing the client to regain a feeling of control over his or her sleep (Zunkel, 2005). They are based on the client's inability to fall asleep or to stay asleep. Generic or nonpharmacologic interventions include reducing noise, avoiding napping during the day, avoiding using the bed and bedroom for activities other than sleep, avoiding caffeinated beverages after midafternoon, limiting fluid intake after din-

1. Answer the questions in the shaded areas.
2. Draw a line through the times you were asleep.
3. Put down (↓) arrows at the times you went to bed and up (↑) arrows at the times you got up.

(Each tick mark represents 1 hour)

Date		9:00 PM	10:00 PM	11:00 PM	12:00 AM	1:00 AM	2:00 AM	3:00 AM	4:00 AM	5:00 AM	6:00 AM	7:00 AM	8:00 AM	9:00 AM	Rate your quality of sleep* (1-3)	Rate your level of daytime alertness (1-3)	I took a nap (If yes, indicate time of nap and length. If no, leave blank.) Time	Length	Rate your mood today (1-3)
	EXAMPLE														1	2	4:00 PM	45 min	2
	NIGHT 1																		
	NIGHT 2																		
	NIGHT 3																		
	NIGHT 4																		
	NIGHT 5																		
	NIGHT 6																		
	NIGHT 7																		
	NIGHT 8																		
	NIGHT 9																		
	NIGHT 10																		
	NIGHT 11																		
	NIGHT 12																		
	NIGHT 13																		
	NIGHT 14																		

*1=poor; 2=fair; 3=good

FIGURE 12.2 Sleep diary. Adapted from Searle. (1994). *A to Zzzz. Easy steps to help you sleep.* Chicago, Il: Author.

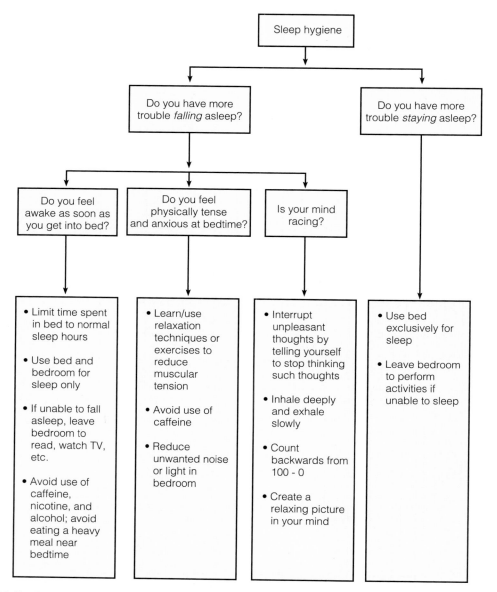

FIGURE 12.3 Treatment selection decision tree to promote sleep hygiene. Adapted from Searle. (1994). *A to Zzzz. Easy steps to help you sleep.* Chicago, IL: Author.

ner to avoid nocturia, avoiding exercise before bedtime, establishing a relaxing routine before bedtime, establishing regular bedtime routines, and maintaining a regular rise time in the morning regardless of sleep duration the previous night. Pharmacologic treatment options include sedating antidepressants, nonbenzodi-azepine hypnotics, and antihistamine drugs. Sleep agents may also include melatonin or over-the-counter herbal preparations (eg, herbal teas). Homeopathic remedies and aromatherapy are also used to treat sleep disorders. (Chapter 16 discusses the use of antianxiety and hypnotic agents. Chapter 18 discusses the use of complementary and alternative medicine to induce sleep.)

In cases when interventions for the treatment of insomnia are unsuccessful, or other serious sleep problems seem probable, formal work-up in a sleep lab is recommended. Candidates for such a work-up include clients with daytime sleepiness, excessive snoring, unusual limb movements such as restless legs syndrome or periodic limb movement disorder, or morbidly obese individuals. Diagnostic tests include objective polysomnographic testing (ie, the monitoring of multiple electrophysiological parameters, including electroencephalographic, electrooculographic, and electromyographic activity), oral or nasal airflow, respiratory effort, chest and abdominal wall movement, and oxyhemoglobin saturation. Actigraphy is a nonintrusive test used to study sleep–wake patterns and circadian rhythms by assessing movement of the wrist (Zunkel, 2005).

Pain Management

Sleep and pain problems are among the most common complaints in our society, so it is not surprising that these conditions frequently coincide in the same individual (Moldofsky, 2004).

Pain is more than a mere sensation. It has two components: sensory and affective. Regardless of the cause of pain, both of these components must be considered. Pain may either cause or exacerbate symptoms such as fatigue or sleep disturbance among clients with mental illness. Pain may also cause or exacerbate anxiety and depression. In chronic pain, anxiety, anger, and even depression are often unwelcome accompaniments to the pain because chronic pain has a negative impact on every aspect of a client's quality of life (McCaffery & Pasero, 2001; Romano, 2001). Examples of pain experienced by clients in the psychiatric–mental health clinical setting include headache (eg, migraine, cluster), back pain (eg, acute or chronic), arthritis, and fibromyalgia (Moldofsky, 2004). Clients who are prescribed antipsychotic medication may develop adverse effects that also produce discomfort or pain.

The JCAHO standards of care for pain management apply to all clinical settings, including psychiatric–mental health settings. The goal of pain management is to reduce or eliminate pain, or make the pain more manageable. According to McCaffery and Pasero (1999), nonpharmacologic methods of pain management can diminish the emotional components of pain, strengthen coping abilities, give clients a sense of control, contribute to pain relief, decrease fatigue, and promote sleep. Nursing interventions focus on acknowledging the presence of pain, listening attentively to the client's description of pain, providing pain management education to establish a comfort-function goal of pain relief, and providing noninvasive pain-relief measures (eg, cognitive behavioral interventions, relaxation techniques, meditation).

As noted in Chapter 7, the World Health Organization (WHO) *Analgesic Ladder* may be followed to effectively manage pain. For example, nonsteroidal anti-inflammatory drugs (NSAIDs) are effective in the treatment of a variety of acute and chronic conditions. Effective treatment of migraine or cluster headaches may require as many as three medications to manage acute episodes, manage breakthrough or residual pain, and to serve as a daily preventive medication. Individuals with persistent moderate to severe pain, such as neuropathic pain or fibromyalgia, may require around-the-clock analgesia or muscle relaxants. Opiates, dopaminergic drugs, or anticonvulsants may be required to minimize pain in clients with restless legs syndrome (Glassroth, 2004; Moldofsky, 2004; Pasero & McCaffery, 2004; see Chapter 16 for additional information).

If the plan for pain management is unsuccessful, a pain evaluation referral to a pain management clinic is considered to determine the cause and appropriate effective treatment of the client's pain (see Chapter 20). Such referrals are made by the attending clinician if approval is granted by the client's insurance carrier.

Protective Care

The potential for violence is inherent in any psychiatric–mental health setting. According to JCAHO standards, the milieu should be purposeful and planned to provide safety, a testing ground for new patterns of behavior, and consistency when setting limits. **Protective nursing care** of the psychiatric–mental health client focuses on providing observation and care so that the client does not injure himself or herself, injure others, or become injured when around other clients. The client must be supervised to prevent use of poor judgment, loss of self-respect, destruction of property, embarrassment of others, or leaving of the clinical setting without permission.

At times, it is necessary to prevent clients from harming themselves or others. The stabilization of clients with dangerous behavior requires the *flexible* use of seclusion and restraints, restricted to situations in which there is an emergency situation resulting in extreme danger to the client or others in the environment.

In 1992, the Food and Drug Administration (FDA) issued a safety alert regarding restraint-related deaths and injuries. It cited a list of guidelines for the correct use of appropriate mechanical and physical restraints, and also promoted restraint-free care when possible. Other regulatory agencies such as the National Alliance for the Mentally Ill (NAMI), the Health Care Financing Administration (HCFA), and JCAHO have also addressed the issue of safety during the use of seclusion and mechanical or physical restraints (Hamilton, 2001; Rogers & Bocchino, 1999).

Following is a summary of the Behavioral Health Care Restraint and Seclusion Standards that apply to all behavioral health settings in which restraint and seclusion is used (eg, free-standing psychiatric hospitals, psychiatric units in general hospitals, and residential treatment centers that are owned by the hospital.):

1. If the facility uses accreditation for deemed status purposes, the physician or other licensed independent practitioner (LIP) must perform a face-to-face assessment of the client within the first hour after emergency application of restraint or seclusion. An initial order is good for 4 hours.
2. After the first 4-hour order expires, a qualified RN or other qualified staff member reevaluates the client's need for continuation of restraint or seclusion.
3. If restraint or seclusion is still deemed clinically necessary, the LIP is notified, and a written or verbal order is given for an additional 4 hours.
4. Following the 8-hour period that the client has been in restraint or seclusion, the LIP conducts another in-person reevaluation of continued need for restraint or seclusion. If necessary, a third 4-hour order is written.
5. This cycle would continue as long as the client requires restraint or seclusion.
6. If a client who is in restraints requires continuous, uninterrupted monitoring to ensure safety, the in-person observer must have direct eye contact with the client. This can occur through a window or doorway if the client is capable of violent behavior or becomes agitated when staff members are present.

7. If a client who is in seclusion requires continuous, uninterrupted monitoring to ensure safety, the in-person observation can progress to audio and visual monitoring after the first hour in seclusion.

In addition to the above standards, nursing interventions are provided to assess and assist the client with signs of injury associated with the application of restraint and seclusion; nutrition and hydration; circulation and range of motion in extremities; vital signs; hygiene and elimination; physical and psychological status and comfort; and readiness for discontinuation of restraint and seclusion. Not all of the interventions may be necessary. Also, visual checks can be done when and if the client is too agitated to approach (JCAHO, 2005).

The issue of seclusion and restraints reached national prominence in 1998 after a series in the *Hartford Courant* documented 142 client deaths associated with restraint use over a 10-year period (Zwillich, 1999). Such tragic and preventable deaths have led federal legislative representatives to present bills restricting the use of seclusion and restraints. In November 1999, the Senate passed legislation limiting the use of seclusion and restraints in *federally funded* health care facilities (Sharfstein, 1999; Zwillich, 1999). This legislation, subsequently passed by the House of Representatives, also forces hospitals and psychiatric treatment facilities to report all deaths that occur while clients are in restraints.

In January 2003, the American Psychiatric Nurses Association (APNA) announced a collaborative publication with the American Psychiatric Association (APA) and the National Association of Public Health Systems (NAPHS) with support from the American Hospital Association (AHA) Section for Psychiatric and Substance Abuse Services titled *Learning From Each Other: Success Stories and Ideas for Reducing Restraint/Seclusion in Behavioral Health*. The document provides ideas on leadership, staff education, assessment, treatment planning, documentation, milieu management, and debriefing. It includes a list of resources, publications, and an appendix of forms, assessment tools, and checklists. The complete text of the publication is available free at the Web sites of the sponsoring organizations.

The use of seclusion and restraints is discussed in more detail in Chapter 31. Specific nursing interventions regarding restraints and seclusion are also discussed in chapters focusing on clinical symptoms such as agitation, disorientation, confusion, and psychotic behavior.

Behavior Therapy

Behavior therapy is a mode of treatment that focuses on modifying observable and, at least in principle, quantifiable behavior by means of systematic manipulation of the environment and variables thought to be functionally related to the behavior (Shahrokh & Hales, 2003). Behavior therapy can be used in two different ways to help clients. First, it aims to eliminate certain clinical symptoms exhibited by clients with a history of alcohol dependence, phobias, or eating disorders, and temper tantrums and bed-wetting in children. Second, behavior therapy is also used to develop desirable behavior. Behaviorists believe that problem behaviors are learned, and therefore can be eliminated or replaced by desirable behaviors through new learning experiences.

General principles of behavior therapy as identified by Rowe (1989) include the following:

- Faulty learning can result in psychiatric disorders.
- Behavior is modified through the application of principles of learning.
- Maladaptive behavior is considered to be deficient or excessive; thus, behavior therapy seeks to promote appropriate behavior or decrease or eliminate the frequency, duration, or place of occurrence of inappropriate behavior.
- One's social environment is a source of stimuli that support symptoms; therefore, it also can support changes in behavior through appropriate treatment measures.

The stress of hospitalization, unexpected medical procedures, unfamiliar hospital routines, and restricted freedom can precipitate a variety of behavioral responses in clients that can impair the nurse–client relationship (Nield-Anderson, Minarik, Dilworth, et al., 1999). For example, the client may receive inadequate care because the nurse feels uncomfortable, afraid, angry, or intimidated by the client's psychiatric diagnosis or presenting clinical symptoms. Behaviors such as noncompliance, manipulation, aggression, and violence are generally treated with behavior therapy.

Behavior therapy techniques include behavior modification and systematic desensitization, aversion therapy, cognitive behavior therapy, assertiveness training, implosive therapy, and limit-setting.

Behavior Modification. Three models of learning theory are used in behavior modification. **Pavlov's Theory of Conditioning** states that a stimulus elicits a response (eg, a red, ripe apple stimulates one's salivary glands). **Skinner's Theory of Operant Conditioning** states that the results of a person's behavior determine whether the behavior will recur in the future. For example, permitting a child to stay home from school because he did not finish his homework assignment leads to further episodes of homework not being completed, whereas sending the child to school and having him face the consequences of incomplete homework diminishes the behavior. **Therapeutic lifestyle change counseling (TLC)** is an important behavior modification tool used in clinical practice. Similar to the Stages of Change Model, TLC counseling utilizes motivational behavioral techniques to implement necessary lifestyle changes of clients with chronic conditions or illnesses. It is indicated as secondary prevention and management for many medical and psychiatric diagnoses such as substance abuse, nicotine abuse, and obesity resulting from overeating or sedentary lifestyle. Clients participate in one or more monthly sessions of high-intensity behavioral counseling for at least 3 months. It is often recommended before pharmacologic intervention and continued even after medication is prescribed (Mackey, 2004). The application of the Stages of Change Model is discussed in Chapter 25.

Systematic desensitization is based on Pavlov's theory. This behavior therapy eliminates the client's fears or anxieties by stressing relaxation techniques that inhibit anxious responses. Clients are taught ways to relax as they vividly imagine a fear. For example, a mail carrier is intensely afraid of dogs because one bit him. He is taught relaxation techniques, and then is asked to visualize a dog several yards away. He is instructed to imagine himself walking toward the dog, and whenever he becomes anxious, he is instructed to divert his attention by using a relaxation technique. This imagined role-playing situation continues until the man no longer experiences anxiety. The next step involves slowly approaching a live dog while using relaxation techniques to decrease anxiety. Therapy is successful if the client loses his intense fear of dogs.

In operant conditioning, good behavior is rewarded with physical reinforcers (eg, food) or social reinforcers (eg, approval, tokens of exchange); the reinforcers are withheld if maladaptive behavior occurs. Such rewards generally encourage positive or good behavior, bringing about a change in attitudes and feelings. Operant conditioning has been successful in teaching language to autistic children, teaching ADL and social skills to cognitively disabled children and adults, and teaching social skills to regressed psychotic clients.

Aversion Therapy. **Aversion therapy** uses unpleasant or noxious stimuli to change inappropriate behavior. The stimulus may be a chemical, such as disulfiram (Antabuse) or apomorphine, used to treat alcoholics; electrical, such as a pad-and-buzzer apparatus, used to treat children who have urinary incontinence while sleeping; or visual, such as films of an auto accident shown to drivers who are arrested for speeding or for driving while under the influence of alcohol or drugs. Aversion therapy has been used in the treatment of alcoholism and compulsive unacceptable or criminal social behavior. This therapy is controversial for many reasons because the form of stimuli used does not always lead to the expected response and can sometimes be positively reinforcing. Aversion therapy has been used with good effect in some cultures in the treatment of opioid addicts (Sadock & Sadock, 2003).

Cognitive Behavior Therapy. **Cognitive behavior therapy** uses confrontation as a means of helping clients restructure irrational beliefs and behavior. In other words, the therapist confronts the client with a specific irrational thought process and helps the client rearrange maladaptive thinking, perceptions, or attitudes. Thus, by changing thoughts, a person can change feelings and behavior. Cognitive behavior therapy is considered a choice of treatment for depression and adjustment difficulties. *Rational emotive therapy* is a type of cognitive therapy that employs the release of

controlled emotions or spiritual experiences as primary vehicles to promote inner growth and achieve self-actualization. Members of a cognitive therapy group share details of personal events in a spontaneous manner (Shahrokh & Hales, 2003).

Assertiveness Training. During **assertiveness training,** clients are taught how to relate appropriately to others using frank, honest, and direct expressions, whether these are positive or negative in nature. The person voices opinions openly and honestly without feeling guilty. One is encouraged not to be afraid to show an appropriate response, negative or positive, to an idea or suggestion. Many people hold back their feelings, being unable to say how they feel. Others may show inconsiderate aggression and disrespect for the rights of others. Assertiveness training teaches one to ask for what is wanted, to take a position on various issues, and to initiate specific action to obtain what one wants while respecting the rights of others. Such training is beneficial to both mentally ill and mentally healthy persons.

Implosive Therapy. **Implosive therapy,** or **flooding,** is the opposite of systematic desensitization. Persons are exposed to intense forms of anxiety producers, either in imagination or in real life. Flooding is based on the premise that escaping from anxiety-provoking experiences reinforces the anxiety through conditioning. Clients are encouraged to face feared situations. Flooding is continued until the stimuli no longer produce disabling anxiety. Although implosive therapy is used in the treatment of phobias and other problems causing maladaptive anxiety, many clients refuse flooding because of the psychological discomfort involved (Sadock & Sadock, 2003). Virtual reality is another example of this type of therapy used to treat clients with phobias.

Limit-Setting. **Limit-setting** is an important aspect of the therapeutic milieu. Limits reduce anxiety, minimize manipulation, provide a framework for client functioning, and enable a client to learn to make requests. Eventually the client learns to control her or his own behavior.

The first step in limit-setting is to give advanced warning of the limit and the consequences that will follow if the client does not adhere to the limit. Choices are provided whenever possible because they allow the client a chance to participate in the limit-setting. For example, the nurse tells a 17-year-old client with substance abuse that he is to keep his room orderly, practice good personal hygiene, and attend therapy sessions twice a week. If he does not follow these rules or regulations, he must forfeit one or more of his privileges. However, he will be allowed to state his feelings about the limits and to decide which of his privileges will be discontinued temporarily.

The consequence of limit-setting should not provide a secondary gain (eg, individual attention) or lower self-esteem. The consequence should occur immediately after the client has exceeded the limit. Consistency must occur with all personnel on all shifts to contribute to a person's security and to convey to the client that someone cares.

Adjunctive or Management Therapy

Occupational, art, music, psychodrama, recreational, play, pet, speech, and nutritional therapies all have psychotherapeutic values and are called *adjunctive* or *management therapy*. The purpose of these therapies is to promote personal change, to develop responsibility and accountability, to express creative needs, and to express feelings or conflicts the client is unable to express verbally (see Table 12-1). The psychiatric-mental health nurse may refer a client to a specific therapist when a specific need or problem is identified. Referrals may also occur during the multidisciplinary treatment team meetings.

In Shape

Kenneth Jue, a social worker in charge of a large community services agency in Keene, New Hampshire, developed an innovative therapeutic milieu program, In Shape, to improve the well-being and quality of life for clients with serious and persistent mental illness. After some research, Jue learned that the life span of mentally ill clients was 10 to 20 years shorter than that of non–mentally ill individuals. Health problems contributing to their early deaths, including diabetes and heart disease, were often related to obesity, an adverse effect of psychotropic medication. The program has been so successful that it is funded, in part, by the Robert Wood Johnson Foundation, local United Way, New Hampshire Endowment for Health, Monadnock Family Services, as well as smaller foundations. Examples of In Shape programs include smoking cessation, nutrition, weight loss, and exercise such as swimming, water aerobics, or racquetball. Experts view In Shape as a model to improve both the lives

and life spans of millions of people with mental illness (Mehren, 2004).

SELF-AWARENESS PROMPT

Which type of behavior therapy do you think would be the hardest for you to implement when caring for a client in your age group: behavior modification, assertiveness training, or limit-setting? Why? What resources or experiences do you think would help you to improve your ability to implement this specific behavioral therapy intervention?

Evaluation of the Therapeutic Milieu

The therapeutic milieu requires periodic evaluation to determine its effectiveness. The **Ward Atmosphere Scale (WAS)** is an instrument that can be used to evaluate the effectiveness of a therapeutic milieu (Moos, 1997). It consists of ten subscales. Each subscale is rated by staff and clients to provide information regarding what actually exists and what should exist in a therapeutic milieu. Subscale items focus on:

1. Staff control of rules, schedules, and client behavior
2. Program clarity of day-to-day routine
3. Measurement of client involvement in social functioning, attitudes, and general enthusiasm
4. Practical preparation of the client for discharge and transition into the community
5. Supportive atmosphere of staff, doctors, and peers toward clients
6. Degree of spontaneity in the environment that allows the client to express feelings freely
7. Promotion of responsibility, self-direction, and independence, as well as staff response to client suggestions or criticisms
8. Order and organization of the unit, including staff and client responses
9. Encouragement of verbalization of personal problems by clients
10. Encouragement of verbalization of feelings such as anger, and the channeling of feelings into appropriate behavior

This instrument is appropriate for evaluating therapeutic milieus in inpatient settings, partial hospitalization programs, day-treatment centers, and community-based mental health programs.

KEY CONCEPTS

◆ The therapeutic milieu, also called the therapeutic environment, is designed to meet the emotional and interpersonal needs of clients, help them control problematic behavior, and assist them in the development of coping skills.

◆ Standards have been set forth by the JCAHO as a guide in developing a therapeutic milieu.

◆ The multidisciplinary psychiatric treatment team is composed of members from several disciplines who discuss each client's progress and review each client's individualized plan of care. The psychiatric–mental health nurse manages and coordinates activities in the milieu.

◆ Interventions in the milieu focus on client education, spiritual needs, personal and sleep hygiene, pain management, protective care, behavior therapy, and adjunctive or management therapies.

◆ Adjunctive or management therapies are also provided to promote personal change, to develop responsibility and accountability, to express creative needs, and to express feelings or conflicts that the client is unable to express verbally.

◆ The Ward Atmosphere Scale (WAS) is an instrument that can be used to evaluate the effectiveness of a therapeutic milieu in inpatient settings, partial hospitalization programs, day-treatment centers, and community-based mental health programs.

For additional study materials, please refer to the Student Resource CD-ROM located in the back of this textbook.

CHAPTER WORKSHEET

CRITICAL THINKING QUESTIONS

1. Consider the WAS subscales identified in the text as you evaluate the area of your current clinical assignment. How many of the 10 subscales are evident on this unit? What are your recommendations for improvement? How might you implement these recommendations?

2. Although assertiveness training is listed as a treatment modality under behavior therapy, it is also a useful method of communication for nurses. Explore assertive communication—assess your communication skills and identify strategies for improving your own assertiveness. Discuss how assertive behavior can help the nursing profession to come into its own.

REFLECTION

Review the quote at the beginning of the chapter and then interview three members of the staff who work with clients in your current clinical area (the staff members may represent different disciplines such as nursing, social services, or occupational therapy). Ask each of them to describe their perceptions of a therapeutic milieu. Do they have similar perceptions? If not, how do their perceptions differ?

NCLEX-STYLE QUESTIONS

1. As part of the milieu therapy, the client has the freedom to do which of the following?
   a. Express feelings in a socially acceptable manner
   b. Select daily schedule based on personal preferences
   c. Revise rules according to individual needs
   d. Vote on policies and procedures of the unit

2. An adolescent client tells the evening-shift nurse that the day-shift nurse promised that she could stay up late to watch a special television program. No specific instructions/alterations have been indicated anywhere on the patient's chart regarding this issue. The evening nurse does which of the following to maintain the therapeutic milieu?
   a. Allows the client to stay up late to promote staff unity
   b. Encourages client to express feelings about staff disagreement on this issue
   c. Maintains the same rules for all clients, therefore refusing client request
   d. Uses staying up late as a reward for this client's good behaviors

3. A client with a psychotic disorder refuses to bathe or change her clothes. Which of the following interventions is congruent with the role of the nurse as a mother surrogate?
   a. Allow the client to make decisions about hygiene
   b. Assist client to bathe and change clothes
   c. Encourage family member to talk to client
   d. Put client in private room to avoid offending others

4. The nurse assesses all of the following factors in a client complaining of insomnia. Which of the following does the nurse encourage the client to modify?
   a. Drinking coffee before midday
   b. Going to bed at the same time each night
   c. Exercising 2 hours before bedtime
   d. Reducing noise at bedtime

5. Virtual reality is to be used to treat a client's phobic response. The nurse interprets this type of treatment as an example of which of the following?
   a. Assertiveness training
   b. Aversion therapy
   c. Implosive therapy
   d. Behavior modification

6. The nurse is preparing an orientation program for a group of new staff members at a community mental health center. As part of the program, the nurse will be describing the therapeutic milieu. Which of the following would the nurse include? Select all that apply.
   a. Use of a multidisciplinary treatment team
   b. Participation of client's family and support persons
   c. Use of limit-setting
   d. Employment of behavioral interventions
   e. Education of the client and family

Selected References

American Nurses Association. (2001). *Code of ethics for nurses—Provisions.* Washington, DC: Author.

Carpenito-Moyet, L. J. (2006). *Handbook of nursing diagnosis* (11th ed.). Philadelphia: Lippincott Williams & Wilkins.

Gallagher, S., & Zeind, S. M. (1998). Bridging patient education and care. *American Journal of Nursing, 98*(8), 16aaa–16ddd.

Glassroth, C. H. (2004). Successful migraine management: Patient-customized care. *Clinician Reviews, 14*(5), 56–62.

Hamilton, M. (2001). Cutting the fuse. *ADVANCE for Nurses, 2*(12), 25–28.

Joint Commission on Accreditation of Healthcare Organizations (JCAHO). (2005). Restraint and seclusion. Retrieved January 13, 2005, from http://www.jcaho.org

Katz, J. R. (1997). Back to basics: Providing effective patient teaching. *American Journal of Nursing, 97*(5), 33–36.

Kearns, M. L. (2002). Managing the spiritual needs of patients. *ADVANCE for Nurse Practitioners, 10*(3), 101–104.

Mackey, S. L. (2004). Therapeutic lifestyle change. *Clinician Reviews, 14*(9), 56–62.

McCaffery, M., & Pasero, C. (1999). *Pain: Clinical manual* (2nd ed.). St. Louis, MO: Mosby.

McCaffery, M., & Pasero, C. (2001). Assessment and treatment of patients with mental illness. *American Journal of Nursing, 101*(7), 69–70.

Mehren, E. (2004, December 25). Program gives mentally ill a workout. *Orlando Sentinel*, A17.

Moldofsky, H. (2004). Pain and insomnia: What every clinician should know. *Medscape Neurology & Neurosurgery, 6*(2). Retrieved December 23, 2004, from http://www.medscape.com/viewarticle/ 494872_print

Moos, R. H. (1997). *Evaluating treatment environments: A social-ecological approach.* Somerset, NJ: Transaction Publishers.

Munro, N. (2002). Sleep deprivation in critically ill patients. *ADVANCE for Nurses, 3*(19), 13–16.

National Center for Education Statistics. (1992). *National Adult Literacy Survey.* Washington, DC: Department of Education. Retrieved February 5, 2004, from http://nces.ed.gov/naal

Nield-Anderson, L., Minarik, P.A., Dilworth, J. M., Jones, J., Nash, P. K., O'Donnell, K. L., et al. (1999). Responding to difficult patients. *American Journal of Nursing, 99*(12), 26–33.

Pasero, C., & McCaffery, M. (2004). Pain control: Comfort-function goals. *American Journal of Nursing, 104*(9), 7–81.

Rogers, P. D., & Bocchino, N. L. (1999). CE: Restraint-free care: Is it possible? *American Journal of Nursing, 99*(10), 27–33.

Romano, T. J. (2001). Essentials of chronic pain management. *Anesthesia Today, 12*(2), 1–14.

Rowe, C. (1989). *An outline of psychiatry* (9th ed.). Dubuque, IA: William C. Brown.

Sadock, B. J., & Sadock, V. A. (2003). *Kaplan & Sadock's synopsis of psychiatry: Behavioral sciences/clinical psychiatry* (9th ed.). Philadelphia: Lippincott Williams & Wilkins.

Schultz, J. M., & Videbeck, S. L. (2005). *Lippincott's manual of psychiatric nursing care plans* (7th ed.). Philadelphia: Lippincott Williams & Wilkins.

Searle. (1994). *A to Zzzz. Easy steps to help you sleep.* Chicago, IL: Author.

Shahrokh, N., & Hales, R. E. (Eds.) (2003). *American psychiatric glossary* (8th ed.). Washington, DC: American Psychiatric Press, Inc.

Sharfstein, S. S. (1999). Seclusion and restraint. *Psychiatric Times, 16*(7), 1, 12.

Sherman, R. (2003). News hour. *ADVANCE for Nurses, 4*(13), 21–22.

Sullivan, H. S. (1968). *The interpersonal theory of psychiatry.* New York: Norton.

Sumner, C. H. (1998). Recognizing and responding to spiritual distress. *American Journal of Nursing, 98*(1), 26–31.

Winslow, E. H. (2001). Patient education materials. *American Journal of Nursing, 101*(10), 33–38.

Zunkel, G. M. (2005). Insomnia: Overview of assessment and treatment strategies. *Clinician Reviews, 15*(7), 37–44.

Zwillich, T. (1999). Movement to minimize seclusion, restraints gains momentum. *Clinical Psychiatry News, 27*(12), 5.

Suggested Readings

Allen, R. P., & Hening, W. A. (2005). Diagnosis and treatment of restless legs syndrome. *Clinician Reviews, 15*(3), 57–68.

American Nurses Association. (2005). *Pain management nursing: Scope and standards of practice.* Washington, DC: Author.

Bourbonneire, M., Stumpf, N. E., Evans, L. K., & Maislin, G. (2003). Organizational characteristics and restraint use for hospitalized nursing home residents. *Journal of the American Geriatrics Society, 51*, 1079–1084.

Champagne, T., & Stromberg, N. (2004). Sensory approaches in inpatient psychiatric settings: innovative alternatives to seclusion and restraint. *Journal of Psychosocial Nursing & Mental Health Services, 42*(9). Retrieved January 24, 2005, from http://www.jpnonline.com

Damaskos, R., & Stewart, M. (2003). Cognitive behavioral interventions for pain management. *Oncology Issues, 18*(5), 40–42.

Huckshorn, K. A. (2004). Reducing seclusion and restraint use in mental health settings: Core strategies for prevention. *Journal of Psychosocial Nursing & Mental Health Services, 42*(9). Retrieved January 24, 2005, from http://www.jpnonline.com

Larson, D. B., Larson, S. S., & Puchalski, C. M. (2000). The once-forgotten factor in psychiatry, Part 1: Residency training addresses religious and spiritual issues. *Psychiatric Times, 17*(1), 18–23.

Palmer, R. S., & Staff. (2003). Managing insomnia. *Geriatric Times, 4*(2), 31–33.

Schaffer, S. D., & Yucha, C. B. (2004). Relaxation & pain management. *American Journal of Nursing, 104*(8), 75–82.

Schutte, S., & Doghramji, K. (2003). Eyes wide open: Update on sleep disorders. *Clinical Advisor, 6*(2), 17–27.

Spittler, K. L. (2006). A look at "biophilia"—How does nature impact physical and mental health? *Neuropsychiatry Reviews, 7*(1), 10–11.

Stahl, S. M. (2005). Finding better answers for sleep disorders. *Psychopharmacology Educational Update, 1*(5), 6–7.

Stanley-Hermanns, M. S., & Miller, J. (2002). Animal-assisted therapy. *American Journal of Nursing, 102*(10), 69–76.

CHAPTER 13 / CRISIS AND DISASTER INTERVENTION

*Any serious interruption in the steady state or equilibrium of a person, family, or group is considered a **crisis**. A crisis is a state of emotional turmoil. It is also considered an emotionally significant event which acts as a turning point for better or worse in a person's life.* —MITCHELL & RESNIK, 1981

AFTER STUDYING THIS CHAPTER, YOU SHOULD BE ABLE TO:

1. Define the terms *crisis* and *disaster.*
2. Distinguish the six classifications of a crisis according to severity.
3. Describe the characteristics of a crisis.
4. Recognize the phases of a crisis.
5. Articulate the five periods of the disaster recovery process.
6. Explain how the following balancing factors can influence the development of a crisis: realistic perception of the event, adequate situational support, and adequate defense and/or coping mechanisms.
7. Compare and contrast crisis intervention and disaster mental health nursing.
8. Interpret the goals of crisis intervention.
9. Verbalize the role of the psychiatric–mental health nurse in crisis intervention and disaster nursing.
10. Use the steps of crisis intervention.
11. Discuss the issue of legal immunity for the crisis worker.

LEARNING OBJECTIVES

KEY TERMS

Crisis
Crisis forensics
Crisis intervention
Crisis response team
Crisis situations
Disaster
Disaster intervention
Disaster mental health nursing
Disaster response team
Maturational crisis
Paradigm of balancing factors
Situational crisis

On December 26, 2004, the world's most powerful earthquake in more than 40 years struck deep under the Indian Ocean in South Asia, triggering massive tsunamis that obliterated seaside communities and holiday resorts, killing tens of thousands of people in a dozen countries. The psychological effects of this natural disaster included feelings of despair, anxiety, and fear for safety and security.

In October 2002, the "beltway sniper" killed several individuals in Maryland, Virginia, and Washington, DC. Residents of these areas responded to this stressful situation by discontinuing their daily routines such as grocery shopping, going to gas stations, eating at restaurants, attending outdoor activities, and taking their children to school. Numerous outdoor events were cancelled. Public schools maintained a lockdown mode and later cancelled classes.

On September 11, 2001, the hijacking of commercial airplanes and subsequent terrorist attacks on the World Trade Center and Pentagon left many Americans feeling numb, frightened, angry, and profoundly sad. The number of individuals classified as missing or dead was high, businesses were destroyed, and many individuals stated that they would never fly again.

The news media refer to such events as **disasters**, or traumatic events that occur suddenly, often without warning; cause great damage; deprive people of their homes and possessions; and generally precipitate **crisis situations**, conditions or periods of emotional instability that can result in a psychiatric disorder. A crisis situation can also threaten the safety, integrity, or reputation of an individual or members of the community. Among those most influenced are survivors or witnesses of the events and those whose friends, family, and acquaintances were survivors or victims. To promote recovery from such situations, it is extremely important to provide crisis or disaster intervention. This chapter focuses on the different aspects of crisis, including examples of precipitating events, and the major interventions used to control or resolve a crisis situation. Information regarding disaster intervention and nursing care is included where appropriate. The legal implications associated with crisis situation and crisis intervention for children/adolescents also are highlighted.

Crises

Most people exist in a state of equilibrium, despite the occurrence of crisis situations. That is, their everyday lives contain some degree of harmony in their thoughts, wishes, feelings, and physical needs. This existence generally remains intact unless there is a serious interruption or disturbance of one's biologic, psychological, spiritual, or social integrity. As undue stress occurs, one's equilibrium can be affected, and one may lose control of feelings and thoughts, thus experiencing an extreme state of emotional turmoil. When this occurs, one may be experiencing a crisis. Individuals respond to crisis in different ways. Table 13-1 summarizes two types of common responses to a crisis, high anxiety–emotional shock or stunned–inactive response.

Types of Crises

A crisis can be situational or maturational. A **situational crisis** refers to an extraordinarily stressful event such as domestic violence or "beltway sniper" incidents that affects an individual, or family regardless of age, socioeconomic status, or sociocultural status. A situational crisis can be personal or public (ie, affect an entire community). Examples of events that can precipitate a *personal situational crisis* include eco-

---

TABLE 13.1 Two Common Responses to a Crisis

TYPE OF RESPONSE	CLINICAL SYMPTOMS
High-anxiety–emotional shock	Hyperactivity
	Loud screaming or crying
	Wringing of the hands
	Rapid speech
	Increased respirations
	Flushed face
	Nausea/vomiting
	Emotionally out of control
Stunned-inactive response	Inactivity
	Aimless wandering
	Pale appearance
	Rapid pulse, low blood pressure
	Cold, clammy skin
	Diaphoresis
	Nausea/vomiting
	Syncope (fainting)

nomic difficulty, medical or psychiatric illness, rape, child abuse or neglect, divorce, or death of a loved one due to a terminal illness. Examples of disasters that can precipitate a *public situational crisis* include workplace violence, school violence, hurricane, tornado, or tsunami.

A **maturational crisis,** on the other hand, is an experience—such as puberty, adolescence, young adulthood, marriage, or the aging process—in which one's lifestyle is continually subject to change. These are the normal processes of growth and development that evolve over an extended period and require a person to make some type of change. Another example of a maturational crisis is retirement, in which a person faces the loss of a peer group as well as loss of a status identity.

Classification According to Severity

Situational and maturational crises also can be classified based on the severity of the precipitating events. A classification system developed by Burgess and Baldwin (1981) systematically describes six types of crises based on the severity of the situation. Each classification is briefly summarized below.

1. *Class 1*: Dispositional or situational crisis in which a problem is presented with a need for immediate action, such as finding housing for the homeless during subzero temperatures
2. *Class 2*: Life transitional or maturational crisis that occurs during normal growth and development, such as going away to college or experiencing a planned pregnancy
3. *Class 3*: Situational crisis due to a sudden, unexpected, traumatic event or disaster, such as the loss of a home during a hurricane or earthquake
4. *Class 4*: Maturational or developmental crisis involving an internal stress and psychosocial issues, such as questioning one's sexual identity or lacking the ability to achieve emotional independence
5. *Class 5*: Situational crisis due to a preexisting psychopathology, such as depression or anxiety, that interferes with activities of daily living (ADL) or various areas of functioning
6. *Class 6*: Psychiatric situational crisis or emergency, such as attempted suicide, drug overdose, or extreme agitation, resulting in unpredictable behavior or the onset of an acute psychotic disorder

Characteristics of a Crisis

A crisis usually occurs suddenly, when a person, family, or group is inadequately prepared to handle the event or situation. Normal coping methods fail, tension rises, and feelings of anxiety, fear, guilt, anger, shame, and helplessness may occur. Most crises, unless the result of a natural or manmade disaster, are generally short in duration, lasting 24 to 36 hours. Crises rarely last longer than 4 to 6 weeks, whereas the period of recovery from a disaster such as a hurricane may involve several years. A crisis situation can cause increased psychological vulnerability, resulting in potentially dangerous, self-destructive, or socially unacceptable behavior, or it can provide an opportunity for personal growth. The outcome of a crisis situation depends on, among other factors, the availability of appropriate help (Mitchell & Resnik, 1981).

Phases of a Crisis

Research involving crisis has led to the identification of specific stages or phases associated with it. Most individuals consider Eric Lindemann (1965) to be the father of crisis theory. His theory evolved from the study of grief responses in families of victims of the Coconut Grove nightclub fire in Boston in 1943. After World War II, Gerald Caplan (1964) contributed to the concept of crisis theory while working with immigrant mothers and children. Each described stages or phases of a crisis. Generally, theorists describe five stages or phases of a crisis:

1. Precrisis
2. Impact
3. Crisis
4. Resolution
5. Postcrisis

The general state of equilibrium in which a person is able to cope with everyday stress is called the *precrisis phase.* When a stressful event occurs, the person is said to be experiencing the *impact phase.* This phase occurs when, for example, a pediatrician tells a young couple that their 5-year-old son has inoperable cancer. After the shock is over, the young parents become acutely aware of their son's critical illness and poor prognosis. This is an extraordinarily stressful event, threatening their child's life and their integrity as a family. With this realization, they are now in the *crisis phase.* They may experience continuing confusion, anxiety, and disorganization because they feel helpless and are unable to cope with their son's phys-

TABLE 13.2 Phases of a Crisis

PHASES	DESCRIPTION
1. **Precrisis**	State of equilibrium or well-being
2. Initial **impact** or shock occurs (may last a few hours to a few days)	High level of stress
	Inability to reason logically
	Inability to apply problem-solving behavior
	Inability to function socially
	Helplessness
	Anxiety
	Confusion
	Chaos
	Possible panic
3. **Crisis** occurs (may last a brief or prolonged period of time)	Inability to cope results in attempts to redefine the problem, avoid the problem, or withdraw from reality
	Ineffective, disorganized behavior interferes with daily living
	Denial of problem
	Rationalization about cause of the situation
	Projection of feelings of inadequacy onto others
4. Recoil, acknowledgment, or beginning of **resolution** occurs	Acknowledges reality of the situation
	Attempts to use problem-solving approach by trial and error
	Tension and anxiety resurface as reality is faced
	Feelings of depression, self-hate, and low self-esteem may occur.
Resolution, adaptation, and change continues	Occurs when the person perceives the crisis situation in a positive way
	Successful problem-solving occurs.
	Anxiety lessens
	Self-esteem rises
	Social role is resumed.
5. **Postcrisis** begins	May be at a higher level of maturity and adaptation due to acquisition of new positive coping skills, or may function at a restricted level in one or all spheres of the personality due to denial, repression, or ineffective mastery of coping and problem-solving skills
	Persons who cope ineffectively may express open hostility, exhibit signs of depression, or abuse alcohol, drugs, or food.
	Symptoms of neurosis, psychosis, chronic physical disability, or socially maladjusted behavior may occur.

ical condition. When the young parents are able to regain control of their emotions, handle the situation, and work toward a solution concerning their son's illness with or without intervention from others, they are in the *resolution phase* of a crisis. If they are able to resume normal activities while living through their son's hospitalization and illness, they are in the *postcrisis phase*. The experience of a crisis and passage through the phases may result in permanent emotional injury or it may make the young parents feel a stronger bond with each other and their son, depend-ing on their ability to cope. These phases are described further in Table 13-2.

Paradigm of Balancing Factors

Various factors can influence an individual's ability to resolve a crisis. Aguilera (1997) describes a **paradigm of balancing factors** that determines the resolution of a crisis. These factors, which can affect an individual's return to equilibrium, are (1) realistic perception of an event; (2) adequate situational support; and (3) adequate defense or coping mechanisms to help resolve a problem. Figure 13-1 incorporates Aguilera's paradigm, depicting a comparison of what could happen in the presence or absence of adequate balancing factors during a stressful situation, specifically, that of the young parents whose son has cancer.

Additional factors may influence the development of a crisis. These factors include the person's physical and emotional status, previous experience with similar situations, and cultural influences.

Realistic Perception

A *realistic perception* occurs when a person is able to distinguish the relationship between an event and feelings of stress. For example, a 45-year-old executive recognizes the fact that her company is on the verge of bankruptcy because of inefficient projected financial planning by the board of trustees. Although she realizes the seriousness of the situation and feels stress, she does not place the blame on herself and view herself as a failure. Her *perception,* rather than the actual event, determines her reaction to the situation.

Situational Supports

Situational supports refers to the resources available in the person's environment. Consider the example of the 45-year-old executive. The executive may discuss the situation with a financial consultant, a lawyer, or the firm's accountant. Such persons available in the environment are considered to be situational supports because they reflect appraisals of one's intrinsic and extrinsic values. Support by these people may prevent a state of disequilibrium and crisis from occurring. When emotional or environmental support systems such as family or friends are not as readily available, a person is more likely to define the event as more overwhelming or hazardous, thus increasing his or her vulnerability to crisis.

Defense Mechanisms

Defense or *coping mechanisms* are those methods usually used by the individual, when dealing with anxiety or stress, to reduce tension in difficult situations (see Chapter 2). Common defense mechanisms utilized during a crisis generally include denial, rationalization, identification, regression, or repression. Behavioral responses such as refusal to face reality, intellectualization about why the situation occurred, productive worrying about how to deal with the cri-

sis, grieving over perceived losses, social withdrawal, or agitation may be exhibited by victims during a crisis. Coping mechanisms are used during early developmental stages and, if found effective in maintaining emotional stability, will become a part of a person's lifestyle in dealing with daily stress. The person who has met developmental tasks and achieved a level of personal maturity usually adapts more readily in a crisis. Recall the example of the executive. She may cope by burying herself in her work, calling an emergency meeting of the board of trustees to discuss the situation, or withdrawing from the situation.

Crisis and Disaster Intervention

Crisis intervention is an active but temporary entry into the life situation of an individual, a family, or a group during a period of stress (eg, divorce, rape, or natural disaster; Mitchell & Resnik, 1981). It is an attempt to resolve an immediate crisis when a person's life goals are obstructed and usual problem-solving methods fail. The client is called on to be active in all steps of the crisis intervention process, including clarifying the problem, verbalizing feelings, identifying goals and options for reaching goals, and deciding on a plan. Crisis intervention can occur in many settings: the home, emergency department, industrial dispensary, classroom, surgical intensive care unit, or psychiatric unit. The generic approach focuses on a particular kind of crisis by directly encouraging adaptive behavior and providing general support, environmental manipulation, and anticipatory guidance. The individual approach focuses on the present, shows little or no concern for the developmental past, and places an emphasis on the immediate causes of disequilibrium. It can be used as secondary or tertiary prevention and can be effective in preventing future crises.

The goals of crisis intervention are:

- To decrease emotional stress and protect the client from additional stress
- To assist the client in organizing and mobilizing resources or support systems to meet unique needs and reach a solution for the particular situation or circumstance that precipitated the crisis, ultimately enabling the individual to understand the relationship of past life experiences to current stress; prevent hospitalization; reduce the risk of chronic maladaptation; and promote adaptive family dynamics

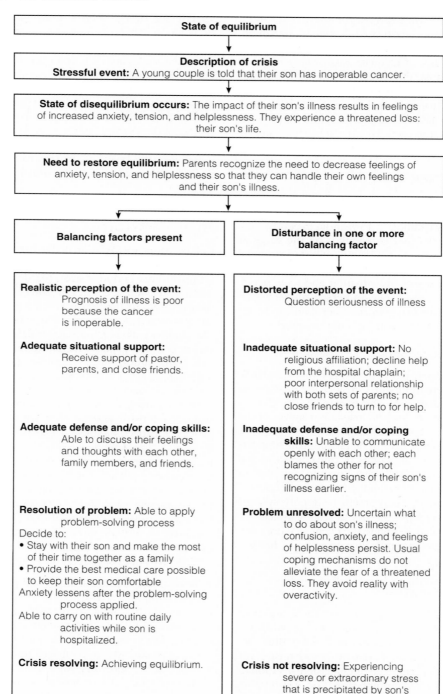

FIGURE 13.1 Crisis situation paradigm.

- To return the client to a precrisis or higher level of functioning

Disaster intervention involves the provision of postdisaster support services during the early phase of a disaster. **Disaster mental health nursing** includes the application of the nursing process to meet the biopsychosocial needs of victims and communities as they experience different periods of the recovery process. A brief summary of the transitional periods and nursing interventions provided follows:

1. Heroic period immediately after the disaster, when victims take action to protect lives and properties. Victims may require medical care as well as crisis intervention to meet their immediate biopsychosocial needs.
2. Honeymoon period 4 weeks to 6 months after the disaster, when victims develop a strong sense of unity through shared experiences of a catastrophic disaster. Clients may require interventions for clinical symptoms of psychiatric disorders such as anxiety, post-traumatic stress disorder (PTSD), or unresolved grief.
3. Period of disillusionment that may last up to 2 years after the disaster. Clients may require psychosocial interventions if patience is exhausted; dissatisfaction, frustration, anger or violence occur; or clinical symptoms of disorders such as depression or alcoholism evolve.
4. Period of reconstruction that may last for several years. Nurses may utilize interventions such as empowerment techniques to help victims regain self-confidence and courage toward restoring their lives (University of Hyogo, 2005).

The psychiatric–mental health nurse may be a member of a crisis or disaster response team. **Crisis response teams** are groups of trained professionals, typically including mental health specialists, victim advocates, public safety individuals, and members of the clergy, among others who volunteer their services. They are on call to provide immediate, short-term, on-scene crisis intervention, emotional support, and referrals to families, neighbors, witnesses and/or survivors who have been traumatized by experiences such as a death, a serious injury, or a violent crime (National Organization for Victim Assistance, 2005). **Disaster response teams** consist of trained professional individuals who provide a combination of physical, psychological, and emotional support for victims of natural or manmade disasters. The support may begin while the disaster is in progress and continue for a period of time until recovery is deemed adequate or completed (University of Hyogo, 2005).

The Role of the Psychiatric–Mental Health Nurse or Nurse Practitioner During a Crisis or Disaster

The most essential element of psychiatric–mental health intervention during a crisis or disaster is the ability of the nurse to provide emotional support while assessing the individual's emotional and physical needs and enlisting his or her cooperation. Whittlesey, Vinekar, and Tucker (1999) discuss the role of the psychiatric–mental health nurse or practitioner in crisis situations, emphasizing the educational preparation of the nurse, because most practitioners have little experience dealing with individual or community crises or disasters. The nurse must understand the effects of severe stress on the average person. Indeed, clients are vulnerable to permanent damage as a result of exposure to continued stress. Clinicians may develop trauma symptoms as a result of secondary exposure. They may experience "compassion fatigue," that is, feel emotionally drained even as they experience a heightened level of physiologic arousal. Thus, secondary exposure can lead to an extreme reaction, such as the development of PTSD (Catherall, 2005).

Preparation for intervening during crisis situations takes on various forms. Role-play exercises, focusing on the possible emotional responses of both client and nurse during a specific crisis situation or disaster, are one example. Preparation also includes attending educational seminars to develop crisis intervention techniques to assist victims experiencing denial, anger, remorse, or grief, and guide the victim toward the resolution phase of the crisis. For example, the Crisis Prevention Institute (CPI) provides a training program, Nonviolent Crisis Intervention, an innovative, holistic system for defusing and safely managing anxious, hostile, violent or physically aggressive behavior, while still protecting the therapeutic relationships with clients. The program is known worldwide for its behavior management practices and is recognized as the international standard for crisis prevention and intervention (CPI, 2005).

The nurse's attitude may affect the outcome of the client's response during intervention. For example, the nurse may give the impression that a particular situation is not a crisis, whereas the client thinks that it is the worst thing that could happen. Here, the nurse's attitude blocks good communication and effective crisis intervention.

Steps in Crisis Intervention

Crisis intervention is not to be confused with traditional psychotherapy. Clients may need to address issues quickly, but may not tolerate frequent sessions. They may not respond to interventions, and may require an extended amount of time to resolve issues. A multidisciplinary approach may facilitate resolution because it provides support and a learning opportunity for both client and nurse.

The process of crisis intervention contains four steps: assessment; planning of therapeutic intervention; implementation of therapeutic intervention; and resolution of the crisis with anticipatory planning and evaluation (Aguilera, 1997). When working with a maturational crisis (also referred to as a *developmental* or *internal crisis*) or a situational crisis (also referred to as an *accidental* or *external crisis*), the crisis worker should be aware of the following usual occurrences (Lego, 1984):

- Most crises occur suddenly, without warning; therefore, there is inadequate prior preparation to handle such a situation.
- The client in crisis may perceive the crisis to be life threatening.
- There is a decrease or loss of communication with significant others.
- Some displacement from familiar surroundings or significant others occurs.
- All crises have an aspect of an actual or perceived loss involving a person, object, idea, or hope.

Assessment

Assessment of a client during crisis intervention depends on several factors, such as the severity of the crisis situation, the client's perception of the crisis, and the accurate interpretation of data to formulate a nursing diagnosis.

Determining Crisis Severity. The first factor in the assessment process is to determine the severity of the crisis situation and to identify the degree of disruption the client is experiencing. Is the individual anxious, depressed, fearful, confused, disoriented, suicidal, or homicidal? Is the crisis a result of an interpersonal or intrapersonal issue? Does the crisis involve one person, several people, or a community? Is this a criminal situation with actual or potential harm or lethality? Individuals who are isolated, are dependent, were previously traumatized, and have physical or mental disorders are considered to be at risk for a high degree of disruption. In addition, the effects of a crisis on children can be compounded if adults express great fear and anger around them, thus being insensitive to children's insecurities or needs. Recognizing the magnitude of physical, emotional, social, and spiritual components of a crisis is essential to helping clients, as well as to intervening so that additional complications do not develop (Davidhizar & Shearer, 2002).

When the nurse assesses the dangerousness of a client's behavior toward self or others, the term **crisis forensics** is used. The word *forensics* is used because the nurse has a responsibility toward society, the liberty interest of the client, and the legal regulation of psychiatry, all of which are operating in a crisis mode (Saunders, 2000).

Assessing Client's Perception. The second factor involves assessing the client's perception of the event. Two major approaches may be used: symptom-focused and constructivist self-development theory (CSDT). The symptom-focused approach focuses on the emotions of the client, whereas the CSDT focuses on one's relationship with oneself and one's relationship with others.

Rosenbloom (1999) compares the symptom-focused approach of crisis intervention to the CSDT of McCann and Pearlman (1990). According to McCann and Pearlman, a symptom-focused approach concentrating on the emotions of the client does not adequately explore root causes of trauma. That is, some individuals are unaware of the significance of the event in their lives. Are the client's perceptions realistic or distorted? Does the client see the situation as a threat to self-esteem, well-being, intimacy, self-control, or ability to trust? As a result of any misperceptions about the severity of the crisis event, the client in crisis may be misdiagnosed and receive inappropriate treatment. With CSDT, identifying a threat can help clients connect to their experiences on an emotional level and make sense of their feelings. Examining symptoms does not necessarily help clients understand what is particularly distressing or destabilizing them. Also using CSDT, attention is given to present coping skills and the availability of support systems on which the individual can rely for continued support.

Formulating Nursing Diagnoses. Formulating nursing diagnoses is the third factor in the assessment of a client in crisis. Examples of nursing diagnoses for clients experiencing a crisis may include the following:

- Anxiety
- Fear
- Ineffective Coping
- Impaired Verbal Communication
- Risk for Injury
- Dysfunctional Grieving
- Disabled Family Coping
- Post-Trauma Response

Planning of Therapeutic Intervention

With information gained through the assessment process and the formulation of one or more nursing diagnoses, several specific interventions are proposed. Connoly and Chandler (1997) state that individuals must learn to ask for help and realize the potential for growth during a crisis situation. They should be involved in the choice of alternate coping methods and encouraged to make as many arrangements as possible by themselves. If significant others are involved, their needs and reactions must also be considered. The nurse should identify strengths and resources of all persons providing support.

Implementation of Therapeutic Interventions

Therapeutic intervention depends on preexisting skills, the creativity and flexibility of the nurse, and the rapidity of the person's response. The nurse helps the person establish an intellectual understanding of the crisis by noting the relationship between the precipitating factor and the crisis. He or she also helps the client explore coping mechanisms, remember or recreate successful coping devices used in the past, or devise new coping skills. Reducing immobility caused by anxiety and encouraging verbalization of feelings is an immediate goal of the nurse. Medication may be required to stabilize clinical symptoms of anxiety or depression if the client does not initially respond to therapeutic interventions. (See Chapter 16 for additional information regarding psychopharmacology.)

Have you ever experienced a crisis situation? If so, describe how you reacted. What effects did you experience? Was the crisis resolved within a short period of time? How was it resolved? What did you learn from this personal experience?

An attempt is also made to establish new supportive and meaningful relationships and experiences, reopening the person's social world. The therapeutic techniques commonly used by nurses performing crisis intervention are listed in Box 13-1.

BOX 13.1 COMMONLY USED THERAPEUTIC TECHNIQUES IN CRISIS INTERVENTION

- Displaying acceptance and concern and attempting to establish a positive relationship
- Encouraging the client to discuss present feelings, such as denial, guilt, grief, or anger
- Helping the client to confront the reality of the crisis by gaining an intellectual—as well as emotional—understanding of the situation; not encouraging the person to focus on *all* the implications of the crisis at once
- Explaining that the client's emotions are a normal reaction to the crisis
- Avoiding false reassurance
- Clarifying fantasies; contrasting them with facts
- Not encouraging the client to place the blame for the crisis on others because such encouragement prevents the client from facing the truth, reduces the client's motivation to take responsibility for behavior, and impedes or discourages adaptation during the crisis
- Setting limits on destructive behavior
- Emphasizing the client's responsibility for behavior and decisions
- Assisting the client in seeking help with the activities of daily living until resolution occurs
- Evaluating and modifying nursing interventions as necessary

Resolution

During resolution, anticipatory planning and evaluation occur. Reassessment is crucial to ascertain that the intervention is reducing tension and anxiety successfully rather than producing negative effects. Reinforcement is provided whenever necessary while the crisis work is reviewed and accomplishments of the client are emphasized. Assistance is given to formulate realistic plans for the future, and the client is given the opportunity to discuss how present experiences may help in coping with future crises.

Crisis Intervention Modes

The steps in crisis intervention presented in the preceding paragraphs usually are evident during individual crisis counseling. Clients also may elect to participate in a crisis group that resolves various crises through use of the group process (seen in self-awareness groups, personal growth groups, or short-term group therapy). Such groups generally meet for four to six sessions. They provide support and encouragement to persons who depend on others for much of their sense of personal fulfillment and achievement. Family crisis counseling includes the entire family during sessions and lasts approximately 6 weeks. This type of counseling is considered the preferred method of crisis intervention for children and adolescents.

Suicide prevention and crisis intervention counseling centers provide telephone hotlines on a 24-hour basis (Fig. 13-2). Volunteers who have had intensive training in telephone interviewing and counseling, and can give the person in crisis immediate help, usually staff such hotlines.

Mental health crisis intervention services are often hospital based or tied to community mental health centers. Mobile crisis response units provide services to the homebound, older adult clients, or individuals who live in rural areas. Behavioral outreach programs designed to provide on-site crisis intervention services to persons with serious and persistent mental illness residing in rural communities have been known to reduce psychiatric hospitalizations by approximately 60% (Crisis Intervention Network, 2001; Hennepin County Medical Center, 2005). Interventions for victims of abuse or violence are included in Chapter 33. Box 13-2 lists some examples of the different types of crisis centers.

Legal Aspects of Crisis Intervention*

Since 1980, the CPI has trained more than 5 million human service professionals (eg, police officers, emergency medical personnel) in the technique of nonviolent crisis intervention. As noted earlier, participants are trained to recognize an individual in crisis and prevent an emotionally or physically threatening situation from escalating out of control. Crisis intervention training helps eliminate staff confusion, develops self-confidence among staff, and promotes teamwork (CPI, 2005).

Most people are not required by law to help a person in crisis. However, certain individuals such as police officers, firefighters, and emergency medical personnel are legally responsible to provide help. In certain states, doctors and nurses are also expected to intervene during an emergency or crisis situation. Generally, these individuals are legally protected as long as they provide reasonable and prudent care according to a set of previously established criteria, and thus do not hesitate to aid people who need their help. (See Doctrine of Charitable Immunity in Chapter 5, Ethical and Legal Issues.)

The criteria or standards of care for a person providing crisis intervention state that the person who begins to intervene in a crisis is obligated to continue the intervention unless a more qualified person relieves him or her. Discontinuing care constitutes abandonment, and the caregiver is liable for any damages suffered as a result of the abandonment. Any unauthorized or unnecessary discussion of the crisis incident by the person intervening is considered a breach of confidentiality. Touching a crisis victim without the victim's permission could result in a charge of battery. However, permission can be obtained verbally or by nonverbal actions that express a desire for help. Consent also can be implied. Implied consent is permission to care for an unconscious crisis victim to preserve life or prevent further injury. Therefore, "failure to act in a crisis carries a greater legal liability than acting in favor of the treatment" (Mitchell & Resnik, 1981, p. 34).

---

*The following information is a summary of simple, broad statements regarding the legal aspects of crisis intervention and in no way is intended to provide legal counsel. The intent of the author is to inform the nurse of the potential for legal liabilities.

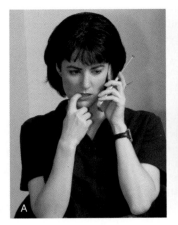 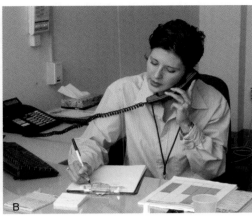

FIGURE 13.2 A client (**A**) calls a 24-hour telephone crisis hotline worker (**B**).

In cases where a client is injured by the actions of a crisis worker, negligence may be charged. However, the client must prove that the worker acted with a blatant disregard for the standard of care. Usually, the charge is dropped if the caregiver can prove that he or she acted in a prudent and reasonable manner.

Crisis Intervention for Children and Adolescents

Childhood and adolescent development can be significantly altered as a consequence of exposure to a disaster or a crisis. The entire family is affected. Trauma can change the way children view their world. Assumptions about safety and security are challenged. Their reactions will depend upon the severity of the trauma, their personality, the way they cope with stress, and the availability of support. It is not uncommon for children to regress both behaviorally and academically after a trauma. The emotional responses of adolescents mirror those of adults. However, differences include profound changes in their attitudes toward life and their future. These attitudes often trigger risk-taking behaviors that, if prolonged, can have secondary effects such as sleep disturbances, poor school performance, and lowered self-esteem (Bensing, 2003).

Assessment of Children and Adolescents in Crisis

To assess a child or adolescent in crisis, the nurse needs to have a working knowledge of the theories of

---

BOX 13.2   EXAMPLES OF CENTERS THAT PROVIDE CRISIS INTERVENTION

Children's Protective Services

Domestic Violence Crisis Center

Kids-in-Crisis Center

Life Crisis Center

Parents-in-Crisis Center

Rape Crisis Center

Sexual Assault Crisis Center

Suicide Crisis Center

Youth Crisis Center

Workplace Crisis Center

SELF-AWARENESS PROMPT

Reflect on your ability to interact with clients in a crisis. Are you able to present a mature, nonjudgmental attitude? Are you able to maintain a calm approach? Do you have a need to rescue others? What preparation do you feel would improve your ability to be a crisis clinician?

personality growth and development (see Chapter 24). Assessment focuses on psychosocial abilities, specifically intellectual, emotional, and social development (Mitchell & Resnik, 1981).

Common Reactions of a Child or Adolescent in Crisis

A child or adolescent in crisis presents a complex challenge. Depending upon the age of a child, individual needs and responses may differ with the same crisis events. Among the many events that produce a crisis state in a child or adolescent's life, injury, illness, and death are considered to be the most disruptive (Mitchell & Resnik, 1981).

It is natural for a child or adolescent to first experience denial that the crisis situation really happened. When the child or adolescent does respond, clinical symptoms are usually correlated to developmental stages. Clinical symptoms commonly exhibited include:

- Excessive fears, worries, self-blame, or guilt
- Irritability, anger, or sadness
- Sleep disturbances or nightmares
- Weight problems resulting from loss of appetite or overeating
- Agitation or restlessness
- Somatic complaints such as headaches or stomachaches
- Behavioral regression or aggression
- Poor concentration and loss of interest in school or activities

These symptoms may range from mild to severe. A child or adolescent who is in crisis should be encouraged to process emotions or reactions within 24 to 36 hours after the traumatic event to prevent the development of PTSD.

Interventions for a Child or Adolescent in Crisis

The major functions of crisis intervention for a child or adolescent in crisis are to:

- Provide safety and security including freedom from fears and terrors associated with the crisis event
- Provide an opportunity for bonding with a professional who displays an atmosphere of open acceptance, encourages verbalization of feelings and emotions, and assists the child or adolescent in practicing coping and communication skills

- Provide stabilization services that will assist a child or adolescent in the return to a precrisis level of functioning
- Assist the child or adolescent and his or her family members in resolving issues or situations that may have precipitated the crisis
- Provide linkages with community services to facilitate aftercare to process trauma and prevent the development of PTSD

Resolution of a Child's or Adolescent's Crisis

Resolution of a crisis may occur in a child's or adolescent's home or school, or in the community. Crisis response teams, also referred to as *mobile acute crisis teams,* are available 24 hours a day, 7 days a week and provide crisis counseling in homes and schools. Family members, teachers, and other concerned adults are encouraged to actively participate in the resolution of a crisis. Emergency shelters or safe houses are provided at confidential locations to provide for basic needs of a child who is the victim of domestic violence. Outreach programs provide individual support and crisis counseling to a child or adolescent experiencing difficulty at home and school because of domestic violence issues (Crossroads, 2003; Life Skills, 2003; Mitchell & Resnik, 1981; Wheeler Clinic, 2003).

KEY CONCEPTS

◆ A crisis situation such as divorce, rape, or a manmade or natural disaster can interrupt or disturb one's biologic, psychological, spiritual, or social integrity and may affect an individual, family, or community.

◆ There are two types of crises: a situational crisis, which refers to an extraordinary stressful event; and a maturational crisis, which can occur as one's lifestyle is continually subject to change. Disasters such as a hurricane or tornado are classified as situational crises.

◆ The onset of a crisis usually occurs suddenly, when normal coping methods fail, tensions rise, and emotional feelings such as fear, anxiety, or helplessness occur.

◆ Crises are classified depending on the degree of disruption or severity of the situation. Class 6, the most severe type, includes psychiatric emergencies, such as suicide or drug overdose.

◆ The individual in crisis generally experiences five phases: precrisis, impact, crisis, resolution, and postcrisis.

◆ Disaster intervention involves the provision of postdisaster support services during the early phase of a disaster. Disaster mental health nursing includes the application of the nursing process to victims and communities as they experience the following transitional periods during the recovery process: heroic period, honeymoon period, period of disillusionment, and period of reconstruction.

◆ Aguilera has described a paradigm of balancing factors. Balancing factors include realistic perception of an event, adequate situational support, and adequate defense or coping mechanisms to help resolve a problem. Assessment of these factors is important during crisis intervention.

◆ The nurse clinician or practitioner who assists in crisis interventions should not confuse crisis intervention with traditional psychotherapy. A multidisciplinary approach may facilitate resolution of crisis.

◆ Crisis intervention consists of assessment, planning therapeutic intervention, implementation of intervention techniques, and resolution of crisis with anticipatory planning for the future.

◆ Crisis intervention modes include counseling of individuals, groups, or families; telephone hotlines; mental health crisis intervention services; mobile crisis or disaster response units; and outreach programs in rural communities.

◆ Legal aspects of crisis intervention focus on which personnel are expected to assist in crisis situations; when legal immunity is granted; when the obligation to continue crisis intervention is expected; and when negligence may be charged.

◆ The focus of assessment of a child or adolescent in crisis centers is on the child's or adolescent's psychosocial abilities, specifically his or her intellectual, emotional, and social development. Reactions to interventions depend upon the severity of the trauma, the child's or adolescent's personality and ability to cope with stress, and the availability of support.

For additional study materials, please refer to the Student Resource CD-ROM located in the back of this textbook.

CHAPTER WORKSHEET

CRITICAL THINKING QUESTIONS

1. You have just completed the most difficult examination of your nursing education. A classmate has been struggling with her grades and is sure she has been unsuccessful. As you listen to her, you realize her perception is distorted and she is exhibiting inadequate coping skills. How might you help her use balancing factors to prevent her from having a crisis?

2. Interview a family member about a family crisis (eg, a death, an illness, an injury, or a divorce). Analyze how the family went through the phases of crisis. Did some family members come to resolution and others remain in crisis longer? What is the difference in the coping abilities of those different family members? What does this tell you about your family's ability to handle crises?

3. Create a fact sheet about the legal aspects of crisis intervention in your state. Prepare a 15-minute presentation and share the information you researched with your classmates.

REFLECTION

Crisis can be a turning point for better or for worse in a person's life. Review the quote at the beginning of the chapter and, applying this quote, cite at least three ways divorce can be a turning point in the life of a middle-aged woman who has been physically and emotionally abused by her husband for several years. State the rationale for your answers.

NCLEX-STYLE QUESTIONS

1. A client who informs the nurse that she has recently filed for divorce complains of feeling confused, helpless, and disorganized for the last 2 days. The nurse identifies that the client is in which crisis phase?
   a. Precrisis
   b. Initial impact
   c. Postcrisis
   d. Resolution

2. A retired couple recently moved to a new state and is now away from their children. The husband is admitted to the critical care unit after an acute myocardial infarction. The wife verbalizes feelings of being overwhelmed by anxiety. Which factor would the nurse identify as having a major impact on the crisis situation experienced by the wife?

   a. Environment of the critical care unit
   b. Fact of her husband's illness
   c. Loss of environmental supports
   d. Poor coping mechanisms

3. An older adult client is admitted to the nursing home for rehabilitation after surgery to repair a fractured hip. The client is fearful that she will not be able to return to her previous independent lifestyle. Which intervention would be the priority?

   a. Collaborating with the physical therapist to motivate the client
   b. Encouraging the client to verbalize feelings and thoughts about the current situation
   c. Providing reassurance that the situation will work out okay
   d. Teaching the client about various community supports available

4. A client comes to the emergency department (ED) after being sexually assaulted. She is fearful and crying. Which intervention would be the best initially?

   a. Assessing whether a supportive relative or friend can come to the ED
   b. Completing the rape crisis protocol for the physical examination
   c. Conveying an attitude of acceptance and concern to establish trust
   d. Referring client to a rape crisis support group

5. A client who has experienced a loss states that she has attempted to use problem-solving approaches by trial and error. She is exhibiting which phase of a crisis?

   a. Postcrisis
   b. Recoil or beginning resolution
   c. Shock
   d. Precrisis

6. A woman is brought to an emergency shelter that has been set up for the victims of a recent category 4 hurricane. She has numerous cuts and bruises on her arms and legs. During the assessment the client reports that her home was severely damaged. "I just moved here 6 months ago and now everything I had is basically gone. What am I going to do?" The nurse interprets the severity of the client's crisis, classifying it as:

   a. Class 1
   b. Class 3
   c. Class 5
   d. Class 6

Selected References

Aguilera, D. C. (1997). *Crisis intervention: Theory and methodology* (7th ed.). St. Louis, MO: C. V. Mosby.

Bensing, K. (2003). Psychology of disaster. *ADVANCE for Nurses, 4*(13), 13–16.

Burgess, A. W., & Baldwin, B. A. (1981). *Crisis intervention: Theory and practice.* Englewood Cliffs, NJ: Prentice-Hall.

Caplan, G. (1964). *Principles of preventive psychiatry.* New York: Basic Books.

Catherall, D. R. (2005). Secondary stress and the professional helper. Retrieved February 12, 2005, from http://www.ctsn-rest.ca/Secondary.html

Connoly, P. M., & Chandler, S. C. (1997). Crisis theory and intervention. In B. S. Johnson (Ed.), *Psychiatric–mental health nursing: Adaptation and growth* (4th ed, pp. 789–806). Philadelphia: Lippincott-Raven.

Crisis Intervention Network. (2001). Outreach programs. Retrieved June 3, 2001, from http://www.crisisintervention network.com/

Crisis Prevention Institute, Inc. (2005). CPI history. Retrieved August 23, 2005, from http://www.crisisprevention.com/about/history.html

Crossroads. (2003). Crisis intervention. Retrieved May 7, 2003, from http://www.fortnet.org/crossroads/service.html

Davidhizar, R., & Shearer, R. (2002). Helping children cope with public disasters. *American Journal of Nursing, 102*(3), 26–33.

Hennepin County Medical Center. (2005). Behavioral emergency outreach program. Retrieved August 23, 2005, from http://www.hcmc.org/depts/psych/cicbeop.htm

Lego, S. (Ed.). (1984). *The American handbook of psychiatric nursing.* Philadelphia: J. B. Lippincott.

Life Skills, Inc. (2003). Crisis services. Retrieved May 7, 2003, from http://www.lifeskills.com/crisis-services.htm

Lindemann, E. (1965). Symptomatology and management of acute grief. In H. J. Pared (Ed.), *Crisis intervention: Selected readings*. New York: Family Service Association of America.

McCann, L., & Pearlman, L. A. (1990). *Psychological trauma and the adult survivor: Theory, therapy, and transformation*. New York: Brunner/Mazel.

Mitchell, J., & Resnik, H. L. P. (1981). *Emergency response to crisis*. Bowie, MD: Robert J. Brady.

National Organization for Victim Assistance. (2005). NOVA's Crisis Response Team. Retrieved August 23, 2005, from http://www.trynova.org

Rosenbloom, D. (1999). Fostering connection with clients through the use of a trauma framework. *Psychiatric Times, 16*(6), 47–48.

Saunders, N. C. (2000). Crisis forensics: Comparative risks. *Psychiatric Times, 17*(2), 16, 20.

University of Hyogo. (2005). *Nurse's handbook: Mental health care in disasters*. Retrieved August 25, 2005, from http://www.coe-cnas.jp/eng/group_psyc/index.asp

Wheeler Clinic. (2003). Emergency mobile psychiatric services for children. Retrieved May 7, 2003, from http://www.wheelerclinic.org/children/emergency_psychiatric.php

Whittlesey, S., Vinekar, S., & Tucker, P. (1999). The Oklahoma City bombing: Learning from disaster. *Psychiatric Times, 16*(6), 43–46.

Benjamin, M. (2000). Home-based care may be best choice for youths in psychiatric crisis. *Psychiatric Times, 17*(3), 21.

Carpenito-Moyet, L. J. (2006). *Handbook of nursing diagnosis* (11th ed.). Philadelphia: Lippincott Williams & Wilkins.

Conner, M. G. (2004). Crisis intervention for teenagers—A family guide. Retrieved August 23, 2005, from http://www.help-for-parents.org/Crisis/CrisisInterventionTeens.htm

JAMA Patient Page. (2000). Helping children cope with violence. *Journal of the American Medical Association, 284*(5), 654.

Kaplan, A. (2001). How will your patients respond to September 11? *Geriatric Times, 2*(6), 4–5.

Peternelj-Taylor, C. A., Huff, A. G., Connolly, P. M., & Peterson, K. (2003). Working with special environments: Forensic clients, crisis intervention and the homeless. In W. K. Mohr (Ed.), *Johnson's psychiatric–mental health nursing* (5th ed., pp. 201–210). Philadelphia: Lippincott Williams & Wilkins.

Rose, C., & Jagim, M. (2003). Psychiatric triage RNs in the ED. *American Journal of Nursing, 103*(9), 101–105.

White, J. (2002, September 30). One year later: The impact and aftermath of September 11: "The American Psychiatric Nurses Association Responds to the September 11 Tragedy." *Online Journal of Issues in Nursing, 7*(3), Manuscript 3. Retrieved August 25, 2005, from http://www.nursingworld.org/ojin/topic19/tpc19_3.htm

Suggested Readings

Antai-Otong, D. (2002, January/February). Overwhelming stressful events: Proactive response key to coping. *American Nurse, 3*.

CHAPTER **14** / INDIVIDUAL PSYCHOTHERAPY

The goal of individual therapy is to alleviate patients' emotional difficulties in living and the elimination of symptomatology. —FROMM-REICHMANN, 1960

LEARNING OBJECTIVES

AFTER STUDYING THIS CHAPTER, YOU SHOULD BE ABLE TO:

1. Define the terms *transference, countertransference, resistance,* and *parataxis.*
2. Compare and contrast the principles of individual psychotherapy for children, adolescents, and adults.
3. Explain the qualifications of a nurse–therapist.
4. Articulate the role of the nurse as counselor.
5. Describe some alternate approaches to conventional psychotherapy.

KEY TERMS

Behavior therapy
Brief cognitive therapy
Brief interpersonal psychotherapy
Cognitive-behavioral therapy
Counseling
Countertransference
Dialectic behavioral therapy
E-therapy
Individual psychotherapy
Parataxis
Psychoanalysis
Psychotherapy
Resistance
Split-treatment psychotherapy
Transference

Psychotherapy has been referred to as the treatment of emotional and personality problems and disorders by psychological means. Many different techniques may be used to treat problems and disorders and to help the client become a mature, satisfied, and independent person. However, an important factor common to all of the techniques is the client–therapist relationship with its interpersonal experiences (Kolb, 1982).

Sigmund Freud (1856–1939) introduced the concept of **psychoanalysis,** the original *talking therapy,* which involved analyzing the root causes of behavior and feeling by exploring the unconscious mind and the conscious mind's relation to it. He was the first to understand and describe the psychotherapeutic process as an interpersonal experience between client and therapist. He thought that our relationships with other people, including clients, are patterned by early infant and childhood relationships with significant people in our environment. These patterns of relationships are repeated later in our lives and may interfere with client–therapist relationships because of **transference,** or the client's unconscious assignment to the therapist of feelings and attitudes originally associated with important figures in his or her early life. Transference can be positive (affectionate) or negative (hostile). The therapist, in turn, may exhibit **countertransference,** or an emotional reaction to the client based on the therapist's unconscious needs and conflicts. Such a response could interfere with therapeutic interventions during the course of treatment. **Resistance,** the conscious or unconscious psychological defense against bringing repressed thoughts into conscious awareness, may also occur and interfere with the client's ability to benefit from psychotherapy. Examples of resistance include remaining silent for a long period of time, being late for a therapy session, or missing appointments (Shahrokh & Hales, 2003; Sadock & Sadock, 2003).

Harry Stack Sullivan, a psychiatrist and psychoanalyst known for his research on the psychotherapy of schizophrenia and for his view of complex interpersonal relationships as the basis of personality development, introduced the term **parataxis.** It refers to the presence of distorted perception or judgment exhibited by the client during therapy. Parataxis is thought to be the result of earlier experiences in interpersonal relationships and occurs as a defense against anxiety (Shahrokh & Hales, 2003; Fromm-Reichmann, 1960).

According to the American Nurses Association (ANA; 2000), psychotherapy may be performed by the certified specialist in psychiatric–mental health nursing. Psychotherapy may also be performed by licensed clinical social workers, clinical psychologists, and psychiatrists. Psychotherapy is a process in which a person who wishes to relieve symptoms, resolve problems in living, or seek personal growth enters into a contract to interact in a prescribed way with the psychotherapist (Shahrokh & Hales, 2003). **Counseling** is a form of supportive psychotherapy in which the nurse and other qualified professionals, such as licensed mental health counselors, offer guidance or assist the client in viewing options to problems that are discussed by the client in the context of the nurse–client relationship (ANA, 2000). The psychiatric–mental health nurse must understand these dynamics while using counseling interventions or providing care to clients involved in psychotherapy. Chapter 3 focused on the development of theory-based psychiatric nursing practice and the various roles the nurse serves, including those of therapist and counselor. This chapter focuses on the application of individual therapy and counseling as they relate to the psychological needs of clients, including children and adolescents. Family, couple, and group therapy are addressed in Chapter 15.

Individual Psychotherapy

The principles of psychotherapy are based in part on the application of concepts by Freud and Sullivan. (Box 14-1 summarizes the major schools of psychotherapy). The psychotherapeutic process is designed to bring about understanding of and insight into the historical and dynamic factors that may be unknown to the client and that are among the causes of the mental disturbance for which the client seeks help (Fromm-Reichmann, 1960). Simply put, the main purpose of individual psychotherapy is to gain control of one's life.

Individual psychotherapy is a confidential relationship between client and therapist that may occur in the therapist's office, outpatient clinic, or mental hospital. Gender is an important and surprisingly neglected variable in the understanding and practice of psychotherapy. Gender can influence the client's

BOX 14.1 SCHOOLS OF
PSYCHOTHERAPY

I. Reconstructive psychotherapy: focuses on emotional and cognitive restructuring of self.
   A. Psychoanalysis (Sigmund Freud): may require several years of therapy and focuses on all aspects of the client's life
   B. Modifications of psychoanalysis: analytic play therapy (Anna Freud), character analysis (Wilhelm Reich), cognitive analysis (Jean Piaget), existential analysis (Ludwig Binswanger), and transactional analysis (Eric Berne)
   C. Group approaches: psychodrama (J. L. Moreno), psychoanalysis in groups (Alexander Wolf), orthodox psychoanalysis (S. R. Slavson)

II. Reeducative therapy: focuses on the exploration of new ways of perceiving and behaving (individual or group). Examples include client-centered therapy (Carl Rogers), behavior therapy (Ivan Pavlov, B. E. Skinner, J. B. Watson), and cognitive-behavior therapy (Aaron Beck).

III. Supportive therapy: focuses on the reinforcement of the client's self-esteem, ability to adapt, and sense of emotional well-being. Therapy may occur over a brief period or intermittently for years (individual or group). Examples include brief cognitive therapy, brief solution-focused therapy, and bereavement therapy, adaptations of the more coventional modes of therapy.

Edgerton, J. E. & Campbell, R. J. (Eds.). (2003). *American psychiatric glossary* (7th ed.). Washington, DC: American Psychiatric Press, Inc; Kolb, L. C. (1982). *Modern clinical psychiatry* (10th ed.). Philadelphia: W. B. Saunders; and Lego, S. (1996). *Psychiatric nursing: A comprehensive reference* (2nd ed.). Philadelphia: Lippincott-Raven.

lish boundaries of the relationship. The client's problems are noted, present coping skills are identified, strengths and attributes are explored, and open communication is established. The working phase occurs when the therapist and client focus on the client's problems and reach an understanding of why the problems have occurred. Ideally, the termination phase occurs when the client has achieved maximum benefit of therapy. However, termination may occur at any time during the sessions if the client is resistant to treatment or relocation occurs (Lego, 1996).

The goals of individual psychotherapy are to alleviate the client's discomfort or pain, alter character structure and strengthen the client's ego, promote emotional and interpersonal maturation, and improve the client's ability to perform or act appropriately. These goals are achieved by:

- Establishing a therapeutic relationship with the client
- Providing an opportunity for the client to release tension as problems are discussed
- Assisting the client in gaining insight about the problem
- Providing the opportunity to practice new skills
- Reinforcing appropriate behavior as it occurs
- Providing consistent emotional support

If a client is also receiving medication prescribed to stabilize clinical symptoms of a psychiatric disorder (eg, anxiety, depression), the therapist may elect to discuss the efficacy of the medication with the client during a therapy session. Some therapists prefer to treat medication management as a separate entity.

Modes of Individual Psychotherapy

In the past, individual psychotherapy typically involved long-term therapy. However, the advent of managed care has had a profound impact on the practice of psychotherapy. To reduce costs, clients who rely on psychiatric–mental health care benefits are limited to short-term or *brief therapy*. Brief therapy is a form of psychotherapy that is defined in terms of the number of sessions (generally not more than 15) or in terms of specified objectives that are usually goal-oriented, active, focused, and directed toward a specific problem or symptom (Shahrokh & Hales, 2003). The conventional intensive individual therapies of the past, such as psychoanalysis and uncovering therapy, are being replaced with brief cognitive therapy, behavior therapy, cognitive-behavioral therapy, and brief

choice of therapist, the "fit" between therapist and client, the sequence and content of the clinical material presented, the diagnosis, and the length and outcome of treatment. Age, race, culture, life experiences, and other variables also play an important role in the development of a therapeutic relationship between client and therapist.

There are three phases of individual psychotherapy: introductory, working, and termination. During the introductory phase, the therapist and client estab-

interpersonal psychotherapy. A summary of these more commonly used therapies is presented in this chapter. Additionally, Table 14-1 summarizes the other modes of individual psychotherapy such as psycho-analysis, uncovering therapy, hypnotherapy, reality therapy, and rational–emotive therapy, as well the interventions utilized by the nurse therapist.

Brief Cognitive Therapy

Brief cognitive therapy uses a time-limited, goal-oriented, problem-solving, here-and-now approach. The therapist assumes an active role while working with individuals to solve present-day problems by iden-tifying distorted thinking that causes emotional dis-comfort, exploring alternate behaviors, and creating change. There is little emphasis on the cause of the problem. Rather, the client and therapist explore why present thinking is causing the client distress. Candi-dates for this mode of therapy are described as edu-cated, verbal, and psychologically minded. They are free of borderline personality characteristics (see Chapter 24, Personality Development and Personality Disor-ders), do not exhibit psychotic symptoms, and often present with depressed mood, anxiety, or anger prob-lems (Lego, 1996; Schuyler, 2003). Couples and families may also benefit from this therapy. Box 14-2 describes the basic principles of brief cognitive therapy.

Behavior Therapy

Behavior therapy focuses on modifying overt symp-toms without regard to the client's private experience or inner conflicts. It is based on the assumption that behaviors or responses are learned and may be relearned. Used by behaviorists Pavlov, Watson, and Skinner, this therapy has been effective in the treat-ment of phobias, eating disorders, substance abuse, schizophrenia, sexual dysfunction, chronic night-mares, and some personality disorders. Chapter 12 provides a detailed discussion of various types of behavior therapy.

The role of the therapist is to help the client analyze behavior, define problems, and select goals. Techniques

TABLE 14.1 Modes of Individual Psychotherapy

MODE	SUMMARY	INTERVENTIONS BY THE NURSE THERAPIST
Psychoanalysis	Lengthy, 3 to 5 years; client talks in an uncontrolled, spontaneous manner of "free association" about anxieties, fears, and childhood images	Explores repressed feelings by interpreting dreams, emotions, and behavior Encourages a reliving experience to deal with once-fearful experiences
Uncovering therapy	Uncovering of conflicts, mainly uncon-scious	Assists client in exploring insight to work through conflict
Hypnotherapy	Adjunct to therapy to effect behavioral change and relaxation, control atti-tudes, and uncover repressed feelings or thoughts	Hypnotizes client Encourages discussion of emotional conflicts
Reality therapy	Based on premise that persons who are mentally unhealthy are irresponsible, cannot meet all of their basic needs, and refuse to face reality	Rejects unrealistic behavior displayed by client Assists the client in assuming responsibility for actions and in making value judgments
Rational–emotive therapy	A form of experiential therapy based on the premise that behavior is con-trolled by values and beliefs	Applies learning principles to question illogi-cal thinking Promotes problem-solving abilities, social skills, and assertiveness Techniques: visual imagery, role playing, modeling, behavior reversal, thought stop-ping, self-assessment, self-monitoring, and assertiveness training

BOX 14.2 BASIC PRINCIPLES OF BRIEF COGNITIVE THERAPY

- Humans are information-processing organisms, taking in data and generating appraisals.
- Feelings and behavior are influenced in the here-and-now by thoughts.
- Humans are capable of altering their thinking by dealing with conscious processes.
- Complicated problems do not require complicated solutions.
- Early learning lays down cognitive distortions by role modeling, feedback, culture, and early experience.
- Psychotherapy is an active collaborative venture between therapist and client.
- The therapist co-creates the problem with the client.
- Psychotherapy harnesses the client's problem-solving skills.
- The focus of cognitive therapy is on the here-and-now.
- Change can occur without directly dealing with transference.

Schuyler, D. (2003). *A practical guide to cognitive therapy.* New York: W. W. Norton.

include limit-setting, promoting positive adaptive behaviors, discouraging the use of maladaptive behaviors, promoting assertiveness, and assisting the client in exploring new ways of adjusting to the environment. Techniques such as assertiveness training, desensitization, role-playing, and self-management training may be used to achieve desired behaviors.

Cognitive-Behavioral Therapy

Cognitive-behavioral therapy combines the individual goals of cognitive therapy and behavioral therapy. It integrates the cognitive restructuring approach of cognitive therapy with the behavioral modification techniques of behavioral therapy. The therapist works with the client to identify both the thoughts and the behaviors that are causing distress, and to change those thoughts in order to readjust the behavior. Examples of techniques used to help clients uncover and examine their thoughts and change their behaviors may include behavioral homework assignments,

conditioning (eg, the use of reinforcement to encourage a specific behavior), and validity testing (eg, the therapist asks the client to produce evidence that a fundamental belief is true and does not require change or modification). Cognitive-behavioral therapy can be employed in any situation in which there is a pattern of unwanted behavior accompanied by distress and impairment. It is recommended as a treatment option for several psychiatric disorders such as affective disorders, personality disorders, anxiety disorders, or substance-related disorders. It is also frequently used as a tool to deal with clients who experience chronic pain (Smith, 2005).

Solution-focused brief therapy is a new and increasingly used therapeutic approach similar to cognitive-behavioral therapy. It focuses on helping clients construct solutions rather than solve problems, noting that change occurs all the time and individuals are capable of adapting and effecting change. The premise is that following a six-step process will enable the client to find quick solutions to whatever problems he or she may be facing. Although it is generally limited to 3 to 8 weeks in length, it can be used over a longer period of time (All About Counseling.Com, 2005).

Brief Interpersonal Psychotherapy

Brief interpersonal psychotherapy (BIPT) is a semistructured, psychodynamically time-limited model of psychotherapy. It is an adaptation of the interpersonal model used by Peplau, Horney, Fromm, and Sullivan and is designed for use in a 3- to 4-month framework. (See Chapter 3 for a discussion of Peplau's Interpersonal theory.)

Assessment focuses on an interpersonal inventory of the client's relationships with members of his or her family of origin. Data collected establishes the overall relationship competency of the client and the client's level of satisfaction with his or her environment. The therapist reinforces the client's self-esteem; employs a conversational, goal-focused approach; reinforces and supports the positive use of defense mechanisms or coping skills; and avoids the use of transference and countertransference.

Four problem areas commonly associated with depression and anxiety respond to BIPT. These include grief related to loss by death or separation, ongoing interpersonal conflict, social role change requiring adaptation, and long-standing interpersonal problems of loneliness or isolation (MacKenzie, 1997). Currently, when psychopharmacology (if indicated) is combined with BIPT, recidivism or recurrence of psychiatric disorders is dramatically reduced.

Split-Treatment Psychotherapy

Split-treatment psychotherapy, also referred to as *dual treatment, triangulated treatment,* or *medication backup,* involves a protocol between a nurse–therapist who provides psychotherapy and a psychiatrist or nurse practitioner who provides pharmacotherapy for the client. Clients with the diagnosis of a mood disorder, dual diagnosis, psychotic disorder, or mental retardation are often seen in split-treatment psychotherapy. Therapists who specialize in certain treatment approaches such as cognitive or behavioral therapy often request that medication be prescribed by another clinician. This type of therapy is deeply rooted and widely practiced in places such as community mental health centers because of the increasing pressure from managed care organizations and third-party payers (Balon & Riba, 2001).

Individual Therapy With Children and Adolescents

The need for psychotherapy for a child or adolescent is based upon such factors as the client's current problem, life history, level of development, ability to cooperate in treatment, and what interventions are most likely to help with the presenting concerns. Psychotherapy is often used in combination with other interventions such as the administration of medication, use of behavior management, or cooperative work with the school. The therapist must have an understanding of the normal development for a child or adolescent of any given age as well as an understanding of the individual's life story. Individual psychotherapy focuses on improving the client's adaptive skills in and outside the family setting (American Academy of Child & Adolescent Psychiatry, 2005; Sadock & Sadock, 2003).

The relationship that develops between the therapist and client is very important. Most pediatric or adolescent clients do not voluntarily seek treatment; they are referred to treatment because of a disturbance noted by a family member, teacher, or pediatrician. If the client feels comfortable, safe, and understood, it is much easier to express his or her thoughts and feelings.

Psychotherapy provides emotional support, helps the client resolve conflicts with people, helps the client understand problems and feelings, and assists the client in trying out new solutions to old problems. Parents may be involved in varying degrees depending upon the age of the client and the nature of the identified conflict or disturbance. The therapist acts as an advocate and may be called upon to make recommendations that affect various aspects of the client's life (American Academy of Child & Adolescent Psychiatry, 2005; Sadock & Sadock, 2003). Individual psychotherapy for children and adolescents, including techniques utilized to help a child express emotions, fears or concerns, are addressed in Chapter 29.

Counseling

The psychiatric nurse uses counseling interventions to assist clients in improving or regaining their previous coping abilities, fostering mental health, and preventing mental illness and disability (ANA, 2000). Counseling interventions may occur in a variety of settings and may include the following:

- Communication and interviewing techniques
- Problem-solving skills
- Crisis intervention
- Stress management
- Relaxation techniques
- Assertiveness training
- Conflict resolution
- Behavior modification

Counseling is an important intervention during one-to-one interactions with clients or during the presentation of psychoeducation groups, medication groups, and discharge planning groups. Clients and their family members and significant others are given an opportunity to verbalize any concerns they may have. The counselor provides reassurance and clarification as the need arises. Reassurance helps the client regain self-confidence and decreases feelings of guilt, anxiety, or fear. Clarification helps the client gain a clearer picture of reality by understanding feelings and behavior. Explaining to a client with depression that the symptoms he or she is experiencing are related to a chemical imbalance in the brain that can be helped by antidepressant medication is an example of clarification of reality. Chapter 12 discusses the nurse's role as a counselor when providing client education, addressing spiritual needs, promoting personal and sleep hygiene, providing pain management, providing protective care, using behavioral therapy, and assisting with adjunctive or management therapies.

Alternate Approaches to Psychotherapy

Online psychotherapy, or **e-therapy,** is a viable alternative source for help when traditional psychotherapy is not accessible. It is effective and private, and is conducted by skilled, qualified, ethical professionals. For some individuals, it may be the only way they are willing to obtain help from a professional therapist. One online service, Therapy 4 Life (http://www.therapy4life.com/), provides therapists for individual therapy, couples therapy, metaphysical or spiritual therapy, and holistic healing.

Other alternatives to psychotherapy currently being used can be identified by a review of the literature. Many of these approaches relate to the therapist's use of technology and the Internet. For example, in England, a psychiatrist conducts psychotherapy with a client in New York by way of cyberspace (Demott, 1999). At Massachusetts General Hospital in Boston, a Psychiatric Tele-Consultation Unit provides electronic consultation to primary care physicians while the client is still in the office (Sherman, 1999b). In Montana, a psychiatrist uses telepsychiatry or video equipment and appropriate computer software to conduct "med checks," consultations, evaluation and treatment planning, and brief short-term psychotherapy for a largely refractory population of clients who are scattered over hundreds of miles. Videophone psychotherapy has been used with clients who received bone marrow transplants that required up to 2 months of isolation in a hospital room (Sherman, 1999c).

Modifications also have been made in the use of psychotherapy. Modified life review therapy, cognitive therapy, and insight-oriented therapy are being used to treat older adult clients with major depression (Finkelstein, 1999). **Dialectic behavioral therapy** (DBT), developed by Linehan for chronically suicidal individuals suffering from borderline personality disorders, is a comprehensive psychosocial treatment modality that blends together the most effective interventions in behavior therapy and balances them with treatment strategies that focus on acceptance and validation. It is effective in the treatment of bipolar disorder (Knowlton, 1999). Linehan received the 1999 research award given by the New York City–based American Foundation for Suicide Prevention. Grills (Rudderow, 1999) uses motivational interviewing to encourage clients with destructive behaviors (eg, alcohol or drug abuse) to express reasons for concern and to present their own arguments for change. Grills claims that this approach works because it brings with it a certain attitude about people, the healing process, behavioral change, and an appreciation of the role clients play in the healing process. The application of basic psychotherapeutic skills to cross-cultural situations has been addressed by McCabe (Sherman, 1999a). According to McCabe, cross-cultural therapy is essential in a society in which ethnic subcultures continue to grow. These subcultures remain underserved in terms of psychiatric–mental health care. The obstacles to psychiatric–mental health care are financial as well as cultural, including language barriers and lack of knowledge (see Chapter 4 for more information). Because it is not always possible to match client and therapist ethnically, therapists are responsible for developing cultural competency to provide care for those of different ethnic and racial backgrounds.

KEY CONCEPTS

◆ Psychotherapy is a process in which a person enters into a contract with a therapist to relieve symptoms, to resolve problems in living, or to seek personal growth.

◆ During psychotherapy, the client may exhibit behaviors such as transference, resistance or parataxis. The therapist may exhibit countertransference. Any of these behaviors can interfere with therapeutic interventions during treatment.

◆ Three phases occur during individual psychotherapy. During the introductory phase, the therapist and client establish boundaries, gather information regarding the client's problems and coping skills, and explore client attributes and strengths. Open communication is also established. During the working phase, the client and therapist focus on the client's problems and their causes. Termination generally occurs when the client has reached maximum benefit from therapy; however, termination may also occur due to resistance to treatment or relocation.

◆ Cost containment by managed care companies has had an effect on the practice of psychotherapy, promoting short-term, brief psychotherapy. Conventional intensive psychotherapies have been replaced by brief cognitive therapy, behavior therapy, cognitive-behavioral therapy, and brief interpersonal psychotherapy.

◆ Psychotherapy also helps children and adolescents in a variety of ways. They receive emotional support, resolve conflicts with people, understand feelings and problems, and try out new solutions to old problems.

◆ Nurses who possess a master's degree in psychiatric nursing and are certified clinical nurse specialists may conduct individual therapy.

◆ Counseling is a form of supportive psychotherapy performed by nurses in the clinical setting to assist clients in improving or regaining previous coping abilities, fostering mental health, and preventing mental illness or disability. Counseling can occur during one-to-one interactions with clients or during the presentation of various groups to address identified needs.

◆ Creative alternate approaches to psychotherapy have occurred as a result of technological advances: cyberspace therapy, telepsychiatry, and videophone psychotherapy. Modifications have also occurred in the use of psychotherapy to treat the older adult, chronically suicidal clients with borderline personality disorders, and clients with destructive behaviors such as alcohol or drug abuse.

◆ Competence in cross-cultural therapy is essential to provide services to individuals of different ethnic and racial backgrounds.

For additional study materials, please refer to the Student Resource CD-ROM located in the back of this textbook.

CHAPTER WORKSHEET

CRITICAL THINKING QUESTIONS

1. Review the modes of individual psychotherapy listed in Table 14.1. Identify which mode(s) you believe would be most appropriate for a 24-year old female client who is exhibiting clinical symptoms of depression secondary to the death of her fiancé. Explain the rationale for your selection of each mode.

2. Develop a 15-minute presentation comparing and contrasting the role of the nurse–therapist and the psychiatric nurse using counseling interventions. Share the presentation with your classmates.

3. Construct an educational tool describing alternative approaches to psychotherapy identified in this chapter. Interview at least three nursing staff members to determine whether they believe alternative approaches are viable sources for help when traditional psychotherapy is not accessible.

REFLECTION

Reflect on the chapter opening quote about the goal of individual therapy. Articulate how split-treatment psychotherapy achieves this goal. Identify clients who might benefit from split-treatment psychotherapy. Explain the rationale for your selection.

NCLEX-STYLE QUESTIONS

1. Which of the following occurs when a therapist has an emotional reaction to the client based on the therapist's unconscious needs and conflicts?
   a. Transference
   b. Parataxis
   c. Psychoanalysis
   d. Countertransference

2. Which example best illustrates the role of the nurse as a counselor?
   a. Assigning responsibilities for running a community meeting to several clients
   b. Conducting a thorough nursing admission assessment for a client
   c. Clarifying reasons for admission with a client having poor reality testing
   d. Teaching a small group about the use of antidepressant medications

3. During which phase of individual therapy would the nurse expect problems to be noted and present coping skills to be identified?

a. Introductory phase
b. Working phase
c. Orientation phase
d. Termination phase

4. Which therapy would the nurse identify as being used when a semistructured, psychodynamically time-limited model of psychotherapy is employed to treat problems such as grief, loneliness, or isolation?
   a. Reality therapy
   b. Uncovering therapy
   c. Brief interpersonal therapy
   d. Cognitive therapy

5. Which of the following modes of the individual psychotherapy focus on the here and now with little emphasis on the cause of the problem?
   a. Brief cognitive therapy
   b. Cognitive–behavioral therapy
   c. Solution-focused therapy
   d. Brief interpersonal therapy

Selected References

All About Counseling.Com. (2005). Counseling approaches. Retrieved August 28, 2005, from http://www.allabout counseling.com/counseling_approaches.htm

American Academy of Child & Adolescent Psychiatry. (2005). What is psychotherapy for children and adolescents? Retrieved September 1, 2005, from http://www.aacap.org/publications/factsfam/therapy.htm

American Nurses Association. (2000). *Scope and standards of psychiatric–mental health nursing practice*. Washington, DC: American Nurses Publishing.

Balon, R., & Riba, M. B. (2001). Improving the practice of split treatment. *Psychiatric Annals, 31*(10), 594–595.

Burgio, L. D., Stevens, A., Burgio, K. L., Roth, D. L., Paul, P., & Gerstle, J. (2002). Teaching and maintaining behavior management skills in the nursing home. *The Gerontologist, 42,* 487–496.

Demott, K. (1999). More psychiatrists on the couch and online. *Clinical Psychiatry News, 27*(3), 17.

Edgerton, J. E. & Campbell, R. J. (Eds.). (1994). *American psychiatric glossary* (7th ed.). Washington, DC: American Psychiatric Press, Inc.

Finkelstein, J. B. (1999). Modify psychotherapy for depressed elderly. *Clinical Psychiatry News, 27*(8), 25.

Fromm-Reichmann, F. (1960). *Principles of intensive psychotherapy.* Chicago: University of Chicago Press.

Knowlton, L. (1999). Marsha Linehan: Dialectic behavioral therapy. *Psychiatric Times, 16*(7), 54.

Kolb, L. C. (1982). *Modern clinical psychiatry* (10th ed.). Philadelphia: W. B. Saunders.

Lego, S. (1996). *Psychiatric nursing: A comprehensive reference* (2nd ed.). Philadelphia: Lippincott-Raven Publishers.

MacKenzie, K. R. (1997). *Time-managed group psychotherapy: Effective clinical applications.* Washington, DC: American Psychiatric Press, Inc.

Rudderow, A. (1999). Therapist serves as a motivational guide. *Clinical Psychiatry News, 27*(4), 22.

Sadock, B. J., & Sadock, V. A. (2003). *Kaplan and Sadock's synopsis of psychiatry: Behavioral sciences/clinical psychiatry* (9th ed.). Philadelphia: Lippincott Williams & Wilkins.

Schuyler, D. (2003). *A practical guide to cognitive therapy.* New York: W. W. Norton.

Shahrokh, N., & Hales, R. E. (Eds.). (2003). *American psychiatric glossary,* (8th ed.). Washington, DC: American Psychiatric Press, Inc.

Sherman, C. (1999a). Bridging the gap: Therapy for patients from other cultures. *Clinical Psychiatry News, 27*(5), 23.

Sherman, C. (1999b). Teleconsults dial psychiatrists into primary care. *Clinical Psychiatry News, 27*(3), 17.

Sherman, C. (1999c). Telepsychiatry dials into primary care. *Clinical Psychiatry News, 27*(2), 1–2.

Smith, J. E. (2005). Cognitive-behavioral therapy. Retrieved August 28, 2005, from http://www.chclibrary.org/micromed/00043200.html

Suggested Readings

Balon, R. (2001). Positive and negative aspects of split treatment. *Psychiatric Annals, 3*(10), 598–603.

Batoosingh, K. A. (1999). Interpersonal psychotherapy: Clock keeps ticking. *Clinical Psychiatry News, 27*(5), 22.

Esposito, J. (2003). Calling all nurses: The 411 about telepath nursing. *Vital Signs, 13*(6), 24.

Fingeld, D. L. (1999). Psychotherapy in cyberspace. *Journal of American Psychiatric Nursing Association, 5*(4), 105.

Franklin, D. (2004). Developer of DBT predicts wider use of modality. *Clinical Psychiatry News, 32*(10), 36.

Johnson, K. (2000). CBT is quicker that IBT in treating bulimia. *Clinical Psychiatry News, 28*(3), 27.

Ko, D. (2001). In schizophrenia, nurse-administered behavioral therapy shows benefit. *CNS News, 3*(10), 1, 18.

London, R. T. (2005). Making dual therapy work. *Clinical Psychiatry News, 33*(2), 19.

CHAPTER 15 / FAMILY, COUPLE, AND GROUP THERAPY

*The phenomena of emotional bonding, role enactment, communication, sexuality,
and the broader system that provides the context for a relationship become the
focus of couple therapy when conflict occurs.* —CHISHOLM, 1996
*Interest in the family of the psychiatric patient has blended over the years to interest in the
family as the psychiatric patient. This conceptual focus on the family as a whole instead of one
individual member is the key element of the family therapy approach.* —JONES, 1980
*Groups are a crucial part of life experience for people .... They constitute a potent force for the
prevention and remediation of personal and social problems.* —BRILL, LEVINE, & BRILL, 2001

LEARNING OBJECTIVES

AFTER STUDYING THIS CHAPTER, YOU SHOULD BE ABLE TO:

1. Describe at least three alternatives to the traditional nuclear family.
2. Articulate the developmental stages of the family according to Duvall's theory of the family life cycle.
3. Compare and contrast characteristics of functional and dysfunctional families.
4. Explain the development of couple, family, and group therapy.
5. Explain the purpose of couple, family, and group therapy.
6. Analyze four different modes of family therapy, stating the role of the therapist in each mode.
7. Compare and contrast the goals of couple and family therapy.
8. Develop a couple or family assessment guide.
9. Formulate a list of the common nursing diagnoses applicable to families participating in family therapy.
10. Construct a genogram and explain its usefulness in family therapy.
11. Recognize the advantages of group therapy.
12. Identify at least six factors considered to be essential components of group therapy.
13. Construct the stages of group development in group therapy.
14. Compare and contrast the nurse–therapist's role in couple, family, and group therapy.

KEY TERMS

Autocratic group leader
Brief couples therapy
Closed groups
Contextual therapy
Couple therapy
Democratic group leader
Dysfunctional families
Families
Family therapy
Group therapy
Healthy functioning family
Laissez-faire group leader
Marital-relations therapy
Object-relations therapy
Open groups

Families are groups of individuals who interact, support, and influence each other in performing basic functions. They are an integral part of society, bound together by intense and long-lasting ties of past experience, social roles, mutual support, and expectations. The family constitutes an interactive milieu in which the exchange of information among individual members continually occurs. The term *couple* is used to describe two adults who have a close or intimate relationship. They may be heterosexual or homosexual, single, married, or in a same-sex union. The term *group* is used to describe at least three individuals who gather together to share or discuss common problems or concerns.

This chapter focuses on the application of couple, family, and group therapy as they relate to the psychosocial needs of clients, families, or significant others. The role of the nurse–therapist is also discussed.

Overview of Families

Families have undergone many changes in the last 50 years. Various lifestyles and arrangements have emerged. Historically, "family" referred to the traditional nuclear family, that of father, mother, and children. Today, alternatives to this traditional nuclear family include single-parent households, blended families involving the remarriage of one parent to someone who may or may not have children, extended families that include the presence of other relatives, and cohabitation between nonmarried persons. Families may consist of married or nonmarried, homosexual or heterosexual couples and may include children.

All family members influence one another as they interact and support each other in performing basic functions necessary for the family's well-being. As women continue to join the workforce in greater numbers, changes occur in child care, childrearing practices, and role sharing. In a dual-career family in which both husband and wife work, the husband must assume some roles that mothers and wives traditionally performed. These changes in the traditional nuclear family have made it necessary for parents to teach their children new skills to help them cope in today's society.

The family also influences personal development. In the family setting, members learn how to relate to and communicate with others. If the family has a positive influence on its members, they will develop a sense of self-worth and positive self-esteem, ultimately becoming productive members of society. Conversely, poor parenting skills, ineffective role-modeling, and the inability of parents to communicate effectively may have negative influences on family members. As a result of these negative influences, family members often have difficulty adjusting to the expectations of society.

The Family Life Cycle

The family is a developing system that must progress in the proper manner for healthy child development. According to Duvall's (1984) theory, there are predictable, successive stages of growth and development in the life cycle of every family. Each stage is characterized by specific tasks to be achieved. These family developmental tasks refer to growth responsibilities achieved by a family as a unit and by individual developmental requisites. However, individual developmental needs and family tasks may not always agree, possibly leading to conflict and resulting in poor interpersonal relationships, the development of individual emotional problems, or a family crisis. Duvall identified eight stages of the family life cycle. Table 15-1 summarizes each of Duvall's eight stages, including the age and school placement of the oldest child, which affects the responsibilities of the family members. An understanding of these stages provides the nurse with guidelines for analyzing family growth and health promotion needs and the ability to provide therapeutic intervention when conflict arises.

Healthy Functioning Families

Finding research on the so-called "normal" family is difficult, although much is published about dysfunctional or pathogenic families. However, healthy families demonstrate specific characteristics:

- The ability to communicate thoughts and feelings
- Parental guidance in determining the functioning level of the total family

In addition, the healthy family expects interactions among its members to be unreserved, honest, atten-

TABLE 15.1 Duvall's Eight Stages of the Family Life Cycle

STAGE	DESCRIPTION OF FAMILY TASKS
I. Beginning families (no children; commitment to each other; referred to as a couple)	Establishing a mutually satisfying marriage by learning to live together and to provide for each other's personality needs Relating harmoniously to three families: each respective family and the one being created by marriage Family planning: whether to have children and when Developing a satisfactory sexual and marital role adjustment
II. Early childbearing (begins with birth of first child and continues until infant is age 30 months)	Developing a stable family unit with new parent roles Reconciling conflicting developmental tasks of various family members Jointly facilitating developmental needs of family members to strengthen each other and the family unit Accepting the new child's personality
III. Families with pre-school children (first-born child $2\frac{1}{2}$ years old; continues until age 5)	Exploring of environment by children Establishing privacy, housing, and adequate space Having husband–father become more involved in household responsibilities Developing of preschooler to a more mature role and assuming responsibilities for self-care Socializing of children such as attending school, church, sports Integrating of new family members (second or third child)
IV. Families with school-aged children (firstborn child ages 6 to 13)	Separating from children as they enter school Promoting school achievement of children Maintaining a satisfying marital relationship, because this is a period when it diminishes Promoting open communication in the family
V. Families with teenagers	Accepting adolescence Maintaining a satisfying marital relationship while handling parental responsibilities Maintaining open communication between generations Maintaining family ethical and moral standards by the parents while the teenagers search for their own beliefs and values
VI. Launching-center families (covers the first child through last child leaving home)	Allowing children to experiment with independence Expanding the family circle to include new members by marriage Accepting the new couple's own lifestyle and values Devoting time to other activities and relationships by the parents Reestablishing the wife and husband roles as the children achieve independent roles Assisting aging and ill parents of the husband and wife
VII. Families of middle years ("empty nest" period through retirement)	Maintaining a sense of well-being psychologically and physiologically by living in a healthy environment Attaining and enjoying a career or other creative accomplishments by cultivating leisure-time activities and interests Sustaining satisfying and meaningful relationships with aging parents and children Strengthening the marital relationship
VIII. Families in retirement and old age (begins with retirement of one or both spouses, continues through loss of one spouse, and terminates with death of the other spouse)	Maintaining satisfying living arrangements Maintaining marital relationships Adjusting to a reduced income Adjusting to the loss of a spouse

tive, and protective, whereas interactions in the unhealthy family tend to be reserved, guarded, or antagonistic (Goldenberg & Goldenberg, 2003).

In the **healthy functioning family,** no single member dominates or controls another. Instead, there is a respect for the individuation of other family members and their points of view and opinions, even if the differences lead to confrontation or altercation. Family members participate in activities together, unlike members of dysfunctional families, who tend to be isolated from one another, possibly trying to control others in the family. Although power is found in healthy families in the parent coalition (union or alliance), it is not used in an authoritarian manner. Children are allowed to express opinions, negotiations are worked out, and power struggles do not ensue. Good communication patterns are paramount (Goldenberg & Goldenberg, 2003).

A healthy functioning family encourages personal autonomy and independence among its members, but individuality is not obscured. Family members are able to adapt to the changes that occur with normal growth and development and to cope with separation and loss.

In a healthy functioning family, each family member typically progresses through specific stages of development, which include bonding, independence, separation, and individuation. Ego boundaries are clearly developed. By the time members reach adolescence, they begin to function more independently. Increased independence requires an adjustment in the relationship of all family members. However, family members should not function so independently of each other that the family system is impaired or the rights of individual family members are violated. Otherwise, distress in the family can result. Other problems that may cause distress include marital disharmony, differing childrearing techniques, and the acute physical or emotional illness of a member. See Supporting Evidence for Practice 15-1 for an overview of the effect of cardiac disease on the family.

Dysfunctional Families

Like mental health and mental illness, family functioning occurs on a continuum. Healthy families can become dysfunctional under stress when issues of power persist and go unresolved; no identified leader or parent helps take control and establish some sense of order. Instead, the family experiences chaos, which results from leadership that may be changing from one member to another over short periods. Control or power is attempted through intimidation instead of open communication and negotiation. The lack of lead-

---

SUPPORTING EVIDENCE FOR PRACTICE 15.1
Adaptations by Client and Family During Illness

PROBLEM UNDER INVESTIGATION / The effects of a medical diagnosis—coronary artery disease—on the life of a client and the client's family

SUMMARY OF RESEARCH / A literature review of 13 research studies published between the years of 1982 and 2000 focused on family adaptation and interventions after a cardiac event. Research revealed that certain themes prevailed within the family unit, including increased anxiety, fear, and mood disturbances; changes in family roles and functioning; and struggles to reduce lifestyle risk factors. Interventions for the clients and families included support groups to provide them with information about coronary artery disease; decrease isolation and anxiety; and share problems, experiences, and solutions. Although individual outcomes such as increased self-esteem, increased self-efficacy, and lowered anxiety occurred, family outcomes were mostly unaffected. Researchers concluded that family functioning during the acute and recovery phases of coronary artery disease involves many complex issues, and families may require interventions of greater intensity and longer duration.

SUPPORT FOR PRACTICE / Recognizing the effect of any serious illness on family functioning is a key nursing responsibility. Nursing interventions for clients with serious medical conditions such as coronary artery disease should address family adaptations and role changes during the acute and recovery phases.

SOURCE: Van Horn, E., Fleury, J., & Moore, S. (2002). Family interventions during the trajectory of recovery from cardiac event: An integrative literature review. Heart & Lung, 31, 186-98.

ership sometimes makes it difficult to determine who fulfills the parental role and who fulfills the child's role. This confusion encourages dependency, not autonomy, and individuation is not enhanced. In contrast, the sharing of similar thoughts and feelings among all family members is viewed as family closeness rather than a loss of autonomy (Goldenberg & Goldenberg, 2003).

In **dysfunctional families,** communication is not open, direct, or honest; usually, it is confusing to other family members. Little warmth is demonstrated. All these experiences tend to undermine each member's individual thoughts, feelings, needs, and emotions so that they are regarded as unimportant or unacceptable. Also, in dysfunctional families, children and adults may perform roles that are inappropriate to their age, sex, or personality. For example, the mother of a 7-year-old daughter and a 3-year-old son may expect the daughter to take care of the son and help prepare meals. This expectation can create distress in the daughter because of the amount of responsibility being placed on her, and because she is being forced to fulfill the role of a mother. If such expectations persist, it could result in a dysfunctional family system.

Culturally Diverse Families

Culture influences family functioning in many ways. Established cultural traditions give families a sense of stability and support from which members draw comfort, guidance, and a means of coping with the problems of life (Andrews & Boyle, 2003). The ability to communicate through the use of the same language is necessary if one is to understand cultural diversity. Duvall's stages of the family life cycle do not apply to all cultures because of differences in family and kinship systems, social life, political systems, language and traditions, religion, health beliefs and practices, and cultural norms. It is imperative for the nurse–therapist to consider these differences when assessing family members for therapy to avoid labeling a family as dysfunctional because of cultural differences.

History of Family and Couple Therapy

In the 1950s, psychotherapists began looking not only at individuals with problems, but also at the pattern of relationships that corresponded with couple and family problems. These psychotherapists included Murray Bowen, Nathan Ackerman, Salvador Minuchin,

Jay Haley, and Virginia Satir. They began changing their approach from treating only the individual to including the couple or family, to help increase therapeutic effectiveness. This change in therapeutic approach was based on the belief that until the pattern of the couple or family was changed, the individual's behavior would remain fixed.

This approach corresponds with another method: viewing the family as a system of relationships, such as that between brother and sister or mother and daughter. Each member of the family must be able to communicate in a productive and healthy way with other members in the system. If there is a breakdown in the system, all members are affected. Thus, a change or disruption in one family member affects the family system and all its members.

When a disruption occurs, members may participate in individual, couple, family or group therapy. Individual therapy was addressed in Chapter 14. Following is a discussion of family, couple, and group therapy.

Family Therapy

Family therapy is a method of treatment in which family members gain insight into problems, improve communication, and improve functioning of individual members as well as the family as a whole. This type of therapy is particularly useful when the family system does not perform its basic functions adequately. Issues such as dysfunction or the acting out of a child, marital conflict, or intergenerational relationship problems can be improved through family therapy. The client in family therapy is considered the family system as a whole, rather than any individual member.

Family therapy differs from individual therapy. Family therapy assumes that outside or external influences play a major role in personality development and the regulation of members' lives. In individual therapy, however, it is believed that internal or intrapsychic thoughts, feelings, and conflicts are the major components of personality development (Goldenberg & Goldenberg, 2003).

Traditionally, in family therapy, the person who seeks treatment is considered the client. If the problem is primarily within the individual and he or she is motivated to change, individual treatment can be helpful and can improve behavior. If the client's behavior is symptomatic of a dysfunctional family system, however, improvement may not be as significant or last as long. Some family therapists believe that if one individual in a family system changes self-functioning, this will eventually have an impact on the functioning of the family, and positive changes will occur in the entire system. Other family therapists believe that if the person who is symptomatic improves, regression to old patterns of behavior or to other dysfunctional behaviors can occur if the family has not changed also. In some situations, family members who are resistant to change become more dysfunctional as the person who seeks treatment responds favorably to therapy.

As the family works through problems, each individual member's role(s) should become clear. Sometimes *scapegoating* occurs. The family needs to maintain a "sick" person in the family, or a scapegoat, to aid in denying the family pathology. Once the family is able to perceive this scapegoating, family therapy focuses on family problems instead of on the individual who was the scapegoat (Cohen & Lipkin, 1979).

Approaches to Family Therapy

Jones (1980) and Sadock and Sadock (2003) describe several orientations or approaches to family therapy. A brief description of the more common approaches follows.

Integrative Approach

Nathan Ackerman, a trained psychoanalyst, considered by some to be the grandfather of family therapy, used the integrative approach, including both individual and family as a cluster. He focused on family values. Ackerman believed in interlocking pathology, which occurs when an individual's problems are entwined into a neurotic interaction with the family and social environment.

Therapists using the integrative approach consider the interactions between the person and his or her social environment and give equal weight to the internal and external influences. The family needs to share concern for each member's welfare. A problem arises when interpersonal conflict is internalized by the client and it becomes an intrapersonal conflict. The overall goals of therapy are to identify and remove the pathogenic or intrapersonal conflict, improve communication and problem-solving, and promote more healthy relationships within the family (Jones, 1980; Sadock & Sadock, 2003). For example, a family of five is having financial difficulty resulting from poor money management. The husband internalizes blame because he is the primary wage earner and head of the household; thus

he develops the intrapersonal conflict of guilt. During family therapy, the wife and children admit to excessive spending and the husband's intrapersonal conflict of guilt is resolved.

Psychoanalytic Approach

Therapists using the psychoanalytic approach base many of their views on Freud's work, believing that family members are affected by each member's psychological makeup. Individual behaviors are regulated by the family's feedback system. Problems arise when there is an internalization process or introjection of parental figures. For example, unresolved conflicts between first- and second-generation family members are internalized (lived out) or projected onto family members in current marital or parental relationships. Simply stated, a 40-year-old woman who observed her mother's difficulty relating to a rigid husband has difficulty relating to her husband when he disciplines their teenage children. She has unconsciously incorporated or internalized an aspect of her mother's personality into her own.

Psychoanalytic therapy is intensive over a long period and focuses on cognitive, affective, and behavioral components of family interaction. One goal is to guide the family members who exhibit pathology into clarifying old misunderstandings and misinterpretations between themselves and parents and members of the family of origin and establishing an adult-to-adult relationship (Jones, 1980; Sadock & Sadock, 2003).

Bowen Approach

Murray Bowen's approach to family therapy or family systems therapy views the family as consisting of both emotional and relational systems. Bowen believed that an individual's behavior is a response to the functioning of the family system as a whole (Bowen, 1994).

One concept from Bowen's theoretical approach is the differentiation of self-concept. This refers to the degree that an individual is able to distinguish between the feeling process and the intellectual process in oneself, thereby making life decisions based on thinking rather than on feeling. Other concepts include the identification of emotional triangles or three-person interactions in a family, the importance of intergenerational family history in understanding dysfunction, and the role of anxiety on functioning of the individual and the family. Dysfunction in the family is related to the method in which families as a whole respond to anxiety. Processes that can be used to handle anxiety include projection to a child, conflict between spouses, and dysfunction in an individual spouse.

Therapy using this approach focuses on guiding one or more family members to become a more solid, defined self in the face of emotional forces created by marriage, children, or the family of origin. Ultimately the result is to gain the clarity and conviction to carry through one's own positions, such as a parent, spouse, or dependent child (Titleman, 1998).

Structural Approach

Structuralists, like the well-known Salvador Minuchin, view the family as a system of individuals. The family develops a set of invisible rules and laws that evolve over time and are understood by all family members. A hierarchical system or structure develops in the family. Problems arise if family boundaries become enmeshed (tangled with no clear individual roles) or disengaged (individual detaches self from the family). Problems also arise when a family cannot cope with change (Jones, 1980).

The structural therapist observes the activities and functions of family members. Therapy is short term and action oriented, with the focus on changing the family organization and its social context. A holistic view of the family is developed, focusing on influences that family members have on one another. Guidance is given toward developing clear boundaries for individual members and changing the family's structural pattern (Sadock & Sadock, 2003).

Interactional or Strategic Approach

The interactional or strategic approach, pioneered by Virginia Satir and Jay Haley, uses communication theory as the foundation. In this approach, the therapist studies the interactions between and among family members, recognizing that change in one family member occurs in relation to change in another family member. Family members develop a calibration or rating and feedback system so that homeostasis is maintained. Interactionists agree with structuralists that a set of invisible laws emerges in the family relationship, and that problems arise if these family rules are ambiguous. When power struggles develop in a family, strategies employed to control the situation may provoke symptoms. These symptoms are interpersonal, with at least one family member contributing to the dysfunction of another (Jones, 1980; Sadock & Sadock, 2003).

Therapy is based on the concept of homeostasis. According to this concept, as one member gains insight and becomes better, another family member may become worse. Communication is considered the basis for all behavior. Therapy deals with the interpersonal relationships among all family members and focuses on why the family is in therapy and what changes each member expects. The family thus helps set goals for the treatment approach.

Social Network or Systemic Approach

Some therapists believe that the family operates as a social network. They believe that healing comes from social relationships. Problems ensue if the family social network loses its ability to recover quickly from illness or change. A systems approach is used, but is not clearly defined. The growth model is used to understand emotional difficulties that arise during different stages of development.

Therapy emphasizes the natural healing powers of the family. It involves bringing several people together as a social network. For the first few meetings, this may encompass people who are outside of the family, but who have similar ideals and goals. Family members are helped to set goals for optimal outcomes or solving of problems (Jones, 1980).

Behaviorist Approach

Behaviorists believe that the family is a system of interlocking behaviors, that one type of behavior causes another. They deny internal motivating forces, but believe individuals react to external factors and influences. The individual learns that he or she obtains satisfaction or rewards from certain responses of other individuals. Behavior is thus learned. Problems arise when maladaptive behavior is learned and reinforced by family members, who respond either positively or negatively. Sometimes a particular behavior is exhibited to gain attention.

Therapy includes interpreting family members' behavior but not necessarily changing it. However, restructuring interpersonal environments may bring about change. Thus, therapy is based on an awareness process as well as on behavioral change. Therapeutic approaches using principles of social learning theory are taught. Approaches are direct and clearly stated. In an effort to bring about change, positive reinforcement is given for desired behavior. The family is involved in goal setting for desired outcomes, and a contract may be established for this purpose (Jones, 1980; Sadock & Sadock, 2003).

Goals of Family Therapy

When meeting with a family or identified client in a family, assessing the family's beliefs, values, and power structure, as well as the family's immediate problem, is important. In addition, the therapist needs to have insight into her or his own value system so as not to influence the assessment or the direction of treatment. What the family identifies as problems may not be what the therapist identifies as problems, because of differences in values, culture, and socioeconomic class. Goals may need to be modified according to the family's value system. The therapist also focuses the work on the problems that the family identifies, and explains to the dysfunctional family why the therapist sees the problems differently. The family, not the therapist, should provide the information for and determine the direction of change when goals are being set. Each family member should state her or his goals and the outcomes expected from the therapy. If the therapist and family are from similar backgrounds, the problems identified and the methods of resolving them tend to be more similar.

A major goal of family therapy is to facilitate positive changes in the family. Other goals include fostering open communication of thoughts and feelings and promoting optimal functioning in interdependent roles. The therapist needs to assess the roles each family member fulfills and determine whether these roles are rigid or inflexible. In addition, the therapist needs to function as a role model, demonstrating how to deal with conflicts. Developing contracts for the family members may be useful in goal setting (eg, keeping a room clean, having fewer quarrels, paying more attention to the needs of other family members).

Initially, the therapist determines which family members need to participate or continue in family therapy and how the problems of the identified client(s) interlock with the relationships of other family members. This interlocking relationship may need to be modified. Finally, the therapist helps family members take a realistic view of their relationships with one another and the overall effect of their behavior on each other.

Stages of Family Therapy

The three main stages of family therapy are the initial interview, the intervention or working phase, and the termination phase.

Initial Interview

Usually, a family therapist is contacted by telephone by the identified client or by another family member regarding the identified client. The caller expresses concern regarding the problem or symptom(s), and the family therapist sets up an appointment for an initial interview with the family. Most therapists ask all family members to be present at this time. Later, the therapist may decide that not all members need to be present at the family sessions. (For example, very young children may be excluded.) The information gleaned from all family members at the initial interview can be invaluable during later sessions.

During the initial interview, some therapists gather data regarding family history; other therapists focus on the present functioning of the family (Goldenberg & Goldenberg, 2003). Confidentiality laws prohibit family involvement without the client's consent. An outline of a family assessment guide that can be used to obtain information during the initial interview is shown in Box 15-1.

If a certain family member is reluctant to come in for the initial interview, it may be helpful if the therapist states the rationale for seeing all family members at that time. For example, the therapist could state that the problem affects all members of the family and that it is important to attend. The therapist can explain that therapy will not be effective without that member's attendance and input.

During the initial interview, the therapist facilitates the process of determining which problems the family has identified as needing attention. This process occurs in stages and includes:

BOX 15.1	**FAMILY ASSESSMENT GUIDE**

I. Construction of a family genogram
II. Description of the family in relation to the community, focusing on ethnicity, socioeconomic class, educational level, and religion
III. Description of presenting problems, focusing on each family member's perception of the identified problems
IV. Identification of communication patterns focusing on who speaks to whom, tone of voice, emotional climate, and manner by which emotions are expressed
V. Identification of roles of family members as supportive, antagonistic, critical, scapegoat, rescuer, or victim. Are there family coalitions, pairings, triangles, or splits?
VI. Developmental history of the family in general and of the presenting problems
VII. Family's expectations of therapy

Goldenberg, 2003). During this phase, the therapist identifies the strengths and problems of the family. The therapist determines which of these strengths are present in the family seeking help, because strengths are useful in helping the family remain stable when other relationships seem threatened by change. Twelve family strengths, identified by Otto (1963), are the ability to:

1. Provide for the physical, emotional, and spiritual needs of each family member.
2. Be sensitive to the needs of family members.
3. Communicate feelings, emotions, beliefs, and values effectively.
4. Provide support, security, and encouragement to enhance creativity and independence.
5. Initiate and maintain growth-producing relationships within and without the family system.
6. Maintain and create constructive and responsible community relationships in the neighborhood, school, town, and local and state governments.
7. Grow with and through children.
8. Help oneself and accept help when appropriate.
9. Perform family roles flexibly.
10. Show mutual respect for the individuation and independence of each family member.
11. Use a crisis as a means of growth.
12. Have a concern for family unity and loyalty, and for cooperation among family members.

- *Engagement stage*: The family meets and is put at ease by the therapist.
- *Assessment stage*: Problem(s) that concern the family are identified.
- *Exploration stage*: The therapist and family explore additional problems that may have a bearing on present family concerns.
- *Goal-setting stage*: The therapist synthesizes all the information, and the family members state what they would like to see changed.
- *Termination stage*: The initial interview ends, an appointment is set for the next session, and it is determined which family members need to attend (Haley, 1991).

During the initial interview, the therapist assesses and synthesizes all the information the family has provided and formulates ideas or interventions for bringing about positive changes to resolve the identified problems. Box 15-2 describes nursing diagnoses specific for families.

Intervention or Working Phase

The goal of the intervention phase is to help the family accept and adjust to change (Goldenberg &

During the intervention or working phase, families do a lot of work, and the therapist participates in the therapeutic process. Usually, family sessions occur once a week for approximately 1 hour. Some family members may be motivated to participate to help the identified client; other members may be reluctant to participate because of fears of having family secrets revealed. It is unusual for all family members to be will-

BOX 15.2	EXAMPLES OF NURSING DIAGNOSES FOR FAMILIES

Compromised Family Coping: The supportive family member or close friend provides insufficient, ineffective, or compromised support, comfort, assistance, or encouragement needed by the client experiencing a health challenge.

Disabled Family Coping: The family demonstrates, or is at risk to demonstrate, destructive behavior in response to an inability to manage internal or external stressors due to inadequate physical, psychological, or cognitive resources.

Readiness for Enhanced Family Coping: A family member involved with the individual's health challenge demonstrates effective management of adaptive tasks to promote enhanced health and growth in relation to the client and in regard to self.

Interrupted Family Processes: The state in which a normally supportive family experiences, or is at risk to experience, a stressor that challenges effective functioning ability of the family.

Dysfunctional Family Processes: Alcoholism: The psychosocial, spiritual, economic, and physiologic functions of the family members and system are disorganized because of alcohol abuse by a family member.

Parental Role Conflict: A parent or primary caregiver experiences or perceives a change in role in response to external factors such as illness, separation, divorce, and so forth.

Impaired Parenting: One or more of the primary caregivers demonstrate real or potential inability to provide a constructive environment to nurture the growth and development of a child or children.

Adapted from Carpenito-Moyet, L. J. (2006). *Handbook of nursing diagnosis* (11th ed.). Philadelphia: Lippincott Williams & Wilkins.

ing and eager to participate in family therapy sessions. The therapist can ask all members their view of the problem, what they would like to see changed, and their thoughts and feelings about other members of the family. Through this technique, the therapist can learn a great deal about the problems and conflicts that are occurring in the family system (Goldenberg & Goldenberg, 2003).

Soon, the family members begin to recognize that the therapist's role is to clarify and interpret communication as well as to offer suggestions and guidance. The therapist does not assume the role of a parent, child, or arbitrator. The therapist facilitates open, honest communication among family members. Learning appropriate methods of expressing themselves may cause some stress in family members, especially if there have been hostility, angry outbursts, or little communication. Also, some sessions—particularly those dealing with conflicts and altercations—may make family members feel uncomfortable. As therapy continues, family members begin to realize that relationships can change. They recognize that roles do not have to be fixed and rigid; they may change as personal growth occurs in the family. Family members become more autonomous as positive changes such as open communication and alterations in behavior (ie,

interdependent roles) occur. They also recognize that change is equal in all family members. It is important that the family members are satisfied with their new level of functioning before terminating therapy (Wright & Leahey, 2005).

Termination Phase

Sometimes, families want to terminate the sessions prematurely. They may indicate this desire through their behavior. For instance, family members may begin to be late or not show up for scheduled appointments, or all members may not continue to participate, as agreed in the initial interview. Such behavior may occur if the family perceives that a certain type of change is threatening to the family's present functioning. At this point, the therapist needs to review the identified problems with the family and renegotiate the contract and number of family sessions. This review is helpful in recognizing problems that remain and goals that have been met.

If the family has achieved the goals and the identified specific problems have been resolved, then it is time to initiate the termination phase. However, the therapist should remember that no family terminates therapy without experiencing some problems. Also, some family members may be somewhat reluctant to terminate the sessions because they fear that dysfunctional behaviors may recur, or because they have become dependent on the therapist. Nevertheless, termination should take place. By the time of termination, typically, the family has learned how to solve its own problems in a healthy manner, has developed its own internal support system, and has learned to communicate openly, honestly, and directly. Power has been appropriately assigned and redistributed, and family members are able to work out and resolve problems at home without the therapist's help or interventions. The original problems or symptoms have been alleviated, and it is time for termination of family therapy sessions (Goldenberg & Goldenberg, 2003).

There are times when it is appropriate for nurses to seek the input of additional resources when problems are complex. For example, a referral may be made to family support groups such as Parents Anonymous, Toughlove, or Families Anonymous. Nurses need to have an extensive knowledge of professional resources within the community to refer families for additional support (Wright & Leahey, 2005).

The Nurse–Therapist's Role in Family Therapy

The clinical nurse specialist or nurse practitioner with a graduate degree in psychiatric–mental health nursing can function in many highly skilled roles, one of which is serving as a family therapist (Cain, 1986).

Involving the family when one of its members becomes ill is not new to nursing. During the initial assessment, regardless of the illness, nurses obtain information about the client's family members, including grandparents, aunts, and uncles. Nurses also include family members in health education and teaching. However, viewing the family as a specialty, in and of itself, is relatively new for psychiatric–mental health nurses.

Nurses functioning in the role of family therapists conduct family assessments, participate in family teaching and education, and provide family therapy (Cain, 1986). The nurse–family therapist obtains a detailed family history of at least three generations to gain information regarding how the family has functioned in the past and how it is currently functioning.

One assessment tool that nurses can use in determining the family's constellation of members is a genogram (Fig. 15-1), a diagram of family-member relationships, usually over three generations. The genogram

is simple to use and can provide a great deal of information about the family.

In a genogram, the names of family members are placed on horizontal lines to indicate separate generations. Vertical lines denote any children. The children are ranked from oldest to youngest, going from left to right. The symbols used to depict each family member are usually squares for males and circles for females. Inside the square or circle is the family member's name and age. Outside of the symbols, pertinent information can be written, such as *cancer, stroke, depression, workaholic*, and so on. Other symbols can be used to denote marriage, death, adoption, divorce, separation, miscarriage, abortion, or twins (Wright & Leahey, 2005).

This simple and easy-to-use tool can provide valuable information in one perusal. A family is often interested in doing a genogram because it gives them a diagram of family relationships, including significant information. The genogram also is useful in teaching the family members about family systems. Family members need to begin to understand the roles they fill, and how their roles influence the family system. After they realize that roles are learned and that they can choose to alter their roles, change can occur. At that point, the family can begin to work on its problems (Cain, 1986).

Couple Therapy

Couple therapy, an intervention involving two individuals sharing a common relationship (a married or nonmarried, homosexual or heterosexual pair), is a way of resolving tension or conflict in a relationship. When two people enter into a relationship, they each bring a set of beliefs about love, intimacy, gender roles, sexuality, and marriage. These beliefs determine the nature and quality of their relationship, the kind of problems they will have, and how they will go about resolving them.

Most couples seek couple therapy to resolve troublesome behavior and/or dysfunctional interaction problems within their relationship. Problems may arise at any time during the development of a couple's relationship, as each person attempts to maintain independence while attempting to experience mutual growth and fulfillment as part of a couple.

Couple therapy may be indicated for several reasons. These include, but are not limited to, the presence of a crisis such as a job loss; medical or mental illness, or death; emotional tension and the inability to

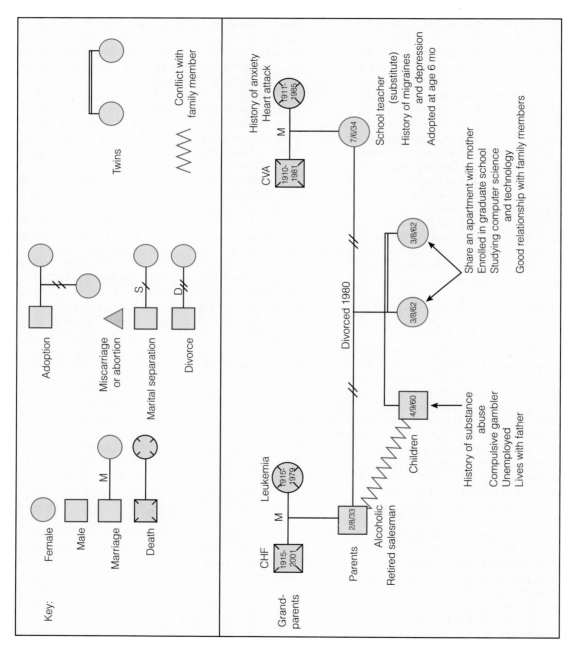

FIGURE 15.1 Sample three-generation genogram.

communicate needs; lack of trust; sexual dissatisfaction or difficulty; disagreement regarding how children or adolescents should be disciplined; or stress related to providing care for dependent elderly parents (Chisholm, 1996).

Traditionally, men are more reluctant to take on the client role. Their help-seeking is often tentative and complicated by conflicting motives. Therapists may not fully understand the male experience, the connection between men's problematic behaviors, and their psychic pain. Brooks (1998) believes that therapists can provide successful couple therapy if they incorporate the following core elements into their therapeutic approach with male clients:

- Anticipate resistance and articulate the benefits of therapy.
- Promote a positive experience during the initial meeting by neither shaming the male client nor excusing his resistance.
- Offer hope that the therapy will be beneficial.
- Highlight the male client's more positive characteristics.
- Urge male clients to see themselves as products, and sometimes victims, of their upbringing in a "gendered" culture.
- Accept male clients where they are and gradually shape their therapy behavior.

Types of Couple Therapy

Several types of therapy are available to couples. Examples include **marital-relations therapy**, **contextual therapy**, and **object-relations therapy**. Marital-relations therapy (also referred to as *conjoint therapy*) is the most common treatment method in couple therapy. It is a form of psychotherapy designed to modify the interactions of two individuals who are in conflict with each other over social, emotional, sexual, or economic issues. Co-therapy with therapists of both sexes is recommended because this approach prevents one partner from feeling overwhelmed when confronted by two members of the opposite sex. Contextual therapy is a nondirective form of couple therapy that addresses changes or imbalances in giving and taking or entitlement and fulfillment that occur within the relationship over time. Through promotion of mutual responsibility, understanding, and trust, contextual therapy fosters a dialogue between couples, thus reestablishing the integrity of the couple's interpersonal relationships. Object-relations therapy is a psychodynamic approach to resolve self-

destructive patterns of relationships with people or objects such as food or alcohol (Chisholm, 1996; Helm, Wynne, & Simon, 1985; Klee, 2002; Sadock & Sadock, 2003). The term *combined therapy* refers to the use of the preceding therapies concurrently or in combination. For example, a partner or couple may begin treatment with an object-relations therapist, continue in therapy with a marital-relations therapist, and terminate therapy after contextual therapy (Sadock & Sadock, 2003).

Another type of couple therapy is **brief couples therapy** as described by Papp (1997). This therapy is based on understanding each partner's belief systems and how these systems interlock to govern their lives and relationships. Beliefs determine the nature and quality of relationships, the kind of problems a couple will have, and how the couple will resolve problems.

When beliefs are acted on over time, they form themes, or highly charged emotional issues, that dominate a relationship. Recurring conflicts may occur as a result of such issues. Techniques that can be used to understand and change dysfunctional relationships of couples include:

- Understanding what each person wants changed and in what way he or she would like to change it.
- Understanding each person's perception of solutions and how he or she intends to bring this about.
- Looking for the constraints that stand in the way of bringing about a desired solution.
- Exploring three-generational and cultural sources of beliefs and constraints, and placing them in their context by tracing them to their source in family of origin or culture.
- Challenging the constraints by introducing an alternate way of perceiving or reacting to a specific situation.
- Exploring the motivating force that would help the couple work toward their desired goal.
- Identifying hidden qualities or values that can be defined as positive, and expanding on them.
- Identifying a negative central theme that can be changed into one that is more constructive.
- Asking future-oriented questions, such as "How would you like your relationship to be different?"

Couple Assessment

Chapter 9 discusses the assessment process. However, couple assessment takes this step a bit further by including the collection of more comprehensive data

---

BOX 15.3 EXAMPLES OF NURSING DIAGNOSES FOR COUPLES

Caregiver Role Strain: The 60-year-old daughter and son-in-law of a man with the diagnosis of heart failure verbalize the presence of emotional and social burdens related to 24-hour responsibilities.

Decisional Conflict: One of the partners in a couple verbalizes uncertainty about whether to continue in the relationship because of the lack of emotional and financial support by the other partner.

Impaired Communication: The male partner of a client describes the inability to communicate with his partner who exhibits disordered, unrealistic thinking at times.

Powerlessness: A husband verbalizes a perceived lack of personal control over finances related to his wife's inability to manage money.

Risk for Loneliness: The female partner of a couple verbalizes loneliness related to frequent separation from her partner, who works long hours and travels frequently.

Adapted from Carpenito-Moyet, L. J. (2006). *Handbook of nursing diagnosis* (11th ed.). Philadelphia: Lippincott Williams & Wilkins.

---

about physical or mental illness in either or both partners, difficulties in interpersonal and/or sexual relationship of the couple, and identification of any developmental issues either partner may be experiencing. A family assessment guide, described later in this chapter in the section on family therapy, is a useful tool to gather data because couples with children are influenced by family life cycle changes. In addition, the developmental demands of children can strain the relationship of partners (Chisholm, 1996). Collection of these data leads to the identification of nursing diagnoses. Examples of nursing diagnoses specific to couples are highlighted in Box 15-3.

Goals of Couple Therapy

The main goal of couple therapy is to resolve problems and conflicts (eg, troublesome behavior and dysfunctional patterns) that couples are unable to handle themselves. Goals may include the establishment of trust and loyalty, enhancement of sexual intimacy, improvement in listening and expressive skills, and the establishment of empathy for each individual. Couple therapy is considered successful when stated goals are met, couples are satisfied with the outcome even if termination of the relationship occurs, and each partner is able to generalize growth to other relationships (Chisholm, 1996).

The Nurse–Therapist's Role in Couple Therapy

The certified clinical nurse specialist or advanced nurse practitioner with a graduate degree in psychiatric–mental health nursing has received supervised clinical experience and has extensive knowledge and skills in providing psychotherapy. The nurse–therapist's role in couple therapy is to assist clients in dealing constructively with thoughts, emotions, and behaviors. Part of the nurse–therapist's role in couple therapy is to persuade each partner in the relationship to take responsibility in understanding the psychodynamic makeup of the personality. Emphasis is placed on each person's accountability for the effects of behavior on his or her own life, the life of the partner, and the lives of others in the environment. Attempts are made to alleviate the disturbances, to reverse or change maladaptive patterns of behavior, and to encourage personality growth and development. Couple therapy does not guarantee the maintenance of the relationship. In some instances the partners are in a nonviable union that should be dissolved (Sadock & Sadock, 2003). Table 15-2 describes the issues or indications for and the therapist's interventions in marital-relations, contextual, and object-relations therapies.

Group Therapy

Group therapy is a method of therapeutic intervention based on the exploration and analysis of both internal (emotional) and external (environmental) conflicts and the group process (Lego, 1996). It is an identifiable system consisting of at least three people who share a common goal (Nudelman, 1986). Yalom (2005), considered to be a leading practitioner in the field of group therapy, believes that therapy groups are composed of many forms, with the major emphasis on the importance of the "here-and-now" experience.

Group therapy as a treatment method has long been effective in resolving psychiatric problems. In the

TABLE 15.2 Types of Couple Therapy

THERAPY	ISSUES	INTERVENTIONS BY NURSE THERAPIST
Marital-relations therapy	Negative interactions Conflicts in problem solving Inability to communicate Sexual dysfunction	Encourages partners to identify their own behavior Provides communication and problem-solving training Encourages imaging and fantasy exercises related to sexual dysfunction
Contextual therapy	Power struggles Abuse of child or spouse Infidelity Impaired development as a couple Parental conflict	Directs concern toward issues involving both partners May include children Focuses on trust, loyalty, and fairness to reduce power struggles and parental conflict
Object-relations therapy	Complaint by child or adolescent Poor self-esteem Recurrent dissatisfaction with partner or spouse Escalating interactions and emotional patterns	Reflects position of partners Focuses on empathy, anger control, vulnerability, and misperceptions

Chisholm, M. M. (1996). Couple therapy. In S. Lego (Ed.), *Psychiatric nursing: A comprehensive reference* (2nd ed., pp. 53–60). Philadelphia: Lippincott-Raven Publishers.

early 1900s, Dr. Joseph Pratt, a physician practicing in Massachusetts, initially treated tuberculosis patients individually. Gradually, he began to meet with them weekly in small groups to educate them about their chronic disease, to help alleviate feelings of depression and hopelessness, and to provide support and encouragement to follow through with their treatment regimen. In 1919, Dr. Cody Marsh, a psychiatrist and ordained minister, became the first practitioner to apply Dr. Pratt's theories to the treatment of institutionalized psychiatric patients. Shortly thereafter, Dr. Jacob Mareno, a Viennese psychiatrist, was credited with first defining the term "group therapy." During the 1930s, many psychologists and psychiatrists became interested in group therapy and began to explore its use in practice. During World War II, group therapy experienced significant growth, providing optimal treatment for both military and civilian populations. In the 1950s and 1960s, therapists expanded the traditional psychoanalytic approach and became creative in employing various types of groups, such as encounter groups, sensitivity-training groups, and self-growth and development groups. Later, social workers, family counselors, nurses, and other professionals began the practice of group therapy.

Group therapy has several advantages including the following:

- Decreased isolation and dependence
- Opportunities for helping others
- Interpersonal learning and development of coping skills
- Decreased transference to the therapist while developing the ability to listen to other group members

Groups can be a valuable treatment element, encouraging members to use one another's assets to foster their own growth. Members of the group become more aware of self, learn what behaviors are more acceptable, develop therapeutic and supportive relationships, and improve communication (Nudelman, 1986).

Characteristics of Group Therapy

Group therapy differs from individual therapy in that it is more effective for treating problems with interpersonal relationships. It also allows psychiatric clients a greater opportunity for reality testing and experiencing mutual concern and support. However, members of groups may feel more vulnerable, frightened, and at risk than clients participating in individual therapy. Moreover, the transference process may be less obvious and overlooked by the nurse–therapist.

Certain essential elements are common to all types of group therapy. Yalom (2005) has identified 11 essential elements of group therapy:

1. *Instillation of hope* is the first and often most important factor. White (1987) describes people participating in the group experience as initially feeling demoralized and helpless, and points out that providing them with hope is therefore a most worthwhile achievement. Clients should be encouraged to believe that they can find help and support in the group and that it is realistic to expect that problems will eventually be resolved.
2. *Universality* can be defined as the sense of realizing that one is not completely alone in any situation. Group members often identify this factor as a major reason for seeking group therapy. During the sessions, members are encouraged to express complex, often very negative feelings in the hope that they will experience understanding and support from others with similar thoughts and feelings.
3. The *imparting of information* includes both didactic instruction and direct advice, and refers to the imparting of specific educational information plus the sharing of advice and guidance among members. The transmission of this information also indicates to each member the others' concern and trust.
4. *Altruism* in therapy groups benefits members through the act of giving to others. Clients have the experience of learning to help others, and in the process they begin to feel better about themselves. Both the group therapist and the members can offer invaluable support, insight, and reassurance while allowing themselves to gain self-knowledge and growth.
5. The *corrective recapitulation of the primary family group* allows members in the group to correct some of the perceptions and feelings associated with unsatisfactory experiences they have had with their family. The participants receive feedback as they discuss and relive early familial conflicts and experience corrective responses. Family roles are explored, and members are encouraged to resolve unfinished family business.
6. The *development of socializing techniques* is essential in the group as members are given the opportunity to learn and test new social skills. Members also receive information about maladaptive social behaviors.
7. *Imitative behavior* refers to the process in which members observe and model their behaviors after one another. Imitation is an acknowledged therapeutic force; a healthy group environment provides valuable opportunities for experimenting with desired changes and behaviors.
8. *Interpersonal learning* includes the gaining of insight, the development of an understanding of a transference relationship, the experience of correcting emotional thoughts and behaviors, and the importance of learning about oneself in relation to others.
9. *Group cohesiveness* is the development of a strong sense of group membership and alliance. The concept of cohesiveness refers to the degree to which a group functions as a supportive problem-solving unit. Ideally, each member feels acceptance and approval from all others in the group. This factor is essential in ensuring optimal individual and group growth.
10. *Catharsis,* similar to group cohesiveness, involves members relating to one another through the verbal expression of positive and negative feelings.
11. *Existential factors* that are constantly operating in the group make up the final component. These intangible issues encourage each group member to accept the motivating idea that he or she is ultimately responsible for his or her own life choices and actions.

Other theorists view group therapy somewhat differently. Taylor (1982) states that members of a group reflect persons in the larger society, and that group conditions replicate reality. Within this structure, group participants present their concerns and problems; in return, they receive direct feedback and resolutions. Sadock and Sadock (2003) view the key elements of group therapy as involving the expression of feelings, the group atmosphere, the various types of member participation, and the skill and expertise of the group leader.

Types of Therapy Groups

A wide variety of therapy groups that use the major theoretical frameworks can exist. Typically, therapy groups may be open or closed. **Open groups** do not have established boundaries; members may join and leave the group at different times. Group cohesion and leadership stability are identified as major elements. **Closed groups** have a set membership, a specific time-frame, or both of these components. Specific membership may address the needs of a particular kind of client, such as a group of female college students who are bulimic or an aftercare group for previously hospitalized clients. Most closed groups require members to start the group at the same time and then terminate the group after a predetermined length of time. Both open and closed therapy groups are used extensively in inpatient and outpatient treatment settings (Lego, 1996).

Group therapy may be provided using various models. Five models of group therapy ranging on a continuum from supportive to psychoanalytic group therapy are commonly described (Marram, 1978):

1. *Support groups* focus on increasing the members' adaptation, self-esteem, and sense of emotional well-being.
2. *Reeducation and remotivation groups* (often very beneficial for psychiatric clients who are withdrawn or socially isolated) attempt to increase communication and interaction among members to foster more acceptable and appropriate behaviors.
3. *Problem-solving therapy groups* focus on the resolution of specific problems that clients have identified.
4. *Insight without reconstruction groups* emphasize interpersonal communication by group leaders while working on effecting change by increasing the members' cognitive and emotional understanding of their problems.
5. *Personality reconstruction groups* use psychoanalytic theory and encourage the members to explore former relationships and problems and their impact on the present.

Establishment of a Group

Typically, group therapy participants are selected on the basis of personal treatment philosophies and individual client needs. In addition, the desired size of the group (usually no larger than ten members), diagnosis of participants, age, gender, intellectual level, verbal or communication skills, motivation, and social skills are important. During the selection process, a decision is made regarding whether the group will be homoge-

nous or heterogeneous in nature. For example, a group focusing on women's issues, such as single parenting, may not be therapeutic for adolescents, women in their 70s, or male clients. Conversely, a group focusing on loss and grief could be suitable for various age groups, either gender, and persons married, widowed, single, or divorced. For example, in a 40-bed adult unit, examples of groups that may be conducted include task-oriented, codependency, loss and grief, medication, spiritual quest, women's issues, men's issues, eating disorders, substance abuse, cognitive skills, and discharge-planning groups. Clients with psychotic disorders who are agitated, confused, fragmented, or experiencing regression in their behavior may benefit from a therapy group, referred to as *focus therapy,* specifically designed to meet their needs and to embrace their level of functioning.

Some concern has been voiced about the lack of therapy programs for certain groups. For example, Ulus (2002) addresses the lack of group therapy programs available for men with mood disorders, relationship difficulties, uncontrollable anger, anxiety, comorbid substance abuse, and employment or legal problems. She identified several obstacles, including the predominance of female therapists, group therapy programs available only during working hours, lack of financial resources to pay for the high cost of therapy, and inadequate insurance coverage for mental health treatment.

The environmental setting also is important when establishing a group. Room temperature, lighting, sound, furnishings, privacy, location, and seating arrangements contribute to an atmosphere conducive to therapeutic group process.

Stages of Group Development

All therapy groups have three major phases: a beginning or orientation phase, a middle or working phase, and an ending or termination phase. During each stage, significant issues concerning group growth and development arise and are dealt with by the group. The key issues involve dependency and interdependency.

The beginning or orientation phase of any type of group therapy is often one of much stress and anxiety for group members. Each person is concerned with how she or he will fit into the group as the group norms and acceptable behaviors are identified. During this phase, frequent testing, minimal disclosure, and periods of awkwardness and uncomfortable silence may occur. The major task is for the group to resolve these initial feelings and to achieve a sense of group

SELF-AWARENESS PROMPT

Reflect on how you interact with people. What type of leadership style do you think you would use? Explain why.

identification and definition of purpose. The tasks of the leader are to create a supportive and accepting environment, to promote unification, and to encourage verbalization of feelings.

Each client has rights as a group member, including not being forced to participate in the group, the freedom to leave the group at any time, and freedom from having someone else's values imposed upon him or her (Bensing, 2001).

During the middle phase—the working phase—the group becomes more cohesive, and members explore relationships and conflicts. Members of the group begin to express both positive and negative feelings, and unhealthy behaviors are openly confronted. Throughout this phase, evidence of continued resistance may continue as increased pressure is placed on members to participate in risk taking. The major tasks for members during the working phase are to develop a sense of reliance on each other, to assume a heightened sense of responsibility for the group direction, and to maintain trust and openness in the group relationships. The therapist's role is to encourage members to explore their conflicts and goals, to identify repetitive behaviors, and continually to clarify the group goals and tasks.

During the final phase of group therapy, termination may occur in several different ways, depending on whether the group is open or closed. As the members prepare to leave, they reflect on the insights and growth that they have made in the group. They share feedback with one another as they experience ambivalence about leaving the group. Most members feel both sadness and optimism as they anticipate the future. They may feel a sense of loss and rejection by the group, and feelings of anger, envy, and hostility may surface. The group therapist assumes a less active role during the termination phase as he or she helps the members to integrate the changes and to say goodbye. Nudelman (1986) recommends that the therapist conduct an exit interview with each group member to review the individual's progress and to make an accurate evaluation of the group experience. As members leave the group, the therapist hopes that the members are more realistic in their perception of themselves, have an increased sense of self-esteem, are more resourceful in resolving problems, and are better able to assume responsibility for all facets of their lives.

Group Leadership Styles

The three basic styles of group leadership are described as autocratic, democratic, and laissez-faire. **Autocratic group leaders** generally do not encourage active participation or interaction among group members. Such leaders maintain authority and control over group members. **Democratic group leaders** encourage active participation, value the input and feedback of group members, and promote cohesiveness among the group members as they develop problem-solving and decision-making skills. **Laissez-faire group leaders** allow much freedom in the group setting. If the group members are not highly motivated, task oriented, or knowledgeable, group tasks or goals may not be met (Crenshaw, 2003).

Role of the Nurse– Therapist in Group Therapy

The primary role of the nurse–therapist in group therapy is to guide individuals through a problem-solving process by anticipating and responding to the needs and concerns of group members. A solid understanding of the basics of group dynamics is essential to becoming a skilled group therapy leader (Bensing, 2001).

To be an effective leader of group therapy, a nurse must meet three major qualifications:

1. Theoretical preparation through lectures, reading, formal coursework, seminars, and workshops
2. Supervised practice in the role of co-leader and leader
3. Personal experience as a group therapy member

In a therapy group, the nurse–therapist has both task and maintenance role functions. Group task functions are concerned with the practical issues of leading a group, whereas group maintenance functions focus on less-tangible group processes (Table 15-3). Nurses need to know about these role functions and to become skillful in their administration.

TABLE 15.3 Nurse–Therapist Task and Maintenance Role Functions in Group Therapy

TASK ROLE FUNCTIONS	MAINTENANCE ROLE FUNCTIONS
• Identify the goals and plans for the group. • Select an appropriate time and place for the group to meet. • Seek necessary administrative permission. • Select appropriate members for the group. • Decide on a cotherapist. • Decide whether the group will be open or closed. • Decide frequency and length of group meetings.	• Orient group members to purpose and goals. • Observe and comment on group process. • Propose questions and interventions based on theoretical framework. • Facilitate creative problem-solving. • Maintain group's direction in pursuit of task. • Act as a support and resource person. • Promote termination.

KEY CONCEPTS

◆ The term *couple* is used to describe two adults who have a close or intimate relationship. They may be heterosexual or homosexual, single, married, or in a same-sex union.

◆ Families may consist of married or nonmarried, homosexual or heterosexual couples with or without children. They are an integral part of society in which members learn how to relate to and communicate with others.

◆ Duvall's theory of the family life cycle describes the family as a system that experiences developmental tasks as it progresses through eight predictable, successive stages of growth.

◆ Like mental health and mental illness, family functioning occurs on a continuum. Healthy families encourage personal autonomy and independence. Healthy families can become dysfunctional under stress when issues of power persist and are not resolved.

◆ Family therapy is a method of treatment in which family members gain insight into problems, improve communication, and improve functioning of individual members and the family as a whole.

◆ Several approaches to family therapy have been identified, including the integrative approach, psychoanalytic approach, Bowen approach, structural approach, interactional or strategic approach, social network or systematic approach, and behavioral approach.

◆ The three main stages of family therapy include the initial interview, the intervention or working phase, and the termination phase.

◆ The family nurse–therapist obtains a detailed family history of at least three generations to provide information regarding the family's current and past levels of functioning. A genogram may be used as an assessment and teaching tool to convey information about family relationships when addressing family issues.

◆ Couple therapy is used to resolve tension or conflict in a relationship by changing troublesome behavior and dysfunctional patterns in the couple.

◆ Several types of therapy are available to couples, including marital-relations therapy, contextual therapy, object-relations therapy, and brief couples therapy.

◆ Group therapy is an effective treatment method used to address the psychiatric problems of persons who share a common goal. The five basic models of group therapy include support groups, reeducation and remotivation groups, problem-solving therapy groups, insight without reconstruction groups, and personality reconstruction groups.

◆ The phases of group development are similar to the phases of individual psychotherapy: orientation, working, and termination stages.

◆ Three leadership styles are noted during group therapy: autocratic, democratic, and laissez-faire.

◆ The primary role of the nurse–therapist in group therapy is to guide individuals through a problem-solving process by anticipating and responding to the needs and concerns of group members.

For additional study materials, please refer to the Student Resource CD-ROM located in the back of this textbook.

CHAPTER WORKSHEET

CRITICAL THINKING QUESTIONS

1. Interview three members of your family, preferably of different genders and ages, referencing Otto's 12 family strengths. How does each member perceive the family? What differences in perception occur with gender and age? How do their perceptions match your own? Does this information provide a picture of strength or dysfunction?

2. Create a genogram of your family, going back as far as possible. What patterns of disease, marriage, and so forth can you assess? What did you learn about roles in your family, and what might you do with this information?

REFLECTION

Reflect on the opening chapter quote by Jones. Do you agree with the current conceptual focus of family therapy? Explain the reason for your response. If you do not agree with the conceptual focus, what changes would you make in your approach as a family therapist?

NCLEX-STYLE QUESTIONS

1. The nurse assesses the family of an adolescent client with a diagnosis of depression. The parents describe believing that family unity and harmony are essential. Disagreement with the family by the adolescent is viewed as betrayal of the parents. The nurse recognizes that this family belief is dysfunctional because it:
   a. encourages adolescent rebellion.
   b. prevents autonomous child development.
   c. provides a united front by the parents.
   d. represents limit-setting that is too strict.

2. Which characteristic would the nurse expect to assess in a family that is considered dysfunctional?
   a. Individual autonomy is encouraged.
   b. Family problems are identified.
   c. Disagreement between spouses is present.
   d. The parent and child exhibit role reversal.

3. The parents of a young adult recently diagnosed with schizophrenia express feelings of being overwhelmed and powerless in coping with the client at home. Which nursing diagnosis would be most appropriate?
   a. Compromised Family Coping
   b. Impaired Social Interaction
   c. Ineffective Family Therapeutic Regimen Management
   d. Deficient Knowledge

4. The community health nurse visits the family of a client with Alzheimer's disease and discusses issues of increasing stress related to the worsening of the client's symptoms. The nurse suggests appropriate referrals to the community agency on aging and the local Alzheimer's Association based on the knowledge that these referrals primarily would:
   a. help the client with Alzheimer's disease improve functioning.
   b. allow the family to vent thoughts and feelings to others.
   c. enhance family's problem-solving ability with help of outside resources.
   d. provide direction to a dysfunctional system.

5. The nurse–therapist uses which assessment method to assist a family to understand the roles they play and how these roles influence the family system?
   a. Family interviews
   b. Family genogram
   c. Determination of communication patterns
   d. Determination of economic and educational functioning

6. A client attending group therapy tells the nurse that she realizes she is not completely alone with her problems. The nurse understands that this realization represents one of the essential components of group therapy, called:

a. altruism.
b. catharsis.
c. transference.
d. universality.

Selected References

Andrews, M. M., & Boyle, J. S. (2003). *Transcultural concepts in nursing care* (4th ed.). Philadelphia: Lippincott Williams & Wilkins.

Bensing, K. (2001). Facilitating groups: An essential part of modern health care. *ADVANCE for Nurses, 2*(11), 27–28.

Bowen, M. (1994). *Family therapy in clinical practice.* Lanham, MD: Rowman & Littlefield Publishers.

Brill, N. I., Levine, J., & Brill, N. (2004). *Working with people. The helping process* (8th ed.). Boston: Allyn and Bacon.

Brooks, G. R. (1998). *A new psychotherapy for traditional men.* San Francisco: Jossey Bass.

Cain, A. (1986, September). Family therapy: One role of the clinical specialist in psychiatric nursing. *Nursing Clinics of North America.*

Carpenito-Moyet, L. J. (2006). *Handbook of nursing diagnosis* (11th ed.). Philadelphia: Lippincott Williams & Wilkins.

Chisholm, M. M. (1996). Couple therapy. In S. Lego (Ed.), *Psychiatric nursing: A comprehensive reference* (2nd ed., pp. 53–60). Philadelphia: Lippincott-Raven Publishers.

Cohen, R., & Lipkin, G. (1979). *Therapeutic group work for health care professionals.* New York: Springer.

Crenshaw, B. G. (2003). Working with groups. In W. K. Mohr (Ed.), *Johnson's psychiatric-mental health nursing* (5th ed., pp. 151–167). Philadelphia: Lippincott Williams & Wilkins.

Duvall, E. (1984). *Marriage and family development* (5th ed.). Philadelphia: J. B. Lippincott.

Goldenberg, I., & Goldenberg, H. (2003). *Family therapy: An overview* (6th ed.). Belmont, CA: Wadsworth Publishing Co.

Haley, J. (1991). *Problem solving therapy* (2nd ed.). Hoboken, NJ: John Wiley & Sons.

Helm, S., Wynne, L. C., & Simon, F. B. (1985). *Language of family therapy—a systematic vocabulary and source book.* Rochester, NY: Family Process.

Jones, S. (1980). *Family therapy: A comparison of approaches.* Bowie, MD: Robert J. Brady.

Klee, T. (2002). Object relations theory. Retrieved June 4, 2003, from http://www.objectrelations.org/overview. htm

Lego, S. (1996). *Psychiatric nursing: A comprehensive reference* (2nd ed.). Philadelphia: Lippincott-Raven Publishers.

Marram, G. (1978). *The group approach in nursing practice* (2nd ed.). St Louis, MO: C. V. Mosby.

Nudelman, E. (September, 1986). Group psychotherapy. *Nursing Clinics of North America.*

Otto, H. (1963). Criteria for assessing family strength. *Family Process, 2(2).*

Papp, P. (1997, November). *Brief couples therapy.* Presentation delivered at the 10th Annual United States Psychiatric and Mental Health Congress Conference, Orlando, FL.

Sadock, B. J., & Sadock, V. A. (2003). *Kaplan and Sadock's synopsis of psychiatry: Behavioral sciences/clinical psychiatry* (9th ed.). Philadelphia: Lippincott Williams & Wilkins.

Taylor, C. M. (Ed.). (1982). *Interventions with groups. Essentials of psychiatric nursing* (4th ed.). St. Louis, MO: C. V. Mosby.

Titleman, P. (Ed.). (1998). *Clinical applications of Bowen family systems theory.* New York: Haworth Press.

Ulus, E. (2002). Group therapy program addresses men's needs. *Psychiatric Times, 19*(2), 75–76.

Van Horn, E., Fleury, J., & Moore, S. (2002). Family interventions during the trajectory of recovery from cardiac event: An integrative literature review. *Heart & Lung,* 31, 186–198.

White, E. (1987, February 18). Well supported. *Nursing Times.*

Wright, L., & Leahey, M. (2005). *Nurses and families: A guide to family assessment and intervention* (4th ed.). Philadelphia: F. A. Davis.

Yalom, I. E. (2005). *The theory and practice of group psychotherapy* (5th ed.). New York: Perseus Books.

Suggested Readings

Ehrlich, F. M. (1998). Psychoanalysis and couple therapy. *Psychiatric Times, 15*(12), 11.

Ellen, E. F. (1999). Group therapy requires good clinical judgment, careful screening. *Psychiatric Times, 16*(10), 1, 9–10.

Goldman, E. L. (1999). Psychotherapy for bipolar disorder: A family affair. *Clinical Psychiatry News, 27*(9), 20.

Minuchin, S. (1974). *Families and family therapy.* Cambridge: Harvard University Press.

Minuchin, S., & Fishman, H. C. (1981). *Family therapy techniques.* Cambridge: Harvard University Press.

Philpot, C. L., Brooks, G. R., Lusterman, D. D., & Nutt, R. L. (1997). *Bridging separate gender worlds: Why men and women clash and how therapists can bring them together.* Washington, DC: American Psychiatric Association Press.

Satir, V. (1991). *Conjoint family therapy* (4th ed.). London: Souvenir Press.

Sherman, C. (1999). Bridging the gap: Therapy for patients from other cultures. *Clinical Psychiatry News, 27*(5), 23.

Sherman, C. (2000). Assessment is good opportunity to change family dynamics. *Clinical Psychiatry News, 28*(3), 25.

Whitfield, C. L. (1989). *Healing the child within: Discovery and recovery for adult children of dysfunctional families.* Deerfield Beach, FL: Health Communications.

CHAPTER 16 / PSYCHOPHARMACOLOGY

In contemporary [psychiatric] treatment, psychological and psychopharmacologic models are highly compatible. When used in a combination or matrix model, the clinical outcomes are positive and powerful in enhancing quality of life for both the client and family and improving functional status. —KRUPNICK, 1996

The use of drugs to treat psychiatric disorders is often the foundation for a successful treatment approach that can also include other types of interventions such as psychotherapy or behavioral therapies. —SADOCK & SADOCK, 2003

LEARNING OBJECTIVES

AFTER STUDYING THIS CHAPTER, YOU SHOULD BE ABLE TO:

1. Articulate how the terms *pharmacodynamics* and *pharmacokinetics* relate to the science of psychopharmacology.
2. Differentiate primary, secondary, and tertiary effects of psychotropic drugs.
3. Identify implications of drug polymorphism, discontinuation syndrome, neuroleptic malignant syndrome, serotonin syndrome and metabolic syndrome in the psychiatric setting.
4. Explain the rationale for the administration of each of the following: antipsychotic agents/neuroleptics, antianxiety agents and hypnotics, antidepressants, stimulants used as mood elevators, antimanic agents used as mood stabilizers, anticonvulsants used as mood and behavior stabilizers, and antiparkinsonism or anticholinergic agents to treat medication-induced movement disorders.
5. Recognize the contraindications for and possible adverse effects of the following: antipsychotic agents/neuroleptics, antianxiety agents and hypnotics, antidepressants, stimulants, antimanic agents, anticonvulsants, and antiparkinsonism or anticholinergic agents.
6. Explain the nursing implications when administering various classifications of psychotropic drugs.
7. Demonstrate an understanding of the importance of client and family education regarding psychotropic drugs.

KEY TERMS

Acute dystonia
Acute dyskinesia
Akathisia
Atypical antipsychotics
Clearance
Clinical efficacy
Clinical psychopharmacology
Conventional antipsychotics
Discontinuation (withdrawal) syndrome
Drug half-life
Drug polymorphism
Extrapyramidal adverse effects (EPS)
First pass effects
Median effective dose
Median toxic dose
Metabolic syndrome
Neuroleptic malignant syndrome (NMS)
Neuroleptics
Parkinsonism

Peak plasma concentration	Primary effects	Tertiary effects
Pharmacodynamics	Psychopharmacology	Therapeutic index
Pharmacokinetics	Secondary effects	Therapeutic window
Potency	Serotonin syndrome	Tolerance
	Tardive dyskinesia (TD)	Typical antipsychotics

Psychopharmacology is the study of the regulation and stabilization of emotions, behavior, and cognition through the interactions of endogenous signaling substances or chemicals in the brain, such as acetylcholine, dopamine, glutamate, norepinephrine, or serotonin, with drugs (Wilcox & Gonzales, 1998). **Clinical psychopharmacology** is the study of drug effects in clients and the expert use of drugs in the treatment of psychiatric conditions. Abnormalities in emotions, behavior, and cognition are assumed to be caused by biochemical alterations of neurotransmitters and their functions in the brain. Clinical symptoms are generally lessened when the biochemical alterations are corrected by pharmacotherapy.

The introduction of new psychotropic agents is perhaps the most rapidly growing area in the fields of psychiatry and clinical pharmacology. In recent years, important new drugs have been introduced, revolutionizing the treatment of various psychiatric disorders. This progress has been made possible through advances in neuroscience and clinical research during the last few decades (Puzantian & Stimmel, 2001).

This chapter focuses on the following classifications of psychotropic agents, also referred to as *psychoactive* or *psychotherapeutic* drugs:

- Antipsychotic agents/neuroleptics
- Antianxiety agents and hypnotics
- Antidepressants
- Stimulants used as mood elevators
- Antimanic agents used as mood stabilizers
- Anticonvulsants used as mood and behavior stabilizers
- Antiparkinsonism or anticholinergic agents that are used to alleviate extrapyramidal symptoms or adverse effects of psychotropic agents

Each classification is discussed with the focus on principles or rationale for therapy; contraindications, precautions, and adverse effects; implications for nursing actions; and client and family education when applicable. Med Alert boxes are included, focusing on drug–drug interactions and unusual adverse effects. Daily dosage ranges for each classification of drugs, listed by both generic and trade name, are also given. Psychotropic agents used to treat specific disorders such as dementia, eating disorders, or substance abuse are discussed in the appropriate chapters. Finally, the back-of-book CD-ROM lists drugs used in the treatment of psychiatric and neurologic disorders.

The Science of Psychopharmacology

The science of psychopharmacology focuses on neurotransmission, the sending of impulses from one neuron to another across the synapse (the region surrounding the point of contact between two neurons or between a neuron and an effector organ) via the aid of specific substances called *neurotransmitters*. The last few decades have seen an explosion in the amount of data concerning the molecular biology of neurotransmission.

Neurotransmitters—chemicals such as acetylcholine, dopamine, glutamate, norepinephrine, and serotonin—reside in tiny sacs at the end of axons, the long tube-like parts of neurons, and are released when electrical impulses pass along the axon. When neurotransmitters cross the synapse, they undergo six steps in synaptic transmission as they bind to receptors on the surface of the next neuron (postsynaptic response; see Figure 16-1 for how neurons communicate). These steps include synthesis, vesicular uptake, transmitter release, receptor binding, cellular uptake, and transmitter metabolism. Each of these steps offers a potential target for therapeutic intervention by a drug. For example, certain drugs

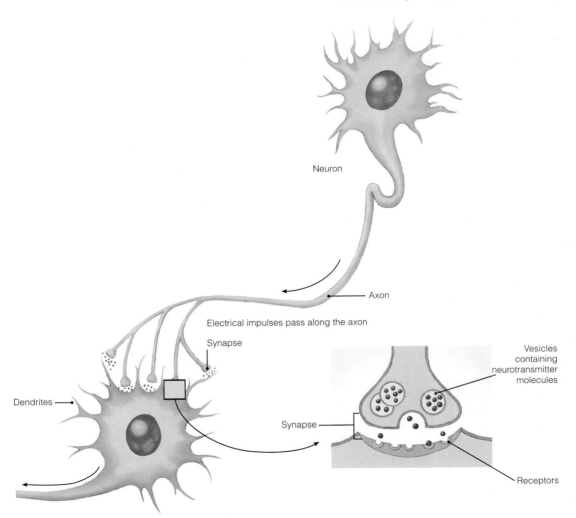

FIGURE 16.1 How neurons communicate.

can enhance the release of neurotransmitters, block neurotransmitter synthesis, or inhibit the cellular uptake of neurotransmitters (Wilcox & Gonzales, 1998).

As more groups and subgroups of neurotransmitter receptors are isolated and categorized, our understanding of psychopharmacology has broadened and has become useful in predicting future lines of research.

The interconnectedness of various neural subsystems is taken into account when attempting to explain pharmacologic data and the pathophysiology of mental illness. For example, typical antipsychotic drugs such as haloperidol (Haldol) block post-synaptic

dopamine receptors; atypical antipsychotic drugs such as risperidone (Risperdal) block both dopamine and serotonin receptors; antidepressant drugs such as sertraline (Zoloft) or paroxetine (Paxil) (selective serotonin reuptake inhibitors, or SSRIs) bind with the serotonin transporter and inhibit reuptake of serotonin into the presynaptic neurons; and anxiolytic drugs such as lorazepam (Ativan) enhance gamma-aminobutyric acid (GABA) neurotransmission (Khan, 1999; Peterson, 2001; Sadock & Sadock, 2003).

The use of psychotropic drugs leads to changes in emotions, behavior, and cognition caused by the drug's primary, secondary, or tertiary effects. **Primary effects** occur as a drug is synthesized, released, and metabolized, and as it acts on the receptor sites of a neurotransmitter system (ie, noradrenaline, acetylcholine, dopamine, serotonin, glutamate, or GABA). **Secondary effects** result from interactions among the neurotransmitters, neuropeptides, and hormones as they influence each other's function in the brain. For example, dopamine exerts a tonic inhibitory effect on the release of acetylcholine. **Tertiary effects** are the final changes in the clinical symptoms induced by a drug, such as the stabilization of anxiety or depression (Khan, 1999).

Two major aspects of pharmacology, including psychopharmacology, are pharmacodynamics and pharmacokinetics.

Pharmacodynamics

Pharmacodynamics is the study of the biochemical and physiologic effects of drugs and the mechanisms by which the effects are produced. Put simply, pharmacodynamics refers to the effects of a drug on the body (TheFreeDictionary.Com, 2005a). *Receptors* for a drug are cellular components to which a drug binds and through which it initiates its pharmacodynamic effects. The drug can be an agonist for a receptor and stimulate the specific biologic activity of the receptor or an antagonist that inhibits biologic activity (Sadock & Sadock, 2003). Several terms are used to describe the effects of a drug on the body. They include:

- **Potency** of a drug refers to the relative dosage of a drug that is required to achieve a desired effect. For example, 10 mg of the antidepressant paroxetine (Paxil) would be considered as potent as 100 mg of the antidepressant sertraline (Zoloft) if it achieved the same effect as sertraline.
- **Clinical efficacy** refers to the maximum clinical response achievable by the administration of a specific drug. For example, a client whose clinical symptoms are stabilized by 10 mg of paroxetine (Paxil) exhibits maximum clinical efficacy, often reported as a percentage such as 90% or 100%.
- **Median effective dose** is the dosage at which 50% of clients experience a specific therapeutic effect when prescribed a certain psychotropic drug. Blood levels below the median effective dose are associated with a poor response to the specific drug.
- **Median toxic dose** is the dosage at which 50% of clients experience a specific toxic effect when taking a prescribed drug. Blood levels above the median dose may precipitate a toxic state.

- **Therapeutic index** or **therapeutic window** has been defined as the ratio of the median effective dose to the median toxic dose.
- **Tolerance** refers to the need for markedly increased amounts of a specific drug over time to achieve the same desired effect (Sadock & Sadock, 2003; Shahrokh & Hales, 2003).

The psychiatric–mental health nurse must be familiar with these terms because they are used in a variety of clinical settings such as substance abuse units; during clinical research studies involving psychotropic agents; and when agents are prescribed for special populations, such as older adults and children.

Pharmacokinetics

Pharmacokinetics is the study of the movement of drugs and their metabolites through the body by the process of drug absorption, distribution, metabolism, and excretion or elimination (TheFree-Dictionary.Com, 2005b). Pharmacokinetics, put simply, refers to how the body handles the drug. After the drug is ingested, it is absorbed into the bloodstream and distributed to various parts of the body in the form of a free or protein-bound drug. Only the free fraction can pass through the blood–brain barrier. The distribution of a drug to the brain is governed by the brain's regional blood blow, the blood–brain barrier, and the drug's affinity for its receptors in the brain. High cerebral blood flow, high lipid solubility, and high receptor affinity promote the therapeutic actions of the drug (Sadock & Sadock, 2003). The unbound protein of the drug is then transported to the liver, the principal site of metabolism, where it is changed into a more readily excreted form that is subsequently excreted from the body (eg, bile, feces, urine). Psychotropic drugs are also excreted in sweat, tears, and breast milk (Sadock & Sadock, 2003).

Most psychotropic drugs are metabolized by the cytochrome P-450 (CYP) hepatic enzyme system, which contains more than 30 isoenzymes referred to as metabolizing subsystems (eg, CYP1A2, CYP2D6, CYP2C9, CYP3A3). The phase 1 enzymatic process of metabolism involves oxidation. During this phase, a specific drug is reduced to form a more water-soluble compound. Smoking, environment, the ethnic origin or age of the client, or pollutants all can influence phase 1 metabolism. The effects of the influence of these factors are unpredictable because they may increase or decrease drug metabolism. During the phase 2 enzymatic process, a compound (such as glucuronide) is added to the parent drug or the phase

1-metabolized drug to enhance water solubility and promote excretion by the kidney or gastrointestinal (GI) tract (Deitch, 2003).

The addition of other drugs may increase or decrease psychotropic drug metabolism. For example, drugs may be identified as substrates, inducers, or inhibitors. *Substrates* are drugs metabolized by an isoenzyme in the CYP hepatic enzyme system. Amitriptyline (Elavil) is an example of a substrate that is metabolized in several of the subsystems. Substrates can be affected by an inducer or inhibitor. *Inducers* are drugs that, when administered at the same time as a substrate in the same metabolic system in the liver, are likely to speed up the metabolism of a substrate. For example, phenobarbital (Barbita) and carbamazepine (Tegretol) are inducers that would speed up the metabolism of the substrate amitriptyline (Elavil). Therefore, amitriptyline is metabolized quicker in the body and eliminated before it has a chance to be most effective. The effects of enzyme induction are sometimes more difficult to predict because these are dependent on drug half-lives, the rate of enzyme production, and individual genetic variations. *Inhibitors* are drugs that compete with another drug such as a substrate for enzyme binding sites. They block the process of metabolism of another drug when given concurrently and metabolized by the same metabolic system in the liver. For example, fluvoxamine (Luvox) and paroxetine (Paxil) are psychotropic inhibitors that slow or block the metabolism of amitriptyline (Elavil). Therefore, toxicity or toxic adverse effects can occur as a result of an elevation of the serum level of amitriptyline. Duration of inhibition corresponds to the half-lives of the respective drugs (Deitch, 2003; Hospitalist.Net, 2005; Peterson, 2001; Sadock & Sadock, 2003).

Four concepts are important to understand regarding the metabolism and excretion of psychotropic drugs: peak plasma concentration, drug half-life, first pass effects, and clearance (Sadock & Sadock, 2003). The **peak plasma concentration** is defined as the greatest accumulation of the drug in the plasma. It varies depending upon the route of administration and rate of absorption of the drug. Parenteral administration of a drug generally achieves peak plasma concentration more rapidly than oral administration. **Drug half-life** refers to the amount of time it takes for metabolism and excretion to reduce the plasma concentration of a specific drug by half. The liver is the principal site of metabolism, and bile, feces, and urine are the primary routes of excretion. **First pass effects** describes the initial metabolism of an orally administered drug within the hepatic circulation and the fraction of the absorbed drug that reaches systemic circulation unmetabolized. For example, drugs administered sublingually enter the bloodstream directly and avoid first pass effects. **Clearance** refers to the amount of a drug excreted from the body in a specific period of time. Figure 16-2 depicts the pharmacokinetics and pharmacodynamics of psychotropic drug therapy.

FIGURE 16.2 Pharmacokinetics and pharmacodynamics of drug therapy.

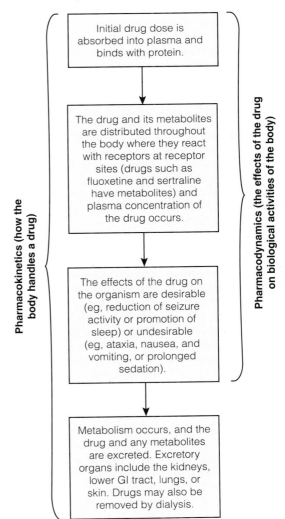

Factors Affecting Pharmacodynamics and Pharmacokinetics

As the U.S. population becomes more ethnically diverse, the nurse must be knowledgeable about the client's cultural beliefs and values regarding health and illness, as well as the client's response to treatment, including drug therapies. The term *ethnopharmacology* describes the study of the effect of ethnicity on responses to prescribed medication. An awareness of characteristic distributions of genotypes (ie, genetic constitution of the client) and phenotypes (ie, observable attributes or physical manifestations of the client) that affect pharmacokinetics can determine decisions about drug choice and dosage (Deitch, 2003; Sherman, 2005.)

The goal of psychopharmacology is to achieve a desired beneficial effect with minimal, if any, adverse effects. The psychiatric–mental health nurse needs to have a basic understanding of factors affecting pharmacodynamics and pharmacokinetics. For example, most drug references list considerations such as contraindications to the use of a specific drug (eg, the presence of renal or liver impairment), precautions (eg, directions regarding the use and administration of a specific drug), and adverse effects (eg, headache, blurred vision, increased blood pressure). The potential for drug–drug and drug–food interactions and indications for use of a specific drug also are listed.

Drug Polymorphism

Drug polymorphism refers to pharmacodynamic and pharmacokinetic variations that occur on the basis of several factors such as a client's age, gender, size, and body composition or genetic endowment (Kudzma, 1999; DeMott, 1999). For example, drug polymorphism may occur in the older adult as a result of age-related changes such as decreased absorption, hepatic function, protein binding, and renal excretion affecting the pharmacokinetics of a drug. The dosage of certain drugs may require calculation according to a client's age and/or weight. The presence of pathophysiology (structural or functional damage to an organ or tissue), such as thyroid, cardiac, hepatic, or renal impairment, can interfere with drug metabolism or excretion and promote drug polymorphism (Sadock & Sadock, 2003; Sherman, 2005).

Environmental, cultural, and genetic factors contribute to drug polymorphism among various ethnic groups. Environmental factors such as diet influence the half-life of a drug and its metabolism. For example, among African American and Hispanic clients, treatment for hypertension (such as low-salt diets and the use of diuretics) can significantly affect the retention of lithium (Eskalith), increase lithium plasma levels, and place the client at risk for lithium toxicity. Cornmeal, a dietary staple for Hispanic clients, inhibits CYP3A4 pathway metabolism of substrates such as amitriptyline (Elavil) or haloperidol (Haldol), resulting in the need to frequently monitor and adjust drug dosages (Sherman, 2005). Smoking acts as an inducer of CYP microsomal enzyme substrates and speeds up the metabolism of antipsychotic agents. Smoking is also thought to increase the metabolism of benzodiazepines. Therefore, clients who smoke may require higher doses of these agents because of reduced plasma concentration of the drugs. The dosages of such drugs should be monitored and adjusted accordingly if the client stops smoking while under treatment (Sadock & Sadock, 2003).

Cultural factors that affect drug response include a client's values and beliefs. For example, the frequent use of herbal and homeopathic remedies in some cultures can alter the body's response to various drugs, placing clients at risk for drug–drug interactions. Many herbal formulations used in Asia contain a black pepper derivative that inhibits metabolism of clozapine (Clozaril) or olanzapine (Zyprexa) by CYP3A4 and CYP1A2 isoenzymes. Drug adverse effects may appear at a lower dosage. Also, clients may not inform clinicians that they are experiencing adverse effects caused by a certain drug because it is not acceptable to report symptoms. Instead, the clients may discontinue taking the prescribed medication (Sadock & Sadock, 2003; Sherman, 2005).

Finally, genetic or biologic factors in certain ethnic groups have an impact on drug efficacy. More than one third of African Americans and Asians produce reduced amounts of CYP2D6 isoenzyme and are, therefore, slow metabolizers of some atypical antipsychotics and antidepressants that are substrates for that enzyme. Because the metabolism of benzodiazepines by the CYP3A4 isoenzyme pathway is slower in Asians, they require lower initial doses of these drugs. African American clients tend to respond better to tricyclic antidepressants, phenothiazines, and anxiolytics than do European American clients. European Americans have higher rates of receptor binding for antidepressants, but respond more slowly to these drugs and require higher doses. Asian clients respond to lower antidepressant levels (Sherman, 2005).

The U.S. Food and Drug Administration (FDA) recently approved the use of a pharmacogenomic diagnostic chip (AmpliChip by Roche) for genotyping. Genotyping for CYP gene variations can identify clients who will not benefit from, or may react badly to, certain psychotropic drugs. The chip provides an accurate genotype for two drug-metabolizing enzymes, 2D6 and 2C19. Examples of psychotropic drugs metabolized by 2D6 enzyme include fluoxetine (Prozac), paroxetine (Paxil), and venlafaxine (Effexor). Examples of drugs metabolized by 2C19 enzyme include amitriptyline (Elavil), citalopram (Celexa), and sertraline (Zoloft). This information can help clinicians improve the response for ultrarapid metabolizers and minimize adverse effects experienced by poor metabolizers of these substrates (Mrazek, 2005; Sherman, 2005).

Discontinuation (Withdrawal) Syndrome

Abrupt discontinuation or reduction in the dosage of a number of psychotropic drugs can precipitate a transient emergence of clinical symptoms, referred to as **discontinuation (withdrawal) syndrome** with rebound or relapse of original symptoms; uncomfortable new physical and psychological symptoms; or physiologic withdrawal at times (Ramaswamy, Malik, & Dewan, 2005). They can occur with tricyclic antidepressants (TCAs) and tetracyclic antidepressants, monoamine oxidase inhibitors (MAOIs), SSRIs, and other newer antidepressants. For example, discontinuation symptoms associated with TCAs are classified as physical (eg, lethargy, headache, tremor, sweating, insomnia, nausea, vomiting) or psychological (eg, irritability, anxiety/ agitation, dysphoria, nightmares, paradoxical agitation). Discontinuation symptoms rarely occur with the use of MAOIs because serious side effects and dietary restrictions discourage clinicians from prescribing them. Serotonin discontinuation syndrome may occur when dosage of SSRIs such as paroxetine (Paxil), sertraline (Zoloft), or fluoxetine (Prozac) is reduced or stopped abruptly. Clinical symptoms may include affective symptoms such as agitation or dysphoria; GI symptoms such as nausea, vomiting, or diarrhea; disequilibrium symptoms such as dizziness, vertigo, or ataxia; sensory symptoms such as paresthesia or numbness; sleep disturbances; or general somatic symptoms such as lethargy, headache, or tremor. Discontinuation symptoms generally emerge within 1 to 3 days, whereas the recurrence of depressive symptoms usually occurs 2 to 3 weeks after an antidepressant is stopped. Discontinuation symptoms generally remit within a few days if the antidepressant is re-started (Ramaswamy, Malik, & Dewan, 2005).

More severe discontinuation syndromes are associated with atypical antipsychotics such as clozapine (Clozaril), mood stabilizers such as lithium (Eskalith), dopamine receptor antagonists such as haloperidol (Haldol), and benzodiazepines such as alprazolam (Xanax). Generally, these clinical symptoms are time limited. In some situations, clinical symptoms may be minimized by restarting the drug if it was discontinued abruptly and then gradually reducing the dosage. Gradual dosage reduction is recommended especially if the client received a high dosage of the drug for a period of at least 2 months (Sadock & Sadock, 2003).

Medicating the Psychiatric–Mental Health Client

According to a 1997 study of 1,228 psychiatric clients, close to 90% were treated with medication. Approximately 75% had psychiatric management (ie, the monitoring of clinical status; client and family education; the prescription, monitoring, and adjustment of medication or other treatments; the establishment of a therapeutic relationship; and the development or modification of a treatment plan). A significantly lower percentage—approximately 45%—underwent psychotherapy. The findings clearly show the psychiatric community's current reliance on medication in treating clients (Pincus, Zarin, Tanielian, & Johnson et al., 1999).

The decision to medicate a client exhibiting clinical symptoms of a psychiatric disorder is often based on consideration of several guidelines (Bernstein, 1998). These guidelines are highlighted in Box 16-1. Some clinicians practice off-label prescribing. For example, the anticonvulsant gabapentin (Neurontin) has been prescribed for the treatment of phantom stump pain after a below-the-knee amputation, and the tetracyclic antidepressant mirtazapine (Remeron) has been administered in small doses to induce sleep. Various anticonvulsant drugs are also used to stabilize behavior in clients with the diagnosis of bipolar disorder or personality disorder. According to a nationwide survey conducted in 2004, 48% of psychiatric clients opposed off-label prescribing compared with 31% who favored

BOX 16.1 PSYCHOPHARMACOLOGIC GUIDELINES: MEDICATING THE CLIENT

- Rational pharmacotherapy requires decisions regarding when and when not to medicate.
- Emotional responses to ordinary life situations should generally not be medicated.
- Psychiatric illnesses such as depression and psychosis generally require pharmacotherapy.
- Failure to medicate properly may prolong the client's illness and suffering.
- Irrational use of medications may lead to simultaneous adverse reactions to multiple drugs.
- Detailed medical and psychiatric history, as well as assessment of client attitudes toward medication, are needed.
- Appropriate medication must be carefully chosen.
- The dose should be titrated according to response and adverse effects; the "standard dose" is seldom optimal.
- All medications should be temporarily withheld if unexplained adverse response occurs.
- It is generally advisable to start only one medication

at a time, and to observe the client before others are added.
- Lack of desired response may indicate that the client is not taking medication as directed.
- The physician must be aware of the possible lack of bioequivalence among generic drug preparations.
- The addicting potential of sedatives such as benzodiazepines should be kept in mind.
- Interactions between various psychotropic drugs and between psychotropic and nonpsychotropic drugs, as well as potential interactions between alcoholic beverages and various medications, must be considered in prescribing medication.
- Physicians must be aware of increased sensitivity and persistence of various drugs in elderly clients, and the interactions between underlying medical conditions and psychotropic drugs.
- Before medication is prescribed, the potential risks and benefits of treatment must be discussed with the client.

it; 22% were uncertain (Foley & Ries, 2004). Off-label prescribing is legal, common, necessary, and recognized in some states by statute and by U.S. Supreme Court review (Kramer & McCall, 2006.) Special treatment considerations are given to children, older adult clients, pregnant and nursing women, persons with hepatic or renal insufficiency, and persons with comorbid medical illnesses. However, even in the most ideal situations, psychopharmacology can result in adverse effects affecting the client's treatment. Table 16-1 summarizes common adverse effects of psychotropic medications and appropriate nursing interventions.

Antipsychotic Agents

Antipsychotic agents are used primarily to treat most forms of psychosis, such as schizophrenia, schizoaffective disorder, delusional disorder, mood disorder with psychosis, and psychoses associated with delirium and dementia. Symptoms may include impaired communication or the inability to relate to others, delusions, hallucinations, lack of responsiveness to external stimuli, and the inability to identify reality. These agents are also used to manage confusion, behavior problems, and personality disorders. Small doses may be used to treat anxiety, tension, agitation, dizziness, intractable

hiccups, nausea and vomiting, and to control pain when combined with other drugs.

Antipsychotic agents that produce significant neurologic adverse effects have been referred to as **neuroleptics**; the terms **conventional antipsychotics** and **typical antipsychotics** are also used to describe these agents. Antipsychotic agents provide symptom control by blocking the dopamine receptors in the brain. Dopamine is a chemical messenger that regulates thinking, emotion, behavior, and perception. Excess amounts of dopamine cause nerve impulses in the brain stem to be transmitted faster than normal, resulting in strange thoughts, hallucinations, and bizarre behavior. Blocking dopamine activity lessens or prohibits the development of such thoughts and behaviors. Examples of typical antipsychotic agents include phenothiazines (eg, thioridazine) and nonphenothiazines (eg, haloperidol).

New-generation antipsychotics, referred to as **atypical antipsychotics**, that block the activity of both serotonin and dopamine have been developed. Thus, they are used to treat both the positive and negative symptoms of disorders such as schizophrenia (see Chapter 22 for discussion of symptoms of schizophrenia). These agents produce fewer motor adverse effects than the typical neuroleptic agents do. Examples of

TABLE 16.1 Nursing Interventions for Common Adverse Effects of Psychotropic Drugs

ADVERSE EFFECT	INTERVENTIONS
Blurred vision	Explain that anticholinergic effects of medication can occur initially, but should clear. Caution client about driving or operating hazardous machinery. If blurred vision continues after 1 to 2 weeks, notify attending practitioner because a dosage reduction or change in medication may be necessary.
Constipation	Assess and monitor bowel movements. Promote adequate fluid intake (2500–3000 cc daily if not medically contraindicated). Promote dietary intake of fresh fruits, vegetables, and bran products. Provide stool softeners or bulk-forming agents prescribed by practitioner.
Drowsiness	Caution client to avoid driving or operating hazardous equipment. Give entire daytime dose of medication at bedtime if drowsiness persists. Explain that drowsiness is usually a transient symptom.
Dry mouth	Encourage the use of low-calorie or sugarless hard candy, mints, gum, or beverages.
Gastrointestinal disturbances	Explain that anorexia, nausea and vomiting, or irritation may present as transient adverse effects. Encourage taking medication with food. Refer to attending practitioner if clinical symptoms do not improve.
Hypo- or hyperglycemia	Monitor blood sugar routinely and establish baseline data if the client is taking a TCA or antipsychotic medication. Report any irregular results to attending practitioner.
Hypotension, orthostatic	Monitor blood pressure to establish baseline data before start of medication and during periods of dosage adjustment. Instruct client to rise slowly when changing from lying to sitting or standing position. Instruct client to avoid hot showers or baths because they promote vasodilation.
Insomnia	Assess sleep pattern and sleep hygiene practice. Advise against use of caffeine. Take medication as prescribed (eg, taking SSRIs at bedtime can cause insomnia; psychostimulants can increase arousal and should be avoided at bedtime).
Libido changes (sexual dysfunction)	Discuss potential adverse effects with client because they vary depending on drug category (can increase or decrease libido). Conduct a sexual history. Provide emotional support.
Tachycardia	Monitor pulse to obtain baseline data if client is taking a TCA, lithium, or anticholinergic medication. Educate client about effects of caffeine. Report any irregularities to attending practitioner.
Urinary retention	Educate client about anticholinergic effects of antipsychotic drugs and TCAs. Instruct client to report any changes in urinary frequency and notify attending practitioner of changes.
Weight gain	Instruct client to monitor weight on a weekly basis. Educate client about dietary measures to avoid weight gain. Refer to dietitian or nutritionist. Encourage development of an exercise program.

atypical antipsychotics include clozapine (Clozaril), risperidone (Risperdal), olanzapine (Zyprexa), quetiapine (Seroquel), aripiprazole (Abilify), and amisulpride (Solian).

Traditionally, typical antipsychotics such as haloperidol (Haldol) are used to treat psychiatric emergency situations involving acute psychosis. However, a study published by Sherman in the October 1999 issue of the *Journal of Clinical Psychiatry* discusses the intramuscular use of droperidol (Inapsine), a dopamine receptor antagonist, to treat psychiatric emergencies such as acute psychosis and delirium. Researchers found that droperidol was more rapidly absorbed with intramuscular injection, was eliminated more quickly from the body, and had adverse effects comparable to, and possibly somewhat less than, haloperidol. Clients who received droperidol showed a more rapid response to the medication and were less likely to need a second injection.

Contraindications and Precautions

Contraindications to the use of antipsychotic agents include a history of drug hypersensitivity, severe depression, bone marrow depression, blood dyscrasias, and brain damage. Clients with a history of impaired liver function, cardiovascular disease, hypertension, glaucoma, diabetes, Parkinson's disease, peptic ulcer disease, seizure disorder, or pregnancy require close observation when taking antipsychotic medication. Although most atypical antipsychotics have not been associated with prolongation of the Q–T interval as evidenced on electrocardiogram (ECG), caution is needed if these agents are prescribed with other drugs known to increase the Q–T interval. Antipsychotic agents are used cautiously in older adult clients.

General Adverse Effects

Adverse effects may occur due to the use of antipsychotic medication or due to a drug–drug interaction if the client is taking other medication to treat a medical problem. For example, delirium or neurotoxicity may occur if a client is taking medications such as haloperidol (Haldol) and diphenhydramine (Benadryl) concurrently. Clozapine (Clozaril) may cause a serious hematologic side effect called agranulocytosis. This side effect can be potentially life threatening and thus the client needs to be closely monitored with weekly blood work initially and at regular intervals thereafter. The newer-generation antipsychotics have been asso-

---

> ### BOX 16.2 MAJOR ADVERSE EFFECTS OF ANTIPSYCHOTIC DRUGS
>
> - Anticholinergic effects such as drowsiness, dry mouth, nasal congestion, blurred vision, constipation, and urinary retention
> - Skin reactions such as urticaria, dermatitis, and pigmentation of the skin
> - Photosensitivity or phototoxicity
> - Gastrointestinal distress such as nausea, heartburn, and cholestatic jaundice
> - Orthostatic hypotension during the first 2 weeks of treatment
> - Weight gain and possible edema
> - Seizures due to a lowering of the seizure threshold
> - Alteration in sexual functioning due to diminished sex drive
> - Alteration in laboratory values: agranulocytosis, neutropenia, hyperglycemia, elevated prolactin, and increased cholesterol
> - Mild ECG changes; sinus tachycardia

ciated with new-onset type 2 diabetes, changes in lipid metabolism and blood concentrations, elevation of prolactin causing galactorrhea or hyperprolactinemia, and arrhythmias. Combining anxiolytics, anticonvulsants, alcohol, or antidepressants with an antipsychotic agent can induce sedation. Major adverse effects of antipsychotic drugs are listed in Box 16-2. Although the list is lengthy, most of the effects usually are mild. They can be annoying, however, and should be treated as soon as they are recognized.

Neuromuscular or Neurologic Adverse Effects

Antipsychotic drugs are associated with neuromuscular and neurologic adverse effects. The major adverse effects include **acute dystonia** (abnormal positioning or spasm of muscles of the head, neck, trunk, or limbs), **acute dyskinesia** (any disturbance of movement), **parkinsonism**, and **akathisia** (motor restlessness), which are collectively called **extrapyramidal adverse effects [EPS]; tardive dyskinesia (TD); and neuroleptic malignant syndrome (NMS)** (Shahrokh & Hales, 2003). A summary of these neuromuscular or neurologic adverse effects and their treatment is presented in Table 16-2. Some of the newer,

TABLE 16.2 Neuromuscular/Neurologic Adverse Effects of Typical Antipsychotics

ADVERSE EFFECT	DEFINITION/SYMPTOMS	ONSET/PREVALENCE	TREATMENT/INTERVENTIONS
Parkinsonism	Motor retardation or akinesia, characterized by masklike appearance, rigidity, tremors, "pill rolling," salivation	Generally occurs after first week of treatment or before second month (2%–90%)	Anticipate dose reduction Administer anticholinergic agent, such as benztropine mesylate
Akathisia (motor restlessness)	Constant state of movement, characterized by restlessness, difficulty sitting still, or strong urge to move about	Generally occurs 2 weeks after treatment begins (35%)	Anticipate dose reduction or change drug class; give benzodiazepine or beta blocker
Acute dystonic reactions (disturbance of movement involving the muscles of the head, neck, trunk, or limbs)	Irregular, involuntary spastic muscle movement; wryneck or torticollis; facial grimacing; abnormal eye movements; backward rolling of eyes in the sockets (oculogyric crisis)	May occur anytime from a few minutes to several hours after first dose of antipsychotic drug (2%–90%)	Anticipate dose reduction or change drug class; give anticholinergic agent, benztropine mesylate, diphenhydramine, or muscle relaxants such as baclofen. IM injection of a drug may be necessary to treat adverse effects.
Tardive dyskinesia (abnormal movements)	Most frequent serious adverse effect resulting from termination of the drug, during reduction in dosage, or after long-term, high-dose therapy. Characterized by involuntary rhythmic, stereotyped movements; tongue protrusion; cheek puffing; involuntary movements of extremities and trunk	Occurs in approximately 3%–5% of clients taking antipsychotics in first 10 years Cumulative prevalence over 10–20 years is about 40%–55%	Reduce dosage to stabilize or minimize adverse effects; discontinue agent if the adverse effects are irreversible and can not be stabilized Give vitamin E, benzodiazepine, beta blocker, or clozapine
Neuroleptic malignant syndrome (NMS)	Idiosyncratic, rare syndrome characterized by hyperpyrexia, severe muscle rigidity, altered consciousness, alterations in blood pressure, elevated creatinine phosphokinase, elevated white blood cell count	May develop within 24–72 hours after first dose or after years of continued drug exposure; more common in persons younger than 20 and older than 60 years of age (0.1%–1%)	Discontinue antipsychotic agent; have cardiopulmonary and renal support available; administer skeletal muscle relaxant (eg, dantrolene) or centrally acting dopamine receptor agonist (eg, bromocriptine), fever reduction, hydration, deep vein thrombosis prophylaxis. Know that the combination of benzodiazepines and electroconvulsive therapy has been successful in relieving NMS after dantrolene or bromocriptine has failed. After stabilization, can restart low dose low-potent neuroleptic in 2–3 weeks.

atypical antipsychotics demonstrate improved adverse effect profiles.

Extrapyramidal adverse effects may occur during the early phase of drug therapy. Acute dystonia (also referred to as tardive dystonia) is diagnosed on the basis of sustained muscle contractions that develop after at least 1 month of antipsychotic treatment, although tardive phenomena usually develop months to years after exposure to antipsychotic drugs (Koller & Cho, 2004). Tardive dyskinesia may occur after short-term use of moderate doses, although it generally occurs after long-term use of high-dose therapy. Neuroleptic malignant syndrome can occur suddenly from 1 to 7 days after neuroleptic therapy is initiated, or can occur as late as 2 months into therapy. It has also occurred when dopamine receptor (dopaminergic) agonists, such as the combination of carbidopa and levodopa (Sinemet) used for Parkinson's disease, are discontinued (Marder & Van Putten, 1995; Herman, 1998). Clozapine (Clozaril), an atypical antipsychotic, does not cause these neuromuscular or neurologic adverse effects; often it is administered to clients who exhibit psychotic symptoms and also have neurologic disorders such as Parkinson's disease.

Nursing Implications

Antipsychotic treatment has changed dramatically during the last 50 years. From their start as pure dopamine D2 antagonists, to serotonin/dopamine antagonists, and now to partial dopamine agonists, these medications have changed in their mechanism of action as well as expected benefits (Littrell, 2004). In 2003, the FDA asked all manufacturers of atypical antipsychotic medications to add a black box warning statement to the prescribing information stating the potential for the development of **metabolic syndrome** (hyperglycemia, dyslipidemia, and abdominal obesity). The risk for these three closely interlinked conditions seems to differ according to the antipsychotic drug used: the risk is the highest with the use of clozapine (Clozaril) and olanzapine (Zyprexa) (Gerson & Margolis, 2004).

Before starting therapy and at periodic intervals as determined by the prescribing clinician, clients receiving antipsychotic drug therapy need an evaluation of blood pressure, complete blood count (CBC), serum glucose level, lipid panel, liver function tests, and vision tests. They also should undergo a thorough baseline screening for personal and family history of meta-bolic problems, hypertension, and cardiovascular disease; assessment of body mass index (BMI) and waist circumference; and nutritional and activity counseling (American Diabetes Association, American Psychiatric Association, American Association of Clinical Endocrinologists, and North American Association for the Study of Obesity, 2004).

When administering antipsychotic drugs, keep in mind the following:

1. If antacids are needed, administer them either 2 hours before or 1 hour after administration of the antipsychotic medication.
2. If a single daily dose is ordered, administer oral form within 1 or 2 hours of bedtime, whenever possible, to aid sleep. Minor adverse effects are less bothersome at this time.
3. Avoid contact with concentrated solutions while preparing them, because they are irritating to the skin and may cause contact dermatitis.
4. When administering liquid concentrates, follow pharmacy recommendations to mask the taste of the concentrate and to avoid irritation of oral mucosa.
5. Do not administer antipsychotic drugs subcutaneously unless specifically ordered. Change needles after filling the syringe and before injecting the medication to avoid tissue irritation. The Z-track method is generally used. Fluphenazine (Prolixin) and haloperidol (Haldol) may be injected in the deltoid or gluteal muscle. Risperidone (Risperdal) is to be injected in the gluteal muscle only.
6. Be aware that both olanzapine (Zyprexa [Zyprexa Zydis]) and risperidone (Risperdal-M-TAB) come in an orally disintegrating form; therefore, monitor the client's compliance to ensure adequate absorption.
7. If a client is noncompliant, expect to administer the antipsychotic drug intramuscularly. Fluphenazine decanoate (Prolixin) may be administered every 1 to 2 weeks, haloperidol decanoate (Haldol LA) is usually administered every 2 to 4 weeks, and risperidone (Risperdal) is administered every 2 weeks to clients who are noncompliant regarding use of prescribed medication.
8. Know that antipsychotic agents may provoke seizures in clients with seizure disorders.
9. Closely observe the client receiving antipsychotic drugs for the following:

- Therapeutic effects of the drugs, such as decreased agitation, decreased hallucinations, and increased socialization
- A decrease in nausea and vomiting if the drug is administered as an antiemetic
- Drug-induced EPS, early signs of TD, and NMS
- Anticholinergic effects, respiratory depression, and hypersensitivity
- Signs of agranulocytosis (eg, sore throat, fever, discomfort)
- Drug-induced, endocrine-related changes such as menstrual irregularities, breast enlargement, lactation, hyperglycemia, and changes in libido
- Signs of weight gain, jaundice, high fever, upper abdominal pain, nausea, diarrhea, and skin rash
- Drug–drug interactions (see Box 16-3) (Abrams, 2007; Karch, 2007)

BOX 16.3 MED ALERT: ANTIPSYCHOTICS/NEUROLEPTICS

Dosages of neuroleptics or antipsychotic drugs are reduced when administered to children, adolescents, or the elderly. Nevertheless, drug interactions can occur. Following is a summary of drug–drug interactions to be considered when providing care to clients receiving neuroleptic drugs:

1. Neuroleptics can potentiate the effects of central nervous system depressants, antidepressants, anticholinergic agents, phenytoin, beta blockers, antibiotics such as tetracycline, thiazide diuretics, antihypertensives, surgical muscle relaxants, and quinidine.
2. Neuroleptics can reduce the effects of lithium, anticonvulsants, antibiotics, postganglionic blocking agents, antiparkinson agents, methyldopa, and hypoglycemic agents.
3. The effects of neuroleptics can be increased by the concomitant use of antidepressants, beta blockers, barbiturates, and methyldopa.
4. The effects of neuroleptics can be reduced by the concomitant use of lithium, cimetidine, antidiarrheal drugs, antacids, and anticholinergic agents and by smoking (cytochrome p-450 induction means that higher doses of neuroleptics may be needed if client smokes).

When assessing clients receiving antipsychotic drugs for evidence of neurologic adverse effects, the Abnormal Involuntary Movement Scale (AIMS) commonly is used. Involuntary movements of the face, extremities, and trunk are rated on a scale from 0 (no adverse effects) to 4 (severe effects). Facial and oral movements, extremity movements, trunk movements, global movements, and denture status are assessed. The assessment takes usually 5 to 10 minutes; the total score may range from 0 to 42. A lower AIMS score indicates that the client is exhibiting fewer neurologic adverse effects.

In long-term care, an Antipsychotic Drug Use Assessment Form is used to monitor appropriate use of psychotropic drugs for psychogeriatric clients. The intent is to limit the use of these drugs to appropriate diagnoses or specific behavior (eg, dementia with agitation); evaluate efficacy of the drug; monitor for adverse effects; attempt gradual dose reduction unless medical contraindication is documented by the physician; and provide therapeutic alternatives such as behavioral intervention, environmental modification, and modification of staff approach.

Client Education

Nurses need to inform clients about the planned drug therapy, drug dosage, length of time it takes to achieve therapeutic results, and possible adverse effects of drug therapy. Table 16-3 highlights the daily dosages of common antipsychotic agents. Clients are instructed to report any physical illnesses or unusual adverse effects. They should be educated about the potential for drug–drug interactions when taking vitamins, minerals, herbs, dietary supplements, and over-the-counter (OTC) drugs or medications prescribed by another physician.

Include the following instructions about antipsychotic drug therapy when teaching a client and family:

- Avoid alcohol and sleeping pills, which can cause drowsiness and decrease one's awareness of environmental hazards, and other medication during drug therapy.
- Refrain from driving or operating hazardous machinery while taking antipsychotic drugs.
- Avoid exposure to direct sunlight for any extended time to prevent sunburn or over-pigmentation of the skin.
- Do not increase, decrease, or cease taking drugs without discussing this step with the physician.

TABLE 16.3 Daily Dosage of Commonly Used Antipsychotics

GENERIC NAME	TRADE NAME	DOSAGE RANGE (mg/day)
acetophenazine	Tindal	60–120 mg
aripiprazole (atypical)	Abilify	10–30 mg
chlorpromazine	Thorazine	25–2000 mg
chlorprothixene	Taractan	30–600 mg
clozapine (atypical)	Clozaril	215–900 mg
fluphenazine	Prolixin	1–40 mg
fluphenazine decanoate	Prolixin Decanoate	5–100 mg q 1–2 wk
haloperidol	Haldol	1–100 mg
haloperidol decanoate	Haldol Decanoate	12.5–200 mg q 2–4 wk
loxapine	Loxitane	10–50 mg
mesoridazine	Serentil	30–400 mg
molindone	Moban	15–200 mg
olanzapine (atypical)	Zyprexa Zyprexa (IM)	5–20 mg 2.5–10 mg q d
perphenazine	Trilafon	4–64 mg
pimozide	Orap	1–20 mg
prochlorperazine	Compazine	5–150 mg
quetiapine (atypical)	Seroquel	25–800 mg
risperidone (atypical)	Risperdal Risperdal (IM)	0.5–16 mg 25–50 mg q 2 wks
thioridazine	Mellaril	10–800 mg
thiothixene	Navane	1–60 mg
trifluoperazine	Stelazine	2–80 mg
ziprasidone (atypical)	Geodon Geodon (IM)	20–160 mg 10–40 mg

Several of the above-listed antipsychotics are also available in liquid form.

Expect to be taken off the drug slowly to avoid nausea or seizures.

- Avoid taking antacids during antipsychotic therapy because antacids might decrease the absorption of antipsychotic drugs from the intestinal tract, thus altering the effects.
- Be aware that dizziness or syncope (caused by a drop in blood pressure with position changes) can occur for about an hour after receiving the drug; take extra caution when walking or moving about to prevent falls or injuries.

- Practice good oral hygiene to minimize the risk of mouth infections, dental caries, and ill-fitting dentures. Follow up with a dentist yearly.
- Keep the drugs in a safe place, especially if children are in the home because they may mistake tablets or capsules for candy.

Antianxiety Agents and Hypnotics

Clients who experience anxiety often have difficulty falling asleep at night because they entertain their worries or concerns 24 hours a day. Conversely, clients who have difficulty sleeping at night may exhibit clinical symptoms of anxiety, fatigue, and a decreased ability to function during normal waking hours (Abrams, 2007). According to a National Sleep Foundation poll conducted in 2002, 58% of the respondents reported experiencing insomnia a few nights each week, whereas 35% reported experiencing insomnia nightly within the last year (National Sleep Foundation, 2002).

Antianxiety and hypnotic agents are central nervous system (CNS) depressants that share many characteristics. Although antianxiety agents are used primarily to treat daytime stress, larger doses may be used to promote sleep. Although hypnotics are used primarily to relieve insomnia, smaller doses produce antianxiety or sedative effects. Antianxiety agents, also referred to as *anxiolytics,* may also be used to manage withdrawal symptoms associated with chronic alcoholism, to control convulsions, and to produce skeletal muscle relaxation. Antianxiety agents are classified as benzodiazepines and nonbenzodiazepines. Certain antihistamines, beta blockers, SSRIs, and atypical antidepressants also have anxiolytic qualities.

Hypnotics

Hypnotics are used to induce a state of natural sleep, reduce periods of involuntary awakenings during the night, and increase total sleep time. Hypnotic medications have seen a dramatic evolution. Initially, barbiturates and non-barbiturates were the major hypnotic drugs of choice. In the 1970s, these agents were replaced by benzodiazepine hypnotic agents. Benzodiazepines resulted in fewer adverse effects than barbiturates in overdose along with a longer duration of hypnotic efficacy. However, concerns remain regarding rebound insomnia and withdrawal, as well as abuse possibility (Stimmel, 1999).

Another evolutionary step improving the pharmacologic treatment of insomnia occurred in the 1990s. Equally effective, shorter half-life drugs with fewer daytime adverse effects, such as temazepam (Restoril), replaced the longer-acting benzodiazepine hypnotics. Currently, several pharmacologic treatment options for insomnia are available: short-acting benzodiazepines such as triazolam (Halcion), intermediate-acting benzodiazepines such as lorazepam (Ativan), and long-acting benzodiazepines such as diazepam (Valium); novel nonbenzodiazepines such as buspirone (BuSpar) or eszopiclone (Lunesta); sedating antihistamines such as hydroxyzine hydrochloride (Atarax); natural products such as melatonin; and a few selected antidepressants such as mirtazapine (Remeron).

Pharmacologic treatment guidelines for insomnia focus on therapy that continues nightly for up to 10 nights or intermittently for 2 or 4 months. The need for continued use is reevaluated at 2- to 4-month intervals (Stimmel, 1999). Two drugs have been approved for long-term use to counter insomnia: the nonbenzodiazepine, eszopiclone (Lunesta), and the noncontrolled melatonin agonist, ramelteon (Rozerem). Indiplon is an investigational nonbenzodiazepine drug that may soon be released for the treatment of insomnia.

Benzodiazepine Anxiolytics and Hypnotics

Benzodiazepines are used primarily as antianxiety agents. However, they also may be used to treat insomnia. Commonly used benzodiazepines include chlordiazepoxide (Librium), clonazepam (Klonopin), diazepam (Valium), oxazepam (Serax), clorazepate (Tranxene), lorazepam (Ativan), prazepam (Centrax), alprazolam (Xanax), and triazolam (Halcion). These benzodiazepines work selectively on the limbic system of the brain, which is responsible for emotions such as rage and anxiety. Benzodiazepines produce tranquilizing effects with possible sedation. They also may numb emotions, taking away one's enthusiasm and zest for life. Adverse effects may also include ataxia and slurred speech. In addition, individuals who take 40 milligrams or more of diazepam (Valium) daily for several months may experience seizures if they stop taking the drug abruptly.

A rebound phenomenon, referred to as *paradoxical excitation,* may also occur after the abrupt discontinuation of benzodiazepines. The client may become more anxious, exhibit aggressive or antisocial behavior, or experience withdrawal symptoms of confusion, toxic psychosis, convulsions, or a condition resembling delirium tremens. This withdrawal syndrome may develop at any time up to 3 weeks after stopping a long-acting benzodiazepine, but may occur within a few hours after abrupt cessation of short-acting benzodiazepines. On rare occasions, this same paradoxical effect can occur in children or geriatric clients with administration of benzodiazepines, causing excitation rather than producing the intended calming effect. Close monitoring of the client is required when initiating therapy to assess for this possible reaction (Sadock & Sadock, 2003).

When used in combination with alcohol, the interactive effects can be lethal. The serum levels of benzodiazepines increase, resulting in respiratory distress or other medical emergencies. Benzodiazepines also interfere with normal coping mechanisms; increase irritability, aggressiveness, and hostility when taken over an extended period of time; and increase the risk for depression. Long-term use of benzodiazepines is not recommended because these drugs can produce dependency. Additionally, benzodiazepines are associated with the phenomenon of tolerance (ie, needing increasing amounts of the drug to achieve the same effect and the occurrence of withdrawal symptoms if it is abruptly discontinued; Sadock & Sadock, 2003).

Nonbenzodiazepine Anxiolytics and Hypnotics

Nonbenzodiazepines include meprobamate (Equanil), which is used to relieve muscle tension associated with anxiety or for insomnia, and buspirone (BuSpar), which is an azasperone or novel anxiolytic.

Meprobamate is a bis-carbamate ester that falls pharmacologically between the barbiturates and benzodiazepines. It causes CNS depression but not anesthesia. Buspirone blocks the release of serotonin and prevents the uptake of dopamine. It is considered to be significantly free of drug–drug interactions and is the preferred drug in the treatment of anxiety when clients have chronic obstructive pulmonary disease. Buspirone produces less sedation with fewer adverse effects that impair cognition and performance (Cole & Yonkers, 1995).

Antihistamines as Anxiolytics and Hypnotics

Many antihistamines are available to treat a wide variety of medical problems, such as allergic and dermatologic or neurodermatologic reactions, motion sickness, nausea and vomiting, and drug-induced EPS. Antihistamines also are one of the most common classes of sleep-inducing agents. The antihistamines most commonly used to treat anxiety and insomnia are hydroxyzine hydrochloride (Atarax), hydroxyzine pamoate (Vistaril), and diphenhydramine hydrochloride (Benadryl). Common adverse effects include drowsiness, dizziness, anticholinergic effects such as dry mouth or blurred vision, gastritis, paradoxical excitement, and hypotension. Older adult clients may exhibit clinical symptoms of delirium secondary to such adverse effects.

Beta Blockers as Anxiolytics

Beta blockers are used to diminish tachycardia, benign essential tremors, impulsivity, and agitation associated with anxiety. The most commonly used beta blockers include propranolol (Inderal), atenolol (Tenormin), metoprolol (Lopressor), and nadolol (Corgard). Adverse effects may include hypotension, bronchospasm, bradycardia, fatigue, dizziness, depression, pharyngitis, agranulocytosis, heart block, and GI upset.

Selective Serotonin Reuptake Inhibitors and Atypical Antidepressants as Anxiolytics

Five SSRI antidepressants—paroxetine (Paxil), sertraline (Zoloft), citalopram (Celexa), fluoxetine (Prozac) and escitalopram (Lexapro)—were recently approved by the FDA for the treatment of anxiety disorders. The atypical antidepressant venlafaxine (Effexor), which is a serotonin and norepinephrine reuptake inhibitor (SNRI), has also been approved for the same use. Although approved for the treatment of anxiety, these drugs are commonly categorized as antidepressants and are discussed in that section of this chapter. Their use is also discussed in the chapters related to anxiety and mood disorders (19, 20, and 21.)

Contraindications, Precautions, and Adverse Effects

Contraindications and precautions to the use of antianxiety and hypnotic agents depend upon the specific agent prescribed and are too numerous to list at this time. However, many of the agents are contraindicated in the presence of acute narrow-angle or open-angle untreated glaucoma, severe renal or hepatic impairment, blood dyscrasias, pregnancy or lactation/nursing, acute post-myocardial infarction, psychosis, or during the use of MAOIs. Precautions are recommended to prevent drug–drug interactions. For example, anxiolytics may lower the seizure threshold when prescribed concurrently with anticonvulsant agents; potentiate CNS depression with the use of alcohol; or affect clotting time in clients undergoing anticoagulant therapy. Elderly clients and clients with a history of seizures, cerebral vascular disease, adrenal disease, diseases that affect metabolism or hemodynamic responses, suicidal tendency, or history of electroconvulsive therapy should be evaluated before use of these agents (Murphy, 2005; Sadock & Sadock, 2003). The more common adverse effects were included during the discussion of each category of the antianxiety agents.

Nursing Implications

Before administering antianxiety agents or hypnotics, assess the client's mental and physical status to avoid the risk of possible adverse effects. Pregnant women or those who are breast-feeding typically are not prescribed antianxiety agents because of the risk of adverse effects. If a client complains of a sleep disturbance, the cause should be identified, if possible. Appropriate nursing interventions such as sleep hygiene measures, relaxation therapy, sleep restriction therapy, and stimulus control are to be tried first as alternatives to the administration of hypnotics.

When administering antianxiety or hypnotic drugs, keep in mind the following:

1. Administer the daily dose at bedtime to promote sleep, minimize adverse effects, and allow more normal daytime activities to occur.
2. Administer intramuscular dosages deeply and slowly into large muscle masses because they are irritating to tissues and can cause pain at the site of injection. The Z-track method is generally used to avoid irritation of tissue.
3. Observe for therapeutic effects.
4. Observe for adverse effects such as oversedation, hypotension, pain at the injection site, skin rashes, and paradoxical excitement such as hostility, rage, confusion, depersonalization, or hyperactivity. Rare adverse effects include GI discomfort, nausea, vomiting, menstrual irregularities, blood dyscrasias, photosensitivity, and nonthrombocytopenic purpura.

5. Monitor for adverse effects of beta blockers, especially hypotension, bronchospasm, bradycardia, and depression.
6. Know that alprazolam (Xanax) is available as an orally disintegrating tablet that has been labeled Niravam; clonazepam (Klonopin) is available in wafer form labeled Klonopin/ Rivotril; and lorazepam (Ativan) can be administered sublingually for rapid absorption.
7. When administering antianxiety agents parenterally, do not administer solutions that are cloudy or contain a precipitate.
8. Be alert for possible drug–drug interactions (see Box 16-4) (Abrams, 2007; Karch, 2007.)

BOX 16.4   MED ALERT: ANTIANXIETY AGENTS AND HYPNOTICS

Dosages of anxiolytics and hypnotics are reduced when given to children, adolescents, or the elderly. Following is a summary of drug–drug interactions and unusual adverse effects to be considered when providing care to clients receiving antianxiety or hypnotic agents:

1. Alcohol, narcotic analgesics, TCAs, and CNS depressants can cause an increase in CNS depression when used concurrently with this classification of psychotropic medication.
2. Displacement of digoxin from serum proteins can occur when taken concurrently with buspirone.
3. Hypertension can occur when buspirone and MAOIs are combined during therapy.
4. Prothrombin times may vary during anticoagulant therapy.
5. The use of cimetidine (Tagamet) reduces the clearance of diazepam and alprazolam.
6. Benzodiazepines may decrease the actions of carbamazepine.
7. Erythromycin may inhibit the metabolism of diazepam and chlordiazepoxide.
8. Beta blockers may decrease the effects of insulin and oral antidiabetic agents.
9. Beta blockers may increase the effects of thyroxine, phenytoin, clonidine, and phenothiazines.
10. Avoid use of alprazolam in clients who have severe pulmonary disorders.
11. Antianxiety agents aggravate the symptoms of acute intermittent porphyria.

Client Education. Tell clients the name of the drug they have been prescribed, the dosage, and the expected course of treatment. Table 16-4 lists daily dosages of common antianxiety agents and hypnotics.

In addition, include the following information in client and family teaching:

- Review the adverse effects of the prescribed medication and instruct the client to report the onset of any adverse effects as well as symptoms such as fever, malaise, sore throat, petechiae, easy bruising or bleeding, and skin rash.
- Instruct the client to avoid the use of alcoholic beverages with antianxiety agents because alcohol can increase the depressant effects of these agents, possibly causing death.
- Instruct the client that smoking can increase the metabolism of benzodiazepine agents and reduce the desired effects of the prescribed drug.
- Instruct the client not to alter the dose of medication and not to drive or operate hazardous machinery or equipment.
- Instruct the client to avoid ingesting large amounts of beverages containing caffeine, a stimulant, because it can decrease the effects of hypnotic agents and increase the effects of beta blockers.
- Instruct the client that grapefruit juice interacts with alprazolam (Xanax), fluvoxamine (Luvox), buspirone (BuSpar), sertraline (Zoloft), and triazolam (Halcion), inhibiting enzyme metabolism that may result in fatal consequences.
- Explain that sudden cessation of benzodiazepines can cause rapid eye movement or rebound effects such as insomnia, nightmares, hyperexcitability, agitation, or convulsions and sudden death.
- Instruct the client to avoid excessive use of these drugs to prevent the onset of substance abuse or addiction.
- Explain that hypnotics are ineffective as analgesics.
- Instruct clients who take hypnotics to keep a sleep diary (see Chapter 12) to determine the efficacy of the prescribed hypnotic.
- Explain rebound insomnia, which is the worsening of insomnia that may occur after discontinuation of medication.

Antidepressants

Antidepressants are used to treat depressive disorders caused by emotional or environmental stressors; losses; drugs; disease states such as cerebral vascular

TABLE 16.4 Daily Dosage of Commonly Used Antianxiety Agents and Hypnotics

GENERIC NAME	TRADE NAME	DOSAGE RANGE (mg/day)
Antianxiety Agents		
atenolol	Tenormin	50–200 mg
alprazolam	Xanax	0.5–8 mg
buspirone*	BuSpar	15–60 mg
chlordiazepoxide	Librium	10–100 mg
citalopram*	Celexa	10–60 mg
clomiprimine hydrochloride	Anafranil	25–250 mg
clonazepam	Klonopin (Rivotril in Canada)	0.5–20 mg
clorazepate dipotassium	Tranxene	7.5–90 mg
diazepam	Valium	2–40 mg
diphenhydramine hydrochloride	Benadryl	25–300 mg
escitalopram oxalate*	Lexapro	10–20 mg
fluoxetine*	Prozac	10–80 mg
fluvoxamine maleate**	Luvox	50–300 mg
hydroxyzine hydrochloride	Atarax	10–100 mg
hydroxyzine pamoate	Vistaril	25–100 mg
lorazepam	Ativan	1.0–10 mg
meprobamate	Miltown/Equanil	200–1200 mg
oxazepam	Serax	30–120 mg
paroxetine*	Paxil	12.5–75 mg
prazepam	Centrax	10–40 mg
propanolol	Inderal	40–120 mg
sertraline*	Zoloft	25–200 mg
venlafaxine*	Effexor XR	37.5–225 mg
Hypnotic Agents		
amobarbital sodium	Amytal	50–300 mg
aprobarbital	Alurate	40–160 mg
diphenhydramine hydrochloride	Benadryl	25–300 mg
eszopiclone	Lunesta	1–3 mg
estazolam	ProSom	1–2 mg
flurazepam	Dalmane	15–30 mg
hydroxyzine hydrochloride	Atarax	10–100 mg
hydroxyzine pamoate	Vistaril	25–100 mg
quazepam	Doral	7.5–15 mg
ramelteon	Rozerem	8 mg
secobarbital	Seconal	100–200 mg
temazepam	Restoril	15–30 mg
trazodone†	Desyrel	25–75 mg
triazolam	Halcion	0.125–0.5 mg
zaleplon	Sonata	5–20 mg
zolpidem	Ambien	5–10 mg
zopiclone in Canada	Imovane	3.75–7.5 mg

* Listed as antidepressant; also effective as an anxiolytic.
**Listed as mood disorder agent; used primarily to treat obsessive-compulsive disorder.
†Listed as antidepressant; also used to treat insomnia. Natural sleep products are listed in Chapter 18.

accidents; or depression that cannot be related to an identifiable cause. These drugs are classified as SSRIs, TCAs, atypical antidepressants, and MAOIs.

SSRIs represent the latest advancement in pharmacotherapy. They inhibit the 5-hydroxytryptamine (5-HT) system uptake of indoleamine (serotonin). Abnormalities in 5-HT function can result in mood disturbances, anxiety, altered cognition, aggressive behavior, or altered sexual drive.

TCAs increase the level of a neurotransmitter, either serotonin or norepinephrine, in the space between nerve endings. A deficiency in either of these transmitters is thought to cause depression. Choice of medication depends on which chemical is thought to be deficient in the nerve endings.

Atypical antidepressants do not readily fit into the familiar categories of TCAs, MAOIs, or SSRIs. At present, the following atypical antidepressants have been identified: trazodone (Desyrel), bupropion (Wellbutrin), venlafaxine (Effexor), mirtazapine (Remeron), maprotiline (Ludiomil), reboxetine (Edronax, Vestro), and duloxetine (Cymbalta). Nefazodone (Serzone) has been removed from the market because it was linked to 55 cases of liver failure.

Trazodone, chemically unrelated to other antidepressants, is a mixed serotonergic agonist and antagonist. Bupropion, which has a different chemical structure than the other antidepressants, appears to block more dopamine reuptake. Venlafaxine and duloxetine are novel bicyclics (SNRIs) unrelated to the TCAs; they inhibit neuronal uptake of serotonin and norepinephrine. Mirtazapine and maprotiline are tetracyclics believed to enhance central noradrenergic and serotonergic activity. Reboxetine is a noradrenaline reuptake inhibitor (NARI).

MAOIs prevent the metabolism of neurotransmitters, but are used less frequently than the TCAs because they are less effective, must be given for longer periods before they are beneficial, are more toxic, have a longer duration of action, and may cause severe adverse reactions if taken with tyramine-rich foods.

Selective Serotonin Reuptake Inhibitors

SSRIs are a popular class of antidepressants, now considered the first line of therapy for treating depression. Although this class of drugs is relatively safe and useful for a broad spectrum of potential indications, the FDA recently recommended that a black box warning be added to drug labels stating that SSRIs increase the risk of suicidal behavior in depressed children and teens. SSRIs depend on neuronal release of serotonin for their action: the blockage of the neuronal uptake of serotonin. By inhibiting the uptake of serotonin into the nerve terminal, the level of the neurotransmitter at the synapse increases, exerting a clinically significant antidepressant effect. The term *chemical imbalance* is often used to describe a deficiency of serotonin and the presence of depression. A chemical imbalance may occur as a result of neurologic or organic changes in the cerebral cortex.

Selective serotonin reuptake inhibitors are used in the treatment of depression alone or in the presence of concurrent disorders such as anxiety, panic attacks, eating disorders, sleep disorders, alcoholism, or schizophrenia. Flexible dosing is another advantage because single doses may be administered in the morning or at bedtime. Dosage titration to achieve a therapeutic level usually occurs slowly. Although a therapeutic response may occur within the first 2 weeks of treatment, clients may not receive full benefit of the antidepressant agent until 8 weeks (Zoler, 2004).

Contraindications, Precautions, and Adverse Effects

Caution is needed when SSRIs are prescribed concurrently with anticoagulants. Monitor prothrombin times closely. The dosages of theophylline and alprazolam are reduced to avoid excessive plasma concentrations of both drugs. Diazepam, alcohol, and tryptophan should be avoided. A recent labeling change for the administration of sertraline warns that the co-administration of sertraline and pimozide (Orap) greatly increases the plasma concentration level of pimozide, which has a very narrow therapeutic index. This could result in significant toxicity.

Concurrent use of the herbal supplement St. John's Wort, a serotonin agonist such as buspirone (BuSpar), or an MAOI such as phenelzine (Nardil) with SSRIs can lead to the accumulation of serotonin. For example, if a client has been taking an MAOI, a 14-day drug clearance is required before initiating SSRI therapy to avoid an accumulation of serotonin and subsequent **serotonin syndrome.** This phenomenon, not to be confused with discontinuation syndrome described earlier in the chapter, occurs as a result of central and peripheral serotonergic hyperstimulation. The clinical presentation of serotonin syndrome is characterized by a variety of symptoms such as confusion, delirium, agitation, irritability, ataxia, incoordination, tremor, seizures, hyperreflexia, diaphoresis, nausea, vomiting, diarrhea, abdominal pain, hypotension or hypertension, tachycardia, hyperthermia, cyanosis, severe respiratory depression, and coma. The incidence of this syndrome appears to be increasing, due in part to the large numbers of serotonergic medications available for the treatment of a variety of neurologic conditions. Symptoms usually develop soon after the addition of a new medication or a dosage increase in current medication. Onset may range from 2 to 24 hours from the time of medication ingestion. Presentation can vary from mild symptoms to coma, which is associated with high morbidity and mortality. Examples of drugs associated with serotonin syndrome include L-tryptophan, MAOIs, amphetamines, cocaine, TCAs, SSRIs, meperidine, trazodone, buspirone, and lithium (Lantz, 2001; Moen, 2002; Sherman, 1999).

Common adverse effects of SSRIs include nausea, diarrhea, constipation, tremor, insomnia, somnolence, dry mouth, headache, nervousness, anorexia, weight loss, sweating, and sexual dysfunction. Mild or moderate hyponatremia is often overlooked in elderly depressed clients who are prescribed SSRIs because the nonspecific symptoms are common in this population; however, such adverse effects can lead to lethal complications if untreated (Moon, 2004).

Nursing Implications

When administering SSRIs, special considerations include advising clients to avoid use if pregnant or lactating; administering the drug once a day, in the morning or evening; arranging for lower doses in older adult clients or clients with hepatic or renal impairment; increasing dosages at intervals of not less than once a week; establishing suicide precautions for clients who are severely depressed; and reporting any unusual adverse effects to the attending physician (Karch, 2007).

Because certain drugs should not be administered concurrently with SSRI therapy, ensure that the client's chart and medication administration record are marked clearly to avoid any adverse drug–drug interactions.

Client Education. Instruct clients who are receiving SSRI drug therapy to do the following:

- Take the drugs exactly as prescribed. Never attempt to alter the dosage. (See Table 16-5 for a listing of daily dosages for SSRI therapy.)
- Avoid taking grapefruit juice with fluvoxamine (Luvox) and sertraline (Zoloft).

TABLE 16.5 ■ Daily Dosage of Selective Serotonin Reuptake Inhibitors

GENERIC NAME	TRADE NAME	DOSAGE RANGE (mg/day)
citalopram	Celexa	10–60 mg
escitalopram oxalate	Lexapro	10–20 mg
fluoxetine	Prozac	10–80 mg
fluvoxamine	Luvox	50–300 mg (used in depression associated with OCD)
paroxetine	Paxil	10–60 mg
sertraline	Zoloft	25–200 mg

Fluoxetine and paroxetine are also available in controlled release tabs.
All but fluvoxamine are available as oral solutions or concentrate.

- Avoid altering the dosage of the medication. Contact the physician before discontinuing use of the drug.
- Report any unusual symptoms such as tremors, nausea and vomiting, anorexia, weight loss, nervousness, or sexual dysfunction.
- Avoid the use of diazepam, alcohol, and tryptophan.
- Inform the physician if taking an anticoagulant or theophylline.
- Avoid operating hazardous machinery, including an automobile, if drowsiness occurs.
- Notify the physician if symptoms of depression worsen.
- Keep the medication out of the reach of children.
- If taking psychostimulants to potentiate antidepressant therapy, report any additional symptoms of irritability, insomnia, headache, palpitations, blurred vision, dry mouth, constipation, or dizziness.
- Have his or her blood pressure and pulse monitored initially and after each dosage change to detect hypotension, hypertension, and irregular heart rates.

Tricyclic Antidepressants

TCAs generally are used to treat symptoms of depression such as insomnia, decreased appetite, decreased libido, excessive fatigue, indecisiveness, difficulty thinking and concentrating, somatic symptoms, irritability, and feelings of worthlessness. These agents are considered effective in 85% of those people who exhibit symptoms of depression. Clients receiving TCAs usually show increased mental alertness and physical activity with mood elevation within a few days after therapy is initiated. Typically, clients receiving antidepressant drug therapy continue taking the medication for up to 1 year to allow neurotransmitters to return to normal levels and to achieve a reversal of the depressive episode. Other disorders that usually respond to TCAs include agoraphobia, borderline personality disorder, dysthymic disorder, obsessive–compulsive disorder, panic disorder, and schizoaffective disorder (Maxmen, Dubovsky, & Ward, 2002). Examples of TCAs commonly used to treat depression include nortriptyline (Pamelor), imipramine (Tofranil), doxepin (Sinequan), desipramine (Norpramin), and protriptyline hydrochloride (Vivactil).

Contraindications, Precautions, and Adverse Effects

Clients who are pregnant or breast-feeding, persons recovering from a myocardial infarction, or those with severe liver or kidney disease should not receive TCAs. Caution is necessary when administering these drugs to clients with asthma, urinary retention, hyperthyroidism, glaucoma, cardiovascular disorders, benign prostatic hypertrophy, alcoholism, epilepsy, and schizophrenia.

Several drugs increase the effects of TCAs; they include antihistamines, atropine, alcohol, narcotic analgesics, benzodiazepines, and urinary alkalizers (eg, sodium bicarbonate). Barbiturates, nicotine, and chloral hydrate decrease the effects of TCAs (Abrams, 2007; Karch, 2007).

Common adverse effects of TCAs include dry mouth, blurred vision, tachycardia, urinary retention, and constipation. Less frequently encountered adverse effects include loss of appetite, insomnia, hypotension, anxiety, and increased intraocular pressure. Potentially dangerous adverse effects of tricyclic drug therapy include agranulocytosis, jaundice, increased seizure susceptibility in clients with epilepsy, and prolongation of atrioventricular conduction time. Acute toxicity due to overdose may occur.

Nursing Implications

Assess the client's level or severity of depression, including the presence of suicidal ideation; note any adverse effects; monitor for drug interactions; and observe for therapeutic effects of TCAs.

Within 2 or 3 weeks after the initial dose, tricyclic drugs should reach a serum plasma level at which optimal response occurs (therapeutic window). Therefore, if no therapeutic response is observed within 4 to 8 weeks, another drug usually is prescribed.

Because these agents may cause urinary retention and constipation, assess the client for abdominal distention. Also, assess the client's vital signs and cardiac status closely. Orthostatic hypotension, tachycardia, or arrhythmias may occur. Report any significant changes immediately and expect the medication dosage to be adjusted accordingly. Monitor clients receiving high doses for signs of seizure activity.

Client Education. Instruct clients receiving tricyclic drug therapy to do the following:

- Take drugs exactly as prescribed. Never attempt to alter the dosage. (See Table 16-6 for daily dosages of commonly used tricyclic antidepressants.)
- Be aware that the therapeutic effects may not occur for 2 to 3 weeks after initial therapy. Check with the physician about the need for follow-up laboratory testing for drug levels to monitor dosage.
- Avoid taking OTC cold remedies or other drugs without the physician's knowledge. Consult with the pharmacist before adding any OTC drug to the regimen.
- Inform other professionals who may be treating you, such as a dentist or surgeon, of the drug therapy.
- Report any adverse effects, such as fever, malaise, sore throat, mouth sores, urinary retention, fainting, irregular heartbeat, restlessness, mental confusion, or seizures.
- Avoid excessive exercise and high temperatures because these drugs (because of their anticholinergic effects) block perspiration.
- Know that these drugs are not addictive, but some clients may have a chronic deficiency in neurotransmitters, requiring them to take these agents over an extended period.

Atypical Antidepressants

Atypical antidepressants represent a conglomeration of agents that elude traditional classification. When clients do not respond to the use of SSRIs or TCAs, atypical antidepressants are considered to be alternatives or second-line therapy.

TABLE 16.6 🔲 Daily Dosage of Commonly Used Tricyclic and Atypical Antidepressants

GENERIC NAME	TRADE NAME	DOSAGE RANGE (mg/day)
Tricyclic Antidepressants		
amitriptyline	Amitril, Elavil, Endep	50–300 mg
desipramine	Norpramin Pertofrane	75–300 mg
doxepin	Sinequan, Adapin	75–300 mg
imipramine	Tofranil	75–300 mg
nortriptyline	Aventyl, Pamelor	50–150 mg
protriptyline	Vivactil	15–60 mg
trimipramine	Surmontil	75–300 mg
Atypical Antidepressants		
bupropion	Wellbutrin	200–450 mg
maprotiline	Ludiomil	25–225 mg
mirtazapine	Remeron	15–45 mg
reboxetine	Edronax, Vestro	4–12 mg
trazodone	Desyrel	25–600 mg
venlafaxine	Effexor	75–375 mg

Contraindications, Precautions, and Adverse Effects

Any comorbid medical condition, including cardiac or neurologic disorders, requires close consideration when atypical antidepressants are ordered. Venlafaxine is contraindicated in the presence of uncontrolled hypertension because of its potential to increase blood pressure. Bupropion is contraindicated in the presence of seizure disorder, bulimia, anorexia, trauma, or lactation. Caution is exercised with the use of bupropion in clients with renal or liver disease, heart disease, or history of a myocardial infarction. Mirtazapine is a tetracyclic with similar qualities and contraindications as those associated with TCAs. Maprotiline is contraindicated in the presence of seizure disorders and acute myocardial infarction. Trazodone is contraindicated in the presence of a recent myocardial infarction and should be used with caution in clients who have a preexisting cardiac disease or abnormal liver function tests. New labeling alerts health care providers to potential drug interactions when trazodone is given with the antifungal, ketoconazole, or with the antivirals ritonavir and indinavir. The anticonvulsant carbamazepine (Tegretol) reduces plasma concentrations of trazodone when coadministered.

Adverse effects vary depending upon which atypical drug is used (Karch, 2007; Peterson, 2001; Sadock & Sadock, 2003). Common adverse effects include drowsiness or somnolence, dizziness, dry mouth, and GI upset. In addition, trazodone may cause CNS overstimulation; mirtazapine causes weight gain; maprotiline may cause EPS; bupropion and certain SSRIs such as duloxetine and fluoxetine may precipitate symptoms of mania or psychosis; and venlafaxine and trazodone may cause sexual dysfunction.

Nursing Implications

Providing care for clients who take atypical antidepressants can be challenging because of the variety of contraindications and potential adverse effects associated with each drug. This is further compounded if the client has an existing comorbid medical disorder. The client may need to undergo a physical exam including laboratory tests, ECG, and electroencephalogram (EEG) to rule out the presence of preexisting cardiac disorder, neurologic disorder, liver disease, or renal impairment. When administering atypical antidepressants, adhere to the following:

1. Monitor vital signs to detect potential adverse effects such as hypertension, hypotension, arrhythmias, or infection during therapy.
2. Establish safety precautions if CNS changes such as confusion, drowsiness, incoordination, or weakness occur.
3. Administer medication with food to decrease adverse GI effects such as anorexia and GI upset.
4. Expect to administer lower doses or administer the drugs less frequently if the client is older or debilitated.
5. Do not administer atypical antidepressants within 14 days of MAOI administration.
6. Ensure that clients who are depressed and potentially suicidal have access to only limited quantities of the prescribed drug.
7. Monitor liver and hepatic function tests in clients with a history of liver or renal impairment (Karch, 2007; Peterson, 2001).

Client Education. Instruct the client receiving atypical antidepressant drug therapy and the family to do the following:

- Take medication exactly as prescribed. Do not combine doses or attempt to make up missed doses. Do not abruptly discontinue taking the drug. (See Table 16-6 for daily dosages of commonly used atypical antidepressants.)
- Report any adverse effects or changes in medical condition.
- Avoid the use of alcohol, sleep-inducing drugs, and OTC drugs while taking this medication.
- Use contraceptives to prevent pregnancy. Consult with your health care provider if pregnancy occurs.
- Avoid prolonged exposure to sunlight or sunlamps when taking mirtazapine.
- Take drug (eg, trazodone, venlafaxine) with food or a snack to enhance absorption and decrease likelihood of dizziness (Karch, 2007; Peterson, 2001).

Monoamine Oxide Inhibitors

MAOIs may be prescribed for clients with treatment-resistant depression; clients who have depression associated with anxiety attacks, phobic attacks, or many somatic complaints; clients who fail to respond to TCAs or who cannot tolerate SSRIs; and clients who are in the depressive phase of bipolar disorder. MAOIs may be superior to TCAs in treating atypical depression (Maxmen, Dubovsky, & Ward, 2002).

Contraindications, Precautions, and Adverse Effects

The list of conditions that prohibit the use of MAOIs is lengthy. Box 16-5 lists these conditions, underscoring the need for caution when prescribing or administering these drugs. Serious drug–drug interactions have occurred when MAOIs are administered concurrently with dextromethorphan, CNS depressants, other antidepressants, antihypertensive medication, antihistaminic preparations, levodopa, or meperidine. Morphine is a safe alternative to meperidine. Caution is needed when treating clients with a history of angina pectoris, pyloric stenosis, epilepsy, and diabetes mellitus. Drugs that increase the effects of MAOIs have been identified as anticholinergics, adrenergic agents, alcohol, levodopa, and meperidine (Abrams, 2007).

Frequently seen adverse effects include abnormal heart rate, orthostatic hypotension, drowsiness or

---

BOX 16.5 | CONDITIONS THAT PROHIBIT THE USE OF MAOIs

- Asthma
- Cerebral vascular disease
- Congestive heart failure
- Hypertension
- Hypernatremia
- Impaired kidney function
- Cardiac arrhythmias
- Pheochromocytoma
- Hyperthyroidism
- Liver disease
- Abnormal liver function tests
- Severe headaches
- Alcoholism
- Glaucoma
- Atonic colitis
- Paranoid schizophrenia
- Debilitated clients
- Age older than 60 years
- Pregnancy
- Age younger than 16 years

---

insomnia, headache, dizziness, blurred vision, vertigo, constipation, weakness, dry mouth, nausea, vomiting, and loss of appetite.

As stated earlier, MAOIs are antidepressants that are well known for their multiple drug and food interactions because they inhibit the enzyme that breaks down the amino acids tyramine and tryptophan. An accumulation of these substances triggers the release of norepinephrine, and a *hypertensive crisis* may occur. Clinical symptoms include elevation of diastolic and systolic blood pressure, headache, diaphoresis, dilation of pupils, rapid heart rate or arrhythmias, and intracerebral hemorrhage (Ahmed & Fecik, 2000). The foods and beverages to be avoided are found in Box 16-6.

Nursing Implications

MAOIs are nonaddictive and are considered safe and effective if taken as directed. As with TCAs, observe the client for signs of therapeutic effects, adverse effects, and drug or food interactions.

To reach a maximum therapeutic effect, MAOIs may require 2 to 6 weeks of therapy. Beneficial response

BOX 16.6 FOODS AND BEVERAGES THAT CONTAIN TYRAMINE AND TRYPTOPHAN

Hypertensive crisis may occur if MAOIs are taken with the following:

- Aged cheese
- Avocados
- Bananas
- Beer
- Caffeine
- Canned figs
- Chicken livers
- Chocolate
- Fava bean pods
- Guacamole dip
- Meat tenderizers
- Pickled herring
- Raisins
- Sauerkraut
- Sour cream
- Soy sauce
- Wine
- Yeast supplements
- Yogurt

TABLE 16.7 Daily Dosage of Commonly Used Monoamine Oxidase Inhibitors

GENERIC NAME	TRADE NAME	DOSAGE RANGE (mg/day)
isocarboxazid	Marplan	10–70 mg
phenelzine	Nardil	15–90 mg
tranylcypromine	Parnate	20–60 mg

should be evident within 3 to 4 weeks. Monitor the client closely for possible overdose and have medications readily available should signs and symptoms occur. Medication for overdose includes phentolamine for excessive pressor response (dilation of blood vessels and lowering of arterial blood pressure) and diazepam for excessive agitation.

Client Education. Instruct the client receiving MAOIs in the following:

- Take the drugs exactly as prescribed. (See Table 16-7 for daily dosages of commonly used MAOIs.) Avoid altering the dosage or discontinuing the use of the drug.
- Avoid the intake of foods containing tyramine and tryptophan, caffeine-containing beverages, and beer and wine.
- Report any symptoms such as severe headache or heart palpitations that may indicate a hypertensive crisis requiring immediate intervention.
- Avoid overactivity because these agents may suppress anginal pain, a warning of myocardial ischemia.
- Have vision checked periodically because optic toxicity may occur if therapy is administered over an extended period.
- Carry a MedicAlert card to inform emergency room staff about therapy with MAOIs.

Box 16-7 lists some important adverse reactions that may occur with antidepressants.

Sustained-Release, Parenteral, and Transdermal Antidepressants

Researchers have found that as many as 50% of clients discontinue taking their antidepressant medications before completing the recommended length of therapy. One of the most important factors cited for medication noncompliance is the inability to tolerate adverse effects such as drowsiness and fatigue, anxiety, headache, nausea, and sexual dysfunction. The need to take medication on a daily basis throughout long-term therapy and the desire to maintain confidentiality about their use of antidepressants were also considered to be contributing factors (Bowes, 2002).

As a result of several studies that focused on the role of medication tolerability in treatment adherence, drug companies have developed various formulations of antidepressants. Examples include orally disintegrating mirtazapine; sustained-release bupropion, methylphenidate hydrochloride, dextroamphetamine and amphetamine; enteric-coated or modified-release fluoxetine; extended-release venlafaxine and methylphenidate; and controlled-release paroxetine (Bowes, 2002; Karch, 2007; Sadock & Sadock, 2003).

Although intravenous clomipramine, imipramine, maprotiline, and citalopram have been widely used throughout Europe, only amitriptyline has been approved for use parenterally in the United States. Research findings indicate that the parenteral route is well tolerated, with no greater incidence of adverse effects than oral medication.

Parenteral administration includes the assurance of drug compliance, provides an option for clients who cannot tolerate oral medication, and is an alternative choice of treatment for severely ill, treatment-resistant clients before the use of electroconvulsive therapy.

BOX 16.7 MED ALERT: ANTIDEPRESSANTS

Assume that there is a potential for drug interactions when treating for depression. Dosages of antidepressants are reduced when given to children, adolescents, or the elderly. Nortriptyline, fluoxetine, and doxepin are available in liquid form. Fluoxetine is now available in a once-a-week dose. Imipramine-PM and amitriptyline are available for intramuscular injection. Uncommon, but potentially serious, adverse effects can occur during the administration of antidepressants. They include:

1. Onset of psychosis, possibly secondary to anticholinergic effects of TCAs
2. Confusional states secondary to anticholinergic effects of TCAs
3. Seizures due to lowering of the threshold as with the use of buproprion
4. Hyperpyretic crisis if TCA is given with fluoxetine
5. Paralytic ileus if TCA is given with an anticholinergic
6. Severe convulsions or death if TCA is given with an MAOI
7. Liver disorder due to trazodone
8. Focal necrotizing vasculitis due to fluoretine
9. Intraocular pressure increase with use of paroxetine
10. Severe hyponatremia linked to use of SSRIs.

Specific drug–drug interactions are listed at the discussion of each classification of antidepressant drugs in the text. The U.S. Government Printing Office released a medical alert (February 1995) stating severe CNS toxicity, hyperpyrexia, and death are recognized consequences when using Eldepryl concurrently with antidepressants (MAOIs, TCAs, and SSRIs).

Transdermal antidepressant therapy, a noninvasive and painless route of administration, requires no technical support, and may make the use of parenteral antidepressants more acceptable (Eakin, Detke, & Bodkin, 2001).

Stimulants as Mood Elevators

Stimulants or psychostimulants, also referred to as *mood elevators,* are used to potentiate antidepressant medications in treatment-resistant depression (ie, in clients who partially respond to antidepressants) and treatment-refractory depression (ie, in clients who do not respond to antidepressants). Research evidence has shown that certain clients may require more dopaminergic effects for therapeutic antidepressant treatment. Stimulants have also been proven effective in reducing depression in medically ill clients, post-stroke clients, and clients with acquired immunodeficiency syndrome (AIDS). Other uses of stimulants include the treatment of narcolepsy, attention-deficit hyperactivity disorder (ADHD) in children, residual ADHD in adults, and obesity (Sadock & Sadock, 2003).

Amphetamine stimulants cause a release of norepinephrine and dopamine into the synapse from the presynaptic nerve cell and block their reuptake. This action stimulates the sympathetic nervous system, resulting in alertness, wakefulness, vasoconstriction, suppressed appetite, and hypothermia. Methylphenidate (Concerta, Ritalin) produces a milder CNS response than amphetamine stimulants (Boyd, 2002).

As stated earlier in the chapter, stimulants can be used alone or in conjunction with antidepressant medication to enhance their therapeutic effects. They are also used in the treatment of narcolepsy, ADHD, and obesity. Daily dosages, included in Table 16-8, may vary depending upon the age of the client (ie, child, adolescent, adult, or geriatric client) and the rationale for treatment (eg, narcolepsy, depression, ADHD, obesity).

TABLE 16.8 Daily Dosage of Commonly Used Stimulants (Mood Elevators)

GENERIC NAME	TRADE NAME	DOSAGE RANGE (mg/day)
dexmethylphenidate HCL	Focalin	2.5–20 mg
dextroamphetamine	Dexedrine	5–60 mg
dextroamphetamine and amphetamine	Adderall	2.5–40 mg
methylphenidate	Ritalin	10–60 mg
methylphenidate HCL	Concerta	18–54 mg
methylphenidate HCL, USP	Metadate CD	20–60 mg
modafinil	Provigil	100–200 mg

Contraindications, Precautions, and Adverse Effects

The use of stimulants is contraindicated during or within 14 days of the administration of MAOIs. Stimulants are not prescribed in the presence of glaucoma, advanced arteriosclerosis, cardiovascular disease, moderate-to-severe hypertension, hyperthyroidism, marked anxiety or agitation, drug or alcohol abuse, or the history of tics or Tourette's syndrome. Stimulants have also been administered to persons with Tourette's syndrome and comorbid ADHD; however, the risks and benefits must be weighed before prescribing them for such clients (Sadock & Sadock, 2003).

Potential adverse effects are too numerous to list in detail; however, the most common adverse effects include appetite suppression and sleep disturbances (drowsiness or insomnia). Occasionally, GI disturbances, mild increases in pulse and blood pressure, and CNS overstimulation have been observed. Arrhythmias can occur with the use of amphetamine stimulants. Stimulant-associated toxic psychosis is rare.

Drug–drug interactions reported include hypertensive crisis when combined with MAOIs. Stimulants also are known to increase levels of anticonvulsants, anticoagulants, TCAs, and SSRIs.

Nursing Implications

When administering stimulants, adhere to the following:

1. Assess the client's blood pressure, pulse, weight, height, and sleep habits initially, then monitor during each visit.
2. Assess CNS activity (eg, abnormal body movements or changes in mental status), growth progression, and appetite of children and adolescent clients taking amphetamine stimulants.
3. Ensure that timed-release tablets are swallowed whole, not chewed or crushed.
4. Monitor CBC and platelet counts periodically in clients undergoing long-term therapy with methylphenidate.
5. Administer stimulants in the morning and then at noon. If it is necessary to give the second dosage of medication later in the day, it should be given no later than 6 PM to avoid insomnia.

Client Education

Teach clients who are receiving stimulants the following:

- Take the drug exactly as prescribed. Do not crush or chew sustained- or timed-release tablets. If the drug appears to be ineffective, notify your health care provider.
- Report any unusual clinical symptoms such as insomnia, abnormal body movements, palpitations, nervousness, vomiting, diarrhea, fever, skin rash, pale stools, or yellowing of the skin or eyes.
- Avoid the use of alcohol or OTC drugs including nose drops and cold remedies to avoid serious drug–drug interactions.
- Avoid pregnancy while taking stimulants because they may cause harm to the fetus.

Antimanic Agents or Mood Stabilizers

Antimanic agents, or mood stabilizers, refer to agents that prevent or diminish the frequency and intensity of manic behavior, mood swings, aggressive behavior, and dyscontrol syndrome. Lithium has long been considered the treatment of choice for the manic phase of bipolar disorder (formerly termed "manic-depressive illness"). It is also used in the treatment of major depressive disorder, schizoaffective disorder, therapy-resistant schizophrenia, and chronic aggression (Sadock & Sadock, 2003).

Research has shown at least three alternate treatment options, especially for those individuals with bipolar disorder who are unable to tolerate lithium salts. They include the use of anticonvulsants such as carbamazepine (Tegretol), carbamazepine extended-release (Equetro), gabapentin (Neurontin), lamotrigine (Lamictal), topiramate (Topamax), and valproate (Depakene); calcium channel antagonists such as norverapamil and nicardipine (Cardene); and antipsychotics such as aripiprazole (Abilify), olanzapine (Zyprexa), olanzapine/fluoxetine (Symbyax), risperidone (Risperdal), and ziprasidone (Geodon). This section of the chapter, however, focuses on the use of lithium salts. Anticonvulsants are discussed in the next section.

The leading current theory hypothesizes that lithium's antidepressant effects result from the augmentation of serotonin function in the CNS. Lithium is thought to balance serotonergic neurotransmission, preventing a decreased activity of nerve impulses that causes depression and preventing an increased activity of nerve impulses that causes mania. In clients exhibiting the manic phase of bipolar disorder, lithium appears to enhance the thyrotropin-releasing hormone–stimulated prolactin response and reduce dopamine transmission.

The body does not metabolize lithium. It is completely absorbed by the GI tract. It does not bind to plasma proteins, is not metabolized, and is distributed nonuniformly throughout body water. Approximately 80% of a lithium dose is reabsorbed in the proximal renal tubules and excreted by the kidneys. The lithium ion, similar to the sodium ion, is thought to maintain a constant sodium concentration in the brain, regulating mood swings as well as impulses traveling along nerve cells. Since lithium behaves as a salt in the body, sodium intake by the client must remain relatively stable during treatment; otherwise, lithium levels will be altered and toxicity or lower-than-therapeutic levels can occur (Sadock & Sadock, 2003).

Contraindications, Precautions, and Adverse Effects

Lithium should not be prescribed during pregnancy or in the presence of severely impaired kidney function. Caution should be used when prescribing lithium for clients who have heart disease; perspire profusely; are on a sodium-restricted diet; are hypotensive; have epilepsy, parkinsonism, or other CNS disorders; or are dehydrated. Serum lithium concentrations may increase in the presence of extreme vomiting, diarrhea, or perspiration, resulting in lithium toxicity.

Common adverse effects include nausea, metallic taste, abdominal discomfort, polydipsia, polyuria, muscle weakness, fine hand tremors, fatigue, and mild diarrhea, as well as edema of the feet, hands, abdominal wall, or face. These effects may occur as early as 2 hours after the first dose is taken. Leukocytosis is a common benign effect of lithium treatment (Sadock & Sadock, 2003.)

Lithium toxicity occurs when serum lithium levels exceed 1.5 to 2.0 mEq/L. Signs and symptoms include drowsiness, slurred speech, muscle spasms, blurred vision, diarrhea, dizziness, stupor, convulsions, and coma. Death has occurred as a result of lithium toxicity.

Nursing Implications

Before beginning therapy with lithium, the client undergoes a complete physical examination including laboratory tests and an ECG to obtain baseline information and to rule out any cardiac, thyroid, hepatic, or renal abnormalities. When administering lithium therapy, be sure to include the following:

1. Give the prescribed drug during or after meals to decrease gastric irritation.
2. Monitor serum lithium levels at least twice a week during the initiation of therapy before stabilization of manic episode. After stabilization, expect to monitor levels every month.
3. Obtain serum samples 12 hours after a lithium dose is administered. The desired levels should reach 1.0 to 1.5 mEq/L.
4. Observe clients for decreases in manic behavior and mood swings; adverse effects; and drug interactions.
5. Recognize that diuretics and anti-inflammatory agents such as indomethacin increase the effects of lithium; that acetazolamide, sodium bicarbonate, excessive amounts of sodium chloride, drugs with high sodium content, and theophylline compounds decrease lithium's effects.
6. To avoid lithium toxicity, obtain electrolyte levels, a thyroid profile, and a liver profile routinely as ordered depending upon the established protocol.

Client Education

Instruct clients receiving lithium therapy to do the following:

- Take the drug exactly as directed. (See Table 16-9 for daily dosage of lithium salts.)
- Do not alter the dosage or cease taking the prescribed drug. Be aware that lithium may require 3 to 5 weeks to be effective.
- Do not decrease dietary salt intake unless instructed to do so by a physician because it increases the risk of adverse effects, including toxicity, due to increased concentration of lithium. Similarly, increased salt intake will lower lithium concentration and may induce symptoms of hypomania or mania.
- Maintain a high intake of fluids (8–10 glasses daily) unless contraindicated because of a physical disorder. Decreases in body fluid intake can lead to dehydration and lithium toxicity.

TABLE 16.9 Daily Dosage of Lithium Salts (Mood Stabilizers)

GENERIC NAME	TRADE NAME	DOSAGE RANGE (mg/day)
lithium carbonate	Eskalith Lithonate Lithobid Lithotabs Eskalith CR	900–1800 mg in divided doses until serum levels reach 1.0–1.5 mEq/L
lithium citrate	Cibalith-S	Begin with 300 mg b.i.d. and gradually increase by 300-mg increments to achieve desired serum lithium level

- Avoid crash or fad diets.
- Avoid excessive exercise in warm weather. Excessive perspiration increases the risk of adverse effects.
- Have blood lithium levels monitored regularly. Blood samples should be taken 12 hours after the previous dose of lithium; therefore, do not take the morning dose until the serum sample has been taken. Keep in mind that other laboratory tests, including blood urea nitrogen, thyroid profile, electrolyte levels, and liver profile, are monitored to avoid adverse effects.
- Avoid taking other medications without a physician's knowledge because these may increase or decrease the effects of lithium.
- Report any unusual symptoms, illnesses, or loss of appetite immediately to a physician.
- Continue to take the drug despite an occasional relapse. Some clients respond slowly to lithium therapy.
- Notify a doctor whenever a change in diet occurs because this may affect the lithium level.
- Do not breast-feed while taking lithium.
- Schedule an annual physical examination.
- Carry a MedicAlert card or wear a MedicAlert bracelet.

Anticonvulsants

Anticonvulsant drugs are used to treat seizure disorders, which are not uncommon among individuals with psychiatric disorders. They may be used to control seizure activity, such as that associated with petit mal (absence), grand mal (tonic–clonic), psychomotor, akinetic and myoclonic, or focal epileptic seizures, or seizures associated with neurosurgery (Bristol-Myers Squibb, 1996). Anticonvulsants are also used to reduce seizure-induced aggressive behavior, and they may have the same effect on persons who exhibit aggressive behavior but do not have epilepsy. Anticonvulsants may be used alone or in combination with an antipsychotic drug to reduce episodes of violent behavior in clients with the diagnosis of schizophrenia. Divalproex (Depakote) and gabapentin (Neurontin) are standard treatment for the manic phase of bipolar disorder. Individuals experiencing acute substance abuse withdrawal may be given sedatives and anticonvulsant medications to prevent or treat seizures and delirium tremens. Other examples of the use of anticonvulsant therapy include treatment of clients with delirium and dementia associated with Axis III physical disorders or conditions such as brain tumor, history of head injury, explosive personality disorder, or epilepsy (Sadock & Sadock, 2003).

Several chemical classifications of anticonvulsants may be used: long-acting barbiturates, benzodiazepines, hydantoins, and succinimides. The newer anticonvulsant agents, such as gabapentin (Neurontin), lamotri-

SELF-AWARENESS PROMPT

Examine your attitude about the use of psychotropic drugs to stabilize clinical symptoms of psychiatric disorders. How would you feel about medicating a child or an older adult? What biases, if any, would come into play? How would you feel about medicating a client in your age group? If your answer to either of these questions reveals discomfort on your part, what measures can be taken to change your attitude or discomfort?

gine (Lamictal), oxcarbazepine (Trileptal), and topiramate (Topamax), are structurally diverse and have multiple CNS effects. They differ in metabolism, drug interactions, and adverse effects. None of them has an identical combination of neurochemical actions (Sadock & Sadock, 2003).

Because of their divergent mechanisms of action, each anticonvulsant may have a unique therapeutic profile outside of epilepsy. Neurotransmitter release from presynaptic nerve terminals is linked to voltage-sensitive sodium channels (VSSCs), voltage-sensitive calcium channels (VSCCs), or the gamma-aminobutyric reuptake pump. Anticonvulsants may bind to VSSC, VSCC, or GABA A receptors to modulate or reduce the release of neurotransmitters. As a result of this activity, some anticonvulsants are effective in the treatment of bipolar disorder, schizophrenia, chronic pain, agitation, aggressive behavior, anxiety disorder, and substance abuse (Grady, 2005; Maxmen, Dubovsky, & Ward, 2002; Sadock & Sadock, 2003). Commonly used anticonvulsants include carbamazepine (Tegretol), clonazepam (Klonopin), gabapentin (Neurontin), lamotrigine (Lamictal), phenytoin (Dilantin), primidone (Mysoline), topiramate (Topamax), and valproic acid (Depakene). Pregabalin (Lyrica) is a new anticonvulsant that is FDA approved to treat diabetic peripheral neuropathy and postherpetic neuralgia as well as seizure activity.

Contraindications, Precautions, and Adverse Effects

Anticonvulsants are contraindicated or must be used cautiously in clients with CNS depression. The presence of hepatic or renal damage, liver disease, or bone marrow depression prohibits the use of anticonvulsants. Increased incidence of birth defects may occur if anticonvulsants are used during pregnancy. Women who are breast-feeding should not take anticonvulsants.

Common adverse effects include dizziness, blurred vision, sedation, and GI upset. Ataxia also may occur. CNS depression increases if alcohol is used during treatment with anticonvulsant medication. The effectiveness of oral contraception is decreased when topiramate is used. The development of a rash while taking lamotrigine could prove to be life threatening (Karch, 2007).

Nursing Implications

When administering anticonvulsant drug therapy, be sure to include the following:

1. Administer the drug on a regular schedule to maintain therapeutic blood levels.
2. Administer oral anticonvulsant drugs with meals or fluid to reduce gastric irritation and decrease adverse GI effects. Anticipate giving ranitidine (Zantac) as ordered to eliminate gastric irritation.
3. Observe for therapeutic effects, which occur approximately 7 to 10 days after drug therapy is started.
4. Monitor for adverse effects including CNS changes (eg, drowsiness, sedation, ataxia), GI irritation, skin disorders, blood dyscrasias, respiratory depression, liver damage, gingival hyperplasia, hypocalcemia, and lymphadenopathy.
5. Observe for drug interactions, such as decreased effects of oral anticoagulants, corticosteroids, beta adrenergic blockers, and theophylline; increased hepatotoxicity with acetaminophen; and increased sedation when administered with other CNS depressants.
6. Arrange for laboratory testing to monitor the client's liver function, blood count including platelets, and serum drug levels (Karch, 2007; Abrams, 2007).

Client Education

Instruct clients receiving anticonvulsant drug therapy to do the following:

- Inform the health care provider of any known physical illnesses or pregnancy, and about any medication or OTC drugs presently being used.
- Take medication exactly as prescribed with food or glass of fluid at the same time each day. (See Table 16-10 for the daily dosage of commonly used anticonvulsants.)
- Avoid drinking grapefruit juice if taking carbamazepine because it interferes with metabolism of the drug and may cause a fatal reaction.
- Avoid the use of antacids because they reduce the serum level of anticonvulsant medication.
- Ask for the same brand and form of drug when renewing prescriptions.
- Follow directions when taking a liquid preparation of phenytoin.
- Report any unusual or adverse effects to the health care provider.
- Refrain from driving or operating heavy machinery if drowsiness occurs.
- Wear a MedicAlert bracelet stating the use of anticonvulsants.

TABLE 16.10   Daily Dosage of Commonly Used Anticonvulsants

GENERIC NAME	TRADE NAME	DOSAGE RANGE (MG/DAY)
carbamazepine	Tegretol	600–1200 mg
clonazepam	Klonopin	1.5–20 mg
ethosuximide	Zarontin	500–1500 mg
gabapentin	Neurontin	300–2400 mg
lamotrigine	Lamictal	25–500 mg
oxcarbazepine	Trileptal	300–1200 mg
phenytoin	Dilantin	300–625 mg
pregabalin	Lyrica	150–600 mg
primidone	Mysoline	500–2000 mg
topiramate	Topamax	25–400 mg
valproate	Depakote	500–1500 mg
sodium valproate	Epival in Canada	
valproic acid	Depakene	500–1500 mg

Antiparkinsonism Agents

Antiparkinsonism agents have been used to treat *medication-induced movement disorders*, such as neuroleptic-induced parkinsonism. Antiparkinsonism agents include anticholinergic agents, some antihistaminergic agents, and dopaminergic agonists and precursors (such as levodopa, a natural precursor of dopamine). (A similar term, *antiparkinsonian agent*, refers to the use of these agents in the treatment of *Parkinson's disease.*) Anticholinergic agents (eg, benztropine [Cogentin], biperiden [Akineton]) block the action of acetylcholine receptors in the brain and peripheral nervous system in an attempt to correct an imbalance between a deficiency of dopamine and an abundance of acetylcholine. Anticholinergics decrease salivation, spasticity, and tremors in persons who have minimal symptoms or cannot tolerate levodopa. Their primary use in clinical psychiatry is the treatment of medication-induced movement disorders, neuroleptic-induced dystonia, and medication-induced postural tremor. Anticholinergic agents are also of limited use in the treatment of neuroleptic-induced akathisia (Sadock & Sadock, 2003).

Certain antihistaminergic agents (eg, diphenhydramine [Benadryl] and orphenadrine [Norflex]) are used in clinical psychiatry to treat neuroleptic-induced parkinsonism, neuroleptic-induced acute dystonia, and neuroleptic-induced akathisia. Antihistaminics also function as hypnotics and anxiolytics. They act by competitively antagonizing histamine at the H_1 histamine receptor. They do not block the release of histamine, but rather antagonize most of its effects (Sadock & Sadock, 2003; Stanilla & Simpson, 1995).

Dopaminergic agonists (eg, amantadine [Symmetrel]) and precursors (eg, levodopa [Dopar, Larodopa]) increase the release of dopamine in the nigrostriatal pathway for clients with parkinsonism, thereby helping to relieve their symptoms (Karch, 2007; Sadock & Sadock, 2003; Stanilla & Simpson, 1995). These agents, along with other agents such as propranolol (Inderal), clonidine (Catapres), clonazepam (Klonopin), and lorazepam (Ativan), are the drugs of choice for treating extrapyramidal disorders and idiopathic or postencephalitic Parkinson's disease.

Contraindications, Precautions, and Adverse Effects

Drugs with anticholinergic and antihistaminergic effects, such as benztropine (Cogentin), biperiden, trihexyphenidyl (Artane), and diphenhydramine (Benadryl), which are used to alleviate acute EPS, are contraindicated in clients with glaucoma, myasthenia gravis, GI obstruction, prostatic hypertrophy, and urinary bladder neck obstruction. These drugs must be used with caution in clients exhibiting symptoms related to cardiovascular disorders.

Dopaminergic agents, such as carbidopa and levodopa (Sinemet), bromocriptine (Parlodel), levodopa (Dopar), pramipexole (Mirapex), pergolide (Trental), and ropinirole (Requip), are contraindicated in the presence of known hypersensitivity to specific drugs; in concomitant use with MAOIs, meperidine (Demerol), and other opioids; and in the presence of uncontrolled hypertension, narrow-angle glaucoma, or breast-feeding (Sadock & Sadock, 2003).

Nursing Implications

When administering antiparkinsonism agents, include the following actions:

1. Administer the agent (except levodopa) with or immediately after food intake to prevent or reduce GI distress.
2. Recognize that a form of carbidopa/levodopa (Parcopa) is available as an orally disintegrating tablet for clients who have difficulty swallowing, or holding a glass of water.
3. Observe for therapeutic effects such as decreased salivation, tremor, and drooling (anticholinergic effects).
4. Observe for improvement in gait, balance, posture, speech, and self-care ability.
5. Monitor for adverse effects of anticholinergic agents such as dry mouth, drowsiness, constipation, and urinary retention.
6. Monitor for adverse effects to antiparkinsonism agents such as psychosis, depression, hallucinations, insomnia, and irritability (Karch, 2007; Abrams, 2007).

Client Education

As is true with other types of drug therapy, the client receiving medication to lessen or reverse EPS of psychotropic drugs needs instructions about following the physician's prescribed dosage (Table 16-11).

Additional instructions for the client and family members include the following:

- Maintain an adequate amount of fluid intake (2000–3000 cc daily unless contraindicated) to prevent excessive dryness of the mouth. Take medication just before meals, chew gum, or suck on hard candies to help alleviate this adverse effect.
- Avoid operating potentially hazardous machinery or driving an automobile if symptoms of blurred vision or drowsiness occur.

TABLE 16.11 Daily Dosage of Commonly Used Antiparkinsonism Agents

GENERIC NAME	TRADE NAME	DOSAGE RANGE (mg/day)
amantadine	Symmetrel	100–300 mg
benztropine	Cogentin	0.5–6 mg
biperiden	Akineton	2–16 mg
bromocriptine	Parlodel	2.5–100 mg
carbidopa/ levodopa	Sinemet	Varies per individual
diphenhydramine	Benadryl	25–200 mg
entacapone	Comtan	200–1600 mg
levodopa	Larodopa or Dopar	1000–8000 mg
pergolide	Permax	0.05–5 mg
pramipexole	Mirapex	0.375–4.5 mg
procyclidine	Kemadrin	10–20 mg
ropinirole	Requip	0.75–24 mg
selegiline	Eldepryl	5–10 mg
tolcapone	Tasmar	300–600 mg
trihexyphenidyl	Artane	2–15 mg

- Report any adverse effects or unusual symptoms to the health care provider.
- Use caution when rising from a sitting or reclining position because of the possibility of postural hypotension and drowsiness.
- Limit strenuous activities in hot weather because anticholinergic drugs may cause anhidrosis (the inability to sweat).
- Have routine vision examinations to reduce the risk of glaucoma.
- Limit use of alcohol, high-protein foods, and vitamin B_6 because they decrease the therapeutic effects of levodopa.

SELF-AWARENESS PROMPT

Review Box 16-1 regarding psychopharmacologic guidelines and medicating the client. Are the guidelines helpful? Do you feel adequately prepared to administer prescribed psychotropic drugs? Please explain your answers.

KEY CONCEPTS

◆ The last few decades have seen an explosion in the amount of data concerning the molecular biology of neurotransmission, broadening our understanding of the science of psychopharmacology.

◆ The importance of drug polymorphism has been researched as clinicians have become more culturally competent in the treatment of psychiatric disorders.

◆ Guidelines have been published regarding the use of psychotropic medications to treat psychiatric disorders in the psychiatric setting.

◆ Antipsychotic agents that produce significant neurologic adverse effects have been referred to as neuroleptics (typical or conventional antipsychotics). New-generation antipsychotic agents (referred to as atypical antipsychotics) act to stabilize positive and negative symptoms and produce fewer adverse motor effects than neuroleptic agents.

◆ Antianxiety agents and hypnotics are central nervous system depressants that share many characteristics, including the ability to reduce anxiety and promote sleep.

◆ Antianxiety agents (anxiolytics) include several drug classifications, including benzodiazepines, non-benzodiazepines, antihistamines, beta blockers, certain selective serotonin reuptake inhibitors, and atypical antidepressants. Research has shown that some of the newer drugs are successful in the treatment of both anxiety and depression.

◆ Drug companies have developed various formulations of antianxiety agents (eg, wafer form, sublingual, orally disintegrating) to enhance medication tolerability and facilitate compliance.

◆ Hypnotic agents are used to induce a state of natural sleep, reduce periods of involuntary awakenings during the night, and increase total sleep time.

◆ Antidepressants include selective serotonin reuptake inhibitors, tricyclic antidepressants, atypical antidepressants, and monoamine oxidase inhibitors.

◆ Drug companies have developed various formulations of antidepressants (eg, sustained-release, parenteral, transdermal, orally disintegrating) to enhance medication tolerability and facilitate compliance.

◆ Stimulants (also referred to as psychostimulants or mood elevators) are used to potentiate the effects of antidepressant medication, although they are also used to treat narcolepsy, ADHD, and obesity.

◆ Although lithium has long been considered the treatment of choice for the manic phase of bipolar disorder, research has shown that certain anticonvulsants and atypical antipsychotics are also effective. These alternative drugs are valuable in the treatment of clients who cannot tolerate lithium salts.

◆ Anticonvulsants are effective in the treatment of seizure disorders, which are common among clients with psychiatric disorders. They are also used to treat symptoms of bipolar disorder, agitation, aggressive behavior, anxiety disorder, pain, and substance abuse.

◆ Antiparkinsonism agents are used to treat medication-induced movement disorders, neuroleptic-induced dystonia, and medication-induced postural tremor as well as idiopathic or postencephalitic Parkinson's disease.

For additional study materials, please refer to the Student Resource CD-ROM located in the back of this textbook.

 CHAPTER WORKSHEET

CRITICAL THINKING QUESTIONS

1. Research and create a lesson plan to teach clients and families about antipsychotic agents. Collaborate with a pharmacy student, and team-teach this material to an appropriate group. How does the pharmacy student's focus differ from yours? What are the strengths you bring to this process, and what are the pharmacy student's?

2. Monoamine oxidase inhibitors (MAOIs) present unique problems for the clients taking them. What member of the health care team would be of great assistance to you as you prepare client education materials for this group of drugs? Why?

3. We know that medications alleviate symptoms and it is necessary for them to be taken to do so. Yet, in many of our large cities, homeless people with mental illness roam the streets with symptoms raging, medications forgotten. What might be done about this problem? What would you envision as the nurse's role in this community mental health issue?

REFLECTION

Reflect on the chapter opening quote by Sadock and Sadock. Explain how the use of drugs provides a foundation for a successful treatment approach for a specific disorder, such as depression. What information could you provide to a client who is resistant to trying a psychotropic drug? How would you present the information? Would you include any other staff members in the presentation? If so, who and why?

NCLEX-STYLE QUESTIONS

1. When administering the neuroleptic haloperidol (Haldol) to a client, the nurse understands that it is decreasing the amounts of which neurotransmitter?
   a. Acetylcholine
   b. Dopamine
   c. Serotonin
   d. Histamine

2. For the client receiving the antipsychotic medication clozapine (Clozaril), which laboratory study would be most important for the nurse to monitor?
   a. Complete blood count
   b. Liver function study
   c. Thyroid profile
   d. Renal function study

3. A client receiving the neuroleptic medication chlorpromazine (Thorazine) exhibits excessive drooling and fine hand tremors. Which medication would the nurse expect the physician to order?
   a. Benztropine (Cogentin)
   b. Acetaminophen (Tylenol)
   c. Lorazepam (Ativan)
   d. Naproxen (Aleve)

4. The nurse instructs a client receiving the MAOI agent phenelzine (Nardil) about dietary restrictions for foods high in tyramine to prevent which adverse effect?
   a. Gastrointestinal upset
   b. Hypertensive crisis
   c. Neuromuscular effects
   d. Urinary retention

5. The nurse advises the client taking lithium carbonate to do which of the following to prevent toxic effects of lithium?
   a. Maintain adequate sodium and water intake.
   b. Avoid foods high in tyramine.
   c. Establish a schedule for regular sleep.
   d. Monitor for increased temperature.

6. Two days ago, a client stopped taking his prescribed paroxetine (Paxil). Which of the following would lead the nurse to suspect that a client is experiencing serotonin discontinuation syndrome? Select all that apply.
   a. Agitation
   b. Dizziness
   c. Paresthesia
   d. Headache
   e. Nightmares
   f. Ataxia

Selected References

Abrams, A. C. (2007). *Clinical drug therapy: Rationales for nursing practice* (8th ed.). Philadelphia: Lippincott Williams & Wilkins

Ahmed, D. S., & Fecik, S. (2000). MAOIs: Still here, still dangerous. *American Journal of Nursing, 100*(2), 29–30.

American Diabetes Association, American Psychiatric Association, American Association of Clinical Endocrinologists, & North American Association for the Study of Obesity. (2004). Consensus development conference on antipsychotic drugs and obesity and diabetes. *Diabetes Care, 27*, 596–601.

Bernstein, J. G. (1998). *Handbook of drug therapy in psychiatry* (2nd ed.). Littleton, CO: PSG Publishing.

Bowes, M. (2002, July/August). Advances in medicine: New sustained-release formulations of antidepressant medications. *Geriatric Times, 3* (Suppl. 4).

Boyd, M. A. (2002). *Psychiatric nursing: Contemporary practice* (2nd ed.). Philadelphia: Lippincott Williams & Wilkins.

Bristol-Myers Squibb. (1996). *Guide to psychotropic agents*. Secaucus, NJ: Pocket Prescribing.

Cole, J. O., & Yonkers, K. A. (1995). Nonbenzodiazepine anxiolytics. In A. F. Schatzberg & C. B. Nemeroff (Eds.), *Textbook of psychopharmacology* (pp. 231–246). Washington, DC: American Psychiatric Press.

Deitch, M. (2003). Drug interactions. *ADVANCE for Nurses, 4*(23), 17–18, 24.

DeMott, K. (1999). Ethnicity can influence psychotropic effectiveness. *Clinical Psychiatry News, 27*(10), 13.

Eakin, M. C., Detke, M. J., & Bodkin, J. A. (2001). Psychopharmacology update: Parenteral antidepressants: Is America ready? *Psychiatric Times, 18*(5), 25–30.

Foley, K., & Reis, A. (2004). Vital signs: Nearly half of patients oppose off-label prescribing. *Clinical Psychiatry News, 32* (12), 1.

Gerson, L., & Margolis, S. (2004). Nursing strategies for the prevention and management of antipsychotic-induced metabolic abnormalities. *Advanced Studies in Nursing, 2*(3), 79–80.

Grady, M. M. (2005, January). Anticonvulsants in psychiatry. *Psychopharmacology Educational Update: Supplement to Clinical Psychiatry News, 1*(1), 3.

Herman, L. (1998). Clinical challenge: One man in a million. *Clinical Advisor, 1*(10), 18–23.

Hospitalist. Net. (2005). Cytochrome p450 drug metabolism and interactions. Retrieved September 12, 2005, from http://www.hospitalist.net/highligh.htm

Karch, A. M. (2007). *2007 Lippincott's nursing drug guide.* Philadelphia: Lippincott Williams & Wilkins.

Khan, A. U. (1999). How do psychotropic medications really work? *Psychiatric Times, 16*(10), 12–20.

Koller, W., & Cho, C. (2004). Tardive dystonia following antipsychotic treatment. *Medscape Neurology & Neurosurgery, 6*(2). Retrieved October 14, 2004, from http://www.medscape.com/viewarticle/489669

Kramer, S. I., & McCall, W. V. (2006). Off-label prescribing: 7 steps for safer, more effective treatment. *Current Psychiatry, 5*(4), 14–16, 21–22, 26–28.

Krupnick, S. L. W. (1996). General nursing roles in psychopharmacology. In S. Lego (Ed.), *Psychiatric nursing: A comprehensive reference* (2nd ed., pp. 499–514). Philadelphia: Lippincott-Raven Publishers.

Kudzma, E. C. (1999). Culturally competent drug administration. *American Journal of Nursing, 99*(8), 46–51.

Lantz, M. S. (2001). Serotonin syndrome: A common but often unrecognized psychiatric condition. *Geriatrics, 56*(1), 52–53.

Littrell, K. H. (2004). Current developments in the pharmacologic treatment of psychosis. *Advanced Studies in Nursing, 2*(1), 9–14.

Marder, S. R., & Van Putten, T. (1995). Antipsychotic medications. In A. F. Schatzberg & C. B. Nemeroff (Eds.), *Textbook of psychopharmacology* (pp. 247–262). Washington, DC: American Psychiatric Press.

Maxmen, J. S., Dubovsky, S. L., & Ward, G. W. (2002). *Psychotropic drugs fast facts* (3rd ed.). New York: W. W. Norton.

Moen, J. C. (2002). Woman with uncontrollable leg movement. *Clinician Reviews, 12*(5), 75–78, 81.

Moon, M. A. (2004). SSRI-induced hyponatremia underrecognized. *Clinical Psychiatry News, 32*(3), 58.

Mrazek, D. A. (2005). Pharmacogenomic DNA chip: Test anticipates adverse response to medication. *Current Psychiatry, 4*(7), 67, 71–73.

Murphy, J. L. (Ed.). (2005). *Nurse practitioners' prescribing reference.* New York, NY: Prescribing References.

National Sleep Foundation. (2002). 2002 Sleep in America poll. Retrieved September 4, 2006, from http://www.sleepfoundation.org/hottpics/index.php?secid=16&id=208

Peterson, A. M. (2001). Depressive disorders. In V. P. Arcangelo & A. M. Peterson (Eds.), *Pharmacotherapeutics for advanced practice: A practical approach* (pp. 591–602). Philadelphia: Lippincott Williams & Wilkins.

Pincus, H. A., Zarin, D. A., Tanielian, T. L., Johnson, J. L., West, J. C., Pettit, A. R., et al. (1999). Psychiatric patients and treatments in 1997. *Archives of General Psychiatry, 56*(5), 441–449.

Puzantian, T., & Stimmel, G. L. (2001). Review of psychotropic drugs. *CNS News, 3*(4), 27–31.

Ramaswamy, S., Malik, S., & Dewan, V. (2005). Tips to manage and prevent discontinuation syndromes. *Current Psychiatry, 4*(9), 29–30, 37–39, 43–44.

Sadock, B. J., & Sadock, V. A. (2003). *Kaplan & Sadock's synopsis of psychiatry: Behavioral sciences/clinical psychiatry* (9th ed.). Philadelphia: Lippincott Williams & Wilkins.

Sherman, C. (1999). Discontinuation symptoms tied to SSRI's half-life. *Clinical Psychiatry News, 27*(10), 1–2.

Sherman, C. (2005). Factor ethnicity into drug treatment—Part 2. *Clinical Psychiatry News, 33*(8), 42.

Shahrokh, N., & Hales, R. E. (Eds.) (2003). *American psychiatric glossary* (8th ed.). Washington, DC: American Psychiatric Press.

Stanilla, J. K., & Simpson, G. M. (1995). Drugs to treat extrapyramidal adverse effects. In A. F. Schatzberg & C. B. Nemeroff (Eds.), *Textbook of psychopharmacology* (pp. 281–299). Washington, DC: American Psychiatric Press.

Stimmel, G. L. (1999). Future directions in the treatment of insomnia. *Psychiatric Times' Monograph, 16*(5), 1–8.

TheFreeDictionary.Com. (2005a). Pharmacodynamics. Retrieved September 13, 2005, from http://encyclopedia.thefreedictionary.com/Pharmacodynamics?p

TheFreeDictionary.Com. (2005b). Pharmacokinetics. Retrieved September 13, 2005, from http://encyclopedia.thefreedictionary.com/Pharmacokinetics?p

Wilcox, R. E., & Gonzales, R. A. (1998). Introduction to neurotransmitters, receptors, signal transduction, and second messengers. In A. F. Schatzberg & C. B. Nemeroff (Eds.), *Textbook of psychopharmacology* (pp. 3–30). Washington, DC: American Psychiatric Press.

Zoler, M. L. (2004). Antidepressants may need 8 weeks to take effect. *Clinical Psychiatry News, 32*(9), 29.

Suggested Readings

Ayd, F. J., Jr. (2000). Evaluating interactions between herbal and psychoactive medications. *Psychiatric Times, 17*(12), 45–47.

Cheng, G. S. (2000). Drug interactions can mar depression tx in the medically ill. *Clinical Psychiatry News, 28*(2), 10.

Fink, M. (1999). Neuroleptic malignant syndrome: Recognition and treatment. *Psychiatric Times, 16*(8), 6.

Fink, M. (2000). Neuroleptic malignant syndrome best treated as catatonia. *Psychiatric Times, 17*(11), 28–29.

Higgins, B. C. (1999). Prochlorperazine-induced dystonia. *American Journal of Nursing, 99*(11), 34.

Jefferson, J. W. (2001). So you thought you knew everything about lithium use in the elderly. *Geriatric Times, 2*(1), 28.

Lauriello, J., & Keith, S. M. (2005). Using IM antipsychotics: Lessons from clinical practice. *Current Psychiatry, 4*(4), 44-46, 51-53.

Leo, R. J. (2001). Movement disturbances associated with SSRIs. *Psychiatric Times, 18*(5), 33-36.

Munoz, C., & Hilgenberg, C. (2005). Ethnopharmacology: Understanding how ethnicity can affect drug response is essential to providing culturally competent care. *American Journal of Nursing, 105*(8), 40-48.

Petit, J. M., & Reynolds, N. C. (2004). Adult-onset focal dystonia: Overview of diagnosis and management. *American Journal of Nurse Practitioners, 8*(11), 45-47, 49-52, 55-57.

Prows, C. A., & Prows, D. R. (2004). Medication selection by genotype. *American Journal of Nursing, 104*(5), 60-70.

Ramadan, M. I., Werder, S. F., & Preskorn, S. H. (2005). Drug-drug interactions: Avoid serious adverse events with mood stabilizers. *Current Psychiatry, 4*(5), 27-29, 33-34, 39-40.

Rose, L. E. (2004). New frontiers in the pharmacotherapy of psychosis: Treating the spectrum of psychotic disorders. *Advanced Studies in Nursing, 2*(1), 7-8.

Sherman, C. (2000). Cultural, genetic factors influence drug response. *Clinical Psychiatry News, 28*(10), 14.

Sherman, C. (2005a). Factor ethnicity into drug treatment—Part 1. *Clinical Psychiatry News, 33*(7), 31.

Sherman, C. (2005b). Patches and sprays are coming to psychiatry. *Clinical Psychiatry News, 33*(7), 27.

Strong, M. J. (2004). Impact of safety and tolerability on treatment outcomes and overall patient health. *Advanced Studies in Nursing, 2*(1), 16-22.

ECT is the most effective and rapidly acting treatment for major depressive disorder and plays an important role in the treatment of geriatric patients, but its use is limited by cognitive and other side effects. —LISANBY, 2006

Despite studies proving efficacy, it [ECT] remains the most controversial treatment in psychiatry. —HALL & BENSING, 2005

LEARNING OBJECTIVES

AFTER STUDYING THIS CHAPTER, YOU SHOULD BE ABLE TO:

1. Compare and contrast the rationale for the use of *electroconvulsive therapy* (ECT), *vagus nerve stimulation* (VNS), *transcranial magnetic stimulation* (TMS), and *magnetic seizure therapy* (MST).
2. Explain the ECT procedure.
3. Identify the indications for using ECT.
4. Explain the conditions associated with increased risk during ECT.
5. Recognize the presence of ECT adverse effects.
6. Describe advances in ECT.
7. Formulate nursing interventions to prepare a client for ECT.

KEY TERMS

Clitoridectomy
Electroconvulsive therapy (ECT)
Electronarcosis
Insulin shock therapy
Lobotomy
Magnetic seizure therapy (MST)
Physiotherapy
Postictal agitation
Psychosurgery
Somatic therapy
Sterilization
Transcranial magnetic stimulation (TMS)
Vagus nerve stimulation (VNS)

The biologic treatment of mental disorders is referred to as **somatic therapy.** In the early 20th century, various somatic procedures, such as lobotomy, sterilization, clitoridectomy, and insulin shock therapy, were performed to treat the mentally ill client. Physiotherapy, a noninvasive procedure, is another type of somatic therapy that was utilized in the psychiatric clinical setting.

Although the potential for major physiologic complications and death existed, physicians performed these techniques in an attempt to minimize disordered behavior by locating their perceived origins in the body (Ginther, 1998).

Lobotomy, also called **psychosurgery,** is a surgical intervention that originated in 1936. This invasive surgery severs fibers connecting one part of the brain with another, or removes or destroys brain tissue. It is designed to affect the client's psychological state, including modification of disturbed behavior, thought content, or mood. Currently, prefrontal lobotomy and transorbital lobotomy are two types of psychosurgery still used in research and treatment centers for clients with chronic disorders and those who have not responded to other recommended approaches.

Sterilization, ligation of the fallopian tubes in a woman and excision of a part of the vas deferens in a man, and **clitoridectomy,** surgical removal of part of the clitoris, were invasive procedures performed predominantly on female clients who exhibited "inappropriate" or aggressive sexual behavior.

Manfred Sakel, who believed that nervous hyperactivity occurring in morphine withdrawal was caused by an excess of epinephrine, developed **insulin shock therapy** in 1928. He postulated that this therapy, which uses large doses of insulin to decrease glucose levels to induce hypoglycemia or insulin coma, would also depress the levels of excess epinephrine and stabilize the hyperactivity. Sakel then expanded his theory to include the treatment of excitation exhibited by clients with the diagnosis of schizophrenia. The use of insulin shock therapy rapidly declined in the 1970s and has since been replaced by clinical psychopharmacology and psychotherapy (Sadock & Sadock, 2003).

Physiotherapy is the application of hydrotherapy and massages to induce relaxation in clients. The effects are short lasting, and the treatments produce few adverse effects if any. In the past, hydrotherapy by the application of wet packs and cold sheets was used to treat agitation and depression. Clients were also placed in tubs of hot or cold water to induce relaxation and decrease agitation. A partial tub cover served as a restraint when the client sat or reclined in the tub. Present-day hydrotherapy includes the use of hot baths, whirlpool baths, showers, and swimming pools.

Present-day somatic therapies include clinical psychopharmacology (see discussion in Chapter 16), phototherapy (see discussion in Chapter 21), electroconvulsive therapy (ECT), and vagus nerve stimulation (VNS). Two investigational therapies that are considered an alternative to ECT are transcranial magnetic stimulation (TMS) and magnetic seizure therapy (MST). This chapter focuses on the history of ECT, use of ECT in the psychiatric clinical setting, including a description of the procedure, indications and conditions associated with increased risk during its use, adverse effects, advances in the technique, guidelines for ECT, and nursing interventions. A discussion of VNS, TMS, and MST is also included.

History of Electroconvulsive Therapy

Hall and Bensing (2005), Fink (2004), and Sadock and Sadock (2003) provide an excellent overview of the discovery and evolution of ECT. Although electric eels were used to ease headaches and camphor-induced seizures were used to treat psychosis as early as the 16th century, most histories of ECT start in 1934, when catatonia and other schizophrenic symptoms were successfully treated with pharmacologically induced seizures. Before the introduction of ECT, intramuscular injections of camphor suspended in oil and then the intravenous administration of pentylenetetrazol were used to induce seizures. In 1938, Cerletti and Bini introduced *electroshock therapy* (EST), but it later became known as ECT. In 1940, the first documented treatment of ECT was administered in the United States. An American psychiatrist, Abram E. Bennett, suggested the use of spinal anesthetics and the use of the muscle relaxant curare to reduce the incidence of fractures. In 1951, succinylcholine (Anectine) became the muscle relaxant of choice during ECT.

Between 1960 and 1970, during the advent of more effective neuroleptics, deinstitutionalization of the mentally ill, and complaints of ECT misuse, the use of ECT declined. Complaints about ECT misuse resulted in the development of ECT task forces by the Commissioner of Mental Health in Massachusetts, the American Psychiatric Association (APA), and the International Psychiatric Association. Between 1985 and 1990, the National Institute of Mental Health (NIMH) and the APA combined efforts to develop guidelines for patient selection and treatment. Although the Surgeon General released a report on mental health favoring the use of ECT in 1999, some well-intentioned activists who received ECT inappropriately suffered side effects that their doctors did not explain, or who were told that the effects of ECT were always permanent, attacked the treatment itself when the doctor who delivered the treatment was at fault. As a result of such complaints, the New Freedom Commission Report released in 2003 cited the need for mental health care reform in the United States. In 2004, the World Health Organization and Mind Freedom cited ECT as a violation of the rights of mental health clients.

These allegations have been countered by the publication of educational articles such as Clinical Science Versus Controversial Perceptions and the National Institutes of Health Consensus Statement on ECT. Although the National Association of the Mentally Ill (NAMI) does not endorse particular forms of treatment, it believes that informed individuals with neurobiologic disorders have the right to receive NIMH-approved treatments such as ECT from properly trained practitioners. NAMI opposes actions intended to limit this right (Papolos & Devanand, 2005).

Electroconvulsive Therapy

Electroconvulsive therapy (ECT) uses electric currents to induce convulsive seizures in neurons in the entire brain to alleviate symptoms such as major depression, acute manic episodes, or schizophrenia. Although the exact mechanism of ECT is unclear, four main theories exist: the *neurotransmitter theory* (the correction of biochemical abnormalities of peptide and neurotransmitters such as serotonin and dopamine produce effects similar to that of tricyclic antidepressants or selective serotonin reuptake inhibitors); *neuroendocrine theory* (a release of hormones by the hypothalamus or pituitary produce antidepressant effects); *anticonvulsant theory* (the treatment itself minimizes or eliminates symptoms); and the *frontal lobe theory* (ECT minimizes or eliminates symptoms of mood or behavioral disorders that originate in the frontal lobe) (Hall & Bensing, 2005; Sadock & Sadock, 2003).

With ECT, electrodes are applied to the client's scalp. Two types of electrode placements, bitemporal or bilateral (BL; one electrode placed on each temporal area) and right unilateral nondominant temporal (RUL; two electrodes placed on the right temporal area), are commonly used during the procedure (Figure 17-1). The left hemisphere is dominant in most persons; therefore, unilateral electrode placement is almost always over the right hemisphere. If a person exhibits right-hemisphere dominance, the polarity of electrode stimulation should be alternated during successive treatments. RUL placement has been described as more advantageous than BL placement because the negative effects on the client's cognition and memory after treatment are lessened. However, clinical efficacy is lower, with at least a 15% greater failure rate compared with BL placement (Fink, 1999; Sadock & Sadock, 2003).

A third type of placement, bifrontal (BF), in which the electrodes are placed on the forehead immediately above each eye, has been studied recently. Ongoing studies of BF placement find equal efficacy to BL placement. BF may be a useful alternative to BL placement (Fink, 1999; Fink, Abrams, Bailine, & Jaffe, 1996). **Electronarcosis** is a type of ECT that produces a sleep-like state without the presence of convulsions. Anesthetics and muscle relaxants are used to prohibit the development of convulsions during electrostimulation.

Indications for Use

Initially, ECT was used to treat clients with depression, schizophrenia, or the depressive phase of bipolar disorder, and clients at risk for suicide. Such use has been broadened to include clients who exhibit therapy-resistant depression, delusional depression, obsessive–compulsive disorder (OCD), acute schizophrenia, schizoaffective disorder, intractable mania, catatonia, pseudodementia, and neuroleptic malignant syndrome. Individuals who cannot take antidepressants because of health problems or who are intent on suicide and who would not wait 3 weeks for an antidepressant to work, would be good candidates for ECT. In addition, clients who were previously treated with ECT and responded well to the procedure often elect to continue with ECT

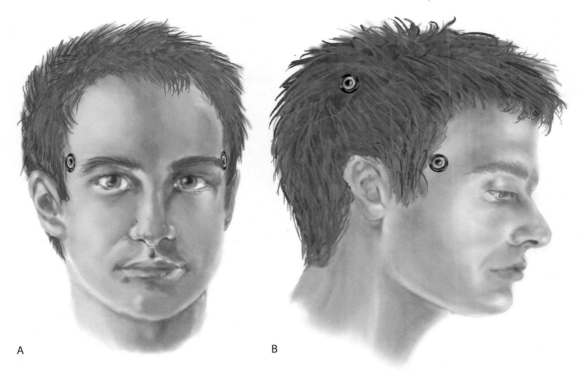

A   B

FIGURE 17.1 (**A**) Bitemporal electrode placement; (**B**) unilateral electrode placement.

during periods of exacerbations of clinical symptoms. Approximately 100,000 Americans elect to undergo ECT treatments each year. The effectiveness of ECT for the short-term benefit of movement disorders, such as Parkinson's disease, remains uncertain. ECT is not effective in somatization disorders (unless accompanied by depression), personality disorders, and anxiety disorders other than OCD (Crowe, 2005; Sadock & Sadock, 2003; MayoClinic.com, 2006).

ECT, initially used to treat adults, has been proven effective in the treatment of special populations, such as pregnant women who are unable to take psychotropic medication; children or adolescents who are depressed, are delusional, or exhibit manic episodes of bipolar disorder; elderly clients with severe depression; and persons with mental retardation who have an underlying mental health condition such as depression, mania, psychosis, or catatonia (DeMott, 1999; Fink & Foley, 1999; Sherman, 1999). Box 17-1 lists indications for ECT in children and adolescents.

Conditions Associated With Increased Risk During ECT

Several contraindications to ECT were cited when it was first introduced in 1938. At that time, the mortality rate was listed as one death per 1,000 procedures. Although serious consideration is still given regarding the use of ECT in the presence of medical conditions such as cardiac disease, expected benefits are weighed against possible risks and the likelihood of morbidity or mortality.

For example, if hypertension is caused largely by emotional factors, it need not be a cause for rejection, but may be an indication for the use of ECT. The use of ECT in the presence of myocardial disease depends on the seriousness and urgency for treatment if agitation exacerbates heart problems. In such situations, the APA guidelines for ECT published in November 2000 state that the ECT procedure can be modified to lower morbidity or augment efficacy. Such modifications may

BOX 17.1 INDICATIONS FOR ECT IN PREPUBERTAL CHILDREN AND ADOLESCENTS

PREPUBERTAL CHILDREN

- Catatonia, pervasive refusal of food and fluids, and/ or the presence of neuroleptic malignant syndrome
- Delirious mania
- Depressive mood disorder, mania, or psychosis with positive symptoms that are unresponsive to psychotherapy and/or other medicines; exhibits moderate to severe functional impairment; and clinical symptoms persist for more than 6 months
- Suicidal attempts or ideation that require a protective environment

ADOLESCENTS

- Catatonia or neuroleptic malignant syndrome
- Delirious mania
- Severe depressive mood disorders requiring hospitalization with failure to respond to two trials of alternative treatments
- Severe depressive mood disorder with prominent weight loss and/or suicidality
- Acute psychosis that is unresponsive after 4 weeks of neuroleptic treatment in adolescents who exhibit good academic achievement and/or when psychosis is precipitated by history of drug use

BOX 17.2 SPECIAL CONSIDERATIONS AND CONDITIONS ASSOCIATED WITH INCREASED RISK DURING ECT

SPECIAL CONSIDERATIONS

- Cardiac decompensation
- Aortic aneurysm
- Tuberculosis
- Recent fractures

CONDITIONS ASSOCIATED WITH INCREASED RISK

- Hypertension
- History of angina
- History of coronary thrombosis
- Recent myocardial infarction
- Bone disease
- Pregnancy
- Space-occupying lesion
- Recent cerebral vascular accident
- Retinal detachment
- Pheochromocytoma
- Bleeding or clotting problem
- Pulmonary conditions such as chronic obstructive pulmonary disease, asthma, or pneumonia

include changing the ECT technique, altering pharmacologic regimens, administering ECT in a different hospital or clinic location, and utilizing additional medical specialists or monitoring procedures (APA, 2000). According to statistics cited by Sadock and Sadock (2003), approximately 100,000 clients annually receive ECT in the United States. The mortality rate is about 0.002% per treatment and 0.01% for each client. Special considerations and conditions associated with increased risk during ECT are listed in Box 17-2.

Adverse Effects

The most common adverse effects reported by clients during ECT include headache, nausea, disorientation, and memory disturbance. Rare skeletal complications, such as vertebral compressions or fractures, have occurred. Although the client may not recall events immediately surrounding treatment, memory gradually returns over several weeks.

The effects of ECT are cumulative. Marked confusion may occur in up to 10% of clients during treatment. As the client progresses through a course of treatment—for example, one treatment two to three times a week for a total of 6 to 12 treatments—cognition may show signs of increased disturbance. Although memory impairment during a course of treatment is common and may be cumulative, follow-up data indicate that almost all clients regain their cognitive baseline function after 6 months. Furthermore, most studies indicate that approximately 80% of clients recover or are much improved. Recovery usually begins after a week and remains quite effective in clients who have not responded to one or more trials of antidepressant drug therapy. Some clients, however, complain of persistent memory difficulties after the discontinuation of ECT. Also, because not all clients respond well to a course of ECT or because they experience relapse within 6 months of treatment, a maintenance treatment of antidepressants, lithium, or ECT may be required. (Crowe, 2005; Mann, 2001; Sadock & Sadock, 2003).

Postictal (Seizure) Agitation

Hyperactive delirium may occur as the client emerges from the anesthesia. Clinical symptoms include marked motor restlessness, agitation, incoherence, disorientation, and a fluctuating level of consciousness. This phenomenon, referred to as **postictal agitation,** may last from a few minutes to an hour. The client may require intravenous diazepam (Valium) to stabilize the symptoms (Fitzsimons & Ramos, 1996; Sadock & Sadock, 2003).

Advances in ECT

In the past, any seizure was thought to be effective in restoring mental health by minimizing clinical symptoms. Research has proven that electrode location and the form and dosage of the electrical stimulus contribute to the clinical efficacy and cognitive effects of seizures (Fink, 1999; Fink & Abrams, 1998). The characteristics of seizures are best seen in the seizure electroencephalogram (EEG). The EEG is examined for duration, characteristics, and endpoint. Seizures, as noted on the EEG, should be longer than 25 seconds for ECT to be effective. Seizures fewer than 25 seconds in duration, without defined periods of EEG activity, and without a sharp endpoint, are considered inefficient treatments.

As noted earlier, when effective treatments are not elicited despite attention to EEG details, augmentation strategies are considered. They include changing the placement of electrodes; selecting an alternate anesthesia; using intravenous caffeine; reducing the impact of benzodiazepines by administering the antagonist flumazenil (Anexate); or adding pindolol (Visken), which blocks serotonin uptake and allows levels of serotonin to rise rapidly to increase response to ECT (Fink, 1999; Finkelstein, 1999). Continuation ECT (ie, repeated episodes of ECT treatment) has been used to prevent relapse in clients who were treatment resistant before the use of ECT.

Guidelines for ECT

Guidelines for treatment frequency, restrictions, systemic examinations, and the role of caretakers were developed in 1996 by the Association of Convulsive Therapy (Fink et al., 1996). As stated earlier, the APA

published a *Provider Handbook of ECT Guidelines* in November 2000. Briefly summarized, the guidelines state that:

- ECT is a major treatment with well-defined indications and it should not be reserved as a last resort.
- The most common use of ECT is with clients who have not responded to alternative treatments such as pharmacotherapy, who exhibit a deterioration in clinical symptoms, or who exhibit suicidality.
- There are no absolute contraindications to ECT; however, consideration is given to the degree of risk to potential benefits of ECT (see Box 17-2 earlier in this chapter).

Role of the Nurse During ECT

The role of the nurse during electroconvulsive therapy includes educating the client about the procedure before treatment, obtaining informed consent, preparing the client for treatment, providing care during the procedure, and assisting with post-treatment recovery.

Client Education Before ECT

Generally, an instruction sheet describing the procedure is given to clients and their significant others. A videotape, such as one produced by Geropsychiatric Education Programs (2003), may be shown during the discussion. The nurse emphasizes that the client will be asleep during the procedure and, although low-voltage current is passed to the brain, the client will not be harmed or feel any pain. Instructions for preparation, such as nothing by mouth (NPO) and the need to void before the procedure, are outlined. Common adverse effects after treatment are listed and reviewed. The client is told to postpone any major decisions until few weeks after the course of treatment is completed. The client and significant others are given an opportunity to ask questions about the procedure, and the nurse clarifies any misunderstanding they may have. Supporting Evidence for Practice 17-1 highlights information about the need for client education about ECT.

Informed Consent

After the client and/or family have been educated about the ECT procedure, including a discussion of the risks and mortality rate, benefits, and alternative treatment options to ECT, and why the treatment has been recommended, the client is given the opportunity to

---

SUPPORTING EVIDENCE FOR PRACTICE 17.1
Student Nurses' and Clients' Attitudes About ECT

PROBLEM UNDER INVESTIGATION / ECT as the primary intervention for severe depression

SUMMARY OF THE RESEARCH / Several randomized trials of severely depressed clients undergoing ECT, simulated or sham ECT, and the combination of ECT with drug therapy were conducted to study the decrease in depressive symptoms after therapy, symptom status at 6-month follow-up, effect on cognitive function, and mortality. On the basis of six trials involving 256 subjects, researchers concluded that ECT was significantly more effective than simulated ECT. In 18 trials enrolling 1,144 subjects, ECT was significantly more effective than pharmacotherapy. Bitemporal ECT was more effective than unitemporal ECT in 22 trials involving 1,408 subjects.

SUPPORT FOR PRACTICE / ECT remains an important treatment option for the management of severe depression. However, negative attitudes of student nurses and clients may act as barriers to the use of ECT in the psychiatric–mental health setting. Many resources provide education about the ECT procedure and its efficacy. Student nurses working with clients who are candidates for ECT could plan an educational program, giving both the students and the clients an opportunity to dispel any myths and improve their attitudes about ECT.

SOURCE: Barclay, L. (2003). Electroconvulsive therapy more effective than medication in depression. Lancet, 361, 799–808.

---

accept or refuse treatment. However, if a client has been deemed legally incapacitated to give an informed consent, the consent may be obtained by a court-appointed guardian, a designated health care surrogate, or an advance directive.

Client Preparation for Treatment

Client preparation for treatment focuses on providing a safe environment, monitoring vital signs, alerting the team to any problems, and providing reassurance to reduce anxiety. The nurse generally has a procedure check list that is completed to ensure that the client is ready to receive ECT and that emergency care is readily available.

Care During ECT and the Recovery Period

During treatment, the nurse observes motor seizure activity (tonic–clonic seizure activity is usually strongest in the muscles of the client's jaw and face), gently protects the client's extremities to prevent injury, and records the length of the motor seizure. The anesthesiologist and physician monitor the seizure (ictal) EEG for duration, defined periods of different seizure activity, and a sharp endpoint. Evidence of seizure activity may also be recorded by electromyelogram (EMG). Pulse oximetry and the client's cardiac

function via electrocardiogram (ECG) are also monitored (Sadock & Sadock, 2003). The nurse assesses the client throughout the procedure for potential adverse effects. Box 17-3 gives a step-by-step description of the nurse's role and accompanying nursing interventions during the ECT. See the accompanying box for examples of North American Nursing Diagnosis Association (NANDA) Nursing Diagnoses related to ECT.

According to ECT guidelines, an ECT recovery nurse, nurse anesthetist, or anesthesiologist provides interventions during the post-treatment period until adequate oxygenation, spontaneous respirations, consciousness, and orientation return. Interventions are provided as needed until the client is awake, alert, and oriented to person, place, and time.

Resources for Client Education

Several Web sites provide education and seek to dispel fears about ECT. Wikipedia, The Free Encyclopedia (http://en.wikipedia.org/wiki/ect) discusses the historical use of ECT; how it works; indications for use, including psychiatric diagnoses; efficacy of treatment; risks and benefits; adverse effects; controversy and fears; and alternative treatment. Other Web sites that provide educational material are Depression ECT (http://familydoctor.org/handouts/058.html); NIMH (www.nimh.nih.gov/events/prmagrec.htm); HealthyPlace.com, Inc. (www.healthyplace.com); and

BOX 17.3 ECT PROCEDURE

1. A thorough physical assessment, including heart, lung, and bone examination, should precede any treatment. A dental exam is advised for the elderly client and clients with inadequate dental care. An examination of the spine is indicated if there is a history of a spinal disorder. Ongoing medications are evaluated to prevent drug interactions with medication used during ECT, because some medications that clients take last 24 hours although the client is NPO 8 hours before ECT. Also, elderly clients do not metabolize medications as readily as younger clients.
2. The client should not eat or drink at least 8 hours before treatment.
3. Vital signs are taken 30 minutes before treatment.
4. Instruct the client to empty the bladder just before or after vital signs are taken.
5. Remove dentures, contact lenses, metal hair accessories, or any prosthesis that may conduct electricity or injure the client during treatment.
6. Apply electrocardiogram electrodes.
7. Insert IV line.
8. A sedative may be given to decrease anxiety.
9. An atropine-like drug, Robinul, is given to dry up body secretions and prevent aspiration.
10. The client is given a quick-acting anesthetic, such as Brevital, after being placed on a padded mat or table.
11. Medication such as Anectine is given to produce muscle paralysis or relaxation and prevent severe muscle contractions.
12. Oxygen may be administered by way of an Ambu bag if spontaneous respirations are decreased. Pulse oximetry is monitored.
13. A plastic airway or bite block is usually in place to prevent obstruction of the airway or biting of the tongue.
14. EEG electrodes are applied to deliver electrical shock.
15. The limbs may be restrained gently to prevent fractures during a severe clonic seizure. Usually the seizure is barely noticeable; slight toe twitching, finger twitching, or goose bumps may occur.
16. The client awakens approximately 20 to 30 minutes after treatment and appears groggy and confused.
17. Vital signs are taken during the recovery stage. The nurse stays with the client until the client is oriented and able to care for him- or herself.

Electroconvulsive Therapy—E.C.T (www.psycom.net/depression.central.ect.html).

Alternative Somatic Therapies

Vagus nerve stimulation (VNS) was approved for the treatment of epileptic seizures by the Food and Drug Administration (FDA) in 1997. On July 18, 2005, the VNS system (a thin, round pulse generator or battery) was approved by the FDA for the treatment of refractory depression in adults. The device is implanted under the skin on the upper left side of the chest. A flexible, insulated plastic tube containing electrodes connects the device to the left vagus nerve on the left side of the neck. Impulses of electrical energy stimulate the vagus nerve that originates in the brain. This stimulation is thought to affect some of the nerve connections to areas in the brain that are prone to seizure activity. A special magnet can be passed over the device to deliver extra electronic stimulation in between cycles. The approval, which is the FDA's first for an implantable device to treat depression, stipulated that the product must carry a black box warning that the device is permanent (RemedyFind.com, 2005).

Transcranial magnetic stimulation (TMS) is an investigational technique that was first developed in 1985. Since 1995, it has been studied in the potential treatment for clients with clinical symptoms of major depression, auditory hallucinations, and other psychiatric and neurologic disorders. TMS utilizes a specialized electromagnet placed on the client's scalp to generate short magnet pulses, similar to the strength of a magnetic resonance imaging scanner's magnetic field, but much more focused. These pulses stimulate the underlying cerebral cortex. Low-frequency stimulation (one pulse per second) has been shown to induce reductions in brain activation; higher frequencies (greater than five pulses per second) have been shown to increase brain activation. TMS is an outpatient procedure that does not require anesthesia or administration of intravenous fluids, and it can be administered in a physician's office or clinic. Each ses-

---

**EXAMPLE OF NANDA NURSING DIAGNOSES/
RELATED TO ECT**

- Acute Pain related to headache or muscle ache secondary to seizure activity and tissue trauma
- Anxiety (moderate) related to memory loss and disorientation secondary to effects of ECT on cerebral function
- Potential for Acute Confusion related to temporary memory loss during recovery stage of ECT
- Potential for Impaired Cognition related to temporary memory loss during a course of ECT
- Risk for Aspiration related to administration of anesthesia during ECT
- Risk for Aspiration related to post-ECT somnolence
- Risk for Injury related to uncontrolled tonic–clonic movements associated with postictal (seizure) agitation during ECT
- Self-Care Deficit related to confusion and fatigue during the recovery stage of ECT
- Situational Low Self-Esteem related to feelings of helplessness during ECT

---

sion takes approximately 30 minutes. Research protocols suggest daily stimulation five times per week for at least 2 weeks or up to 6 weeks. Although the FDA has not approved the use of TMS in the United States at this time, it has been approved in Canada and Israel as an alternative for ECT (National Alliance for the Mentally Ill, 2005).

Magnetic seizure therapy (MST) is a novel convulsive therapy for depression. MST is conducted in an ECT suite where clients are anesthetized in a similar fashion to ECT. High-intensity repetitive TMS (rTMS) is

---

SELF-AWARENESS PROMPT

Examine your feelings and attitude about the use of ECT. Do you have any biases or objections to this form of treatment? Have you ever witnessed ECT? Do you feel capable of providing nursing interventions to clients who receive ECT? If not, how could you prepare yourself to be a member of an ECT team?

---

used to induce focal seizures. The use of MST allows researchers to administer smaller amounts of electricity than the amount used in ECT to more precisely target regions of the cortex. Compared with ECT, MST has a shorter duration, lower ictal EEG amplitude, and less postictal suppression. During investigational studies, clients had fewer subjective side effects and recovered orientation more quickly. Although MST was found to be superior to ECT on measures of attention, retrograde amnesia, and category fluency, it is at a very early stage of clinical testing and has not been approved for use by the FDA (Moore, 2004).

KEY CONCEPTS

◆ Somatic procedures were performed in the early 20th century to treat psychiatric clients. They included lobotomy, sterilization, clitoridectomy, and insulin shock therapy. Present-day somatic treatments include clinical psychopharmacology, phototherapy, electroconvulsive therapy (ECT), and vagus nerve stimulation (VNS).

◆ ECT is the application of electric currents to induce convulsive seizures. It is used to treat the clinical symptoms of depression, obsessive–compulsive disorder, acute schizophrenia, schizoaffective disorder, intractable mania, catatonia, pseudodementia, and neuroleptic malignant syndrome as well as for individuals who cannot take antidepressants because of health problems or who are at high risk for suicide.

◆ Research has focused on improving the clinical efficacy and cognitive effects of ECT-induced seizures. It has proven that depressed children, the elderly, and persons with mental retardation can benefit from ECT. Although clients with movement disorders secondary to Parkinson's disease are also treated with ECT, the efficacy has not been established.

◆ Common adverse effects of ECT include headache, nausea, disorientation, and memory disturbance.

◆ Postictal agitation or hyperactive delirium may occur as the client emerges from anesthesia and may last from a few minutes to an hour.

◆ Prior to ECT, expected benefits, possible risks, and the likelihood of morbidity or mortality are discussed with the client and/or family members.

◆ Nursing interventions include pre-ECT teaching, ensuring that informed consent is obtained, preparing the client for treatment, providing care during the procedure, and assisting with post-treatment recovery.

◆ VNS is a somatic therapy that has been approved by the FDA for the treatment of refractory depression in adults. Transcranial magnetic stimulation (TMS) and magnetic seizure therapy (MST) are two somatic therapies that are under investigation as alternatives to ECT.

For additional study materials, please refer to the Student Resource CD-ROM located in the back of this textbook.

 CHAPTER WORKSHEET

CRITICAL THINKING QUESTIONS

1. Interview a psychiatric nurse about the use of ECT. Has the nurse provided care for clients who received ECT? Why did the clients undergo ECT? How many treatments did the clients receive? What responses, both physiologically and emotionally, did the clients exhibit post-therapy?
2. A 45-year-old severely depressed female client is scheduled for ECT. Develop an educational tool to be used to instruct the client and family members about the treatment protocol. What concerns do you think they might verbalize? What knowledge do you possess to reassure them that ECT is a safe procedure?

REFLECTION

The chapter opening quotes present pro and con views of ECT that provide a topic for debate. Which view would you defend? If your answer is "con," what additional information would you offer to defend your choice? If your answer is "pro," explain the rationale for your choice.

NCLEX-STYLE QUESTIONS

1. The nurse understands that ECT treatments are thought to alleviate symptoms of depression by which action?

a. Altering serotonin levels
b. Causing memory loss
c. Enhancing the efficacy of psychotropic drugs
d. Stimulating the thyroid gland

2. The nurse in the outpatient ECT clinic reviews the client's history for which of the following that might increase the client's risk during ECT?

a. Degenerative joint disease
b. Insulin-dependent diabetes mellitus
c. Recent myocardial infarction
d. Use of multiple medications

3. The nurse teaches the client scheduled for ECT treatment that preparation includes which of the following?

a. Eating a light breakfast at least 3 hours before treatment
b. Limiting intake of carbohydrates at least 3 days before treatment
c. Refraining from food and fluids for at least 8 hours before treatment
d. Washing hair the morning of treatment

4. Which intervention would be the priority during the ECT procedure?

a. Assessing EEG
b. Assisting the physician
c. Monitoring seizure actions
d. Protecting the client

5. In the post-ECT recovery period, which finding would alert the nurse to a possible problem?

a. Sleepiness
b. Lack of seizure activity
c. Urinary incontinence
d. Vital sign alterations

6. Which of the following conditions would be an indication for an adolescent to receive ECT? Select all that apply.

a. Neuroleptic malignant syndrome
b. Severe depression with suicidality
c. Delirious mania
d. Somatization disorder
e. Movement disorders

Selected References

American Psychiatric Association (2000). *Provider handbook of ECT guidelines.* Washington, DC: Author.

Barclay, L. (2003). Electroconvulsive therapy more effective than medication in depression. *Lancet, 361,* 799–808.

Crowe, R. (2005). Electroconvulsive therapy. Retrieved September 21, 2005, from http://www.vh.org/adult/patient/psychiatry/electroconvulsivetherapy/

DeMott, K. (1999). Electroconvulsive therapy may improve refractory bipolar disorder in children. *Clinical Psychiatry News, 27*(12), 19.

Fink, M. (1999). *Electroshock: Restoring the mind.* New York: Oxford University Press.

Fink, M. (2004). Rethinking electroconvulsive therapy. *Clinical Psychiatry News, 32*(10), 16.

Fink, M., & Abrams, R. (1998). EEG monitoring in ECT: A guide to treatment efficacy. *Psychiatric Times, 15*(5), 70–72.

Fink, M., Abrams, R., Bailine, S., & Jaffe, R. (1996). Ambulatory electroconvulsive therapy. *Task Force Report No. 1 of the Association for Convulsive Therapy, 12,* 42–55.

Fink, M., & Foley, C. A. (1999). Pediatric ECT: An update. *Psychiatric Times, 16*(9), 63–65.

Finkelstein, J. B. (1999). ECT may be enhanced with pindolol adjunct. *Clinical Psychiatry News, 27*(8), 11.

Fitzsimons, L. M., & Ramos, F. (1996). Electroconvulsive therapy. In S. Lego (Ed.), *Psychiatric nursing: A comprehensive reference* (2nd ed., pp. 477–483). Philadelphia: Lippincott-Raven.

Geropsychiatric Education Programs (2003). Electroconvulsive therapy (ECT). The treatment, questions, and answers [videotape]. Retrieved September 25, 2005, from http://www.gpep.ca/gpep_videos.html#videoindex

Ginther, C. (1998). Book takes unflinching look at somatic therapies of the early 20th century. *Psychiatric Times, 15*(5), 54.

Hall, J. M., & Bensing, K. (2005). Electroconvulsive therapy. *ADVANCE for Nurses, 6*(18), 13–17.

HealthyPlace.com, Inc. (2002/2003). All about ECT: Electroconvulsive therapy. Retrieved September 25, 2005, from http://www.healthyplace.com/communities/depression/treatment/ect/index.asp

Henderson, C. (2002). What is ECT? Retrieved November 8, 2002, from http://www.javascript:%20ci0

Lisanby, S. H. (2006). Magnetic seizure therapy: Development of a novel treatment for geriatric depression. Retrieved April 15, 2006, from http://www.beeson.org

Mann, A. (2001). Earlier use of antidepressants, tapered doses reduce relapse rate post ECT. *Clinical Psychiatry News, 29*(12), 41.

MayoClinic.com. (2006). Electroconvulsive therapy: Dramatic relief for severe mental illness. Retrieved April 15, 2006, from http://www.mayoclinic.com/print/electroconvulsive therapy

Moore, H. W. (2004). A novel convulsive therapy for depression. *Neuropsychiatry News, 5*(7), 6, 8.

National Alliance for the Mentally Ill (NAMI). (2005). Transcranial magnetic stimulation. Retrieved September 23, 2005, from http://www.nami.org

Papolos, D., & Devanand, D. P. (2005). All about ECT. Retrieved September 21, 2005, from http://www.psycom.net/depression.central.ect.html

RemedyFind.com. (2005). Vagus nerve stimulation. Retrieved September 25, 2005, from http://www.remedyfind.com/rem.asp?ID=4173

Sadock, B. J., & Sadock, V. A. (2003). *Kaplan & Sadock's synopsis of psychiatry: Behavioral sciences/clinical psychiatry* (9th ed.). Philadelphia: Lippincott Williams & Wilkins.

Sherman, C. (1999). ECT often a good choice for depressed elderly. *Clinical Psychiatry News, 27*(6), 19.

Suggested Readings

Abrams, R. (2002). *Electroconvulsive therapy* (4th ed.). Oxford, United Kingdom: Oxford University Press.

Carpenito-Moyet, L. J. (2006). Handbook of nursing diagnosis (11th ed.). Philadelphia: Lippincott Williams & Wilkins.

Diamond, E. A. (1999). Web site offers valuable information on ECT. *Psychiatric Times, 16*(9), 23.

Doskoch, P. (2000). Is rTMS as effective as ECT? *NeuroPsychiatry, 1*(6), 1, 9–10.

George, M. S., Lisanby, S. H., & Sackheim, H. A. (1999). Transcranial magnetic stimulation. *Archives of General Psychiatry, 56,* 300.

Kellner, C. H., Pritchett, J. T., Beale, M. D., & Coffey, C. E. (1997). *Handbook of ECT.* Washington, DC: American Psychiatric Press.

Prudic, J., & Sackheim, H. A. (1999). Electroconvulsive therapy and suicide risk. *Journal of Clinical Psychiatry, 60,* 104.

Swartz, C. M. (2006). 4 ECT electrode options: Which is best for your patient? *Current Psychiatry, 5*(3), 115–116.

Complementary or alternative medical (CAM) practices in the United States have grown dramatically in the last decade in popularity. One in every three persons in the United States now resorts to the use of CAM therapy or employs a CAM practitioner to treat a variety of maladies from pain to stress management. —REILLY, 2000

LEARNING OBJECTIVES

AFTER STUDYING THIS CHAPTER, YOU SHOULD BE ABLE TO:

1. Discuss complementary and alternative medicine therapies as classified by the National Institutes of Health's National Center for Complementary and Alternative Medicine.
2. Differentiate the concepts of curing and healing.
3. Articulate the components of the holistic model of nursing.
4. Construct a list of complementary and alternative medicine therapies to treat insomnia, pain, stress and anxiety, depression, and cognitive decline.
5. Discuss the roles assumed by the client and the holistic nurse during the nursing process.
6. Identify the importance of client education during the practice of holistic nursing and use of complementary and alternative medicine therapies.
7. Formulate a set of guidelines to be given to a client receiving complementary and alternative medicine therapy.

KEY TERMS

Aromatherapy
Cellopathy
Complementary and
    alternative medicine
    (CAM)
Curing
Essential oils
Healing
Holism
Holistic nursing
Homeopathic remedies
Homeopathy

Complementary and alternative medicine (CAM) refers to various disease-treating and disease-preventing practices or therapies that are not considered to be conventional medicine taught in medical schools, not typically used in hospitals, and not generally reimbursed by insurance companies (National Center for Complementary and Alternative Medicine [NCCAM], 2002). Other terms used to describe these therapeutic approaches include *integrative medicine* and *holistic medicine*. During the last 30 years, public interest in the use of CAM systems, approaches, and products has risen steadily. Depending on how CAM is defined, an estimated 6.5% to as much as 43% of the U.S. population has used some form of CAM. Furthermore, it has been estimated that one person in three uses these therapies for clinical symptoms of anxiety, depression, back problems, and headaches. Reasons for this dramatic change include dissatisfaction with increasing health care costs, managed care restrictions, and the focus on management of clinical symptoms rather than etiology (Jancin, 2000; Sadock & Sadock, 2003). As a result of the surge in interest and usage of CAM, the National Institutes of Health (NIH) provided a $50 million budget to support the NCCAM (Jancin, 2000).

Further evidence of the popularity and increasing use of CAM is the addition of such services to benefits packages offered by third-party reimbursement agencies and managed care organizations. This addition is in direct response to the demand by insured clients. Moreover, approximately one half to two thirds of the medical schools in the United States now offer elective courses in CAM therapies such as acupuncture, massage therapy, hypnosis, and relaxation techniques (White, 1999).

In March 2000, the White House Commission on Complementary and Alternative Medicine Policy (WHCCAMP) was established to address issues related to the practice of CAM. The Commission's primary task was to provide, through the Secretary of Health and Human Services, legislative and administrative recommendations for ensuring that public policy maximizes the potential benefits of CAM therapies to consumers. The Commission developed 29 recommendations and actions that addressed education and training of health care practitioners in CAM; coordination of research about CAM products; the provision of reliable and useful information on CAM to health care professions; and provision of guidance on the appropriate access to and delivery of CAM (WHCCAMP, 2005). Box 18-1 lists examples of key recommendations by the Commission.

Integrating CAM therapies into nursing practice to treat physiologic, psychological, and spiritual needs requires differentiation of the concepts of curing and healing clients. **Curing** is described as the alleviation of symptoms or the suppression or termination of a disease process through surgical, chemical, or mechanical intervention. This restoration of function, referred to as **cellopathy,** reflects the medical model of care. **Healing** is defined as a gradual or spontaneous awakening that originates within a person and results in a deeper sense of self, effecting profound change. Nurses who integrate CAM into clinical practice and help their clients access their greatest healing poten-

---

BOX 18.1 KEY RECOMMENDATIONS BY WHITE HOUSE COMMISSION ON COMPLEMENTARY AND ALTERNATIVE MEDICINE POLICY (FINAL REPORT, 2005)

- Federal agencies should receive increased funding for clinical, basic, and health services research on complementary and alternative medicine (CAM).
- Increased efforts should be made to strengthen the emerging dialogue among CAM and conventional medicine practitioners.
- Education and training of CAM and conventional medicine practitioners should be designed to ensure public safety, improve health, and increase the availability of qualified and knowledgeable CAM and conventional medicine practitioners to enhance collaboration among them.
- Quality and accuracy of CAM information on the Internet should be improved by establishing a voluntary standards board, public education campaigns, and actions to protect consumer privacy.
- Information on training and education of providers of CAM services should be accessible to the public.
- CAM products should be safe and meet appropriate standards of quality and consistency.

tial practice holistic nursing. This client-oriented approach fits well with the culture of the many CAM therapies used to treat the psychological, spiritual, and physical needs of clients.

This chapter describes holistic nursing and discusses the common CAM therapies that may be used in the psychiatric–mental health clinical setting. Box 18-2 lists therapies identified by the NIH as appropriate for use with psychiatric–mental health clients.

Holistic Nursing

Holism is a way of viewing health care in terms of patterns and processes instead of medication, technol-

---

BOX 18.2 COMPLEMENTARY AND ALTERNATIVE THERAPIES USED IN THE PSYCHIATRIC–MENTAL HEALTH CLINICAL SETTING

Acupressure: Based on the concept of *chi* or *qi*, the essential life force, this Chinese practice uses finger pressure at the same points that are used in acupuncture to balance chi and achieve health.

Acupuncture: Based on the concept of energy fields and chakras (centers in the body located in the pelvis, abdomen, chest, neck, and head), Chinese acupuncture identifies patterns of energy flow and blockage. Hair-thin needles are inserted to either stimulate or sedate selected points going from the head to the feet to correct imbalance of *chi* or *qi*.

Aromatherapy: Initially used by Australian aborigines, essential plant oils are used to promote health and well-being by inhalation of their scents or fragrances, essential oil massage, or application of the liquid oil into an electronic infusor, which turns oil into vapor.

Art therapy: Clients are encouraged to express their feelings or emotions by painting, drawing, or sculpting.

Biofeedback: This therapy teaches clients how to control or change aspects of their bodies' internal environments.

Chinese herbal medicine: An ancient science in modern times, herbs are used to treat a variety of maladies. They may be taken as tea from barks and roots, through the addition of white powders or tinctures to food and juice, or as herbal tonics.

Dance and movement therapy: This therapy enables the client to use the body and various movements for self-expression in a therapeutic environment.

Guided imagery: Clients use consciously chosen positive and healing images to help reduce stressors, to cope with illness, or to promote health.

Homeopathy: Based on the law of "similars," this system of healing, developed in the 18th century, states that a much-diluted preparation of a substance that can cause symptoms in a healthy person can cure those same symptoms in a sick person. Homeopathic medicines (remedies) are made from plant, animal, and mineral substances and are approved by the Food and Drug Administration.

Hypnosis: Hypnosis is used to achieve a relaxed, yet heightened, state of awareness during which clients are more open to suggestion.

Massage therapy: Massage therapy is considered to be a science of muscle relaxation and stress reduction and includes techniques such as healing touch, Rolfing, and Trager therapy.

Meditation: During this therapy, clients sit quietly with eyes closed and focus the mind on a single thought. Chanting or controlled breathing may be used.

Spiritual healing: Spiritual healing addresses the spirit, which is the unifying force of an individual, and may occur as the direct influence of one or more persons on another living system without using known physical means of intervention.

Therapeutic or healing humor: Based on the belief that laughter allows one to experience joy when faced with adversity, therapeutic humor is positive, loving, and uplifting. It connects the usual with the unusual and conveys compassion and understanding. Humor may be found in movies, stories, pantomime, mime, cartoons, and the like.

Therapeutic touch: This therapy is based on the premise that disease reflects a blockage in the flow of energy that surrounds and permeates the body. A four-step process of centering, healing intent, unruffling, and energy transfer occurs as a practitioner attempts to detect and free the blockages.

ogy, and surgery. Consciousness is considered to be real and influential in illness and wellness. The assessment of thoughts, emotions, beliefs, and attitudes is paramount in the holistic approach. **Holistic nursing** involves caring for the whole person, and is based on the philosophy that there is an interrelationship among biologic, psychological, social, and spiritual dimensions of the person. It focuses on searching for patterns and causes of illness, not symptoms; viewing pain and disease as processes that are a part of healing; treating the person as a whole, autonomous client rather than a fragmented, dependent individual; emphasizing the achievement of maximum health and wellness; and equating prevention with wholeness. Holistic nurses use body–mind, spiritual, energetic, and ethical healing (Clark, 1999–2000).

The American Holistic Nurses' Association (AHNA), established in 1981 by Charlotte McGuire, has devel-

oped standards of care that define the discipline of holistic nursing, which has been considered a specialty since 1992 (Box 18-3). A three-tiered program is now available for nurses to obtain national certification through the AHNA. It includes application to qualify for certification, completion of a qualitative assessment of the applicant's ability to integrate foundation concepts of holistic nursing in one's life and practice, and the successful completion of a quantitative assessment (ie, national examination). Many alternative medical therapies require certification programs within their scope of practice (Falsafi, 2004). Hospitals across the country are increasingly aware of the importance of holistic nursing and certification for excellence in nursing practice. In hospitals employing certified holistic nurses, there are fewer lawsuits, patients experience fewer complications, and care outcomes are significantly better (Keefe, 2004).

BOX 18.3 SUMMARY OF THE AMERICAN HOLISTIC NURSES' ASSOCIATION CORE VALUES OF STANDARDS OF CARE

CORE VALUE 1. HOLISTIC PHILOSOPHY AND EDUCATION

1.1 **Holistic Philosophy:** Holistic nurses develop and expand their conceptual framework and overall philosophy in the art and science of holistic nursing to model, practice, teach, and conduct research in the most effective manner possible.

1.2 **Holistic Education:** Holistic nurses acquire and maintain current knowledge and competency in holistic nursing practice.

CORE VALUE 2. HOLISTIC ETHICS, THEORIES, AND RESEARCH

2.1 **Holistic Ethics:** Holistic nurses hold to a professional ethic of caring and healing that seeks to preserve wholeness and dignity of self, students, colleagues, and the person who is receiving care in all practice settings, be it in health promotion, birthing centers, acute or chronic health care facilities, end-of-life care centers, or in homes.

2.2 **Holistic Nursing Theories:** Holistic nurses recognize that holistic nursing theories provide the framework for all aspects of holistic nursing practice and transformational leadership.

2.3 **Holistic Nursing and Related Research:** Holistic nurses provide care and guidance to persons

through nursing interventions and holistic therapies consistent with research findings and other sound evidence.

CORE VALUE 3. HOLISTIC NURSE SELF-CARE

3.1 **Holistic Nurse Self-Care:** Holistic nurses engage in self-care and further develop their own personal awareness of being an instrument of healing to better serve self and others.

CORE VALUE 4. HOLISTIC COMMUNICATION, THERAPEUTIC ENVIRONMENT, AND CULTURAL DIVERSITY

4.1 **Holistic Communication:** Holistic nurses engage in holistic communication to ensure that each person experiences the presence of the nurse as authentic and sincere; there is an atmosphere of shared humanness that includes a sense of connectedness and attention reflecting the individual's uniqueness.

4.2 **Therapeutic Environment:** Holistic nurses recognize that each person's environment includes everything that surrounds the individual, both the external and the internal (physical, mental, emotional, social, and spiritual) as well as patterns not yet understood.

4.3 **Cultural Diversity:** Holistic nurses recognize each person as a whole body–mind–spirit being and mutually create a plan of care consistent with cultural background, health beliefs, sexual orientation, values, and preferences.

CORE VALUE 5. HOLISTIC CARING PROCESS

5.1 **Assessment:** Each person is assessed holistically using appropriate traditional and holistic methods while the uniqueness of the person is honored.

5.2 **Patterns/Problems/Needs:** Actual and potential patterns/problems/needs and life processes related to health, wellness, disease or illness which may or may not facilitate well-being are identified and prioritized.

5.3 **Outcomes:** Each person's actual or potential patterns/problems/needs have appropriate outcomes specified.

5.4 **Therapeutic Care Plan:** Each person engages with the holistic nurses to mutually create an appropriate plan of care that focuses on health promotion, recovery or restoration, or peaceful dying so that the person is as independent as possible.

5.5 **Implementation:** Each person's plan of holistic care is prioritized, and holistic nursing interventions are implemented accordingly.

5.6 **Evaluation:** Each person's responses to holistic care are regularly and systematically evaluated, and the continuing holistic nature of the healing process is recognized and honored.

Reprinted with permission from the American Holistic Nurses' Association. (2000). *Summary of AHNA core values.* Flagstaff, AZ: Author.

Summary of Holistic Nursing Process

The holistic nurse teaches the client self-assessment skills related to emotional status, nutritional needs, activity level, sleep–wake cycle, rest and relaxation, support systems, and spiritual needs. Nurses need to be aware that clients may self-prescribe herbs or medications for serious underlying physiologic or psychological conditions that have not been previously brought to the attention of a health care provider. If such a situation occurs, the nurse discusses with the client the importance of seeking appropriate medical attention to prevent potential medical complications, adverse reactions to self-prescribed herbs, or adverse herb–drug interactions.

After the client completes self-assessment, problems (diagnoses) are identified, and guidelines are provided to assist the client with problem-solving skills. The client and nurse discuss mutually agreed-on goals and outcomes. For example, suppose the client identifies the problem of overeating related to the inability to express anxiety. The client's goal may be to develop positive coping skills when experiencing anxiety. Specific outcomes are developed with the client's input and might include identifying events that contribute to anxiety, reporting which coping skills were used, and reporting fewer episodes of overeating. After

the nurse and client agree on goals and outcomes, the client is encouraged to assume responsibility for making these changes. The nurse remains a support, coach, and assessor as the client actively participates in the intervention process. The nurse helps the client by reinforcing self-esteem, confidence, a sense of self-worth, and a positive outlook. Client self-evaluations and subjective comments are used to assess progress toward goals. It is important to remember that the client is a partner in all aspects of the holistic nursing process (Clark, 1999–2000).

Use of Complementary and Alternative Therapies in the Psychiatric–Mental Health Setting

Public interest in holistic health care has prompted providers of psychiatric–mental health care to include both traditional and CAM therapies in their practices. Various studies have indicated that 50% of adults and 20% of children are seeing nonphysician practitioners and are availing themselves of CAM (Mulligan, 2003).

The NCCAM defines CAM as those health care and medical practices that are not currently an integral part of conventional medicine. It also notes that CAM practice changes continually and that therapies proven safe and effective often become accepted as part of general health care practices (Mulligan, 2003). Although other entities may define CAM and classify interventions differently, the NCCAM divides CAM therapies into five major categories: alternative or whole medical systems, mind–body medicine, biologically based practices, manipulative and body-based practices, and energy medicine (NCCAM, 2002; Poss, 2005). A brief discussion of the more common CAM therapies utilized in the psychiatric–mental health setting follows.

Homeopathy (Alternative Medical System)

Homeopathy, also called *vitalism,* is classified by the NCCAM as an *alternative medical system* that evolved independently of and prior to the conventional biomedical approach. (Other examples of alternative or whole medical systems include traditional Chinese medicine, Ayurvedic medicine, non-Western cultural medical traditions, and naturopathy.) Homeopathy is a specific healing therapy started in the late 1700s to early 1800s by Samuel Hahnemann, a German physician and chemist. He formulated the theory that the body possesses the power to heal itself. Therefore, a substance creating certain symptoms in a healthy person would cure an ill person exhibiting the same particular set of symptoms. For example, the symptoms of arsenic poisoning include abdominal discomfort, such as stomach cramping with burning pain, nausea, and vomiting. Arsenicum album is a homeopathic remedy used to treat people with symptoms of food poisoning, such as nausea, vomiting, and abdominal discomfort. The remedy "cancels out" the illness (O'Brien, 2002).

Aromatherapy (Biologically Based Practice)

Aromatherapy, named by the French chemist Maurice René-Maurice Gattefosse in 1928, is classified as a *biologically based practice.* (Other examples of biologically based practices include herbal, special dietary, orthomolecular, and individual biological therapies.) Aromatherapy is the controlled, therapeutic use of **essential oils** for specific measurable outcomes. Essential oils are volatile, organic constituents of aromatic plant matter that trigger different nerve centers in the brain to produce specific neurochemicals (Mulligan, 2003).

Mind–Body Medicine

Mind–body medicine includes techniques that assist in the mind's ability to affect bodily functions and symptoms. Examples of these interventions include meditation, spiritual healing and prayer, and music therapy.

Mindfulness-based stress reduction (MBSR), a form of mind–body medicine, was introduced in 1979 by Jon Kabat-Zinn at the University of Massachusetts Medical School. Mindfulness is described as paying nonjudgmental purposeful attention in the present moment of time. Concentration is enhanced by focusing one's attention on the physical sensations that accompany breathing. Clients are introduced to different forms of MBSR including breathing meditation, body scanning, walking meditation, and hatha yoga. MBSR has proven effective in the treatment of fibromyalgia, anxiety disorders, chronic pain, and recurrent depression. Approximately 240 academic medical centers, hospitals, university health services, and free-standing clinics use the MBSR model (Poss, 2005).

Manipulative and Body-Based Practices

Manipulative and body-based practices include therapies that are applied to improve health and restore function. Examples include Tai Chi, massage therapy, chiropractic treatments, and yoga.

Energy Medicine

Energy medicine includes techniques that focus on energy fields originating in the body (biofields) or from other sources, such as electromagnetic fields. Biofield techniques are said to affect energy fields around the body. Examples include therapeutic touch, healing touch, and Reiki. Bioelectromagnetic-based techniques, which are a form of energy therapy, use electromagnetic fields to treat conditions such as asthma, migraine headaches, or other pain.

Indications for Use of Complementary and Alternative Therapy

Clients in search of low-cost, safe, and effective treatment for clinical symptoms such as insomnia, pain, stress and anxiety, depression, and cognitive decline

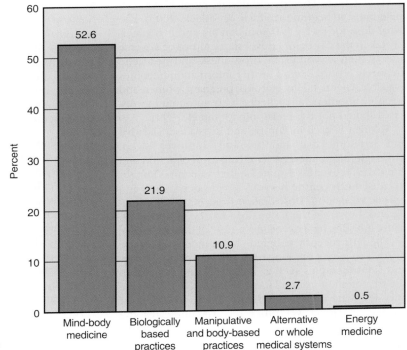

CAM Domain and Whole Medical Systems

FIGURE 18.1 Most frequently used categories of complementary and alternative medicine (CAM) domain and whole medical systems.

have turned to nonpharmaceutical, CAM therapies for symptom relief. Figure 18-1 displays the most frequently used CAM therapies to treat these clinical symptoms.

Information regarding the safety and efficacy of selected herbs discussed in this section is not all-inclusive. Research continues to focus on herb–drug and herb–herb interactions, therapeutic dosages of various herbs, and potential adverse effects of herbal therapy. For example, the American Herbal Products Association has grouped common medicinal herbs into the following four safety classes:

- Class 1: Herbs that are considered safe when used appropriately
- Class 2: Herbs with specific restrictions for external use only; not to be used during pregnancy; not to be used while nursing; and herbs with other specific restrictions
- Class 3: Herbs labeled with instructions that use should occur under supervision of an expert regarding dosage, contraindications, potential adverse

effects, drug interactions, and other relevant information related to the safe use of the specific herbal substance
- Class 4: Herbs for which insufficient data are available for safety classification (McGuffin, Hobbs, Upton, & Goldberg, 1997).

Insomnia

Psychologic stress commonly causes clients to experience problems sleeping. Clients often rely on homeopathic remedies or aromatherapy.

Homeopathy

Two herbal or **homeopathic remedies** (herbal medicines used in homeopathy) helpful in treating insomnia and jet lag are melatonin and valerian (*Valeriana officinalis*). In 1995 alone, there were 20 million new melatonin users in the United States. Melatonin is a neurohormone secreted by the pineal gland that helps set the body's circadian cycle, thus triggering the onset of sleep. This hormone is available in powder, capsules, or tablets. Therapeutic dosage range is 0.2 to 5 milligrams at bedtime (Sadock & Sadock, 2003). The usual dose for jet lag is 0.5 milligrams, and it is generally taken the day before travel starts. Although adverse effects such as confusion, drowsiness, and headache are rarely reported, until further information becomes available, clients taking steroids, pregnant women and lactating mothers, and clients with autoimmune diseases should not use melatonin (Stimmel, 1999).

Valerian is used in Europe and Russia as a sedative and hypnotic that induces and improves sleep. Although information on its mechanism of action and clinical effectiveness is quite limited, valerian is known to cause both central nervous system depression and muscle relaxation. Doses range from 300 to 900 milligrams; however, the latter dose has been known to cause morning hangover (Bilger, 1997a; Stimmel, 1999).

The NIH recently concluded that more studies are needed to assess the long-term efficacy of new drugs and CAM therapies such as melatonin and valerian in the treatment of insomnia. According to NIH, there are very few data regarding efficacy in the treatment of chronic insomnia, yet other research indicates the potential for substantial adverse effects. Other alternative treatments for insomnia include light therapy, acupuncture, yoga, and Tai Chi, but none of these have been evaluated sufficiently (Splete, 2005).

Aromatherapy

Some clients find that aromatherapy relaxes them and induces sleep. Essential oils may be applied directly to the skin, where they are absorbed into the bloodstream; administered with a compress; diluted with water or alcohol for massage; or released into the air for inhalation. English lavender, orange blossom, and marjoram stimulate the release of serotonin and the production of melatonin to serve as a hypnotic to induce sleep. Roman chamomile, clary sage, sandalwood, and rose are also used to treat insomnia.

Ethnicity and learned memory of smell do much to influence the choice of essential oil. For example, often Hispanics and Latinos prefer sweet marjoram, African Americans prefer cardamom, and Asians prefer ylang-ylang (Buckle, 2002; Hilton, 2000).

Pain

Clients may have numerous somatic complaints, may be hypochondriacal, or may have pain disorders associated with psychological or general medical conditions. Several forms of CAM therapies are used to reduce pain. Some of them (eg, acupressure, aromatherapy, homeopathy, imagery, therapeutic touch) can be learned quickly and have little or no risk to their use. Other unconventional therapies (eg, acupuncture, nutritional supplements, osteopathic manipulations) require extensive training and have some risks associated with their use (Milton, 2001). Examples of CAM therapies used to control pain may include:

- Homeopathic remedies consisting of herbs or minerals, such as Arniflora Arnica Gel or Traumed cream, may relieve pain, swelling, and stiffness in clients who exhibit chronic pain syndrome secondary to arthritis, fibromyalgia, or neuropathy.
- Hypnosis, an excellent way to mobilize a client's resources to alter physical sensations such as pain, allows clients to concentrate on competing sensations or simply to detach themselves.
- Relaxation therapy, guided imagery, biofeedback, and meditation also use the client's ability to concentrate on focal points, thus reducing painful sensations.
- Aromatherapy stimulates the brain to release endorphins for pain control.
- Acupuncture or acupressure relieves pain by correcting imbalances of *qi* or *chi* (vital energy) and improving the flow of energy (see Box 18-2 for a complete definition); massage therapy relieves pain through manipulation of soft tissue and surfaces of the body, increasing blood and lymph flow and improving musculoskeletal tone; therapeutic touch and healing touch involve the transfer of energy over specific body parts to relieve pain and promote healing. All have been used in the psychiatric–mental health clinical setting to minimize pain (Evans, 1999; Hilton, 2000; Hutchinson, 1999; Milton, 2003).

An analysis of the records of 5,750 chronic pain clients treated at the University of Michigan Pain Center between 1993 and 2000 concluded that white clients are more likely to use selected CAMs such as manipulation, biofeedback, relaxation training, or acupuncture than are African American clients (Perlstein, 2004).

Stress and Anxiety

Several CAM therapies are used to relieve stress and anxiety. Homeopathic remedies, massage therapy, and therapeutic humor are commonly used. Other therapies may include hypnosis, biofeedback, therapeutic touch, meditation, and aromatherapy (eg, calming oils such as lavender, chamomile, and neroli).

Homeopathy

Homeopathic remedies (herbal medicines) such as kava-kava (*Piper methysticum*), passion flower (*Passiflora incarnata*), and valerian are frequently used to treat clinical symptoms of anxiety and stress (Astin, 1998).

Kava-kava, a green, leafy member of the pepper family, is considered to be the most potent anxiolytic available without a prescription. It is nonaddictive, and clients who use it rarely develop tolerance. It does not alter mental clarity or interfere with reaction time, alertness, or other cognitive abilities. It is particularly useful in the management of daytime anxiety. The average daily dosage for general anxiety ranges from 60 to 300 milligrams per day in divided doses. It is administered in a single dose at bedtime for treatment of insomnia secondary to anxiety. Various adverse effects have been noted, including dermatitis, shortness of breath, visual disturbances such as sensitivity to light and hallucinations, exacerbation of Parkinson's disease, torticollis, and tardive dyskinesia (Waddell, Hummel, & Sumners, 2001; Zal, 2000). It has been removed from the market in Europe and Canada because of adverse drug interactions and hepatotoxicity risk (Edie & Dewan, 2005). Passion flower is a mild herb that can be used as a sedative, hypnotic, or antispasmodic. Administered to relieve anxiety, it is available in tincture form (one dropperful in warm water every 6 hours as needed) or capsule form (200–300 mg) from the freeze-dried plant (two capsules every 6 hours as needed). Nighttime hypnotic doses to treat insomnia secondary to anxiety range from 200 to 300 milligrams of the extract 1 hour before bedtime. Adverse effects include hypersensitivity, vasculitis, and altered consciousness. Excessive use of this herb should be avoided during pregnancy and lactation (Zal, 2000).

Valerian, dubbed "God's Valium," acts as an anxiolytic as well as a hypnotic. It is sold as a tea, tincture, or extract, and is available in capsule form. Daytime dosage to decrease anxiety is one half to one teaspoonful of the fluid extract in warm water, or one 150- or 300-milligram capsule daily (Zal, 2000). Daily dosage may be increased to 600 or 900 milligrams. It is considered to be a food additive that is safe in usual amounts found in food. When taken in therapeutic amounts, the most common adverse effects are resid-

ual morning drowsiness and headache (Edie & Dewan, 2005).

Massage Therapy

Approximately 80 different types of massage therapy are available for clients who prefer this form of therapy to reduce stress and anxiety. Massage therapy promotes relaxation, has a sedative effect on the central nervous system, and promotes the release of energy and emotions. Minor adverse effects caused by force, allergies to oils applied during massage, or psychological conditions such as the fear of being touched may lead to discomfort and pain during massage. Although the application of too much force can result in fractures, ruptured liver, or damaged nerves, these complications are rare. Massage therapy is contraindicated in numerous medical conditions such as deep vein thrombosis, infection, and advanced osteoporosis (Reilly, 2005).

Therapeutic Humor

Therapeutic humor also has been identified as a form of CAM used to relieve stress and anxiety. Beneficial effects include improved immune function, increased pain tolerance, and decreased stress response. It acts as a healthy coping mechanism, serves as an outlet for hostility and anger, provides a healthy escape from reality, and relieves anxiety and sadness related to loss. Therapeutic humor also promotes attention, facilitates communication, builds relationships, and energizes (Buxman, 2001; MacDonald, 2004; Salameh & Fry, 1987).

Depression

Herbal remedies such as St. John's wort (*Hypericum perforatum*), SAM-e (*S*-adenosyl-L-methionine), therapeutic touch or massage therapy, acupuncture, and aromatherapy are frequently used to minimize the clinical symptoms of depression. Meditation also may be used.

Homeopathy

The herbal medicine St. John's wort is the most popular antidepressant in Germany. The mechanisms of action in the treatment of depression remain unclear. However, pharmacologically, St. John's wort has been shown to affect neurotransmitters. It is an option for clients who exhibit low levels of depression; it also may be used for clients who are more seriously depressed but have not experienced success with conventional antidepressant therapy. It appears to be effective treatment for depression in children, adolescents, and adults (Bilger, 1997a; Sherman, 1999). Dosages range from 500 to 2000 milligrams per day. For children, the usual dose is 300 milligrams per day; for adolescents and adults, the usual dose is 300 milligrams three times a day. Adverse effects include nausea and vomiting, dry mouth, fatigue, skin rash, phototoxicity, and acute neuropathy, which generally subside after the herb is discontinued. St. John's wort can induce hypomania and mania in clients with bipolar disorder and exacerbate psychosis in clients with the diagnosis of schizophrenia. Its use is limited by the negative interactions that have resulted when it is coadministered with certain medications. St. John's wort is contraindicated during pregnancy or concurrent therapy with other antidepressants (Assemi, 2000; Ayd, 2001; Baker, 2000; Bilger, 1997a; Cuccinelli, 1999b, Edie & Dewan, 2005; Waddell et al., 2001).

SAM-e is a naturally occurring compound in the human body formed from methionine and adenosine triphosphate. SAM-e is found in many mammalian tissues, especially the liver and brain. It regulates the secretion of neurotransmitters, such as serotonin and dopamine, but it has not been compared directly with selective serotonin reuptake inhibitors (SSRIs). SAM-e has been approved as a prescription drug in Italy, Germany, Spain, and Russia, and must be taken with folic acid and vitamin B_{12} daily to be effective. It is available as a stable, enteric-coated tablet. Starting daily dosage is 400 milligrams, but research indicates therapeutic dosages range from 800 to 2000 milligrams per day for severe depression. No apparent adverse effects have been noted, except for gastric distress, restlessness, headache, and insomnia. SAM-e may precipitate manic episodes in clients prone to bipolar disorder (Baker, 2000; Boschert, 1999; Keller, 2001; Knowlton & Staff, 2001; Pies, 2000).

Meditation

Meditation is particularly indicated for clients with stress-related disorders or any condition exacerbated by stress, such as depression, chronic illness or pain, or terminal illness. The benefits of meditation include relaxation, reduced stress, normalized blood pressure, increased energy, improved overall health, increased mental clarity and concentration, enhanced creativity, and an increased sense of emotional balance and well-being. Clients who practice meditation state that they experience positive physical, emotional, cognitive, behavioral, attitudinal, and spiritual changes, a state of "open stillness" (Edwards, 2003; Sklar, 2004).

Cognitive Decline

Clients who experience short-term memory loss or progressive memory loss, or who want to slow the progression of cognitive decline, often request homeopathic remedies. The herbal remedy ginkgo (*Ginkgo biloba*) is the best-studied and most popular herb used to treat cognitive decline. Its primary biologic activity appears to be inhibition of platelet-activating factor. The extract also functions as an antioxidant to neutralize free radicals, possibly affecting norepinephrine, serotonin, monoamine oxidase, acetylcholine, and nitric oxide (Cuccinelli, 1999a). Research has shown that it can improve blood flow in the brain and the extremities and alleviate vertigo and ringing in the ears. Ginkgo is often referred to as a "smart pill" that is used to improve cognitive functions in individuals with cerebral insufficiency or cognitive decline caused by vascular dementia or senile dementia of the Alzheimer's type. Ginkgo should not be used in individuals with hemophilia or other bleeding disorders, or in clients taking anticoagulant or antiplatelet agents. Use during pregnancy and lactation is to be avoided. Adverse effects are mild and include gastrointestinal symptoms, headache, allergic skin reactions, irritability, restlessness, and peripheral visual disturbances. Daily dosage ranges from 120 (40 mg three times a day) to 240 milligrams (80 mg three times a day). It may take up to 6 weeks of therapy before therapeutic effects are seen (Bilger, 1997a, 1997b; Cuccinelli, 1999a; Victoroff, 2000; Waddell, et al., 2001).

Other herbal remedies may be used to improve mental function. These include ginseng (dosages vary according to whether liquid or root extract is used); guarana (not recommended for use in the United States); and rosemary tincture (at a 1:5 ratio) administered in amounts of 2 to 4 milliliters three times a day (Cline, 2003).

Implications for Nursing

In an attempt to improve health and/or combat illness, numerous Americans have resorted to the use of CAM therapy. Figure 18-2 indicates the use of CAM therapy by U.S. adults in the year 2002. Figure 18-3 reflects CAM use by race/ethnicity. This flurry of interest has

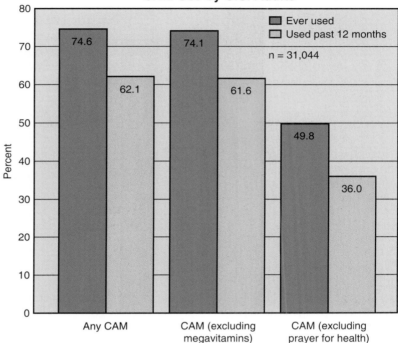

FIGURE 18.2 Complementary and alternative medicine (CAM) use in U.S. adults.

stimulated a movement to integrate CAM into the conventional health care system. Not only will nurses be questioned about CAM therapies, but they will need to be proactive and engage in open dialogue with clients about their use of CAM to address safety issues.

Adverse Effects

Clients using alternative and complementary therapies such as aromatherapy, herbal remedies, and nutritional supplements have been referred to as members of the "over-the-counter" culture. Concern has been expressed regarding adverse effects of the combination of various herbs; the interactions of herbs and prescription or over-the-counter drugs; high doses of nutritional supplements taken by consumers; and the potential for serious psychiatric sequelae (Ayd, 2001; Rand, 2001). Table 18-1 highlights some selected drug interactions and adverse effects of commonly used remedies.

Following are a few examples of adverse effects associated with the use of herbal remedies. In one instance, a client was seen because of feeling tired.

When laboratory work was completed, liver function tests were abnormally high. The client's husband asked his wife if she had told the nurse about the various herbal remedies she had self-prescribed. Upon further investigation, the nurse informed the client that the abnormal test results were caused by abuse of herbal remedies. The client agreed to abstain from taking the

SELF-AWARENESS PROMPT

How informed are you about alternative therapies? Do you know anyone who has used this type of therapy? Do you believe clients with psychiatric disorders would benefit from this type of treatment? Would you feel comfortable providing supportive care to a client who requested herbal remedies instead of antidepressant medication? Explore your reasons for your answers to these questions.

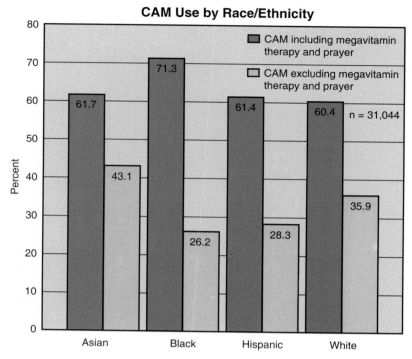

FIGURE 18.3 Complementary and alternative medicine (CAM) use by race/ethnicity.

TABLE 18.1 Potential Drug Interactions of Commonly Used Remedies

REMEDY	USE	POTENTIAL DRUG INTERACTIONS
Ginkgo (Ginkgo biloba)	Herb used to increase memory in dementia	Aspirin, ergotamine, warfarin, thiazide diuretics, phenobarbital, NSAIDs
Kava-kava	Herb used to decrease anxiety	Levodopa, dopamine, alprazolam, ethanol
Melatonin	Hormone used to treat insomnia and jet lag	Verapamil, steroids, immunosuppressant drugs
Passion flower	Herb used as a sedative, hypnotic, or antispasmodic	Alcohol, other central nervous system depressants
SAM-e	Amino acid supplement used to treat depression	Reports of drug interactions nearly nonexistent
St. John's wort	Herb used to treat depression and anxiety	Cyclosporine, warfarin, MAOIs, SSRIs, theophylline, digoxin, narcotics, reserpine, photosensitizing drugs
Valerian	Herb used as a sedative and hypnotic	Barbiturates, alcohol, central nervous system depressants

Adapted from Coleman (2001), Rand (2001), and Stimmel (1999).

remedies, and her liver function test results returned to within normal limits. In another situation, a client was combining St. John's wort with a prescribed antidepressant because she could not tolerate higher doses of the antidepressant. During a routine medication check, she complained of several adverse effects and admitted to the nurse that she had self-prescribed the herbal remedy.

An article in *The Orlando Sentinel* (Diet Herb, 2000) noted the link between a specific diet herb and kidney cancer. The cancer-causing chemical was found in a weight-loss product that contained the Chinese herb *Aristolochia fangchi,* which is often substituted for another herb, *Stephania tetrandra*. Belgium banned the herb when cases of kidney failure and urinary tract cancer began to appear. Clients were advised to undergo surgery to remove their kidneys and ureters.

Additionally, the shelf life of some herbal remedies has not been established, further adding to the concern about the development of potential adverse effects. Moreover, standardized dosages of some herbal drugs have not been established because of lack of research, and the components of some preparations have not been the same when prepared in different areas or countries.

Psychiatric Manifestations

The use of herbal remedies has been associated with the development of or exacerbation of psychiatric problems. Sherman (2002) discusses the potential for serious psychiatric problems associated with the use of herbal products such as St. John's wort, dehydroepiandrosterone (DHEA), and ma huang. St. John's wort may precipitate mania during the treatment of depression. DHEA, an adrenocortical hormone used by some clients to increase libido and prevent memory loss, may precipitate agitation, irritability, and delusions. Ma huang, an extract of ephedra used by some clients to increase energy, may precipitate affective disturbances and psychosis. Additional research may lead to issues involving the use of these products regarding competence to stand trial, criminal responsibility, and litigation.

Client Education and Resources

Findings reinforce the idea that the use of natural herbal medicine may not be without risk (Sego, 2006).

With these concerns in mind, the nurse should instruct the client to:

- Inform health care providers of all therapies being used, whether self-prescribed or prescribed by a practitioner. Clients may not consider home remedies to be CAM therapies (see Supporting Evidence for Practice 18-1).
- Follow directions regarding storage of remedies or supplements.
- Follow instructions regarding prescribed dosages and type of preparation (eg, powder, oil, tincture).
- Report any unusual symptoms, allergic reactions, or concerns while undergoing therapy.
- Recognize that the sources of herbal products are as varied as the label names, and that quality has been shown to be widely inconsistent even when there is only one manufacturer.
- Utilize the "Rule of Gs" that states herbs beginning with the letter G are likely to interfere with warfarin metabolism.
- Recognize that the use of more than one herb product makes it impossible to determine allergies or other serious interactions.
- Maintain all scheduled appointments.
- Read any instructional information provided by the practitioner, and request clarification of information as needed.

Various Web sites provide information related to the clinician and client education. For example, the International Bibliographic Information on Dietary Supplements (IBIDS) database offers physicians, researchers, and clients one-stop shopping for scientific information on dietary supplements (http://ods.od.hih.gov/showpage.aspx?pageid=146). The goal of this database is to help clinicians decide whether they should recommend dietary supplements, to inform the public about the use of supplements, and to guide researchers in planning supplement-related studies.

ADVANCE for Nurse Practitioners has committed a Web site—Complementary Care Forum, consisting of a panel of experts who represent a variety of complementary care disciplines—to answer questions about complementary care techniques and to clarify information about alternative therapies (www.advancefornp.com). Friedman (2001) lists the name, address, and services offered by several worthwhile alternative medicine Web sites (pp. 87–88).

PROBLEM UNDER INVESTIGATION / Assessment of geographic, social, cultural and health status factors affecting the use of health care services.

SUMMARY OF THE RESEARCH / According to researchers at Wake Forest University Baptist Medical Center in Winston-Salem, N. C., almost half of the adults in 12 rural counties in western North Carolina use home remedies rather than complementary and alternative medicine (CAM) for specific ailments and to enhance their mental health and general well-being. Remedies involving honey, lemon, vinegar, or whiskey, used alone or in combination were the most prevalent, followed by herbs, teas, and other traditional cures. Respondents described 238 distinct remedies that researchers categorized into eight groups: honey-lemon-vinegar-whiskey, used alone or in combination; herbs; teas; traditional remedies involving substances such as baking soda or turpentine; vitamins and minerals; food; over-the-counter products; and products bought from health food stores. An estimated 45.7% of the rural adult population used home remedies. Statistics indicated that rural adults ages 30 to 44 years are most likely to use home remedies (56%), whereas white people ages 65 years and older are least likely (35.7%). More women (50%) than men (39%) use home remedies; whereas 7% of women use vitamins and minerals compared with 3% of men. Respiratory and throat and mouth conditions most often were treated with honey, lemon, vinegar, and whiskey remedies, whereas cardiovascular conditions, infections, allergies, and mental health typically were treated with herbs. Researchers concluded that the widespread use of home remedies contrasts sharply with the use of alternative therapies such as acupuncture, chiropractic, and herbal medicine, which was estimated at only 8.6%.

SUPPORT FOR PRACTICE / Knowledge of geographic, social, cultural, and health care practices of clients has become increasingly important because these factors create unique challenges for nurses who must balance between today's care standards and traditional cultural or religious beliefs while providing care. During the assessment process, clients may not consider home remedies to be classified as CAM, and the nurse may not think to ask about specific home remedies that may interfere with treatment or cause adverse effects. It is the responsibility of nurses who provide care for clients in rural or culturally diverse settings to familiarize themselves with the health care practices of their clients so that they are able to anticipate unique client needs.

SOURCE: ADVANCE Newsmagazines for Nurse Practitioners staff. (2004). Home Remedies.Retrieved November 24, 2004, from http://nurse-practitioners.advanceweb.com/common/Editorial

KEY CONCEPTS

◆   Complementary and alternative medicine (CAM) refers to various disease-treating and disease-preventing practices or therapies that are not considered to be conventional medicine.

◆   Public interest in, and use of, alternative and complementary therapies is ever-growing. The National Institutes of Health (NIH) has funded the development of the National Center for Complementary and Alternative Medicine (NCCAM).

◆   Nurses who integrate alternative and complementary therapies into clinical practice and help their clients access their greatest healing potential practice holistic nursing.

◆   Clients are active participants in the holistic nursing process. The holistic nurse teaches the client self-assessment skills, discusses mutually agreed-on goals and outcomes with the client, encourages the client to assume responsibility for making decisions and changes, supports the client as changes are made, and promotes self-evaluation by the client.

◆   During the educational process, the holistic nurse and client discuss the importance of open communication regarding, for example, self-prescribing therapies and following directions regarding the storage and dosage of remedies and supplements.

◆   Alternative and complementary therapies are classified by the NCCAM into five categories: alternative or whole medical systems, mind–body medicine, biologically based practices, manipulative and body-based practices, and energy medicine.

◆ Common symptoms in the psychiatric setting that have responded to alternative and complementary therapies include insomnia, pain, stress and anxiety, depression, and cognitive decline. Various therapies used to treat symptoms include homeopathic remedies, aromatherapy, acupuncture, acupressure, massage therapy, therapeutic humor, and meditation.

◆ Herbal remedies have been associated with adverse reactions and the development of psychiatric problems. The American Herbal Products Association has developed a safety classification system for use of common medicinal herbs. Client education is essential.

For additional study materials, please refer to the Student Resource CD-ROM located in the back of this textbook.

 ## CHAPTER WORKSHEET

CRITICAL THINKING QUESTIONS

1. A 20-year-old male client describes clinical symptoms of anxiety. He informs you that he does not want to take anxiolytic medication, but is willing to try CAM therapies. What interventions would you plan for this client?

2. Interview a clinical nurse specialist or advanced nurse practitioner in private practice. Ask the nurse to explain his or her view about CAM. What assessment tools does the nurse use to obtain data about the client's interest in or use of CAM therapies? What educational materials does he or she have available for clients who express an interest in this therapy?

REFLECTION

According to the quote at the beginning of the chapter, one in every three persons in the United States uses some form of CAM therapy. Does your nursing program include a course on this topic? If so, does it address the application of CAM therapies in the psychiatric–mental health clinical setting? If not, do you feel that the clients are receiving adequate care to help them access their greatest healing potential? Please explain your answer.

NCLEX-STYLE QUESTIONS

1. A nurse is asked to present a class on holistic nursing. Which phrase would the nurse integrate into the presentation to best describe this practice?
   a. Alleviation of disease symptoms
   b. Facilitation of medical treatment methods
   c. Focus on the spiritual needs of clients
   d. Achievement of maximum health and wellness

2. The nursing plan of care for a female client complaining of severe pain from chronic rheumatoid arthritis incorporates the use of guided imagery and relaxation therapy. The nurse understands that these techniques achieve pain relief by which mechanism?
   a. Allows client to detach herself from the pain
   b. Promotes concentration on sensations other than pain
   c. Stimulates brain to release endorphins
   d. Corrects the imbalance of vital energy

3. The client tells the nurse about her regular use of the remedy kava-kava. Further assessment would reveal that this remedy is used to relieve which of the following?
   a. Anxiety
   b. Depression
   c. Fatigue
   d. Pain

4. A client taking physician-prescribed antidepressant medications is taught by the nurse to avoid which of the following herbal remedies?
   a. Kava-kava
   b. Lavender
   c. St. John's wort
   d. Valerian

5. The nurse would instruct a client interested in taking the herb *Ginkgo biloba* to improve cognitive function that it cannot be used with which of the following medications?

a. Anticoagulant agents
b. Antidepressant medications
c. Antihypertensive agents
d. Antidiarrheal medications

6. A client considering CAM therapy asks the nurse about energy medicine. Which of the following would the nurse include as examples of this type of CAM? Select all that apply.

a. Ayurvedic medicine
b. Therapeutic touch
c. Music therapy
d. Reiki
e. Tai Chi

Selected References

ADVANCE Newsmagazines for Nurse Practitioners staff. (2004). Home remedies. Retrieved November 24, 2004, from http://nurse-practitioners.advanceweb.com/common/Editorial

American Holistic Nurses' Association. (2000). *Summary of AHNA core values.* Flagstaff, AZ: Author.

Assemi, M. (2000). Herbal preparations: Concerns for operative patients. *Anesthesia Today, 10*(3), 17–23.

Astin, J.A. (1998). Why patients use alternative medicine: Results of a national study. *Journal of the American Medical Association, 279*(19), 1548–1553.

Ayd, F. J. (2001). Interactions between prescription drugs and herbs or other natural remedies. *Geriatric Times, 2*(5), 28–31.

Baker, B. (2000). SAMe for depression: Efficacy, safety still unproven. *Clinical Psychiatry News, 28*(1), 27.

Bilger, B. (1997a). Natural remedies. *Hippocrates, 12*(11), 25–27.

Bilger, B. (1997b). Nature's pharmacy. *Hippocrates, 12*(11), 20–24.

Boschert, S. (1999). SAMe cuts depression, but is costly. *Clinical Psychiatry News, 27*(10), 9.

Buckle, J. (2002). Clinical aromatherapy: Therapeutic uses for essential oils. *ADVANCE for Nurse Practitioners, 10*(5), 67–68, 88.

Buxman, K. (2001). Nurses jest for stress: Making humor a habit can lighten the stress in any department. *ADVANCE for Nurses, 2*(10), 23–24, 34.

Clark, C. C. (1999–2000). Holistic nursing. In Rodgers, B. & Rodgers, L. J. (Eds.), *Continuing education for Florida nurses* (pp. 201–225). Sarasota, FL: Bert Rodgers Schools of Continuing Education.

Cline, J. (2003). Complementary and alternative medicine. In W. K. Mohr (Ed.), *Johnson's psychiatric-mental health nursing* (5th ed., pp. 275–289). Philadelphia: Lippincott Williams & Wilkins.

Coleman, S. (2001). Proceed with caution: Recognizing adverse effects of alternative medicine on prescriptive drugs. *ADVANCE for Nurses, 2*(14), 21–22, 28.

Cuccinelli, J. H. (1999a). Alternative medicine: Ginkgo biloba. *Clinician Reviews, 9*(8), 93–97.

Cuccinelli, J. H. (1999b). Alternative medicine: Saint-John's-wort. *Clinician Reviews, 9*(4), 102–103.

Diet herb is linked to kidney cancer. (2000, June 8). *The Orlando Sentinel.*

Edie, C. F., & Dewan, N. (2005). Which psychotropics interact with four common supplements. *Current Psychiatry, 4*(1), 17–18, 23–25, 29–30.

Edwards, L. (2003). Meditation as medicine. *ADVANCE for Nurse Practitioners, 11*(5), 49–52.

Evans, B. M. (1999). Complementary therapies and HIV infection. *American Journal of Nursing, 99*(2), 42–45.

Falsafi, N. (2004). Holistically speaking. Retrieved April 18, 2004, from http://www.advancefornurses.com/common/editorial

Friedman, Y. (2001). Navigating the world of alternative medicine. *American Journal of Nursing, 101*(3), 87–89.

Hilton, L. (2000). Scent therapy relieves stress. *Vital Signs, 10*(4), 24.

Hutchinson, C. P. (1999). Healing touch: An energetic approach. *American Journal of Nursing, 99*(4), 43–48.

Jancin, B. (2000). Alternative medicine experiences growing pains. *Clinical Psychiatry News, 28*(2), 44.

Keefe, S. (2004). Holistic nursing 101. Retrieved December 21, 2004, from http://nursing.advanceweb.com/common/editorial.

Keller, L. (2001). SAM-e: More research, more uses. *ADVANCE for Nurses, 2*(21), 21–22.

Knowlton, L., & Staff. (2001). Investigating SAM-e. *Geriatric Times, 2*(5), 23–24, 26.

MacDonald, C. M. (2004). A chuckle a day keeps the doctor away: Therapeutic humor and laughter. *Journal of Psychosocial Nursing & Mental Health Services, 42*(3). Retrieved January 24, 2005, from http://www.jpnonline.com.

McGuffin, M., Hobbs, C. Upton, R., & Goldberg, A. (1997). Botanical safety handbook. Boca Raton, FL: CRC Press.

Milton, D. (2001). Alternative therapies for pain management. *ADVANCE for Nurses, 2*(21), 25–26.

Milton, D. (2003). Pain management. *ADVANCE for Nurses, 4*(23), 13–16.

Mulligan, M. (2003, April). Alternative medicine. *M. D. News Central Florida,* 10–11.

National Center for Complementary and Alternative Medicine (NCCAM) Report. (2002). *Alternative Therapies in Health and Medicine, 8*(2), 20–28.

National Center for Complementary and Alternative Medicine (NCCAM) & National Center for Health Statistics (NCHS). (2002). The use of complementary and alternative medicine in the U.S. Retrieved October 20, 2005, from http://nccam.nih.gov/news/camsurvey_fs1.htm.

O'Brien, S. B. (2002). Healing with homeopathy: An introduction to basic tenets. *ADVANCE for Nurse Practitioners, 10*(5), 63-64, 66.

Perlstein, S. (2004). CAM use assessed in patients who have chronic pain. *Clinical Psychiatry News, 32*(6), 81.

Pies, R. (2000). SAM-e and the over-the-counter culture. *Psychiatric Times, 17*(2), 7.

Poss, J. E. (2005). Mindfulness-based stress reduction: Applications for nurse practitioners. *American Journal for Nurse Practitioners, 9*(7/8), 9-11, 15-18.

Rand, V. E. (2001). Complementary medicine: Herbal products and uses. *Geriatric Times, 2*(5), 21-22.

Reilly, A. M. (2005). Massage therapy. *ADVANCE for Nurse Practitioners, 13*(5), 37-38, 40, 42.

Reilly, M. (2000). An overview of the role of acupuncture within pain management and anesthesia practice. *Anesthesia Today, 10*(3), 1-5.

Sadock, B. J., & Sadock, V. A. (2003). *Kaplan & Sadock's synopsis of psychiatry: Behavioral sciences/clinical psychiatry* (9th ed.). Philadelphia: Lippincott Williams & Wilkins.

Salameh, W. A., & Fry, W. (1987). *Handbook of humor and psychotherapy: Advances in the clinical use of humor.* Sarasota, FL: Professional Resource Press.

Sego, S. (2006). What clinicians should know about herbals. *Clinical Advisor, 9*(1), 46-51.

Sherman, C. (1999). St. John's wort seems effective, safe in children, adolescents. *Clinical Psychiatry News, 27*(11), 6.

Sherman, C. (2002). Many herbs can carry serious psychiatric risks. *Clinical Psychiatry News, 30*(1), 14.

Sklar, D. L. (2004). Stressed out? Relax and read on. Some alternatives to living with stress for you and your patients. *Central Florida M.D. News, 6*(4), 17-19.

Splete, H. (2005). NIH panel assesses treatments for insomnia. *Clinical Psychiatry News, 33*(9), 62.

Stimmel, G. L. (1999). Future directions in the drug treatment of insomnia. *Psychiatric Times Monograph, 16*(5), 1-8.

Victoroff, J. (2000). The genie is waiting in the bottle. *Psychiatric Times, 17*(3), 68-70.

Waddell, D. L., Hummel, M. E., & Sumners, A. D. (2001). Three herbs you should get to know. *American Journal of Nursing, 101*(4), 48-53.

White House Commission on Complementary and Alternative Medicine Policy. (2005). White House Commission on Complementary and Alternative Medicine Policy: Final Report. Retrieved October 18, 2005, from http://www.whcamp.hhs.gov/fr1.html

White, V. (1999). Alternative medicine becoming mainstream, study finds. *Vital Signs, 9*(5), 12.

Zal, H. M. (2000). Alternative medicine: Herbal medicine and the treatment of anxiety. *Psychiatric Times, 17*(3), 63-67.

Suggested Readings

Begley, S. S. (2002). The energetic language of therapeutic touch. *ADVANCE for Nurse Practitioners, 10*(5), 69-71.

Blumenthal, M. (2001). Asian ginseng: Potential therapeutic uses. *ADVANCE for Nurse Practitioners, 9*(2), 26, 28, 33.

Davision, R. T., & Connor, K. M. (2000). *Herbs for the mind: What science tells us about nature's remedies for depression, stress, memory loss, and insomnia.* New York: Guilford Publications.

Launer, K. (2002). Hypnosis, pain, and surgery: How hypnosis can decrease the perception of pain during and after surgery. *ADVANCE for Nurses, 3*(19), 25-26.

Levitt, R. (2000). Herbal medicine: An ancient science in modern times. *Vital Signs, 10*(1), 19, 26.

Ott, M. J. (2002). Yoga as a clinical intervention: Pain control and stress reduction may be just a breath away. *ADVANCE for Nurse Practitioners, 10*(1), 81-83, 90.

Pettit, J. L. (2000). Alternative medicine: Melatonin. *Clinician Reviews, 10*(6), 87-91.

Tedesco, P., & Cicchetti, J. (2001). Like cures like: Homeopathy. *American Journal of Nursing, 101*(9), 43-48.

Varlas, K. (2001). The power of imagination: Using guided imagery to reduce stress. *ADVANCE for Nurse Practitioners, 9*(5), 51-54.

CHAPTER 19 / ANXIETY DISORDERS

Anxiety disorders are among the most prevalent of mental disorders. Although their importance, from a public health perspective, was relatively ignored until recently, it has become increasingly clear that these disorders are common and disabling. —STEIN, 2004

LEARNING OBJECTIVES

AFTER STUDYING THIS CHAPTER, YOU SHOULD BE ABLE TO:

1. Articulate the difference between anxiety and fear.
2. Explain the following terms: *signal anxiety, anxiety trait, anxiety state,* and *free-floating anxiety.*
3. Discuss the following theories of anxiety: psychoanalytic, cognitive behavior, biologic, genetic, and social–cultural (integrated).
4. Compare the different levels of anxiety.
5. Construct a list of the more common physiologic, psychological or emotional, behavioral, and intellectual or cognitive symptoms of anxiety.
6. Identify the clinical symptoms of panic disorder, agoraphobia, social phobia, specific phobia, generalized anxiety disorder, and obsessive–compulsive disorder.
7. Distinguish between post-traumatic stress disorder and acute stress disorder.
8. Integrate an understanding of cultural differences when assessing clients for clinical symptoms of an anxiety disorder.
9. Describe the role of the nurse providing care for a client with an anxiety disorder.
10. Formulate a nursing plan of care for a client with clinical symptoms of generalized anxiety disorder.

KEY TERMS

Agoraphobia
Anxiety
Anxiety state
Anxiety trait
Compulsion
Fear
Free-floating anxiety
Ideational compulsion
Obsession
Phobia
Secondary traumatization
Signal anxiety

Anxiety disorders are the most common psychiatric–mental health disorder in the United States and in most other populations studied. They affect approximately 19.1 million individuals in the United States or 13.3% of the U.S. population between the ages of 18 and 54 years. Anxiety disorders frequently co-occur with depressive disorders, eating disorders, or substance abuse, and produce inordinate morbidity, use of health care facilities, and functional impairment (National Institute of Mental Health [NIMH], 2005; Sadock & Sadock, 2003). According to *The Economic Burden of Anxiety Disorders*, a study commissioned by the Anxiety Disorders Association of America (ADAA), almost one third of the yearly mental health bill of $148 billion (approximately $42 billion) is used to treat anxiety disorders. The study also revealed that a person with an anxiety disorder is three to five times more likely to go to the doctor and six times more likely to be hospitalized for psychiatric disorders than nonsufferers are (ADAA, 2003).

Like adults, children and teens experience anxiety and can develop anxiety disorders (see Chapter 29 for more information). Some of the disorders tend to be specific to age development. For example, children between the ages of 6 and 9 years may experience a separation anxiety disorder. Generalized anxiety disorder and social anxiety disorder are more common in middle childhood and adolescence. Panic disorder also can occur in adolescence. Depression commonly occurs with anxiety among teenagers (ADAA, 2003).

Until recently, the belief was that anxiety disorders declined with age. However, experts now believe that aging and anxiety are not mutually exclusive. Most older adults with an anxiety disorder experienced anxiety when they were younger. Stresses and vulnerabilities unique to the aging process (eg, chronic physical problems, cognitive impairment, and significant emotional losses) contribute to the development of increased anxiety, possibly causing an exacerbation of a previous anxiety disorder (ADAA, 2003).

As long as anxiety disorders are viewed as individual burdens restricted to individual clients, it is difficult to convince society to treat anxiety disorders with the same concern accorded other psychiatric–mental health disorders. Anxiety disorders are costly. These costs are not restricted to individual clients. They also involve employers, health insurance providers, and the national economy. The true costs of treating anxiety disorders cannot be fully determined without an assessment of the adequacy of available treatments (Sheehan, 1999). This chapter focuses on the theories, clinical symptoms, and nursing process related to the spectrum of anxiety disorders.

Overview of Anxiety
Historical Perspectives

Anxiety was first recognized as a medical diagnostic entity in the late 1800s. Before this time, anxiety was considered a feature of many medical conditions. In 1871, Jacob DaCosta described a chronic cardiac syndrome that included many psychological and somatic symptoms exhibited by soldiers. This "irritable heart syndrome" due to autonomic cardiac symptoms was later referred to as the *DaCosta syndrome*. World War II veterans and other survivors of combat exhibited a similar cluster of symptoms due to severe stresses that was eventually identified as post-traumatic stress disorder (PTSD; Sadock & Sadock, 2003).

Sigmund Freud first introduced the concept of anxiety in the early 1900s. He referred to it as a danger signal that a person exhibits in response to the perception of physical pain or danger. He recognized anxiety as a central component of mental diseases.

Related Terminology

The term **anxiety** is used to describe feelings of uncertainty, uneasiness, apprehension, or tension that a person experiences in response to an unknown object or situation. A "fight-or-flight" decision is made by the person in an attempt to overcome conflict, stress, trauma, or frustration.

Fear is different from anxiety. It is the body's physiologic and emotional response to a known or recognized danger. A person whose car stalls on a railroad crossing experiences fear of injury or death as the train approaches the crossing. The client who undergoes emergency exploratory surgery may be afraid of the surgery and develop symptoms of anxiety because the client is uncertain what the outcome will be.

Several terms have been used to describe different types of anxiety. They include signal anxiety, anxiety trait, anxiety state, and free-floating anxiety. **Signal anxiety** is a response to an anticipated event. For example, a father who normally is relaxed exhibits tachycardia, dizziness, and insomnia when his child attends school for the first time. He is experiencing signal anxiety.

An **anxiety trait** is a component of personality that has been present over a long period and is measurable by observing the person's physiologic, emotional, and cognitive behavior. The person who responds to various nonstressful situations with anxiety is said to have an anxiety trait. For example, a 25-year-old secretary frequently complains of blurred vision, dizziness, headaches, and insomnia in a relatively stress-free job.

An **anxiety state** occurs as the result of a stressful situation in which the person loses control of her or his emotions. A mother who is told that her son has been injured in a football game and has been taken to the emergency room may exhibit an anxiety state by becoming hysterical, complaining of tightness in the chest, and insisting on seeing her injured son.

Free-floating anxiety is anxiety that is always present and is accompanied by a feeling of dread. The person may exhibit ritualistic and avoidance behavior (phobic behavior). A woman who is unable to sleep at night because she is certain someone will break into her home goes through a complicated ritual of checking all the windows and doors several times. She also avoids going out after dark because she fears coming back to a dark, empty home.

Etiology of Anxiety

The etiology of anxiety can be addressed from several perspectives using various theories. These include genetic, biologic, psychoanalytic, cognitive behavior, and social–cultural theories.

Genetic Theory

Genetic studies have produced solid evidence that at least some genetic component contributes to the development of anxiety disorders (Sadock & Sadock, 2003). In 1996, researchers at the National Institute of Mental Health determined that the gene 5-HTTP influences how the brain makes use of serotonin. Statistics indicated that the gene caused a 3% to 4% difference in the degree of anxiety or tension the subjects experienced. Findings from this same study were also used to explore the origins of normal and pathological personality patterns.

Family studies have been conducted to determine the prevalence of anxiety in relatives. Two methods are generally used: the family history, which relies on indirect interviews with an informant, and the family study, which is based on direct interviews of family members. These methods have been used to explore theories regarding various classifications of anxiety (Nicolini, Cruz, Camarena, Paez, & De La Fuente, 1999). For example, almost half of all clients with panic disorder have at least one affected relative; about 15% to 20% of individuals with obsessive–compulsive disorder (OCD) come from families in which another immediate family member has the same problem; and about 40% of people with agoraphobia have a relative with agoraphobia (Sadock & Sadock, 2003).

Some studies have suggested that a relatively simple genetic model may explain the genetic or inheritance pattern of anxiety. The hypothesis states that there are some genes that play a major role, contributing to the manifestation of clinical symptoms of anxiety. For example, recent data provide strong evidence that chromosome 9 may be linked to the development of panic disorder; chromosome 13q may be linked to a potential subtype of panic disorder called "panic syndrome"; and significant linkage was found at chromosome 14 for simple phobia, and possible linkages for social phobias, panic disorder, and agoraphobia. Data regarding potential linkages at chromosome 1 for panic disorder, chromosome 3 for agoraphobia, chromosome 11 for panic disorder, and chromosome 16 for social and simple phobia have also been reported (Norton, 2004).

Biologic Theory

In general, studies have evaluated the links between anxiety and the following: catecholamines; neuroendocrine measures; neurotransmitters such as serotonin, γ-aminobutyric acid (GABA), and cholecystokinin; and autonomic reactivity. Neuroimaging studies have also been performed (Sadock & Sadock, 2003).

Studies evaluating catecholamine levels (eg, epinephrine and norepinephrine) have shown that these levels in clients with anxiety appear to be similar to those of normal control clients. Neuroendocrine studies have been inconclusive.

Neurotransmitter studies have revealed that serotonin plays a role in causing anxiety. Specifically, excessive serotonin activity in critical brain areas such as the raphe nucleus, hypothalamus, thalamus, basal ganglia, and limbic system may relate to anxiety. Agents such as buspirone and benzodiazepines inhibit serotonin transmission, which leads to the relief of anxiety symptoms (Roerig, 1999).

Neuroimaging research focuses on normal anatomy and neurochemistry, and behavioral, pharmacologic, and cognitive challenge theories to understand the biologic basis of anxiety. Research focuses on identifying potential predictors of treatment response. For example, positron emission tomography (PET) studies have shown increased metabolic activity and blood flow in the frontal lobes, basal ganglia, and the cingulum of clients with the diagnosis of OCD (Holman & Devous, 1992; Sadock & Sadock, 2003).

Laboratory studies have shown that a panic attack is characterized by a sudden increment in tidal volume rather than in respiratory frequency. In these studies, a computerized, calibrated body suit (Respitrace) was used to allow 24-hour recordings. Results have shown that clients who have spontaneous panic attacks experience a tripling of respiratory tidal volume.

Studies also have attempted to study the correlation between anxiety and heart disease. Kawachi, Sparrow, Vokonas, and Weiss (1994) examined the relationship between anxiety symptoms and the risk of coronary heart disease. This study concluded that there is a strong association between symptoms of anxiety and the presence of coronary artery disease.

Psychoanalytic Theory

Psychoanalytic theory originates in the work of Sigmund Freud, who suggested that anxiety is the result of unresolved, unconscious conflicts between impulses for aggressive or libidinal gratification and the ego's recognition of the external damage that could result from gratification. For example, unconscious conflicts of childhood, such as fear of losing a parent's love or attention, may emerge and result in feelings of discomfort or anxiety in childhood, adolescence, or early adulthood (Roerig, 1999).

A newer psychodynamic theory proposes that anxiety is an interaction between temperament and environment. Clients enter the world with an inborn physiologic reactivity that predisposes them toward early fearfulness. As they struggle with dependency conflicts, they develop weak representations of themselves and use poor strategies, such as avoidance, to cope with life stresses. Their feelings of safety decrease, and they develop a loss of control along with an increase of negative emotions, culminating in anxiety and an initial panic attack (Medscape, 2000).

Cognitive Behavior Theory

The cognitive behavior theory, developed by Aaron Beck, suggests that anxiety is a learned or conditioned response to a stressful event or perceived danger. According to this theory, conceptualization or faulty, distorted, or counter-productive thinking patterns accompany or precede the development of anxiety. For example, individuals may perceive certain somatic sensations, such as heart palpitations or jittery feelings, as considerably more dangerous than they truly are. The individuals then interpret these sensations as indicating that they are about to experience sudden, imminent danger. Further, these misinterpretations may arise from fear and other emotions or from stimuli such as caffeine or exercise (Roerig, 1999). Clinical Example 19-1 illustrates two different cognitive reactions to the same stressful event.

Social–Cultural Theory (Integrated Theory)

Social–cultural theorists believe integrated social or cultural factors cause anxiety. As a person's personality develops, his or her impression of self may be negative

---

CLINICAL EXAMPLE 19.1

TWO DIFFERENT COGNITIVE REACTIONS TO THE SAME STRESSFUL EVENT

JB and SV, two college roommates, received probationary notices because of failure to complete a required course successfully. JB made an appointment to discuss her grades with her advisor, whereas SV was unable to sleep and complained of a headache, lightheadedness, and shortness of breath and began to doubt her ability to continue in college.

JB exhibited effective coping skills and accepted responsibility for her actions, thereby showing a positive response to the stress of probationary action. SV exhibited signs of anxiety, a maladaptive response to the stress of probationary action. As a child, she may have had limited opportunity to condition herself to stress, her parents may have fostered dependency by making decisions for her, or this may have been her first experience with what she considered a failure.

(low self-concept). The person experiences difficulty adapting to everyday social or cultural demands because of this low self-concept and inadequate coping mechanisms. The stressful stimuli of society and one's culture pose a psychological threat for such a person, possibly resulting in the development of maladaptive behavior and the onset of an anxiety disorder. For example, a 19-year-old man has difficulty maintaining a C average in high school and does not fit in with his peers. He works as a delivery person for a pizza company. As he makes a delivery, he receives a traffic ticket for driving with a faulty muffler. The police officer informs him that he will not be fined if he replaces the defective muffler within 24 hours. The young man makes an appointment to have his car fixed. However, his employer says he cannot allow him to take the time off. The young man becomes tense and experiences feelings of dizziness, tachycardia, and shortness of breath as he responds to his employer's comment. Because of inadequate coping mechanisms, he is unable to consider alternate options, such as asking the employer to use the company car for a day or suggesting that he change work schedules with another employee. His low self-concept prevents him from pointing out to his employer that he has been a faithful employee with a good work record, and therefore his request should receive special consideration due to the nature of the problem. Unless this young man develops a positive self-concept and adequate coping mechanisms, he will continue to experience difficulty dealing with the stress of daily social or cultural problems.

Clinical Symptoms and Diagnostic Characteristics

The clinical symptoms of anxiety are numerous. They are generally classified as physiologic, psychological or emotional, behavioral, and intellectual or cognitive responses to stress. (See the accompanying Clinical Symptoms and Diagnostic Characteristics box). The clinical symptoms may vary according to the level of anxiety exhibited by the client.

Anxiety occurs on a continuum, ranging from normal to panic. This range is often referred to as the *levels of anxiety.*

- Normal: The client may experience periodic warnings of a threat—such as uneasiness or apprehension—that prompt the client to take necessary steps to prevent a threat or lessen its consequences (Sadock & Sadock, 2003).

CLINICAL SYMPTOMS AND DIAGNOSTIC CHARACTERISTICS / ANXIETY

CLINICAL SYMPTOMS

Physiologic Symptoms
- Elevated pulse, blood pressure, and respiration
- Dyspnea or hyperventilation
- Diaphoresis
- Vertigo or lightheadedness
- Blurred vision
- Anorexia, nausea, and vomiting
- Frequency of urination
- Headache
- Insomnia or sleep disturbance
- Weakness or muscle tension
- Tightness in the chest
- Sweaty palms
- Dilated pupils

Psychological or Emotional Symptoms
- Withdrawal
- Depression
- Irritability
- Crying
- Lack of interest or apathy
- Hypercriticism
- Anger
- Feelings of worthlessness, apprehension, or helplessness

Behavioral Symptoms
- Pacing
- Inability to sit still
- Fingering hair continuously or other nervous habits
- Hypervigilance

Intellectual or Cognitive Symptoms
- Decreased interest
- Inability to concentrate
- Nonresponsiveness to external stimuli
- Decreased productivity
- Preoccupation
- Forgetfulness
- Orientation to past rather than present or future
- Rumination

DIAGNOSTIC CHARACTERISTICS
- Vary based on anxiety disorder diagnosed

- Euphoria: The client experiences an exaggerated feeling of well-being that is not directly proportional to a specific circumstance or situation. Euphoria usually precedes the onset of mild anxiety. However, many individuals experience episodic euphoria without transitioning to mild anxiety.
- Mild anxiety: The client has an increased alertness to inner feelings or the environment. At this level, an individual has an increased ability to learn, experiences a motivational force, may become competitive, and has the opportunity to be individualistic. Feelings of restlessness may also be present, and the individual may not be able to relax. Individuals working under stress to meet certain deadlines may experience an acute state of mild anxiety until their work is completed. Clients with a history of chronic anxiety may experience frequent episodes of restlessness, tremulous motor activity, rigid posture, and the inability to relax.
- Moderate anxiety: The client experiences a narrowing of the ability to concentrate, with the ability to focus or concentrate on only one specific thing at a time. Pacing, voice tremors, increased rate of speech, physiologic changes, and verbalization about expected danger occur. Clients who seek treatment for anxiety generally present with these symptoms during an acute phase.
- Severe anxiety: The ability to perceive is further reduced, and focus is on small or scattered details. Inappropriate verbalization, or the inability to communicate clearly, occurs because of increased anxiety and decreased intellectual thought processes. Lack of determination or the ability to perform occurs as the person experiences feelings of purposelessness. Questions such as "What's the use?" or "Why bother?" may be voiced. Physiologic responses also occur as the individual experiences a sense of impending doom. Severe anxiety may occur before a client seeks help.
- Panic state: Complete disruption of the ability to perceive takes place. Disintegration of the personality occurs as the individual becomes immobilized, experiences difficulty verbalizing, is unable to function normally, and is unable to focus on reality. Physiologic, emotional, and intellectual changes occur as the individual experiences a loss of control. A client may experience all levels of anxiety during treatment before clinical symptoms are stabilized.

The *Diagnostic and Statistical Manual of Mental Disorders, 4th Edition, Text Revision (DSM-IV-TR)* identifies several different anxiety disorders, each with its own set of criteria (American Psychiatric Association [APA], 2000). Anxiety disorder due to a medical condition is discussed in Chapter 20. Substance-induced anxiety disorder is included in Chapter 25 along with other substance-abuse disorders.

Panic Disorder With or Without Agoraphobia

Panic disorder is a real illness with both a physical and a psychological component. This debilitating condition affects approximately 1.7% (2.4 million) of the adult U.S. population and has a very high comorbidity rate with major depression. The onset usually begins during the late teens or early twenties. Although it can occur in both men and women, women are twice as likely to be afflicted as are men (ADAA, 2003).

Three types of panic attacks have been identified. Typically, an individual's first panic attack seems to occur "out of the blue" while the person is engaged in some ordinary activity such as grocery shopping, driving a car, or doing housework. The individual suddenly experiences frightening and uncomfortable symptoms that may include terror, a sense of unreality, or a fear of losing control. Such *unexpected panic attacks* occur without warning and for no discernable reason, as noted above.

Situational panic attacks occur in response to specific environmental stimuli or events that are anxiety producing (eg, riding in an elevator or flying on an airplane). *Situationally predisposing panic attacks* refer to an attack with the likelihood or potential to reoccur when an individual's anxiety level increases. If the client is able to utilize anxiety-reducing coping skills, the likelihood of a panic attack's reoccurring decreases (Richards, 2003).

The differential diagnosis for a client with panic disorder includes a large number of medical disorders (eg, cardiovascular, pulmonary, endocrine, or neurologic diseases, or electrolyte imbalances) and many psychiatric–mental health disorders (eg, drug intoxications, drug withdrawal, eating disorders, or cognitive disorders). After the presence of an immediately life-threatening condition is ruled out, the clinical suspicion is panic disorder (Sadock & Sadock, 2003).

According to *DSM-IV-TR* diagnostic criteria, panic attacks are not caused by the direct physiologic effects of a substance or a general medical condition, and they are not better accounted for by another mental disorder. Panic attacks usually last between 1 minute and 1 hour. The intensity of the attacks may fluctuate considerably in the same person (NIMH, 2000). See the accompanying Clinical Symptoms and Diagnostic Characteristics box.

The client develops these symptoms suddenly, with the symptoms increasing in intensity within minutes of awareness of the first sign. For example, chest pain occurs, followed by three other symptoms that increase in intensity within 10 minutes of the onset of chest pain. (The diagnosis here would be Panic Disorder Without Agoraphobia.) See Clinical Example 19-2.

During the panic attack, the individual may experience a fear of being alone in a public place (**agoraphobia**). Most researchers believe agoraphobia develops as a complication in clients with panic disorder; that is, clients have a fear of having a panic attack in a public place from which escape would be difficult (Sadock & Sadock, 2003). (See discussion of

---

CLINICAL EXAMPLE 19.2

THE CLIENT WITH PANIC DISORDER

MJ, a 21-year-old woman who lived in New York, recently became engaged to a marine stationed in California. On four separate occasions 2 weeks after her engagement, MJ experienced episodes of dizziness, fainting, fatigue, chest pain, and choking sensations while at work. At the suggestion of her employer, she scheduled an appointment with her family physician to discuss her physical symptoms. After a negative physical examination, the family physician asked MJ if she was excited about her engagement. She hesitated at first, then stated that she loved her fiancé but was reluctant to leave her job, friends, and family to move to California. MJ was able to relate the onset of her symptoms to the time of her engagement. The family physician helped MJ to explore feelings of ambivalence about her engagement and suggested that she seek the help of a therapist. After several weeks of counseling, the panic attacks subsided, and she was able to discuss her feelings with her fiancé.

CLINICAL SYMPTOMS AND DIAGNOSTIC CHARACTERISTICS /
PANIC ATTACK

CLINICAL SYMPTOMS
- Palpitations, pounding heart, or accelerated heart rate
- Diaphoresis
- Tremors
- Shortness of breath or smothering sensation
- Feeling of choking
- Chest pain or discomfort
- Nausea or abdominal distress
- Vertigo
- Feelings of unreality or of being detached from oneself
- Fear of losing control or of going crazy
- Fear of dying
- Numbness or tingling sensations (paresthesia)
- Chills or hot flashes

DIAGNOSTIC CHARACTERISTICS
- Period of intense fear or discomfort
- Evidence of at least four clinical symptoms
- Sudden onset of symptoms, peaking within 10 minutes

---

phobias in the next section.) The diagnosis then would be Panic Disorder With Agoraphobia. After a panic attack, the individual exhibits concern about having additional panic attacks, worries about implications of the attack or its consequences, or displays a significant change in behavior (APA, 2000). About one in three people with panic disorder develop agoraphobia (NIMH, 2005).

Phobias

Phobias are the most common form of mental disorders among women and second among men, affecting 8% (11.5 million) of adult Americans (ADAA, 2003; Sadock & Sadock, 2003). A **phobia** is described as an irrational fear of an object, activity, or situation that is out of proportion to the stimulus and results in avoidance of the identified object, activity, or situation. The person unconsciously displaces the original internal source of fear or anxiety, such as an unpleasant childhood experience, to an external source. Avoidance of the object or situation allows the person to remain free of anxiety.

A *phobic reaction* can be so mild that it hardly affects a person's life. The feared object or situation may enter the person's life so rarely that the phobia does not interfere with daily functioning. Other phobias, such as fear of water, may prohibit common activities such as taking a shower or brushing one's teeth. Three major types of phobias are described here.

Agoraphobia

Recognized as the most common phobic disorder, *agoraphobia* is the fear of being alone in public places from which the person thinks escape would be difficult or help would be unavailable if he or she were incapacitated. Normal activities become restricted and individuals refuse to leave their homes.

Approximately 3.2 million American adults ages 18 to 54 years have agoraphobia. Two thirds of those exhibiting clinical symptoms are women, in whom symptoms develop between the ages of 18 and 35 years. Because some cultural or ethnic groups restrict the participation of women in public life, this practice must be considered before diagnosing an individual with agoraphobia. Onset of symptoms may be sudden or gradual. Clients are likely to develop depression, fatigue, tension, and spontaneous obsessive or panic disorders (APA, 2000; NIMH, 2005).

Social Phobia

Social phobia, also referred to as *social anxiety disorder,* is a compelling desire to avoid situations in which others may criticize a person. Social phobia begins in childhood or adolescence, interferes with development, predisposes one to depression and substance abuse, and prevents one from working, dating, or getting married. Early identification is important. (See Supporting Evidence for Practice 19-1.) Social phobia is considered to be the third largest psychological problem in the United States, affecting approximately 5.3 million (3.7%) Americans yearly (ADAA, 2003). First-degree relatives of persons with social phobia are about three times more likely to be affected with social phobia than are first-degree relatives of those without psychiatric–mental health disorders. Because onset usually begins in childhood or adolescence, it is important that social phobia be differentiated from appropriate fear and normal shyness (ADAA, 2003).

Examples of social phobias include fears of performing in public, of public speaking, of eating or drinking in public, of using public restrooms, or of using public transportation. The person realizes that the fear is excessive or disproportionate to the activity or situation. Social phobia rarely is incapacitating, but may cause considerable inconvenience. The abuse of alcohol and other drugs may occur as the person with social phobia attempts to reduce anxiety. Other comorbid disorders, including major depression, body dysmorphic disorder (Chapter 20), or a medical condition, may exist.

The person with clinical symptoms of social phobia experiences persistent, irrational fear of criticism, humiliation, or embarrassment. Because they avoid social situations and often experience a disruption in school, academic achievement, or job performance, clients are misdiagnosed 90% of the time with disorders such as schizophrenia, bipolar disorder, avoidant personality disorder, or depression. It is rare for clinical symptoms to develop after a person reaches the mid-twenties (ADAA, 2003; Richards, 2003; Sadock & Sadock, 2003).

In certain cultures, such as Japanese or Korean, individuals may develop persistent and excessive fears of giving offense to others in social situations instead of being embarrassed themselves. Such fears may cause extreme anxiety and avoidance of social interactions.

Specific Phobia

A specific phobia is defined as an excessive fear of an object, an activity, or a situation that leads a person to avoid the cause of that fear. Approximately 6.3 million (4.4%) Americans are affected yearly. Women are twice as likely to be affected as are men (ADAA, 2003).

The *DSM-IV-TR* lists five subtypes of this disorder: animal, natural environment, blood–injection–injury, situational, and other (eg, fear of space, sound, or costumed characters). Overall, there are approximately 700 identified phobias. Some of the more common ones are listed in Box 19-1.

SUPPORTING EVIDENCE FOR PRACTICE 19.1
Identifying Social Phobia in the Primary Care Setting

PROBLEM UNDER INVESTIGATION / How to identify the prevalence of social phobia, psychiatric comorbidity, the relationship of social phobia to functional impairments, and patterns of health care use in primary care practice

SUMMARY OF RESEARCH / There were 511 adult subjects, 341 of whom were women, most (55.2%) of whom were white, and 41.2% of which had >3 years of college education. Thirty-six of the subjects, who screened positive for social phobia by use of the Social Phobia Questionnaire, were invited for a follow-up interview using the Comprehensive International Diagnostic Interview. The subjects were then asked to rate anxiety and avoidance related to 10 social situations (eg, public speaking or party attendance). The results of the survey indicated that 10 of the 36 respondents with social phobia met criteria for generalized subtypes of social phobia. Comorbid psychiatric disorders of major

depression (58%), generalized anxiety (30.6%), panic disorder (27.8%), and substance abuse within 12 months (25%) were identified. Functional impairment, emergency room visits, primary care appointments, and mental health care visits were more prevalent in subjects with social phobia than in the subgroup of respondents who did not meet *DSM-IV* criteria for the disorders being evaluated and used for comparison.

SUPPORT FOR PRACTICE / Many psychiatric disorders (eg, depression and anxiety) are identified in the primary care setting; however, social phobia is not as well known and therefore may go undetected. Psychiatric–mental health nurses may want to screen for social phobia in clients who present with clinical symptoms of depression or panic attacks.

SOURCE: Stein, M. B., McQuaid, J. R., Laffaye, C., & McCahill, M. E. (1999). Social phobia in the primary care medical setting. Journal of Family Practice, 49(7), 514–519.

BOX 19.1 | **COMMON PHOBIAS**

- Acrophobia: fear of heights
- Agoraphobia: fear of open places
- Algophobia: fear of pain
- Androphobia: fear of men
- Astrophobia: fear of storms, lightning, or thunder
- Autophobia: fear of being alone
- Aviophobia: fear of flying
- Claustrophobia: fear of enclosed places
- Entomophobia: fear of insects
- Hematophobia: fear of blood
- Hydrophobia: fear of water
- Iarrophobia: fear of doctors
- Necrophobia: fear of dead bodies
- Nyctophobia: fear of night
- Ochlophobia: fear of crowds
- Ophidiophobia: fear of snakes
- Pathophobia: fear of disease
- Pyrophobia: fear of fire
- Sitophobia: fear of flood
- Thanatophobia: fear of death
- Topophobia: fear of a particular place
- Zoophobia: fear of animals

The content of phobias as well as their prevalence varies with culture and ethnicity. A specific phobia must be diagnosed only if the fear is excessive in the context of the specific culture and the fear causes a significant impairment or distress. See Clinical Example 19-3.

Generalized Anxiety Disorder

Generalized anxiety disorder (GAD) is characterized by unrealistic or excessive anxiety and worry occurring more days than not in a 6-month period. The concern is about several events, such as job or school performance, and the individual is unable to control the worry. At least three of the following six symptoms are reported: restlessness, fatigue, impaired concentration, irritability, muscle tension, and sleep disturbance. The anxiety interferes with social, occupational, or other important areas of functioning and is not the direct result of a medical condition or substance abuse. GAD can begin across the life cycle, but the risk is highest between childhood and middle-age (ADAA, 2003; APA, 2000).

GAD, commonly seen in the primary care setting, is associated with disability, medically unexplained symptoms, and overuse of health care resources

THE CLIENT WITH A PHOBIA DISORDER

MS, 19 years old, was attending a movie when she began to perspire profusely, tremble, breathe rapidly, and feel nauseated. She left the movie before it ended. Her symptoms became more common when she was around a group of people. As a result of these feelings, MS began to avoid crowds, and her daily activity consisted of going to work and returning home immediately after work. Within a month, MS became housebound. She attempted to relieve her anxiety by using alcohol to relax, but did not experience any relief. MS was encouraged by her family to seek psychiatric help. Counseling revealed that she had been lost in a crowd as a child while attending a circus and had been separated from her parents for several hours. Recently, she had moved into an apartment. The therapist explored her feelings about moving away from the family home. Memories of being separated from her parents as a child were identified as the underlying cause of her phobic reaction.

THE CLIENT WITH GENERALIZED ANXIETY DISORDER

RP, a 50-year-old man, was admitted to the psychiatric hospital for treatment of a generalized anxiety disorder. As the student nurse completed the initial assessment form, she noted that RP was quite restless, sitting on the edge of his bed and fidgeting with his gown. He constantly rearranged his personal items on the bedside stand. Complaints of dizziness, an upset stomach, insomnia, and frequency of urination were noted. RP appeared to be easily distracted as various people walked into the room to care for another client and was rather impatient with the student nurse as she took the admitting vital signs. The client's hands were cold and clammy and the radial pulse was 120 while the client sat on the edge of his bed.

During postclinical conference, the student nurse shared her feelings of irritation about RP. She also stated that the client's anxiety was "infectious" and that she found herself becoming tense although she tried to remain calm during the admission procedure. Another student stated that she would have given RP a sedative first to allow him to settle down and then would have attempted to carry out the initial assessment. The group discussed interpersonal reactions with persons who exhibit clinical symptoms of generalized anxiety and how easy it would be to avoid contact with the client.

(Roerig, 1999). Approximately 2.8% (4 million) of the adult U.S. population is affected. Women are twice as likely as men to be afflicted (ADAA, 2003). The comorbidity of GAD and other disorders is very likely (ADAA, 2003). See Clinical Example 19-4.

Obsessive–Compulsive Disorder

OCD is characterized by recurrent **obsessions** (a persistent, painful, intrusive thought, emotion, or urge that one is unable to suppress or ignore) or **compulsions** (the performance of a repetitive, uncontrollable, but seemingly purposeful act to prevent some future event or situation), or a combination of both, that interferes with normal life. Currently, OCD is recognized as the fourth most common mental health diagnosis in the world, after depression, substance abuse, and phobia. Approximately 2.3% (3.3 million) of the U.S. adult population in all socioeconomic classes is afflicted with this disorder.

Approximately one third of afflicted adults had their first symptoms in childhood. Although the mean age of onset is 20 years, OCD can occur as early as 2 years of age (ADAA, 2003; APA, 2000; Pavlovich-Danis, 2000).

Common obsessive thoughts involve religion, sexuality, violence, the need for symmetry or exactness, and contamination. Everyone has experienced recurrent thoughts at one time or another. Lines of a song or poem may invade one's thoughts and continually run through one's mind. The difference is that obsessions are considered senseless or repugnant, and they cannot be eliminated by logic or reasoning. A repetitive thought of killing one's mate is an example of a violent obsession (APA, 2000).

Common compulsions include handwashing, avoidance of touch, ritualistic sexual behavior, swallowing, stretching, rocking, and hoarding. For example, a client may wash his or her hands 100 times a day to avoid contamination or illness. An **ideational compulsion** is an urge to carry out an act within one's mind. Examples of this type of compulsion are replicating words or speech in one's mind or drawing in one's mind. Such actions are common in children and adolescents. Resistance to the act increases anxiety. Yielding to the compulsion decreases anxiety, the primary gain (APA, 2000).

Approximately 18% to 42% of clients with OCD exhibit hoarding and saving compulsions. Such behavior may be part of a broader clinical syndrome that includes indecisiveness, perfectionism, procrastination, difficulty organizing tasks, and avoiding routine daily activities (Frost & Hanl, 1996; Steketee & Frost, 2003). People with OCD generally have considerable insight into their own problems. Most of the time, they know their symptoms are senseless or exaggerated and not really necessary. However, this insight into their illness is not sufficient to enable them to control their thoughts or behavior. Some individuals are able to keep their symptoms under control during the hours when they are at work or attending school. However, resistance weakens when symptoms persist over months or years. Several comorbid psychiatric disorders, such as major depressive disorder, alcohol-use disorders, eating disorders, and personality disorders, may exist with OCD (Sadock & Sadock, 2003). Indeed, OCD may become incapacitating. See Clinical Example 19-5.

Post-Traumatic Stress Disorder

PTSD is a syndrome that develops after an individual sees, is involved in, or hears about a traumatic experience, such as the terror attacks on the World Trade Center in New York City and Pentagon in Virginia on September 11, 2001. Although PTSD can appear at any age (children have also experienced PTSD), it is most prevalent in young adults, because they tend to be exposed to precipitating situations. Approximately 3.6% (5.2 million) of the adult U.S. population is afflicted (ADAA, 2003; Sadock & Sadock, 2003).

The more common antecedents of PTSD include sexual abuse; assaultive violence; accidents; traumatic losses such as the sudden death of a spouse; diagnosis of a life-threatening illness in self or loved ones; acts of terrorism; witnessing a violent act; natural disaster; and war-related trauma (Davidson, 2001; Mellman, 1999). Women appear to be more susceptible to PTSD because they are exposed to more personal violence

---

CLINICAL EXAMPLE 19.5

THE CLIENT WITH OBSESSIVE–COMPULSIVE DISORDER

AY, a 56-year-old client, was observed performing the following ritualistic behavior continuously. The only time she would interrupt the activity was to go to the clients' dining room for meals, to attend to personal hygiene at the insistence of the staff, and to sleep. AY would begin by standing at the nurses' station for a few moments, mumbling incoherently at the staff, and then continue by starting on a ritualistic pathway. As she left the nurses' station she would walk 10 steps to the right, touch the wall with her right hand, flicker the light switch, and then proceed to her next objective, approximately 20 steps away. There she would touch another wall, do a 360° turn, and again mumble a few incoherent words. She then headed back to the nurses' station, repeating the behavior on the opposite side of the room. If there were any intrusions during this ritualistic performance, AY would exhibit signs of extreme anxiety. This behavior dominated her life and interfered with her role and social functioning.

Students who observed AY were amazed at the energy she possessed because she never seemed to tire. They were hesitant to approach her during this ritualistic activity because they were uncertain what she might do. One student stated, "I know this sounds foolish, but I'm afraid she might get upset and become hostile toward me." Another student said she felt foolish trying to walk with AY as she attempted to show AY that she wanted to help her and be with her. A third student observed that the behavior was accepted by other clients on the unit and that no one seemed to interrupt AY.

---

than are men. Individuals with a history of a psychiatric disorder who lack social support, respond negatively to life events, perceive themselves as helpless, or have a history of a prior trauma exposure are at risk for the development of PTSD (Davidson, 2001; Mellman, 1999).

Kaiman (2003), a nurse practitioner and clinical specialist, initiated a psychotherapy group for clients with the diagnosis of PTSD. He discusses in detail the clinical symptoms of four aging World War II combat veterans who exhibited clinical symptoms of delayed-onset or exacerbated PTSD. Symptoms include isolation secondary to self-perceived or actual feelings of rejection by peers; unpredictable outbursts of rage; exaggerated startle response; avoidance of feelings; survival guilt; sleep disturbances and nightmares; intrusive thoughts of combat and lost buddies; marital discord resulting in divorce; and the presence of alcohol abuse and depression. See the accompanying Clinical Symptoms and Diagnostic Characteristics box.

The diagnosis of *acute onset* refers to symptoms that last fewer than 3 months. If symptoms persist beyond 3 months, the diagnosis of *chronic onset* is used. *Delayed onset* is used to describe the onset of symptoms that occur at least 6 months after exposure to the initial stressful situation or trauma. Impaired role and social functioning may occur. In addition, the client experiences interference with occupational and recreational functioning. Low self-concept and suicidal ideation or thoughts may occur, along with substance abuse, because the individual has difficulty coping with the recollections of the traumatic experience.

PTSD is associated with a greater burden of medical illness than is seen with depression alone. Clinical symptoms may be exacerbated by physical disabilities of the nervous system and the cardiovascular system (eg, head injury, reduced cerebral blood flow, failing vision, or arrhythmias). Furthermore, comorbidity rates are high among clients with PTSD, with approximately 66% of clients having at least two other disorders such as depressive disorder, substance-related disorder, bipolar disorder, or other anxiety disorders. Approximately one third of the comorbid cases persist for many years (Sadock & Sadock, 2003).

Acute Stress Disorder

Acute stress disorder is differentiated from PTSD in that symptoms occur during or immediately after the trauma, last for at least 2 days, and either they resolve within 4 weeks after the conclusion of the event or the diagnosis is changed to PTSD. For example, nurses providing direct or indirect care to clients are at risk for an occupational acute stress disorder. The nurse is exposed to the traumatic event through contact with the client, a phenomenon referred to as **secondary traumatization**. Clinical symptoms may include recurrent images or nightmares about the traumatic event. Repeated exposure to trauma can compromise the client's ability to cope with stress and precipitate

---

CLINICAL SYMPTOMS AND DIAGNOSTIC CHARACTERISTICS /
POST-TRAUMATIC STRESS DISORDER

CLINICAL SYMPTOMS

- Recurrent and intrusive distressing recollection
- Recurrent distressing dreams
- Acting or feeling as if the event were recurring
- Intense psychological distress to internal or external cues symbolizing an aspect of the event
- Physiologic reactions on exposure to stimuli that resemble an aspect of the event
- Avoidance of thoughts, feelings, or conversations associated with the trauma
- Avoidance of activities, places, or people associated with the trauma
- Inability to recall an important aspect of the trauma
- Feeling of detachment or estrangement from others
- Restricted affect
- Insomnia
- Labile emotion
- Decreased concentration
- Hypervigilance
- Exaggerated startle response

DIAGNOSTIC CHARACTERISTICS

- Exposure to traumatic event involving:
  - Experience or witness of, or confrontation with, events involving death (actual or threatened) or serious injury to self or others
  - Resultant feelings of intense fear, helplessness, or horror
- Persistent re-experience of trauma
- Consistent and persistent avoidance of stimuli associated with trauma, such as avoiding thoughts or places, being unable to remember aspects of trauma, or experiencing feelings of detachment
- Persistently heightened feelings of arousal
- Symptoms occurring for longer than 1 month
- Evidence of impairment in functioning

an acute stress disorder (Figley, 1995; Badger, 2001; Schwartz, 2005).

Clients with the diagnosis of acute stress disorder experience dissociative symptoms such as numbness or detachment; a reduction in awareness of surroundings; derealization; depersonalization; or dissociative amnesia. The traumatic event is experienced persistently, although the individual avoids stimuli that arouse recollections of the trauma. Marked symptoms of anxiety or increased arousal occur. Social and occupational functioning are significantly impaired. The individual is unable to pursue necessary tasks (APA, 2000).

Acute stress disorder requires timely diagnosis and treatment to prevent the development of PTSD. Approximately 80% of clients who experience clinical symptoms of acute stress disorder will meet the diagnostic criteria for PTSD 6 months later. Of this group, 75% will continue to meet the diagnostic criteria 2 years after the traumatic event (Bryant, 1999; Harbert, 2002).

Atypical Anxiety Disorder

Atypical anxiety disorder is a catch-all category for clients who exhibit signs of an anxiety disorder, but do not meet criteria for any of the previously described conditions listed in this classification.

THE NURSING PROCESS

ASSESSMENT

Anxiety disorders can be complex, presenting with confounding comorbidities that challenge even the most experienced nurse. The first step in the assessment process is to identify the client's level of anxiety and to determine whether a threat of self-harm or harm to others exists. Obtain a thorough history, if possible, focusing on the client's physiologic, emotional, behavioral, and cognitive functioning, keeping in mind that the client's chief complaint and presenting problem may not be anxiety but one of vague physical or emotional complaints. If possible, use a screening tool or assessment scale.

Screening Tools and Assessment Scales

Various screening tools are available for use in the clinical setting. The mnemonic DREAMS (Box 19-2) and the acronym HARM (Box 19-3) are used to assist nurses in

the recognition of PTSD. The Yale-Brown Obsessive Compulsive Scale (Y-BOCS) also is useful in facilitating diagnosis by identifying thought processes and behavior patterns common to OCD. The Beck Anxiety Inventory (BAI) is commonly used to screen for generalized anxiety disorder and the Fear Questionnaire (FQ) is used to screen for phobias. The Faces Anxiety Scale (FAS) is used in settings such as intensive care units when clients are unable to speak due to the use of mechanical ventilation. Other examples of assessment tools used to evaluate the presence of anxiety include the Hamilton Anxiety Rating Scale, the Liebowitz Social Anxiety Scale, the Sheehan Disability Scale, the Global Assessment Scale, and the Obsessive–Compulsive Disorder Screener (Davidson, 2001; Morgan & Bober, 2005; Pavlovich-Danis, 2000; Silver & Gound, 2002).

Clients with anxiety disorders often receive unnecessary medical tests that lead to excessive costs, misdiagnosis, and unnecessary procedures and treatments. However, a true medical illness must be ruled out. As noted earlier in this chapter, anxiety can occur secondary to a medical condition such as emphysema, hyperthyroidism, or cardiac arrhythmias, or as an adverse effect to medication.

General Description and Appearance

The client with an anxiety disorder may be in severe distress or be immobilized. Alternatively, the client may be engaged in purposeless, disorganized, or aggressive activity. Feelings of intense awe, dread, or terror may occur. The client may express the fear that he or she is "losing control." Clients who exhibit such signs of acute anxiety or panic state may harm themselves or others and need to be supervised closely until the level of anxiety is decreased. Such individuals may need to be placed in a general hospital, mental health center, or inpatient psychiatric hospital to ensure a protective environment, stabilize clinical symptoms of anxiety, evaluate for the presence of a comorbid medical or psychiatric–mental health disorder, promote a therapeutic relationship, and develop a plan of care. The stabilization of a serious or life-threatening comorbid medical condition takes precedence.

Communication and Cognitive Ability

During the assessment process, ask the client what he or she believes is causing the problem and if any particular stressor can be linked to the onset of symp-

---

BOX 19.2 DREAMS: A MNEMONIC TOOL FOR SCREENING CLIENTS FOR POST-TRAUMATIC STRESS DISORDER

Detachment: Does the individual detach from the traumatic event or personal relationships?

Re-experiencing: Is the client re-experiencing nightmares, recollections, or flashbacks of the traumatic event?

Event: As a result of the traumatic event, does the client exhibit significant distress accompanied by fear or helplessness?

Avoidance: Does the client avoid close friends or places associated with the traumatic event?

Month: Has the client experienced the identified clinical symptoms for at least 1 month?

Sympathetic: Is the client experiencing sympathetic hypervigilance or hyperarousal symptoms?

Source: Adapted from Lange, J.T., Lange, C. L., & Cabaltica, R. B. G. (2000). Primary care treatment of post-traumatic stress disorder. *American Family Physician, 62,* 1035–1040, 1046.

BOX 19.3 HARM: AN ACRONYM TOOL FOR SCREENING CLIENTS FOR POST-TRAUMATIC STRESS DISORDER

Hyperarousal: Does the client exhibit irritability, difficulty concentrating, insomnia, or a heightened startle reflex?

Avoidance: Does the client avoid people or activities, lack feelings, or feel detached from others?

Re-experiencing: Does the client frequently experience nightmares, recollections, or flashbacks about the traumatic event?

Month: Has the client experienced related symptom clusters for at least 1 month? Did the onset of symptoms occur at least 6 months after the traumatic event?

Source: Adapted from Silver, M., & Gound, M. (2002). Posttraumatic stress disorder: Recognition and recovery. *ADVANCE for Nurse Practitioners, 10*(11), 65–68, 80.

---

toms. The client's response will give firm clues about the acuity of the situation. Many clients, when asked what is going on in their life, will relate information in great detail. Therefore, exercise caution to ensure that the client provides adequate information to facilitate the assessment process but not so much as to overwhelm the nurse and prolong the process.

Assessing the client's cognitive abilities is also important because an impairment in cognitive ability may interfere with the client's ability to communicate accurate information to the nurse or to participate in the development of the plan of care. Clients experiencing anxiety may be oriented to past events rather than present or future, have difficulty concentrating, exhibit the inability to recall recent or past events, verbalize recurrent or obsessive thoughts, or demonstrate nonresponsiveness to external stimuli.

Mood, Affect, and Feelings

Asking a question such as "How do you feel about what is happening in your life?" gives the client an opportunity to get in touch with and label his or her feelings. Clients who are anxious commonly state that they are angry, fearful, or depressed. It is important to determine whether similar symptoms have occurred in the past;

what happened to cause the past distress; the frequency and duration of the symptoms; and how the client coped with them (Smith-Alnimer, 1996; Storz, 1999).

If possible, also obtain information from a significant other or family member to validate the client's responses. Perceptions can be distorted in the presence of severe anxiety.

Behavior

Common behavioral symptoms of anxiety include pacing, the inability to sit still, hypervigilance, and sleep disturbances. Sleep disturbances may include sleep-onset insomnia, sleep-maintenance insomnia, re-experiencing symptoms (eg, nightmares related to trauma), or a hyperarousal state (eg, difficulty initiating and maintaining sleep). Also assess the client for the presence of nervous habits (eg, nail biting or finger tapping), an exaggerated startle response, avoidance behavior due to a phobia or associated with a traumatic event, or compulsive behavior. Occupational functioning and social or family relationships may be impaired. Ask the client how long the symptoms have persisted and what he or she has done to minimize them. For example, does the client self-medicate with over-the-counter drugs, take prescription drugs, or use alcohol or other substances that have a potential for abuse? Be sure to obtain a list of all medications the client takes for the management of clinical symptoms of medical and/or psychiatric disorders.

Transcultural Considerations

Considerable cultural variation exists in the expression of anxiety. When assessing clinical symptoms exhibited by a client, consider the cultural context, cultural norms, and environmental setting.

Epidemiologic studies have demonstrated panic disorder occurring throughout the world. In some cultures, panic attacks may involve intense fear of witchcraft or magic. Exposure to trauma is more common in cultural settings such as Palestine, Israel, Algeria, Ethiopia, and Cambodia, where rape, combat, politically motivated torture, or genocide are prevalent. Approximately one third of individuals exposed to severe trauma develop PTSD. The risk for the development of clinical symptoms increases proportionately with the duration and severity of the trauma. Rape is the most common trigger of PTSD.

Immigrants from some countries, such as Cuba, Mexico, or Middle Eastern countries, may be reluctant to discuss experiences of torture or PTSD due to fear of reprisal as they seek political asylum. Research studies have shown that displaced individuals such as Cambodian refugees relocated in the United States may exhibit PTSD symptoms for decades. The effects depend on the economic, social, and cultural conditions from which refugees are displaced and in which refugees are placed. In addition to trauma, other factors that may contribute to PTSD include having poor English skills; being unemployed, retired or disabled; living in poverty; or being older (Kilgore, 2005).

When establishing the diagnosis of a specific phobia, the fear must be considered excessive when compared to cultural norms. Moreover, culturally prescribed ritualistic behavior that exceeds cultural norms, that occurs at times and places judged to be inappropriate by others of the same culture, and that interferes with social role functioning meets the criteria for OCD.

Some cultures, especially those of the Middle East such as Afghani and Pakistani, restrict participation of women in public life. This cultural norm must be distinguished from the diagnosis of agoraphobia (APA, 2000).

NURSING DIAGNOSES

Formulating nursing diagnoses for clients exhibiting clinical symptoms of anxiety is challenging because subjective data may be difficult to validate due to the client's increased level of anxiety. Consider factors that necessitate nursing care, such as activity level, communication, sleep pattern, self-perception, relationship with others, sexuality, and coping skills. The possibility that a medical problem could be causing the symptoms also must be considered. Some Examples of North American Nursing Diagnosis Association (NANDA) Nursing Diagnoses are listed in the accompanying box.

OUTCOME IDENTIFICATION

When identifying appropriate outcomes, consider factors such as the client's physical status and activity tolerance; severity of clinical symptoms; presence or absence of support systems; and the clinical setting in which treatment occurs. Examples of Stated Outcomes are highlighted in the accompanying box.

PLANNING INTERVENTIONS

Interventions are planned based on the severity of symptoms, presence of comorbid (medical diagnosis or psychiatric diagnosis such as depression) conditions, and the client's motivation for treatment. Focusing on six areas for the client can help the client develop an increased tolerance of anxiety and an increased awareness of strengths and limitations (Johnson, 1997). These areas are:

1. Acceptance that the experience of anxiety is natural and inevitable
2. Understanding that one's level of anxiety may fluctuate
3. Understanding that shame is a self-imposed response to anxiety
4. Ability to learn and apply self-help techniques to reduce anxiety
5. Ability to remain calm in anxiety-producing situations
6. Development of problem-solving and coping skills

IMPLEMENTATION

Maintain a calm, nonjudgmental approach to convey acceptance toward the client. Initially, during interactions, use short, simple sentences to reduce the client's heightened response to environmental stimuli. Remember that clients with anxiety are often unable to screen stimuli and may become overwhelmed in unfamiliar surroundings.

EXAMPLES OF NANDA NURSING DIAGNOSES/ ANXIETY DISORDERS

- Anxiety related to impending divorce as evidenced by client's apprehension, lack of self-confidence, and statement of inability to relax
- Impaired Verbal Communication related to decreased attention secondary to obsessive thoughts
- Ineffective Coping related to poor self-esteem and feelings of hopelessness secondary to chronic anxiety
- Post-Trauma Syndrome related to physical and sexual assault
- Powerlessness related to obsessive–compulsive behavior
- Disturbed Sleep Pattern related to excessive hyperactivity secondary to recurring episodes of panic
- Impaired Social Interaction related to high anxiety secondary to fear of open places

---

EXAMPLES OF STATED OUTCOMES/ ANXIETY DISORDERS

- The client will verbalize feelings related to anxiety.
- The client will relate decreased frustration with communication.
- The client will demonstrate an improved ability to express self.
- The client will express optimism about the present.
- The client will socialize with at least one peer daily.
- The client will express confidence in self.
- The client will verbalize a reduction in frequency of flashbacks.
- The client will identify factors that can be controlled by self.
- The client will identify stimuli that precipitate the onset of acute anxiety.

Assistance in Meeting Basic Needs

Assist the client in meeting basic needs and encourage verbalization of feelings. Use a firm approach to provide external controls for the client who may be at risk for self-harm or harm to others. Clients with severe anxiety may elicit responses from peers who are unable to tolerate the client's anxiety state. Encourage the client to eat a well-balanced diet. Restlessness, irritability, and inability to concentrate may sometimes be the result of poor nutrition or use of caffeinated beverages. Attempt to channel the client's behavior by engaging the client in physical activities that provide an outlet for tension or frustration and promote sleep.

Medication Management

Psychotropic drugs are generally reserved for moderate-to-severe symptoms of anxiety, especially when the disorder significantly impairs function. A multidimensional pharmacologic treatment approach may be necessary when comorbid medical or psychiatric–mental health disorders exist.

Commonly, the classes of pharmacologic agents prescribed to treat clinical symptoms of anxiety include benzodiazepines, antidepressants, and beta blockers.

Certain anticonvulsants and atypical antipsychotics are also being used. Prior to the advent of short-acting benzodiazepines, other medications such as selective serotonin reuptake inhibitors (SSRIs), and serotonin–norepinephrine reuptake inhibitors (SNRIs), tricyclic antidepressants (TCAs), long-acting benzodiazepines, monoamine oxidase inhibitors (MAOIs), and antihistaminic agents were frequently used.

Benzodiazepines such as clonazepam (Klonopin) and lorazepam (Ativan) are prescribed for anxiety disorders because they work quickly, they are well-tolerated, their dosage may be adjusted rapidly, and they can be used as needed for situational or performance anxiety. However, these agents are no longer recommended as the first line of treatment for most classifications of anxiety. Dependence and difficulties with withdrawal when used long term may occur. In addition, benzodiazepines are associated with the potential for abuse. Antidepressants, particularly SSRIs such as paroxetine (Paxil) and sertraline (Zoloft) and the SNRI venlafaxine (Effexor) are frequently the agents of choice because of their demonstrated effectiveness and lack of abuse and dependence liabilities. The non-benzodiazepine buspirone (BuSpar) may be used to enhance the efficacy of SSRIs. Studies have shown that beta blockers such as propranolol (Inderal) or atenolol (Tenormin), as centrally and peripherally acting agents, are effective in treating social phobia and prevent the development of PTSD in acutely traumatized individuals. Anticonvulsants such as gabapentin (Neurontin) and tiagabine (Gabitril) have also proven effective in the treatment of anxiety disorders. Atypical antipsychotic agents such as risperidone (Risperdal) are generally prescribed when clinical symptoms cause extreme functional impairment or reach paranoid or delusional proportions. They are also used when clients are unable to tolerate benzodiazepines or the newer SSRIs approved for treating various anxiety disorders. Hypnotics also may be prescribed temporarily to alleviate insomnia (Pollack, 2004; Sadock & Sadock, 2003; Storz, 1999).

Many therapists believe that psychotropic agents should be prescribed for short-term use only. Drug Summary Table 19-1 lists the common psychoactive drugs used to treat anxiety disorders. Chapter 16 discusses the nurse's role in psychopharmacology.

Interactive Therapies

After the client's level of anxiety is stabilized, discuss expected outcomes with the client. The six areas stated earlier in planning interventions are also addressed during participation in various interactive therapies and treatment modalities.

Individual psychotherapy can be effective when the client's symptoms do not affect functioning to a significant degree. Clients with the diagnosis of GAD and PTSD often benefit from this form of therapy, which includes educational and supportive counseling. The client is provided with informational literature; taught relaxation techniques; encouraged to participate in diversional activities and hobbies; and encouraged to express his or her feelings and concerns.

DRUG SUMMARY TABLE 19-1 ❦ Drugs Used for Anxiety Disorders

GENERIC (TRADE) NAME	DAILY DOSAGE RANGE	IMPLEMENTATION
Drug Class: Benzodiazepines		
alprazolam (Xanax) GAD, panic disorder	0.5–8 mg	Instruct client to avoid use of alcohol and sleep-inducing or over-the-counter drugs and not to drive a car if dizziness or drowsiness occurs; instruct client about the potential for drug dependence and withdrawal syndrome if drug is discontinued abruptly.
clonazepam (Klonopin) GAD, panic disorder, performance anxiety	0.5–20 mg	Monitor liver function and blood count in clients receiving long-term therapy; monitor for mild paradoxical excitement during the first 2 weeks of therapy, respiratory distress, palpitations, and constipation; instruct client to avoid use of alcohol and sleep-inducing or over-the-counter drugs.
lorazepam (Ativan) GAD, performance anxiety	1.0–10 mg	Inform client of increased central nervous system depression when taken with alcohol; monitor for transient mild drowsiness or sedation, and mild paradoxical excitement during first 2 weeks of therapy; instruct client to report constipation, dry mouth, or nausea; discuss potential for drug dependence and withdrawal syndrome with client.
Drug Class: SSRIs, SNRIs, and Atypical Agents		
buspirone (BuSpar)* GAD	15–60 mg	Provide sugarless lozenges or ice chips if dry mouth or altered taste occurs; arrange for analgesic if headache or musculoskeletal aches are reported; monitor for dizziness, nervousness, GI disturbances, dreams, nightmares, or excitability.
citalopram (Celexa) OCD	10–60 mg	Limit amount of drug given in prescription to potentially suicidal clients; give in the morning with food if desired; monitor for GI disturbances, diaphoresis, dizziness, insomnia or somnolence, and palpitations; instruct male client that medication may cause ejaculatory disorders.

(Continued on following page)

DRUG SUMMARY TABLE 19-1 🍸 **Drugs Used for Anxiety Disorders** *(Continued)*

GENERIC (TRADE) NAME	DAILY DOSAGE RANGE	IMPLEMENTATION
Drug Class: SSRIs, SNRIs, and Atypical Agents		
escitalopram (Lexapro) GAD	10–20 mg	Contraindicated with use of MAOIs or until after 2 weeks of discontinuation; avoid use in third trimester of pregnancy; do not give with citalopram (Celexa) or alcohol; monitor with use of lithium, oral anticoagulants, NSAIDS, aspirin; monitor for nauseas, sleep disturbance, decreased appetite, abnormal bleeding, and diaphoresis.
fluoxetine (Prozac) GAD, OCD, panic disorder	20–50 mg	Give drug in the morning; give in divided doses if taking 20 mg/day; not to be given concurrently with or until after 2 weeks of discontinuation of an MAOI; avoid use of alcohol; monitor client's response closely in the presence of hepatic or renal impairment or diabetes as well as for headache, nervousness, abnormal sleep pattern, GI disturbances, and weight loss
fluvoxamine (Luvox) OCD	50–300 mg	Give at bedtime; if dose is 100 mg, divide dose and give larger dose at h.s.; limit quantity of dispensed drug to clients at risk for suicide; monitor for dizziness, drowsiness, insomnia, GI disturbances, mania, rash, seizures, and weight loss.
paroxetine (Paxil) GAD, OCD, PTSD, panic disorder, social anxiety disorder	10–60 mg	Give in the morning; not to be given concurrently with or until after 2 weeks of discontinuation of an MAOI; contraindicated with use of pimozide (Orap) or thioridazine (Mellaril); avoid use of alcohol; monitor digoxin, phenytocin, phenobarbital, theophylline, or warfarin levels; do not give St. John's wort concomitantly as it may cause serotonin syndrome; monitor for hyponatremia, abnormal bleeding, tremor, and decreased appetite.
sertraline (Zoloft) GAD, OCD, PTSD, panic disorder, social anxiety disorder	25–200 mg	Give once daily in AM or PM, do not give concurrently with or until after 2 weeks of discontinuation of an MAOI; contraindicated with use of pimozide (Orap); monitor for mania or hypomania, suicidal ideation, hyponatremia, weight loss, tremor, serotonin syndrome, or GI upset
venlafaxine (Effexor)** GAD, social anxiety disorder	75–375 mg	Monitor BP and reduce dose or discontinue if hypertension occurs; monitor for dreams, tremor, dizziness, somnolence, GI disturbance, and dry mouth.
Drug Class: Beta Blockers		
atenolol (Tenormin) Performance anxiety, panic disorder	50–200 mg	Give with meals if GI disturbances occur; obtain baseline vital signs and monitor for any changes while taking drug; monitor for dizziness, loss of appetite, nightmares, depression, and sexual impotence.
propranolol (Inderal) Performance anxiety panic disorder	40–120 mg	Give with meals to facilitate absorption; monitor BP and pulse while taking drug; monitor for dizziness, drowsiness, blurred vision, GI disturbances, nightmares, sexual impotence, and difficulty breathing.

*Atypical agent

**SNRI

Insight-oriented psychotherapy, which focuses on helping clients understand the unconscious meaning of anxiety, the symbolism of the avoided situation, the need to repress impulses, and the secondary gains of symptoms, is used in the treatment of panic disorder and agoraphobia (Sadock & Sadock, 2003).

Some anxiety disorders, such as GAD, PTSD, social phobia, performance anxiety, panic disorder, and OCD, also respond to cognitive-behavioral therapy. This approach involves teaching the client to recognize and change certain negative or faulty cognitions, and acts by using behavioral techniques to desensitize fears or anxiety. For example, a young woman with the diagnosis of a specific phobia (fear of heights) agrees to participate in cognitive-behavioral therapy. The nurse–therapist plans interventions with the woman's input to desensitize her fear by gradually exposing the woman to various heights. The client also is educated about phobic reactions and is taught relaxation techniques.

Other interactive therapies that have been effective in the treatment of anxiety disorders include virtual reality, group therapy, family therapy, and environmental modification. See Chapters 14 and 15 for a discussion of these therapies and the role of the psychiatric–mental health nurse.

Alternative and Behavioral Therapies/Techniques

Several alternative therapies have proven effective in the reduction of anxiety. Consider the following when caring for clients:

- Visual imagery: This technique has been used effectively to reduce anxiety experienced by clients with cancer. As clients relax, they engage in a fantasy in which they visualize the identified cause of anxiety, such as pain caused by cancer or the cancer itself. A person who has an unresolved conflict, such as not attending the funeral of a loved one, could use this technique in an attempt to work through guilt or unresolved grief.
- Eye movement desensitization and reprocessing: This technique requires the client to watch rapid rhythmic movements of the therapist's hand or a set of lights to distract attention from the stress the client experiences when visualizing the traumatic event such as sexual assault, combat, or a disaster.
- Change of pace or scenery: Walking in the woods or along the beach, listening to music, caring for a pet, or engaging in a hobby are a few ways to change pace or scenery in an attempt to decrease anxiety by removing oneself from the source or cause of stress.
- Exercise or massage: Exercise can be a release or outlet for pent-up tension or anxiety. Massage is soothing and helps to relax one's muscles. Expectant mothers who practice the Lamaze technique for prepared childbirth use effleurage, or a massage of the abdominal muscles during uterine contractions, to promote relaxation.
- Transcendental meditation: The four components of this relaxation technique include a quiet environment, a passive state of mind, a comfortable position, and the ability to focus on a specific word or object. Physiologic, psychological, and spiritual relaxation occurs.
- Biofeedback: In this technique, the client is able to monitor various physiologic processes by auditory or visual signals. This technique has proven effective in the management of conditions such as migraine headaches, essential hypertension, and pain that is the result of increased stress and anxiety.
- Systematic desensitization: Simply stated, this technique refers to the exposure of a person to a fear-producing situation in a systematized manner to decrease a phobic disorder. A behavioral therapist usually works with the client.
- Exposure and response prevention: Clients with OCD and PTSD are exposed several times a week to anxiety situations that trigger clinical symptoms. Positive responses include reduced symptoms maintained over time. This approach is considered to be a form of cognitive-behavioral therapy.
- Relaxation exercises: Various methods are used to help people learn to relax. Common steps to relaxation include taking a deep breath and exhaling (similar to the cleansing or relaxing breathing of Lamaze technique); tensing and then relaxing individual muscles, starting with the head and progressing to the toes; and finally, relaxing all parts of the body simultaneously. Some methods suggest that the person imagine a peaceful scene before doing the exercise.
- Therapeutic touch (TT): This technique is designed to restore balance to a client's energy field.
- Healing touch (HT): This technique is designed to consider how client empowerment, practitioner self-care, and the nature of the therapeutic relationship come to bear on healing (Hutchinson, 1999). Although these therapies are controversial, many nurses practice either TT or HT.
- Hypnosis: Some behavioral therapists use hypnosis to enhance relaxation or imagery. People have also been taught self-hypnosis to decrease anxiety.

- Implosion therapy (flooding): In this behavioral technique, the client imagines or participates in real-life situations that cause increased levels of anxiety or panic sensations. These therapy sessions are rather lengthy and are terminated when the client demonstrates considerably less anxiety than at the start of the session.

Client Education

Nurses play a vital role in educating clients and their family members or significant others about realistic goals and expectations of treatment. Ideally, client education is usually initiated at the time of diagnosis. Several approaches can be used to help clients better understand the wide array of clinical symptoms; prevalence; predisposing factors; prognosis; and treatment of anxiety disorders. The nurse may meet with the client on a one-to-one basis, educational classes may be held, and support groups may be provided. Family members or significant others may also gain access to resources and support groups that can aid in the recovery process. Feedback provided by the nurse or peers enables the client to understand that he or she is not alone in feeling shame, frustration, anger, or rage. Self-help techniques, problem-solving skills, and coping skills are also explored (Davidson, 2001).

EVALUATION

Whether the client requires hospitalization or participated in outpatient treatment, evaluation focuses on the client's response to treatment. Clients who respond to treatment generally self-disclose an understanding of their clinical symptoms, are able to identify causes, and exhibit coping skills to promote behavioral change. The client's understanding of medication management is reviewed if the client is taking psychotropic agents.

Discuss the continuum of care with the client, stressing the importance of maintaining contact with support people and with those who must be contacted if clinical symptoms of anxiety increase and panic or a crisis occur. An example is provided in Nursing Plan of Care 19-1: The Client With Generalized Anxiety Disorder.

M**VIE** viewing **GUIDES**

NURSING PLAN OF CARE 19.1

THE CLIENT WITH GENERALIZED ANXIETY DISORDER

Cindy, a 24-year-old female client, was admitted to the emergency room with complaints of dyspnea, chest pain, rapid pulse, and a feeling of "something stuck in her throat." She stated that the symptoms started approximately a week ago, interfering with her ability to work. Before that time, she had been in good health. Her last physical examination, approximately 6 months ago, was within normal limits. The tentative diagnosis by the emergency room physician was acute respiratory infection.

As she was undergoing different laboratory tests, Cindy's nonverbal behavior included fingering the sheets as she talked, clearing her throat frequently, and shaking her right foot as she sat on the edge of the examining table.

During the nursing assessment, Cindy related feelings of low self-esteem and stated that she felt pressured at times as she attempted to work full-time and take care of an invalid mother who lived with her. She further related that she had no time to herself and was beginning to resent the fact that her mother had to live with her.

DSM-IV-TR DIAGNOSIS: Generalized Anxiety Disorder

ASSESSMENT: Personal strengths: Alert, oriented in all spheres; employed full-time; good physical condition according to last physical examination

Weaknesses: Inability to communicate her feelings to her mother; feelings of low self-esteem and resentment

NURSING DIAGNOSIS: Anxiety related to responsibility of providing care for an invalid mother

OUTCOME: The client will develop effective coping skills or patterns to reduce anxiety.

Planning/Implementation	Rationale
Encourage the client to describe present feelings.	Addressing feelings directly may help diminish the client's anxiety.
Assist the client in identifying positive coping skills.	Identifying positive coping skills may help reduce the client's anxiety and promote self-confidence.
Teach the client relaxation exercises.	Relaxation exercises are effective ways to reduce anxiety.

NURSING DIAGNOSIS: Impaired Verbal Communication related to resentment

OUTCOME: The client will relate feelings verbally and understand the cause of resentment.

Planning/Implementation	Rationale
Encourage verbalization of feelings about client's role reversal as caretaker for an aging mother and the role's impact on her social life.	The more specific the client can be about her feelings, the better she will be able to deal with her present situation.
Assist the client in identifying a support person or group with whom she can openly discuss her feelings.	Supportive therapy may help the client resolve anger and resentment toward her mother.

NURSING DIAGNOSIS: Situational Low Self-Esteem related to change in lifestyle that involves caring for an invalid mother

OUTCOME: The client will verbalize increased feelings of self-worth.

Planning/Implementation	Rationale
Review with the client her strengths and abilities.	The client may not have had feedback about her strengths and abilities.
Encourage the client to reflect on past and present interactions with her mother.	The client may not be aware of the relationship between emotional issues and low self-esteem.
	Reflecting on interactions gives the client an opportunity to explore factors contributing to her situational low self-esteem.
Give positive feedback for sharing of feelings and concerns.	Positive feedback enhances the client's self-worth.

EVALUATION: Prior to discharge from the emergency room, review the discharge plan of care with the client, including follow-up supportive therapy and community resources for home health care for her mother. Ask the client to summarize her understanding and expectations of the suggested interventions.

KEY CONCEPTS

◆ Anxiety is an emotional response to an unknown object or situation, whereas fear is a response to a known or recognized danger.

◆ Anxiety may be experienced in different forms: signal anxiety, anxiety trait, anxiety state, or free-floating anxiety.

◆ The etiology of anxiety is addressed by various theories: genetic, biologic, psychoanalytic, cognitive behavior, and social–cultural or integrated.

◆ Clinical symptoms of anxiety are classified as physiologic, psychological or emotional, behavioral, and intellectual or cognitive.

◆ Anxiety occurs on a continuum from normal to panic state. This range is often referred to as the different levels of anxiety.

◆ The *DSM-IV-TR* classification of anxiety disorders includes panic disorder with or without agoraphobia, phobias, generalized anxiety disorder, obsessive–compulsive disorder, post-traumatic stress disorder, acute stress disorder, anxiety disorder due to a medical condition, substance-induced anxiety disorder, and atypical anxiety disorder.

◆ Nursing interventions for a client with an anxiety disorder are based on the severity of symptoms, presence of comorbid (medical or other psychiatric) conditions, and the client's motivation for treatment. Interventions focus on assisting the client to develop an increased tolerance of anxiety and an increased awareness of strengths and limitations.

◆ Nursing interventions include providing a safe environment in which the client feels accepted, is able to channel behavior in an acceptable manner, and is able to verbalize feelings while meeting basic needs. The nurse uses various interventions and treatment modalities including assistance with meeting basic needs, medication management, interactive therapies such as individual psychotherapy and cognitive-behavioral therapy, alternative and behavioral therapies to reduce anxiety, and client education to assist the client in reaching identified outcomes.

◆ Evaluation focuses on the client's ability to self-disclose an understanding of anxiety, exhibit coping skills to promote behavioral change, and exhibit an understanding of medication management if psychotropic agents are prescribed.

For additional study materials, please refer to the Student Resource CD-ROM located in the back of this textbook.

CHAPTER WORKSHEET

CRITICAL THINKING QUESTIONS

1. Assess your own feelings of anxiety. What causes you anxiety? What physical and cognitive responses occur when you are anxious? At what level do you experience most of your anxiety?
2. Interview a Vietnam veteran about his or her experiences during the war. Are symptoms of post-traumatic stress disorder evident? How might a veteran's experiences compare with those of an experienced inner-city emergency-room nurse? Is PTSD a disorder we should research related to its potential in nurses?
3. Pick four of the eight relaxation techniques discussed in this chapter and experience them yourself. Which provided you with the most relaxation? How might you incorporate some of these techniques into your own life?

REFLECTION

According to the chapter opening quote, clients with anxiety disorders often present with various vague physical complaints. Develop a self-reporting assessment checklist for a client to complete to rule out the possibility of an anxiety disorder. If the client identified several clinical symptoms of anxiety, what interventions would you propose?

NCLEX-STYLE QUESTIONS

1. The nurse assesses a client with the diagnosis of generalized anxiety disorder for which clinical symptoms?
   a. Fear and avoidance of specific situations or places
   b. Persistent obsessive thoughts
   c. Re-experience of feelings associated with traumatic events
   d. Unrealistic worry about a number of events in one's life

2. The nurse understands that which of the following represents the primary gain experienced by a client when giving in to a compulsion?

   a. Attention from others
   b. Decrease in anxiety
   c. Disability payments
   d. Relief from responsibility

3. A client with the diagnosis of obsessive–compulsive disorder is admitted to the psychiatric inpatient unit for treatment when ritualistic behaviors become incapacitating. During the initial phase of treatment, which intervention would be best?

   a. Accepting client rituals
   b. Challenging client rituals
   c. Limiting client rituals
   d. Teaching prevention of rituals

4. A client with post-traumatic stress disorder has symptoms of isolation and avoidance of feelings. He states, "I know that everyone thinks that I'm cold and unfeeling and that's OK with me. I really don't need to become involved with anyone after my experiences." Which nursing diagnosis would be the priority?

   a. Ineffective Role Performance related to persistent fear of trauma
   b. Ineffective Coping related to use of defense mechanisms secondary to post-trauma
   c. Impaired Social Interaction related to self-perceived feelings of rejection by peers
   d. Spiritual Distress related to feelings of guilt secondary to surviving traumatic event

5. The technique of exposing a client to a fear-producing sensation in a gradual manner is called:

   a. Biofeedback
   b. Imaging
   c. Relaxation techniques
   d. Systematic desensitization

6. A client is to receive medication therapy for an anxiety disorder. To reduce the risk of dependence and problems with withdrawal, which of the following agents would the nurse most likely anticipate as being prescribed? Select all that apply.

   a. Paroxetine (Paxil)
   b. Sertraline (Zoloft)
   c. Lorazepam (Ativan)
   d. Venlafaxine (Effexor)
   e. Clonazepam (Klonopin)

Selected References

American Psychiatric Association. (2000). *Diagnostic and statistical manual of mental disorders* (4th ed., text revision). Washington, DC: Author.

Anxiety Disorders Association of America. (2003). Statistics and facts about anxiety disorders. Retrieved November 20, 2003, from www.adaa.org/mediaroom/index.cfm

Badger, J. M. (2001). Understanding secondary traumatic stress. *American Journal of Nursing, 101*(7), 26-32.

Bryant, R. A. (1999, Winter). The acute stress disorder scale: A tool for predicting post-traumatic stress disorder. *Australian Journal of Emergency Management,* 13-15.

Davidson, M. R. (2001). The nurse practitioner's role in diagnosing and facilitating treatment in patients with post-traumatic stress disorder. *American Journal for Nurse Practitioners, 5*(9), 10-17.

Figley, C. R. (1995). Compassion fatigue as secondary traumatic stress disorder: An overview. In C. R. Figley (Ed.), *Compassion fatigue: Coping with secondary stress disorder in those who treat the traumatized* (pp. 1-20). New York: Brunner/Mazel.

Frost, R. & Hanl, T. (1996). A cognitive-behavioral model of compulsive hoarding. *Behavioral Research Therapy, 34,* 341-50.

Harbert, K. (2002). Acute traumatic stress: Helping patients regain control. *Clinician Reviews, 12*(1), 50-58.

Holman, B. L., & Devous, M. D. (1992). Functional brain SPECT: The emergence of a powerful clinical method. *Journal of Nuclear Medicine,* (10).

Hutchinson, C. P. (1999). Healing touch: An energetic approach. *American Journal of Nursing 99*(4), 43-48.

Johnson, B. S. (1997). *Psychiatric-mental health nursing: Adaptation and growth* (4th ed.). Philadelphia: Lippincott-Raven.

Kaiman, C. (2003). Combat veteran. *American Journal of Nursing, 103*(11), 33-42.

Kawachi, I., Sparrow, D., Vokonas, P. S., & Weiss, S. T. (1994). Symptoms of anxiety and risk of coronary heart disease: The normative aging study. *Circulation,* (11).

Kilgore, C. (2005). PTSD symptoms persist in refugees for decades. *Clinical Psychiatry News, 33*(9), 39.

Lange, J. T., Lange, C. L., & Cabaltica, R. B. G. (2000). Primary care treatment of post-traumatic stress disorder. *American Family Physician, 62*(9), 1035-1040, 1046.

Medscape, Inc. (2000). Theories of panic disorder. Psychiatry & mental health clinical management, Section II. Retrieved February 24, 2004, from www.medscape.com/viewarticle/419254_2

Mellman, T. A. (1999, November). Emerging clinical strategies for the comprehensive treatment of PTSD. In CME, Inc. (Ed.),

New approaches to the management of PTSD and panic disorder (p. 5). King of Prussia, PA: SmithKline Beecham Pharmaceuticals.

Morgan, C. D., & Bober, J. F. (2005). Psychological testing: Use do-it-yourself tools or refer? *Current Psychiatry, 4*(6), 56–60, 66.

National Institute of Mental Health. (2000). Facts about generalized anxiety disorder. Retrieved February 23, 2004, from http://www.nimh.nih.gov/publicat/gadfacts.cfm

National Institute of Mental Health. (2005). The numbers count: Mental disorders in America. Retrieved October 27, 2005, from http://www.nimh.nih.gov/publicat/numbers.cfm

Nicolini, H., Cruz, C., Camarena, B., Paez, F., & De La Fuente, J. R. (1999). Understanding the genetic basis of obsessive-compulsive disorder. *CNS Spectrums, 4*(5), 32–34, 47–48.

Norton, P. G. W. (2004). Chromosome 9q may be linked to panic disorder. *Clinical Psychiatry News, 32*(8), 19.

Pavlovich-Danis, S. J. (2000). Obsessive-compulsive disorder, obsessive-compulsive disorder, obsessive-compulsive disorder. *Nursing Spectrum, 10*(20), 12–15.

Pollack, M. H. (2004). Treating anxiety: Current therapies and beyond. *Clinical Psychiatry News Supplement, 32*(8), 10–13.

Richards, T. A. (2003). What is social anxiety/social phobia? Retrieved February 23, 2004, from http://www.anxietynetwork.com/spwhat.html#top

Roerig, J. L. (1999). Diagnosis and management of generalized anxiety disorder. *Journal of American Pharmaceutical Association, 39*(6), 811–821.

Sadock, B. J., & Sadock, V. A. (2003). *Kaplan & Sadock's synopsis of psychiatry: Behavioral sciences/clinical psychiatry* (9th ed.). Philadelphia: Lippincott Williams & Wilkins.

Schwartz, T. (2005). PSD in nurses. *American Journal of Nursing, 105*(3), 13.

Sheehan, D. V. (1999, November). Treatment of the spectrum of anxiety disorder. In CME, Inc. (Ed.), *New milestones in treating anxiety and depression* (p. 13). King of Prussia, PA: SmithKline Beecham Pharmaceuticals.

Silver, M., & Gound, M. (2002). Posttraumatic stress disorder: Recognition and recovery. *ADVANCE for Nurse Practitioners, 10*(11), 65–68, 80.

Smith-Alnimer, M. C. (1996). The client who is anxious. In S. Lego (Ed.), *Psychiatric nursing: A comprehensive reference* (2nd ed., pp. 195–200). Philadelphia: Lippincott-Raven.

Stein, M. B., McQuaid, J. R., Laffaye, C., & McCahill, M. E. (1999). Social phobia in the primary care medical setting. *Journal of Family Practice, 49*(7), 514–519.

Steketee, G., & Frost, R. (2003). Compulsive hoarding: current status of the research. *Clinical Psychiatry Review, 23,* 905–27.

Storz, D. R. (1999). Getting a grip on anxiety. *Clinical Advisor, 2*(3), 17–26.

Suggested Readings

Alper, B. S., & Raglow, G. (2005). Generalized anxiety disorder. *Clinical Advisor, 8*(5), 71–73.

Baker, B. (1999). Virtual reality Tx reduces anxiety. *Clinical Psychiatry News, 27*(4), 1–3.

Black, D. W. (1999). Epidemiology of obsessive-compulsive disorder: Cross culture and economy. *CNS Spectrums, 4*(5), 6–12.

Carpenito-Moyet, L. J. (2006). *Handbook of nursing diagnosis* (11th ed.). Philadelphia: Lippincott Williams & Wilkins.

Chard, K. M., & Gilman, R. (2005). Counseling trauma victims: 4 brief therapies meet the test. *Current Psychiatry, 4*(8), 50, 55–58, 61–62.

Girgenti, J. R. (2004). Hurricane anxiety. *ADVANCE for Nurses, 5*(21), 18–19.

Grinfield, M. J. (1999). When Johnny comes marching home again: POWs face emotional challenges. *Psychiatric Times, 16*(8), 1–4.

Karch, A. M. (2007). *2007 Lippincott's nursing drug guide.* Philadelphia: Lippincott Williams & Wilkins.

Kelly, V. C., & Saveanu, R. V. (2005). Performance anxiety: How to ease stage fright. *Current Psychiatry, 4*(6), 25–28, 33–34.

Knowlton, L. (1999). Screening tools for social anxiety disorder. *Psychiatric Times, 16*(8), 22.

London, R. T. (2004). When thoughts are obsessive. *Clinical Psychiatry News, 32*(8), 32.

Mahoney, D. (2004). Social phobia eased by cognitive-behavioral tx. *Clinical Psychiatry News, 32*(3), 28.

Mason, M. (1999). Weighed down with worry. *Hippocrates, (7),* 15–20.

Norton, P. G. W. (2004). Soldiers' mental health needs are not being met. *Clinical Psychiatry News, 32*(8), 1, 4.

Norton, T. (2004). Strategies for treating PTSD. *Clinical Psychiatry News, 32*(12), 20.

Stein, M. B., McQuaid, J. R., Laffaye, C., & McCahill, M. D. (1999). Social phobia in the primary care medical setting. *Journal of Family Practice, 49*(7), 514–519.

Wiegartz, P. S., & Rasminsky, S. (2005). Treating OCD in patients with psychiatric comorbidity. *Current Psychiatry, 4*(4), 57–58, 61, 65–68.

Yaryura-Tobias, J. A. (1999). Exploring old and new symptoms in obsessive-compulsive disorder. *Psychiatric Times, 16*(6), 30–31.

CHAPTER 20 / SOMATOFORM AND DISSOCIATIVE DISORDERS

These disorders encompass mind–body interactions in which the brain, in ways still not well understood, sends various signals that impinge on the patient's awareness, indicating a serious problem in the body. —SADOCK & SADOCK, 2003
If worrying were harmless, it would not be much of a problem. But worrying does take its toll. And if you stress your system with excessive worry, it is likely to wear out earlier. —TWERSKI, 1995

AFTER STUDYING THIS CHAPTER, YOU SHOULD BE ABLE TO:

1. Discuss the following factors or theories related to somatoform disorders: biologic or genetic factors, organ specificity theory, Selye's general adaptation syndrome, familial or psychosocial theory, and learning theory.
2. Explain the following theories related to dissociative disorders: state-dependent learning theory and psychoanalytic theory.
3. Compare and contrast the clinical symptoms of somatization and conversion disorders.
4. Distinguish between dissociative amnesia and dissociative fugue.
5. Differentiate between anxiety disorder due to a general medical condition and psychological factors affecting a medical condition.
6. Relate the importance of addressing medical issues and cultural differences when assessing a client with a somatoform or dissociative disorder.
7. Articulate at least five common nursing diagnoses appropriate for clients exhibiting somatoform or dissociative disorders.
8. Develop a list of interventions to reduce stress.

LEARNING OBJECTIVES

KEY TERMS

Depersonalization disorder
Dissociative amnesia
Dissociative disorder
Dissociative fugue
Dissociative identity disorder
Dysmorphobia
General adaptation syndrome (GAS)
La belle indifference
Primary gain
Pseudoneurologic manifestation
Secondary gain
Somatoform disorders

Anxiety can occur under many guises that are not readily recognized by the nurse or practicing clinician. For example, clients may experience anxiety as the result of a specific medical condition (eg, hyperparathyroidism), as a result of treatment for a specific medical condition (eg, thyroid medication), or as a result of changes in employment or lifestyle due to a medical condition (eg, myocardial infarct). Anxiety can also precipitate somatic complaints without a physical basis (eg, back pain or gastrointestinal [GI] symptoms) or interfere with the ability to recall important personal information, usually of a traumatic or stressful nature, that is too extensive to be explained by normal forgetfulness. Moreover, the emotional dimensions of medical conditions are often overlooked when medical care is given.

Chapter 19 described the more commonly seen anxiety disorders. This chapter provides an overview of the relationship between anxiety and real or perceived medical conditions and dissociative reactions such as amnesia, fugue, identity disorder, and depersonalization. Possible etiologic theories are discussed, and an overview of each disorder is presented. The steps of the nursing process focus on the more prominent clinical symptoms for each disorder.

Etiology of Somatoform and Dissociative Disorders

Several theories and research studies have attempted to explain the role of stress or emotions in the development or exacerbation of somatoform and dissociative disorders. Following is a brief discussion of these theories.

Theories Regarding Somatoform Disorders

Somatoform disorder is the diagnosis given to individuals who present with symptoms suggesting a physical disorder without demonstrable organic findings to explain the symptoms (American Psychiatric Association [APA], 2000). Theories regarding the etiology of somatoform disorders include biologic and genetic factors, the organ specificity theory, Selye's general adaptation syndrome, the familial or psychosocial theory, and the learning theory.

Biologic and Genetic Factors

Research has suggested that biologic and genetic factors are responsible for the development of certain somatoform disorders. A limited number of brain-imaging studies of clients with clinical symptoms of somatoform disorders have reported decreased metabolism in the frontal lobes and in the nondominant hemisphere (Sadock & Sadock, 2003). Some studies point to a neuropsychological basis for the development of somatization disorder. These studies propose that clients have attention and cognitive impairments that result in faulty perception and assessment of somatosensory inputs.

Genetic data indicate that somatization disorder tends to run in families, occurring in 10% to 20% of the first-degree female relatives of clients with somatization disorder. Research into cytokines (messenger molecules of the immune system that communicate with the nervous system, including the brain) indicates that abnormal regulation of the cytokine system may contribute to the development of nonspecific symptoms of somatoform disorders (eg, hypersomnia, anorexia, fatigue, and depression) (Sadock & Sadock, 2003).

Organ Specificity Theory

In 1953, Lacey, Bateman, and Van Lehn studied characteristic physiologic response patterns that they believed to be present since childhood. They concluded that a person responds to stress primarily with physical manifestations in one specific organ or system, thereby showing susceptibility to the development of a specific disease. This theory is referred to as the *organ specificity theory.* For example, when faced with an emotional conflict, a 25-year-old woman experiences the sudden onset of lower abdominal pain and diarrhea (conversion disorder). The pain and diarrhea give the client a legitimate reason to avoid conflict and persist until the conflict is resolved. She has the potential for development of irritable bowel syndrome if she continues to experience frequent episodes of stress. Other persons may be prone to low back pain, asthmatic attacks, or skin rashes, depending on their susceptible organ or system.

Selye's General Adaptation Syndrome

According to Hans Selye (1978), an individual who copes with the demands of stress experiences a "fight-

or-flight" reaction. The body puts into effect a set of responses that seeks to diminish the impact of a stressor and restore homeostasis. This reaction, termed **general adaptation syndrome (GAS),** occurs in three stages: alarm reaction; resistance in which adaptation is ideally achieved; and exhaustion, in which acquired adaptation or resistance to the stressor is lost. If adaptation occurs, stress does not have a negative effect on an individual's emotional or physical well-being (ie, the "fight" has been won). However, emotional disorders such as anxiety, physical deterioration secondary to a somatoform disorder, or death can occur as a result of continued stress in the presence of a weakened physical condition (ie, the "fight" is lost because the body could not restore homeostasis) (Sadock & Sadock, 2003).

Familial or Psychosocial Theory

Proponents of the familial or psychosocial theory assert that characteristics of dynamic family relationships, such as parental teaching, parental example, and ethnic mores, may influence the development of a somatoform disorder. According to family therapist Salvador Minuchin (1974), role modeling is an important factor in personality development. He identified the "psychomatogenic family" as a group of individuals who internalize feelings of anxiety or frustration rather than express their feelings in a direct manner. As a result of this internalization, they develop physiologic symptoms rather than face or resolve conflict. Children of such families observe the coping mechanisms of their parents and other family members, developing similar behaviors when the need arises, thereby avoiding conflict and experiencing positive reinforcement.

Learning Theory

According to the learning theory, a person learns to produce a physiologic response (somatization) to achieve a reward, attention, or some other reinforcement. Jeanette Lancaster (1980) states that the following dynamics occur during the development of this learned response:

1. The learning is of an unconscious nature.
2. There was a reward or reinforcement in the past when the person experienced specific physiologic symptoms.
3. Reinforcement can be positive or negative. Negative reinforcement is considered better than no reinforcement at all.

4. The person is unable to give up the disorder willfully.

For example, a child stays home from school when he is ill and receives attention from his mother as she reads to him, fixes his favorite meals, and monitors his vital signs. As a result of this experience, he unconsciously learns to produce physiologic symptoms of a migraine headache or an upset stomach as he feels the need for attention. This behavior may continue throughout his life as he attempts to satisfy unmet needs.

Theories Regarding Dissociative Disorders

The diagnosis of **dissociative disorder** is given to individuals who exhibit the separation of an idea or mental thoughts from conscious awareness or from emotional significance and affect (APA, 2000). Some examples of dissociative disorders are **dissociative amnesia** (the inability to recall important personal details because of a psychological or physical trauma), **dissociative fugue** (a person's sudden and unexpected departure from home or work and inability to recall the past), **dissociative identity disorder** (also known as multiple personality disorder), and **depersonalization disorder** (patient experiences a distorted perception of self, body, and life, associated with a feeling of unreality). Theories regarding the etiology of dissociative disorders include the state-dependent learning theory and psychoanalytic theory. Various causative factors have also been identified. Specific disorders will be discussed at length later in the chapter; below are some brief examples to illustrate each theory.

State-Dependent Learning Theory

The theory of state-dependent learning states that dissociative amnesia is caused by stress associated with traumatic experiences endured or witnessed (eg, abuse, rape, combat, natural disasters); major life stresses (eg, abandonment, death of a loved one, financial troubles); or tremendous internal conflict (eg, turmoil over guilt-ridden impulses, apparently unresolvable interpersonal difficulties, criminal behaviors). Memory of the event is laid down during the event, and the emotional state may be so extraordinary that it is hard for an affected person to remember information learned during the event. Furthermore, some individuals are believed to be more predisposed to the development of dissociative amnesia (eg, those who are easily hypnotized) (Merck Manual of Diagnosis and Therapy, 2005; Sadock & Sadock, 2003).

Theorists believe the cause of dissociative fugue is similar to that of dissociative amnesia, with some additional factors. Fugue is thought to remove an individual from accountability for one's actions and may absolve one of certain responsibilities, remove one from an embarrassing situation or intolerable stress, reduce one's exposure to a perceived hazard such as a dangerous, risk-taking job, or protect one from suicidal or homicidal impulses (Merck Manual of Diagnosis and Therapy, 2005).

Psychoanalytic Theory

According to psychoanalytic theory, dissociative amnesia is considered to be a defense mechanism whereby an individual alters consciousness as a way of dealing with an emotional conflict or an external stressor. Secondary defenses include repression, which blocks disturbing impulses from consciousness and denial which allows the conscious mind to ignore external reality (Sadock & Sadock, 2003).

Other Factors

The cause of dissociative identity disorder is unknown; however, four types of causative factors have been identified: a traumatic life event (usually childhood physical or sexual abuse), vulnerability for the disorder to develop, environmental factors, and the absence of external support. Death of a close relative or friend during childhood or witnessing a trauma or death are also traumatic events that can precipitate the development of dissociative identity disorder.

Depersonalization disorder frequently occurs in life-threatening danger such as accidents, assaults, and serious illnesses and injuries. Although it has not been studied widely, depersonalization disorder may be caused by psychological, neurologic, or systemic disease. It has been associated with epilepsy, brain tumors, sensory deprivation, and emotional trauma as well as with an array of abused substances (Merck Manual of Diagnosis and Therapy, 2005; Sadock & Sadock, 2003).

Clinical Symptoms and Diagnostic Characteristics

The more common physiologic, psychological or emotional, behavioral, and intellectual or cognitive

symptoms of anxiety were discussed in Chapter 19. The features, clinical symptoms, and diagnostic characteristics specific to somatoform and dissociative disorders, as well as the relationship between anxiety and medical conditions, based on the information described in the *Diagnostic and Statistical Manual of Mental Disorders, 4th Edition, Text Revision (DSM-IV-TR)*, are presented in this chapter (APA, 2000).

Somatoform Disorders

According to the *DSM-IV-TR*, somatoform disorders are reflected in disordered physiologic complaints or symptoms, are not under voluntary control, and do not demonstrate organic findings. Although symptoms in all of the somatoform disorders cause impairment in social or occupational functioning or create significant emotional distress, the complaints are not fully explained by the objective physical findings (Adams, 2003).

Somatoform disorders are often encountered in general medical settings. There are seven types of somatoform disorders:

1. Body dysmorphic disorder
2. Somatization disorder
3. Conversion disorder
4. Pain disorder
5. Hypochondriasis
6. Undifferentiated somatoform disorder
7. Somatoform disorder, not otherwise specified

Body Dysmorphic Disorder

Individuals with body dysmorphic disorder (BDD) have a pervasive subjective feeling of ugliness and are preoccupied with an imagined defect in physical appearance or a vastly exaggerated concern about a minimal defect. The person believes or fears that he or she is unattractive or even repulsive. The fear is rarely assuaged by reassurance or compliments. If a slight physical abnormality exists (eg, hair, skin, or facial flaws), the person displays excessive concern about it. This preoccupation causes clinically significant distress or impairment in social, occupational, or other important areas of functioning. Obsessive–compulsive traits (Figure 20-1) and a depressive syndrome are frequently present. The most common age of onset of BDD is from adolescence through the third decade of life. Prognosis is unknown because this disorder can persist for several years (Phillips, 2000; Sadock & Sadock, 2003). Previous research suggests this group has poor mental health–related quality of life and high

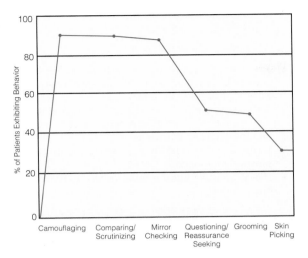

FIGURE 20.1 Ritualistic behaviors, including obsessive–compulsive traits, in body dysmorphic disorder.

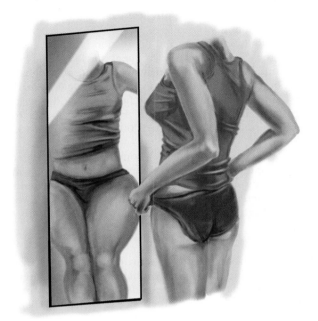

FIGURE 20.2 Client with body dysmorphic disorder.

lifetime rates of psychiatric hospitalization, suicidal ideation, and suicide attempts (Phillips, Siniscalchli, & McElroy, 2004).

The prevalence of BDD (historically known as **dysmorphobia**) in the community is unknown. However, reported rates in clinical mental health settings range from under 5% to approximately 40%. Reported rates in cosmetic surgery and dermatology settings range from 6% to 15% (APA, 2000). According to the American Society of Plastic Surgeons (ASPS), the top five cosmetic surgery procedures in 2003 included nose reshaping, liposuction, breast augmentation, eyelid surgery, and face-lift (ASPS, 2004). Cultural concerns about physical appearance and the importance of proper physical appearance may influence preoccupation with an imagined physical deformity (Figure 20-2). BDD may be equally common in women and men of various cultures. Average age of onset is 16, although diagnosis often doesn't occur for another 10 to 15 years (APA, 2000).

Somatization Disorder

Somatization (Briquet's) disorder was originally described by Briquet in 1859. It is a chronic, severe anxiety disorder in which a client expresses emotional turmoil or conflict through significant physical complaints (including pain and GI, sexual, and neurologic symptoms), usually with a loss or alteration of physical

functioning. Such a loss or alteration is not under voluntary control and is not explained as a known physical disorder. Somatization disorder differs from other somatoform disorders because of the multiple complaints voiced and the multiple organ systems affected.

This disorder is often familial. Although etiology is unknown, it is believed that marked dependency and intolerance of frustration contribute to the verbalization of physical complaints representing an unconscious plea for attention and care. The prevalence of this disorder varies from 5% to 10% in primary care populations, with a female predominance ratio of 20 to 1 (APA, 2000). The onset usually occurs before age 25 years. It is considered a chronic illness in persons demonstrating a dramatic, confusing, or complicated medical history, because they seek repeated medical attention. The physical symptoms or complaints that occur in the absence of any medical explanation govern the person's life, influencing the person to take medication, alter lifestyle, or see a physician. The symptoms are not intentionally produced or feigned. When there is a related general medical condition, the physical complaints or resulting social or occupational impairment are in excess of what would be expected from history, physical examination, or laboratory findings.

In addition, anxiety and depression often are seen, and the client may make frequent suicide threats or attempts. The person also may exhibit antisocial behavior or experience occupational, interpersonal, or marital difficulties. Because the client constantly seeks medical attention, he or she frequently submits to unnecessary surgery (APA, 2000; Sadock & Sadock, 2003).

The type and frequency of somatic symptoms differ across cultures. For example, there is a higher reported frequency of somatization disorder in Greek and Puerto Rican men than in men in the United States. Therefore, the symptom reviews must be adjusted to the culture.

Conversion Disorder

Conversion disorder is a somatoform disorder that involves motor or sensory problems suggesting a neurologic condition. It has been described as an adaptation to a frustrating life experience in which the client utilizes pantomime when direct verbal communication is blocked (Ford & Folks, 1985; Maldonado, 1999). Anxiety-provoking impulses are converted unconsciously into functional symptoms.

The phrase **la belle indifference** is used to describe client reactions such as showing inappropriate lack of concern about the symptoms and displaying no anxiety. This is because the anxiety has been relieved by the conversion disorder. Clients may also exhibit a **pseudoneurologic manifestation** (sensory or motor loss that does not follow neurologic function but rather comes and goes with stress or a functional need). For example, when suddenly awakened or startled, the sensory or motor loss is briefly gone.

Four subtypes of conversion disorder have been identified, based on the nature of presenting symptoms or deficit. These subtypes are highlighted in Box 20-1.

Although the disturbance is not under voluntary control, the symptoms occur in organs that are voluntarily controlled. Conversion symptoms serve four functions:

- Permit the client to express a forbidden wish or impulse in a masked form
- Impose punishment via the disabling symptom for a forbidden wish or wrong-doing
- Remove the client from an overwhelming life-threatening situation (**primary gain**)
- Allow gratification of dependency (**secondary gain**) (Maldonado, 1999).

BOX 20.1 SUBTYPES OF CONVERSION DISORDERS

1. Motor symptoms or deficit such as impaired balance, paralysis of an upper or lower extremity, dysphagia, or urinary retention
2. Sensory symptoms or deficit such as anesthesia or loss of touch or pain sensation, double vision, blindness, or hallucinations
3. Seizures or convulsions with voluntary motor or sensory components
4. Mixed presentation if symptoms are of more than one category

---

Primary gain allows relief from anxiety by keeping an internal need or conflict out of awareness. Secondary gain refers to any other benefit or support from the environment that a person obtains as a result of being sick. Examples of secondary gain are attention, love, financial reward, and sympathy.

Malingering and factitious disorder must be differentiated from conversion disorder, which occurs as a result of unconscious motivation. Malingering is the production of false or grossly exaggerated physical or psychological symptoms that are consciously motivated by external incentives to avoid an unpleasant situation (eg, to avoid work or to obtain drugs). Malingering may also represent adaptive behavior to avoid a traumatic situation (eg, feigning illness to avoid incarceration). Factitious disorder is the consciously motivated production or feigning of physical or psychological symptoms to assume the sick role. External incentives such as economic gain or avoidance of legal responsibility are absent (APA, 2000; Maldonado, 1999).

Several studies have reported that 5% to 15% of psychiatric consultations in the general hospital population and 25% to 40% of Veterans Administration hospital consultations involve clients with conversion disorder. Conversion disorder occurs in 1% to 3% of clients referred to mental health clinics. The onset can occur at any time; however, it is more common in adolescents and young adults. Comorbid psychiatric disorders include major depressive disorder, other anxiety disorders, and schizophrenia (Sadock & Sadock, 2003). Conversion disorder occurs more frequently in the rural population, in individuals of lower socioeconomic status, and in individuals less knowledgeable about medical and psychological concepts. Higher rates are also reported in developing regions (APA, 2000).

Although the disorder may occur for the first time during middle age or later maturity, the typical age of onset is usually late childhood or early adulthood. Such a disorder frequently impairs normal activities, possibly leading to the development of a chronic sick role. Studies suggest that a considerable number of clients diagnosed with conversion disorder may develop a disease process at some time in the future, which may explain the pathological findings presented initially (Maldonado, 1999). See Clinical Example 20-1: The Client Exhibiting Conversion Disorder.

CLINICAL EXAMPLE 20.1

THE CLIENT EXHIBITING CONVERSION DISORDER

BJ, a 45-year-old female, lived on a farm with her husband and three children ages 17, 15, and 12 years. The 17-year-old son assisted his father with several chores, including driving the farm equipment while harvesting crops.

One afternoon, BJ's husband and son did not return for dinner. BJ was quite concerned and asked her daughters to go to the field where her husband was harvesting wheat to see why they were late. Approximately 20 minutes later, both daughters returned and informed their mother that their brother had been injured in an accident and was taken to the hospital by neighbors. They were told that their brother had "mangled" his right arm in the farm equipment.

As BJ listened to her daughters, she became quite upset. When her husband returned from the hospital, BJ complained of localized weakness and double vision, and exhibited an unsteady gait. Her husband insisted that she be seen in the emergency room prior to visiting with her son. BJ was given a thorough physical examination, which ruled out any physiologic cause. The emergency room physician spoke to BJ about her son's accident and determined that BJ was exhibiting clinical symptoms of conversion disorder secondary to anxiety related to her son's traumatic injury.

Pain Disorder

The International Association for the Study of Pain defines pain as "an unpleasant sensory and emotional experience associated with actual or potential tissue damage, or described in terms of such damage" (Victoroff, 2001, p. 20). The diagnosis of pain disorder is given when an individual experiences significant pain without a physical basis for pain or with pain that greatly exceeds what is expected based on the extent of injury. In order for there to be a diagnosis of pain disorder, the pain must disrupt social and/or occupational functioning. For example, an individual who has a history of a back injury verbalizes an increase in pain during the course of financial difficulties and informs his employer that he is unable to work. External factors may amplify the client's clinical symptoms (Adams, 2003).

Although pain disorder may occur at any stage of life, it occurs more frequently in the fourth or fifth decade of life; is more frequent in women who complain of chronic pain such as headaches and musculoskeletal pain; is more common in persons with blue-collar occupations; and occurs in approximately 40% of those individuals who complain of pain. Approximately 10% to 15% of adults in the United States have some form of work disability due to back pain. Comorbid psychiatric disorders include depression, anxiety, and substance abuse (Sadock & Sadock, 2003).

The *DSM-IV-TR* lists two subtypes of pain disorder to clarify further the factors involved in the etiology of pain. The two subtypes are: Pain Disorder Associated With Psychological Factors, and Pain Disorder Associated With Both Psychological Factors and General Medical Condition (see Box 20-2).

Hypochondriasis

Hypochondriasis is a somatoform disorder in which a client presents with unrealistic or exaggerated physical complaints. Minor clinical symptoms are of great concern to the person and often result in an impairment of social or occupational functioning. Preoccupations usually focus on bodily functions or minor physical abnormalities. Such persons are commonly referred to as "professional patients" who shop for doctors because they feel they do not get proper medical attention. Such clients often elicit feelings of frustration and anger from health care providers.

This disorder usually is accompanied by anxiety, depression, and compulsive personality traits. It gener-

BOX 20.2 SUBTYPES OF
PAIN DISORDER

- Pain Disorder Associated With Psychological Factors: Psychological factors are judged to have a major role in the onset, severity, exacerbation, or maintenance of pain. The individual may have a valid reason for pain, but the pain becomes worse in association with life events and/or internal emotional conflicts. General medical conditions play either a minimal or no role in the onset of this disorder.
- Pain Disorder Associated With Both Psychological Factors and General Medical Condition: Diagnostic criteria state that the pain due to a general medical condition is the predominant focus of the clinical presentation and is severe enough to warrant clinical attention. It causes distress or impairment in social, occupational, or other important areas of functioning; however, psychological factors affect the onset, severity, exacerbation, or maintenance of the pain.

ally occurs in early adulthood and usually becomes chronic, causing impaired social or occupational functioning. The person may adopt an invalid's lifestyle, possibly becoming actually bedridden. This disorder is found equally in men and women (APA, 2000).

The disorder can occur at any age, but is more common in the second and third decade of life. Approximately 2% to 7% of clients seen in general medical practice are diagnosed with this disorder. The client becomes preoccupied with the fear of developing or already having a disease or illness in spite of medical reassurance that such an illness does not exist (APA, 2000; Sadock & Sadock, 2003).

Undifferentiated Somatoform Disorder

The diagnosis of undifferentiated somatoform disorder is used when one or more physical complaints, such as fatigue, pain, or loss of appetite, last 6 months or longer and, after appropriate evaluation, cannot be explained by a known general medical condition or the direct effects of a substance. For example, the client may have concurrent conversion, hypochondri-

acal, and somatoform pain symptoms (Adams, 2003). If a medical condition does exist, the complaints or resulting social or occupational impairment are in excess of what should be expected on the basis of a comprehensive physical examination. This is a residual category for presentations that do not meet the full criteria for the disorders previously discussed (APA, 2000; Sadock & Sadock, 2003).

Somatoform Disorder, Not Otherwise Specified

The diagnosis of somatoform disorder, not otherwise specified is used when somatoform symptoms do not meet the criteria for any specific somatoform disorder. Examples include pseudocyesis or a false belief that one is pregnant, nonpsychotic hypochondriasis of fewer than 6 months, and unexplained physical complaints of fewer than 6 months not caused by another mental disorder (APA, 2000; Sadock & Sadock, 2003).

Dissociative Disorders

The essential feature of dissociative disorders is a disruption of integrated functions of consciousness, memory, identity, or perception of the environment. Onset may be sudden, gradual, transient, or chronic.

The *DSM-IV-TR* lists five clinical types of dissociative disorders: dissociative amnesia, dissociative fugue, dissociative identity disorder, depersonalization disorder, and dissociative disorder, not otherwise specified. Dissociative disorder, not otherwise specified is a category in which the predominant feature is a dissociative symptom but it does not meet the criteria for any specific dissociative disorder, such as loss of consciousness not attributable to a general medical condition. Dissociated amnesia, dissociative fugue, dissociative identity disorder, and depersonalization disorder are discussed below.

Dissociative Amnesia

Dissociative amnesia (formerly known as *psychogenic amnesia*) is characterized by the inability to recall an extensive amount of important personal information because of physical or psychological trauma. It is not the result of delirium or dementia. Predisposing factors include an intolerable life situation, unacceptability of certain impulses or acts, and a threat of physical injury or death. Most cases are seen in the hospital emergency department, where the client is taken after a traumatic event or after being found wandering the streets. Dissociative amnesia can be described as:

1. Circumscribed or localized: Occurrence a few hours after a traumatic experience or major event
2. Selective: Inability to recall part of the events of a specific time
3. Generalized: Inability to recall events of one's entire life
4. Continuous: Inability to recall events after a specific event up to and including the present

Clinical features include perplexity, disorientation, and purposeless wandering. Although the client may experience a mild or severely impaired ability to function, it is usually temporary because rapid recovery generally occurs. The condition is more common during natural disasters or wartime. It is most common among young adults. The number of reported cases has increased related to previously forgotten early childhood trauma such as incest or sexual abuse. This increase in reported cases may be caused by the increased awareness of the diagnosis among mental health professionals or an overdiagnosis in individuals who are highly suggestible (APA, 2000; Sadock & Sadock, 2003). See Clinical Example 20-2: The Client With Dissociative Amnesia.

Dissociative Fugue

Dissociative fugue (formerly known as *psychogenic fugue*) differs from dissociative amnesia in that the person suddenly and unexpectedly leaves home or work and is unable to recall the past. Assumption of a new identity, either partial or complete, may occur after relocating to another geographic area where the person is unable to recall his or her previous identity. During the fugue, the person may appear normal and attract no attention. The person may engage in complex social interactions; however, at some point, confusion about one's identity or the return of the original identity may make the person aware of amnesia or cause distress. Fugue is a rare occurrence that may be seen during times of extreme stress such as war, severe conflicts, or natural disasters, and may last days or months. Excessive use of alcohol may contribute to the development of this rare disorder. The person generally must receive psychiatric care because of amnesia regarding recent events or lack of awareness of

---

CLINICAL EXAMPLE 20.2

THE CLIENT WITH DISSOCIATIVE AMNESIA

VW, a 32-year-old male, was carpooling with other employees because his car was in the repair shop. As they left for home on a Wednesday evening, it began to snow heavily. The roads were slippery and visibility was limited. Approximately 2 miles from home, a moving van entered the highway from a shopping center. The driver of the moving van lost control of the truck and hit the driver's side of the automobile in which VW was a passenger. The driver of the automobile was seriously injured, as was the front seat passenger. VW and another employee who was seated in the back seat survived the accident with minor injuries. The driver of the automobile died en route to the hospital. The driver of the moving van escaped injuries. As VW was examined in the hospital emergency room, he was unable to recall the details of the accident and could not recall how he arrived in the emergency room. He also could not recall the names of the passengers in the car.

A thorough physical examination was performed, and a neurologic consult was requested. The results of both examinations revealed that VW was exhibiting clinical symptoms of localized dissociative amnesia.

---

personal identity. Rapid recovery can occur (APA, 2000; Merck Manual, 2005; Sadock & Sadock, 2003).

Dissociative Identity Disorder

Sybil and *The Three Faces of Eve* are popular media representations of persons with dissociative identity disorder (DID), formerly known as *multiple personality disorder*, in which a person is dominated by at least one of two or more definitive personalities that alternatively take over the person's behavior. Emergence of various personalities, or "alters," occurs suddenly and often is associated with psychosocial stress and conflict. When two or more alters exist, each is aware of the other(s) to varying degrees. One personality can interact with the external environment at any given moment. However, one or any number of the other personalities actively perceives all that is occurring. The individual personalities are usually quite different and frequently appear to be opposites. Each is complex and integrated, with its own unique behavior patterns and social relationships. For example, a shy, middle-aged bachelor may present himself as a gigolo on weekends. Passive identities tend to have incomplete or less complex memories. Controlling, hostile, or protective identities have more complete or complex memories.

This disorder may occur in early childhood or later, but rarely is diagnosed until adolescence. The degree of impairment may vary from moderate to severe, and may lead to disability or incapacity, depending on the persistence, number, and nature of the various alters. This disorder can be difficult to identify unless the person is observed closely. It is seen more frequently in adult women than in adult men and has been estimated to occur in approximately 5% of all psychiatric disorders. It is associated with a high incidence of suicide attempts and is believed to be more likely to end in suicide than any other mental disorder (APA, 2000; Merck Manual, 2005; Sadock & Sadock, 2003).

Depersonalization Disorder

The client who exhibits symptoms of depersonalization disorder experiences an uncomfortable, distorted perception of self, body, and one's life that is associated with a sense of unreality. This temporary loss of one's own reality includes feelings of being in a dreamlike state, out of the body, mechanical, or bizarre in appearance. Predisposing factors include fatigue, meditation, hypnosis, anxiety, physical pain, severe stress, and depression. Depersonalization may occur as an occasional isolated incident and is not necessarily pathological (Sadock & Sadock, 2003).

Clinical diagnosis includes documentation of frequent prolonged episodes that impair occupational and social functioning. Dizziness, depression, anxiety, fear of "going insane," and a disturbance in the subjective sense of time are common associated features. Adolescents and young adults are more likely to experience this disorder, which rarely occurs after age 40 years.

Voluntarily induced experiences of depersonalization can occur during the meditative practices of many cultures and religions and should not be confused with this disorder.

Although prognosis is good for the disorder with an acute onset, the person may need to be removed from a threatening situation or environment to prevent the development of a chronic depersonalization disorder that may wax and wane in intensity during future actual or perceived stressful events (APA, 2000).

Anxiety Disorder Due to a General Medical Condition

The essential features of anxiety disorder due to a general medical condition include prominent anxiety, panic attacks, or obsessions or compulsions that are judged to be caused by the direct physiologic effects of a medical condition. Studies indicate that the noradrenergic or the serotonergic system may be the underlying etiology for the diverse medical conditions causing symptoms of this disorder (Sadock & Sadock, 2003).

A comprehensive assessment of multiple factors is necessary to make this diagnosis. The clinician considers the relationship of anxiety with the onset, exacerbation, or remission of the general medical condition. The clinician also rules out the presence of a primary anxiety disorder, a substance-induced anxiety disorder, or other primary mental disorders such as delirium (APA, 2000; Sadock & Sadock, 2003). Box 20-3 lists examples of selected medical problems that can cause anxiety.

Psychological Factors (Anxiety) Affecting Medical Condition

The essential feature of psychological factors affecting medical condition is the presence of one or more specific psychological or behavioral factors such as anxiety or depression that adversely affect a general medical condition. The factors may influence the course of the general medical condition, precipitate or exacerbate symptoms of the general medical condition, constitute an additional health risk for the individual, or interfere with treatment of the medical condition. Psychological or behavioral factors such as anxiety; the presence of "type A" personality which is characterized by an excessive competitive drive, impatience, aggressiveness, and a sense of urgency; or stress-related physiologic responses may significantly affect the course of almost every major category of disease. This diagnostic category is intended for any medical condition caused by or influenced by psychological factors (APA, 2000; Sadock & Sadock, 2003).

BOX 20.3	SELECTED MEDICAL PROBLEMS THAT CAN CAUSE ANXIETY

Cardiovascular:	Arrhythmia, congestive heart failure, ischemic heart disease, mitral valve prolapse, pulmonary embolism
Endocrine:	Addison's disease, Cushing's syndrome, hypothyroidism, hyperthyroidism, hyperglycemia, hyperparathyroidism, hyper-adrenocorticism
Hematologic:	Anemia, cancer, pheochromocytoma
Neurologic:	Cerebrovascular accident (CVA), encephalopathy, neoplasms, encephalitis
Nutritional:	Vitamin B_{12} deficiency, folate deficiency, iron deficiency, porphyria
Respiratory:	Chronic obstructive pulmonary disease (COPD), pneumonia, hyperventilation

Box 20-4 lists possible medical problems and conditions caused by anxiety. See Clinical Example 20-3 for an example of a client with essential hypertension secondary to anxiety.

BOX 20.4	POSSIBLE MEDICAL PROBLEMS AND CONDITIONS CAUSED BY PSYCHOLOGICAL FACTORS (ANXIETY)

- Allergies: Asthma; hay fever
- Cardiovascular: Arrhythmia and an increased possibility of stroke distress of coronary arteries high blood pressure
- Immune: Reduced number of white blood cells, which fight infection
- Gastrointestinal: Colitis, diarrhea, nausea, ulcers
- Genitourinary: Menstrual problems, sexual dysfunction
- Locomotor: Rheumatoid arthritis
- Muscular: Backaches, headaches, migraines
- Skin: Acne, dermatitis, eczema

CLINICAL EXAMPLE 20.3

THE CLIENT WITH ESSENTIAL HYPERTENSION SECONDARY TO ANXIETY

JB, a 54-year-old male executive, was seen by the company's attending physician for his annual physical examination. As the office nurse assessed him, she noted that his face was flushed, his blood pressure was 160/110, and he stated that he had only 30 minutes until he had to attend a meeting. After his physical examination was completed, the physician instructed JB to return to his office twice a week to have his blood pressure monitored and placed him on antihypertensive medication. JB returned as directed for the next few weeks, but continued to present with symptoms of hypertension. Although the nurse continued to stress preventive measures, JB did not alter his lifestyle. Approximately 4 months later, JB was admitted to the intensive care unit of the local community hospital with the diagnosis of a cerebral vascular attack. As a result of this condition, JB is a right-sided hemiplegic with expressive aphasia. He had to retire early and was engaged in a rehabilitative program to restore maximum functional ability.

A student nurse caring for JB commented, "He could be my father. He's so young to spend the rest of his life as a disabled person." After reading the history and admission forms, the same student stated, "Why didn't he follow his doctor's advice to prevent his attack? Didn't he care what happened?" JB eventually answered this question, stating, "I didn't think this would happen to me. I never lost my temper when I was upset. Maybe I should have said what I thought rather than worry about hurting the other guy's feelings."

THE NURSING PROCESS

ASSESSMENT

Chapters 9 and 19 discussed the importance of assessing the client's general appearance, communication skills, and observable behavior, as well as obtaining a thorough biopsychosocial and cultural history, and validating data obtained from the client. The assessment of clients with somatoform and dissociative disorders can be difficult and complex because of the presence of a comorbid medical condition, somatic complaints that cannot be validated, amnesia or fugue, an identity disorder, or depersonalization.

Assessment of Clients With a Comorbid Medical Diagnosis

It is not unusual for a client with anxiety to verbalize clinical symptoms of a comorbid medical diagnosis. As stated earlier, a comprehensive assessment is necessary to determine whether the medical condition is the result of anxiety, the medical condition causes anxiety, or the client has a history of chronic anxiety and has developed a medical condition unrelated to the presence of anxiety (eg, resulting from physiologic or organic changes).

Ask clients presenting with anxiety and medical conditions (eg, eczema, arrhythmia, cerebral vascular accident, or chronic obstructive pulmonary diseases) to be specific about the onset of their clinical symptoms. Use the following questions to help assess the client:

- Who diagnosed the medical condition and when?
- Did the anxiety occur before or after the development of the medical condition?
- Are you taking medication that can contribute to anxiety?
- Are you able to perform your usual activities of daily living?

The Holmes and Rahe (1967) Social Readjustment Rating Scale can be used as an assessment tool to determine the amount of stress experienced by clients exhibiting clinical symptoms of disorders such as psychological factors affecting medical condition. This scale ranks 43 critical life events according to the severity of their impact on a person. Each event has a point value: the death of a spouse is considered the most significant life event and minor violations of the law are considered the least significant. The point values of events a person experiences in a single year are totaled, thus indicating the severity of environmental stressors and the potential for a health change within 2 years of the onset of stressors. For example, an individual could experience anxiety exacerbating asthma, stress-related exacerbation of an ulcer, or delayed recovery from a myocardial infarction if the rating score is above 200.

Assessment of Clients With Somatoform Disorders

Assessing clients with somatoform disorders such as hypochondriasis, somatization disorder, or conversion disorder is challenging. Clients are often unaware that their basic problem is psychological, so they press their physicians for medical tests and treatments. As a result of their insistence, they may undergo many physical examinations and tests to determine that no physical disorder exists. Referrals to specialists for consultations are common, even when the client has developed a reasonably satisfactory relationship with one physician.

BDD causes clients great distress and disability but is difficult to assess. Such clients do not reveal their symptoms probably because of poor insight or shame about their appearance. Clients who present with pain, especially chronic pain and headaches, are also difficult to assess because, in some cases, the pain may exist without apparent cause or it may be perpetuated by factors that are remote from the initial cause (American Pain Society, 2001). Various assessment tools or screening scales for BDD or pain may be effective, depending upon the client's willingness to cooperate during the assessment process. Examples include the Body Dysmorphic Disorder Questionnaire, a 5-minute, client-rated screen scale; the Body Dysmorphic Disorder Examination to diagnose BDD, survey symptoms, and measure severity; the Wong-Baker Faces Pain Rating Scale; the Numeric Rating Scale used to measure both acute and chronic pain; the Brief Headache Screen developed by the American Academy of Neurology; and the McGill Pain Questionnaire (MPQ). Additional assessment tools and screening tests are listed in Chapter 19.

During the assessment process, be sure to obtain a history of the following regarding somatic complaints:

- Repeated visits to physicians or emergency rooms
- Admissions to hospitals (general or psychiatric)
- Any surgical interventions
- List of current medications (Clients with somatoform disorders often seek medication and self-prescribe over-the-counter drugs.)

The client's denial of any emotional problems; self-preoccupation; inability to express self and feelings; reliance on medications; and manipulative behavior can make it difficult to assess the client's degree of insight and judgment.

Assessment of Clients With Dissociative Disorders

Clients who present with clinical symptoms of dissociative disorders require a thorough physical examination to rule out organic causes such as a brain tumor. Sadock and Sadock (2003) suggest that the assessment focuses on clinical features such as:

- Client's level of orientation and ability to maintain contact with reality
- History of a precipitating emotional trauma
- Client's ability to recall recent and past events or the use of confabulation to cover up memory gaps
- Client's level of anxiety and possible coexistence of depression
- Client's degree of impaired social functioning (eg, stormy relationships, drug and alcohol abuse)
- Client's degree of occupational functioning (eg, inability to hold a job due to changes in personality)
- History of suicidal gestures or self-mutilation
- Evidence of other psychiatric disorders that are difficult to differentiate from dissociative disorder (eg, psychosis and personality disorders)

Lego (1996) lists specific questions to ask during the assessment process to determine the presence of DID, which is difficult to differentiate from other dissociative states, psychotic states, and personality disorders. These questions relate to symptom categories such as unexplainable time loss, feelings of depersonalization or derealization, presence of flashbacks or intrusive images, unexplained changes in one's home environment, unknown abilities, or feelings of being controlled by an internal force.

EXAMPLE OF NANDA NURSING DIAGNOSES/ SOMATOFORM AND DISSOCIATIVE DISORDERS

- Activity Intolerance related to increased physical complaints secondary to hypochondriasis
- Acute Confusion related to amnesia secondary to dissociative fugue
- Adult Failure to Thrive related to diminished coping abilities secondary to dissociative amnesia
- Ineffective Health Maintenance related to lack of motivation secondary to chronic pain disorder
- Anxiety related to dysphagia secondary to cerebral vascular accident (anxiety disorder due to a medical condition)
- Impaired Social Interaction related to effects of multiple somatic complaints that interfere with relationships
- Ineffective Coping related to unrealistic fear of having a disease despite reassurance to the contrary (hypochondriasis)
- Fatigue related to extreme stress secondary to imagined defect in appearance (body dysmorphic disorder)
- Impaired Physical Mobility related to leg pain secondary to conversion disorder

---

NURSING DIAGNOSES

Nursing diagnoses for clients exhibiting somatoform or dissociative disorders vary, given the possibility of a real or perceived comorbid medical condition. Examples of North American Nursing Diagnosis Association (NANDA) Nursing Diagnoses for clients who present with clinical symptoms of somatoform or dissociative disorders are listed in the accompanying box.

OUTCOME IDENTIFICATION

Stated outcomes focus on the client's ability to recognize his or her own anxiety; to identify stressors related to the present physical condition; to identify ways to modify or eliminate the stressors; to relate an increase in psychological and physiologic comfort; and to develop effective coping skills to avoid exacerbation of any comorbid medical conditions, somatoform disorders, or dissociative disorders. Examples of Stated Outcomes are highlighted in the accompanying box.

EXAMPLES OF STATED OUTCOMES/
SOMATOFORM AND
DISSOCIATIVE DISORDERS

- The client will report a reduction in symptoms of activity intolerance secondary to multiple somatic complaints of pain.
- The client will have diminished episodes of confusion related to amnesia as fugue improves.
- The client will identify at least three positive coping abilities to decrease adult failure to thrive.
- The client will increase social relatedness as amnesia improves.
- The client will describe lifestyles that promote health maintenance.
- The client will describe his or her own anxiety and coping patterns related to dysphagia.
- The client will verbalize fewer somatic complaints as social interactions improve.
- The client will demonstrate a decrease in exaggerated gastrointestinal physical complaints.
- The client will verbalize and demonstrate acceptance of appearance.
- The client will verbalize a decrease in the level and frequency of pain.
- The client will demonstrate measures to increase physical mobility.

PLANNING INTERVENTIONS

The nurse uses a holistic, individualized approach when planning care for clients with somatoform or dissociative disorders. Physical symptoms, whether real or imagined, can be quite distressing to the client. Clients with dissociative disorders may not be able to care for themselves as they present with impaired judgment. Immediate medical attention or hospitalization may be required to provide traditional medical treatment such as bed rest, diet as tolerated, physical therapy, pain medication, or psychotropic medication. Laboratory tests and x-ray examinations may be ordered to rule out organicity (Schultz & Videbeck, 2005).

After the client's medical condition is stabilized, interventions are planned to help the client develop insight into his or her condition; to help the client develop effective coping skills to reduce anxiety and avoid exacerbation of any coexisting medical condition; and to help the client identify supportive therapies that will reduce anxiety. The six areas in which to help the client develop an increased tolerance of anxiety and an increased awareness of strengths and limitations (listed in Chapter 19) are also considered when planning interventions for clients with somatoform or dissociative disorders (Johnson, 1997; Schultz & Videbeck, 2005).

IMPLEMENTATION

A variety of levels of care can be provided for clients with the diagnosis of somatoform or dissociative disorders depending upon the degree of disability the client exhibits, the presence of any comorbid medical or psychiatric disorders, the client's motivation for treatment, the availability of community resources, and insurance and managed care considerations. Interventions focus on stabilizing and resolving crises; managing symptoms; identifying and modifying maladaptive coping skills; teaching effective self-management techniques; and improving lifestyles. As always, client education is extremely important and included when appropriate in the following interventions (Schultz & Videbeck, 2005).

Assistance in Meeting Basic Needs

Be aware of your verbal and nonverbal responses to the client to avoid appearing judgmental when emphasizing the importance of identifying the source of stress or conflict that forms the basis of the symptom(s) and preventing secondary gain. Building a trust relationship with the client encourages the client to stay with one nurse or health care provider as the client develops alternative ways to deal with anger, anxiety, stress, or other feelings (Schultz & Videbeck, 2005).

Nursing interventions may warrant assisting clients with activities of daily living until physical symptoms are stabilized because these symptoms are quite real to clients with hypochondriasis, conversion disorder, pain disorder, or somatization disorder. Provide detailed explanations about the importance of taking prescribed medications, adhering to a specific diet, and following through with prescribed treatments such as physical therapy.

Clients with dissociative disorders who experience a distorted perception of the environment or who present with more than one personality may require placement in a structured clinical setting. Here, interventions would focus on relieving anxiety, promoting feelings of safety and security because clients may be at risk for self-mutilation, and improving ability to function in usual activities. Reality orientation is utilized to provide the client with pertinent information that he or she is unable to recall. It may be necessary to involve family members or significant others to validate information.

Medication Management

The use of psychoactive medication to manage clinical symptoms of somatoform or dissociative disorders is governed by the presence of a comorbid anxiety disorder, major depressive disorder, or psychotic disorder. Drug Summary Table 20-1 highlights examples of the major drugs used for symptoms associated with somatoform and dissociative disorders. Consideration must also be given to the treatment of a comorbid medical condition and the potential for any drug–drug interactions. A brief summary of approaches used is presented here.

Medication Management for Somatoform Disorders.
Clients with the diagnosis of hypochondriasis usually resist the use of medication. Conversely, clients with the diagnosis of depersonalization or conversion disorder have responded well to anxiolytics, and clients with the diagnosis of pain disorder have benefited from the use of selective serotonin reuptake inhibitors (SSRIs) and tricyclic antidepressants (TCAs). Relatively high doses of SSRIs and TCAs have also proven effective in the treatment of BDD (Sadock & Sadock, 2003).

Medication Management for Dissociative Disorders.
Although psychoactive medication is not considered the treatment of choice for clients with the diagnosis of dissociative disorders, medication is utilized to treat comorbid anxiety disorders (see Chapter 19) or psychosis (see Chapters 22 and 28).

Medication may be used to conduct drug-assisted interviews. Short-acting barbiturates such as thiopental (Pentothal) or sodium amobarbital (Amytal) are given intravenously during the interviews. Benzodiazepines may help clients with dissociative amnesia or dissociative fugue to recall forgotten memories. Although little attention has been given to the treat-

ment of clients with depersonalization disorder, clinical symptoms usually respond to antianxiety agents (Sadock & Sadock, 2003).

Interactive Therapies and Behavioral Interventions

Several types of interactive therapies such as individual, group, insight-oriented, and cognitive therapy (see Chapters 14 and 15) have proven effective in treating somatoform and dissociative disorders. Hypnosis may be used as a means of relaxing clients with dissociative disorders enough for them to recall what has been forgotten. Interactive therapy provides the client with a primary therapist who can encourage the client to express feelings, to focus on coping with somatic complaints, and to develop alternative ways to express emotion. Clients with the diagnosis of somatization disorder, hypochondriasis, conversion disorder, BDD, or depersonalization disorder benefit the most from interactive therapies (Maldonado, 1999; Norton, 2004; Ruane, 2005; Sadock & Sadock, 2003).

Behavioral interventions (see Chapter 12) are also used in the treatment of somatoform disorders. For example, if a client with the diagnosis of hypochondriasis has been told by a physician following a physical examination that he or she has no life-threatening or severe illness, but the client continues to verbalize clinical symptoms, limit-setting is used because physical complaints may be expressed to avoid responsibilities, gain attention, handle conflict, manipulate others, or meet dependency needs. Family members or significant others may be advised to employ limit-setting also. When limit-setting is employed, be aware—and alert family members to be aware—of the possible transference the client may display because the client views the limit-setting individual as an authority figure. Transference can also occur when clients of a different culture view the nurse as oppressive or racist. The nurse may react with countertransference due to unconscious ethnic prejudices or unrealistic expectations that the client adopt mainstream white American middle-class values (Louie, 1996; see Chapter 11 for a discussion of transference and countertransference).

Holistic Approach

Some therapists prefer to use a holistic approach (see Chapter 18) in the treatment of somatoform and dissociative disorders. The client's role is to attempt to

DRUG SUMMARY TABLE 20-1 ▼ **Drugs Used for Somatoform and Dissociative Disorders**

GENERIC (TRADE) NAME	DAILY DOSAGE RANGE	IMPLEMENTATION
Drug Class: SSRIs		
citalopram (Celexa)	10–60 mg	Limit amount of drug given in prescription to potentially suicidal clients; give in the morning with food if desired; monitor for GI disturbances, diaphoresis, dizziness, insomnia or somnolence, and palpitations; instruct male client that medication may cause ejaculatory disorders.
fluoxetine (Prozac)	20–50 mg	Give drug in the morning; give in divided doses if taking 20 mg/day; should not be given concurrently with or until after 2 weeks of discontinuation of an MAOI; avoid use of alcohol; monitor client's response closely in the presence of hepatic or renal impairment or diabetes as well as for headache, nervousness, abnormal sleep pattern, GI disturbances, and weight loss.
fluvoxamine (Luvox)	50–300 mg	Give at bedtime; if dose is 100 mg, divide dose and give larger dose at bedtime; limit quantity of dispensed drug to clients at risk for suicide; monitor for dizziness, drowsiness, insomnia, GI disturbance, mania, rash, seizures, and weight loss.
paroxetine (Paxil)	10–50 mg	Contraindicated during or within 14 days of MAOI therapy; limit amount of drug given to potentially suicidal clients; administer in the morning; use cautiously in the presence of hepatic or renal impairment; monitor for drowsiness, tremor, somnolence, GI disturbances, and sexual dysfunction in males.
sertraline (Zoloft)	50–200 mg	Contraindicated during or within 14 days of MAOI therapy, or with pimozide (Orap) or disulfiram (Antabuse); if given in concentrated form, dilute just before giving in 4 oz water, ginger ale, orange juice, etc.; monitor for increase in uric acid and hyponatremia, GI disturbances, tremor, weight loss, and anxiety.
Drug Class: TCAs		
amitriptyline (Elavil)	25–150 mg	Monitor for lethargy, sedation, blurred vision, dry eyes, dry mouth, arrhythmias, hypotension, constipation; contraindicated during or within 14 days of MAOI therapy. Use cautiously with elderly clients.
protriptyline (Vivactil)	5–40 mg	Monitor for blurred vision, decreased appetite, difficulty urinating, dizziness, drowsiness, dry mouth, sensitivity to sunlight and temperature, weight gain, seizures; avoid use after acute MI; contraindicated during or within 14 days of MAOI therapy.
Drug Class: Atypical Agents		
buspirone (BuSpar)	15–60 mg	Provide sugarless lozenges or ice chips if dry mouth or altered taste occurs; arrange for analgesic if headache or musculoskeletal aches are reported; monitor for dizziness, nervousness, GI disturbances, dreams, nightmares, or excitability. Avoid use of grapefruit juice.

NOTE: Although SSRIs and TCAs are used to control pain experienced by clients with somatoform disorders, pain control also includes the use of medication such as NSAIDs, sustained-release oral forms of oxycodone and morphine, and transdermal fentanyl.

identify any stressors related to the present physical condition, discuss ways to modify or eliminate the stressors, and then state specific changes that can be made. After anxiety-producing stressors are identified, nursing interventions may include the following:

- Separating the client from a specific environmental or familial stressor that increases anxiety or causes emotional conflict
- Assisting the client to identify personal strengths and weaknesses
- Assisting the client to identify positive or alternate coping mechanisms such as music, art, or dance therapy to reduce stress or anxiety, express him- or herself, and enhance self-concept
- Helping the client identify support systems, such as a close friend, family member, professional counselor, member of the clergy, or community support group
- Reviewing age-related developmental tasks with the client to promote insight and explore ways to handle difficult or unmet tasks successfully
- Teaching the client relaxation techniques or exercises
- Identifying alternative methods to decrease anxiety such as biofeedback, visualization techniques, hypnosis, meditation, behavior modification, psychotherapy, and family counseling
- Providing access to interventions specific to a client's culture such as home remedies, trips to religious shrines, or faith healers
- Providing family education to help family members develop alternate approaches or responses to the client's behavior or needs
- Administering prescribed medication for physical or psychological needs, recognizing the potential for drug dependency or abuse in clients with somatoform disorders

These interventions are problem oriented or situation centered to promote insight into the development of somatoform or dissociative disorders. They are also tailored to meet the needs of culturally diverse clients.

Project Smart

An innovative program to help clients with the diagnosis of a somatoform or dissociative disorder cope with stressful life events was developed in the 1980s. Focusing on the resistance phase of Selye's GAS and building on the work of Hinkle, Maslow, Maddi, and Kobasa, the Stress Resistance Project followed up with 1,200 men and women over a 12-year period to observe who coped well with stressful life events and what mechanisms they used to accomplish this. They concluded that stress-resistant persons displayed six characteristics that facilitated adaptive problem solving:

1. Use of reasonable mastery skills
2. Commitment to some meaningful project
3. Making of wise lifestyle choices
4. Seeking out social support
5. Maintenance of a sense of humor
6. Demonstration of concern for the welfare of others

Recognizing that these characteristics did not appear to be genetic, the Stress Resistance Project designed a program to teach these skills to persons who did not routinely use them when faced with stressful events. Project Stress Management and Relaxation Training (SMART) advocates the gradual reduction of dietary stimulants, use of relaxation exercises, participation in aerobic exercise, and stress inoculation procedures in which adaptive solutions to common problems are considered. Project SMART can be done individually or as a group for mastering life stress (Flannery, 1994).

EVALUATION

Evaluation begins with a review of the client's role in the individualized, holistic approach to care. The client is given an opportunity to compare pretreatment clinical symptoms, including those related to a comorbid medical condition, with changes that have occurred as a result of nursing interventions employed during treatment. Clients who respond to treatment are able to identify anxiety-producing stressors and demonstrate insight into their specific disorder. Effective coping skills are exhibited.

Post-treatment continuum of care is discussed. The client is strongly encouraged to maintain contact with an attending physician, who manages medical problems, as well as a support person or group. See Nursing Plan of Care 20-1: The Client With Anxiety Due to a Medical Condition.

M**○**VIE viewing **GUIDES**

THE CLIENT WITH ANXIETY DUE TO A MEDICAL CONDITION

Lourdes, a 53-year-old female, was admitted to the general hospital for treatment of chronic obstructive pulmonary disease (COPD). During the assessment, Lourdes related that she had a history of smoking at least one pack of cigarettes daily since she was a teenager. Approximately 2 years ago, she experienced her first hospitalization because she felt short of breath and could not stop coughing. A complete physical evaluation revealed the diagnosis of chronic bronchitis and emphysema. She has stopped smoking, but still craves cigarettes.

Lourdes stated that she has been hospitalized twice since her initial hospitalization and requires oxygen on a regular basis when she is at home. Lourdes also stated that she refuses to take any "unnecessary medication" but has agreed to take albuterol, brethine, vanceral, and prednisone when prescribed by her pulmonologist.

Just prior to this most recent hospitalization, Lourdes experienced nervousness, the inability to fall asleep, and a rapid heart rate while at rest. She has also felt "shaky all over" and becomes nauseated when she eats. She commented, "I get butterflies in my stomach" and "I feel like something terrible is going to happen to me."

Lourdes related that her husband has been supportive and their three adult children stop by frequently to visit with her. She hopes to go home within a few days.

DSM–IV–TR DIAGNOSIS: Anxiety disorder due to COPD (COPD includes diagnoses such as chronic bronchitis, emphysema), and possible side effects of medication

ASSESSMENT: Personal strengths: Alert, oriented in all spheres; has stopped smoking; uses prescribed medication; demonstrates insight into her medical condition; supportive family

Weaknesses: None identified

NURSING DIAGNOSIS: Anxiety related to unpredictable nature of chronic bronchitis and emphysema as evident by complaints of rapid pulse, nausea, trembling, insomnia, and "butterflies"

OUTCOME: The client will demonstrate an understanding of anxiety due to her medical condition.

Planning/Implementation	Rationale
Discuss the relationship between COPD and anxiety.	The client may be unaware of the relationship between COPD and anxiety.
Encourage the client to express her feelings about her medical diagnosis.	Verbalization of feelings can help identify symptoms of anger, fear, or anxiety.
Make observations to the client about her anxiety and help her to see the relationship between her medical condition and anxiety.	The sooner the client recognizes the cause of her anxiety, the more quickly she will be able to alter her response.

NURSING DIAGNOSIS: Ineffective Coping related to presence of physical illness of chronic bronchitis

OUTCOME: The client will take action to deal with anxiety independently and effectively.

Planning/Implementation	Rationale
Teach the client to monitor for objective and subjective manifestations of anxiety (eg, insomnia, tachycardia, "shaky feeling").	Recognizing the manifestations of anxiety gives the client confidence in having an understanding of anxiety.
Teach the client to use relaxation techniques and pursed-lip breathing independently.	These interventions are effective, non-chemical ways for the client to independently control her anxiety.
Assist the client to anticipate future problems that may provoke an anxiety response (eg, progression of medical condition).	Having a plan for managing anticipated difficulties may reduce the client's anxiety.

EVALUATION: Prior to discharge from the hospital, ask client to describe level of anxiety and frequency of symptoms. Review effectiveness of coping skills during hospitalization. Explore client's understanding of physiologic and psychologic response to COPD. Review the discharge plan of care with the client and availability of outpatient follow-up regarding anxiety.

KEY CONCEPTS

◆ Several theories explain the role of stress or emotions in the development of somatoform and dissociative disorders. Theories regarding the etiology of somatoform disorders include biologic and genetic factors, organ specificity theory, Selye's general adaptation syndrome, familial or psychosocial theory, and learning theory. Theories regarding the etiology of dissociative disorders include the state-dependent theory and psychoanalytic theory. Several causative factors have also been identified.

◆ Anxiety disorder due to a general medical condition differs from the diagnosis of psychological factors affecting medical condition. The former disorder is due to the direct physiologic effects of a medical condition; the latter refers to psychological factors having an adverse effect on a medical condition. For example, anxiety may be the result of a cerebral vascular accident (an anxiety disorder due to a general medical condition), or anxiety may exacerbate the physiologic symptoms of a stroke victim (psychological factors affecting medical condition).

◆ Clients with somatoform disorders experience disordered physiologic complaints or symptoms that are not under voluntary control and do not demonstrate organic findings; clients with dissociative disorders exhibit a disruption of consciousness, memory, identity, or perception of the environment.

◆ The assessment of a client with clinical symptoms of a somatoform or dissociative disorder can be difficult and complex because of the presence of a comorbid medical condition, somatic complaints, or the presence of dissociative symptoms. Assessment of clients with somatoform disorders focuses on general appearance, communication skills, observable behavior, biopsychosocial history, cultural history, and validation of data obtained from the client.

◆ The nursing diagnosis generally addresses clinical symptoms of medical problems as well as anxiety.

◆ Nursing interventions focus on assisting the client in meeting basic needs, medication management, stabilizing the client's medical condition, helping the client develop insight into his or her condition, helping the client develop effective coping skills to reduce stress and anxiety, and assisting the client in identifying supportive therapies to enhance continuum of care. Family education is provided throughout to assist family members in developing alternate approaches or responses to the client's behavior or needs.

For additional study materials, please refer to the Student Resource CD-ROM located in the back of this textbook.

CHAPTER WORKSHEET

CRITICAL THINKING QUESTIONS

1. Ask three of your clients with recent health changes to identify any critical life events that occurred within the past 2 years. What coping skills did they use to reduce stress related to these events? Did the recent health changes occur prior to or after the critical life events? How can you increase their understanding of the effect that life events may have on health?

2. It is generally recommended that nursing interventions for somatoform disorders consist of a holistic approach. How holistic are you with any client? How holistic are you in your own health maintenance routines? How might a holistic approach reduce health care costs?

REFLECTION

Reflect on the chapter opening quote by Sadock and Sadock. Explain the phrase stating that the brain "sends various signals that impinge on the patient's awareness, indicating a serious problem in the body." Cite at least three examples of possible stress- or anxiety-induced medical problems. What interventions would you provide for each of these medical problems to minimize the effect of further stress or anxiety?

NCLEX-STYLE QUESTIONS

1. The client tells the nurse, "I know that these headaches mean I have a serious disease like cancer. The tests are not correct, since they did not pick it up." The client has been diagnosed with hypochondriasis, which the nurse understands is characterized by which of the following?

    a. Predominant complaints of pain
    b. Preoccupation with fear of serious disease
    c. Symptoms that are associated with motor function
    d. Symptoms that are concocted to avoid situations

2. The nurse establishes which nursing diagnosis for a client with conversion disorder characterized by pain and the inability to move his left leg?

    a. Fatigue related to difficulty moving left leg secondary to pain
    b. Ineffective Health Maintenance related to chronic disability
    c. Impaired Physical Mobility related to leg pain secondary to conversion disorder
    d. Chronic Low Self-Esteem related to the presence of conversion disorder

3. A client with somatization disorder is assessed for which of the following symptoms?

    a. Family relationships in which arguments are frequent and vocal
    b. Physical symptoms for which no medical explanation exists
    c. Stressful lifestyle handled by frequent use of substances of abuse
    d. Severe chronic illness associated with immune system dysfunction

4. A client with body dysmorphic disorder is assessed for complaints of which of the following?

    a. Anxiety attacks
    b. Excessive fatigue
    c. Preoccupation with body defect
    d. Symptoms of mild depression

5. Which intervention would be most effective for a client with a somatoform disorder if the client continues to verbalize physical symptoms related to unmet dependency needs?

    a. Confrontation
    b. Limit-setting
    c. Reflection
    d. Reality orientation

6. A community group is developing a program that is based on the ideas of Project SMART to help the clients cope with stressful life events. Which of the following activities would most likely be included? Select all that apply.

    a. Rapid reduction in caffeine products
    b. Multiple drug therapy regimens
    c. Use of relaxation exercises
    d. Participation in aerobic exercises
    e. Identification of adaptive solutions

Selected References

Adams, D. B. (2003). Somatoform disorders. Retrieved November 9, 2005, from http://psychological.com/somatoform_disorders.htm

American Pain Society. (2001). Pain: Current understanding of assessment, management, and treatments. Retrieved September 6, 2005, from http://www.jcaho.org/news+room/health+care+issues/pain_mono_npc.pdf

American Psychiatric Association. (2000). *Diagnostic and statistical manual of mental disorders* (4th ed., text revision). Washington, DC: Author.

American Society of Plastic Surgeons (ASPS). (2004). Cosmetic surgery popular in 2003. *Clinician News, 8*(4), 23.

Flannery, R. B., Jr. (1994). *Becoming stress resistant through the Project SMART program.* New York: Crossroad Press.

Ford, C. V., & Folks, D. G. (1985). Conversion disorders: An overview. *Psychosomatics, 26,* 371–383.

Holmes, T. H., & Rahe, R. H. (1967). The social readjustment rating scale. *Journal of Psychosomatic Research,* (11), 213–218.

Johnson, B. S. (1997). *Psychiatric-mental health nursing: Adaptation and growth* (4th ed.). Philadelphia: Lippincott-Raven.

Lacey, J., Bateman, D., & Van Lehn, R. (1953). Autonomic response specificity. *Psychosomatic Medicine,* (8).

Lancaster, J. (1980). *Adult psychiatric nursing.* New York: Medical Examination Publishing.

Lego, S. (1996). The client with dissociative identity disorder. In S. Lego (Ed.), *Psychiatric nursing: A comprehensive reference* (2nd ed., pp. 246–252). Philadelphia: Lippincott-Raven.

Louie, K. B. (1996). Cultural issues in psychiatric nursing. In S. Lego (Ed.), *The American handbook of psychiatric nursing* (2nd ed., pp. 608–615). Philadelphia: Lippincott Williams & Wilkins.

Maldonado, J. R. (1999, November 11–14). *The somatoform disorders.* Paper presented at the 12th Annual United States Psychiatric & Mental Health Congress, Session #421, Atlanta, GA.

Merck Manual of Diagnosis and Therapy. (2005). Dissociative disorders. Retrieved November 10, 2005, from http://www.merck.com/mrkshared/mmanual/section15/chapter188

Minuchin, S. (1974). *Families and family therapy.* Cambridge: Harvard University Press.

Norton, P. G. W. (2004). Somatization severity reduced a year after CBT. *Clinical Psychiatry News, 32*(9), 66.

Phillips, K. A. (2000). *Body dysmorphic disorder (BDD)* (Case Studies in OCD Management, Case Study #4, 7–9). [A CME Activity]. St. Louis, MO: Solvay Pharmaceuticals.

Phillips, K. A., Siniscalchi, J. M., & McElroy, S. L. (2004). Depression, anxiety, anger, and somatic symptoms in patients with body dysmorphic disorder. *Psychiatric Quarterly, 75*(4), 309–320.

Ruane, J. J. (2005). On the front line: Providing optimal management of pain. *Supplement to the Clinical Advisor: A Practical Approach to Pain Management: A Therapeutic Update,* (10), 3–8.

Sadock, B. J., & Sadock, V. A. (2003). *Kaplan & Sadock's synopsis of psychiatry: Behavioral sciences/clinical psychiatry* (9th ed.). Philadelphia: Lippincott Williams & Wilkins.

Schultz, J. M., & Videbeck, S. L. (2005). *Lippincott's manual of psychiatric nursing care plans* (7th ed.). Philadelphia: Lippincott Williams & Wilkins.

Selye, H. (1978). The stress of life (2nd ed.). New York: McGraw-Hill.

Twerski, A. J. (1995). *When do the good things start?* (4th ed.). New York: St. Martin's Press.

Victoroff, J. (2001). When pain goes on and on. *Psychiatric Times, 18*(4), 19–21.

Suggested Readings

Barsky, A. J., & Ahern, D. K. (2004). Literature monitor: Psychosocial therapy may ease hypochondriasis. *Clinician Reviews, 14*(5), 43–44.

Boschert, S. (2004). Chronic pain interventions avoid surgery, drugs. *Clinical Psychiatry News, 32*(10), 56.

Carpenito-Moyet, L. J. (2006). *Handbook of nursing diagnosis* (11th ed.). Philadelphia: Lippincott Williams & Wilkins.

Feusner, J., Winograd, A., & Saxena, S. (2005). Beyond the mirror: Treating body dysmorphic disorder. *Current Psychiatry, 4*(10), 69–74, 81–83.

Friedman, M., & Rosenman, R. (1981). *Type A behavior and your heart.* New York: Knopf.

Karch, A. M. (2007). *2007 Lippincott's nursing drug guide.* Philadelphia: Lippincott Williams & Wilkins.

Leahy, R. (2005). The way of the worrier. *Psychology Today, 32*(6), 68–71.

MacReady, N. (2005). Tests show complexity of dissociative disorder. *Clinical Psychiatry News, 33*(1), 33.

Mahoney, D. (2005). Compulsive tanning may mean body dysmorphobia. *Clinical Psychiatry News, 33*(9), 38.

McNamara, D. (2005). Body dysmorphic disorder is often chronic and undertreated. *Clinical Psychiatry News, 33*(8), 36.

Merck Manual of Diagnosis and Therapy. (2005). Somatoform disorders. Retrieved November 10, 2005, from http://www.merck.com/mrkshared/mmanual/section15/chapter186

Miller, V. A. (2005). Misunderstood and misdiagnosed: The agony of migraine headache. *ADVANCE for Nurse Practitioners, 13*(10), 55-62.

Prescribing Reference, Inc. (2005, Fall). *Nurse practitioners' prescribing reference.* New York: Author.

Selye, H. (1991). *Stress without distress.* New York: New American Library.

Turkus, J. A., Cohen, B. M., & Courtois, C. A. (2003). The spectrum of dissociative disorders: An overview of diagnosis and treatment. Retrieved November 10, 2005, from http://www.voiceofwomen.com/VOW2_11950/center.html

Watkins, C. E. (2005). Body dysmorphic disorder. Retrieved November 10, 2005, from http://www.ncpamd.com/body_dysmorphic_disorder.htm

CHAPTER 21 / MOOD DISORDERS

Mood disorders encompass a large group of disorders in which pathological mood and related disturbances dominate the clinical picture. Previously referred to as affective disorders, the term mood disorders is preferred because it refers to sustained emotional states, not merely the external or affective expression of a transitory emotional state. —SADOCK & SADOCK, 2003

LEARNING OBJECTIVES

AFTER STUDYING THIS CHAPTER, YOU SHOULD BE ABLE TO:

1. Briefly describe the historical perspective of mood disorders.
2. Explain the following theories of mood disorders: genetic, biochemical, biologic, psychodynamic, behavioral, cognitive, and life events and environmental.
3. Recognize the primary risk factors for developing mood disorders.
4. Differentiate among the clinical symptoms of major depressive disorder, bipolar I disorder, and bipolar II disorder.
5. Articulate the rationale for the use of the diagnosis mood disorder due to a general medical condition.
6. Compare and contrast the clinical symptoms of dysthymic disorder, cyclothymic disorder, premenstrual dysphoric disorder, and mood disorder with postpartum onset.
7. Articulate the rationale for each of the following modes of treatment for mood disorders: medication management, somatic therapy, interactive therapy, and complementary and alternative therapy.
8. Formulate an education guide for clients with a mood disorder.
9. Construct a sample plan of care for an individual exhibiting clinical symptoms of major depressive disorder.

KEY TERMS

Affective disorders
Anaclitic depression
Anergia
Anhedonia
Apathy
Asthenia
Bipolar disorder
Depressive disorders
Dysthymia
Elation
Endogenous depression
Euphoria
Hypomania
Mania
Poverty of speech content
Psychomotor agitation
Psychomotor retardation
Rapid-cycling
Residual symptoms

Mood disorders (previously referred to as **affective disorders**) encompass a large group of disorders involving pathological mood and related disturbances. The *Diagnostic and Statistical Manual of Mental Disorders, 4th Edition, Text Revision (DSM-IV-TR)* divides mood disorders into two main categories: depressive disorders and bipolar disorders (American Psychiatric Association [APA], 2000). Mood disorders are one of the most commonly occurring psychiatric–mental health disorders. Only alcoholism and phobias are more common. Mood disorders impose an enormous burden on the individual, the family, and society as a whole (Grant & Morrison, 2001; Sadock & Sadock, 2003).

The National Institute of Mental Health (NIMH, 2005) and the National Association for Research on Schizophrenia and Depression (NARSAD, 2005), have released the following statistics regarding the prevalence of mood disorders affecting American adults 18 years of age or older in any given year. Approximately 18.8 million adults (or 9.5% of the U.S. population) experience depressive disorders. Furthermore, major depression is the leading cause of disability worldwide. It affects approximately 9.9 million adults (or about 5.0 percent of the U.S. population). Nearly twice as many women (6.5 %) as men (3.3 %) suffer from a major depressive disorder. Statistics also reveal that more than 2.3 million adults (or about 1.2 % of the U.S. population) are diagnosed with bipolar disorder (BPD). Men and women are equally likely to develop BPD. By the year 2020, mood disorders are estimated to be the second most important cause of disability worldwide.

The direct costs of treatment for a major mood disorder, combined with the direct costs from lost productivity, are significant and have been estimated to account for approximately $12 billion to $16 billion per year in the United States. Indirect cost, including mortality, work absenteeism, and disability, have been estimated to exceed $32 billion per year (Grant & Morrison, 2001).

Mood disorders can occur in any age group. Infants may exhibit signs of **anaclitic depression** (withdrawal, nonresponsiveness, depression, and vulnerability to physical illness) or *failure to thrive* when separated from their mothers. School-aged children may experience a mood disorder along with anxiety, exhibiting behaviors such as hyperactivity, school phobia, or excessive clinging to parents. Adolescents experiencing depression may exhibit poor academic performance; abuse substances; display antisocial behavior, sexual promiscuity, truancy, or running-away behavior; or attempt suicide (for more information, see Chapters 29 and 31).

Although mood disorders are less common in the older adult than in younger individuals, symptoms of depression are present in approximately 15% to 25% of all older-community residents (ie, age 60 years and older), particularly those living in long-term care facilities. In recent years, marked progress has been made in the diagnosis and treatment of mood disorders in nursing home residents. In 1987, only 10% of nursing home residents were receiving antidepressant medication for clinical symptoms of mood disorders. By 1999, 25% of all residents were receiving antidepressants as a result of more comprehensive assessments and better diagnosis of mood disorders (Katz, Streim, Parmelee, & Datto, 2001).

Despite the high prevalence of major mood disorders in clients of all ages, these disorders are commonly under-diagnosed and under-treated by primary care and other non-psychiatric practitioners, the individuals who are most likely to see clients initially. For example, the incidence of a major mood disorder in primary care clients is approximately 10%, suggesting that clinical symptoms may go undiagnosed or untreated (Sadock & Sadock, 2003). In addition, the social stigma attached to mood disorders contributes to this rate of under-diagnosis and under-treatment. Clients may resist seeking treatment or the practitioner may be reluctant to formally diagnose mood disorders. In addition, poor adherence by clients to long-term treatment of a chronic mood disorder, and client reluctance to reveal the presence of a mood disorder when applying for a driver's license, seeking employment, or seeking security clearance also plays a role in under-diagnosis and under-treatment.

Despite the tendency to underestimate the importance and prevalence of mood disorders, their devastating effects on people's work and personal lives are better understood now than they have been in the past. Researchers are exploring more fully the biologic basis of mood disorders, such as the role of neurotransmitters and neuroendocrine regulation. The data reported are most consistent with the hypothesis that mood disorders are associated with varied impairments in the regulation of norepinephrine and sero-tonin (Sadock & Sadock, 2003).

This chapter discusses the historical perspective of mood disorders, the theories of mood disorders, including the primary risk factors for developing mood disorders, and clinical symptoms and diagnostic characteristics of the major mood disorders diagnosed. Using the nursing process, the chapter presents information about important areas for assessment, and key intervention strategies when providing care for a client with a mood disorder.

Historical Perspective of Mood Disorders

Few disorders throughout history have been described with such consistency as mood disorders. Symptoms that characterize the disorders can be found in medical literature throughout the centuries from the ancient Greeks to the present era. As early as the 4th and 5th centuries BC, the term *melancholia* was used by ancient Greeks to describe the dark mood of depression. Hippocrates used the term melancholia to describe depression and *mania* to describe mental disturbances in clients. During the 2nd century AD, Arteaeus of Cappadocia described *cyclothymia* as a form of mental disease with alternating periods of depression and mania. For centuries, melancholia and cyclothymia were regarded to be separate disease entities rather than diverse expressions of mood disorders. By 1880, four categories of mood disorders existed: mania, melancholia, monomania, and dipsomania. In 1882, a German psychiatrist, Karl Kahlbaum described melancholia and mania as a continuum of the same illness. In 1899, Emil Kraepelin, another psychiatrist, reinforced Kahlbaum's theory about the continuum of depression. Kraepelin introduced the category of *manic-depressive psychosis*, citing most of the criteria now used to establish the diagnosis of bipolar I disorder. He also introduced the category of *involutional melancholia*, now viewed as a mood disorder that occurs in late adulthood (Emental-health.com, 2005a, b; Sadock & Sadock, 2003).

Etiology of Mood Disorders

In the past, causes of a mood disorder were classified as genetic, biochemical, and environmental. In addition, several medical illnesses are highly correlated with mood disorders. Moreover, individuals of any age

---

BOX 21.1 **RISK FACTORS FOR MOOD DISORDERS**

The following risk factors for mood disorders have been established as clinical practice guidelines for primary care practitioners.
- Prior episodes of depression
- Family history of depressive disorders
- Prior suicide attempts
- Female gender
- Age of onset younger than 40 years
- Postpartum period
- Medical comorbidity associated with a high risk of depression
- Lack of social support
- Stressful life events
- Current alcohol or substance abuse or use of medication associated with a high risk of depression
- Presence of anxiety, eating disorder, obsessive-compulsive disorder, somatization disorder, personality disorder, grief, adjustment reactions. Depression may coexist with other psychiatric conditions.

---

may experience changes in mood or affect as an adverse effect of medication. However, older adults are more likely than younger adults to experience medication-related mood disorders. Risk factors for the development of mood disorders have been identified as clinical practice guidelines for primary care practitioners. These are highlighted in Box 21-1. In addition, several theories about mood disorders have been postulated.

Genetic Theory

According to statistics from the National Institute of Mental Health (2005), studies involving adoptees revealed higher correlations of mood disorders between depressed adoptees and biologic parents than adoptive parents. Studies of twins have shown that if an identical twin develops a mood disorder, the other twin has a 70% chance of developing the disorder, too. The risk decreases to about 15% with siblings, parents, or children of the person with the mood disorder. Grandparents, aunts, or uncles have about a 7% chance of developing a mood disorder.

Theorists believe that a dominant gene may influence or predispose a person to react more readily to experiences of loss or grief, thus manifesting symptoms of a mood disorder. For example, Medina (1995) discusses the history of BPD (previously referred to as manic-depressive disorder) research since 1987. He cites the various pseudogenetic studies dealing with the linkage between human genes and human behaviors. "No gene for bipolar disorder has been isolated....There is strong disagreement as to the number of genes actually involved in the disease.The ups and downs of the published literature illustrate the enormous problems researchers encounter attempting to describe human behavior in terms of genetic sequence" (p. 30).

Biochemical Theory

Biogenic amines, or chemical compounds known as norepinephrine and serotonin, have been shown to regulate mood and to control drives such as hunger, sex, and thirst. Increased amounts of these neurotransmitters at receptor sites in the brain cause an elevation in mood, whereas decreased amounts can lead to depression. Although norepinephrine and serotonin are the biogenic amines most often associated with the development of a mood disorder, dopamine has also been theorized to play a role (Figure 21-1).As with norepinephrine and serotonin, dopamine activity may be reduced in depressed mood and increased in mania,the two phases of BPD.These explanations are termed the *biogenic amine hypothesis* (Sadock & Sadock, 2003).

Neuroendocrine Regulation

High levels of the hormone cortisol have been observed in persons with clinical symptoms of a mood disorder. Normally, cortisol levels peak in the early morning, level off during the day, and reach the lowest point in the evening. Cortisol peaks earlier in persons with a depressed mood and remains high all day.

Mood is also affected by the thyroid gland. Approximately 5% to 10% of clients with abnormally low levels of thyroid hormones may suffer from a chronic mood disorder. Clients with a mild, symptom-free form of hypothyroidism may be more vulnerable to depressed mood than the average person (Sadock & Sadock, 2003).

Research studies continue to focus on neuroendocrine abnormalities described in clients with mood disorders.These abnormalities include decreased nocturnal secretion of melatonin; decreased levels of prolactin, follicle-stimulating hormone, testosterone, and somatostatin; and sleep-induced stimulation of growth hormone (Sadock & Sadock, 2003).

Biologic Theory

It has long been believed that there is a biologic relationship between various medical conditions (eg, pain or cardiovascular disease in women) and depression. Following is a brief summary of theories regarding the biologic connections between depression and certain medical conditions.

Neurodegenerative Diseases

A variety of neurodegenerative diseases are associated with depressive manifestations. Depression is the most common psychiatric symptom encountered in clients who have Alzheimer's disease, affecting approximately 25% to 50% of the clients. The relationship between dementia and depression is complex. Some clients become depressed because they are aware of the prognosis of their diagnosis; whereas other clients are depressed due to degenerative changes in the neural system. Depression is also estimated to afflict 40% to 50% of individuals with Parkinson's disease. Postmortem examinations have revealed low levels of norepinephrine and serotonin due to degeneration of both frontocortical circuits and the brainstem regions. Multiple sclerosis (MS) is a third neurodegenerative disorder commonly associated with depressive symptoms. Degenerative effects of widespread areas of the brain, as in stroke, are believed to be the cause of neuropsychiatric symptoms. Various studies have indicated that approximately 25.7 % of clients with MS had the diagnosis of major depression; 30% of individuals studied had contemplated suicide; and more than 6% had attempted suicide (Feinstein, 2002; Patten, Beck, & Williams, 2003).

Immunotherapy

Depression is linked biologically to the use of immunotherapeutic agents in the treatment of certain diseases. Research by Dantzer and Kelley revealed that about one third of clients who receive cytokine therapy develop depression. Symptoms of depression began within days to weeks of therapy and disappeared when the treatment ended (Stong, 2004).

Pancreatic tumors release high levels of cytokine. Research findings revealed that clients with pancreatic tumors exhibited clinical symptoms of depression whereas other cancer clients were not depressed. Additionally, cancer drugs such as procarbazine inhibit dopamine beta-hydroxylase, while vincristine and vinblastine decrease conversion of dopamine to

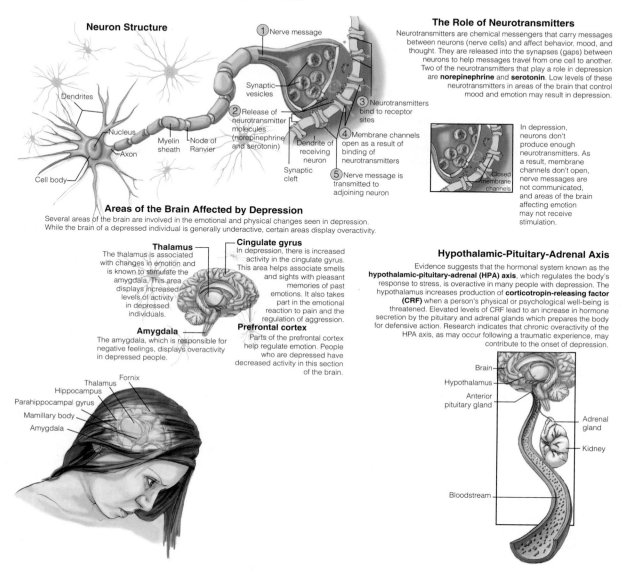

Neuron Structure

① Nerve message

Synaptic vesicles

② Release of neurotransmitter molecules (norepinephrine and serotonin)

③ Neurotransmitters bind to receptor sites

④ Membrane channels open as a result of binding of neurotransmitters

⑤ Nerve message is transmitted to adjoining neuron

Dendrites

Nucleus

Myelin sheath

Node of Ranvier

Axon

Cell body

Dendrite of receiving neuron

Synaptic cleft

The Role of Neurotransmitters

Neurotransmitters are chemical messengers that carry messages between neurons (nerve cells) and affect behavior, mood, and thought. They are released into the synapses (gaps) between neurons to help messages travel from one cell to another. Two of the neurotransmitters that play a role in depression are **norepinephrine** and **serotonin**. Low levels of these neurotransmitters in areas of the brain that control mood and emotion may result in depression.

In depression, neurons don't produce enough neurotransmitters. As a result, membrane channels don't open, nerve messages are not communicated, and areas of the brain affecting emotion may not receive stimulation.

Closed membrane channels

Areas of the Brain Affected by Depression

Several areas of the brain are involved in the emotional and physical changes seen in depression. While the brain of a depressed individual is generally underactive, certain areas display overactivity.

Thalamus
The thalamus is associated with changes in emotion and is known to stimulate the amygdala. This area displays increased levels of activity in depressed individuals.

Amygdala
The amygdala, which is responsible for negative feelings, displays overactivity in depressed people.

Cingulate gyrus
In depression, there is increased activity in the cingulate gyrus. This area helps associate smells and sights with pleasant memories of past emotions. It also takes part in the emotional reaction to pain and the regulation of aggression.

Prefrontal cortex
Parts of the prefrontal cortex help regulate emotion. People who are depressed have decreased activity in this section of the brain.

Fornix
Thalamus
Hippocampus
Parahippocampal gyrus
Mamillary body
Amygdala

Hypothalamic-Pituitary-Adrenal Axis

Evidence suggests that the hormonal system known as the **hypothalamic-pituitary-adrenal (HPA) axis**, which regulates the body's response to stress, is overactive in many people with depression. The hypothalamus increases production of **corticotropin-releasing factor (CRF)** when a person's physical or psychological well-being is threatened. Elevated levels of CRF lead to an increase in hormone secretion by the pituitary and adrenal glands which prepares the body for defensive action. Research indicates that chronic overactivity of the HPA axis, as may occur following a traumatic experience, may contribute to the onset of depression.

Brain

Hypothalamus

Anterior pituitary gland

Adrenal gland

Kidney

Bloodstream

FIGURE 21.1 Pathophysiologic basis of depression.

norepinephrine. Higher depression rates have also been reported in clients who receive tamoxifen and interferon-alpha (MacNeil, 2005).

Medical Conditions

Studies describe the relationship between depression and certain medical conditions. In clients with chronic inflammation, such as occurs with coronary heart dis-ease or type 2 diabetes mellitus, the prevalence of depression increases between 12% and 30% (Stong, 2004). Hypotheses vary regarding the physiologic basis for the higher incidence of depression in people with diabetes. Barden (2004) discusses the implication of increased activity within the hypothalamic–pituitary–adrenal (HPA) axis as one characteristic of depression. Such activity has also been seen as a factor in maintaining glycemic balance. The effects of the

BOX 21.2 MEDICATIONS AND MEDICAL ILLNESSES CORRELATED WITH DEPRESSION

MEDICATIONS

- Analgesics and nonsteroidal anti-inflammatory drugs: opioids, ibuprofen, and indomethacin
- Antimicrobials: sulfonamides and isoniazide
- Antineoplastic agents: asparaginase and tamoxifen
- Antiparkinson agents: levodopa and amantadine
- Cardiac medications and antihypertensives: digoxin, procainamide, reserpine, propranolol, methyldopa, clonidine, guanethidine, and hydralazine
- Central nervous system agents: alcohol, benzodiazepines, meprobamate, flurazepam, haloperidol, barbiturates, and fluphenazine
- Histamine blockers: cimetidine and ranitidine
- Hormonal agents: corticosteroids, estrogen, and progesterone

MEDICAL ILLNESSES

- Central nervous system: Parkinson's disease, strokes, tumors, hematoma, neurosyphilis, and normal pressure hydrocephalus
- Nutritional deficiencies: folate or B_{12}, pernicious anemia, and iron deficiency
- Cardiovascular disturbances: congestive heart failure and subacute bacterial endocarditis
- Metabolic and endocrine disorders: diabetes, hypothyroidism or hyperthyroidism, hypoglycemia or hyperglycemia, parathyroid disorders, adrenal diseases, hepatic or renal disease and premenstrual syndrome
- Fluid and electrolyte disturbances: hypercalcemia, hypokalemia, and hyponatremia
- Infections: meningitis, viral pneumonia, hepatitis, and urinary tract infections
- Miscellaneous: rheumatoid arthritis, cancer (particularly of the pancreas or intestinal tract), tuberculosis, tertiary syphilis, and fibromyalgia

---

increased HPA activity in both diabetes and depression may partly explain the link between the two. Box 21-2 lists medications and medical illnesses that are highly correlated with the development of depression.

Pain

The association between depression and pain is very high. It has been hypothesized that not all pain is linked to an identifiable medical condition such as arthritis or fibromyalgia, but rather it can be biologic in origin (eg, undetected cellular changes) and create a vicious circle in which the pain leads to psychomotor agitation, agitation leads to irritability, irritability leads to aggression, and aggression leads to depression and more pain, often resulting in disability (Finn, 2004).

Psychodynamic Theory

The psychodynamic theory of depression, based on the work of Sigmund Freud, Karl Abraham, Melanie Klein, and others, begins with the observation that bereavement normally produces symptoms resembling a mood disorder. That is, people with a depressed mood are like mourners who do not make a realistic adjustment to living without the loved person. In childhood, they are bereft of a parent or other loved person, usually the result of the absence or withdrawal of affection. Any loss or disappointment later in life reactivates a delayed grief reaction that is accompanied by self criticism, guilt, and anger turned inward. Because the source and object of the grief are unconscious (from childhood), symptoms are not resolved, but rather persist and return later in life (Sadock & Sadock, 2003).

Additionally, several theorists, such as Karl Abraham, Bertram Lewin, and Melanie Klein, have attempted to explain the psychodynamic factors of mania. Manic episodes are viewed as a defense reaction against underlying depression due to the client's inability to tolerate a developmental tragedy, such as the loss of a parent. These episodes also may be the result of a tyrannical superego, producing intolerable self-criticism that is replaced by euphoric self-satisfaction, or an ego overwhelmed by pleasurable impulses such as sex or by feared impulses such as aggression (Sadock & Sadock, 2003).

Behavioral Theory: Learned Helplessness

Behavioral theorists regard mood disorders as a form of acquired or learned behavior. For one reason or another, people who receive little positive reinforcement for their activity become withdrawn, overwhelmed, and passive, giving up hope and shunning responsibility. This, in turn, leads to a perception that things are beyond their control. This perception promotes feelings of helplessness and hopelessness, both hallmarks of depressed states. Behaviorists who subscribe to this theory believe that a client's depressed mood could improve if the client develops a sense of control and mastery of the environment (Sadock & Sadock, 2003).

Cognitive Theory

Cognitive or cognitive-behavioral theorists believe that thoughts are maintained by reinforcement, thus contributing to a mood disorder. People with a depressed mood are convinced that they are worthless, that the world is hostile, that the future offers no hope, and that every accidental misfortune is a judgment of them. Such reactions are the result of assumptions learned early in life and brought into play by disappointment, loss, or rejection. For example, a young child may be told by one parent that the child is not athletic enough to play basketball in grade school. As the child approaches high school, he may assume that he lacks talent and, although he would like to play basketball, he does not try out for the team. Cognitive distortions or self-defeating thoughts become part of a destructive cycle in which the individual exhibits apathy, sadness, and social withdrawal (Sadock & Sadock, 2003).

Life Events and Environmental Theory

Complex etiology based on interacting contributions from life events and the environment may ultimately result in clinical symptoms of depression. For example, stressful life events such as the loss of a parent or spouse, financial hardship, illness, perceived or real failure, and midlife crises are all examples of factors contributing to the development of a mood disorder. Certain populations of people including the poor, single persons, or working mothers with young children seem to be more susceptible than others to stressful events and the development of mood disorders. The life event most often associated with the development of a mood disorder is the loss of a parent before the age of 11 years. The environmental stressor most often

associated with an episode of depressed mood is loss of a spouse. Additionally, dramatic changes in one's life can trigger depressive episodes. For instance, relocation, loss or change of employment, and retirement can all produce symptoms that may or may not be temporary. Some theorists believe that early life events such as abuse and neglect experienced by a client results in a long-lasting change in the brain's biology, affecting the functional states of neurotransmitters and intraneuronal signaling systems (Gillespie & Nemeroff, 2005; Sadock & Sadock, 2003).

Clinical Symptoms and Diagnostic Characteristics of Depressive Disorders

The clinical symptoms of **depressive disorders**, one of the two major types of mood disorders, have been categorized in many ways. One method is by placing depressive behaviors on a continuum from mild or transitory depression to severe depression. Mild depression is exhibited by affective symptoms of sadness or "the blues"—an appropriate response to stress. The person who experiences such depression may be less responsive to the environment and may complain of physical discomfort. However, the person usually recovers within a short period. For example, a person may become disappointed when told that he or she was not chosen as a representative to a conference that the person hoped to attend. During this time, the person may be unable to concentrate, may communicate less with coworkers, may appear less productive than normal, and may isolate him- or herself at work and at home.

Clinical symptoms of moderate depression (**dysthymia**) are less severe than those experienced in a major depressive disorder and do not include psychotic features; e.g., individuals with dysthymia usually complain that they have always been depressed. They verbalize feelings of guilt, inadequacy, and irritability. They exhibit a lack of interest and lack of productivity. Persons with severe depression exhibit psychotic symptoms such as delusions and hallucinations.

Major depressive disorders are referred to as **endogenous depression** when the depressed mood appears to develop from within a client, and no apparent cause or external precipitating factor is identified. Depression caused by a biochemical imbalance is such an example.

CLINICAL SYMPTOMS AND DIAGNOSTIC CHARACTERISTICS /
MAJOR DEPRESSIVE DISORDER

CLINICAL SYMPTOMS

- Depressed mood
- Significant loss of interest or pleasure
- Marked changes in weight or significant increase or decrease in appetite
- Insomnia or hypersomnia
- Psychomotor agitation or retardation
- Fatigue or loss of energy
- Feelings of worthlessness or excessive or inappropriate guilt
- Reduced ability to concentrate or think, or indecisiveness
- Recurrent thoughts of death, suicidal ideation, suicide attempt, or plan for committing suicide

DIAGNOSTIC CHARACTERISTICS

- Evidence of at least five clinical symptoms in conjunction with depressed mood or loss of interest or pleasure
- Symptoms occurring most of the day and nearly every day during the same 2-week period representing an actual change in person's previous level of functioning
- Significant distress or marked impairment in person's functioning, such as in social or occupational areas
- Symptoms not related to a medical condition or use of a substance

CLINICAL EXAMPLE 21.1

THE CLIENT WITH MAJOR DEPRESSIVE DISORDER

AS, a 25-year-old professional basketball player, complained of fatigue during practice. He had a few episodes of vertigo the previous week and also stated that he could not remember the different plays the coach recently designed. The team physician examined AS. During the examination, AS revealed that he did not enjoy playing basketball anymore, had no interest in socializing with his peers or fiancée, and felt as if he "didn't belong" or fit in with other members of the team. The physician noted that despite no physiologic reason for a weight loss, AS had lost 15 pounds since his last physical examination. AS described a lack of appetite for approximately 2 weeks. The team physician was able to determine that AS was exhibiting clinical symptoms of major depressive disorder without psychotic features or suicidal ideation and subsequently prescribed an antidepressant medication and supportive psychotherapy.

The *DSM-IV-TR* categorizes depressive disorders as major depressive disorder; dysthymic disorder; and depressive disorder, not otherwise specified (NOS). The *DSM-IV-TR* diagnostic criteria for prepubertal, adolescent, and adult depression are identical. Information regarding childhood and adolescent depression is provided in Chapter 29. Late-life depression is discussed in Chapter 30.

Major Depressive Disorder

According to NIMH (2005) major depressive disorder has been identified as the fourth leading cause of worldwide disease in 1990, causing more disability than either ischemic heart disease or cerebral vascular disease. According to the *DSM-IV-TR*, persons with a major depressive disorder do not experience momentary shifts from one unpleasant mood to another. During a 2-week period, the individual exhibits five or more of the nine clinical symptoms of a major depressive episode in conjunction with a depressed mood or loss of interest or pleasure (see the accompanying Clinical Symptoms and Diagnostic Characteristics box). The clinical symptoms interfere with social, occupational, or other important areas of functioning. Symptoms are not due to effects of a substance, nor are they caused by a general medical condition. See Clinical Example 21-1.

Major depressive disorder may be coded as mild, moderate, or severe; with or without psychotic features; and as in partial or full remission. Reference also is made to identify it as a single or recurrent episode. The specifier "with seasonal pattern" can be applied to the pattern of major depressive episodes if the clinical symptoms occur at characteristic times of the year. For example, most episodes begin in fall or winter and remit in the spring, although some clients experience it during the summer. Clinicians often refer to this type of mood disorder with seasonal pattern as *seasonal affective disorder (SAD)*. The prevalence of SAD is approximately 7.8% of the U.S. population. This disorder is nearly twice as prevalent in women (10.4%) as in men (5.3%) and usually occurs in women between the ages of 20 and 40 years. Individuals who live in areas where seasonal changes occur are more prone to the development of SAD (eg, Vermont, 16%; Montana, 14%; and North Dakota, 14%). The prevalence of SAD across southern states is approximately 6.7%, suggesting that it is relatively common in the southern U.S. (Stong, 2005).

Dysthymic Disorder

The client with the diagnosis of dysthymic disorder typically exhibits symptoms that are similar to those of major depressive disorder or severe depression. However, they are not as severe and do not include symptoms such as delusions, hallucinations, impaired communication, or incoherence. Clinical symptoms usually persist for 2 years or more and may occur continuously or intermittently with normal mood swings for a few days or weeks. Persons who develop dysthymic disorder are usually overly sensitive, often have intense guilt feelings, and may experience chronic anxiety. Dysthymic disorder affects approximately 5.4% of the U.S. population age 18 years and older (or 10.9 million adults) during their lifetime. Dysthymic disorder often begins in childhood, adolescence, or early adulthood (NIMH, 2005).

According to *DSM-IV-TR* criteria, the individual, while depressed, must exhibit two or more of six clinical symptoms of a major depressive episode, including poor appetite or overeating, insomnia or hypersomnia, low energy or fatigue, low self-esteem, poor concentration or difficulty making decisions, and feelings of hopelessness. Clinical symptoms interfere with functioning and are not caused by a medical condition or the physiologic effects of a substance.

Depressive Disorder, Not Otherwise Specified

The diagnosis of depressive disorder, NOS, is used to identify disorders with depressive features that do not meet the criteria for major depressive disorder, dysthymic disorder, adjustment disorder with depressed mood, or adjustment disorder with mixed anxiety and depressed mood (see Chapter 29 for more information on adjustment disorders).

Clinical Symptoms and Diagnostic Characteristics of Bipolar Disorder

Various descriptive terms are used to describe the labile affect or mood changes of clients with the diagnosis of **bipolar disorder**. These terms include:

- **Euphoria,** an exaggerated feeling of physical and emotional well-being
- **Elation,** a state of extreme happiness, delight, or excitability
- **Hypomania,** a psychopathological state and abnormality of mood falling somewhere between normal euphoria and mania, characterized by unrealistic optimism, pressure of speech and activity, and a decreased need for sleep (some clients show an increase in creativity during hypomanic states, whereas others show poor judgment, irritability, and irascibility). Individuals with hypomania are able to function socially, academically, and occupationally although their behavior is significantly different from their baseline.
- **Mania,** a state characterized by excessive elation, inflated self-esteem, and grandiosity
- **Rapid-cycling,** a state characterized by the occurrence of four or more mood episodes during the previous 12 months; a course modifier for the differential diagnosis of BPD

These changes may be placed on a continuum, from mild to severe, the same as those of depressive behaviors.

The client with mania generally exhibits hyperactivity, agitation, irritability, and accelerated thinking and speaking. Behaviors may include pathological gambling, a tendency to disrobe in public places, wearing excessive attire and jewelry of bright colors in unusual combinations, and inattention to detail (Figure 21-2). The client may be preoccupied with religious, sexual, financial, political, or persecutory thoughts that can develop into complex delusional systems. Flight of ideas, as well as other psychotic symptoms discussed in Chapter 9, may persist (Sadock & Sadock, 2003; Shahrokh & Hales, 2003).

BPD is generally underdiagnosed because of underrecognition of manic and hypomanic episodes. The complex nature of BPD makes an accurate differential

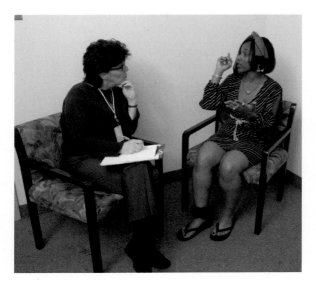

FIGURE 21.2 A client with mania. Note the exaggerated dress and hand movements.

diagnosis a challenge, even for experienced clinicians. Although many clients present to a health care provider within 1 year of symptom onset, there is usually a 5- to 10-year delay from symptom onset to formal diagnosis. Many clients report that they have not been correctly diagnosed until they were seen by three or more health care professionals (St. John, 2005).

As noted earlier, BPD affects approximately 2.3 million American adults (or about 1.2%) age 18 years and older in a given year. Men and women are equally likely to develop BPD. The average age of onset is in the early twenties (NIMH, 2005). The clinical presentation of BPD in children and adolescents is often different from that seen in adults. Moods in children and adolescents tend to be more irritable than euphoric. In addition, adolescents often have greater difficulty with mood liability, explosive outbursts of anger followed by remorse, and prolonged emotional response to stimuli. They often perform poorly academically and exhibit abrupt switches between good and bad behavior. Mania in adolescents is commonly misdiagnosed as antisocial personality disorder (see Chapter 24) or schizophrenia (see Chapter 22). Although BPD is less common with increasing age, the first episode can occur in older adults. The estimated prevalence of mania in elders is 5% to 19%. The mortality rate for untreated BPD is higher than for most types of heart disease and some types of cancer (St. John, 2005).

The category of BPD includes bipolar I disorder; bipolar II disorder; cyclothymic disorder; and BPD, NOS. BPD, NOS, is used to code disorders with features of BPD when these features do not meet the criteria for any specific BPD. Bipolar I, bipolar II, and cyclothymic disorders are discussed in the following sections.

Bipolar I Disorder

Bipolar I disorder occurs less commonly than major depressive disorder with a lifetime prevalence of about 1%, similar to the statistics for schizophrenia (Sadock & Sadock, 2003). It is characterized by one or more manic or mixed episodes in which the individual experiences rapidly alternating moods accompanied by symptoms of a manic mood and a major depressive episode. The specifier *single manic episode* is used when a client experiences the first manic episode. The specifier *recurrent episode* is used to describe the most recent episode when episodes are separated by at least 2 months without clinical symptoms of mania or hypomania (APA, 2000).

During a manic episode, the individual exhibits an abnormal, persistently elevated, or irritable mood that lasts for at least 1 week. Impairment in various areas of functioning, psychotic symptoms, and the possibility of self-harm exist. Psychiatric comorbidities that are common in clients with bipolar I disorder include adult antisocial behavior, alcohol dependence, drug dependence, anxiety disorders, and conduct disorders. See Clinical Example 21-2 and the accompanying Clinical Symptoms and Diagnostic Characteristics box.

Bipolar II Disorder

Bipolar II disorder is characterized by recurrent major depressive episodes with hypomanic (a mood between euphoria and excessive elation) episodes occurring with a particular severity, frequency, and duration. These characteristics were established to decrease the overdiagnosis of hypomanic episodes and the incorrect classification of clients with major depressive disorder as having bipolar II disorder (Sadock & Sadock, 2003). According to the *DSM-IV-TR*, the client with bipolar II disorder has a presence or history of one or more major depressive episodes, alternating with at least one hypomanic episode. The symptoms, which may include psychotic, catatonic, melancholic, or atypical features, can cause significant impairment in various areas of functioning.

CLINICAL EXAMPLE 21.2

THE CLIENT WITH BIPOLAR I DISORDER

MS, a 45-year-old homemaker, was admitted to the psychiatric unit with a diagnosis of bipolar I disorder. The student nurse who assisted with the admission procedure noted that MS was wearing excessive rouge, eye shadow, and lipstick. Her purple dress was adorned with several necklaces, two neck scarves, and two belts. MS's fingernails and toenails were covered with purple nail polish. Every time the nurse attempted to question her, she would respond in a rapid, loud voice. The nurse noted that MS was easily distracted and appeared to jump from one idea to another while talking. She also described herself as an "indispensable" member of her church's governing board and stated, "I need to get home so that I can help the pastor make some important decisions." During the next several days, the nurse noted that MS was unable to sleep at night. Although she participated in numerous activities during the day, MS was not able to complete any projects successfully, due to a short attention span and distractability. She would approach various clients and share intimate personal secrets with them.

During the postclinical conference, student nurses who had attempted to relate to MS made comments such as, "I can't believe someone really dresses like that," "Does she really believe she is needed by the pastor to make decisions?" and "How can I communicate with someone who talks so fast? I have difficulty understanding her."

Bipolar II disorder is believed to occur more frequently in women than in men. Statistics cited in the *DSM-IV-TR* indicate approximately 0.5% of the U.S. population will experience this disorder. Of this group, approximately 85% are fully functional between episodes, while approximately 15% exhibit rapid-cycling (APA, 2000).

Cyclothymic Disorder

The symptoms of cyclothymic disorder are identical to the symptoms of bipolar II disorder, except that they are generally less severe. In cyclothymic disorder, the changes in mood are irregular and abrupt, sometimes

CLINICAL SYMPTOMS AND DIAGNOSTIC CHARACTERISTICS /
MANIC EPISODE

CLINICAL SYMPTOMS

- Mood that is abnormally and persistently elevated, expansive, or irritable lasting at least 1 week
- Inflated self-esteem or grandiosity
- Decrease in need for sleep
- Increased talking or increased pressure to keep talking
- Flight of ideas or subjective feeling of "racing thoughts"
- Easily distractible
- Increased goal-directed activity or psychomotor agitation
- Excessive overinvolvement in pleasurable activities usually associated with a high potential for painful consequences

DIAGNOSTIC CHARACTERISTICS

- Mood disturbance occurring in conjunction with at least three or more clinical symptoms
- Marked and significant impairment in activities or relationships with potential for self-harm or injury to others
- Symptoms not related to a medical condition or use of a substance

occurring within hours. This disorder occurs equally in men and women, possibly accounting for 3% to 5% of all psychiatric outpatients. The lifetime prevalence is estimated to be 0.4% to 1.0% of the U.S. population. Approximately 90% of the individuals with this disorder experience recurrent episodes. Clients with cyclothymia have a 15% to 50% chance of developing bipolar I or II disorder (St. John, 2005). Alcohol abuse and other substance abuse are common in clients with the diagnosis of cyclothymic disorder (APA, 2000; Sadock & Sadock, 2003).

The diagnosis of cyclothymic disorder is used when an individual displays numerous periods of hypomanic symptoms and depressive symptoms that do not meet the criteria for a major depressive episode. Such symptoms occur for at least 2 years, during which they do not subside for more than 2 months at a time. The symptoms are not caused by a general medical condition or

THE CLIENT WITH CYCLOTHYMIC DISORDER

WB, a 35-year-old plumber, was repairing a water heater when he began to talk rapidly and tell one joke after another to the homeowner. He laughed inappropriately and began to brag about his ability to "outwork" other employees. When WB returned to the company warehouse, his supervisor told him that the homeowner had called to inform him about WB's job performance and behavior. The supervisor expressed concern about WB's actions: during the last several months, he had noted that WB appeared to be either very happy or depressed. He described WB's mood as similar to the tracks of a roller coaster, with several ups and downs. WB was advised to see his family physician before he would be permitted to continue to work. After a physical examination by his physician, WB was referred to the local mental health clinic, where the diagnosis of cyclothymic disorder was confirmed. WB was assigned to a case manager and was allowed to return to work within 2 weeks.

the physiologic effects of a substance. Significant distress causes impairment in functioning. Cyclothymic disorder, like dysthymic disorder, frequently coexists with borderline personality disorder (Sadock & Sadock, 2003). See Clinical Example 21-3.

Clinical Symptoms and Diagnostic Characteristics of Other Mood Disorders

Mood disorder due to a general medical condition; substance-induced mood disorder; and mood disorder, NOS, are used to identify mood disorders that do not meet the criteria for major depressive disorder, bipolar I disorder; bipolar II disorder; cyclothymic disorder; or BPD, NOS. Premenstrual dysphoric disorder is a new category suggested for possible inclusion in the *DSM-IV-TR* after research studies have been completed and evaluated. The specifier *with postpartum onset* can be applied to the current or most recent mood disorder if

the onset occurs within 4 weeks after childbirth. A brief discussion of mood disorder due to a general medical condition, premenstrual dysphoric disorder, and mood disorder with postpartum onset is included below. See Chapter 25 for a discussion of substance-induced mood disorder.

Mood Disorder Due to a General Medical Condition

As stated previously, a mood disorder can occur as the result of adverse medication effects or as the direct physiologic consequence of a medical condition. The prevalence of this disorder is 25% to 40% of individuals with certain neurologic conditions (APA, 2000). The client exhibits a prominent and persistent disturbance in mood, which is depressed, markedly diminished, elevated, expansive, or irritable. History, physical examination, or laboratory findings confirm the diagnosis of mood disorder in the absence of delirium. Symptoms cause clinically significant impairment in areas of functioning. See Clinical Example 21-4.

Premenstrual Dysphoric Disorder

Premenstrual dysphoric disorder (PMDD) is a recurring and severe form of premenstrual syndrome (PMS)

THE CLIENT WITH MOOD DISORDER DUE TO A GENERAL MEDICAL CONDITION (CEREBRAL VASCULAR ACCIDENT [CVA])

CD, a 55-year-old woman, was admitted to the sub-acute unit of a long-term care facility for rehabilitation. Before the CVA, she had taught school for 30 years. During hospitalization, CD exhibited a flat affect, labile emotion, anger, loss of appetite, and insomnia, and would respond "I don't know" to questions posed by the staff. The clinical symptoms continued and appeared to interfere with physical therapy. A swallow study was conducted to rule out dysphagia. The results were negative. A psychiatric consultation was requested. The diagnosis confirmed the presence of a mood disorder secondary to a CVA.

causing impaired social and occupational functioning, influencing interpersonal relationships with family and friends. It affects approximately 3% to 7% of menstruating women in the United States. Severe PMDD can affect women at any age between menarche and menopause. Symptoms cease during pregnancy and after menopause (Young, 2001). Although the cause of PMDD has not been established, researchers believe that it is the result of a response to abnormally high estrogen and progesterone levels in women. Other hypotheses suggest that the biogenic amine neurons of women with PMDD are abnormally affected by changes in hormones, that the disorder is an example of chronobiologic phase disorder, or that it is the result of abnormal prostaglandin activity (Sadock & Sadock, 2003).

PMDD, a generally recognized syndrome, involves mood symptoms, behavior symptoms, and physical symptoms. Symptoms commonly experienced include dramatic monthly mood swings accompanied by irritability, anxiety, sleep disturbance, difficulty concentrating, and angry outbursts. Physical symptoms include breast tenderness, abdominal bloating, headache, and edema. Symptoms occur the week before the onset of menstruation and generally end a few days after menses begins (APA, 2000; Patient Information, 2002; Sadock & Sadock, 2003).

Mood Disorder With Postpartum Onset

Harris (2002) describes a dramatic increase in the incidence of mood disorder after childbirth, with the largest risk within 90 days after delivery and an associated increase in risk that continues for approximately 2 years postpartum. Reports indicate increased rates of depression of 12% to 16% during a period of 6 to 12 weeks after delivery.

Postpartum depression disorders are divided into three categories, which include postpartum "blues" (ie, mild changes, characterized by mild mood change 3 to 5 days postpartum), postpartum major depression (ie, clinical symptoms of major depression occurring within 5 weeks after delivery), and postpartum psychosis (ie, major depression with psychotic features or, BPD with depressive or mixed features). Women with postpartum psychosis are at risk for suicide and/or infanticide and require aggressive treatment in a controlled setting with careful supervision. Postpartum psychosis occurs in 0.1% of all postpartum women (Warnock, 2004).

THE NURSING PROCESS

ASSESSMENT

Depression is one of the most common psychiatric conditions seen in primary care practice. It is important that clinicians know how to assess clients with the diagnosis of depression and any coexisting medical condition. Failure to recognize and treat these conditions can exacerbate or limit effective treatment of existing non-psychiatric illnesses such as diabetes, emphysema, or cardiovascular disease (Trivedi, 2005). The nurse should also keep in mind that clients with clinical symptoms of BPD may have psychiatric comorbidities such as anxiety or substance abuse. When conducting an assessment of a client with a mood disorder, maintain eye contact, display empathic listening, and communicate interest and concern in an unhurried manner. Focus the assessment on the client's general description or appearance; ability to communicate; mood, affect, and feelings; and behavior, as well as the presence of risk factors or medical comorbidity.

Screening Tools and Assessment Scales

Many formal screening tools or assessment scales are available to determine the presence of mood disorder. Some of the more common ones are highlighted in Box 21-3.

Although many screening tools can help identify clients with depression, they do not distinguish between major depressive disorder and BPD. The Mood Disorder Questionnaire (MDQ) has been validated as a screening tool for BPD and can be completed in less than 5 minutes. It can correctly identify seven of ten clients with BPD (Hirschfeld, 2004). Also,

BOX 21.3   SCREENING TOOLS AND ASSESSMENT SCALES

Numerous tools and scales can be used to assess a client for a mood disorder. These tools and scales provide qualitative and quantitative evidence of the client's severity of symptoms. Commonly used assessment tools or scales include:

- Hamilton Rating Scale for Depression (HAM-D-17): A 17-item observer-rated scale that assesses depressive symptoms; one of the most widely used instruments for the clinical assessment of depressive states
- Hamilton Rating Scale for Depression (HAM-D-7): A shorter version of the HAM-D-17. It is considered to be a simpler and quicker method to assess depression in clients.
- Global Assessment Scale: A single-item rating scale for evaluating the overall functioning of a client during a specific period on a continuum from psychiatric illness to health
- Zung Self-Assessment Scale: A 20-item self-rating scale that assesses the client's feelings; focuses on clinical symptoms of depression within the last 2 weeks
- Wakefield Questionnaire: A 12-item self-reporting questionnaire that asks a client to identify personal feelings at the time the questionnaire is completed; each item rated on a scale of 0 to 3; score of 15 or higher possibly indicative of depression
- Beck Depression Inventory: A 5-minute, 21-item scale that assesses the intensity of depression in individuals between the ages of 13 and 80 years
- Geriatric Depression Scale: A 30-item basic screening scale for depression in older adults; depression rated as none present, mild, moderate, or severe
- General Health Questionnaire (GHQ): Self-administered screening instrument to detect psychiatric disorders in community settings and non-psychiatric clinical settings
- Young Mania Rating Scale: An 11-item scale that rates the severity of the client's condition over the previous 48 hours; behavioral observations by clinician during the interview also rated
- Manic State Rating Scale: A 26-item nurse-rated scale for assessing manic behavior that might typically be seen in an inpatient unit
- Behavior and Symptom Identification Scale: A comprehensive measure of self-reported symptoms and functional health status that may indicate the need for inpatient psychiatric treatment

---

pain is a highly prevalent, under-appreciated element of depression symptoms, yet most depression assessment instruments pay relatively little attention to pain. Chapter 9 discusses the importance of self-reporting of pain and the use of a pain intensity rating scale during assessment. Therefore, choose the method that best fits personal preference, the client population served, and the practice setting. Also be aware of the potential harms of screening, such as false-positive screening results, the inconvenience of further diagnostic work-up, the adverse effects and costs of treatment for clients who are incorrectly identified as having a mood disorder, and the potential adverse effects of labeling (Berg, 2002).

The U.S. Preventive Services Task Force (2002) recommends asking two specific questions when screening a client for a mood disorder. These two questions about mood and **anhedonia** (the inability to experience pleasure from activities that normally produce pleasurable feelings) may be as effective as using longer instruments and are as follows:

- Over the last 2 weeks, have you felt down, depressed, or hopeless?
- Over the last 2 weeks, have you felt little interest or pleasure in doing things?

Regardless of whether a tool, scale, or the two recommended questions are used, when completed, validate impressions with the client to avoid an incorrect interpretation of data and to allow the client time to provide any additional information that he or she deems important. Input by family members or significant others may be necessary to complete the assessment process and to determine an appropriate nursing diagnosis.

General Description or Appearance

Clients with clinical symptoms of a major depressive disorder are often difficult to approach or assess. The client with major depression may avoid eye contact, dress in dull- or drab-colored clothing or pay little attention to appearance, assume a stooped posture, and exhibit **psychomotor retardation** (a generalized slowing of physical and emotional reactions) or **psychomotor agitation** (excessive motor activity associated with a feeling of inner tension).

Clients with clinical symptoms of BPD are generally excited, talkative to the point of being intrusive, and dressed in bizarre fashion. They are often very friendly and invasive of the territorial space of others (Sadock & Sadock, 2003). Assessment data must reflect which phase of BPD the client is presently exhibiting and describe the frequency with which the symptoms cycle from depressed mood to hypomanic or manic episode (eg, hours, days, or months). Remember that rapid-cyclers have four or more episodes per year.

Communication

In clients with mood disorders, body language may replace communication skills because the client is unable to convey feelings or thoughts. For example, clients with depression may respond to questions with single words, and exhibit delayed responses to questions—requiring the nurse to wait 2 or 3 minutes for a response. Conversely, clients with manic features generally exhibit hyperactivity, in which speech is pressured and considered a nuisance to those around them. They cannot be interrupted while they are speaking.

The inability of clients to relate to the nurse may hinder the development of a therapeutic relationship and the formulation of accurate nursing diagnoses. Consequently, it may be necessary to obtain additional information from family members or employees who bring or send clients for treatment, due to clients' social withdrawal as evidenced by decreased communication or verbalization of suicidal or homicidal thoughts.

Mood, Affect, and Feelings

Feelings of isolation, ambivalence, hostility, guilt, or concern about memory are often noted during the assessment process. Clients who are depressed may have negative views of their environment and of themselves as they reflect on topics of loss, guilt, suicide, and death. They may also exhibit clinical symptoms of thought blocking and **poverty of speech content** (the content of the answer is vague or obscure).

Clients exhibiting the manic phase of BPD are euphoric. However, they also can be irritable. They often demonstrate a low frustration tolerance; anger; hostility; and emotional lability (eg, exhibiting laugh-ter, irritability, and depressed mood within minutes to hours) (APA, 2000; Sadock & Sadock, 2003).

Ask the client to describe the intensity and duration of any changes in mood, affect, and feelings, and what meaning he or she attaches to these changes. Also assess for possible stressors such as changes in physical health, dissatisfaction with marital status, alteration in family dynamics or economic status, cultural or ethnic issues, sexual identity issues, and disappointment with life interests or pursuits. The availability of support systems, community ties, and a spiritual framework should also be assessed.

Behavior

The client's behavior is influenced by thought content, level of cognition, judgment and insight, impulse control (eg, presence of aggressive, destructive, suicidal, or homicidal behavior), and the presence of perceptual disturbances (eg, delusions or hallucinations). Clients with psychotic depression generally exhibit psychomotor agitation, guilt, hallucinations (eg, auditory, visual, or somatic), cognitive impairment (eg, slowed mental processing, impaired attention, and delusions), and more suicidal preoccupation compared with clients suffering from nonpsychotic depression (Gitlin, 2005).

Nursing assessment focuses on the client's ability to meet daily needs, follow directions, and remain compliant with the plan of care. Ask questions regarding sensitivity of mood to changes in the sleep/wake cycle, diet, exercise, work shifts, season, time-zone travel, and postpartum and menstrual symptoms if appropriate (St. John, 2005). Assessment should also focus on the presence of psychotic or suicidal thoughts (see Chapter 31).

Risk Factors

Assess for the presence of risk factors such as pain, medical comorbidity, or the use of medication associated with behavioral changes and a high risk of a mood disorder (see Box 21-2 earlier in this chapter). Prepare the client for a physical examination if a medical doctor has not seen the client within the last year. Thyroid function studies, blood glucose, and drug and alcohol screens may be conducted to rule out common secondary etiologies. The necessity for other studies, such as computed tomography scan or magnetic resonance imaging of the brain, electroencephalogram, and chemical panels is determined by the history and thorough physical exam (St. John, 2005).

Because the client may have a history of a mood disorder, obtain information about prior treatment, including the use of and response to antidepressant medication or other psychotropic medication and any alternative therapies. Obtain a family history to rule out the presence of genetic or biologic predisposition to depression. Clients who exhibit treatment-resistant depression should be evaluated for the presence of psychotic symptoms. Research has shown that clients with moderate-to-severe depression exhibit negative symptoms of schizophrenia (See Chapter 22) and that clients with moderate-to-severe mania exhibit disorganized speech and behavior. Clients diagnosed with severe mood disorders may exhibit psychotic symptoms such as hallucinations, delusions, paranoia, and catatonia continuously for 2 years to life (Lake & Hurwitz, 2006). Clients with psychotic depression often hide delusional beliefs, cognitive deficits, or suicidal ideation. Ask for permission to talk with significant others if psychotic depression is suspected (Boschert, 2005).

Transcultural Considerations

Culture can influence the experience of mood disorder symptoms and methods for communicating how one feels. Consider the Latino, African American, and gay communities. Research has shown that despite lower incomes, lower education levels, poorer access to health care, and higher levels of depression, Latino populations in the United States experience a lower adult mortality rate than whites. In one study, 315 Mexican American women living in California were surveyed. The results indicated that the Latino women who spent their childhoods in Mexico before immigrating to the United States showed lower levels of depression and higher levels of satisfaction with their lives. Intrinsic strengths such as having a sense of mastery, life satisfaction, and resilience contributed to lower depression scores in the Latino women (Heilemann, Lee, & Kury, 2002).

Interviews with depression experts and African Americans who have depression were shown in a video, *Black and Blue: Depression in the African-American Community*. According to the experts, African Americans are less likely to seek help for depression, but they are more likely than whites to be exposed to stressors that put them at a higher risk of developing the condition. They also have higher rates of illnesses (eg, heart disease, stroke, AIDS) that put them at a higher risk for depression. One of the clients interviewed stated he did not want anyone to think of him as being weak and seeking treatment for depression carried additional shame (Frieden, 2004).

According to the results of four different studies, (ie, Urban Men's Health Study, National Comorbidity Sample, Midlife Development in the United States Study, and National Health and Nutrition Examination Survey), although gay men are significantly more likely than adult U.S. men in general to be clinically depressed or distressed, they are often reluctant to seek professional help. Predictors of depression among gay men included anti-gay violence or threats, community alienation rated as "very high," lack of a domestic partner, and not identifying oneself as gay (Perlstein, 2004).

In culturally diverse settings, keep in mind that depression may be experienced in somatic terms rather than as sadness or guilt. For example, Latinos may speak of "having nerves," Asians of being "out of balance" and African Americans of "feeling evil" or "being angry." Judging the seriousness of clinical symptoms also may differ among cultures. Culturally distinctive experiences may be under-diagnosed or misdiagnosed as psychotic symptoms (APA, 2000).

NURSING DIAGNOSES

Before making a nursing diagnosis/diagnoses, be sure that an underlying medical condition does not go unrecognized. This is a crucial point because otherwise the planned interventions may be ineffective. Several factors influence the formulation of nursing diagnoses. They include the client's medical condition (assuming that the medical condition has been evaluated and a diagnosis has been established if a comorbid medical condition exists), ability to perform activities of daily living, level of depression or manic state (including the presence or absence of psychotic symptoms), and the client's admission to or denial of suicidal ideation or plan. Examples of North American Nursing Diagnosis Association (NANDA) Nursing Diagnoses related to mood disorders are presented in the accompanying box.

OUTCOME IDENTIFICATION

Outcome identification for the client with major depression focuses on the client's needs, such as safety and security, physical health, acceptance, belonging, positive self-concept, and empowerment. In addition to those for the client with depression, outcomes for

EXAMPLE OF NANDA NURSING DIAGNOSES/ MOOD DISORDER	EXAMPLES OF STATED OUTCOMES/ MOOD DISORDERS
• Activity Intolerance related to inactivity secondary to depression • Imbalanced Nutrition: Less than Body Requirements related to anorexia secondary to depression or manic state of bipolar disorder • Fatigue related to hyperactivity secondary to manic state of bipolar disorder • Hopelessness related to poor self-concept secondary to depression • Impaired Verbal Communication related to inability to concentrate secondary to depression • Ineffective Coping related to delusions of grandeur secondary to manic state of bipolar disorder • Situational Low Self-Esteem related to feelings of failure secondary to depression • Disturbed Sleep Pattern related to hyperactivity secondary to manic state of bipolar disorder • Social Isolation related to fear of rejection secondary to low self-concept	• The client will identify factors that reduce activity tolerance. • The client will report a reduction of symptoms of activity intolerance. • The client will describe causative factors of anorexia when known. • The client will describe rationale for the use of an appetite stimulant. • The client will discuss the causes of fatigue. • The client will demonstrate improved ability to express self. • The client will identify personal coping patterns and the consequences of the behavior that results. • The client will identify two positive attributes about self. • The client will describe factors that prevent or inhibit sleep. • The client will demonstrate an improved ability to socialize with peers or staff. • The client will differentiate between reality and fantasy.

the manic client will focus on opportunities to channel energy and to accurately perceive reality. Examples of Stated Outcomes related to mood disorders are listed in the accompanying box.

PLANNING INTERVENTIONS

Planning interventions for clients with mood disorders can be done with a feeling of optimism and satisfaction, because most mood disorders are time-limited or can be stabilized with medication and other therapies that enable the client to achieve a healthier state of functioning (Antai-Otong, 2001). For example, clients exhibiting clinical symptoms of a mood disorder secondary to a stressful life event often experience a time-limited mood disorder that responds positively to therapeutic interventions. Conversely, clients with the diagnosis of BPD often do well when taking medication but are at risk for an exacerbation of clinical symptoms if they discontinue taking prescribed medication.

Be alert to a personal vulnerability to depressive disorders. Working with such clients may cause one to react to the atmosphere of depression, and in turn, experience symptoms of depression. When planning care for clients with the diagnosis of depression or BPD, strive to attain and maintain the following personal attitudes:

• Acceptance: Clients with depression are not always able to express their feelings and may exhibit peculiar behavior or low self-esteem. Clients with manic behavior may be manipulative and demanding.
• Honesty: Clients with low self-esteem are less able to tolerate disappointment.
• Empathy: Any attempts to cheer up a client with depression or to minimize negative, painful feelings will be viewed as an inability to understand the client's feelings or problems. Doing so may lead to further withdrawal, isolation, or depression.
• Patience: Clients with depression may be unable to make decisions as simple as what to eat for breakfast or what clothing to wear. Clients who exhibit manic behavior may elicit feelings of irritation, frustration, or anger on the part of the caregiver.

Clients with depression may attempt self-inflicted harm or suffer injury due to severe depression, lack of interest, psychomotor retardation, the inability to concentrate, or the inability to defend themselves against aggressive persons. Be aware of the potential for self-destructive behavior. Such an action may occur as the client's psychomotor retardation lessens, the ability to concentrate returns, and the person is able to formulate a plan of action. Instituting protective care is essential (see Chapters 12 and 31).

Protective care may be necessary for the client with mania as well as for the client with depression. Persons who exhibit manic behavior may injure themselves as a result of excessive motor activity, inability to concentrate, distractibility, or poor judgment. Their destructive tendencies, often caused by poor impulse control, may include self-inflicting behavior and accidental injury. They may provoke self-defensive actions unintentionally from others who fear injury. If the client is experiencing psychotic symptoms, the potential for homicidal behavior could exist.

Planning care may require a multidisciplinary team approach to address additional risk factors such as a medical condition that may or may not contribute to the client's clinical symptoms; dual diagnosis such as the presence or history of alcohol or substance abuse; history of treatment-resistant depression; lack of social support; or a stressful life event such as the death of a spouse or divorce. A thorough knowledge base about psychotropic medication and a proficiency in administration; firm foundational understanding about the current use of somatic therapies; and the ability to provide client and family education are key elements of planning care.

IMPLEMENTATION

Implementing appropriate nursing interventions can occur in a variety of settings. Typically, hospitalization is recommended for clients who are severely depressed, display suicidal ideation, or require medical care secondary to depression. Clients displaying symptoms of acute manic behavior require hospitalization as well. Providing a safe environment is of the utmost importance.

Assistance in Meeting Basic Needs

The severity of the client's symptoms directly influences the degree of importance for physical care. The more severe the depression or mania is, the more important physical care becomes because the client loses interest in self-care and may have difficulty making decisions. Assistance with bathing, grooming, personal hygiene, and selection of appropriate attire may be necessary.

Dietary needs also require close monitoring. The client with depression may exhibit lack of appetite or anorexia, whereas the client with mania may be too hyperactive to eat. Nutritional supplements, dietary snacks, or finger foods may be necessary. Also monitor intake and output daily until the client is able to take the responsibility of meeting nutritional needs.

Evaluate the client's periods of rest and activity. Up to 80% of depressed clients experience difficulties in falling asleep, interrupted nocturnal sleep, or early morning awakening (Doghramji, 2006). The client with depression may sleep continuously in an attempt to avoid the problems and anxieties of reality. Dysthymic depression is characterized by increased feelings of depression as the day progresses. Such clients generally "feel better in the morning" and are more productive at that time. As the day progresses, clinical symptoms of depression become more pronounced. Clients tend to withdraw and lose interest in their environment and self-care. Clients with major depressive disorder or psychotic depression fall asleep early, awaken early, and feel better as the day progresses. The client with mania may experience sleep deprivation due to hyperactivity. A client exhibiting manic behavior commonly stays awake for a few days and then succumbs to physical exhaustion. Good sleep hygiene is an important self-management tool that clients can use to help control their disease course. Encourage clients to keep strict sleep–wake cycles, avoid naps except if a shift worker or elderly, avoid caffeine and over-the-counter stimulants, avoid the use of alcohol, exercise early in the day, spend time in bright light while awake, avoid stimulating activities prior to bedtime, don't watch the clock, eat a light snack before bedtime if hungry, and use the bedroom primarily for sleeping and intimate relations (Doghramji, 2006).

For the client with a short attention span or one who is unable to concentrate, engage the client in simple activities, such as a card game or a short walk. These activities are most effective because the client's self-esteem is enhanced when the tasks are completed. Also consider the client's energy level for activities. The more energy the task requires, the less energy the client will have to engage in hostile, aggressive behavior.

Displaying acceptance can be challenging when a client exhibits hyperactivity, anger, hostility, or demanding, manipulative behavior. Limit-setting may be necessary as the client attempts to express feelings and emotional needs.

Medication Management

Monitoring a client's medication compliance and observing for potential adverse effects is a challenging intervention. Clients who are new to antidepressant therapy are at the greatest risk of discontinuing therapy, and that risk is greatest at the time of first prescription refill. The length of time a client will be receiving antidepressant therapy, the possibility of requiring more than one medication, and the management of adverse effects that may occur should be dis-

cussed with the client (Brunk, 2005). Clients with the diagnosis of a depressive disorder may require an antidepressant (eg, sertaline [Zoloft]) in combination with psychotropic agents to treat clinical symptoms of psychosis (eg, risperidone [Risperdal]). It may be necessary to administer an antidepressant that is also effective in the treatment of underlying anxiety (eg, fluoxetine [Prozac]) or insomnia (eg, mirtazapine [Remeron]). There are several options for medication management of clients with the diagnosis of BPD depending upon the client's presenting symptoms. A client with BPD may require a mood stabilizer (eg, lithium [Eskalith]) as well as a neuroleptic (eg, olanzapine [Zyprexa]) or anticonvulsant (eg, valproic acid [Depakene]) to stabilize aggressive behavior secondary to psychotic symptoms (see Drug Summary Table 21-1).

DRUG SUMMARY TABLE 21-1 Drugs Used for Mood Disorders

GENERIC (TRADE) NAME	DAILY DOSAGE RANGE	IMPLEMENTATION
Drug Class: Antidepressants		
bupropion (Wellbutrin)	150–450 mg	Give in divided doses; monitor for CNS stimulant effects (eg, agitation, increased motor activity), dry mouth, headache, nausea and vomiting, and constipation; avoid use of alcohol.
fluoxetine (Prozac)	10–80 mg	Administer drug in the morning; give in divided doses if taking >20 mg per day; contraindicated during or within 14 days of MAOI therapy; avoid use of alcohol; monitor client's response closely in the presence of hepatic or renal impairment or diabetes mellitus as well as for headache, nervousness, abnormal sleep pattern, GI disturbances, and weight loss.
mirtazapine (Remeron)	15–45 mg	Contraindicated during or within 14 days of MAOI therapy; can be given at night to induce sleep; avoid use of alcohol; monitor for drowsiness, increased appetite and weight gain, dizziness, dry mouth, and constipation.
paroxetine (Paxil)	10–50 mg	Contraindicated during or within 14 days of MAOI therapy; limit amount of drug given to potentially suicidal clients; administer in the morning; use cautiously in the presence of renal or hepatic impairment; monitor for drowsiness, tremor, somnolence, GI disturbances, and sexual dysfunction in males.
sertraline (Zoloft)	50–200 mg	Contraindicated during or within 14 days of MAOI therapy, or with pimozide (Orap) or disulfiram (Antabuse); if given in concentrated form, dilute just before giving in 4 oz water, ginger ale, orange juice, etc.; monitor for increase in uric acid and hyponatremia, GI disturbances, tremor, weight loss, and anxiety.

GENERIC (TRADE) NAME	DAILY DOSAGE RANGE	IMPLEMENTATION
venlafaxine (Effexor)	75–375 mg	Contraindicated during pregnancy; should not be taken concurrently with MAOIs; monitor BP and reduce dose or discontinue if hypertension occurs; monitor for dreams, tremor, dizziness, somnolence, GI disturbance, and dry mouth.
Drug Class: Anticonvulsants as Mood Stabilizers for Bipolar Disorder		
divalproex (Depakene)	500–1500 mg	Give with food if GI disturbances occur; monitor liver function, platelet count, and ammonia levels per protocol; discontinue drug if rash occurs; advise client to wear medical ID alert bracelet; monitor for bruising, jaundice, sedation, and tremor.
gabapentin (Neurontin)	300–3600 mg	Give with food to prevent GI disturbance; advise client to wear medical ID alert bracelet; monitor for dizziness, insomnia, somnolence, and ataxia.
lamotrigine (Lamictal)	25–500 mg	Monitor renal and hepatic function before and during therapy per protocol; if rash occurs, discontinue immediately and be prepared with appropriate life support if needed; monitor for dizziness, drowsiness, GI disturbance, and headache; advise client to wear medical ID alert bracelet.
topiramate (Topamax)	25–400 mg	Give with food if GI disturbances occur; maintain adequate fluid intake in the presence of renal disease; advise client to avoid use of alcohol because serious sedation can occur; monitor for ataxia, somnolence, dizziness, nystagmus, and fatigue.
Drug Class: Lithium Salts		
lithium carbonate (Eskalith)	900–1800 mg	Give with food or milk after meals; ensure adequate daily intake of fluid (2500–3000 cc) and salt unless medically contraindicated; monitor for ECG changes, hand tremor, lethargy, slurred speech, muscle weakness, GI disturbances, and polyuria; follow protocol regarding obtaining lithium levels, thyroid tests, CBC and differential, and baseline ECG.
Drug Class: Atypical Antipsychotics		
aripiprazole (Abilify)	10–30 mg	Monitor for adverse effects.*
olanzapine (Zyprexa)	5–20 ml	Monitor for weight gain and adverse effects.*
risperidone (Risperdal)	0.5–16 mg	Mix oral solution with water, juice, low-fat milk, or coffee; monitor for galactorrhea, weight gain, and adverse effects.*

NOTE: The use of SSRIs and atypical antidepressants listed above are considered to be the first line of antidepressant drugs used in the treatment of major depression because they are better tolerated and produce fewer adverse effects in overdoses than older drugs such as TCAs and MAOIs. Anticonvulsants, lithium (Eskalith), and olanzapine (Zyprexa) are standard treatments for the manic phase of bipolar disorder; however, adjunctive use of benzodiazepines or other antipsychotics may be necessary to stabilize clinical symptoms. See Chapters 16, 19, and 22.

*Adverse effects: Agranulocytosis, changes in blood sugar and lipid serum levels, constipation, dehydration in the elderly, dry mouth, movement disorders (eg, EPS, TD, and NMS), orthostatic hypotension, seizures, sexual dysfunction, and somnolence.

Unfortunately, most antidepressant medication does not become effective or reach a therapeutic level for at least 3 weeks. Thus, additional dosage adjustments may be required to achieve the desired effect. Clients may become frustrated during this time because they expect immediate relief from their clinical symptoms. They may interpret the need for additional dosage adjustments as a poor response to the medication and discontinue taking it. Compliance with medication therapy also may be negatively affected if the client experiences transitory or untoward adverse effects and then refuses to continue with the prescribed medication. Further compounding this problem is the issue involving blood samples to monitor the client's blood drug levels. Clients may refuse to take the medication because they object to having blood drawn to monitor laboratory values. A new finger-stick lithium test approved by the Food and Drug Administration (FDA) can eliminate the inconvenience that often discourages clients who take lithium. New strategies are also being proposed for monitoring serum valproate levels in medically healthy clients who take valproate as the present APA-suggested routine monitoring may not be necessary (Jefferson, 2005; Kaneria, Patel, & Keck, 2005). Moreover, clients with the diagnosis of BPD often stop taking medication when they begin to feel better.

Rapid-cycling BPD can be more difficult to treat effectively. Lithium, which is often considered first-line treatment for non-rapid cycling BPD, is significantly less effective in rapid-cycling clients. Anticonvulsive agents such as valproate (Depakote), divalproex (Depakene), and lamotrigine (Lamictal) are considered to be more efficacious. Atypical antipsychotics such as aripiprazole (Abilify) and olanzapine (Zyprexa) recently received FDA approval to stabilize clinical symptoms of BPD and possibly reduce relapse or rapid-cycling. For the great majority of clients with rapid-cycling BPD, lifetime pharmacotherapy is required (Marcotte, Hussain, & Solomon, 2001; Sherman, 2004).

Pain Management

The neurobiologic substrate of pain symptoms appears to involve both serotonergic and noradrenergic descending pathways. These pathways play a role in buffering pain sensations, and dysfunctions in the two neurotransmitter systems result in amplification of pain. Dual-action agents that modulate noradrenergic as well as serotoninergic systems (serotonin–norepinephrine reuptake inhibitors such as venlafaxine [Effexor], mirtazapine [Remeron], and duloxetine [Cymbalta]) seem to be more effective in reducing pain associated with depression. This is not to say that all clients need dual-action antidepressant treatment; however, the presence of pain suggests that dual-action agents should be considered in the plan of care for clients with a mood disorder (Sherman, 2004).

Somatic Therapies

Electroconvulsive therapy (ECT) has been used for clients who experience treatment-resistant or severe depression. Chapter 17 discusses the nurse's role in ECT. Transcranial magnetic stimulation (TMS) was recently introduced as an alternative somatic therapy to conventional unipolar or bipolar ECT. In this therapy, stimulation is applied over the left dorsolateral prefrontal cortex to minimize the occurrence of a seizure. During the procedure, clients are awake, may sit upright, and are able to move and to interact with staff. Upon completion of the procedure, they can immediately go about their daily routine without supervision. This procedure is advantageous because anesthesia and seizure induction are not needed. In addition, the client experiences minimal to no cognitive disruption. Currently, this somatic approach is used primarily as a research tool (Janicak, Krasuski, Beedle, & Ayd, 1999; Sadock & Sadock, 2003).

Phototherapy—or the exposure to bright artificial light—can markedly reverse the symptoms of seasonal affective disorder (SAD), which occurs in the fall and winter. Phototherapy presumably works by shifting the timing or phase of the circadian rhythms of clients with depression. Morning light advances the timing, whereas evening light delays the timing of circadian rhythms. Thus, using artificial light to simulate morning light can be effective for clients with SAD and, in some instances, with treatment-resistant depression (Kaplan, 1999; Williams, 2005).

Vagus nerve stimulation (VNS) is a new surgical option for treatment-resistant depression. A pacemaker-like device surgically implanted in the left side of the chest sends tiny electric pulses to the left vagus nerve in the neck every few seconds. The nerve then relays messages deep into the brain (ie, key areas of serotonergic and noradrenergic innervation relevant to depression). It is believed that VNS helps regulate the release of neurotransmitters in the brain. Preliminary data suggests that VNS also could help manage anxiety disorders, obesity, pain syndromes, and Alzheimer's disease. Adverse effects include voice alteration or hoarseness, headache, cough, shortness of breath, neck pain, dysphagia, and other pain. There is a small risk for infection and nerve damage. Clients may deactivate the device with a magnet if they are uncomfortable. Pulse stimulation stops when a magnet is held against the left upper chest and resumes when the magnet is removed (Rado & Janicak, 2005; Sadock & Sadock, 2003).

Interactive Therapies

Cognitive, interpersonal, group, family, or behavioral psychotherapy may be utilized according to each client's particular condition and coping capacity. Cognitive psychotherapy is as effective as antidepressant medication in the treatment of mild-to-moderate depression. The approach chosen is influenced by client preference, stage and severity of illness, concurrent life situations, and psychological traits. The frequency of the therapy chosen depends on the need to monitor medication compliance and suicide risk; severity of the illness; the client's own support network; and the nature of the psychotherapeutic goals.

Clients with mania should show some response to medication, such as decreased agitation and restlessness and an increased attention span, before therapy sessions begin. Clients with depression do not benefit from therapy if they display psychomotor retardation. See Chapters 14 and 15 for a discussion of the nurse's role in interactive therapies.

In addition, occupational and recreational therapy may be used to channel the activity level of clients exhibiting manic behavior or psychomotor agitation. Clients with depression may exhibit an increase in self-esteem as they participate in these therapies.

Complementary and Alternative Therapies

The increased interest in complementary and alternative therapies has led to the growing use of natural remedies in the management of mood disorders. These remedies include St. John's wort, SAM-e, valerian, kava-kava, and black cohosh.

Although the exact mechanism of action is unknown, research studies indicate that St. John's wort affects dopaminergic, serotonergic, noradrenergic, and gabaminergic systems, whereas SAM-e increases levels of dopamine and serotonin (Milton, 2001; Resnick, 2001). Unfortunately, St. John's wort and SAM-e may interact with other antidepressants and produce adverse effects such as lethargy, incoherence, or increase in the effects of monoamine oxidase inhibitors (MAOIs) and selective serotonin reuptake inhibitors (SSRIs). Both St. John's wort and SAM-e may induce hypomania or mania in clients with BPD (see Chapter 18).

Valerian is an oral sedative-hypnotic used to reduce anxiety associated with depression. Kava-kava is taken to decrease restlessness. When kava-kava is combined with alprazolam (Xanax), coma may result. Black cohosh root is used to relieve the clinical symptoms of PMDD and PMS.

The effectiveness of acupuncture as a treatment for major depression in women has been investigated. The results of a controlled clinical trial indicate that acupuncture provides significant symptom relief at rates comparable with standard treatments such as psychotherapy or pharmacotherapy (Allen, 2000). These results suggest that a larger clinical trial is warranted. For a more in-depth discussion of other alternative therapies used to treat mood disorders, see Chapter 18.

Client Education

Client education, an ongoing process, begins as soon as the client exhibits the ability to concentrate and process information. Education focuses on teaching clients to recognize the onset or recurrence of clinical symptoms of depression or mania; understand the dynamics of mood disorders; recognize the adverse effects of prescribed medication; and understand the consequences of medication noncompliance and the importance of establishing a support system (see Supporting Evidence for Practice 21-1).

Caution clients who exhibit manic behavior to not assume too many responsibilities or overextend themselves. Instruct clients with depression to contact a support person if feelings of depression return or increase in intensity.

Clients and their families need to understand that BPD is a syndrome and not a single symptom. Some clients, especially teenagers, may have trouble distinguishing bipolar symptoms from their personalities. Several reputable Web sites are available as educational resources to help clients and their families or care-

---

SUPPORTING EVIDENCE FOR PRACTICE 21.1
The Use of Psychoeducation as an Intervention in the Treatment of Bipolar Disorder

PROBLEM UNDER INVESTIGATION / Recurrence of clinical symptoms in bipolar disorder

SUMMARY / The study consisted of 120 outpatient subjects with the diagnosis of Bipolar Disorder who had been in remission for at least 6 months and who scored less than 6 on the Young Mania Rating Scale and less than 8 on the Hamilton Depression Rating Scale. Subjects, after matching for age and sex, were randomly assigned to receive 21 sessions of group psychoeducation (experimental group) or 21 sessions of nonstructured group meetings (control group), in addition to standard psychiatric care. Group psychoeducation focused on the early detection of symptoms, enhancement of treatment compliance, and lifestyle. Researchers concluded that 23 subjects (38%) in the psychoeducation group had significantly fewer relapses and recurrences per subject and demonstrated an increased time span between recurrences of depres-

sion, manic, hypomanic, or mixed episodes than did 36 subjects (60%) in the control group. At 2-year follow-up, 55 subjects (92%) in the control group met criteria for recurrence of bipolar disorder, compared with 40 subjects (67%) in the psychoeducation group. The number of hospitalizations and days of hospitalization per subject were significantly lower in the psychoeducational group compared with the control group.

SUPPORT FOR PRACTICE / Group psychoeducation, when used as a nursing intervention for clients with the diagnosis of bipolar disorder being treated with psychopharmacologic agents, may facilitate early detection of a recurrence of symptoms and thereby decrease the severity of the episode.

SOURCE: Colon, E, et al. (2003). A random trial on the efficacy of group psychoeducation in the prophylaxis of recurrences in bipolar patients whose disease is in remission. Archives of General Psychiatry, 4(60), 402-407.

---

givers recognize disease symptoms and distinguish them from ordinary emotions, cognitions, and behaviors so that relapse can be recognized and treated early (Miklowitz, 2004).

EVALUATION

The client's response to interventions is evaluated based on the attainment of desired outcomes. The nurse compares the client's clinical symptoms as initially seen when entering treatment with symptoms exhibited following completion of a plan of care. Input by family members and members of the treatment team is important.

An important aspect of evaluation involves determining the resolution of clinical symptoms. Not all clinical symptoms improve at the same time. **Residual symptoms** (the phase of an illness that occurs after the remission of the initial clinical symptoms) have been identified in some clients on antidepressant therapy. These symptoms include **anergia** (sluggishness or listlessness), **apathy** (indifference), **asthenia** (pro-

found fatigue with loss of motivation and short-term memory problems), excessive daytime somnolence, fatigue, and hypersomnia.

Although SSRIs are employed to treat an array of mood disorders because they generally produce fewer adverse effects and are usually well tolerated, clients have been known to develop movement disorders similar to those produced by neuroleptics; serotonin syndrome; and serotonin withdrawal syndrome (see Chapter 16). Be alert for evidence of these adverse effects during the evaluation process.

If evaluation reveals an inadequate response to interventions, the nurse reevaluates the nursing diagnosis, inquires about medication adherence, evaluates the degree and nature of response, and determines an appropriate time to reevaluate the client's progress. Evaluation is an ongoing process as the client continues to progress toward optimal health. Nursing Plan of Care 21-1 illustrates the nursing process, focusing on the client with bipolar I disorder.

MOVIE viewing **GUIDES**

NURSING PLAN OF CARE 21.1

THE CLIENT WITH BIPOLAR I DISORDER

By age 31, Carl had already achieved a high-level position as a computer programmer/analyst for a large computer-manufacturing firm. He exhibited endless energy and unrelenting drive. By the time he turned 35, Carl was facing the loss of his career. His early success was overshadowed by a pattern of excess. Over the course of 9 months, Carl had purchased an enormous house, a sports car, a variety of exotic pets, and was faced with credit problems due to his spending spree. During the same time, Carl spent prolonged periods, as much as 5 days at a time, in his home with the shades drawn. He would not answer the telephone and would not answer the doorbell when friends stopped by to check on his well-being. His physical appearance had changed, as his hair had grown long and shaggy. He exhibited a 25-pound weight loss, and he neglected his personal hygiene.

Carl's boss approached him with concern about the changes that he had observed. He offered support by arranging for Carl to participate in the employee assistance program, which was staffed by a psychiatric nurse practitioner. Carl accepted his offer and scheduled an appointment.

DSM–IV–TR DIAGNOSIS: Bipolar I disorder: most recent episode mixed

ASSESSMENT: Personal strengths: Alert and oriented, intelligent, employed, supportive employer, willing to seek treatment, absence of psychotic symptoms

Weaknesses: Poor coping skills, self-neglect, avoided social contact with peers

---

NURSING DIAGNOSIS: Ineffective Individual Coping related to poor impulse control secondary to manic behavior

OUTCOME: Client will identify at least three positive coping measures that can be used when feeling increased stress and/or the impulse to spend money.

Planning/Implementation	Rationale
Explore ways to relieve stress.	Verbalization of feelings may help relieve stress.
Discuss the events that lead to impulsive spending and buying.	Identification of precipitating events may prepare the client to avoid similar circumstances in the future.
Explore the need for medication and/or supportive therapy to improve coping skills.	Involving the client facilitates his understanding and acceptance of responsibility to stabilize his behavior.

NURSING DIAGNOSIS: Imbalanced Nutrition: Less than Body Requirements as evidenced by a 25-pound weight loss related to self-neglect secondary to mixed episodes of bipolar disorder

OUTCOME: Client will increase oral intake as evidenced by eating three meals daily.

Planning/Implementation	Rationale
Consult with dietitian to determine daily caloric requirements and ideal body weight range.	The client's increased activity level during a manic episode increases the need for nutrients. The client may also neglect nutritional needs during a depressed episode.

(Continued on following page)

Planning/Implementation	Rationale
Encourage client to eat meals with others when able.	Eating meals with others increases socialization and provides an opportunity for the client to eat balanced, nutritional meals.
Obtain daily weights until weight is stable.	The client's increased activity level increases the need for nutrients to stabilize weight, avoid continued weight loss, and achieve the appropriate body weight range.

NURSING DIAGNOSIS: Dressing and Grooming Self-Care Deficit related to mixed episodes of depressed mood and manic behavior

OUTCOME: Client will demonstrate an increased interest in personal hygiene and appearance.

Planning/Implementation	Rationale
Provide positive feedback about appearance.	The client may lack interest in personal hygiene and appearance. Positive feedback can foster feelings of well-being and promote self-esteem.
Discuss employee dress code.	The client may be unaware of an employee dress code. Encouraging compliance facilitates responsibility for appropriate dressing and grooming.

NURSING DIAGNOSIS: Social Isolation related to loneliness secondary to mixed episodes of depression and manic behavior

OUTCOME: Client will socialize with at least one peer daily at work.

Planning/Implementation	Rationale
Identify at least one person with whom the client feels comfortable enough to socialize.	The client is more likely to socialize if the surroundings are familiar.
Identify community support groups for clients with bipolar disorder.	The client will need to develop social skills with others to facilitate relationships at work.

EVALUATION: Prior to termination of participation in the employee assistance program, client will meet stated outcomes and demonstrate an improvement in mood, affect, and behavior. Appearance and personal hygiene will improve. Client will also verbalize an understanding of his diagnosis, recognize clinical symptoms of relapse, and understand the need for continuum of care.

KEY CONCEPTS

◆ Mood disorders (eg, depressive disorders and bipolar disorders) are considered one of the most widespread psychiatric disorders. Approximately 18.8 million American adults (or 9.5% of the U.S. population) at least 18 years of age or older have a mood disorder in a given year. Mood disorders affect clients of all ages and are under-diagnosed and under-treated.

◆ Symptoms of mood disorders were described in medical literature as early as the 4th and 5th centuries BC. In 1889, Emil Kraepelin introduced the criteria now used in the classification of bipolar

I disorder and a mood disorder that occurs in late adulthood.

◆ Various theories describe the causes of mood disorders. Certain risk factors for mood disorders have been established, serving as clinical practice guidelines that require review during the assessment of a client who exhibits clinical symptoms of a mood disorder.

◆ Mood disorders can be caused by a medical illness or can result from the adverse effects of certain medications. Women may experience premenstrual dysphoric disorder or mood disorder with postpartum onset during childbearing years.

◆ Several screening tools and assessment scales are used to assess a client for evidence of a mood disorder. Assessment focuses on the client's general description or appearance; ability to communicate; mood, affect, and feelings; and behavior. Possible stressors and risk factors such as a comorbid medical condition or the presence of pain also are explored. Availability of support systems is identified.

◆ During the assessment process, nurses should acknowledge the fact that culture can influence the experience of mood disorder symptoms and methods for communicating how one feels.

◆ Nurses need to exhibit acceptance, honesty, empathy, and patience throughout the nursing process to prevent experiencing symptoms of depression when working with clients diagnosed with mood disorders. Additionally, nurses need to validate their impressions with the client to avoid an incorrect interpretation of data. This validation also allows the client time to provide any additional information the client deems important.

◆ Nursing interventions focus on providing assistance in meeting basic needs; medication management; assisting with somatic therapy; providing interactive therapy or complementary and alternative therapy; and providing client education.

◆ Evaluation, an ongoing process as the client progresses toward optimal health, includes comparing clinical symptoms noted when entering treatment with symptoms exhibited following completion of a plan of care. Input by family members and members of the treatment team is important.

For additional study materials, please refer to the Student Resource CD-ROM located in the back of this textbook.

CHAPTER WORKSHEET

CRITICAL THINKING QUESTIONS

1. As winter progresses, you notice that a classmate seems depressed and unmotivated. Attempts to discuss a mutual class project are met with disinterest. At first you are confused, but after several weeks, you notice she is not dressed as neatly as usual, is eating all the time, and is sleepy in class. What depressive disorder do you suspect? What questions should you ask her to ascertain if your conclusion is correct? What recommendations can you make to her?

2. Observe the population in a homeless shelter or community group home. What behaviors do you observe? Interview some of the staff. Are they prepared for managing client behaviors? What changes might improve their therapeutic effectiveness?

3. Your client with depression confides in you that her new medication, amitriptyline (Elavil), isn't working and she is going to stop taking it. On checking her medication Kardex, you notice she has been taking this drug for 5 days. Prepare a client education plan to teach her about this drug and her depression.

REFLECTION

Reflect on the chapter opening quote by Sadock and Sadock. In your own words, explain what is meant by the phrase "not merely the external or affective expression of a transitory emotional state." During the assessment of a client with the diagnosis of major depressive disorder, what sustained emotional responses would you expect to observe? Please explain.

NCLEX-STYLE QUESTIONS

1. While teaching a group of clients with a mood disorder about causation of the illness, the nurse explains the biogenic amine hypothesis as involving which of the following?

   a. Alterations in the neurotransmitters norepinephrine and serotonin affecting mood

b. Alterations in the neurotransmitters dopamine and acetylcholine affecting mood

c. Foods that contain elevated amounts of tyramine contributing to mood disorders in susceptible people

d. Hormones from the thyroid gland that are produced in lesser amounts contributing to mood disorders

2. The nurse assesses a client with a mood disorder for which factor associated with an increased incidence of this problem?

a. Family history

b. Lack of trust

c. Male gender

d. Poor appetite

3. When attempting to differentiate dysthymic disorder from a major depressive disorder, which findings would the nurse expect to assess if the client is experiencing dysthymic disorder? Select all that apply.

a. Delusions

b. Incoherence

c. Hallucinations

d. Poor appetite

e. Sleeping difficulties

f. Feelings of hopelessness

4. The nurse would assess a client diagnosed with cyclothymic disorder for which behaviors?

a. Feelings of grandiosity and increased spending

b. Feelings of depression and decreased sleep

c. Periods of hypomania and depressive symptoms

d. Periods of depression accompanied by anxiety

5. A client with the diagnosis of major depressive disorder, single episode, without psychotic features, is admitted to the inpatient psychiatric unit. Which question would be best to assess the magnitude of the client's depression?

a. "How long have you felt depressed?"

b. "Have you ever experienced depression before?"

c. "What are your feelings of depression like for you?"

d. "How would you rate your depression on a scale of 1 to 10?"

6. A female client with bipolar I disorder is noted to wear excessive make-up, brightly colored evening clothes that do not match, a vest, three different scarves, and several necklaces and bracelets. Several peers on the unit have been laughing about her appearance. Which nursing action would be best to preserve the client's self-esteem?

a. Help the client change into more appropriate attire.

b. Explain to the peer group that the client has bipolar disorder.

c. Discuss issues of good grooming at the community meeting.

d. Tell the client that she must select less flamboyant clothing.

Selected References

Allen, J. J. B. (2000). Depression and acupuncture: A controlled clinical trial. *Psychiatric Times, 17*(3), 72–75.

American Psychiatric Association. (2000). *Diagnostic and statistical manual of mental disorders* (4th ed., text revision). Washington, DC: Author.

Antai-Otong, D. (2001). Dark days: Treating major depression. *ADVANCE for Nurse Practitioners, 9*(3), 32–39.

Barden, N. (2004). Implication of the hypothalamic-pituitary-adrenal axis in the physiopathology of depression. *Journal of Psychiatry & Neuroscience, 29*(3), 185–193.

Berg, A. O. (2002). Screening for depression: Recommendations and rationale, U.S. Preventive Services Task Force. *American Journal for Nurse Practitioners, 6*(7), 27–30.

Boschert, S. (2005). Look for rigid thinking in psychotic depression. *Clinical Psychiatry News, 33*(10), 25.

Brunk, D. (2005). Antidepressant 'rookies' are more likely to quit. *Clinical Psychiatry News, 33*(11), 1, 8.

Colon, F., Vieta, E., Martinez-Arán, A., Reiners, M., Goikolea, J. M., Benabarre, A., et al. (2003). A randomized trial on the efficacy of group psychoeducation in the prophylaxis of recurrences in bipolar patients whose disease is in remission. *Archives of General Psychiatry, 4*(60), 402–407.

Doghramji, K. (2006). When patients can't sleep. *Current Psychiatry, 5*(1), 49–52, 57–60.

Emental-health.com. (2005a). Historical perspective of depression. Retrieved December 7, 2005, from http://www.emental-health.com/depr_history.htm

Emental-health.com. (2005b). History of bipolar disorder. Retrieved July 2, 2005, from http://www.emental-health.com/bipo_history.htm

Feinstein, A. (2002). An examination of suicidal intent in patients with multiple sclerosis. *Neurology, 59*, 674–678.

Finn, R. (2004). Ask MDD patients about chronic pain. *Clinical Psychiatry News, 32*(8), 1, 66.

Frieden, J. (2004). Minority patients express depression differently. *Clinical Psychiatry News, 32*(7), 32.

Gillespie, C. F., & Nemeroff, C. B. (2005). Early life stress and depression. *Current psychiatry, 4*(10), 15–16, 22, 24, 27–30.

Gitlin, M. (2005, June). Beyond major depressive disorder. *Supplement to Clinical Psychiatry News,* 9–11.

Grant, M., & Morrison, V. (2001). Primary care of major depression: Psychopharmacology strategies. *American Journal for Nurse Practitioners, 5*(7), 39–48.

Harris, B. (2002). Postpartum depression. *Psychiatric Annals, 32,* 405–415.

Heilemann, M. S. V., Lee, K. A., & Kury, F. S. (2002). Depression in Mexican American women. Retrieved December 7, 2005, from http://www.medscape.com/viewarticle/438822_8

Hirschfeld, R. M. A. (2004, July). Strategies for bipolar disorder diagnosis. *Current Psychiatry Bipolar Depression Bulletin,* 1–3.

Janicak, P. G., Krasuski, J., Beedle, D., & Ayd, F. J. (1999). Transcranial magnetic stimulation for neuropsychiatric disorders. *Psychiatric Times, 16*(2), 56–63.

Jefferson, J. W. (2005). Finger-stick lithium test. *Current Psychiatry, 4*(10), 111–112, 117.

Kaneria, R. M., Patel, N. C., & Keck, P. E. (2005). Bipolar disorder: New strategy for checking serum valproate. *Current Psychiatry, 4*(12), 31–32, 37–38, 43–44.

Kaplan, A. (1999). Chronobiology: Light treatment for nonseasonal depression. *Psychiatric Times, 16*(3), 59–62.

Katz, I. R., Streim, J. E., Parmelee, P., & Datto, C. (2001). Treatment of depression in the nursing home: Progress on older problems and emerging new ones. *Long-term Care Interface, 2*(6), 46–52.

Lake, C. R., & Hurwitz, N. (2006). 2 names, 1 disease: Does schizophrenia = psychotic bipolar disorder? *Current Psychiatry, 5*(3), 42–44, 47–48, 52–54, 57–60.

MacNeil, J. S. (2005). Identify, treat depression in cancer patients. *Clinical Psychiatry News, 33*(11), 4.

Marcotte, D. B., Hussain, M. Z., & Solomon, D. A. (2001, November). Challenge of the future: The diagnosis and management of rapid-cycling bipolar disorder. *Clinical Courier, 19*(19), 1–8.

Medina, J. (1995). Pseudogenetics, part II. *Psychiatric Times, 12*(2), 30.

Miklowitz, D. J. (2004, October). Psychosocial therapies for bipolar disorder. *Current Psychiatry Bipolar Depression Bulletin,* 1–4.

Milton, D. (2001). Escaping the "Prozac syndrome." *ADVANCE for Nurses, 2*(6), 23–24.

Murray, C. J., & Lopez, A. D. (1996). *Global burden of disease.* Cambridge, MA: Harvard University Press.

National Association for Research on Schizophrenia and Depression (NARSAD). (2005). Depression. Retrieved January 13, 2005, from http://www.narsad.org/dc/

National Institute of Mental Health. (2005). The numbers count: Mental disorders in America. Retrieved October 27, 2005, from http://www.nimh.nih.gov/pubicat/numbers.cfm?output=print

Patient Information. (2002). Understanding premenstrual dysphoric disorder. *ADVANCE for Nurse Practitioners, 10*(3), 80.

Patten, S. B., Beck, C. A., & Williams, J. V. (2003). Major depression in multiple sclerosis: A population-based perspective. *Neurology, 61,* 1524–1527.

Perlstein, S. (2004). Gay men at increased risk for developing depression, distress. *Clinical Psychiatry News, 32*(7), 48.

Rado, J., & Janicak, P. G. (2005). Vagus nerve stimulation. *Current Psychiatry, 4*(9), 78–82.

Resnick, B. (2001). Depression in older adults. *ADVANCE for Nurses, 2*(14), 23–26.

Sadock, B. J., & Sadock, V. A. (2003). *Kaplan & Sadock's synopsis of psychiatry: Behavioral sciences/clinical psychiatry* (9th ed.). Philadelphia: Lippincott Williams & Wilkins.

Shahrokh, N., & Hales, R. E. (Eds.) (2003). *American psychiatric glossary* (8th ed.). Washington, DC: American Psychiatric Press, Inc.

Sherman, C. (2004). Make pain resolution a key issue in depression tx. *Clinical Psychiatry News, 32*(3), 75.

St. John, D. (2005). Bipolar affective disorder: Diagnosis and current treatments. *Clinician Reviews, 14*(6), 43–50.

Stong, C. (2004). Is there a biologic connection between inflammatory disease and depression? *Neuropsychiatry Reviews, 5*(7), 1, 13.

Stong, C. (2005). Seasonal affective disorder—Prevalence, demographics, and environmental predictors. *Neuropsychiatry Reviews, 6*(7), 9.

Trivedi, M. (2005, October). Comorbid anxiety and depression in the primary care setting. *Self-Study Supplement to Clinician Reviews,* 4–10.

United States Preventive Services Task Force. (2002). Screening for depression: Recommendations and rationale. Retrieved December 7, 2005, from http://www.ahrq.gov/clinic/uspstfix.htm

Warnock, J. K. (2004). Major depression in women: Unique issues. *University of Virginia School of Medicine Reports on Psychiatric Disorders, 1*(1), 1–8.

Williams, G. (Ed.) (2005). Light therapy effectively treats mood disorders. *Neuropsychiatry Reviews, 6*(5), 12.

Young, M. (2001). PMS and PMDD: Identification and treatment. *Patient Care, 35*(2), 29–50.

Suggested Readings

Altman, L. S. (2005). Antidepressants for bipolar depression: Tips to stay out of trouble. *Current Psychiatry, 4*(7), 21–22, 25–29.

Andrews, M. M., & Boyle, J. S. (2003). *Transcultural concepts in nursing care* (4th ed.). Philadelphia: Lippincott Williams & Wilkins.

Carpenito-Moyet, L. J. (2006). *Handbook of nursing diagnosis* (11th ed.). Philadelphia: Lippincott Williams & Wilkins.

Culpepper, L. (2004). Management of comorbid depression and anxiety in the primary care setting. *Clinician Reviews, 14*(4), 103–114.

Dantzer, R. (2004). Is there a connection between inflammatory disease and depression? *Neuropsychiatry Reviews, 5*(7), 1, 13.

Jaques, S. H. (2004). Diabetes and depression. *American Journal of Nursing, 104*(9), 56–59.

Kupfer, D. J. (Ed.). (2004). Bipolar depression: The clinician's reference guide (BD-CRG). Montvale, NJ: Current Psychiatry, LLC.

Locke, C. J. (2003). Premenstrual symptoms: Today's theories and treatments. *ADVANCE for Nurse Practitioners, 11*(2), 77–80.

Lopez, J. F. (2005). The neurobiology of depression. Retrieved January 8, 2005, from http://www. thedoctorwillseeyounow. com/articles/behavior/ depressn_5/

Merriam, A. E. (2005, June). The etiology of depression remains elusive. *Supplement to Clinical Advisor,* 3–8.

Schultz, J.M., & Videbeck, S. L. (2005). *Lippincott's manual of psychiatric nursing care plans* (7th ed.). Philadelphia: Lippincott Williams & Wilkins.

Spader, C. (2005). Erasing myths about postpartum disorders. *Nursing Spectrum.* Retrieved February 21, 2005, from http://community.nursingspectrum.com/MagazineArticles/article.cfm?AID=13606

St. John, D. D. (2005, March). Bipolar disorder: Diagnosing a devastating illness. *Clinical Advisor Supplement,* 3–10.

Tugrul, K. C. (2004, March). Evolving role of antipsychotic therapy in the management of bipolar disorder. *Advanced Studies in Nursing, 2*(1), 24–32.

Willig, J. (2004). Depression in the Hispanic population. *ADVANCE for Nurses, 5*(6), 33–34.

CHAPTER 22 / SCHIZOPHRENIA AND SCHIZOPHRENIC-LIKE DISORDERS

The burden of psychiatric conditions has been heavily underestimated.
Disability caused by active psychosis in schizophrenia produces disability
equal to quadriplegia. —NATIONAL INSTITUTE OF MENTAL HEALTH, 2001

LEARNING OBJECTIVES

AFTER STUDYING THIS CHAPTER, YOU SHOULD BE ABLE TO:

1. Compare at least three current theories contributing to the understanding of the development of schizophrenia.
2. Articulate the classification of the five phases of schizophrenia.
3. Interpret Bleuler's 4 A's.
4. Differentiate the positive, negative, and disorganized symptoms of schizophrenia.
5. Distinguish the five subtypes of schizophrenia.
6. Analyze why an antidepressant drug and an atypical antipsychotic agent may be necessary to stabilize the clinical symptoms of schizophrenia.
7. Articulate the criteria that indicate the presence of metabolic syndrome.
8. Compare and contrast the rationale for the use of the following interactive therapies generally effective when providing care for clients with schizophrenia: group therapy, cognitive behavioral therapy, and personal therapy.
9. Discuss the purpose of including the client and family in multidisciplinary treatment team meetings.
10. Comprehend the importance of continuum of care for clients with schizophrenia.
11. Construct therapeutic nursing interventions when planning care for a client with the diagnosis of schizophrenia, paranoid type.

KEY TERMS

Affective disturbance
Ambivalence
Autistic thinking
Awakening phenomena
Awareness syndrome
Dementia praecox
Disorganized symptoms
Dopamine hypothesis
Double-bind situation
Echolalia
Echopraxia
Looseness of association
Metabolic syndrome
Negative symptoms
Pica
Positive symptoms
Psychogenic polydipsia
Schizophrenia

Schizophrenia is considered the most common and disabling of the psychotic disorders. Although it is a psychiatric disorder, it stems from a physiologic malfunctioning of the brain. This disorder affects all races, and is more prevalent in men than in women. No cultural group is immune, and persons with intelligence quotients of the genius level are not spared. Schizophrenia occurs twice as often in people who are unmarried or divorced as in those who are married or widowed. People with schizophrenia are more likely to be members of lower socioeconomic groups.

The onset of schizophrenia may occur late in adolescence or early in adulthood, usually before the age of 30. Although the disorder has been diagnosed in children, approximately 75% of persons diagnosed as having schizophrenia develop the clinical symptoms between the ages of 16 and 25 years. Schizophrenia usually first appears earlier in men, in their late teens or early twenties, than in women, who are generally affected in their twenties or early thirties.

Clinical symptoms can be draining on both the person with schizophrenia and his or her family because it is considered a chronic syndrome that typically follows a deteriorating course over time. Clients experience difficulty functioning in society, in school, and at work. Family members often provide the financial support, possibly assuming the responsibility for monitoring medication compliance.

Approximately 2.2 million people, or 1% of the earth's population, suffer from schizophrenia or schizophrenic-like disorders (disorders similar to schizophrenia). Schizophrenia impairs self-awareness for many individuals so that they do not realize they are ill and in need of treatment. Statistics indicate that approximately 40% of these individuals (or 1.8 million people) do not receive psychiatric treatment on any given day, resulting in homelessness, incarceration, or violence (National Advisory Mental Health Council, 2001).

Deinstitutionalization and cost shifting by state and local governments to the federal government, namely Medicaid, have contributed greatly to this crisis situation. Additionally, changes in state laws (advocated by civil liberties groups) have made it very difficult to assist in the treatment of psychotic individuals unless they pose an imminent danger to themselves or others. Consequently, individuals with psychotic disorders have been relocated into nursing homes, general hospitals, or prisons, or have been forced to live in the streets or homeless shelters (see Chapter 35).

Schizophrenia has been linked to violence. Predictors of violence among persons with psychotic disorders include failure to take medication, drug or alcohol abuse, delusional thoughts, command hallucinations, or a history of violence. Approximately 50% of schizophrenic clients have a substance-abuse disorder (Sullivan, 2004).

In response to this crisis situation and because of the heterogeneity and complexities of this illness, the National Institute of Mental Health has given the highest priority to training, research, and education about schizophrenia and schizophrenic-like disorders. For example, phase I results of the three-phase Clinical Antipsychotic Trials of Intervention Effectiveness (CATIE) in schizophrenia have recently been released. The 18-month study included nearly 1,500 subjects. During the study, researchers compared the efficacy of the newer atypical antipsychotics olanzapine (Zyprexa), quetiapine (Seroquel), risperidone (Risperdal), and ziprasidone (Geodon) with each other and with a typical first-generation antipsychotic, perphenazine (Trilafon). The purpose of the study is to determine which medications are most effective and, as a result, improve the quality of life for people with schizophrenia. A disappointingly high discontinuation rate (74% of the subjects) occurred within a few months of the study. In addition, 42% of the subjects met the criteria for metabolic syndrome (diabetes, hyperlipidemia, or hypertension), placing them at risk to die of cardiovascular causes within 10 years. The results of phase II findings, which have not yet been released, will focus on clients who did not improve with phase I regimens because of efficacy or tolerability problems and were switched to other antipsychotic therapies (Hillard, 2006; Nasrallah, 2006). Given the information released during the CATIE study, one can see that the role of the nurse can be quite challenging as client and family education is provided to promote health maintenance, lifestyle modifications, and client empowerment.

This chapter discusses the history, etiology, clinical symptoms, and diagnostic characteristics associated with schizophrenia and schizophrenic-like disorders. The different classifications of schizophrenia are presented, and the role of the psychiatric–mental health nurse is described, emphasizing the importance of medication management.

History of Schizophrenia

Written descriptions of schizophrenia have been traced back to Egypt during the year 200 BC. At that time, mental and physical illnesses were regarded as symptoms of the heart and the uterus and thought to originate from blood vessels, fecal matter, a poison, or demons. Ancient Greek and Roman literature indicated that the general population had an awareness of schizophrenia. Greek physicians blamed delusions and paranoia on an imbalance of bodily humors. Hippocrates believed that insanity was caused by a morbid state of the liver. By the 18th century, an understanding about the relationship between nerves and organs increased, and it was finally decided that disorders of the central nervous system were the cause of insanity.

Although the term *schizophrenia* (from the Greek roots *schizo* [split] and *phrene* [mind]) is less than 100 years old, it was first described as a specific mental illness in 1887 by a psychiatrist, Emil Kraepelin. Eugene Bleuler, a Swiss psychiatrist, coined the term in 1911. He was also the first individual to describe the positive and negative symptoms of schizophrenia. Both Kraepelin and Bleuler subdivided schizophrenia into three categories based on prominent symptoms and prognoses: disorganized, catatonic, and paranoid. *Diagnostic and Statistical Manual of Mental Disorders, 4th Edition, Text Revision (DSM-IV-TR)* lists five classifications originally described by *DSM-III* in 1980: disorganized, catatonic, paranoid, residual, and undifferentiated.

The 19th century saw an explosion of information about the body and mind. Evidence was mounting that mental illness was caused by disease in the brain. As a result of research during the last two decades, the evidence that schizophrenia is biologically based has accumulated rapidly. Furthermore, research in the genetics of human disease is also helping to develop more effective therapies and eventually cures for this potentially disabling mental disorder (Schizophrenia.com, 2006).

Etiology of Schizophrenia

Recent research suggests that schizophrenia involves problems with brain chemistry and brain structure.

However, no single cause has been identified to account for all cases of schizophrenia. Scientists are currently investigating possible factors contributing to the development of schizophrenia. Examples of possible factors include genetic predisposition; biochemical and neurostructural changes in the brain; organic or pathophysiologic changes of the brain; environmental or cultural influences; perinatal influences; and psychological stress. Research is rapidly progressing beyond the level of simple transmitters to define neuroanatomical and neurophysiological circuits that lie at the heart of cerebral dysfunction in schizophrenia. Furthermore, brain-imaging technology has demonstrated that schizophrenia is as much an organic brain disorder as is Parkinson's disease or multiple sclerosis (Brier, 1999; Kennedy, Pato, Bauer, et al., 1999; Sherman, 1999a; Spollen, 2005). Numerous theories about the cause of schizophrenia have been developed. Some of the more common theories are described here.

Genetic Predisposition Theory

The genetic, or hereditary, predisposition theory suggests that the risk of inheriting schizophrenia is 10% to 20% in those who have one immediate family member with the disease, and approximately 40% if the disease affects both parents or an identical twin. Researchers have recently identified three patient groups considered to be at "ultra-high risk" for the development of schizophrenia. The risk factors for one group include a family history of psychosis, schizotypal personality disorder (see Chapter 24), and the presence of functional decline for at least 1 month and not longer than 5 years. The conversion rate for this group is considered to be 40% to 60%. Approximately 60% of people with schizophrenia have no close relatives with the illness (Narasimhan & Buckley, 2005; Sherman, 1999a).

The first true etiologic subtype of schizophrenia, the consequence of a chromosome deletion referred to as the *22q1 deletion syndrome,* has been identified. Persons with this syndrome have a distinct facial appearance, abnormalities of the palate, heart defects, and immunologic deficits. The risk of developing schizophrenia in the presence of this syndrome appears to be approximately 25%, according to Dr. A. Bassett of the University of Toronto (Baker, 1999; Kennedy, Pato, Bauer, et al., 1999; Sherman, 1999d).

Scientists also may be close to identifying genetic locations of schizophrenia, believed to be on human chromosomes 13 and 8. One study found that mothers of clients with schizophrenia had a high incidence of the gene type H6A-B44 (Kennedy, Pato, Bauer, et al., 1999; Sherman, 1999d).

Research is now exploring how to proceed with genome scanning and DNA marker technology. To date, seven genes have been confirmed by at least several groups of investigators worldwide as increasing the risk for schizophrenia. Over the next 2 to 3 years, it is likely that between 10 and 20 genes will be implicated (Weinberger, 2004). The reader is referred to resources in the field of neuropsychiatric medicine for additional information.

Biochemical and Neurostructural Theory

The biochemical and neurostructural theory includes the **dopamine hypothesis:** that is, that an excessive amount of the neurotransmitter dopamine allows nerve impulses to bombard the mesolimbic pathway, the part of the brain normally involved in arousal and motivation. Normal cell communication is disrupted, resulting in the development of hallucinations and delusions, symptoms of schizophrenia (Fig. 22-1).

The cause of the release of high levels of dopamine has not yet been found, but the administration of neuroleptic medication supposedly blocks the excessive release. Other neurotransmitters or chemicals in the brain, such as the amino acids glycine and glutamate, and proteins called SNAP-25 and a-fodrin, are also being studied. For example, glutamate is considered to be the most prevalent excitatory neurotransmitter in the brain. Dysfunction of glutamate receptors, which are likely present on every cell in the brain, may be the cause of many neurologic and psychiatric disorders (Kennedy, Pato, Bauer, et al., 1999; Spollen, 2005).

Abnormalities of neurocircuitry or signals from neurons are being researched as well. Supposedly, a neuronal circuit filters information entering the brain and sends the relevant information to other parts of the brain for determining action. A defective circuit can result in the bombardment of unfiltered information, possibly causing both negative and positive symptoms. Overwhelmed, the mind makes errors in perception and hallucinates, draws incorrect conclusions, and becomes delusional. To compensate for this barrage, the mind withdraws and negative symptoms develop (Kennedy, Pato, Bauer, et al., 1999; Well-Connected, 1999). Cognitive deficits, impairments of attention and executive function, and certain types of

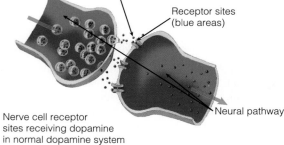

FIGURE 22.1 Dopamine receptors (the dopamine hypothesis).

memory deficits may be the result of abnormal circuitry in the prefrontal cortex (Moore, 2005).

Organic or Pathophysiologic Theory

Those who suggest the organic or pathophysiologic theory offer hope that schizophrenia is a functional deficit occurring in the brain, caused by stressors such as viral infection, toxins, trauma, or abnormal substances. They also propose that schizophrenia may be a metabolic disorder. Extensive research needs to be done, because the case for this theory rests mainly on circumstantial evidence (Well-Connected, 1999).

Environmental or Cultural Theory

Proponents of the environmental or cultural theory state that the person who develops schizophrenia has a faulty reaction to the environment, being unable to respond selectively to numerous social stimuli. Theorists also believe that persons who come from low socioeconomic areas or single-parent homes in deprived areas are not exposed to situations in which they can achieve or become successful in life. Thus they are at risk for developing schizophrenia. Statistics are likely to reflect the alienating effects of this disease rather than any causal relationship or risk factor associated with poverty or lifestyle (Kolb, 1982).

Perinatal Theory

Experts suggest that the risk of schizophrenia exists if the developing fetus or newborn is deprived of oxygen during pregnancy or if the mother suffers from malnutrition or starvation during the first trimester of pregnancy. The development of schizophrenia may occur during fetal life at critical points in brain development, generally the 34th or 35th week of gestation. The incidence of trauma and injury during the second trimester and birth has also been considered in the development of schizophrenia (Well-Connected, 1999).

Psychological or Experiential Theory

Although genetic and neurologic factors are believed to play major roles in the development of schizophrenia, researchers also have found that the prefrontal lobes of the brain are extremely responsive to stress. Individuals with schizophrenia experience stress when family members and acquaintances respond negatively to the individual's emotional needs. These negative responses by family members can intensify the individual's already vulnerable neurologic state, possibly triggering and exacerbating existing symptoms.

Stressors that have been thought to contribute to the onset of schizophrenia include poor mother–child relationships, deeply disturbed family interpersonal relationships, impaired sexual identity and body image, rigid concept of reality, and repeated exposure to double-bind situations (Kolb, 1982). A **double-bind situation** is a no-win experience, one in which there is no correct choice. For example, a parent tells a child who is wearing new white tennis shoes that he may go out to play in the park when it stops raining but that he is not to get his shoes dirty. At the same time, the parent's body language and facial expression convey the message that the parent prefers that the child stay indoors. The child does not know which message to follow.

Clinical Symptoms and Diagnostic Characteristics

Symptoms of schizophrenia may appear suddenly or develop gradually over time. It is a disorder that currently is not curable. Five phases of schizophrenia have been identified. They include the premorbid, prodromal (ie, beginning), onset, progressive, and chronic or residual phases. No clinical symptoms of schizophrenia are expressed during the *premorbid phase*. Gradual, subtle behavioral changes appear during the *prodromal phase*. For example, tension, the inability to concentrate, insomnia, withdrawal, or cognitive deficits may be present. These changes worsen and become recognizable as the symptoms that characterize schizophrenia. Cognitive deficits have been proven to exist 20 years before the third phase, referred to as the *onset phase* of schizophrenia, occurs. Once the symptoms of schizophrenia manifest, the illness evolves into the *progressive phase*. During this phase, clients may recover from the first episode and experience repeated relapses. The end stage of schizophrenia is referred to as the *chronic* or *residual phase*, during which time the client has experienced repeated episodes and relapses for a number of years (Lieberman, 2004; Moon, 1999).

In 1896, Emil Kraepelin introduced the term **dementia praecox,** a syndrome characterized by hallucinations and delusions. As noted earlier, Eugene Bleuler introduced the term schizophrenia and cited symptoms referred to as *Bleuler's 4 A's:* affective disturbance, autistic thinking, ambivalence, and looseness of association. **Affective disturbance** refers to the person's inability to show appropriate emotional responses. **Autistic thinking** is a thought process in which the individual is unable to relate to others or to the environment. **Ambivalence** refers to contradictory or opposing emotions, attitudes, ideas, or desires for the same person, thing, or situation. **Looseness of association** is the inability to think logically. Ideas expressed have little, if any, connection and shift from one subject to another.

Clinical symptoms fall into three broad categories: positive symptoms, negative symptoms, and disorganized symptoms. **Positive symptoms** reflect the presence of overt psychotic or distorted behavior, such as hallucinations, delusions, or suspiciousness, possibly caused by an increased amount of dopamine affecting the cortical areas of the brain. **Negative symptoms** reflect a diminution or loss of normal functions, such as affect, motivation, or the ability to enjoy activities;

these symptoms are thought to result from cerebral atrophy, an inadequate amount of dopamine, or other organic functional changes in the brain. The category of **disorganized symptoms** was recently added. This category refers to the presence of confused thinking, incoherent or disorganized speech, and disorganized behavior such as the repetition of rhythmic gestures. These symptoms and diagnostic characteristics are listed in the accompanying Clinical Symptoms and Diagnostic Characteristics box.

CLINICAL SYMPTOMS AND DIAGNOSTIC CHARACTERISTICS /
SCHIZOPHRENIA

CLINICAL SYMPTOMS

Positive Symptoms

- Excess or distortion of normal functions
- Delusions (persecutory or grandiose)
- Conceptual disorganization
- Hallucinations (visual, auditory, or other sensory mode)
- Excitement or agitation
- Hostility or aggressive behavior
- Suspiciousness, ideas of reference
- Pressurized speech
- Bizarre dress or behavior
- Possible suicidal tendencies

Negative Symptoms

- Diminution or loss of normal functions
- Anergia (lack of energy)
- Anhedonia (loss of pleasure or interest)
- Emotional withdrawal
- Poor eye contact (avoidant)
- Blunted affect or affective flattening
- Avolition (passive, apathetic, social withdrawal)
- Difficulty in abstract thinking
- Alogia (lack of spontaneity and flow of conversation)
- Dysfunctional relationship with others

Disorganized Symptoms

- Cognitive defects/confusion
- Incoherent speech
- Disorganized speech
- Repetitive rhythmic gestures (such as walking in circles or pacing)
- Attention deficits

DIAGNOSTIC CHARACTERISTICS

- Evidence of two or more of the following:
  Delusions
  Hallucinations
  Disorganized speech
  Grossly disorganized or catatonic behavior
  Negative symptoms
- Above symptoms present for a major portion of the time during a 1-month period
- Significant impairment in work or interpersonal relations, or self-care below the level of previous function
- Demonstration of problems continuously for at least a 6-month interval
- Symptoms unrelated to schizoaffective disorder and mood disorder with psychotic symptoms and not the result of a substance-related disorder or medical condition

---

Two diagnostic categories have been developed to describe the etiology and onset of schizophrenia: type I and type II. In *type I schizophrenia,* the onset of positive symptoms is generally acute. Type I symptoms generally respond to typical neuroleptic medication. Theorists believe that an increased number of dopamine receptors in the brain, normal brain structure, and the absence of intellectual deficits contribute to a better prognosis than for those identified with type II schizophrenia.

Type II schizophrenia is characterized by a slow onset of negative symptoms caused by viral infections and abnormalities in cholecystokinin. Intellectual decay occurs. Enlarged ventricles are present. Response to typical neuroleptic medication is minimal. However, negative symptoms generally respond to atypical antipsychotic medication (Sherman, 1999c).

As noted earlier, the *DSM-IV-TR* identifies five subtypes of schizophrenia: paranoid, catatonic, disorganized, undifferentiated, and residual (American Psychiatric Association, 2000). A brief summary of each subtype and a clinical example of each of the first three subtypes are given in the following paragraphs. Box 22-1 summarizes the five subtypes of schizophrenia.

Paranoid Type

Clients exhibiting paranoid schizophrenia tend to experience persecutory or grandiose delusions and

BOX 22.1   CLASSIFICATION OF SUBTYPES OF SCHIZOPHRENIA

PARANOID:

1. Preoccupation with one or more delusions or frequent auditory hallucinations
2. None of the following is prominent: disorganized speech, disorganized or catatonic behavior, or flat or inappropriate affect

CATATONIC:

At least two of the following are present:
1. Motor immobility (ie. rigidity), waxy flexibility, or stupor
2. Excessive motor activity that is purposeless
3. Extreme negativism or mutism
4. Peculiarities of voluntary movement as evidenced by posturing, stereotyped movements, prominent mannerisms or prominent grimacing
5. Echolalia (repeats all words or phrases heard) or echopraxia (mimics actions of others)

DISORGANIZED:

All of the following are prominent and criteria are not met for catatonic type:
1. Disorganized speech
2. Disorganized behavior
3. Flat or inappropriate affect

UNDIFFERENTIATED:

Meets diagnostic characteristics but not the criteria for paranoid, disorganized, or catatonic subtypes

RESIDUAL:

1. Absence of prominent delusions, hallucinations, disorganized speech, and grossly disorganized or catatonic behavior
2. Continuing evidence of, in attenuated form, the presence of negative symptoms or two or more symptoms of diagnostic characteristics

Reprinted with permission from the *Diagnostic and Statistical Manual of Mental Disorders, 4th Edition, Text Revision.* Copyright 2000, American Psychiatric Association.

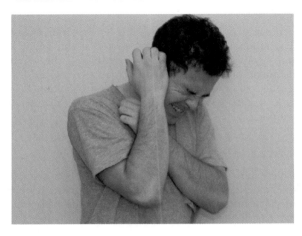

FIGURE 22.2   The client with paranoid schizophrenia experiencing auditory hallucinations.

Example 22-1:The Client With Schizophrenia, Paranoid Type.) Prognosis is more favorable for this subtype of schizophrenia than for the other subtypes of schizophrenia. Clients in whom schizophrenia occurs in their late twenties and thirties usually have established a social life that may help them through their illness. In addition, ego resources of paranoid clients are greater than those of clients with catatonic and disorganized schizophrenia (Sadock & Sadock, 2003).

The student nurse's reaction to paranoid or delusional behavior may be that of overzealousness in

CLINICAL EXAMPLE 22.1

THE CLIENT WITH SCHIZOPHRENIA, PARANOID TYPE

BW, a 35-year-old mechanic, was brought to the admissions office by his wife because he had exhibited strange behavior for several months. He accused his wife of poisoning his food, spending all his money, having an affair with his boss, and telling stories about him. He displayed no facial expressions during his initial interview and became quite argumentative when questioned about his job. At the end of the interview, BW confided in the interviewer that he had been receiving messages from Jesus Christ while watching television.

auditory hallucinations (Fig. 22-2). They also may exhibit behavioral changes such as anger, hostility, or violent behavior. Clinical symptoms may pose a threat to the safety of self or others. (See Clinical

attempting to convince the client that the student is genuinely concerned about his or her well-being. The student may become frustrated if the client is unreceptive to interventions focusing on the establishment of trust. The student may experience fear if the client exhibits unpredictable behavior. Fear is a normal response that results in the exercise of caution.

Catatonic Type

Psychomotor disturbances, such as stupor, rigidity, excitement, or posturing, are the prominent feature of catatonic schizophrenia. **Echolalia,** the pathological parrot-like repetition of a word or phrase, and **echopraxia,** the repetitive imitation of movements of another person, are also features of catatonic schizophrenia. Clients are at risk medically because of extreme withdrawal, which can result in a vegetative condition or excessive motor activity that could produce exhaustion or self-inflicted injury. (See Clinical Example 22-2: The Client With Schizophrenia, Catatonic Type.)

The student nurse may feel challenged when the client with catatonic schizophrenia is unresponsive to interventions and continues to exhibit selective mutism or refuses nursing care, food, and medication. Purposeless movements of hands and feet or extreme catatonic excitement that could result in harm to the caretakers may elicit fear in the student.

CLINICAL EXAMPLE 22.2

THE CLIENT WITH SCHIZOPHRENIA, CATATONIC TYPE

CS, a 25-year-old engineer, was admitted to the hospital as result of dehydration because of refusing to eat. During his hospitalization, CS was negativistic, refusing nursing care, food, and medication. He rarely spoke and assumed uncomfortable positions in bed for long periods. When placed in various positions by the nurse during the morning bath or shower, CS remained in the positions until the nurse changed them. He also exhibited purposeless movements of his hands and feet while sitting in a chair.

CLINICAL EXAMPLE 22.3

THE CLIENT WITH SCHIZOPHRENIA, DISORGANIZED TYPE

MJ, a 19-year-old waitress, was seen in the admitting office of a psychiatric hospital. During the initial interview, she giggled inappropriately. Her long, uncombed hair fell over her face, concealing her facial expressions. She mumbled incoherently at times and displayed the behavior of a 13- or 14-year-old adolescent. She complained of numerous aches and pains and stated that voices told her she was being punished for not cleaning her room. MJ's mother stated that she remained in her room at home and did not socialize with friends. Her parents sought help when they noticed her behavior regressing during the last 2 months.

Disorganized Type

The clinical symptoms of disorganized schizophrenia are considered the most severe of all subtypes. The client experiences a disintegration of personality and is withdrawn. Speech may be incoherent. Behavior is uninhibited, along with a lack of attention to personal hygiene and grooming. Prognosis is poor. (See Clinical Example 22-3: The Client With Schizophrenia, Disorganized Type.)

Because most clients who are diagnosed with schizophrenic disorder, disorganized type, are of a young age, student nurses' reactions may vary from shock to disbelief. Students may identify with the client who is close to their age or resembles someone they know. This reaction could interfere with the development of a therapeutic relationship. Such feelings need to be shared and explored with the clinical instructor.

Undifferentiated Type

Undifferentiated schizophrenia usually is characterized by atypical symptoms that do not meet the criteria for the subtypes of paranoid, catatonic, or disorganized schizophrenia. The client may exhibit both positive and negative symptoms. Odd behavior, delusions, hallucinations, and incoherence may occur. Prognosis is favorable if the onset of symptoms is acute or sudden.

The student nurse may feel uncomfortable or fearful in the presence of a client diagnosed with undifferentiated schizophrenia. The presence of atypical, disorganized clinical symptoms may prevent the student from attempting to communicate with the client.

Residual Type

Residual schizophrenia is the subtype used to describe clients experiencing negative symptoms following at least one acute episode of schizophrenia. Clinical symptoms may persist over time, or the client may experience a complete remission.

Schizophrenic-Like Disorders

The *DSM-IV-TR* lists five subtypes of schizophrenic-like disorders: schizoaffective disorder, schizophreniform disorder, brief psychotic disorder, psychotic disorder due to a general medical condition, and shared psychotic disorder. The first four disorders are discussed briefly here. See Chapter 28 for discussion of shared psychotic disorders.

Schizoaffective disorder is characterized by an uninterrupted period of illness during which, at some time, the client experiences a major depressive, manic, or mixed episode along with the negative symptoms of schizophrenia. During that same period of illness, in the absence of prominent mood symptoms, the individual exhibits delusions or hallucinations for at least 2 weeks.

The diagnosis of *schizophreniform disorder* is used when the client exhibits features of schizophrenia for more than 1 month but fewer than 6 months. Impaired social or occupational functioning does not necessarily occur.

Brief psychotic disorder is a disturbance that involves the sudden onset of at least one of the positive symptoms of psychosis such as hallucinations, delusions, disorganized speech, or grossly disorganized or catatonic behavior. The disturbance occurs for at least 1 day but for less than 1 month, as the individual eventually exhibits a full recovery or return to the former level of functioning.

Psychotic disorder due to a general medical condition is the diagnosis used to describe the presence of prominent hallucinations or delusions determined as resulting from the direct physiologic effects of a specific medical condition. For example, olfactory hallucinations may be experienced in the presence of temporal lobe epilepsy. A right parietal brain lesion

may cause an individual to develop delusions. Evidence from history, physical examination, or laboratory findings is necessary to confirm the diagnosis.

THE NURSING PROCESS

ASSESSMENT

Assessing clients exhibiting clinical symptoms of schizophrenia can be challenging. For example, clients may refuse to communicate or may communicate ineffectively as a result of impaired cognition or the presence of psychotic symptoms such as hallucinations or delusions.

According to L. A. Opler, a physician at Columbia University, the symptoms of schizophrenia should act as a guide during the assessment and development of a plan of care. In other words, he suggests the question to be asked during assessment is, "What's the problem here?" (Sherman, 2004). Along the same line, Sullivan (2004) discusses the use of a schizophrenia treatment algorithm or decision tree meant to be an educational tool and guide for health care professionals conducting assessments. The schizophrenia algorithm, available at http://www.ipap.org, classifies clients by pre-existing condition, comorbid disorder, and presenting symptoms. Both Opler and Sullivan suggest that assessment should focus on the presence or absence of the following clinical symptoms:

- Suicidality: 25% to 50% of individuals with schizophrenia attempt suicide at least once, and 5% to 9% succeed.
- Positive, negative, and disorganized symptoms
- Behavioral changes such as aggression or violent tendencies

- Substance abuse: 40% to 60% of individuals with schizophrenia abuse alcohol and/or stimulants.
- Nicotine use: Individuals with schizophrenia use nicotine to self-medicate to alleviate adverse effects of neuroleptic medication, dysphoric mood, and attentional deficits. Nicotine lowers blood levels of neuroleptics.
- Compliance if the client has a history of prior treatment. Noncompliance, which varies from 30% to 50%, is generally a result of adverse effects of medication.
- Adverse effects of medication
- Metabolic syndrome: Metabolic syndrome may be present as an inherent characteristic in clients with schizophrenia or resulting from the use of antipsychotic medication (see Chapter 16).

Assessment tools such as the Positive and Negative Syndrome Scale (PANSS), the Scale for Assessment of Negative Symptoms (SANS), the Brief Psychiatric Rating Scale (BPRS), or the Mental Status Examination (MSE) may or may not be useful for collecting data about orientation, memory, thought and perceptual processes, intellectual function, judgment, insight, affect, and mood.

History and Physical Examination

If appropriate, obtain subjective data from family members, significant others, or assigned caretakers. Answers to questions such as "What is the client's legal status?," "Where does the client live?," and "Has the client received psychiatric care in the past?" provide pertinent data. The client may not be able to state what, if any, medication has been prescribed and by whom. Therefore, focus additional questions on whether the client has experienced any adverse effects to previously prescribed medication, whether the client has an active support system, whether the client is able to perform activities of daily living, and whether the client displays any bizarre eating habits such as **pica** (eating non-nutritive substances) or compulsive overeating.

Approximately 25% of clients with schizophrenia have major symptoms of depression. It can be difficult to distinguish depression from the negative symptoms of schizophrenia (Sherman, 1999b). Be aware that depressive symptoms are frequent, often severe, and clinically meaningful in schizophrenia. They may indicate a first episode or be a predictor of a relapse of schizophrenia. As stated earlier, attempted suicide

among clients with the diagnosis of schizophrenia is relatively high. Clients with few negative symptoms who have a higher level of intelligence, can think abstractly, and can reflect on their illness are at the highest risk for suicide (Meltzer, 2005; Zoler, 1999).

Another key area of assessment is the client's fluid intake. Ask the client how much water is consumed daily. **Psychogenic polydipsia,** the compulsive behavior of drinking 3 L or more of fluid per day, occurs in a small percentage of clients with schizophrenia. Polydipsia may also occur when clients with multiple psychiatric diagnoses are given several medications to control clinical symptoms. Hyponatremia, electrolyte imbalance, and seizures may occur. Additional symptoms of psychogenic polydipsia include muscle cramps and changes in mental status, such as confusion and disorientation (DeMott, 2000).

Document the client's physical condition noted during the assessment. Comorbid medical problems that are commonly seen in older clients with psychotic disorders include obesity, hypertension, type 2 diabetes, and hepatitis. Also note the presence of any abnormal body movements, disturbance of gait, or unusual behavior. Additionally, document any hallucinations or delusions and other disorders such as anxiety, substance abuse, or depression that are assessed. A complete physical exam may be necessary to differentiate schizophrenia versus acute psychosis resulting from an organic disease. Suspicion of medical illness on the basis of vital signs, physical exam, or history should be thoroughly evaluated. Necessary lab work may include head computed tomography scan, alcohol level, drug screen, electrolytes, complete blood count, liver function tests, blood urea nitrogen (BUN)/creatinine, and tests of endocrine function (Clinician Reviews, 2005).

Transcultural Considerations

According to the *DSM-IV-TR*, clinicians have a tendency to overdiagnose schizophrenia in some ethnic groups. Persons with the diagnosis of schizophrenia in developing nations tend to experience a more acute course with a better outcome than do individuals in industrialized nations.

In the paper, *Infusing Culture Into Psychopathology: A Supplement for Psychology Instructors,* Ritts (1999) discusses the prevalence and cultural diversity of clinical symptoms of schizophrenia in China, Japan, Korea, India, Islamic culture, Israel, Nigeria, Hispanic culture, Germany, and Native American culture. For example, the prevalence of schizophrenia is higher in China compared with its prevalence in Western countries. Catatonic schizophrenia is more common in Asia, Africa, and developing countries. This may be due to the presence of strong family systems and social structures that place lower demands on sick individuals. In the Hispanic culture, hallucinations take the form of ghosts, spirits, or animals. Individuals with the diagnosis of schizophrenia in Germany exhibit delusions related to sexual, homosexual, or technical content.

Always consider cultural differences when assessing clinical symptoms in clients with suspected psychotic disorders. Ideas that appear delusional in one culture may be acceptable in another. For example, speaking in tongues or the presence of visual or auditory hallucinations with religious content may be considered a normal religious experience or a special sign to some individuals. (See Chapter 4 for a more complete discussion.)

NURSING DIAGNOSES

After data have been collected and prioritized, the nursing diagnoses are made. Always consider whether the client is exhibiting an acute onset of symptoms, is exhibiting decompensation of symptoms secondary to failure to take prescribed medication, or is being seen for case management. Examples of North American Nursing Diagnosis Association (NANDA) Nursing Diagnoses used while planning care of clients with clinical symptoms of schizophrenia are highlighted in the accompanying box.

OUTCOME IDENTIFICATION

Expected outcomes are stated for each nursing diagnosis. The statement of outcomes is influenced by several factors, such as the client's present coping strategies and level of cognitive function, the presence or absence of support systems and adequate income, and the clinical setting in which each treatment occurs. Examples of Stated Outcomes are highlighted in the accompanying box.

PLANNING INTERVENTIONS

The nurse's role in planning interventions varies as biologic, cognitive, perceptual, behavioral, and emotional disturbances are considered. Medical interventions

---

EXAMPLES OF NANDA NURSING DIAGNOSES/ SCHIZOPHRENIA

- Disturbed Thought Processes related to the presence of persecutory delusions
- Disturbed Sensory Perception related to the presence of visual hallucinations
- Self-Care Deficit related to poor personal hygiene
- Impaired Verbal Communication related to thought disturbance (looseness of association)
- Noncompliance related to refusal to take prescribed psychotropic medication
- Disturbed Sleep Pattern related to the presence of auditory hallucinations
- Social Isolation related to homelessness
- Ineffective Coping related to fear

---

may be necessary to meet biologic or physical needs. Diagnostic studies may be performed to rule out organicity. Medication may be required to treat depression, anxiety, or hostility, as well as psychotic symptoms. Cognitive therapy, behavioral techniques, and other supportive therapies may be used to empower clients to monitor their thoughts; overcome tendencies

---

EXAMPLES OF STATED OUTCOMES/ SCHIZOPHRENIA

- The client will communicate with members of the treatment team.
- The client will verbalize his or her physical needs.
- The client will exhibit compliance with medication management.
- The client will demonstrate the ability to perform personal hygiene on a daily basis with minimal assistance or prompting.
- The client will verbalize a decrease in the frequency of visual hallucinations.
- The client will verbalize a decrease in the presence of persecutory delusions.
- The client will exhibit an increase in the ability to socialize.
- The client will exhibit an accurate perception of reality.

to withdraw; increase their ability to concentrate; take responsibility for self-care; and cope with guilt, sadness, humiliation, and aggressive impulses. Electroconvulsive therapy may be necessary for treatment-resistant symptoms. Client and family education also focuses on empowerment and health maintenance.

The effects of schizophrenia and schizophrenic-like disorders are profoundly emotional. Clients may reflect a lack of separate identity; react negatively to perceived intrusion of privacy or closeness of personal space; exhibit low self-esteem, self-derogation, and lack of self-worth; display lack of trust; exhibit lack of self-control; and display profound depression (Peplau, 1996). Experts generally agree that treatment should include an integrated approach focusing on clients as well as their family members or significant others.

Continuum of care also must be addressed in the planning phase to avoid relapse or recidivism. Community treatment programs and vocational rehabilitation are highly beneficial and cost effective. According to the National Institute of Mental Health report to Congress on treatment efficacy (2001), the acute treatment success rate for schizophrenia at 6 months was 65%. Relapse rate at 2 years in clients who received antipsychotic medication plus psychosocial therapy specific to schizophrenia was 25%, compared to 63% in clients given medication alone (Jancin, 1998). The failure to provide comprehensive treatment for clients with a dual diagnosis has also been cited as a cause of recidivism. (See Chapter 32, Clients With a Dual Diagnosis.)

IMPLEMENTATION

Implementation focuses on establishing a trusting relationship; establishing clear, consistent, open communication; providing a safe environment; alleviating positive, negative, and disorganized symptoms; and maintaining biologic integrity. Interventions may differ depending on the client's clinical symptoms (ie, acute, rehabilitative, or chronic phase of illness), prognosis, and the clinical setting.

Remember that all behavior is meaningful to the client, if not to anyone else. Clients may refuse to communicate or may communicate ineffectively as a result of self-contradictory or conflicting statements, frequent changes in subject, inconsistency in verbalization, the use of incomplete sentences or fragmented phrases, or the presence of delusions or hallucina-

tions. Encouragement such as "Help me to understand how you feel" has been therapeutic when communicating with clients. Communicate in simple, easy-to-understand terms, directed at the client's present level of functioning. See Chapter 11 for additional information regarding therapeutic interactions.

Assistance in Meeting Basic Needs

Clients with the diagnosis of schizophrenia often exhibit cognitive and behavioral impairment; loss of initiative; low energy; poor concentration; sleep disturbance; social isolation; and withdrawal (Mahoney, 2005). Providing a safe, structured environment is important to maintain biologic integrity and to protect the client from potential self-harm caused by command hallucinations, irrational behavior, disorientation, or poor safety awareness. Clients may require help with activities of daily living because of self-care deficits. Limit-setting, time-out, or physical restraints may be necessary during the acute phase of schizophrenia to decrease agitation or aggressive behavior, or to prevent physical injury to self or others. Box 22-2 lists specific nursing interventions for clients exhibiting agitation, hallucinations, and delusions. See Chapter 12 for additional discussion of the therapeutic milieu.

Medication Management. Clients with schizophrenia often have serious comorbid medical conditions such as cardiovascular disease, respiratory disease, asthma, chronic obstructive pulmonary disease, diabetes, obstructive sleep apnea, obesity, cancer, and HIV/AIDS. Furthermore, schizophrenia is associated with behaviors and lifestyle issues that increase the risk for serious medical conditions. Obesity, binge eating, substance abuse, smoking, lack of exercise, and poor nutrition are widespread among clients (National Center for Health Statistics, 2005). Clients who receive four or more medications concomitantly are, statistically speaking, at very high risk for a drug interaction. In these situations, appropriate references or a pharmacist should be consulted regarding the risk of potential drug interactions (Crimson, 2005).

Medication management of schizophrenia focuses on stabilizing acute symptoms and then maintaining therapeutic plasma levels of the medications to avoid a relapse or exacerbation of clinical symptoms. Drug Summary Table 22-1 lists the major antipsychotic agents prescribed. The use of second-generation

| BOX 22.2 | INTERVENTIONS FOR AGITATION, HALLUCINATIONS, AND DELUSIONS |

AGITATION

- Remove clients from, or avoid, situations known to cause agitation.
- Decrease stimulants such as caffeine, bright lights, and loud noise or music.
- Avoid display of anger, discouragement, or frustration when interacting with client.
- Avoid criticism and do not argue with client.
- Set limits and follow through with consequences if a violation occurs.
- Monitor for physical discomfort such as pain or physical illness.
- Administer prescribed medication as ordered.

HALLUCINATIONS

- Decrease environmental stimuli such as loud noise, extremely bright colors, or flashing lights. If visual hallucinations occur, ask the client to describe what is seen.
- Attempt to identify precipitating factors by asking the client what happened before the onset of hallucinations. If auditory hallucinations occur, ask the client what the voices are saying. Suggest humming, listening to music, exercising, or talking to others.
- Monitor television programs to minimize external stimuli that may precipitate hallucinations.
- Monitor for command hallucinations that may precipitate aggressive or violent behavior.
- Administer prescribed medication as ordered.

DELUSIONS

- Do not whisper or laugh in the presence of the client.
- Do not argue with the client or attempt to disprove delusional or suspicious thoughts.
- Explain all procedures and interventions, including medication management.
- Provide for personal space and do not touch the client without warning.
- Maintain eye contact during interactions with client.
- Provide consistency in care and assigned caregivers to establish trust.

---

antipsychotics has improved the quality of life for clients by relieving a greater spectrum of clinical symptoms of schizophrenia and schizophrenic-like disorders. Not only are these new agents efficacious; they are safer and better tolerated, and thus more effective. Table 22-1 lists the characteristics of second-generation antipsychotics.

The nurse's role during medication management includes administering medication, monitoring responses to the prescribed medication, and reporting any adverse effects. Management of adverse drug effects can be challenging because they can involve many organs and systems in the body. As noted in Chapter 16, clients taking atypical antipsychotics are at risk for the development of **metabolic syndrome** (hypertension, hyperlipidemia, obesity, and hyperglycemia). The following mnemonic, PHATS, is used to monitor metabolic syndrome risk factors:

- Blood **P**ressure greater than 130/85 mm HG
- Serum **H**DL cholesterol less than 40 mg/dL in men and 50 mg/dL in women

- **A**bdominal obesity indicating waist circumference of greater than 102 cm in men and 88 cm in women
- **T**riglycerides equal to or greater 150 mg/dL
- Fasting blood glucose (**S**ugar) equal to or greater than 110 mg/dL

The presence of 3 of the 5 positive criteria indicate metabolic syndrome (Grove, 2006).

Sleepiness and lethargy generally occur at the beginning of therapy. Other adverse effects include allergic reactions, dry mouth, weight gain, menstrual irregularities, and sexual dysfunction. Table 22-2 lists nursing interventions for these common adverse effects that may contribute to the client's noncompliance. Additional interventions, as well as client education regarding the use of antipsychotic drugs, are discussed in Chapter 16. The nurse also plays a major role in developing a therapeutic relationship and educating the client and family about prescribed medication to promote compliance. Factors that contribute to noncompliance include the client's dysfunctional belief about medication (eg, taking medication indicates weakness

DRUG SUMMARY TABLE 22.1 ![icon] Antipsychotic Drugs Used for Schizophrenia

GENERIC (TRADE) NAME	DAILY DOSAGE RANGE	IMPLEMENTATION
aripiprazole (Abilify)	10–30 mg	Monitor for adverse effects*.
clozapine (Clozaril)	75–700 mg	Follow Clozaril Client Management protocol (ie, dispense only 1 week's supply at a time; monitor WBC and cholesterol levels); monitor for weight gain, seizures, and adverse effects*.
haloperidol (Haldol)	4–16 mg	Monitor for refractory arrhythmias, abnormal BUN and WBC lab results, increased motor activity, and adverse effects*.
olanzapine (Zyprexa)	5–20 mg	Monitor for weight gain and adverse effects*.
quetiapine (Seroquel)	25–800 mg	Administer small quantity to any client with suicidal ideation; monitor for adverse effects*.
risperidone (Risperdal)	0.5–16 mg	Mix oral solution with water, juice, low-fat milk, or coffee; monitor for galactorrhea, weight gain, and adverse effects*.
ziprasidone (Geodon)	20–160 mg	Monitor EKG for Q-T changes; monitor for adverse effects*.

NOTE: If the client does not respond adequately to the prescribed antipsychotic agent, adjunctive medication such as lithium (Eskalith); an anticonvulsant such as carbamazepine (Tegretol) or valproate (Depakene); or a benzodiazepine such as clonazepam (Klonopin) may be added. Refer to Chapter 16, Psychopharmacology, for additional information.

*Adverse effects: Agranulocytosis, changes in blood sugar and lipid serum levels, constipation, dehydration in the elderly, dry mouth, movement disorders (eg, EPS, TD, and NMS), orthostatic hypotension, seizures, sexual dysfunction, somnolence, and prolactin elevation

TABLE 22.1 ![icon] Characteristics of Second-Generation Antipsychotics

DRUG (YEAR OF BEGINNING USE)	TRADE NAME	DAILY DOSAGE	THERAPEUTIC PLASMA LEVEL	COMPARISON OF ADVERSE EFFECTS
haloperidol (1970s)	Haldol	4–16 mg/day	4–16 mg/mL	Increased motor activity No weight gain
clozapine (1988)	Clozaril	75–700 mg/day	350–500 mg/mL	No increased motor activity Weight gain Multiple adverse effects Effect on cholesterol metabolism leading to decreased serum cholesterol levels
risperidone (1992)	Risperdal	0.5–16 mg/day	5–30 mg/mL	Minimal increase in motor activity Minimal weight gain Galactorrhea
olanzapine (1994)	Zyprexa	5–20 mg/day	21–54 mg/mL	Minimal increase in motor activity Weight gain Effect on cholesterol metabolism leading to decreased serum cholesterol levels

Drug (Year of Beginning Use)	Trade Name	Daily Dosage	Therapeutic Plasma Level	Comparison of Adverse Effects
quetiapine (mid-1990s)	Seroquel	25–800 mg/day	45–100 mg/mL	No increase in motor activity Minimal adverse effects even with higher doses
ziprasidone (late 1990s)	Geodon	20–160 mg/day	Not established	Minimal increase in motor activity No weight gain Changes in QT segment of EKG (prolongation)
aripiprazole (2002, Dec.)	Abilify	10–30 mg/day	Not established	Anxiety Headache Insomnia Considered to cause minimal adverse effects

or dependency), lack of insight regarding the need to take medication, forgetting to take medication, and the lack of an understanding about the diagnosis of schizophrenia (Pinninti, Stolar, & Temple, 2005). (See Supporting Evidence for Practice 22-1.)

The earlier schizophrenia is treated, the better the outcome is. The use of antipsychotic drugs during the first episode is thought to decrease the frequency of hospitalization and to decrease the time required to control symptoms fully. Dosages vary depending on the age of the client, weight, extent of presenting clinical symptoms, physiologic status, and use of additional medication. Generally, higher doses are used to treat acute episodes and lower doses are administered during the periods of remission. Improvement in psychotic symptoms may be evident within 1 or 2 days. However,

TABLE 22.2 Nursing Interventions for Common Adverse Effects of Antipsychotic Medications

Adverse Effect	Nursing Interventions
Allergic reaction	Educate client to report any rashes, edema, or other unusual symptoms to rule out an allergic reaction.
Dry mouth	Encourage the use of low-calorie or sugarless hard candy, mints, gum, or beverages.
Menstrual irregularity	Inform the client that menstrual irregularity may occur. Encourage her to report any changes in menses, including the possibility of pregnancy.
Somnolence or lethargy	Explain that drowsiness is usually a transient symptom. Caution client to avoid driving or operating hazardous equipment.
Sexual dysfunction	Inform the client that sexual dysfunction has been identified as a potential adverse effect of neuroleptic medication. Conduct a sexual history. Provide emotional support.
Weight gain	Instruct client to monitor weight on a weekly basis. Educate client about dietary measures to avoid weight gain.

SUPPORTING EVIDENCE FOR PRACTICE 22.1
Medication Compliance in Clients With the Diagnosis of Schizophrenia

PROBLEM UNDER INVESTIGATION / How clients with the diagnosis of schizophrenia perceive their illness and the use of medication

SUMMARY OF RESEARCH / The compliance of 102 clients receiving clozapine (Clozaril) for schizophrenia was assessed at time of discharge from treatment using a semi-structured interview based on the Subjective Illness theory. Components of the theory focus on whether clients see themselves as being ill, how they describe their situation, what they believe to be the cause of their illness, and what treatment they think will improve their mental health. Data collected included gender, living arrangement, length of illness, the presence of grandiose delusions or unpleasant adverse effects of medication, attitudes towards medication, and the client's satisfaction with the psychiatrist. Findings indicated that 56.4% of the clients felt they were ill; 14.1% felt they had been ill; and 21.8% denied being ill. In addition, 25% of the clients expected their mental health to improve; 25%

expected some relapses; and another 25% expected their condition to stabilize or possibly get worse. At time of discharge and after 3 months, 33% of the clients had not been taking medication as prescribed and approximately 16% had changed their dosage. None of the components of Subjective Illness theory appeared to have a significant influence on medication compliance; however, the most significant predictor of adherence was the presence of a therapeutic alliance between the client and psychiatrist.

SUPPORT FOR PRACTICE / This study underscores the importance of establishing a therapeutic relationship with a client. For clients diagnosed with schizophrenia, establishment of this therapeutic relationship increases the probability of medication compliance and potential for stabilization of clinical symptoms.

SOURCE: Holzinger, A., Loffler, W., Muller, P., et al. (2002). Subjective illness theory and antipsychotic medication compliance by patients with schizophrenia. Journal of Nervous and Mental Disease, 190, 597–603.

the full benefit evolves over approximately 6 to 8 weeks. Additional medication may be prescribed to treat depression or another comorbid psychiatric disorder.

After symptoms are stabilized, clients may exhibit what has been referred to as the **awareness syndrome** or **awakening phenomena**. For example, after clinical symptoms such as hallucinations, confusion, and ideas of reference are stabilized, the client may begin to experience inner emotions such as anxiety and fear as he or she regains an awareness of reality. Ineffective or dysfunctional coping mechanisms no longer shield the client from environmental stress. Conversely, therapeutic levels of medication may enable clients to assume responsibility for themselves and to participate in various treatment modalities such as individual, group, cognitive, behavioral, supportive, or family therapy.

Over time, treatment resistance may occur due to several factors such as inherent biologic factors; inadequate dose or plasma level of the prescribed drug;

missed diagnosis of a comorbid medical or psychiatric disorder; or inappropriate psychosocial treatment. The following interventions have been used as an approach to treatment-resistant symptoms exhibited by clients with the diagnosis of schizophrenia:

1. Reassessing the diagnosis and degree of compliance
2. Monitoring serum blood levels to optimize the dosage of the neuroleptic
3. Switching to another neuroleptic if the first drug is ineffective
4. Adding a benzodiazepine to reduce agitation resulting from high levels of anxiety or an antidepressant if moderate to severe depression or suicidal ideation is present
5. Adding an anticonvulsant to improve tension, excitement, mood, or agitated behavior
6. Using clozapine if the client has not responded favorably to the use of two different neuroleptics

Interactive Therapies

Three interactive therapies are generally effective when providing care for clients with schizophrenia: group therapy, cognitive behavioral therapy (CBT), and personal therapy (a flexible form of individual therapy). Group therapy focuses on real-life plans, problems, and relationships. It may be behaviorally oriented, insight oriented, or supportive. Group therapy reduces social isolation, increases the sense of cohesiveness, and improves the client's reality testing ability. CBT is thought to improve cognitive distortions, reduce distractibility, and correct errors in judgment. Clients with some insight into their illness are good candidates for CBT. The goal of personal therapy is to enhance personal and social adjustment and forestall relapse (Sadock & Sadock, 2003).

According to Ronald Diamond, MD, a professor of psychiatry at the University of Wisconsin, Madison, most individuals with schizophrenia whose clinical symptoms are stabilized have much the same goals as anyone else (eg, a new car, more money, and a nice house); however, until recently, few clinicians have asked clients what they want from life. In the past, individual therapy between client and therapist has focused on the goals of the therapist rather than those of the client. Diamond proposes a collaborative *recovery approach* similar to that of personal therapy between the therapist and client. He believes that clients will participate in treatment if they trust the therapist and feel they are accomplishing their personal goals (Hughes, 2005).

Psychosocial Therapies

Social skills training, family-oriented therapy, case management (Chapter 8), and assertive community treatment (ACT; Chapters 8 and 35) are forms of psychosocial therapies provided for clients with the diagnosis of schizophrenia. Social skills training focuses on stabilization of behavior, improvement of social performance within family and with peers, improvement of social perception with the family, and the enhancement of extrafamilial relationships (Sadock & Sadock,

2003). Family-oriented therapy is usually a brief but intensive course that focuses on identifying and avoiding potentially troublesome situations. If a problem does emerge with the client, the aim of the therapy is resolve the problem quickly.

Client and Family Education

The client and his or her family members and/or significant others are all involved in the plan of care. They are encouraged to attend multidisciplinary treatment team meetings, where they are introduced to members of the team and given an opportunity to discuss any concerns. During team meetings, the client is encouraged to participate in goal-setting, allowing the client to set the pace. Realistic expectations of the client and family are explored. Stressful situations that might trigger relapse are identified. The efficacy of medication management is discussed, including the importance of recognizing early signs of serious adverse effects. Continuum of care is planned to lessen the chance of recidivism. (See Chapters 8 and 35 for additional information regarding continuum of care, case management, and ACT.)

EVALUATION

The purpose of evaluation is to compare the client's current mental status with stated desirable outcomes identified. If the outcomes have not been met, consider the reasons why. For example, outcomes may not be achieved because of the client's lack of belief in success, or unrealistic expectations regarding recovery. Lack of social support or income, or a cognitive deficit that limits the client's insight regarding his or her illness, may also be factors. Depression may occur because of a decline in dopamine level as the client ages. Additional specific nursing interventions and changes in outcomes may be necessary. See Nursing Plan of Care 22-1: The Client With Schizophrenia, Undifferentiated Type.

M**VIE** viewing **GUIDES**

THE CLIENT WITH SCHIZOPHRENIA, UNDIFFERENTIATED TYPE

Janet, a 47-year-old white female, was brought to the mental health center by her sister, who expressed concern about recent behavioral changes exhibited by Janet. She stated that Janet was diagnosed with schizophrenia, undifferentiated type, at age 40 and was placed on Risperdal 1.0 mg bid.

Janet lived with her sister. She was unemployed but received Social Security Disability compensation. Janet was able to perform activities of daily living independently until recently, when she discontinued taking her medication. As a result of medication non-compliance, Janet became overly concerned about insects and bugs that she believed were in her room. She began to wear gloves to protect her hands as she sprayed insect repellant on all the furniture. She also turned the water on in her bathroom sink because she believed the bugs contaminated the sink. Unfortunately, she neglected to turn the water off and flooded the bathroom.

Although she was oriented to person, place, and time, Janet's speech had become incoherent at times. Janet stated that she felt better while taking medication and, therefore, believed that she was cured of her illness. Consequently, she stopped taking the medication. When Janet's sister confronted her about her recent behavioral changes, Janet was insightful enough to tell her sister that she needed help and agreed to see the nurse at the center where she received follow-up care.

DSM–IV–TR DIAGNOSIS: Schizophrenia, undifferentiated type

ASSESSMENT: Personal strengths: Alert; oriented to person, place, and time; insightful; motivated for treatment; good support system; receives disability payments

Weaknessess: Visual hallucinations; delusional thoughts; noncompliance regarding medication management; incoherent speech at times

---

NURSING DIAGNOSIS: Noncompliance regarding medication management

OUTCOME: Within 24 hours, client will resume taking prescribed medication.

Planning/Implementation	Rationale
Instruct client and sister that medication restores biochemical imbalance and reduces psychotic symptoms.	Clients who are educated about their illness and treatment are more likely to remain compliant with their plan of care.
Educate client and sister about recidivism secondary to noncompliance.	Client stopped taking medication because she thought she was cured.

NURSING DIAGNOSIS: Disturbed Sensory Perception related to the presence of visual hallucinations and delusional thoughts

OUTCOME: Within 48–72 hours of medication compliance, client will voice the absence of hallucinations and delusions.

Planning/Implementation	Rationale
Explore stressors contributing to psychotic symptoms.	Identification of stressors may increase insight into client's fears and reduce anxiety.
Ask client to notify clinic of response to medication within 3 days.	Client is to assume responsibility for resuming medication compliance.
Instruct sister not to confront client about delusions.	Confrontation may exacerbate client's symptoms and result in mistrust of her primary support system.
Encourage participation in reality-based activities at home with sister.	Reinforcement of reality helps client resume prior level of independence.

NURSING DIAGNOSIS: Impaired Verbal Communication related to disordered thinking secondary to schizophrenia

OUTCOME: Within 48–72 hours of medication compliance, client will demonstrate an improved ability to express self.

Planning/Implementation	Rationale
Provide alternative methods of communication if necessary, such as pointing or gesturing.	Client may have difficulty expressing self verbally due to visual hallucinations or fears.
Provide a nonrushed, quiet environment to decrease frustration.	Environmental stimuli may exacerbate psychotic symptoms.
Instruct sister in repetitive approaches to improve communication.	Repetitive communication approaches are less stressful to cognitively impaired clients.

EVALUATION: Client and sister will verbalize an understanding of the plan of care. A follow-up visit is scheduled in 1 week. A community support group for clients and families of clients with schizophrenia has been identified. Sister will return with client to provide supportive data regarding behavior, mood, affect, communication, and medication compliance.

KEY CONCEPTS

◆ Approximately 2.2 million people suffer from schizophrenia and schizophrenic-like disorders.

◆ As a result of deinstitutionalization and changes in financial reimbursement for care, approximately 1.4 million of those individuals who suffer from schizophrenia and schizophrenic-like disorders do not receive psychiatric treatment.

◆ Recent research suggests that schizophrenia is caused by chemical or organic changes in the brain. The most widely held theory is the dopamine hypothesis.

◆ Five phases of schizophrenia have been identified. They include the premorbid, prodromal, onset, progressive, and chronic or residual phases.

◆ Clinical symptoms of schizophrenia are described as positive, negative, or disorganized.

◆ The five subtypes of schizophrenia are paranoid, catatonic, disorganized, undifferentiated, and residual.

◆ Assessment of objective clinical symptoms of schizophrenia can be challenging; therefore, the nurse also uses subjective data presented by family members, significant others, or representatives from the client's support system.

◆ Current treatment of schizophrenia and schizophrenic-like disorders involves an integrated multidisciplinary approach that focuses on nursing interventions occurring in a therapeutic milieu. Treatment modalities include the use of psychopharmacology; medical interventions to meet biologic or physical needs; interactive and psychosocial therapies; and supportive therapies to empower clients. Client and family education is included in the plan of care. Continuum of care must be addressed to decrease recidivism.

For additional study materials, please refer to the Student Resource CD-ROM located in the back of this textbook.

CHAPTER WORKSHEET

CRITICAL THINKING QUESTIONS

1. As you take the first bite of your burger in a fast-food restaurant, you notice a disheveled, dirty man in the booth across from you. He is talking to himself and gesturing wildly. Describe your thought processes as you assess this man. What interventions, if any, would be appropriate?
2. Observe a psychiatric treatment milieu and analyze how the unit is therapeutic for a client with schizophrenia.
3. Develop a presentation for families of clients with schizophrenia that includes the following points: theories of causality, symptoms of disorder, relationship between stress and symptoms, use of medications in treatment, and helpful responses to symptomatic behavior.

REFLECTION

Reread the chapter opening quote. In what manner does active psychosis in schizophrenia produce disability equal to quadriplegia? Cite two or three examples to substantiate your explanation. How would these examples of disability affect the family of a client with schizophrenia? Identify what support systems the family and client could use.

NCLEX-STYLE QUESTIONS

1. A client with schizophrenia, disorganized type, is admitted to the inpatient unit. He frequently giggles and mumbles to himself. He hasn't taken a shower for the last 3 days, presenting a disheveled, unkempt appearance. Which statement would be most appropriate for the nurse to use in persuading the client to shower?
   a. "Clients on this unit take showers daily."
   b. "It's time to shower. I will help you."
   c. "You'll feel better if you shower."
   d. "Would you like to take a shower?"

2. The nurse expects to assess which of the following in a client with the diagnosis of schizophrenia, paranoid type?
   a. Anger, auditory hallucinations, persecutory delusions
   b. Abnormal motor activity, frequent posturing, autism
   c. Flat affect, anhedonia, alogia
   d. Silly behavior, poor personal hygiene, incoherent speech

3. The nurse identifies the nursing diagnosis of Disturbed Thought Processes related to exhibiting delusions of reference for a client with schizophrenia. Which outcome would be most appropriate?
   a. Client will talk about concrete events in the environment without talking about delusions.
   b. Client will state three symptoms that occur when feeling stressed.
   c. Client will identify two personal interventions that decrease intensity of delusional thinking.
   d. Client will use distracting techniques when having delusions.

4. Which nursing response would be most appropriate when a client talks about hearing voices?
   a. "I do not hear the voices that you say you hear."
   b. "Those voices will disappear as soon as the medicine works."
   c. "Try to think about positive things instead of voices."
   d. "Voices are only in your imagination."

5. During a community meeting, a client with schizophrenia begins to shout and gesture

in an angry manner. Which nursing intervention would be the priority?

a. Determining reasons for client agitation
b. Encouraging appropriate behavior in group
c. Facilitating group process in responding to client
d. Maintaining safety of client and others

6. After a class on schizophrenia and its phases, the students identify the following phases. Place the phases in the correct sequence from first to last.

a. Prodromal
b. Premorbid
c. Residual
d. Progressive
e. Onset

Selected References

American Psychiatric Association. (2000). *Diagnostic and statistical manual of mental disorders* (4th ed., text revision). Washington, DC: Author.

Baker, B. (1999). Human genome to debut on Internet this spring. *Clinical Psychiatry News, 27*(12), 10.

Brier, A. (1999). Cognitive deficit in schizophrenia and its neurochemical basis. *British Journal of Psychiatry, 174*(37), 16-18.

Clinician Reviews. (2005). In a page: Acute psychosis. *Clinician Reviews, 15*(4), 59.

Crimson, M. L. (2005, March). Disclaimer. Schizophrenia: The clinician's guide to pharmacotherapy for patients with co-occurring medical conditions. *Supplement to Current Psychiatry, 4*(3), x.

DeMott, K. (2000). Polydipsic patients suffer four times as many comorbidities. *Clinical Psychiatry News, 28*(1), 28.

Grove, G. A. (2006). Beware of PHATS in metabolic syndrome. *Current Psychiatry, 5*(4), 98.

Hillard, J. R. (2006). What shall we do about CATIE? *Current Psychiatry, 5*(2), 11.

Holzinger, A., Loffler, W., Muller, P., Priebe, S., & Angermeyer, M. C. (2002). Subjective illness theory and antipsychotic medication compliance by patients with schizophrenia. *Journal of Nervous and Mental Disease, 190*, 597-603.

Hughes, D. (2005). "A life that's more than just illness". Schizophrenic patients and psychiatrists have divergent goals. *Neuropsychiatry News, 6*(1), 18-19.

Jancin, B. (1998). Schizophrenic outcomes. Not doing too bad. *Clinical Psychiatry News, 26*(10), 31.

Kennedy, J. L., Pato, J., Bauer, A., Carvalho, C., & Pato, D. (1999). Genetics of schizophrenia: Current findings and issues. *CNS Spectrum, 4*(5), 17-21.

Kolb, L. C. (1982). *Modern clinical psychiatry*. Philadelphia: W. B. Saunders.

Lieberman, J. A. (2004). New findings in schizophrenia. Long-term management: A phase approach. *Supplement to Clinical Psychiatry, 32*(7), 7-10.

Mahoney, D. (2005). Schizophrenia prodrome therapies show promise. *Clinical Psychiatry News, 33*(10), 22.

Meltzer, H. Y. (2005). Targeting cognition to improve outcomes in schizophrenia. *Supplement to Clinical Psychiatry News, 33*(8), 2.

Moon, M. A. (1999). Cognitive processing speed slows before schizophrenia. *Clinical Psychiatry News, 27*(7), 1.

Moore, H. W. (2005). Cognitive dysfunction in schizophrenia: Probing pathophysiology and pathogenesis. *Neuropsychiatry News, 6*(8), 12, 14-15.

Narasimhan, M., & Buckley, P. F. (2005). Psychotic prodrome: Are antipsychotics effective? Ethical? *Current Psychiatry, 4*(3), 32-34, 37-38, 45-46.

Nasrallah, H. A. (2006). CATIE's surprises. In antipsychotics' square-off, were there winners or losers? *Current Psychiatry, 5*(2), 48-50, 53-56, 61-62, 65.

National Advisory Mental Health Council. (2001). When someone has schizophrenia. Retrieved January 4, 2006, from http://www.nimh.nih.gov/publicat/schizsoms.cfm

National Center for Health Statistics: Centers for Disease Control and Prevention. (2005). Retrieved February 2, 2005, from http://www.cdc.gob/nchs/faststats/deaths.htm

National Institute of Mental Health. (2001). Mental health: Culture, race, and ethnicity. A report of the surgeon general. Retrieved January 4, 2006, from http://www.surgeongeneral.gov/library/reports.htm

Pinninti, N. R., Stolar, N., & Temple, S. (2005). 5-minute first aid for psychosis. *Current Psychiatry, 4*(1), 36-38, 41-44, 47-48.

Peplau, H. E. (1996). The client diagnosed as schizophrenic. In S. Lego (Ed.), *Psychiatric nursing: A comprehensive reference* (2nd ed., pp. 291-295). Philadelphia: Lippincott-Raven.

Ritts, V. (1999). *Infusing culture into psychopathology: A supplement for psychology instructors*. Retrieved November 20, 2003, from http://www.stlcc.cc.mo.us/mc/users/vrits/psychopath.htm

Sadock, B. J., & Sadock, V. A. (2003). *Kaplan & Sadock's synopsis of psychiatry: Behavioral sciences/clinical psychiatry* (9th ed.). Philadelphia: Lippincott Williams & Wilkins.

Schizophrenia.com. (2006). The history of schizophrenia. Retrieved January 3, 2006, from http://www.schizophrenia.com/history.htm

Sherman, C. (1999a). Brain defects linked to schizophrenia. *Clinical Psychiatry News, 27*(4), 32.

Sherman, C. (1999b). Depressive symptoms significant in schizophrenia. *Clinical Psychiatry News, 27*(3), 29.

Sherman, C. (1999c). Olanzapine or clozapine for resistant schizophrenia. *Clinical Psychiatry News, 27*(8), 13.

Sherman, C. (1999d). The first genetic subtype of schizophrenia is described. *Clinical Psychiatry News, 27*(8), 22.

Sherman, C. (2004). Let symptoms guide schizophrenia treatment. *Clinical Psychiatry News, 32*(5), 23.

Spollen, J. J. III. (2005). The latest theories on the neurobiology of schizophrenia. Retrieved January 8, 2005, from http://www.schizophrenia.com/newsletter/allnews/2002/newnuero6-02.htm

Sullivan, M. G. (2004). Online schizophrenia algorithm almost ready. *Clinical Psychiatry News, 32*(11), 1, 22.

Well-Connected: In-Depth Health Information. (1999). What causes schizophrenia? Retrieved February 10, 2004, from http://nhfpl.adam.com/pages/wci/articles/000047_2.htm

Weinberger, D. R. (2004). Genetics, neuroanatomy, and neurobiology. *Clinical Psychiatry News Supplement: New Findings in Schizophrenia. An Update of Causes and Treatment, 32*(7), 4–6.

Zoler, M. L. (1999). Good function is suicide risk for schizophrenics. *Clinical Psychiatry News, 27*(4), 32.

Suggested Readings

Carpenito-Moyet, L. J. (2006). *Handbook of nursing diagnosis* (11th ed.). Philadelphia: Lippincott Williams & Wilkins.

Knowlton, L., & Staff. (2001). Decreasing suicide in schizophrenia. *Psychiatric Times, 18*(5), 20–21.

McEvoy, J. P. (2005). Managing health risks in psychiatric patients: Practical clinical interventions. Cigarette smoking and schizophrenia. *Supplement to Clinical Psychiatry News, 33*(12), 12–15.

Miller, A. L. (2005). Treatment-resistant psychosis. Are 2 antipsychotics more effective than 1? *Current Psychiatry, 4*(7), 13–16, 19–20.

Pies, R. (2000). The role of psychosocial treatments in schizophrenia. *Psychiatric Times, 17*(3), 17–20.

Schultz, J. M., & Videbeck, S. L. (2005). *Lippincott's manual of psychiatric nursing care plans* (7th ed.). Philadelphia: Lippincott Williams & Wilkins.

Sherman, C. (2004). Cognitive deficits and schizophrenia. *Clinical Psychiatry News, 32* (4), 16.

Torrey, E. F. (2001). *Surviving schizophrenia: A manual for families, consumers, and providers* (4th ed.). London: Collins Publishing Co.

Weiden, P. J. (2004). Advances in the treatment of bipolar disorder and schizophrenia: Switching medications in schizophrenia patients: Considering goals and optimizing outcomes. *Supplement to Clinical Psychiatry News, 32*(12), 7–12.

CHAPTER 23 / EATING DISORDERS

Eating disorders are fascinating, confusing, challenging and deeply disturbing. Physicians, nurses, psychotherapists and other medical and mental health providers frequently find themselves confused and feel overwhelmed when dealing with these disorders. —SOBEL, 2005

AFTER STUDYING THIS CHAPTER, YOU SHOULD BE ABLE TO:

1. Differentiate the terms *anorexia nervosa*, *bulimia nervosa*, and *obesity*.
2. Explain why obesity is not categorized as an eating disorder.
3. Discuss the following theories of eating disorders: genetic or biochemical; psychological or psychodynamic; and family systems.
4. Discuss the following theories of obesity: genetic or biologic, and behavioral.
5. Describe at least five clinical symptoms shared by clients with anorexia nervosa and clients with bulimia nervosa.
6. Differentiate the three personality prototypes of clients with eating disorders that should be considered when planning interventions.
7. Articulate the rationale for medical evaluation of a client with an eating disorder or the diagnosis of obesity.
8. State the criteria for inpatient treatment of a client with an eating disorder.
9. Identify the medical complications of anorexia nervosa, bulimia nervosa, and obesity.
10. Construct an assessment tool to identify clinical symptoms of an eating disorder.
11. Formulate a plan of care for a client with the diagnosis of bulimia nervosa.

LEARNING OBJECTIVES

KEY TERMS

Binge eating
Body mass index (BMI)
Cachexia
Developmental obesity
Obesity
Purging
Reactive obesity
Russell's sign

Eating disorders such as anorexia nervosa, bulimia nervosa, and obesity are among the most challenging illnesses confronting the mental health profession. They are frequently under-diagnosed and, when diagnosed, clients are often treated incorrectly. Unfortunately, a surprising number of individuals do not seek help. Others will remain ill or die, even after years of treatment (Sobel, 2005).

According to statistics released by Anorexia Nervosa and Related Eating Disorders (ANRED), Inc., about 1% or 1 out of 100 female adolescents between the ages of 10 and 20 years has anorexia. Additionally, approximately 4% or 4 out of 100 college-aged women have bulimia or bulimic patterns. There seems to be an increase in the incidence of middle-aged women with anorexia and bulimia, possibly because this group has consistently considered image to be of major importance. Statistics on males with eating disorders are difficult to find, but estimates are that about 5% to 10% of the individuals diagnosed with anorexia and 10% to 15% diagnosed with bulimia are male. Over the next decade, as public awareness of dieting and eating disorders increases, the number of males seeking treatment for eating disorders is likely to increase. Reliable statistics regarding the prevalence of eating disorders in young children or older adults are limited. Although such cases do occur, they are not common (ANRED, 2006; Frieden, 2004).

At the same time, medical experts warn that America's weight problem is reaching epidemic proportions. In the United States, approximately 60% of adult Americans, both male and female, are overweight. About 34% are considered to be obese, and many of these individuals have binge eating habits. Furthermore, about 31% of American teenage girls and about 28% of boys are overweight (ANRED, 2006).

The American Heart Association recognizes obesity as a distinct risk factor for heart disease. In 1998, The National Heart, Lung, and Blood Institute released a report stating that obesity is a complex chronic disease requiring clinician assessment and intervention (Sharp, 1998).

All three disorders may have serious medical consequences if clients remain untreated. However, with proper help, persons with an eating disorder can often learn to stabilize their eating patterns, maintain a healthy weight, and become less preoccupied with food.

Eating disorders are characterized by severe disturbances in eating behavior. Three specific diagnoses exist: anorexia nervosa; bulimia nervosa; and eating disorder, not otherwise specified (American Psychiatric Association [APA], 2000b). The *Diagnostic and Statistical Manual of Mental Disorders, 4th Edition, Text Revision* (*DSM-IV-TR*) has not identified obesity as a psychiatric diagnosis (APA, 2000a). Obesity is considered to be a general medical condition because a consistent association with a psychological or behavioral syndrome has not been established. When there is evidence that psychological factors are of importance in the etiology or course of a particular case of obesity, the diagnosis is listed under psychological factors affecting medical condition. Disorders of feeding and eating that are usually first diagnosed in infancy or early childhood are included in Chapter 29.

Although anorexia is not commonly seen among older adults, the results of the National Diet and Nutrition Survey in London in 1998 revealed that 43% of independent elderly persons consumed fewer than 1,500 calories per day, and 16% to 18% consumed fewer than 1,000 calories per day. This group of individuals are at risk for developing anorexia because of physiologic changes related to aging, pathological conditions (eg, stroke, dental problems), adverse effects of medications (eg, levothyroxine, theophylline), social factors (eg, dependency on others to meet needs), environmental factors (eg, poverty), or psychological conditions (eg, depression) (Endoy, 2005). The issue of involuntary weight loss in the elderly is addressed in Chapter 30.

This chapter focuses on the history of eating disorders; etiology of anorexia, bulimia, and obesity; and addresses the clinical symptoms and diagnostic characteristics of each. Using the nursing process approach, the chapter describes the care of a client with an eating disorder.

History of Eating Disorders

Egyptian hieroglyphics, Persian manuscripts, and Chinese scrolls describe disorders very like what we now call anorexia nervosa and bulimia nervosa. Ancient Romans used *vomitoriums* (lavatory chambers that accommodated vomiting) to relieve themselves after overindulging at lavish banquets. African lore describes *voluntary restrictors* who refused to eat during times of famine so that their children would be able to eat. When the famine passed, some of these individuals, who were admired by peers, continued to refuse to eat in spite of the danger of dying. During the 9th century, followers of St. Jerome, who starved themselves in the name of religion, became thin and stopped having menstrual cycles. In Europe, the first formal description of anorexia nervosa in medical literature was made by Richard Morton in 1689. Two other physicians, Lasegue in 1873 in France and Gull in 1874 in England, wrote articles about anorexia nervosa in modern medical literature. During the 19th century, the term *anorexia* was used, and the psychological aspects of the disease were described. Significant work was provided by the writing and the insight of Hilda Bruch, a physician who assisted in the categorization of anorexia nervosa and began to separate it from other diseases associated with weight loss (ANRED, 2006; Sobel, 2005.)

Etiology of Anorexia Nervosa and Bulimia

The prevalence of eating disorders is at an all-time high. Preoccupation with body image, a component of self-concept, has increased over the years as the diet and fitness industry has emphasized that "thin is in." Pop stars' clothing styles reinforce the thin, sexy ideal girls strive for. In addition, more skin is shown on television and in the movies than ever before (Irvine, 2001; Tumolo, 2003). The dissatisfaction with body image (ie, a negative self-concept) commonly seen in older children, adolescents, and young adults appears to be fully developed in girls as young as 5 years (Moon, 2001).

Four separate elements of body image as described by Schilder (1950) include:

- The actual, subjective perception of the body that an individual forms related to physical appearance and function
- A mental picture of one's body that the individual develops based on internalized feelings and attitudes related to past experiences (eg, a woman who successfully loses 50 pounds and achieves a dress size of 9 still refers to herself as "fat")
- Social experiences or societal stereotype regarding acceptable physical appearance (eg, an adolescent subscribes to a "fitness" magazine and determines that he must reduce his caloric intake and increase his exercise to develop a muscular physique similar to that of the male model in magazine)

- An idealized body image that an individual incorporates into one's mental picture

Body image is changed as one progresses through the different developmental stages of life. Persistent preoccupation with one's body image can impair emotional and cognitive development, interfere with interpersonal relationships, and place an individual at risk for the development of an eating disorder (Bensing, 2003).

Theories of eating disorders are categorized as genetic or biochemical theories, psychological or psychodynamic theories, and family systems theories. The information presented here summarizes the major concepts discussed in the Harvard Mental Health Letter (Grinspoon, 1997), the Internet Mental Health Web site (http://www.mentalhealth.com/), the Anorexia Nervosa and Related Eating Disorders, Inc., Web site (http://www.anred.com/stats.html), and the National Eating Disorders Association Web site (http://www.nationaleatingdisorders. org/). Other references are cited when additional relevant information was located in literature.

Genetic or Biochemical Theories

Several theories have attempted to describe the causes of eating disorders. According to a study published in the May 2001 issue of *Molecular Psychiatry*, researchers in Germany and the Netherlands have found that one form of a gene for Agouti-related protein (AGRP), a chemical messenger that stimulates appetite, occurs more frequently among anorexic persons. This discovery suggests that disruptions of the brain's system for governing food intake contribute to eating disorders (Associated Press, 2001; Sobel, 2005).

A second theory states that eating disorders, including obesity, could be caused by abnormalities in the activity of hormones such as thyroid-stimulating hormone, gonadotropin-releasing hormone, and corticotropin-releasing factors and neurotransmitters such as serotonin, dopamine, and norepinephrine that preserve the balance between energy output and food intake. According to this theory, nerve pathways descending from the hypothalamus control levels of sex hormones, thyroid hormones, and the adrenal hormone cortisol, all of which influence appetite, body weight, mood, and responses to stress. Research has concluded that genetics is 80% responsible for determining the tendency to become obese (Sadock & Sadock, 2003; Sharp, 1998). Studies of twins indicate that 50% to 90% are at risk for anorexia and 35% to 83% are at risk for bulimia (DiscoveryHealth.com Disease Center, 2003). Furthermore, individuals with a mother or sister who has anorexia are considered to be 12 times more likely than others with no family history of anorexia to develop it themselves and they are four times more likely to develop bulimia (ANRED, 2006).

A third theory speculates that high levels of enkephalins and endorphins, opiate-like substances produced in the body, influence eating disorders. Opioids act on the central nervous system, producing analgesia, change in mood, drowsiness, and mental slowness. Gastrointestinal tract motility and appetite are diminished. These biologic changes may contribute to the denial of hunger in clients with anorexia nervosa. Euphoria is not uncommon because plasma endorphin levels are raised in some clients with bulimia nervosa after vomiting (Sadock & Sadock, 2003).

A fourth theory postulates that anorexia results from an imbalance of hormones caused by excessive physical activity. A self-perpetuating cycle develops in which restricted food intake heightens the urge to move, and constantly increasing exercise releases hormones that depress interest in eating.

A fifth theory links the presence of obsessive-compulsive behavior with eating disorders. According to this theory, elevated levels of vasopressin, neuropeptide Y, peptide YY, or a decreased level of cholecystokinin contribute to obsessive-compulsive eating behavior patterns commonly seen in anorexia nervosa.

Recent research has focused on etiological factors including birth trauma (eg, cephalohematoma); preterm birth (eg, less than 32 completed gestational weeks); infection (streptococcus anorexia nervosa); and activity of brain functioning in the right inferior and superior prefrontal lobe and the right parietal regions in women diagnosed with anorexia nervosa, purging type. Further research is needed to verify the role these factors may play in the development of eating disorders (Moore, 2004a; Sobel, 2005).

Psychological and Psychodynamic Theories

A wide range of psychological influences contributing to the development of an eating disorder have been suggested. One theory addresses the theme of starvation as a form of self-punishment, with the unacknowledged purpose of pleasing an introjected or internalized parent. This parent is seen as imposing harsh restrictions on the otherwise well-behaved, orderly, perfectionistic, hypersensitive individual.

A second theory suggests that fasting restores a sense of order to a female who fears the independence of adult femininity (eg, social and sexual functioning) and fears becoming like her mother. Fasting allows the client to exert control over herself and others. The ability to lose weight is a substitute for independence as well as an avoidance of acknowledging one's sexual desires (Sadock & Sadock, 2003).

A third theory notes that individuals starve themselves to suppress or control feelings of emotional emptiness. They struggle for perfection to prove that they do not depend on others to validate their self-concept or self-esteem. Conversely, teenagers with problems managing anger are more likely to engage in bulimic behavior without purging than those who manage anger appropriately (Finn, 2004).

A final theory postulates that females develop an eating disorder because they believe their parents have never responded adequately to their initiatives or recognized individualities. Anorectic females have difficulty distinguishing personal wants from those of others and fear abandonment if they take independent action. Rather than allowing outside influences, including food, to invade them, anorectics deny their needs and will not permit anyone else to control them.

Family Systems Theories

Parents wield a great deal of influence over children's self-concepts and perceptions of the world. The desire to please parents, on whom we are totally dependent as children, is also extremely powerful. Three theories about family relationships and the development of eating disorders have emerged: conflict between parent-child expectations, family preoccupation with weight and appearance, and "enmeshed" families.

The first theory focuses on parental expectations of children. Parents may emphasize intellectual abilities or athletic talents while ignoring emerging emotional needs of their children. Unfortunately, some children try endlessly to gain the approval of an over-controlling, authoritative, passive, or emotionally distant parent while refusing to acknowledge feelings or ideas that may conflict with or contradict those of the family. Anorectics use the avoidance of food to gain attention and satisfy emotional needs. Bulimic individuals soothe themselves with food.

According to the second theory, both anorectic and bulimic individuals are insecure about their physical shape and size. Preoccupation with weight by parents or siblings close to them can inadvertently set into motion a chain of feelings and events emphasizing external appearances. Thinking that life would be perfect if only they were thinner or more attractive, the individuals assume nurturing or caretaking roles toward siblings or other family members. They fail to see that they want or need nurturing. The family may indirectly encourage this behavior by praising the individual for being strong (Bruch, 2003).

The enmeshed family theory states that families with anorectic daughters are smothering toward their members. The responsibilities of each person and the boundaries among them are indistinct. Everyone is said to be over-responsive to and overprotective of everyone else. Individual needs are not met, feelings are not honestly acknowledged, and conflicts are not openly resolved. As the daughter reaches puberty, the parents are reluctant to make necessary changes in the family rules and roles. Anorexia is considered to be a symptom of a rigid family system's need and inability to change (Minuchin, 1974).

Researchers have recently focused on the relationship between maladaptive parental behavior and eating disorders. Johnson, Cohen, Kasen, and Brook (2002) investigated childhood adversities, including the issue of childhood sexual abuse, and their role in the development of an eating disorder during adolescence and early adulthood. They identified several experiences that placed children at risk: physical neglect or sexual abuse; low parental affection; low parental communication with the child; low parental time spent with the child; poverty; and low parental education. Living in such a negative environment created an "empty" feeling and loss of control over one's environment. Consequently, individuals who experienced childhood adversities sought perfection to control their environment in a favorable fashion. Unfortunately, the development of an eating disorder became a solution to the problem.

Etiology of Obesity

Obesity is not a simple problem of will power or self-control, but rather a complex, multifactorial disease. Increasing evidence reveals that genetic, gender, physiologic, psychological, environmental, and cultural factors play a part in the development of obesity (Crouch, 2005). Theories regarding the etiology of obesity are generally grouped into the following categories: genetic or biologic and behavioral theories.

Genetic or Biologic Theories

The first theory, referred to as the *set-point theory,* proposes that body weight is physiologically regulated like pulse or body temperature. Body weight is maintained as the body self-adjusts its metabolism and its release of hormones (Keesy & Hirvonen, 1997).

A second theory states that heredity or genetic predisposition plays a part in the development of obesity. On the basis of studies of identical and fraternal twins and adopted children, theorists postulate that if a person has one obese parent, the chance of that child becoming obese is 60%; if both parents are obese, the chances increase to 90%. Furthermore, identical twins raised apart are more likely to have similar amounts of body fat than fraternal twins raised separately (Foreyt & Poston, 1997).

A third theory, referred to as the *leptin theory,* states that an obesity gene directs the formation of leptin (a protein produced by fat cells), which acts on the hypothalamus and influences hunger and satiety. Most obese individuals experience a resistance to leptin's satiety effect (Albu, Allison, Boozer et al., 1997).

A fourth theory describes the role of medical problems in the development of obesity. Hormonal syndromes such as hypothyroidism, hypercortisolism (Cushing's syndrome), pseudohypoparathyroidism, and primary hyperinsulinism have been identified as risk factors for obesity, especially in childhood and adolescence (Dietz & Gortmaker, 1984; Faust, 2001).

Recent obesity research at the Monell Chemical Senses Center in Philadelphia focused on the biology of craving and its influence on nutritional status and the development of obesity. The premise of the research questioned whether food craving is caused by nutrient or caloric deficit. Research findings indicated that nutritional and caloric deprivation were not necessary to create food cravings. They also found that there was almost a tripling or quadrupling of food cravings during the trial when subjects could eat whatever they wanted (Moore, 2004b).

Behavioral Theories

Inactivity has long been recognized as a contributor to obesity. Most clients who have been obese for some time suffer from an inherited low metabolic rate or resting energy expenditure (REE). One behavioral theory suggests that people may be obese not because they eat too much but because they expend too little energy. This low energy expenditure, coupled with an inactive lifestyle, may cause weight gain or a difficulty in maintaining a healthy weight (White, 2000).

According to research, more than one third of the overweight population, when surveyed, reported that they did not engage in any physical activity during their leisure time. Furthermore, surveys have indicated that children and adolescents participate in fewer than three sessions of vigorous activity per week. Exercise is known to reduce body fat and build healthy muscle mass. Conversely, lack of exercise contributes to obesity (Centers for Disease Control and Prevention, 1996; Whitaker, Pepe, Seidel, & Dietz, 1997; White, 2000).

A second behavioral theory, referred to as the *external cue theory,* suggests that people eat in response to environmental stimuli. Therefore, as stimuli increase (eg, television commercials regarding food or drink, passing a fast-food restaurant, or certain times of the day associated with eating), individuals eat when they aren't hungry and they do not stop eating when they are full (James, 2001).

A third behavioral theory focuses on psychosocial factors. An individual may eat in response to emotions such as loneliness, sadness, anger, or celebration. Stressful interpersonal or family dynamics may also be contributing factors (Epstein, Wisniewski, & Weng, 1994).

Clinical Symptoms and Diagnostic Characteristics of Eating Disorders

Clients with eating disorders share similar clinical symptoms or warning signs including unusual thoughts, feelings, and behavior around food as well as an unhealthy amount of body fat or unhealthy **body mass index (BMI).** The BMI, an indicator of physical fitness, identifies whether a person is overweight or underweight based on height in relation to weight. Individuals who exhibit a BMI less than 18.4 are considered to be underweight. A normal BMI range is 18.5 to 24.9. An individual with a BMI of 25 to 29.9 is considered to be moderately overweight or preobese. An individual with a BMI of 30 to 34.9 is considered to be moderately obese (Class I Obesity), whereas an indi-

vidual with a BMI of 35 to 39.9 is considered to be severely obese (Class II Obesity). An individual with a BMI of more than or equal to 40 is deemed to be extremely obese (Class III Obesity) (National Heart, Lung, & Blood Institute, 1998). Box 23-1 provides a formula for calculating BMI and a chart to determine BMI using height and weight.

Examples of clinical symptoms shared by clients with eating disorders include:

- Focus on body weight and lack of fat to measure one's worth
- Constant dieting on low-calorie, high-restriction diets (clients who were obese and tried dieting without success)
- Impaired body image
- Preoccupation with food or refusal to discuss it
- Use of food to satisfy negative feelings such as anger, rejection, or loneliness
- Compulsive exercising (clients who were obese and tried dieting without success)
- Fear of not being able to stop eating
- Abuse of drugs or alcohol before bingeing
- Stealing, shoplifting, or prostitution to obtain money for food

Clinical symptoms specific to each disorder are discussed within each classification.

Anorexia Nervosa

The client with anorexia nervosa refuses to maintain a normal body weight, intensely fears weight gain, and exhibits a disturbed perception about his or her body. See the accompanying Clinical Symptoms and Diagnostic Characteristics box.

Statistics indicate that anorexia occurs 10 to 20 times more frequently in females than in males. Most females with anorexia are teenaged girls or women who usually are bright achievers. However, the incidence of males suffering from this disorder has increased. Age has little significance: the diagnosis been made in male clients spanning from as young as 5 years to as old as 70 years (Tumolo, 2003). Characterized by an aversion to food, intense fear of becoming obese, and distorted body image, this disorder may result in death due to serious malnutrition. Of diagnosed anorectic clients, 10% to 20% die. Half of these deaths are due to suicide (Jancin, 1999).

Various methods are used to lose weight. Methods include **purging,** or attempts to eliminate the body of

BOX 23.1 DETERMINING BMI

$$BMI = \frac{Weight\ (pounds)}{Height\ (inches)^2} \times 703$$

Example: A person who weighs 150 lb and is 5′5″ (65 inches) tall.

$$BMI = \frac{150\ lb}{65\ in \times 65\ in} \times 703 = \frac{150}{4225} \times 703 = 24.95$$

BODY MASS INDEX CHART

HEIGHT (INCHES)	19	20	21	22	23	24	25	26	27	28	29	30	31	32	33	34	35
								BODY WEIGHT (POUNDS)									
58	91	96	100	105	110	115	119	124	129	134	138	143	148	153	162	167	173
59	94	99	104	109	114	119	124	128	133	138	143	148	153	158	163	168	173
60	97	102	107	112	118	123	128	133	138	143	148	153	158	163	168	174	179
61	100	106	111	116	122	127	132	137	143	148	153	158	164	169	174	180	185
62	104	109	115	120	126	131	136	142	147	153	158	164	169	175	180	186	191
63	107	113	118	124	130	135	141	146	152	158	163	169	175	180	186	191	197
64	110	116	122	128	134	140	145	151	157	163	169	174	180	186	192	197	204
65	114	120	126	132	138	144	150	156	162	168	174	180	186	192	198	204	210
66	118	124	130	136	142	148	155	161	167	173	179	186	192	198	204	210	216
67	121	127	134	140	146	153	159	166	172	178	185	191	198	204	211	217	223
68	125	131	138	144	151	158	164	171	177	184	190	197	203	210	216	223	230
69	128	135	142	149	155	162	169	176	182	189	196	203	209	216	223	230	236
70	132	139	146	153	160	167	174	181	188	195	202	209	216	222	229	236	243
71	136	143	150	157	165	172	179	186	193	200	208	215	222	229	236	243	250
72	140	147	154	162	169	177	184	191	199	206	218	221	228	235	242	250	258
73	144	151	159	166	174	182	189	197	204	212	219	227	235	242	250	257	265
74	148	155	163	171	179	186	194	202	210	218	225	233	241	249	256	264	272
75	152	160	168	176	184	192	200	208	216	224	232	240	248	256	264	272	279
76	156	164	172	180	189	197	205	213	221	230	238	246	254	263	271	279	287

SOURCE: National Heart, Lung, and Blood Institute. Body Mass Index Table, retrieved from http://wwww.nblbi.nih.gov/guidelines/obesity/bmi.tbl.htm.

excess calories by induced vomiting; abuse of laxatives, enemas, diuretics, diet pills, or stimulants; excessive exercise; or a refusal to eat. Deceitful behavior may prevail as the anorectic client disposes of food that he or she is supposed to eat. Although the following symptoms may occur as the disorder progresses (not all persons who are anorectic exhibit all symptoms), clients rarely seek help unless a medical crisis occurs:

- Dry, flaky, or cracked skin
- Brittle hair and nails; hair beginning to fall out
- Amenorrhea or menstrual irregularity
- Constipation
- Hypothermia due to loss of subcutaneous fat
- Decreased pulse, blood pressure, and basal metabolic rate
- Skeletal appearance; BMI of 16 or below
- Presence of lanugo (downy-soft body hair seen on newborn infants)
- Loss of appetite
- Callus formation on finger (**Russell's sign**) due to self-induced purging
- Dental caries
- Total lack of concern about symptoms

CLINICAL SYMPTOMS AND DIAGNOSTIC CHARACTERISTICS/ ANOREXIA NERVOSA

CLINICAL SYMPTOMS

- Refusal to maintain a minimally normal body weight
- Intense fear of gaining weight, even with preoccupation with thoughts of food
- Significant distortion in perception of body size or shape
- Amenorrhea (in women who have established a menstrual cycle)
- Depressed mood
- Social withdrawal
- Irritability
- Insomnia
- Decreased interest in sex
- Inflexible thinking
- Strong need to control one's environment

DIAGNOSTIC CHARACTERISTICS

- Maintenance of body weight of less than 85% of what is expected for age and height, or failure in attaining expected weight during growth period
- Extreme influence of body weight or shape on one's self-perception
- Denial of seriousness of current extremely low body weight
- Absence of three consecutive menstrual cycles

Restricting type: Engagement in activities such as dieting, fasting, or excessive exercise

Binge-eating/purging type: Engagement in binge eating, purging, or both via self-induced vomiting or misuse of laxatives, diuretics, or enemas

The pre-anorectic person is generally considered to be a "model child and student" who is meek, compliant, perfectionistic, and overachieving. The individual usually is overly sensitive, fears independence and sexual relationships, has a low self-concept, and is resistant to growing up and maturing. Starvation is an attention-getting device that permits the anorectic client full control of his or her body, allowing the individual to remain in or revert to a prepubertal state.

Warning signs that should alert parents, teachers, or others to the possibility of anorexia nervosa include the following:

- Drastic weight loss in the presence of unusual eating habits, such as fasting, bingeing, or refusal to eat except tiny portions
- Obsession with neatness or personal appearance, including frequent mirror gazing. The person constantly checks on his or her appearance, fearing unattractiveness and obesity.
- Hostility and the desire to control others
- Calorie counting, dieting, and excessive exercise or hyperactivity
- Weighing self several times daily
- Depressed mood
- Amenorrhea or irregular menses
- Wearing of loose-fitting clothing to hide physical appearance as it changes (Figure 23-1)
- Denial of hunger

As the eating disorder progresses, the anorectic person displays behaviors such as manipulation, stubbornness, hostility, and deceitfulness. Defense mechanisms

FIGURE 23.1 The client with anorexia nervosa. Note the layered, baggy clothing to conceal the weight loss.

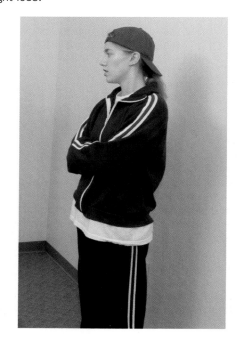

used include denial, displacement, projection, rationalization, regression, isolation, and intellectualization. Comorbid psychiatric disorders that occur with anorexia nervosa include depression (65%), social phobia (34%), and obsessive–compulsive disorder (26%) (Sadock & Sadock, 2003).

According to Erikson's stages of emotional development, food may become a power struggle between mother and child between the ages of 2 and 3 years. Children between the ages of 4 and 5 years use food to sedate feelings of guilt and powerlessness. A love/trust relationship with food becomes solidified between the ages of 6 and 12 years. Between the ages of 13 and 18 years, food can be controlled with no interference (Erikson, 1993, 1994).

Living in an environment that may be overprotective, rigid, or lacking in conflict resolution, the anorectic person achieves secondary gains such as love and undue attention because he or she is considered to be a special or unique person. See Clinical Example 23-1, The Client With Anorexia Nervosa.

Bulimia Nervosa

Episodic **binge eating,** a rapid consumption of a large amount of food in less than 2 hours, is classified as *bulimia nervosa.* The person is aware that the behavior is abnormal, fears the inability to stop eating voluntarily, is self-critical, and may experience depression after each episode. See the accompanying Clinical Symptoms and Diagnostic Characteristics box.

Bulimia nervosa is significantly more common in women than in men (10:1 ratio). The age of onset is usually between 17 and 25 years (APA, 2000a). The BMI of clients with bulimia varies due to fluctuations in weight. If underweight, the BMI usually ranges from 16 to 19. Others may be slightly overweight.

Certain traits are found among individuals with bulimia, who often view themselves as unlovable, inadequate, and unworthy. The desire to please becomes very powerful as the adolescent strives to be perfect, thin, loved, and accepted. Also, many adolescents feel insecure about their physical shape and size in a society that places value on external appearance and nurturing. The psychiatric implications are significant because approximately 50% of clients with bulimia nervosa also experience depression and require antidepressant medication. Other comorbid psychiatric disorders include substance-related, personality, anxiety, bipolar I, and dissociative disorders. Bulimia nervosa may develop into a chronic disorder

---

CLINICAL EXAMPLE 23.1

THE CLIENT WITH ANOREXIA NERVOSA

MJ, 19 years old, was a sophomore in college when her psychology professor noted a change in her classroom behavior as well as a sudden weight loss. When questioned about her behavior, MJ told the professor that she was losing weight to compete for a position on the track team, although she was unable to give him a specific goal regarding her desired weight. She began to wear loose-fitting clothing and would refer to herself as overweight although others commented on her thinness. MJ's meek, compliant behavior changed to that of a deceitful, hostile, and manipulative person. She isolated herself at mealtimes and engaged in various exercises after eating. At times, she would eat large amounts of food and then induce vomiting. A close friend observed MJ taking large amounts of over-the-counter diet pills as well as laxatives. In an effort to continue her weight loss, MJ would set her alarm so that she could exercise during the night and also awaken for early morning jogging. She became obsessed with exercising. Her physical appearance deteriorated as her hair began to fall out, her skin became quite dry, and acne developed. MJ also complained of being chilly all the time and wore layered clothing. During track practice, MJ became lightheaded, felt irregular heartbeats, perspired profusely, and experienced severe fatigue. The track coach took her to the college health clinic to be examined by the physician. Physical examination revealed poor skin turgor and other symptoms of dehydration. The physician also suspected a potassium and protein deficit, although MJ denied any eating problems. Her weight was approximately 15 pounds under the desired weight for her height and body build. She had lost 25 pounds in a 4-month period and experienced amenorrhea for 3 months. The college physician recommended that MJ see the school counselor regarding her concern about weight loss.

---

and occur intermittently over several years (Sadock & Sadock, 2003).

Serious medical consequences may occur because of alternating bingeing and purging. However, the indi-

CLINICAL SYMPTOMS AND DIAGNOSTIC CHARACTERISTICS/
BULIMIA NERVOSA

CLINICAL SYMPTOMS

- Binge eating
- Excessive influence of body shape and weight on self-evaluation
- Use of self-induced vomiting; misuse of laxatives, diuretics, or enemas; fasting or excessive exercise
- Low self-esteem
- Mood disturbance
- Possible stimulant use

DIAGNOSTIC CHARACTERISTICS

- Evidence of recurrent episodes of binge eating occurring on the average of at least two times per week over a period of 3 months
  - Consumption of food in amounts significantly greater in a specific period of time than that which others would consume in that same specific period of time
  - Feelings of lack of control over eating during the binge period
- Recurrent use of inappropriate measures to compensate for binge eating and prevent weight gain
- Demonstration of undue influence of body shape and weight on self-perception
- Episode occurrences not limited to episodes of anorexia nervosa

Purging type: Regular participation in self-induced vomiting or misuse of medications or enemas to rid body of food during binge-eating episode

Nonpurging type: Regular participation in fasting or excessive exercising during binge-eating episode; no use of purging activities

vidual may not seek treatment until a medical emergency occurs. These situations include:

- Chronic inflammation of the lining of the esophagus
- Rupture of the esophagus
- Dilation of the stomach
- Rupture of the stomach
- Electrolyte imbalance or abnormalities, leading to arrhythmias of the heart and metabolic alkalosis
- Heart problems, irreversible heart failure, and death due to abuse of ipecac syrup
- Chronic enlargement of the parotid glands
- Dehydration
- Irritable bowel syndrome or abnormal dilation of the colon
- Rectal prolapse, abscess, or bleeding
- Rupture of the diaphragm, with entrance of the abdominal contents into the chest cavity
- Dental erosion; gum disease
- Chronic edema
- Fungal infections of the vagina or rectum

See Clinical Example 23-2, The Client With Bulimia Nervosa.

CLINICAL EXAMPLE 23.2

THE CLIENT WITH BULIMIA NERVOSA

LR, a 22-year-old computer programmer, was seen in the emergency room of a local community hospital with complaints of weakness, rapid pulse, dizziness, and difficulty swallowing. A physical assessment disclosed symptoms of dehydration with a possible electrolyte imbalance. On being questioned further, LR confided to the physician that she was concerned about her weight and had tried various measures to control her appetite. She found herself craving sweets and other high-calorie foods. When such feelings occurred, she would devour everything in sight that was easily ingested, eating for 1 to 2 hours at times. Her grocery and restaurant bills were quite high, over $150.00 per week, because of such cravings. After such bingeing episodes, LR would induce vomiting to avoid weight gain. She stated that she felt out of control and anxious when she binged. Her main fear was of becoming fat, and when she vomited, she was able to relieve herself of guilt feelings due to overeating. Recent publicity about anorexia and bulimia had caused her to seek help for physical symptoms that had been present for several weeks. LR agreed to a complete physical examination and referral to a counselor who had experience working with bulimic clients.

Eating Disorder, Not Otherwise Specified

This category is for disorders of eating that do not meet the criteria for any specific eating disorder. For example, a client would be diagnosed with eating disorder, not otherwise specified, if the client repeatedly chewed and spit out—but not swallowed—a large amount of food. Another example of this diagnosis is a female client who meets all of the criteria for anorexia nervosa except that she has regular menses.

Obesity

Although **obesity** (increased body weight resulting from an excess accumulation of stored body fat) is not classified as a *DSM-IV-TR* disorder, individuals exhibiting clinical symptoms of obesity and coexisting diagnoses such as anxiety or depression have been treated in the psychiatric setting. Such individuals frequently refer to themselves as bulimics who experience recurrent episodes of binge eating but who do not purge. They admit to a lack of control over eating and relate a history of repeated attempts to lose or stabilize their weight. According to a new diagnostic category proposed for inclusion in the next revision of the *DSM-IV-TR*, these individuals may meet the criteria for Binge Eating Disorder.

The prevalence of obesity in America has tripled since the early 1900s. Weight gain is most pronounced in both sexes between the ages of 25 and 44 years. After age 50 years, weights of men stabilize and may even decline between the ages of 60 and 74. Women continue to gain in weight until age 60; then weight begins to decline. (APA, 2000a; Sadock & Sadock, 2003).

Developmental obesity begins in childhood with overeating, and **reactive obesity** occurs in later life, when compulsive eating is used to cope with stress. Comorbid psychiatric disorders may include depression, anxiety, or a psychotic disorder in which an individual develops an abnormal eating pattern.

Obesity has increased by approximately 54% in children 6 to 11 years of age over the last 20 years. Childhood and adolescent obesity is distinct from obesity in other life stages because psychosocial and biologic changes accompanying puberty influence interventions (James, 2001).

Obesity in childhood has been addressed by numerous researchers. According to the National Health and Nutrition Examination Survey, 25% to 30% of children are obese. Furthermore, approximately 39% of children 6 to 17 years of age weigh 20% more than their ideal body weight (Klish, 1998). Children who live in the Northeastern region of the United States, reside in densely populated areas, watch television rather than exercise, and whose parents are both obese are at greater risk for obesity (James, 2001). Obesity in children is usually caused by a combination of excessive caloric intake and insufficient exercise; however, it is also a feature of various congenital and acquired syndromes such as Down, Klinefelter's, and Prader-Willi syndromes.

The social stigma of being overweight can have long-term, devastating effects on self-esteem because obese children are often teased and rejected by their peers. For example, in August 1996, a 12-year-old-boy in central Florida hung himself the morning that school was to start. His parents stated that he had tried all summer to lose weight before he was scheduled to enter middle school. His pediatrician stated that the boy's body frame was large and, genetically, he was predisposed to develop faster than his peers.

An initiative, *Healthy People 2010,* published by the Department of Health and Human Services (2000), identifies the 10 leading health goals and their importance as public health concerns. Two of the goals which will be used to measure the health of the nation over the next 10 years address activity and obesity. They state:

- Reduce the proportion of children and adolescents who are overweight or obese.
- Increase from 75% to 85% the proportion of children and adolescents aged 6 through 17 who engage in vigorous physical activity that promotes cardio-respiratory fitness 3 or more days per week for at least 20 minutes per occasion.

SELF-AWARENESS PROMPT

Reflect on the style of clothing that you prefer to wear (eg, casual, sport, business). Why do you prefer this style of clothing? When you look at your reflection in the mirror, are you satisfied with your appearance? If not, how would you change it? What measures would you take?

THE NURSING PROCESS

ASSESSMENT

It is not uncommon for a client with clinical symptoms of a psychiatric disorder (eg, depression, delusions, delirium, eating disorder) to refuse to eat, be uninterested in eating, or be unaware of the need or desire to eat. A client may be experiencing physical or psychological problems that interfere with appetite or that make it difficult for the client to eat (Schultz & Videbeck, 2005).

The assessment of clients with clinical symptoms of an eating disorder is a complex process focusing on the client's medical status, physical appearance, ability to meet basic needs, mood and affect, cognitive abilities, interpersonal skills, and behavioral manifestations. Skill is needed in eliciting feelings and thoughts from clients who are generally secretive about their illness and who often use intellectualization to defend their behaviors. A firm but caring approach is used. When obtaining a history, responses to questions such as "What do you think about your weight?" or "What do you think would be a good weight for you?" often reveal information about body image disturbance and the client's perception of ideal body weight (Kameg, Mitchell, & Chmielewski, 2003). Using an assessment tool is helpful in determining whether a psychiatric problem underlies the individual's abnormal eating habits, inability to eat, or refusal to eat.

Assessment Tools

Several assessment guides can be used to collect data about the client with an eating disorder.

The Eating Attitudes Test (EAT-26), developed in 1982, is probably the most widely used standardized measure of symptoms and concerns characteristic of eating disorders. It was selected as the screening instrument used in the 1998 National Eating Disorders Screening Program. The EAT-26 alone does not yield a specific diagnosis of an eating disorder; however, studies have shown that it can be an efficient screening instrument as part of a two-stage screening process. A cut-off score of 20 indicates a potential eating disorder and the need for a follow-up interview. The EAT-26 takes 10 minutes to complete. It is available at http://www.stuaff.niu.edu/csdc/EAT26.htm (Eating Disorder Referral and Information Center, 2006).

A new tool, the SCOFF questionnaire (acronym for Sick, Control, One, Fat, and Food), can be used to assess a client for an eating disorder (Moore, 2000; Morgan, Reid, & Lacey, 1999). The client is asked five questions:

- Do you make yourself **S**ick because you feel uncomfortably full?
- Do you worry that you have lost **C**ontrol over how much you eat?
- Have you recently lost more than the equivalent of **O**ne stone (13–14 pounds) in a 3-month period?
- Do you believe yourself to be **F**at when others say you are too thin?
- Would you say that **F**ood dominates your life?

If the client answers yes to two or more questions, a referral is necessary for further evaluation to determine the presence of an eating disorder. Additional eating disorder assessment tools are available for use in the clinical setting. Conant (1996) and Muscari (1998) have developed assessment guides to use when collecting biopsychosocial data about clients with anorexia nervosa, bulimia nervosa, or obesity. Abraham (2004) lists several questions that are appropriate for obesity assessment in children. Regardless of the specific tool used, the focus is on the following:

- Weight history and what the client thinks an ideal weight would be
- Perception of body appearance, including self-concept and sexuality
- Lifestyle, including living arrangements, meal preparation, financial resources, neighborhood resources, occupation, and available support
- Eating habits or pattern, including kinds, amounts, and frequency of food used or avoided
- Dieting history, including date of onset and what prompted dieting
- Bingeing and purging rituals surrounding food consumption such as the use of diet pills, diuretics, laxatives, or herbal remedies
- Physical activities or exercise used to achieve ideal weight
- Sleep–wake pattern, including the use of sleep remedies
- Interpersonal relationships with family, peers, or authority figures, including history of physical or sexual abuse
- Spiritual difficulties resulting from excessive preoccupation with food or body
- Behavioral changes such as the presence of mood swings or withdrawal from others to eat or starve

- Psychiatric history regarding any prior treatment for an eating disorder as well as the absence or presence of a comorbid psychiatric disorder (eg, depression, anxiety, obsessive–compulsive behavior, substance abuse, suicide attempts)

Physical Examination

A physical examination is conducted to rule out any serious or potentially life-threatening medical complications. Record data about the client's height and weight and assess the client's BMI (Figure 23-2). Although most health care providers use clinical impression and weight-for-age and weight-for-height percentiles, the U.S. Preventive Services Task Force (USPSTF) recommends that BMI should be used to determine whether an individual is underweight, overweight, or obese (Abraham, 2004; USPSTF, 2004). Clients with a history of anorexia nervosa may wear layered clothing to conceal weight loss. The physical examination may reveal clinical symptoms of **cachexia** (eg, malnourishment and emaciation) due to extreme weight loss. Conversely, clients with a history of bulimia nervosa generally appear to be within their ideal body weight range or even slightly above ideal body weight.

Muscari (1998) suggests that a systems review address symptoms specific to eating disorders such as cold intolerance, fatigue, irregular menses, constipation, lethargy, dental problems (eg, discoloration, dental caries), and a history of electrolyte or fluid imbalances. Be alert for possible medical complications of anorexia nervosa, bulimia nervosa, and obesity. For example, metabolic syndrome (ie, pre-diabetes, abdominal obesity, an unfavorable lipid profile, and hypertension) is common, particularly in the overweight and obese population (Table 23-1).

Laboratory Tests

Additional tests may be necessary depending on the client's medical status. They include:

- Electrocardiogram (ECG) to detect bradycardia, arrhythmias, prolonged Q–T interval
- Comprehensive metabolic panel (including serum sodium, potassium, amylase, blood glucose, magnesium and phosphate levels) to rule out electrolyte imbalance, hypoglycemia, and other abnormalities
- Hemogram to rule out anemia, leukopenia, neutropenia, or thrombocytopenia

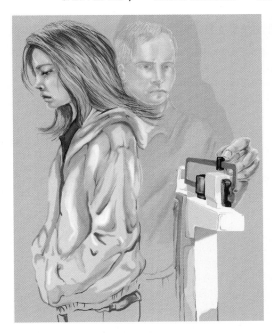

FIGURE 23.2 The nurse weighing the client with anorexia nervosa.

- Endocrine studies such as growth hormone level, cortisol level, and thyroid profile to rule out medical abnormalities
- Ultrasonography to rule out gallstones, blood urea nitrogen, creatinine, and urinalysis to rule out dehydration, kidney stones, ketonuria
- Electroencephalogram (EEG) to rule out any neurologic causes for clinical symptoms
- Drug screen such as for benzodiazepine or psychostimulant use

In the assessment of obesity, if Cushing's syndrome is suspected, a 24-hour urine cortisol level assessment followed by a low-dose dexamethasone suppression test may be beneficial. Clients with signs, symptoms, or laboratory studies consistent with a secondary cause for obesity may be referred to a specialist such as an endocrinologist or specialist in internal medicine for a more complete evaluation to rule out a comorbid medical condition (Hensrud, 1999).

Transcultural Considerations

As with any assessment, be sure to address the client's cultural and ethnic background. Anorexia nervosa is

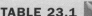
TABLE 23.1 Medical Complications of Anorexia Nervosa, Bulimia Nervosa, and Obesity

ORGAN/SYSTEM	ANOREXIA	BULIMIA	OBESITY
Cardiovascular	Arrhythmias, hypotension, congestive heart failure, mitral valve prolapse, ECG abnormalities, fluid and electrolyte imbalance, peripheral vasoconstriction with acrocyanosis, sudden cardiac death	Cardiomyopathy, peripheral myopathy, hypotension, fluid and electrolyte imbalance	Hypertension, coronary artery disease, varicose veins, left ventricular hypertrophy, heart failure
Endocrine/ metabolic	Delayed onset of puberty, amenorrhea, growth retardation, elevated growth hormone levels, hypothermia, elevated serum cortisol levels, severe hypoglycemia	Fluid and electrolyte imbalance (eg, dehydration, hypokalemia, metabolic acidosis or alkalosis, hypocalcemia), irregular menses, abnormal serotonin metabolism, elevated serum cortisol levels, disordered thermoregulation, decreased estrogen levels	Adult-onset diabetes, complications with pregnancy, gout
Gastrointestinal	Delayed gastric emptying, gastric dilatation and rupture, refeeding pancreatitis, chronic constipation, abdominal hernia, elevated liver enzymes	Salivary and parotid gland hypertrophy, pancreatitis, esophageal perforation, esophagitis, gastritis, gastric dilatation and rupture, abdominal hernia, constipation, hypokalemic ileus, steatorrhea, abnormal liver enzymes, tooth enamel erosion, dental caries, periodontal disease	Cholelithiasis, cholecystitis, colon cancer, hepatosteatosis, hypertriglyceridemia, low HDL cholesterol
Genitourinary	Decreased glomerular filtration rate, renal calculi, elevated blood urea nitrogen (BUN), hypovolemic nephropathy, candida infection	Reduced glomerular filtration rate, elevated BUN, pyuria, hematuria, proteinuria, polyuria, candida infection	Urinary incontinence; breast cancer; endometrial cancer; risk of cancer of colon, rectum, and prostate in men; renal vein thrombosis; gall bladder and biliary cancer in women
Hematologic	Anemia, leukopenia, thrombocytopenia, low erythrocyte sedimentation rate, folate and iron deficiency, clotting factor abnormalities, hypofibrinogenemia, impaired immune response	Vitamin K–deficient coagulopathy	None
Integumentary	Hair loss, lanugo-like hair, dry skin, brittle hair and nails, petechiae, purpura, edema	Russell's sign (finger calluses and abrasions), increased risk for acne	Skin irritation or breakdown
Musculoskeletal	Muscle enzyme abnormalities, pathologic stress fractures, osteopenia, osteoporosis, arrested skeletal growth, loss of muscle mass	Stress fractures, osteoporosis	Arthritis, limited mobility, bone spurs on heels

Organ/System	Anorexia	Bulimia	Obesity
Respiratory	Pulmonary edema secondary to heart failure	Aspiration pneumonitis, pulmonary edema	Obstructive sleep apnea, restrictive lung disease
Neurologic	Significant loss of brain tissue and abnormal electrical activity, seizures, ventricular enlargement	Seizures, ventricular enlargement	None

considered to be prevalent in industrialized societies with an abundance of food and where physical attractiveness is linked to being thin. Such societies include the United States, Canada, Europe, Australia, Japan, New Zealand, and South Africa. Bulimia nervosa occurs with roughly similar frequencies as anorexia nervosa in the industrialized societies listed herein. This disorder affects primarily white individuals, but has been reported among other ethnic groups (APA, 2000a).

A report in the Harvard Mental Health Letter (Grinspoon, 1998) suggests that eating disorders are not chiefly a feature of Western or white culture. Fifteen hundred black, white, Asian, and mixed-race social science students at six universities answered questions about their weight, height, and eating habits. Sixty percent of the men and 45% of the women thought that their weight was normal, whereas 19% of the men and 41% of the women felt they were overweight. Black students were more likely than white students to have some symptoms of bulimia or anorexia. Asian students had fewer symptoms; the results for mixed-race students resembled those for white students. It was concluded that nothing in their culture or social circumstances seems to protect South African black students against eating disorders.

Several studies have reported information about obesity in children and adolescents (James, 2001). According to the Centers for Disease Control and Prevention, obesity is more prevalent in Native American schoolchildren living on or near reservations compared with U.S. children of all ages and genders. The National Center for Health Statistics reported that the percentage of obesity (56%) in certain subgroups of Latino children (eg, Mexican Americans, Puerto Ricans, and Cubans) and in African American children (41%) is greater than that in Caucasian children (29%).

The International Obesity Task Force estimates that the prevalence of obesity in developed countries is similar to that in the United States. The most dramatic increase has been in the United Kingdom, where the prevalence of obesity doubled between 1980 and 1995. In Japan, obesity has doubled among men in the last two decades, and almost doubled for young women ages 20 to 29 years. Obesity in China is more common in urban areas and among women (Jain, 2004).

NURSING DIAGNOSES

When formulating nursing diagnoses, consider several factors such as the client's physical health, nutritional status, developmental level, coping skills, emotional status, behavioral responses, and family dynamics. A coexisting psychiatric disorder such as substance abuse, alcoholism, or obsessive–compulsive disorder may be present. Psychotic symptoms or delirium may occur in severe cases. See the accompanying North American Nursing Diagnosis Association (NANDA) nursing diagnoses box for examples.

OUTCOME IDENTIFICATION

Outcome identification for clients with eating disorders may be stated in the form of short-term and long-term outcomes (Decker, 2003). Short-term outcomes focus on stabilizing any existing medical condition including weight loss; normalizing eating behaviors; and decreasing clinical symptoms of a comorbid psychiatric disorder such as anxiety or depression. Long-term outcomes focus on helping the client develop more constructive coping mechanisms and helping the client and family resolve any psychological issues that precipitated the eating disorder. According to a study of the outcomes for clients with anorexia nervosa, about 50% achieved complete recovery, 21% had an intermediate outcome, and 26% had an outcome that was poor, with an overall mortality rate of 9.8% (Sullivan, Bulik, Fear, & Pickering, 1998). In a similar study of clients with bulimia nervosa, 50% were

EXAMPLES OF NANDA NURSING DIAGNOSES/ EATING DISORDERS

- Imbalanced Nutrition Less than Body Requirements related to refusal to eat
- Imbalanced Nutrition More than Body Requirements related to undesirable eating patterns
- Anxiety related to inadequate coping mechanisms
- Disturbed Body Image related to fear of being overweight
- Constipation related to inadequate food and fluid intake
- Diarrhea related to laxative abuse
- Fatigue related to excessive exercise
- Deficient Fluid Volume related to refusal to drink fluids
- Impaired Social Interaction related to regressive behavior
- Compromised Family Coping related to enabling behaviors
- Risk for Impaired Skin Integrity related to low body mass secondary to malnutrition
- Chronic Low Self-Esteem related to body-image distortion

EXAMPLES OF STATED OUTCOMES/ EATING DISORDERS

- The client will increase caloric and nutritional intake.
- The client will establish regular nutritional eating patterns.
- The client will verbalize feelings of self-worth, guilt, anger, or anxiety.
- The client will demonstrate decreased obsessive–compulsive behavior.
- The client will be free of self-inflicted injury.
- The client will participate in a treatment program.
- The client will evidence improvement in physical status related to complications of obesity or bulimia.
- The client will acknowledge problems with socialization.
- The client will identify the reasons for feelings of isolation.
- The client will identify appropriate diversional activities.
- The client will verbalize fears related to health needs.
- The client will identify alternatives to present coping patterns.
- The client will acknowledge self-harm thoughts.

reported to have recovered fully, 30% experienced occasional relapse, and almost 20% continued to exhibit the full criteria for bulimia nervosa (Keel & Mitchell, 1997). See the accompanying box for Examples of Stated Outcomes for clients with eating disorders.

PLANNING INTERVENTIONS

Planning involves the client and family and, in many settings, a multidisciplinary approach. Members of the multidisciplinary team directed by the nurse include a physician or internist, dietitian, psychotherapist, social worker, and occupational therapist. Dance, music, art, and drama therapy have also been used in planning care for clients with eating disorders.

According to research data presented by Dr. Drew Westen, clients with the same eating disorder may have different personality prototypes and comorbidities that affect treatment responses. He described three personality prototypes that should be considered when planning interventions. The first prototype is a *high-functioning/perfectionistic* client who is articulate, conscientious, empathic, and able to use one's talents effectively. This individual tends to be self-critical, perfectionistic, guilt ridden, and anxious. The second prototype is described as being *constricted/ overcontrolled.* This individual exhibits a limited range of emotions; is passive and unassertive; has difficulty acknowledging or expressing wishes; and displays little psychological insight into his/her own motives or behavior. The third prototype is described as being *emotionally dysregulated/undercontrolled.* This individual has emotions that spiral out of control and change rapidly or unpredictably; expresses emotions in exaggerated ways; shows inappropriate intense anger; is irrational; feels inferior or victimized; and is unable to engage in healthy interpersonal relationships. Dr. Westen concluded that emerging data suggest that treating clinicians tend to adjust their treatment style based on the personality prototype of the client (Worcester, 2004).

GUIDELINES FOR PLANNING INTERVENTIONS

Appropriate planning needs to consider where interventions will occur (Finkelstein, 1999). The client's weight, eating behavior, attitude about food, cognition, physiologic symptoms, and associated psychiatric symptoms determine whether interventions should occur in the hospital, in a partial-hospitalization program, in an intensive outpatient program, or in a private outpatient clinical setting. Special consideration is given to pregnant women, high-school or college students, female athletes, men, diabetic clients, very young clients, older clients with chronic eating disorders, and individuals with comorbid conditions. Outpatient interventions for clients with eating disorders are the preferred approach. Inpatient interventions are highly problematic because clients often deny the illness, evade therapeutic interventions, and engender negative reactions in health care professionals.

Criteria for Hospitalization

Clients are usually hospitalized when the following criteria are met: suicidal ideation is exhibited; severe purging or self-destructive behavior is out of control; psychosis is evident; family is demonstrating crisis; environment is nonsupportive; client fails to respond to outpatient interventions; or any life-threatening condition based on laboratory data monitored during treatment is occurring. The primary goal of inpatient care is weight gain under medical supervision and stabilization of any life-threatening medical conditions or behavior. Table 23-2 summarizes the criteria for hospitalization based on data provided by the APA (2000a, 2000b) and Sadock and Sadock (2003).

Clients may be admitted to a general hospital, intensive care unit, medical–psychiatric unit, or psychiatric hospital, depending on the severity of clinical symptoms. Length of stay is determined by response to interventions as well as certification by the client's insurance company.

IMPLEMENTATION

A holistic approach is recommended when providing care for clients with the diagnosis of an eating disor-

---

TABLE 23.2 Criteria for Hospitalization

CRITERIA	ADULTS	CHILDREN
Weight	<75% of ideal body weight	Acute weight loss due to refusal to eat
Vital signs		
Pulse	<40 bpm	<50 bpm
Blood pressure	<90/60 mmHg	<80/50 mmHg
Temperature	<97.0° F (36.1° C)	<97.0° F (36.1° C)
Laboratory values	Abnormal hepatic, renal, or cardiovascular profiles	Abnormal hepatic, renal, or cardiovascular profiles
	Serum glucose <60 mg/dL	Serum glucose <60 mg/dL
	Serum K <3 meq/l	Hypokalemia
		Hypophosphatemia
ECG	Abnormal	Abnormal
Suicidal	Ideation or attempt	Ideation or attempt

SOURCES: American Psychiatric Association. (2000). *Diagnostic and statistical manual of mental disorders* (4th ed., Text Revision). Washington, DC: Author; American Psychiatric Association. (2000). *Practice guidelines for the treatment of patients with eating disorders* (2nd ed.). Washington, DC: American Psychiatric Press; Sadock, B. J., & Sadock, V. A. (2003). *Kaplan & Sadock's synopsis of psychiatry: Behavioral sciences/clinical psychiatry* (9th ed.). Philadelphia: Lippincott Williams & Wilkins.

der. Depending on symptom severity, the nurse may provide care in a variety of settings (eg, inpatient, partial hospitalization, or outpatient). Adjusting to mood swings and changes of behavior can be quite challenging as the nurse assists the client with meeting basic needs; provides medication management; engages the client in interactive therapies; promotes self-help; and provides client education.

Assistance With Meeting Basic Needs

Be cognizant of any transference by the client and use caution to avoid the response of countertransference. As noted earlier, clients may have difficulty relating to individuals they perceive to be mother, father, or authority figures. The following is a list of approaches that have been used successfully to avoid conflict and develop a trusting relationship with a client when providing assistance to meet the client's basic needs:

- Be matter-of-fact, friendly, patient, and casual if the client is withdrawn or sullen.
- Avoid statements that indicate shock, disbelief, or disgust at the eating or purging behaviors.
- Set limits to avoid manipulative behavior.
- Remain uninvolved when the client is indecisive or ambivalent.
- Avoid confrontation and be nonjudgmental when the client exhibits hostility or anger.
- Avoid discussions or explanations about food, diet, or the body unless these issues are linked with feelings.
- Approach the client with positive expectations despite negative behavior.
- Allow the client to maintain some control; for example, in decision-making.
- Avoid comparing the client's behavior or appearance with others.

Creation of a Safe Environment. Clients with eating disorders may display impulsive, unpredictable, obsessive–compulsive, ritualistic, or self-abusive behavior. Living in a safe, structured environment minimizes the chance of injury to self or others. It also permits assessment for suicidal thoughts or other signs of depression as behavioral change or weight gain occurs. Partial hospitalization (Chapter 8) is designated for clients who are between 75% and 90% of ideal body weight, who do not have laboratory abnormalities, and who are

not at an immediate risk for self-destructive behavior. If the client remains an outpatient, the family or support system is involved in maintaining a safe environment. (See Chapter 31 for a discussion of nursing interventions for clients who exhibit self-abusive or suicidal behavior.)

Stabilization of Medical Condition. After a comprehensive medical evaluation, nursing interventions focus on providing care for physical problems and meeting the basic needs of the client. Collaborate with the client to devise an eating plan that will provide adequate nutrition and retention of food. Total parenteral nutrition, tube feedings, liquid diet, or a special diet recommended by the dietitian may be chosen. Re-feeding syndrome is a potential problem for all eating-disordered clients who are reintroducing fluids and food. They are at risk for severe metabolic imbalances, resulting in cardiovascular, pulmonary, neurologic, hepatic, and bone marrow dysfunction. Re-feeding also unmasks many nutritional deficiencies such as electrolyte and fluid imbalances, glucose intolerance, liver dysfunction, and thiamine deficiency. Once the client's medical condition has been stabilized, a determination is made whether the client should remain hospitalized or be discharged and followed on an outpatient basis. Most clients fare well, some have a moderate challenge, and a few have very severe or even fatal consequences (Johnson, 2005).

Also monitor intake and output, vital signs, weight, elimination patterns, and activity level, and assist with obtaining laboratory data as ordered. Perform or assist with skin care as necessary because the client is at risk for skin breakdown due to lack of muscle and subcutaneous tissue. Provide adequate clothing and bedding to prevent hypothermia. Encourage good dental hygiene. Clients who engage in purging are at risk for the development of dental caries or periodontal disease. Purging also contributes to the erosion of dental enamel secondary to the presence of gastric acid in emesis.

Stabilization of Behavior. Effective treatment programs use behavioral methods to stabilize clinical symptoms of eating disorders. Anorectic clients can be quite manipulative as they attempt to divert attention from their eating habits. Such manipulation may include eating slowly, hiding food, or giving food to other persons. Limiting mealtimes decreases the amount of time the client is dealing with issues of food and eating. After meals, supervise the client for a specified amount of time to prevent bingeing or purging. The chance of successful treatment is better if the client maintains a body weight greater than 90 pounds. That weight appears to be a critical turning point in a client's response to therapy.

The mere act of hospitalization or the development of a behavioral contract implies that compliance is expected and necessary if recovery is to occur. Assigning one member of the multidisciplinary staff to be the client's contact person minimizes the possibility of staff-splitting or manipulation.

Explore alternate methods to minimize compulsive exercise habits that were used by anorectic clients to promote weight loss. Clients with bulimia or obesity can achieve weight loss with exercise plans and diets implemented by the staff. Exercise has been proven to boost self-esteem and body image, relieve stress and anxiety, improve mood and cognition, provide social opportunity, and decrease fatigue. It also improves general fitness by lowering diastolic blood pressure, promoting fat loss, raising HDL and lowering LDL cholesterol, and strengthening immune function (Kenny, 2001).

Expect to implement limit-setting or similar interventions to decrease regressive or negativistic behavior. Consequences are established with input from the client. For example, certain privileges are earned if the client completes a daily schedule, and they are taken away if the client chooses not to participate in the schedule.

Medication Management

Most research related to psychopharmacologic treatment of eating disorders during the last 15 years has focused on bulimia nervosa. Statistics reveal that of 100 clients with bulimia nervosa, some 77 will persevere with a course of medication treatment, and 25 will be in remission at the end of treatment with a single antidepressant. Tricyclic antidepressants such as imipramine (Tofranil); selective serotonin reuptake inhibitors (SSRIs) such as fluoxetine (Prozac); and naltrexone (an opiate antagonist) are considered effective in stabilizing bingeing, obsessive–compulsive behavior, and any underlying depression (Cote, 2001; Grady, 1997; Sadock & Sadock, 2003). Caution is exercised with the use of monoamine oxidase inhibitors (MAOIs) because of the potential for food–drug interaction during binge eating.

Apart from the treatment of comorbid psychopathology such as delirium, phobias, substance abuse, impulse control disorder, major depression, or obsessive–compulsive behavior, the role for psychopharmacologic agents in the treatment of anorexia nervosa is limited (Cote, 2001). For the nonpurging anorectic client, appetite stimulants such as cyproheptadine (Periactin), megestrol acetate (Megace), or dronabinol (Marinol) may be used to accelerate weight gain during initial refeeding phases of treatment. Multivitamins, vitamin D, oral contraceptives, and calcium supplements are recommended to prevent further bone loss in clients with anorexia. The SSRI fluoxetine (Prozac) may be used in the maintenance phase of treatment after a weight gain has occurred and physiologic and psychological functions are restored. The use of other SSRIs such as sertraline (Zoloft) and paroxetine (Paxil) is being explored. Pre-meal anxiolytics may be prescribed because clients are usually extremely phobic and anxious about eating. Other agents that have been used include tricyclic antidepressants (TCAs), MAOIs, and atypical antipsychotics. Unfortunately, TCAs have adverse effects such as the prolongation of the Q-T interval that can cause cardiac arrhythmias. Atypical antipsychotics are used to decrease body image disturbance and anxiety. They also have the potential to promote weight gain. (Cote, 2001; Grady, 1997; Kameg, Mitchell, & Chmielewski, 2003; Sadock & Sadock, 2003). Drug Summary Table 23-1 highlights the major drugs used for eating disorders.

Clients with anorexia or bulimia often are resistant to taking any medication because they fear a loss of control and possible weight gain. They may exhibit behaviors such as palming or cheeking medication and disposing of it when out of the watchful eye of nursing staff. Suicidal clients may save medication to overdose if they feel a loss of control and have tunnel vision regarding a positive response to nursing interventions and therapy. Administering medication before weight is restored and medical problems are stabilized may precipitate a medical crisis such as cardiac arrhythmias or seizures.

Drug therapy is considered for clients with obesity who are unable to control their urge to eat, who have a BMI of 30 or above, or who have a BMI of at least 27 and other risk factors such as hypertension, diabetes mellitus, or elevated cholesterol or triglyceride levels. Most weight loss occurs in the first 6 to 8 months, followed by a plateau period or weight regain after cessation of medication (Sharp, 1998).

DRUG SUMMARY TABLE 23-1 Drugs Used For Eating Disorders

GENERIC (TRADE) NAME	DAILY DOSAGE RANGE	IMPLEMENTATION
Drug Class: SSRIs		
fluoxetine (Prozac) anorexia, bulimia	10–80 mg	Give in the morning; give in divided doses if taking 20 mg per day; should not be given concurrently with or until after 2 weeks of discontinuation of an MAOI; avoid use of alcohol; monitor client's response closely in the presence of hepatic or renal impairment or diabetes mellitus as well as for headache, nervousness, abnormal sleep patterns, GI disturbance, and weight loss.
Drug Class: TCAs		
amitriptyline (Elavil) bulimia	50–300 mg	Contraindicated during or within 14 days of MAOI therapy; may be given in divided doses or daily at h.s.; monitor for alteration in vital signs, anticholinergic effects, confusion, EPS, and CNS overstimulation.
desipramine (Norpramin) bulimia	75–300 mg	Contraindicated during or within 14 days of MAOI therapy; may be given daily in single or divided doses; monitor for symptoms of adverse effects similar to those of amitriptyline.
imipramine (Tofranil) bulimia	75–300 mg	Contraindicated during or within 14 days of MAOI therapy; give total dose at h.s. if drowsiness occurs; monitor for signs and symptoms of infection and obtain CBC if infection is suspected; instruct client to avoid prolonged exposure to sunlight or sunlamps and to use sunscreen or protective garments; monitor for anticholinergic effects and orthostatic hypotension.
Drug Class: Appetite Stimulants		
cyprohepatadine (Periactin) anorexia during re-feeding	4–20 mg	Give syrup form if unable to take tablets; instruct client to avoid taking with alcohol and to report difficulty breathing, thickening of bronchial secretions, hallucinations, tremors, loss of coordination, unusual bleeding or bruising, visual disturbances, or irregular heartbeat.
megestrol acetate (Megace) anorexia during re-feeding	80–320 mg	Give in divided doses q.i.d.; monitor for bleeding, rash, fluid retention, and edema; monitor weight gain according to established weight goals; discontinue drug and notify physician if signs of thromboembolic disease (eg, leg pain, swelling, shortness of breath, and so forth) occur.
Drug Class: Atypical Antipsychotics		
olanzapine (Zyprexa) anorexia	2.5–20 mg	Usually given at night. Monitor for occasional anticholinergic effects such as constipation; weight gain; hyperglycemia; orthostatic hypotension; EPS; TD; NMS
risperidone (Risperdal) anorexia	0.5–8 mg	Mix oral solution with water, juice, low-fat milk, or coffee; monitor for galactorrhea, weight gain, EPS, TD, and NMS.

Dexfenfluramine (Redux) and fenfluramine (FenPhen) have been withdrawn from the market because of an association with valvular heart disease. Two drugs have Food and Drug Administration approval for extended weight loss treatment: sibutramine (Meridia) and orlistat (Xenical). Although sibutramine, a serotonin–norepinephrine reuptake inhibitor, has not been linked to valvular heart disease or pulmonary hypertension, it can increase blood pressure. Clients who take SSRIs, venlafaxine (Effexor), erythromycin, ketoconazole (Nizoral), or alcohol should be monitored for drug–drug interactions with sibutramine. Adverse effects also include constipation, dry mouth, insomnia, anorexia or increased appetite, and nervousness. Orlistat is a lipase inhibitor that blocks the absorption of about one third of ingested dietary fat. Adverse effects include fecal urgency, fatty/oily stools, increased defecation, and fecal incontinence. Clients taking warfarin or cyclosporine should be monitored for potential drug-drug interactions with orlistat (Hensrud, 1999; Sharp, 1998; Bartlett, Lancaster, & New, 2005). Other agents include off-label use of topiramate (Topamax), phentermine hydrochloride (Adipex-P), phendimetrazine tartrate (Bontril PDM), benzphetamine hydrochloride (Didrex), and diethylpropion hydrochloride (Tenuate) (Murphy, 2003).

Interactive Therapies

Several approaches have been documented as effective in the treatment of eating disorders. See Supporting Evidence for Practice 23-1. These approaches include cognitive–behavioral therapy (CBT), interpersonal psychotherapy (IPT), solution-focused brief therapy (SFBT), and family or couple therapy. They are generally included as part of inpatient and outpatient treatment protocols as well as continuum of care. (See Chapters 14 and 15.)

CBT and IPT. On the basis of research findings, the efficacy of CBT and IPT have been compared (Johnson, 2000). Beneficial effects of CBT were evident sooner, by about week 6. However, both treatments were equally effective in the long term. Both therapies focused on binge eating, purging, concerns about shape and weight, and thinking patterns. CBT was found to pro-

---

SUPPORTING EVIDENCE FOR PRACTICE 23.1
The Use of Guided Self-Change as an Intervention in the Treatment of Bulimia Nervosa

PROBLEM UNDER INVESTIGATION / Does a guided self-change approach incorporating the use of a self-care model manual motivate clients with the diagnosis of bulimia nervosa to change behavior?

SUMMARY OF RESEARCH / This study conducted in Germany included 62 subjects over the age of 15 years (average age, 28.7 years) who have suffered from bulimia nervosa for an average of 8.5 years. Two treatment interventions, cognitive–behavioral therapy (CBT) and guided self-change (GSC), were utilized. The group receiving CBT participated in 16 weekly sessions with a trained therapist. Sessions focused on problem-solving skills, concepts about weight, behavior modification, and correcting erroneous ideas about bulimic behavior. The group receiving GSC received a self-help manual and participated in eight semimonthly sessions with a trained therapist. Sessions focused on motivation, biologic and cultural influences, food diaries, strategies for regaining control, and learning to like one's body. Data were collected immediately after and up to 2 years following the intervention. Results indicated that both groups had significant improvement in vomiting, dietary restraint, overeating, and shape.

SUPPORT FOR PRACTICE / This study provides support for psychiatric–mental health nursing interventions for clients with the diagnosis of bulimia nervosa. Issues such as motivation for treatment and recovery, biologic and cultural influences on eating behavior, self-concept, problem-solving skills, strategies for regaining control, and dietary restraint are important components.

SOURCE: Thiels, C. M., Schmidt, U., Treasure, J., Garthe, R., & Troop, N. (1998). Guided self-change for bulimia nervosa incorporating use of a self-care manual. American Journal of Psychiatry, 155(7), 947–953.

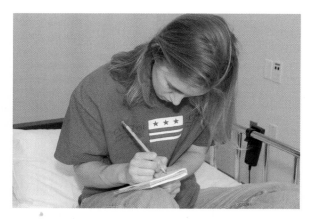

FIGURE 23.3 The client with anorexia nervosa writing in a food diary.

duce interpersonal change after the client overcame binge eating and purging and no longer felt ashamed of such behavior.

With CBT, the nurse–therapist plays an important role guiding clients as they focus on meal planning, impulse control, relaxation or distraction techniques, and problem-solving. Detailed eating and behavioral diaries are often a requirement (Figure 23-3).

During CBT, clients are expected to eat some meals together under supervision. Cognitive strategies focus on dysfunctional beliefs about food, body shape, and weight; the intense link between self-concept and physical appearance; body image distortions; and interpersonal sensitivity. Group participation is used primarily for its supportive qualities.

The nurse–therapist can conduct IPT on an individual or group basis. The goal of this model is to identify the connections among realistic thinking; self-esteem; expression of emotions and needs; control and autonomy; life events; and the onset or maintenance of the eating problem. Four key issues are addressed: grief, interpersonal disputes, role transitions, and long-standing avoidance of relationships (Decker, 2003; MacKenzie, 1997).

SFBT. SFBT empowers clients to recognize and acknowledge their own abilities and resourcefulness. The nurse–therapist views the client as basically healthy, resourceful, and able to solve problems. The client is challenged with two key questions: "How would your life be different if you did not have an eating disorder?" and "How is your life different when your

eating behavior is under control?" The clinician's role during SFBT is to learn the client's view of the problem and what changes need to occur as a result of treatment (Decker, 2003).

Family Therapy. Family therapy has proven effective for the treatment of adolescents with bulimia and anorexia according to data presented at an international conference sponsored by the Academy for Eating Disorders (Worcester, 2004). Family therapy is recommended because family members are often confused about what to do. Like alcoholism or drug abuse, eating disorders affect the entire family. Family members may initially ignore the client's preoccupation with diet, exercise, and weight loss or gain until clinical symptoms are evident. Endless arguments over food may occur as the client's mood and behavior change and the client socially withdraws from the family. Therapy addresses the client's need to control others, the family members' ways of communicating with each other, and what must be done to restore healthy family relationships. Issues such as enmeshment, overprotectiveness, rigidity, and lack of conflict resolution are addressed during the sessions. Siblings and members of an extended family may also be asked to attend. Relapse may occur when the families of clients are conflicted and disengaged.

Sullivan (2005) discusses a unique parent skills-training program that has been implemented in the eating disorders program at Duke University, Durham, NC. The focus of the program is to explore the vital role of parents as part of the treatment team for adolescents with eating disorders and to develop specific parenting skills aimed at helping modify eating behavior. Parents address three barriers that potentiate mealtime conflict: negative perfectionism, expressed negative emotion, and poor self-efficacy. They learn how to create a home environment that doesn't foster negative perfectionism; work diligently on avoiding negative verbal communication with their children; and they learn to model positive coping strategy so that their children will learn new adaptive skills when they experience anger or similar emotions.

Self-Help and Support Groups

Self-help groups can give the client information and support during lifelong recovery. Names and addresses of support groups and meeting times can generally be obtained from local mental health centers, local hospitals, employee assistance programs, the Internet, or national organizations such as Overeaters Anonymous, the American Dietetic Association Consumer Nutrition Hotline, and the National Association of Anorexia Nervosa and Associated Disorders.

In addition, several educational tools are available in the form of seminars, workbooks, pamphlets, diaries, videos, and Internet Web sites. For example, "Shape Up America" is a campaign founded by former Surgeon General C. Everett Koop to promote healthy weight and physical activity. A free interactive Web site, Cyber Kitchen, sponsored by the National Heart, Lung, and Blood Institute is available at http://nhlbi support.com for clients to input health data and obtain menus complete with recipes that match the client's nutritional needs. E-therapy is available for individuals who are resistant to conventional face-to-face treatment (Sherman, 2000).

Client Education

Psychoeducational groups are generally recommended for all but the most severely ill clients at an early point in treatment. The format is that of a classroom. Personal self-disclosure is neither expected nor encouraged. The nurse, who is the leader of the group, promotes discussion about the material being presented and encourages opinions. Family involvement is encouraged. The goal is to provide information and to begin the correction of erroneous notions about food and eating.

Individual client education focuses on the client's understanding of the dynamics of a specific eating disorder. Review the medical complications of the disorder and discuss positive coping skills, as well as an emergency plan to respond to emotional triggers. Assist with developing nutritional plans and a healthy exercise program with the input of the dietitian and activity-therapy staff.

The purpose of self-help and support groups is discussed. The client identifies one or two confidants with whom he or she can relate without fear of rejection. The client learns that recovery involves coping with negative feelings without bingeing or purging; effectively communicating with others; and rebuilding family and social relationships.

EVALUATION

The treatment of clients with eating disorders is time consuming, emotionally charged, and lengthy. Recovery does not occur overnight. It is a lifelong process. Statistics cited indicate that 25% of clients with anorexia nervosa are expected to recover, 25% remain chronically ill, and 50% achieve partial improvement. Forty percent of those who recover will relapse. Ten-year mortality rate is 6.7%; 30-year mortality rate is 18% to 20%. Recovery and relapse rates are not much better for clients with bulimia nervosa (Sherman, 2001).

The prognosis for weight reduction in clients with obesity is poor. Ninety percent of clients who are obese and lose significant amounts of weight regain it eventually. The prognosis for juvenile-onset obesity is poor, and juvenile clients are more likely to have a comorbid emotional disturbance than adult clients (Sadock & Sadock, 2003).

Surgical intervention may be a last resort for severely obese clients who are unable to control their weight and who are at high risk for obesity-related morbidity or mortality. Various types of weight loss surgery are available, and all use gastric resection or intestinal malabsorption (or a combination) to induce and sustain weight loss. Candidates for surgical intervention must meet strict criteria and be committed to maintenance counseling, dietary therapy, behavior therapy, and physical therapy (Crouch, 2005).

Evaluation is also an ongoing process as the client progresses through a treatment program. Continuum of care may include attending a specific support group, keeping scheduled appointments with a therapist or community mental health nurse, or participating in family therapy. See Nursing Plan of Care 23-1: The Client With Anorexia Nervosa, Binge-Eating/Purging Type.

M**�VIE** viewing **GUIDES**

THE CLIENT WITH ANOREXIA NERVOSA, BINGE-EATING/PURGING TYPE

May, a high school senior, voluntarily comes to the high school health clinic because of dizziness, weakness, and abdominal cramping the past 3 days. Her vital signs are within normal range, but she appears to be below her ideal body weight. Initially, May refuses to be weighed, but on further questioning she reveals that she is 5 feet 7 inches tall and weighs 112 pounds. With some encouragement, she relates the following information.

After nearly 4 years of playing competitive high school sports, she has quit the softball, volleyball, and soccer teams and has given up all hope of making the track and cross-country teams. She feels the sports were not supplying her with the amount of exercise she needs to keep her weight "down" as she perceives herself to be fat. She is unable to state what she perceives to be an ideal or "safe" body weight.

May began dieting in 9th grade. During the first month, she lost 25 pounds. Since then, she has maintained a rigorous exercise program by participating in sports, riding a stationary bike 20 minutes a day, using the Stairmaster for 35 minutes, and using Nautilus weights. She has also begun bingeing and purging. She relates that food, losing weight, and exercise are constantly on her mind. She would like to stop bingeing and purging but doesn't know how.

DSM–IV–TR DIAGNOSIS: Anorexia nervosa, binge-eating/purging type

ASSESSMENT: Personal strengths: High school senior, intelligent, motivated for treatment

Weaknesses: Obsessive–compulsive exercising, binge–purge activity, weight loss below ideal body weight, low self-concept

---

NURSING DIAGNOSIS: Imbalanced Nutrition: Less than Body Requirements due to binge–purge activity and excessive exercising

OUTCOME: The client will increase nutritional and caloric intake while restricting binge–purge activity and excessive exercise.

Planning/Implementation	Rationale
Establish a contract with client regarding oral intake and limiting activity to lose weight.	Contracting promotes a sense of control and self-responsibility while establishing goals.
Supervise client during mealtime and after meals. Do not allow client to use the bathroom until at least 30 minutes after each meal.	Supervision prevents the client from hiding, spilling, or discarding food, or using the bathroom to vomit or dispose of concealed food.
Request a dietary consult.	The client needs to discuss beliefs about food, weight, and nutrition.
Educate the client about medical complications associated with anorexia nervosa.	The client may have little knowledge about the potential for medical complications caused by bingeing and purging.

Planning/Implementation	Rationale
Discuss the types of foods that the client eats to relieve anxiety or stress.	The client has the opportunity to discuss the use of food as an ineffective coping behavior.
Encourage the client to explore non–food-related coping skills.	The client learns to separate emotional issues from food and eating behaviors.
Educate the client about problem-solving.	The ability to problem-solve promotes self-confidence and the development of effective coping skills.

NURSING DIAGNOSIS: Disturbed Body Image related to a negative self-concept and the perception of being fat

OUTCOME: The client will verbalize a realistic body image perception.

Planning/Implementation	Rationale
Using a nonjudgmental approach, encourage the client to express feelings, especially about the way she views herself.	Using a nonjudgmental approach gives the client permission to discuss personal feelings without fear of rejection.
Be realistic when providing feedback to the client about her body image perceptions (eg, "safe" body weight for her height).	The client's perception of her body image is closely related to her negative self-concept. Providing honest feedback may help clarify the client's perceptions of her body image.

EVALUATION: May agreed to be seen on an outpatient basis. Evaluation would occur during each scheduled appointment, because relapse can occur at any time during treatment. Evaluation focuses on May's compliance with her behavioral contract, her ability to express her feelings, her self-concept, and any changes she has made to develop a healthy lifestyle. The client agreed to be seen by her attending physician for a physical evaluation, to meet with a dietitian for nutritional education, and to allow family members to be involved in the plan of care. A multidisciplinary team meeting would also be scheduled with May to discuss her continuum of care while attending school.

KEY CONCEPTS

◆ Although eating disorders are among the most challenging illnesses confronting mental health professionals, a surprising number of individuals do not seek help. Others remain ill or die, even after years of treatment.

◆ Although statistics indicate that more females than males are affected by eating disorders, the number of males seeking treatment for eating disorders is likely to increase over the next decade as public awareness of dieting and eating disorders increases.

◆ Although obesity is not categorized as an eating disorder, the diagnosis is included under the category of psychological factors affecting medical condition when there is evidence that psychological factors are of importance in the etiology or course of obesity.

◆ Theories regarding the development of eating disorders focus on genetic or biochemical factors, psychological or psychodynamic factors, and family interactions or relationships. Theories regarding the development of obesity focus on genetic or biologic, and behavioral factors.

◆ Clinical symptoms of eating disorders are reflected in unusual thoughts, feelings, and behavior around food, as well as an unhealthy amount of body fat (unhealthy BMI).

◆ Anorexia nervosa is characterized by an aversion to food and may result in death due to serious malnutrition or other medical complications.

◆ Bulimia nervosa is characterized by the rapid consumption of a large amount of food within a 2-hour period. Serious medical consequences may occur because of alternating bingeing and purging.

◆ Individuals with a BMI of 25 to 29.9 are considered to be moderately overweight or pre-obese. Class I Obesity is diagnosed when a client exhibits a BMI of 30 to 34.9. Individuals with a BMI of 35 to 39.9 are considered to be severely obese (Class II Obesity). Individuals with a BMI of 40 or greater are deemed to be extremely obese (Class III Obesity).

◆ Assessment of a client with an eating disorder is a complex process that focuses on the client's medical status, physical appearance, ability to meet basic needs, mood and affect, cognitive abilities, interpersonal skills, and behavioral manifestations.

◆ The primary goal of inpatient care is weight gain under medical supervision and stabilization of any life-threatening medical conditions or behaviors.

◆ Nursing interventions focus on creating a safe environment; stabilizing the client's medical condition and behavior; managing medication; providing or assisting with interactive therapies; encouraging the use of self-help and support groups; and providing education for the client and family.

◆ Evaluation of the client's response to interventions and treatment is an ongoing process. Recovery is considered a life-long process in which relapses may occur. Surgical intervention may be a last resort for severely obese clients who are at high risk for obesity-related morbidity or mortality.

For additional study materials, please refer to the Student Resource CD-ROM located in the back of this textbook.

CHAPTER WORKSHEET

CRITICAL THINKING QUESTIONS

1. While performing an admission health assessment on a 21-year-old woman admitted for a breast biopsy procedure, you find the following: dry, flaky skin; brittle nails and hair; low blood pressure; slow pulse; and very visible bony prominences. Your questions uncover amenor-rhea and a distorted body image. What nursing interventions are appropriate?

2. Contact a nurse practitioner at a local college health center. What materials about eating disorders does she have available for students? Ask the nurse practitioner to discuss her view of her role in caring for this population.

3. Search the literature for a body image assessment tool developed by a nurse. Administer the tool to classmates who appear thin, average, and overweight. What are your findings?

REFLECTION

Reflect on the chapter opening quote by Sobel. Why do you think Sobel stated that eating disorders are fascinating? How are they confusing? Why are they challenging? In what way are they deeply disturbing?

NCLEX-STYLE QUESTIONS

1. The nurse assesses the family of a 16-year-old client with anorexia as being characterized by over-responsiveness and overprotectiveness. Which term would the nurse use to document this family characteristic?

   a. Chaotic
   b. Enablement
   c. Enmeshment
   d. Functional

2. Which personality characteristic would the nurse expect to find in a client with anorexia nervosa?

   a. Anger
   b. Compliance
   c. Rebellion
   d. Suspicion

3. An adolescent client tells the nurse that she frequently feels compelled to eat a large amount of food in a small amount of time. The nurse identifies this problem as characteristic of which condition?

   a. Anorexia
   b. Bulimia
   c. Overeating
   d. Compulsiveness

4. The nurse understands that a client with reactive obesity generally overeats for which reason?
   a. Providing for self-nurturing
   b. Reducing feelings of stress
   c. Relieving boredom
   d. Satisfying feelings of hunger

5. Which of the following questions would be most appropriate for the nurse to ask a client who is suspected of having the eating disorder anorexia nervosa?
   a. "Do you feel you have a problem controlling your weight?"
   b. "Do you use diet pills, diuretics, laxatives, or purging to lose weight?"
   c. "Do people tell you that you are too fat?"
   d. "Do you eat only when you are hungry?"

6. A 21-year-old female is diagnosed with anorexia nervosa. Which findings would indicate the need for the client to be hospitalized? Select all that apply.
   a. Blood pressure of 100/60 mm Hg
   b. Blood glucose level of 54 mg/dL
   c. Pulse rate of 60 beats per minute
   d. Oral temperature of 96.4°F
   e. Suicidal ideation
   f. Serum potassium of 5 mEq/L

Selected References

Abraham, K. (2004). Recognizing and treating childhood obesity. *American Journal for Nurse Practitioners, 8*(9), 31–32, 35–38.

Albu, J., Allison, D., Boozer, C.N., et. al. (1997). Obesity solutions: Report of a meeting. *Nutrition Reviews, 55,* 150–156.

American Psychiatric Association. (2000a). *Diagnostic and statistical manual of mental disorders* (4th ed., text revision). Washington, DC: Author.

American Psychiatric Association. (2000b). *Practice guidelines for the treatment of patients with eating disorders* (2nd ed.). Washington, DC: American Psychiatric Press.

Anorexia Nervosa and Related Eating Disorders, Inc. (ANRED). (2006). Statistics: How many people have eating disorders? Retrieved January 10, 2006, from http://www.anred.com/stats.html

Associated Press. (2001, April 1). Researchers connect mutated gene to anorexia. *Orlando Sentinel,* p. A9.

Bartlett, T., Lancaster, R., & New, N. (2005). Pediatric obesity: Use a team approach. *Clinical Advisor, 8*(1), 22, 25–28, 31.

Bensing, K. (2003). Unveiling the mystery of body image. *ADVANCE for Nurses, 4*(7), 13–17.

Bruch, H. (2003). *Eating disorders: Obesity, anorexia nervosa, and the person within.* New York: Basic Books.

Centers for Disease Control and Prevention. (1996). Prevalence of physical inactivity during leisure time among overweight persons—1994. *Morbidity and Mortality Weekly Report, 45,* 185–188.

Conant, M. (1996). The client with an eating disorder. In S. Lego (Ed.), *Psychiatric nursing: A comprehensive reference* (2nd ed.). Philadelphia: Lippincott-Raven.

Cote, C. E. (2001). Dying to be thin. *ADVANCE for Nurse Practitioners, 9*(6), 67–74.

Crouch, J. (2005). Adult obesity in the United States. *ADVANCE for Nurse Practitioners, 33*(1), 57–60.

Decker, S. D. (2003). The client with an eating disorder. In W. K. Mohr (Ed.), *Johnson's psychiatric-mental health nursing* (5th ed., pp. 455–477). Philadelphia: Lippincott-Raven.

Department of Health and Human Services. (2000). *Health People 2010.* Washington: Author.

Dietz, W. I. T., & Gortmaker, S. L. (1984). Factors within the physical environment associated with childhood and adolescent obesity in the United States. *American Journal of Clinical Nutrition, 39,* 619–624.

DiscoveryHealth.com Disease Center. (2003). Genetics of eating disorders. Retrieved July 28, 2003, from http://health.discovery.com/minisites/dna/eating.html

Eating Disorder Referral and Information Center. (2006). Assessment tools: Eating Attitudes Test (EAT-26). Retrieved January 13, 2006, from http://www.edreferral.com/assessment.htm

Endoy, M. P. (2005). Anorexia among older adults. *American Journal for Nurse Practitioners, 9*(5), 31–38.

Epstein, L. I. T., Wisniewski, L., & Weng, R. (1994). Child and parent psychological problems affect weight control. *Odyssey Research, 2,* 509–515.

Erikson, E. H. (1993). *Childhood and society* (3rd ed.). New York: W. W. Norton.

Erikson, E. H. (1994). *Identity: Youth and crisis.* New York: W. W. Norton.

Faust, M. (2001). Nutritional problems. In S. Nettina (Ed.), *Lippincott manual of nursing practice* (7th ed., pp. 659–681). Philadelphia: Lippincott Williams & Wilkins.

Finkelstein, J. B. (1999). APA updates eating disorders guideline. *Clinical Psychiatry News, 27*(9), 7.

Finn, R. (2004). Weight problems may be tied to anger habits. *Clinical Psychiatry News, 32*(6), 39.

Foreyt, J. P., & Poston, W. S. C., II. (1997). Diet, genetics, and obesity. *Food Technology, 51,* 70–73.

Frieden, J. (2004). Eating disorders missed, misdiagnosed in men. *Clinical Psychiatry News, 32*(9), 67.

Grady, T. A. (1997, November 13–15). *An update on eating disorders.* Paper presented at the 10th Annual United States Psychiatric & Mental Health Congress, Orlando, FL.

Grinspoon, L. (Ed.). (1997). Eating disorders–Part I. *Harvard Mental Health Letter, 14*(4), 1-4.

Grinspoon, L. (Ed.). (1998). Race and eating disorders. *Harvard Mental Health Letter, 15*(9), 6-7.

Hensrud, D. D. (1999). Managing obesity. *Clinical Advisor* (1), 52-56.

Irvine, M. (2001, July 17). Younger kids are worried about weight. *Florida Today*, p. 1E.

Jain, A. (2004). What works for obesity? A summary of the research behind obesity interventions. London: BMJ Publishing Group Limited.

James, K. S. (2001). All in the family: Treating obesity in children and adolescents. *ADVANCE for Nurse Practitioners, 9*(1), 26-31.

Jancin, B. (1999). A psychological portrait of anorexia nervosa patients. *Clinical Psychiatry News, 27*(7), 24.

Johnson, J. G., Cohen, P., Kasen, S. & Brook, J. S. (2002). Childhood adversities associated with risk for eating disorders or weight problems during adolescence or early adulthood. *American Journal of Psychiatry, 159*, 394-400.

Johnson, K. (2000). CBT is quicker than IBT in treating bulimia. *Clinical Psychiatry News, 28*(3), 27.

Johnson, K. (2005). Refeeding syndrome looms for patients with eating disorders. *Clinical Psychiatry News, 33*(12), 60.

Kameg, K. M., Mitchell, A. M., & Chmielewski, J. (2003). Recognizing and managing eating disorders in primary care. *American Journal for Nurse Practitioners, 7*(6), 9-12, 15-17.

Keel, P., & Mitchell, J. E. (1997). Outcome in bulimia nervosa. *American Journal of Psychiatry, 154*, 313-321.

Keesy, R. E., & Hirvonen, M. D. (1997). Body weight set-points: Determination and adjustment. *Journal of Nutrition, 127*, 1875S-1883S.

Kenny, T. (2001). Get moving: Exercise counseling for sedentary patients. *ADVANCE for Nurse Practitioners, 9*(6), 95-98.

Klish, W. (1998). Childhood obesity. *Pediatrics in Review, 19*(9), 312-315.

MacKenzie, K. R. (1997, November 13-16). *Group psychotherapy for bulimia nervosa.* Paper presented at the 10th Annual United States Psychiatric & Mental Health Congress, Orlando, FL.

Minuchin, S. (1974). *Families and family therapy.* Cambridge, MA: Howard University Press.

Moon, M. A. (2001). Negative self-concept hits overweight girls as early as age 5. *Clinical Psychiatry News, 29*(4), 26.

Moore, A. S. (2000). A new screening tool for eating disorders. *RN, 63*(2), 14.

Moore, H. (2004a). Can anorexia nervosa be triggered by an infection? *Neuropsychiatry Review, 5*(9), 1, 25.

Moore, H. (2004b.) Obesity research focuses on the biology of craving. *Neuropsychiatry Reviews, 5*(7), 10.

Morgan, J. F., Reid, F., & Lacey, J. H. (1999). The SCOFF questionnaire: Assessment of a new screening tool for eating disorders. *British Medical Journal, 319*(7223), 1467-1468.

Murphy, J.L. (Ed.). (2003, Summer). *Nurse practitioners' prescribing reference.* New York: Prescribing Reference.

Muscari, M. E. (1998). Adolescent health: Screening for anorexia and bulimia. *American Journal of Nursing, 98*(11), 22-24.

National Eating Disorders Association. (2002). *Statistics: Eating disorders and their precursors.* Seattle, WA: Author.

National Heart, Lung, and Blood Institute. (1998). Clinical guidelines on the identification, evaluation, and treatment of overweight and obesity in adults—The evidence report. Retrieved January 14, 2006, from http://nhlbisupport.com

Sadock, B. J., & Sadock, V. A. (2003). *Kaplan & Sadock's synopsis of psychiatry: Behavioral sciences/clinical psychiatry* (9th ed.). Philadelphia: Lippincott Williams & Wilkins.

Schilder, P. (1950). *The image and appearance of the human body.* New York: International Universities Press.

Schultz, J. M., & Videbeck, S. D. (2005). *Lippincott's manual of psychiatric nursing care plans* (7th ed.). Philadelphia: Lippincott Williams & Wilkins.

Sharp, D. (1998). Obesity control. *Hippocrates,* (12), 20-27.

Sherman, C. (2000). Eating disorder patients receptive to e-mail therapy. *Clinical Psychiatry News, 28*(7), 23.

Sherman, C. (2001). Eating disorder relapse linked to self-esteem and motivation. *Clinical Psychiatry News, 29*(12), 41.

Sobel, S.V. (2005). Eating disorders. In *Continuing Education for Florida Nurses 2005, Course #9609* (pp. 67-109). Sacramento, CA: Continuing Medical Education Resource.

Sullivan, M. G. (2005). Parents of eating disorder patients join forces. *Clinical Psychiatry News, 33*(1), 42.

Sullivan, P. F., Bulik, C. M., Fear, J. L., & Pickering. (1998). Outcome of anorexia nervosa: A case-control study. *American Journal of Psychiatry, 155*, 939-946.

Thiels, C. M., Schmidt, U., Treasure, J., Garthe, R., & Troop, N. (1998). Guided self-change for bulimia nervosa incorporating use of a self-care manual. *American Journal of Psychiatry, 155*(7), 947-953.

Tumolo, J. (2003). Not just for women anymore: Eating disorders in men. *ADVANCE for Nurse Practitioners, 11*(4), 35-36.

U. S. Preventive Services Task Force (USPSTF). (2004). Screening for obesity in adults: Recommendations and rationale statement. *American Journal for Nurse Practitioners, 8*(10), 47-48, 51-54.

Whitaker, J.A., Pepe, M. S., Seidel, K. D., & Dietz, W. I. T. (1997). Predicting obesity in young adulthood from childhood and parental obesity. *New England Journal of Medicine, 337*(14), 869-873.

White, J. H. (2000). Improving outcomes for obesity. *American Journal for Nurse Practitioners, 4*(10), 9-13, 17-18.

Worcester, S. (2004). Personality may affect eating disorder treatment. *Clinical Psychiatry News, 32*(8), 56.

Suggested Readings

Brunk, D. (2001). Adolescents with eating disorders often turn to herbal remedies. *Clinical Psychiatry News, 29*(6), 17.

Carpenito-Moyet, L. J. (2006). *Handbook of nursing diagnosis* (11th ed.). Philadelphia: Lippincott Williams & Wilkins.

Cloak, N. L., & Powers, P. S. (2005). Are undiagnosed eating disorders keeping your patients sick? *Current Psychiatry, 4*(12), 65-68, 71-72, 75.

Crouch, J. (2005). Comfort, safety, and self-esteem: Meeting the needs of severely obese patients. *ADVANCE for Nurse Practitioners, 13*(4), 43-46.

Gesto, K. (2002). Looks can be deceiving: An overview of bulimia nervosa. *ADVANCE for Nurse Practitioners, 10*(9), 22-27.

James, K. S., & Kohlbry, P. (2004). Adult obesity. *ADVANCE for Nurses, 5*(6), 19-22.

James, K. S., & Cook, L. M. (2006). Anorexia nervosa: Guidelines for recognition and treatment. *ADVANCE for Nurses, 7*(2), 15-19.

Maayan, L. A., & Woolston, J. L. (2005). Eating disorders. In K. Cheng & K. M. Meyers (Eds.), *Child and Adolescent Psychiatry, The Essentials* (pp. 247-265). Philadelphia: Lippincott Williams & Wilkins.

Melville, N. A. (2004). Antidepressants boost eating disorders tx. *Clinical Psychiatry News, 32*(5), 82.

Meszaros, L. (2005). Metabolic syndrome: A new definition for a growing condition. *Central Florida M. D. News, 7*(9), 19-21.

Orbanic, S. (2001). Understanding bulimia: Signs, symptoms, and the human experience. *American Journal of Nursing, 101*(3), 35-42.

Tumolo, J. (2001). Slim pickings: The facts about fad diets. *ADVANCE for Nurse Practitioners, 9*(6), 83-88.

Yager, J. (2001). New strategies for the management of anorexia nervosa. *CNS News, 3*(5), 9-12.

CHAPTER 24 / PERSONALITY DEVELOPMENT AND PERSONALITY DISORDERS

Personality disorders are among the least understood and recognized disorders in both psychiatry and general medical care. They are among the most common of the severe mental disorders and occur frequently with other illnesses (eg, substance use disorders, mood disorders, anxiety disorders). —PERSONALITY DISORDERS FOUNDATION, 2005

LEARNING OBJECTIVES

AFTER STUDYING THIS CHAPTER, YOU SHOULD BE ABLE TO:

1. Define the terms *personality* and *personality disorder.*
2. Summarize the concepts of the following theories of personality development: Freud's psychoanalytic theory, Erikson's psychosocial theory, and Piaget's cognitive developmental theory.
3. Discuss the importance of a working knowledge of personality growth and development in the mental health setting.
4. Identify factors that may contribute to the development of behavioral disturbances in a client with paranoid personality disorder.
5. Identify the characteristics of schizoid personality disorder.
6. Explain the importance of recognizing cultural diversity in clients who exhibit disturbances in cognition, affect, interpersonal relationships, and impulse control.
7. Articulate four outcomes to reduce behavioral disturbances in a client with the diagnosis of borderline personality disorder.
8. Reflect on nonproductive reactions a nurse may exhibit when working with clients who exhibit clinical symptoms of antisocial personality disorder.
9. Develop an educational tool to use when interacting with an elderly client who has clinical symptoms of dependent personality disorder.
10. Construct a nursing plan of care for a client with the diagnosis of histrionic personality disorder.

KEY TERMS

Ego
Egocentrism
Id
Personality
Personality disorder
Projective identification
Schemata
Splitting
Superego

Personality refers to a distinctive set of traits, behavior styles, and patterns that make up our character and individuality (National Mental Health Association, 2006). Personality is the total of a person's internal and external patterns of adjustment to life, determined in part by the individual's genetic make-up and by life experiences. Thus, the dynamics of personality development become increasingly complex throughout the lifespan as one continually interacts with the environment and experiences various stages of physical and psychological maturation. Factors influencing psychological maturation include genetic endowments such as inherited traits, potentials, and characteristics; environmental stressors including parental relationships, peer relationships, and cultural and social experiences; individual accomplishments that are the results of learning and adaptation; and one's mental health status at each developmental stage. Thus, a newborn or infant reacts differently to a given environmental stimulus than does an adolescent, a young adult, or an elderly person.

Personality is believed to occur along a continuum, with healthy traits at one end, personality styles at different gradations along the continuum, and personality disorders at the opposite end. **Personality disorder** is defined as a pervasive pattern of experience and behavior that is abnormal with respect to thinking, mood, personal relations, and the control of impulses (Lebelle, 2006). Personality disorders are long term and can lead to enormous personal and societal costs, including lost productivity, hospitalizations, significant unhappiness, imprisonment, and suicide.

Researchers analyzed data from the 2001-2002 National Epidemiologic Survey on Alcohol and Related Conditions. An estimated 30.8 million adult Americans (or 14.8%) met the *Diagnostic and Statistical Manual of Mental Disorders, 4th Edition, Text Revision (DSM-IV-TR)* criteria for at least one personality disorder. Of these 30.8 million, 16.4 million had obsessive–compulsive personality disorder; 9.2 million had paranoid personality disorder; 7.6 million had antisocial personality disorder; 6.5 million had schizoid personality disorder; 4.9 million had avoidant personality disorder; 3.8 million had histrionic personality disorder; and 1.0 million had dependent personality disorder (Grant, Hasin, & Stinson, 2004).

This chapter focuses on the theories of personality development and the etiology, clinical symptoms, and diagnostic characteristics of personality disorders. It also addresses the effects of a personality disorder on the client and his or her family, and health care providers. The chapter uses the nursing process to provide information about providing care to clients diagnosed with a specific personality disorder.

Theories of Personality Development

Various theories of personality maturation are presented in developmental psychology classes as part of the curriculum in nursing programs. Generally, these theories are categorized as psychoanalytic, cognitive, behavioristic, and interpersonal. A summary of the more common theories, such as those of Sigmund Freud, Eric Erikson, and Jean Piaget, are presented in this chapter.

Freud's Psychoanalytic Theory of Personality Development

Freud's theory of personality development describes three major categories: the development of personality, the organization or structure of personality, and the dynamics of personality. Freud explains the development of the personality by describing three levels of consciousness: the unconscious, preconscious (subconscious), and conscious. The *unconscious level* consists of drives, feelings, ideas, and urges outside of the person's awareness. This is the most significant level of consciousness because of its effect on behavior. A considerable amount of psychic energy is used to keep unpleasant memories stored in the unconscious level of the mind. The *preconscious* or *subconscious level,* midway between the conscious and unconscious levels, consists of feelings, ideals, drives, and ideas that are out of one's ongoing awareness but can be recalled readily. The *conscious level* of the personality is aware of the present and controls purposeful behavior.

The organization or structure of the personality (Freud, 1960) consists of the **id,** which is an unconscious reservoir of primitive drives and instincts dominated by thinking and the pleasure principle; the **ego,** which meets and interacts with the outside world as an integrator or mediator and is the executive function of the personality that operates at all three levels of consciousness; and the **superego,** which acts as the censoring force or conscience of the personality and is composed of morals, mores, values, and ethics largely derived from one's parents. The superego operates at all three levels of consciousness.

According to Freud's explanation of the dynamics of the personality, each person has a certain amount of psychic energy to cope with the problems of everyday living. The id's energy is used to reduce tension and may be exhibited, for example, by frequency of urination, daydreaming, or eating. The ego's energy controls the impulsive actions of the id and the moralistic and idealistic actions of the superego. One whose energy is controlled primarily by the superego generally behaves in an overly moralistic manner because the structure of the personality (eg, superego) monopolizes the psychic energy that governs the person's behavior.

In his psychosexual theory, Freud also describes five phases of the psychobiologic process that have a great impact on personality development: oral, anal, phallic or oedipal, latency, and genital.

- The oral phase (0 to 18 months) is a period in which pleasure is derived mainly through the mouth by the actions of sucking or biting.
- During the anal phase (18 months to 3 years), attention focuses on the excretory function, and the foundation is laid for the development of the superego.
- In the phallic or oedipal stage (3 to 7 years), a stage of growth and development, the child identifies with the parent of the same sex, forms a deep attachment to the parent of the opposite sex, develops a sexual identity of male or female role, and begins to experience guilt.
- During the latency phase (7 years to adolescence), the person learns to recognize and handle reality, has a limited sexual image, develops an inner control over aggressive or destructive impulses, and experiences intellectual and social growth.
- In the genital phase (puberty or adolescence into adult life), the final stage of psychosexual development, the individual develops the capacity for object love and mature sexuality, and establishes identity and independence.

Erikson's Psychosocial Theory of Personality Development

Erik Erikson (1968) emphasizes the concept of identity or an inner sense of sameness that perseveres through external changes, identity crises, and identity confusion in the dynamics of personality development. He posits that there are eight psychosocial stages in one's lifespan. Table 24-1 highlights these stages, focusing on each stage's area of conflict and resolution, basic virtues or qualities acquired, and positive and negative behavior.

According to Erikson, these developmental stages consist of a series of normative conflicts that every person must handle. The two opposing energies (developmental crisis) must be synthesized in a constructive manner to produce positive expectations for new experiences. If the crisis is unresolved, the person does not develop attitudes that will be helpful in meeting future developmental tasks. Failure to resolve a challenge or conflict also results in negative behavior or developmental problems. An opportunity to resolve such conflicts recurs later in one's lifespan.

Piaget's Cognitive Developmental Theory

Jean Piaget's (1963) theory views intellectual development as a result of constant interaction between environmental influences and genetically determined attributes. Piaget's research focused on four stages of intellectual growth during childhood, with emphasis on how a child learns and adapts what is learned from the adult world. The four stages are sensorimotor, preoperational thought, concrete operational, and formal operational.

During the *sensorimotor stage* (0 to 2 years), the infant uses the senses to learn about self and the environment by exploring objects and events and by imitating. The infant also develops **schemata,** or methods of assimilating and accommodating incoming information; these include looking schema, hearing schema, and sucking schema.

The *preoperational thought stage* (2 to 7 or 8 years) is subdivided into the preconceptual and intuitive phases. The preconceptual phase, which occurs between the ages of 2 and 4 years, involves the child's learning to think in mental images, and the development of expressive language and symbolic play. In the intuitive phase, which occurs between the ages of 4 and 7 years, the child exhibits **egocentrism,** seeing things from his or her own point of view. The child is unable to comprehend the ideas of others if they differ from his or her own. As the child matures, he or she realizes that other people see things differently.

The *concrete operational stage* begins at approximately 8 years of age and lasts until age 12 years. The

TABLE 24.1 Summary of Erikson's Psychosocial Theory

DEVELOPMENTAL SPACE	AREA OF CONFLICT AND RESOLUTION	VIRTUES OR QUALITIES	POSITIVE BEHAVIOR OR RESOLUTION OF CONFLICT	NEGATIVE BEHAVIOR
Sensory–oral or early infancy (birth to 18 mos)	Trust vs mistrust	Drive and hope	Displays affection, confidence, gratification, recognition, and the ability to trust others	Suspicious of others, fears affection, projection
Muscular–anal or later infancy (18 mos–3 yrs)	Autonomy vs shame and doubt	Self-control and willpower	Cooperative, expresses oneself, displays self-control, views self apart from parents	Self-doubt, denial, dependency and co-dependency, low self-esteem, loss of self-control
Locomotor-genital or early childhood (3–5 yrs)	Initiative vs guilt	Direction and purpose	Tests reality. Shows imagination, displays some ability to evaluate own behavior, exerts positive controls over self	Excessive guilt, feels victimized, passive, apathetic
Latency or middle childhood (6–11 yrs)	Industry vs inferiority	Method and competence	Develops a sense of duty, and scholastic and social competencies. Displays perseverance and interacts with peers in a less infantile manner	Feels inferior, lacks motivation, uncooperative, incompetent, unreliable
Puberty and adolescence (12–18 yrs)	Identity vs role confusion	Devotion and fidelity	Displays self-certainty, experiments with role, expresses ideologic commitments, chooses a career or vocation, and develops interpersonal relationships	Self-doubt, dysfunctional relationships, rebellion, substance abuse
Young adulthood (19–40 yrs)	Intimacy vs isolation	Affiliation and love	Establishes mature relationship with a member of the opposite sex, chooses a suitable marital partner, performs work and social roles in socially acceptable manner	Self-imposed isolation, emotionally jealous, possessive
Middle adulthood (41–64 yrs)	Generativity vs stagnation	Productivity and ability to care for others	Spends time wisely by engaging in helpful activities such as teaching, counseling, community activities and volunteer work; displays creativity	Egocentric, disinterested in others, overinvolved in activities
Late adulthood or maturity (65 yrs to death)	Ego integrity vs despair	Renunciation or "letting go," and wisdom	Reviews life realistically, accepts past failures and limitations, helps members of younger generations view life positively and realistically, accepts death with dignity	Feels hopeless and helpless, fears death, dwells on past failures and disappointments, unable to adjust to aging process

child is able to think more logically as the concepts of moral judgment, numbers, and spatial relationships are developed.

The *formal operational stage* begins at age 12 years and lasts to adulthood. The person develops adult logic and is able to reason, form conclusions, plan for the future, think abstractly, and build ideals.

Etiology of Personality Disorders

During the process of personality development, the person establishes certain traits that enable him or her to observe, interact with, and think about the environment and oneself. If the person develops a positive self-concept, body image, and sense of self-worth, and is able to relate to others openly and honestly, she or he is said to have characteristics of a healthy personality. Should the person develop inflexible, maladaptive behaviors (eg, manipulation, hostility, lying, poor judgment, and alienation) that interfere with social or occupational functioning, the person exhibits signs and symptoms of a personality disorder.

Personality disorders exist on a continuum. They can range from mild to more severe based on how pervasive the symptoms of a particular personality disorder are, and to what extent a person exhibits these symptoms. Although most individuals can live fairly normal lives with mild symptoms of personality disorders, during times of increased stress or external pressures (eg, caused by work, family, or a new relationship), the symptoms will be exacerbated and begin to seriously interfere with the individual's emotional and psychological functioning. Personality disorders are usually recognizable by adolescence or earlier (ie, borderline personality disorder [BPD] can start as early as age 5), continue throughout adulthood, and become less obvious throughout middle age (National Mental Health Association, 2006).

The potential causes of personality disorders are as numerous as the people who suffer from them. Genetic and biologic factors, as well as a combination of one's personality, social development, and parental upbringing, are associated with these disorders. Environmental factors may cause a person who is already genetically vulnerable to develop a personality disorder (National Mental Health Association, 2006; Sadock & Sadock, 2003). A discussion of the more common theories regarding the development of personality disorders follows.

Genetic Factors

Although research has not isolated the cause of any specific factor at this time, investigations of 15,000 pairs of twins in the United States revealed that monozygotic twins, living together or apart, develop personality disorders much more frequently than dizygotic twins do. Cluster A personality disorders (eg, paranoid, schizoid, or schizotypal) occur more frequently in biologic relatives of clients with schizophrenia than in control groups. Cluster B personality disorders (eg, antisocial, borderline, histrionic, or narcissistic) apparently have a genetic basis as well. Antisocial personality disorder is associated with alcohol use disorder. Depression is common in the family backgrounds of clients with BPDs. Cluster C personality disorders (eg, obsessive-compulsive or dependent) also may have a genetic basis. Clients with avoidant personality disorders often exhibit clinical symptoms of anxiety and depression (Sadock & Sadock, 2003).

Biologic Factors

Research has also indicated that individuals with high levels of hormones such as testosterone, 17-estradiol, and estrone are thought to be biologically predisposed to the development of a personality disorder. Studies of dopaminergic and serotonergic systems indicate that, although in many persons dopamine and serotonin reduce depression and produce a sense of general well-being, high levels of these neurotransmitters have produced impulsive and aggressive behaviors. Furthermore, changes in electrical conductance on electroencephalograms have been noted in clients with antisocial and BPDs (Sadock & Sadock, 2003).

Psychoanalytic Factors

Each human being's personality is largely determined by his or her characteristic defense mechanisms. According to Sadock and Sadock (2003), underlying defensive behaviors or mechanisms that are used to resolve conflict include fantasy, dissociation, isolation, projection, splitting, passive aggression, and acting out. When these behaviors or mechanisms are effective, they can abolish anxiety and depression. Therefore, individuals with personality disorders are reluctant to abandon them.

According to Freud's theory, socially deviant persons have defective egos through which they are unable to control their impulsive behavior. Additionally, a weak superego results in the incomplete development or lack of a conscience. Persons with immature superegos feel no guilt or remorse for socially unacceptable behavior. The drive for prestige, power, and possessions can result in exploitative, manipulative behavior. Moreover, urban societies—such as inner cities—are characterized by a low degree of social interaction, thereby fostering the development of personality disorders.

Childhood Experiences

As noted earlier, according to the various theories of personality development, negative or maladaptive behavior can occur during childhood. Following are examples of childhood experiences that could contribute to the development of a personality disorder:

- Parental rewarding of behavior such as a temper tantrum encourages acting out (ie, the parent gives in to a child's wishes rather than setting limits to stop the behavior).
- Creativity is not encouraged in the child; therefore, the child does not have the opportunity to express him- or herself or learn to relate to others. The ability to be creative could provide the child with the opportunity to develop a positive self-concept and sense of self-worth.
- Rigid upbringing also has a negative effect on the development of a child's personality because it discourages experimentation and promotes the development of low self-esteem. It may also cause feelings of hostility and alienation in the child–parent relationship.
- Parental fostering of dependency discourages personality development and allows the child to become a conformist, rather than an independent being with an opportunity to develop a positive self-concept.
- Parents or authority figures display socially undesirable behavior and the child identifies with them. As a result of this identification process, the child imitates behavior that he or she believes to be acceptable by others. Such behavior frequently puts the child in direct conflict with society.

Characteristics of Personality Disorders

A personality disorder is described as a nonpsychotic illness characterized by maladaptive behavior, which the person uses to fulfill his or her needs and bring satisfaction to him- or herself. Most personality-disordered people experience a permanent stage of anger as a result of frustration, perceived or actual rejection, conflict, or resentment. Their anger is often suppressed or repressed; however, it can be sudden, raging, frightening, and without an apparent provocation by an outside agent. The anger is manifested only when the individual's defenses are down, incapacitated, or adversely affected by internal or external circumstances. The individual is unable to redirect his or her primitive pent-up anger (Vaknin, 2006). Maladaptive behaviors begin during childhood or adolescence as a way of coping and remain throughout most of adulthood, becoming less obvious during middle or old age. As a result of his or her inability to relate to the environment, the person acts out his or her conflicts socially. Emotional, economic, social, or occupational problems are often seen as a result of maladaptive behavior (American Psychiatric Association [APA], 2000).

Individuals with personality disorders have many common characteristics. They include:

- Inflexible, socially unacceptable behaviors
- Self-centeredness
- Manipulative and exploitative behavior
- Inability to tolerate minor stress, resulting in increased inability to cope with anxiety or depression
- Lack of individual accountability for behavior, blaming others for their problems
- Difficulty dealing with reality because of a distorted or superficial understanding of self and the perceptions of others
- Vulnerability to other mental disorders such as obsessive–compulsive tendencies and panic attacks

Individuals with personality disorders rarely seek psychiatric help because the person lacks insight regarding his or her behaviors and does not view them to be maladaptive, contributing to a personality disorder (Lebelle, 2006). Refer to Box 24-1 for a summary of The National Epidemiologic Survey on Alcohol and Related Conditions study on individuals at risk for personality disorders.

Clinical Symptoms and Diagnostic Characteristics of Personality Disorders

The *DSM-IV-TR* groups personality disorders into three clusters or descriptive categories (APA, 2000). Persons

BOX 24.1 RESULTS OF NATIONAL EPIDEMIOLOGIC SURVEY

The National Epidemiologic Survey on Alcohol and Related Conditions (Grant, Hasin, & Stinson, 2004), mentioned earlier in this chapter, surveyed individuals at risk for the development of personality disorders. Trained personnel conducted face-to-face interviews with 43,093 noninstitutionalized U.S. adults. A summary of their findings follows:

- Women were more likely than men to have avoidant, dependent, and paranoid personality disorders.
- Men were three times more likely than women to have antisocial personality disorders.
- Separated/divorced/widowed or never-married individuals were more likely than their counterparts to have avoidant, dependent, paranoid, schizoid, and histrionic personality disorders.
- Native Americans were more likely than whites to have avoidant, paranoid, schizoid, and antisocial personality disorders.
- White persons were more likely than Asian or Hispanic persons to have obsessive–compulsive personality disorder.
- Paranoid, schizoid, and histrionic personality disorders were more prevalent among black persons than among white persons.

CLINICAL SYMPTOMS AND DIAGNOSTIC CHARACTERISTICS / PERSONALITY DISORDERS

CLINICAL SYMPTOMS

Changes in the Following Areas:
- Cognition
- Emotional responses (affect)
- Interpersonal functioning
- Impulse control

DIAGNOSTIC CHARACTERISTICS

- Evidence of an enduring pattern of behavior and inner experience in at least two of the areas above
- Stable, long-lasting pattern exhibited as a marked deviation from that which is expected in the individual's culture
- Onset most likely traceable to adolescence or early adulthood
- Pattern widespread, occurring over personal and social situations
- Resultant distress in important areas of functioning
- Pattern not associated with or due to a medical condition or another mental disorder

who exhibit paranoid, schizoid, and schizotypal personality disorders are considered "odd" or eccentric in the vernacular and are grouped in the first cluster, Cluster A. Persons with disorders in the second cluster, Cluster B—antisocial, borderline, histrionic, and narcissistic personality disorders—are considered to be emotional, erratic, or dramatic in behavior. Anxious or fearful behaviors are often present in the third cluster, Cluster C, which includes obsessive–compulsive, dependent, and avoidant personality disorders. The category Personality Disorder, Not Otherwise Specified (NOS), is reserved for those disorders that do not fit into any of the three clusters. See the accompanying Clinical Symptoms and Diagnostic Characteristics box.

Although factors that may contribute to the development of a personality disorder were discussed earlier in this chapter, additional information regarding a specific personality disorder is included with each disorder to clarify the development of clinical symptoms unique to the disorder.

Cluster A Disorders: Odd, Eccentric Behavior

Paranoid Personality Disorder

Individuals who develop a paranoid personality disorder have chronic hostility that is projected onto others. This hostility develops in childhood as a result of poor interpersonal family relationships. As a result, the person who has experienced much loneliness becomes unwarrantedly suspicious and mistrusts people. The person may suspect attempts to trick or harm him or her, question the loyalty of others, display pathological jealousy, observe the environment for any signs of threat, display secretiveness, become hypersensitive, or display excessive feelings of self-importance. The person also may appear to be unemotional, lack a sense of humor, and lack the ability to relax. Paranoid personality disorder can usually be differentiated from delusional disorder because features such as fixed delusions and hallucinations are absent. Interpersonal relationships are poor, especially when relating to authority figures or co-workers, contributing to lifelong interpersonal, marital, and occupational problems. See Clinical Example 24-1: The Client With a Paranoid Personality Disorder.

Clients with paranoid personality thrive in an environment in which caution and wariness are rewarded and in which individuals are not required to reveal themselves or otherwise make themselves vulnerable. They falter in environments and relationships that require high levels of trust and interdependence (Paul, 2005). The prevalence of paranoid personality disorder is 0.5% to 2.5% of the general population. This disorder is seen more frequently in men (APA, 2000; Lebelle, 2006; Sadock & Sadock, 2003).

Schizoid Personality Disorder

Synonyms for someone with a schizoid personality disorder include "introvert" and "loner" because the person has no desire for social involvement. The clinical symptoms include a pervasive pattern of detachment from social relationships and a restricted range of emotional expression in interpersonal settings. The individual avoids close relationships with family or others, chooses solitary activities, has little interest in sexual experiences, does not take pleasure in activities, lacks close friends or confidants, appears indifferent to praise or criticism, and exhibits emotional coldness such as detachment or flattened affect. Attention is usually focused on objects such as books and cars rather than people.

The client with schizoid personality disorder manages to get ahead in chaotic or challenging environments that do not make emotional demands. He or she may function well in vocations where one generally works alone and is indifferent to approval or criticism of others. The client does not thrive well in corporate environments in which one is expected to be intimate or closely connected to others (Paul, 2005). The prevalence of schizoid personality disorder is estimated to be approximately 7.5% of the general population; some studies report that males are twice as likely to develop this type of personality disorder (APA, 2000; Sadock & Sadock, 2003).

Schizotypal Personality Disorder

The classification of schizotypal personality disorder is used to diagnose persons whose symptoms are similar to, but not severe enough to meet, the criteria for schizophrenia. Clients generally exhibit a disturbance in thought processes referred to as *magical thinking, superstitiousness,* or *telepathy* (a "sixth sense"). They experience ideas of reference, limit social contacts to those involved in the performance of everyday tasks, describe perceptual disturbance such as illusions or depersonalization, demonstrate peculiarity in speech but no loosening of association (shifting of speech from one frame of reference to another), and appear aloof or cold because they exhibit an inappropriate affect. Paranoid ideation, odd or eccentric behavior or appearance, and excessive social anxiety associated with paranoid fears are generally present.

Clients with the diagnosis of schizotypal personality disorder succeed in unconventional environments in which their embrace of the unusual or fantastic is applauded. They are unsuccessful in corporate environments that require adherence to conventional codes of behavior (Paul, 2005). This disorder first may be apparent in childhood or adolescence. It has been

---

CLINICAL EXAMPLE 24.1

THE CLIENT WITH A PARANOID PERSONALITY DISORDER

JV, a 43-year-old Cuban immigrant who worked for a local utility company, was admitted to the hospital for surgery due to a work-related knee injury. During the assessment, the nurse noted that JV was hesitant to answer personal questions related to his medical history and appeared reluctant to provide information about his family. JV's oldest daughter, who had accompanied him to the hospital, offered to provide the necessary information. She also informed the nurse that her father frequently warned the members of the family to lock the doors and windows because he did not trust his neighbors. He refused to allow his wife to leave the house while he was at work and insisted that his children notify him of their activities when they left home. The nurse learned that JV had emigrated from Cuba when he was 20 years old "to get away from the Castro regime." According to JV's daughter, he was a good father who provided well for his family and attended church regularly. Although JV did not verbalize any fixed delusional thoughts, he was very suspicious of strangers or new neighbors.

reported in approximately 3% of the population but the sex ratio is unknown. Only a small percentage of individuals with this disorder develop schizophrenia or other psychotic disorders (APA, 2000; Sadock & Sadock, 2003).

Cluster B Disorders: Emotional, Erratic, or Dramatic Behavior

Individuals with Cluster B personality disorders have the greatest risk for suicide when compared with individuals with Cluster A or Cluster C disorders. The risk is similar for individuals with a major mood disorder but without a personality disorder. Factors contributing to an increased risk of suicide include the presence of comorbid mood or addiction disorders, severity of childhood sexual abuse, degree of antisocial or impulsive characteristics, and a history of irregular psychiatric discharges (Lambert, 2003).

Antisocial Personality Disorder

Synonyms for antisocial personality disorder include *sociopathic, psychopathic,* and *semantic disorder.* Several factors have been proposed to explain the development of the antisocial personality, although the exact cause is unknown. These factors include the following:

- Genetic or hereditary factors interfere with the development of positive interpersonal relationships during childhood. The child therefore does not learn to respect the rights of others.
- Biologic factors such as low levels of serotonin may combine with environmental factors and place the individual at risk for a personality disorder.
- The child may become self-indulgent and expect special favors from others, but does not display appreciation or reciprocal behavior.
- Brain damage or trauma precipitates the development of antisocial behavior. (See Supporting Evidence for Practice 24-1.)
- Low socioeconomic status encourages the development of an antisocial personality; people may turn to maladaptive behaviors, such as stealing, lying, or cheating, just to survive.
- Parents unconsciously foster antisocial behavior in children during developmental years. If parents are too involved in their own personal problems or lifestyle and neglect to spend time with the child or be available when help is needed, the child learns to fend for him- or herself.

SUPPORTING EVIDENCE FOR PRACTICE 24.1
The Impact of Spanking on Children

PROBLEM UNDER INVESTIGATION / Is there a possible causal relationship between punishment by spanking and antisocial behavior in children?

SUMMARY OF RESEARCH / A study, the National Longitudinal Survey of Youth-Child Supplement, was conducted at the Ohio State University Center for Human Resource Research. The subjects were 807 mothers of 910 children aged 6 to 9 years. The mothers were interviewed between 1988 and 1990 regarding the frequency of spanking of their children as a form of punishment for antisocial behavior (eg, disobedience, cheating, lying, and lack of remorse). Analysis controlled for the amount of antisocial behavior at the study onset, maternal emotional warmth, cognitive stimulation, and socioeconomic status. Results indicated that 44% of the mothers spanked their children the week preceding the beginning of the study. Not only did children with greater frequency of spanking in 1988 have higher antisocial behavior scores, but, as the frequency of spanking continued between 1988 and 1990, so did the antisocial behavior scores. Spanking was more likely to be related to increased scores in boys and in European-American children than in children of ethnic minority status.

SUPPORT FOR PRACTICE / Although not everyone who is physically disciplined will develop antisocial behavior, psychiatric–mental health nurses can educate families and communities that alternative forms of discipline of children (eg, limit-setting, time-out, or the use of a behavioral contract) need to be established.

SOURCE: Straus, M. A., Sugarman, D. B., & Giles-Sims, J. (1997). *Spanking by parents and subsequent antisocial behavior of children.* Archives of Pediatrics and Adolescent Medicine, 8(151), 761–767.

- Any behavior that results in a secondary gain of attention, security, or love is tried. If desirable results are obtained, the child continues to use the maladaptive behavior to meet his or her needs.

Antisocial behavior is usually seen in clients between the ages of 15 and 40 years. The diagnosis of *conduct disorder* is given to clients who exhibit clinical symptoms before age 18. Clinical symptoms of conduct disorder usually include truancy, misbehavior at school resulting in suspension or expulsion, delinquency, substance abuse, vandalism, cruelty, and disobedience. See Chapters 29 and 33 for additional information.

Clients with antisocial behavior demonstrate lack of remorse or indifference to persons whom one has hurt or mistreated, or from whom one has stolen; expectation of immediate gratification; failure to accept social norms; impulsivity; consistent irresponsibility; aggressive behavior; lack of respect for social norms; repeated lying; and reckless behavior that disregards the safety of others (APA, 2000; Lebelle, 2006; Sadock & Sadock, 2003).

Clients with the diagnosis of antisocial personality disorder survive in exciting, fast-paced environments in which they are forced to live by their wits. They have difficulty surviving in tightly constrained environments in which they must follow the rules and customs of others (Paul, 2005). Statistics show that 80% to 90% of all crime is committed by individuals with antisocial personality disorder. Cessation of criminal activities tends to occur at around age 40 years. This disorder is more prevalent in men (3%) than in women (1%). In prison populations, the prevalence may be as high as 75% (Sadock & Sadock, 2003.) See Clinical Example 24-2.

Borderline Personality Disorder

Latent, ambulatory, and *abortive schizophrenics* are examples of previous labels for the *DSM-IV-TR* classification of BPD. The client has symptoms that fall between moderate neurosis and frank psychosis, and he or she almost always appears to be in a state of crisis (Sadock & Sadock, 2003).

Theorists state that BPDs may be a result of a faulty parent–child relationship in which the child does not experience a healthy separation from mother and therefore is unable to interact appropriately with the environment. Parent and child share negative feelings and are bound together by mutual feelings of guilt. Another possible cause is trauma experienced at a specific stage of development, usually 18 months, weak-

CLINICAL EXAMPLE 24.2

THE CLIENT WITH AN ANTISOCIAL PERSONALITY DISORDER

MS, a 19-year-old male, was referred to the local community mental health center for a psychiatric–mental health evaluation. According to his parents, who accompanied MS to the center, MS had shown a lack of remorse after he had seriously injured his cousin in a fight. They noted that MS frequently displayed a lack of respect for his parents and repeatedly lied about his involvement with other friends who were stealing items from local department stores. He dropped out of school at the age of 16 years after he obtained his driver's license. MS was recently arrested for driving under the influence of alcohol. He agreed to attend a driver's education class to remove the points from his driving record. However, he failed to attend the class. When confronted by his parents, he lied to them, stating that the class had been canceled. The result of the psychiatric–mental health evaluation revealed the *DSM-IV-TR* diagnosis of antisocial personality disorder.

ening the person's ego and ability to handle reality. A third theory states that the person experiences an unfulfilled need for intimacy. As a result of attempting to establish an ideal relationship, the person becomes disillusioned and experiences rage, fear of abandonment, and depression. In addition, research has shown that individuals with BPD have a biologic defect in the amygdala, the area of the brain that helps to regulate emotions, causing severe mood swings and abnormal behavior (Epigee.Org, 2006).

Individuals with BPD may exhibit impulsive, unpredictable behavior related to gambling, shoplifting, sex, and substance abuse. Contributing to unstable, intense interpersonal relationships are inappropriate, intense anger; unstable affect reflecting depression, dysphoria, or anxiety; disturbance in self-concept, including gender identity; and the inability to control one's emotions. Behaviors such as paranoid ideation, severe dissociation, masochism, frantic efforts to avoid real or imagined abandonment, and suicidal ideation may occur. The client often reports feeling empty, lonely, unable to experience pleasure, and unable to maintain

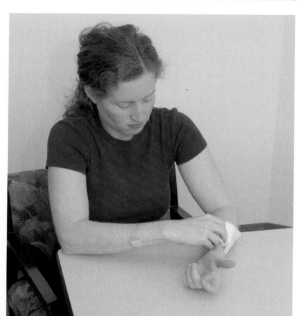

FIGURE 24.1 The client with a borderline personality disorder who exhibits self-mutilating behavior.

employment. Self-mutilating behavior also may occur (Fig. 24-1).

The defense mechanisms most commonly used include denial, projection, splitting, and projective identification. **Splitting** (the inability to integrate and accept both positive and negative feelings at the same moment) and **projective identification** (ability to project uncomfortable or aggressive aspects of one's own personality onto external objects or another person) may be identified as primitive defenses (Rowe, 1989). With splitting, the person can handle only one type of feeling at a time, such as pervasive negativism or anger. This characteristic is opposite to the feeling of ambivalence, in which a person can simultaneously experience feelings of love and hate for another person. During projective identification, the person projects uncomfortable aspects of oneself (eg, hostility toward women) onto someone else. The projector then tries to coerce the other person into identifying with the aspect that has been projected (eg, hostility toward women). Finally, the recipient of the projection and the projector feel a sense of union or oneness

(eg, they both acknowledge hostility toward women). Once the projective identification has occurred, the projector no longer experiences internal conflict. Other examples of uncomfortable aspects of oneself that clients with BPD may project to resolve internal conflict include guilt, helplessness, and suspiciousness (Sadock & Sadock, 2003).

Clients with BPD exist fairly well in creative, permissive environments in which they are free to pursue their passions. They have difficulty existing in environments in which they imagine or feel abandoned by a loved one(s). BPD occurs in all races; is thought to affect about 1% to 2% of the population; is prevalent in women (female-to-male ratios as high as 4:1); and typically presents by late adolescence (APA, 2000; Lebelle, 2006; Paul, 2005; Sadock & Sadock, 2003).

Histrionic Personality Disorder

Histrionic personality disorder is characterized by a pattern of theatrical or overly dramatic behavior. Individuals commonly display discomfort in situations in which they are not the center of attention. The client uses physical appearance, inappropriate sexually seductive or provocative behavior, and self-dramatization and emotional exaggeration to draw attention to self. Style of speech is excessively impressionistic and lacking in detail as the client exhibits labile emotions. The client is easily influenced by others or by circumstances and considers relationships to be more intimate than they really are.

Clients with the diagnosis of histrionic personality disorder enjoy living in artistic environments in which they receive attention and admiration for expressing themselves. They have difficulty living in environments in which they are treated like ordinary workers or they are forced to confront their own failures. Although they may be creative and imaginative, they exhibit dependency and helplessness and handle feelings of criticism poorly (Paul, 2005). This condition is diagnosed more frequently in women and occurs in approximately 2% to 3% of the general population. Comorbid psychiatric disorders may include somatization disorder and alcohol use disorder (APA, 2000; Sadock & Sadock, 2003).

Narcissistic Personality Disorder

The main characteristic of a narcissistic personality disorder is an exaggerated or grandiose sense of self-importance. Clinical symptoms usually develop in early childhood. Typically, the client is preoccupied with fantasies of unlimited success, power, and beauty, believing that he or she is unique and should associate with other high-status individuals. The client requires excessive admiration and envies others, believing that they are envious of him or her. The client also displays arrogance and may display a sense of entitlement and lack empathy as he or she exploits others (APA, 2000; Lebelle, 2006).

Clients who exhibit clinical symptoms of narcissistic personality disorder thrive well in competitive entrepreneurial environments in which they can match wits with others and emerge on top. They have difficulty accepting criticism and existing in environments in which they are treated like ordinary workers or forced to confront their own failures (Paul, 2005). Because clients value beauty, strength, and youthful attributes, aging is handled poorly. Although this disorder is prevalent in less than 1% of the general population and occurs predominantly in men, the number of cases reported is increasing steadily. Furthermore, because the client is prone to extreme mood swings, the risk for suicide is considered to be higher in individuals with narcissistic personality disorder compared with individuals with other personality disorders. Offspring of clients with this disorder may have a higher than usual risk for the development of this disorder themselves (National Mental Health Association, 2006; Sadock & Sadock, 2003).

Cluster C Disorders: Anxious, Fearful Behavior

Obsessive–Compulsive Personality Disorder

Many professionals such as nurses, accountants, and bank tellers may exhibit obsessive–compulsive traits as they attempt to avoid errors or mistakes when they perform task-oriented duties. Conversely, individuals with obsessive–compulsive personality disorder are preoccupied with rules and regulations, are overly concerned with organizational and trivial detail, and are excessively devoted to their work and productivity.

The individual is preoccupied with details, lists, and rules to the extent that the major point of the activity is lost. Perfectionism interferes with task completion, as the client is overly conscientious, scrupulous, inflexible, and reluctant to delegate duties to others. Leisure activities and friendships are excluded because of the client's excessive devotion to work and productivity. The inability to discard worn-out or worthless objects

that have no sentimental value is reflective of the client's miserly spending style (APA, 2000; Lebelle, 2006).

Clients with obsessive–compulsive personality disorder enjoy organized, orderly environments in which conscientiousness and attention to detail are rewarded. They have difficulty living in unstructured, chaotic environments with few rules or customs (Paul, 2005). They commonly experience depression. Interpersonal relationships are affected when a significant other experiences feelings of resentment or hurt. Although the prevalence of this disorder is unknown, it is more common in men and is diagnosed most often in first-born children. It also occurs more frequently in first-degree biologic relatives of clients with the disorder than in the general population (Sadock & Sadock, 2003).

Dependent Personality Disorder

Clients with the diagnosis of dependent personality disorder (also referred to as *passive–dependent personality disorder*) are thoughtful and considerate, faithful and devoted, and agreeable and cooperative; however, they lack self-confidence and are unable to function in an independent role. Such persons allow others to become responsible for their lives because they experience difficulty making everyday decisions, disagreeing with others, and initiating projects or doing things independently. Clients go to excessive lengths to obtain nurturance and support from others. As a result of dependency on others, the client is unrealistically preoccupied with fears of being left alone to care for him- or herself.

Clients with dependent personality disorder are more successful in secure, soothing environments in which they can lean on others as they attempt to make their own choices and decisions. They have difficulty surviving in challenging, go-it-alone environments in which they are forced to rely only on themselves. They urgently seek another relationship when a close relationship ends (Paul, 2005). Persons with recurrent or chronic illness in childhood are considered to be most prone to this disorder, which occurs more frequently in women than in men. See Clinical Example 24-3. It is the most frequently seen personality disorder in mental health clinics (APA, 2000; Lebelle, 2006; Sadock & Sadock, 2003).

Avoidant Personality Disorder

The client with avoidant personality disorder is highly sensitive to rejection, criticism, humiliation, disapprov-

CLINICAL EXAMPLE 24.3

THE CLIENT WITH A DEPENDENT PERSONALITY DISORDER

AJ, a 35-year-old married woman, is seen in the primary care practitioner's office for treatment of a severe upper respiratory infection. During the initial assessment, the client defers the questions to her husband, who has accompanied her. The husband informs the nurse practitioner that his wife has a history of respiratory infections dating back to early childhood. The nurse practitioner observes AJ's dependency on her husband when AJ is asked to change into a gown for her physical examination. AJ insists that the husband remain in the room during the examination. After the examination, the nurse practitioner discusses the treatment options with AJ and her husband. Again, AJ asks her husband for his opinion and tells the nurse practitioner that her husband makes all the "difficult" decisions. The nurse practitioner notes that AJ is exhibiting clinical symptoms of a dependent personality disorder.

BOX 24.2 PERSONALITY DISORDERS: COMMON DESCRIPTIVE BEHAVIORS*

Antisocial personality: Impulsive, aggressive, manipulative

Avoidant personality: Shy, timid, "inferiority complex"

Borderline personality: Impulsive, self-destructive, unstable

Dependent personality: Dependent, submissive, clinging

Histrionic personality: Emotional, dramatic, theatrical

Narcissistic personality: Boastful, egotistical, "superiority complex"

Obsessive–compulsive personality: Perfectionistic, rigid, controlling

Paranoid personality: Suspicious, distrustful

Schizoid personality: Socially distant, detached

Schizotypal personality: Odd, eccentric

*Personality Disorder, Not Otherwise Specified (NOS) is not listed. Individuals with this diagnosis exhibit mixed features and do not meet the full criteria for any one personality disorder.

al, or shame, appearing devastated by the slightest amount of disapproval. This extreme sensitivity interferes with participation in occupational activities, development of interpersonal relationships, and the ability to take personal risks or engage in new activities. Social withdrawal occurs because the client views him- or herself as socially inept, personally unappealing, or inferior to others.

Clients with avoidant personality disorder are more successful in structured, stable environments with a minimum of new experiences and new people. They have difficulty adjusting to loose, unpredictable environments, especially those requiring social activities or public appearances (Paul, 2005). Feelings of anxiety, anger, and depression are common. Social phobia may occur when withdrawal and hypersensitivity persist over time. This disorder is prevalent in 1% to 10% of the general population and in approximately 10% of clients seen in mental health clinics (APA, 2000; Lebelle, 2006; Sadock & Sadock, 2003). Box 24-2 summarizes common descriptive behaviors of the different personality disorders discussed in the preceding paragraphs.

Personality Disorder, Not Otherwise Specified

Two personality disorders are now listed in the category of personality disorder, NOS. These are passive–aggressive personality disorder and depressive personality disorder.

Passive–Aggressive Personality Disorder

Also referred to as *negativistic personality disorder,* an individual with passive–aggressive personality disorder exhibits covert obstructionism through manipulative behavior, procrastination (finds excuses for delays), stubbornness, and inefficiency due to dependency upon others. These behaviors are a manifestation of passively expressed underlying aggression. Clients lack self-confidence and are pessimistic about the future. No epidemiologic data are available at this time (Sadock & Sadock, 2003).

Depressive Personality Disorder

Clients diagnosed with depressive personality disorder exhibit life-long depressive symptoms similar to those seen in dysthymic disorder and major depressive disorder. They are chronically unhappy and exhibit a low self-esteem. They are also self-critical and denigrating about their work, themselves, and their relationships with others. They exhibit poor posture, raspy or hoarse voice, flat or blunted affect, and psychomotor retardation. No epidemiologic data are available at this time (APA, 2000; Sadock & Sadock, 2003).

> ## SELF-AWARENESS PROMPT
>
> Review the clinical symptoms of the different personalities listed in Cluster B of the *DSM-IV-TR* classification of personality disorders. Which personality disorder do you feel would be the most challenging to you as a nurse? Why? Do you feel that your level of tolerance would interfere with providing care for client with the disorder you identified? Explain your answer.

THE NURSING PROCESS

ASSESSMENT

A thorough assessment, including a nursing history and physical examination, is particularly important for clients with personality disorders, to determine the severity of the disorder and ascertain the presence of any underlying biologic disturbances or comorbid, potentially treatable syndromes. For example, individuals with personality disorders are more likely to have a history of an eating disorder or significant trauma. Because personality disorder often manifests in adolescence, a detailed history of the client's childhood and adolescent behavioral patterns is essential.

According to the diagnostic criteria for a personality disorder, disturbances of cognition, affect, interpersonal functioning, and impulse control are present and deviate markedly from the expectations of the individual's culture. These criteria provide the guidelines for a systematic assessment.

Screening and Assessment Tools

Various screening and assessment tools have been utilized in the diagnosis and treatment of clients with personality disorders. Two of the more common instruments are the Millon Clinical Multiaxial Inventory (MCMI-III) and the Structured Interview for DSM-IV Personality (SIDP-IV).

The MCMI-III, based on the theories of personality and psychopathology, is specifically designed to help assess both Axis I disorders (clinical disorders and conditions such as anxiety and depression) and Axis II disorders (personality disorders and mental retardation). The test contains 175 items that, for the most part, can be self-administered by an individual with at least an eighth-grade education within 20 to 30 minutes. This instrument can assist in the diagnosis and development of a treatment approach that takes into account the client's personality style and coping behavior (Millon, 2005).

The SIDP-IV is a semistructured interview that uses questions to examine behavior and personality traits from the client's perspective. It is organized by topics rather than disorders to allow for a more natural conversational flow. This instrument helps distinguish lifelong behavior from temporary states that can result from an episodic psychiatric disorder. Similar to the MCMI-III, this instrument can assist in the diagnosis and development of a treatment approach to improve the client's quality of life (Pfohl, Blum, & Zimmerman, 1997).

Disturbance of Cognition

Clients with personality disorders are in contact with reality, but may have difficulty coping with stress. Cognitive ability may be difficult to assess if the client is suspicious or distrustful; exhibits distorted perceptions of self, other people, or events; or displays impoverished thoughts. Illusions or feelings of depersonalization (complaint of feeling strange or unreal) may be exhibited by clients with schizotypal personality disorder. Insight and judgment may be impaired because maladaptive coping behaviors have become a way of life. Anticipate the need to obtain additional data from family or friends, because clients may exhibit denial and minimize clinical symptoms.

Disturbance of Affect

Pay particular attention to the intensity, degree of lability, and appropriateness of the client's affect. He or she may be irritable; indifferent; exhibit emotional coldness such as flat affect or detachment; exhibit anger; or exhibit dysphoria. Clinical symptoms of anxiety or depression may be present. Obtaining information about the onset of symptoms and history of any previous treatment is significant. Also inquire whether the client has ever attempted suicide or exhibited self-mutilation and whether the client relies on alcohol or drugs to "feel good."

Disturbance of Interpersonal Functioning

Collect data regarding the client's interpersonal functioning. He or she may be reserved, introverted, socially withdrawn, lonely, lack close friends or confidants, or display indifference toward others. Pose questions to family members and friends such as, "Has the client ever been able to maintain a satisfactory interpersonal relationship?" to help provide insight into the client's interpersonal skills.

Dysfunctional Behavior: Lack of Impulse Control

Families commonly endure episodes of explosive anger and rage, self-mutilation, and suicide attempts by clients. These individuals are often referred to treatment by loved ones who recognize a troubling pattern, or who have reached their personal limit in trying to cope with the client's behavior. Displays of unpredictable behavior by the client with a personality disorder are possible during the assessment. Therefore, perform the assessment in a structured environment. Focus the assessment on the client's behavior, such as:

- Which maladaptive behaviors does the client exhibit that lead to lack of impulse control?
- Does the client have a history of being aggressive, disrespectful, reckless, or destructive?
- Are any legal charges pending due to illegal activities such as gambling, shoplifting, or dealing in drugs?
- Has the client been arrested in the past?

Individuals with histrionic behavior are prone to conflict with the law, given their inappropriate sexually seductive or provocative behavior. Clients with antisocial behavior are frequently treated in forensic settings because they fail to comply with social norms when meeting their needs for immediate gratification.

Transcultural Considerations

Culture is an important variable in the development of personality. To understand an ethnic group and work effectively with clients or family members, be aware of a culture's distinctive qualities and the lifestyles, values, and structures within it that influence the development of personality. Poor communication, interpersonal tension, the inability to work effectively, and a poor assessment of health problems can result if cultural differences are ignored. Therefore, pay attention to the client's racial identity, religious preferences, and unique cultural experiences.

As stated in the *DSM-IV-TR*, judgments about personality functioning must take into account the individual's ethnic, cultural, and social background. Do not confuse personality disorders with problems associated with acculturation after immigration, or with the expression of habits, customs, or religious and political values professed by the individual's culture of origin. For example, members of ethnic minority groups, immigrants, or political and economic refugees who display guarded or defensive behaviors because of unfamiliarity with, or in response to, the perceived neglect or indifference of the majority of society may be labeled as having paranoid personality disorder. Others may exhibit defensive behavior and interpersonal styles similar to that of schizoid personality disorder. Always obtain additional information from informants who are familiar with the client's cultural background and determine whether behaviors are culturally sanctioned. See Chapter 4, which addresses cultural and ethnic considerations in psychiatric nursing in greater detail.

NURSING DIAGNOSES

Nursing diagnoses also focus on disturbances of cognition, affect, interpersonal functioning, and impulse control. See the accompanying box for Examples of North American Nursing Diagnosis Association (NANDA) Nursing Diagnoses related to personality disorders.

OUTCOME IDENTIFICATION

Outcome identification for clients who exhibit clinical symptoms of personality disorders generally focuses on improving their ability to differentiate reality from fantasy, developing positive coping skills to reduce stress, improving impulse control and decreasing dysfunctional behavior, developing skills to improve inter-

EXAMPLES OF NANDA NURSING DIAGNOSES/ PERSONALITY DISORDERS	EXAMPLES OF STATED OUTCOMES/ PERSONALITY DISORDERS
• Disturbed Thought Processes related to auditory hallucinations • Disturbed Thought Processes related to distorted perceptions of self and others • Anxiety related to unsatisfactory interpersonal relationships • Hopelessness related to low self-esteem • Ineffective Coping related to lack of impulse control • Ineffective Coping related to lack of insight • Impaired Social Interaction related to manipulation of rules for personal gain • Impaired Verbal Communication related to lack of desire for interaction • Risk for Other-Directed Violence related to low frustration tolerance • Disturbed Sleep Pattern related to agitation • Social Isolation related to socially or legally unacceptable behavior • Social Isolation related to lack of consideration of others	• The client will verbalize increased insight into his or her behavior. • The client will demonstrate decreased manipulative behavior. • The client will exhibit increased impulse control. • The client will not harm others or destroy property. • The client will communicate directly and honestly with other clients and staff about personal feelings. • The client will demonstrate satisfactory, effective relationships with support people. • The client will use the support system without becoming overly dependent on it. • The client will demonstrate alternate ways to deal with frustration. • The client will be free of self-inflicted harm. • The client will verbally recognize that others do not see his or her belief as real. • The client will establish an adequate balance of rest, sleep, and activity. • The client will stop acting on the delusional belief.

personal relationships, and developing insight into their illness. See the accompanying Examples of Stated Outcomes box related to personality disorders.

PLANNING INTERVENTIONS

A working knowledge of personality development and differences in cultural norms and patterns is important for developing an effective plan of care. Personality disorders are chronic, pervasive illnesses that may show exacerbations and complications. As such, it is important to keep in mind that individuals with a personality disorder often require a longer time in treatment, and although a cure is not realistic, personality disorders are definitely treatable. When developing the plan of care, focus on the client's developmental needs that have not been resolved. Interventions are planned to assist the client in understanding identified problems and to anticipate possible future developmental stressors (Personality Disorders Foundation, 2005).

Nursing interventions are directed at the specific behaviors, characteristics, and symptoms that are common to an identified disorder. Clients may exhibit dependent, helpless, childlike behaviors resulting from feelings of abandonment. Clinical symptoms of chronic depression may be present. Planning interventions is challenging because the client may distort ideas and perceptions of others, lack motivation for change, exhibit stubbornness or procrastination, attempt to manipulate or split staff, exhibit distrust, or become completely dependent on assigned caregivers.

Be aware of personal reactions to the client when planning interventions. The subject of nonproductive reactions of nursing staff to clients with BPD was identified by Lego (1996). Many of these reactions could occur when planning and providing interventions for clients with any of the personality disorders. For example, the nurse may feel responsible for the welfare of the client with schizotypal or dependent personality disorder, express guilt because of failure to develop certain interventions to help the client who is exhibiting histrionic or avoidant behavior, or feel disappointment because specific interventions were not discussed by staff or included in the plan of care. Such reactions should be discussed with members of the nursing staff because each member brings a different experience to the attention of the group. When combined, these pieces of information help provide a more comprehensive view of each nurse's responsibilities and relieve the individual nurse of the perceived burden of being the only viable caretaker (Lego, 1996).

IMPLEMENTATION

Establish an environment in which the client, but not the maladaptive behavior, is accepted. Examining one's own feelings about such behavior is crucial to ensure that these feelings do not interfere with therapeutic nursing interventions. Personal feelings, beliefs, and attitudes must be identified, discussed, and accepted before one can work effectively with clients in the clinical setting. Also, be aware of the potential for transference and countertransference to occur. It is neither necessary nor particularly desirable for the client to like you personally. Your purpose is not to be the client's friend. Maintaining a professional role with the client provides a firm basis on which to establish a therapeutic relationship in the best interests of the client. Additionally, remember that clients usually enter treatment because increased anxiety has disrupted social interaction; the client has developed an awareness of and dissatisfaction with his or her unsatisfactory lifestyle; or a significant other has insisted that psychiatric care be sought.

Assistance in Meeting Basic Needs

Clients with the diagnosis of a personality disorder may neglect self-care, have difficulty sleeping, display ineffective coping, exhibit unpredictable aggressive or self-destructive behavior resulting from poor impulse control, isolate themselves from others, or demonstrate noncompliance with the nursing plan of care. Ensure a safe environment, promote trust, and provide consistency when providing assistance in meeting the client's basic needs.

Symptom Management

Some examples of nursing interventions that have proven effective in managing the symptoms of clients with personality disorders are highlighted in Box 24-3 (Carpenito-Moyet, 2006; Sadock & Sadock, 2003; Schultz & Videbeck, 2005). Always be sure to individualize the interventions to meet each client's needs.

Medication Management

According to the Collaborative Longitudinal Personality Disorders Study, about 81% of clients with personality disorders are receiving psychopharmacologic medications. A second study shows that 78% of clients with BPD and 68% of clients with other personality disorders received medication during more than 4 years of a 6-year period. At the end of 6 years, 71% of the clients with BPD and 54% of clients with other personality disorders were still taking medications (Evans, 2005).

Pharmacotherapy is not used exclusively to treat personality disorders. Rather, medications are used as adjunctive therapy, with psychotherapy, psychoeducation, and family support playing a much larger and more dominant role. When medication seems indicated, the usual approach is to let the problematic manifestation (eg, anxiety, behavioral disturbances, depression, distorted perceptions, impulsivity) guide the choice of the medication to be prescribed and administered (Doskoch, 2001; Sadock & Sadock, 2003; Sherman, 2001). Various psychopharmacologic agents facilitate the client's capacity to use psychotherapy by addressing issues of biologic factors such as high levels of neurotransmitters and the presence of mood disorders or anxiety (Gabbard, 1998). For example, psychotropic drugs, which are individualized on the basis of the client's needs, may be prescribed for specific clinical symptoms or behaviors, such as depression, paranoid thoughts, or aggression. Drug Summary Table 24-1 highlights the common drugs used for the client's specific symptoms.

Whenever psychotropic medication is used, exercise caution because clients with antisocial, borderline, paranoid, and schizoid personality disorders may not be compliant with this mode of treatment. In addition, a history of substance abuse or drug dependency may also negate this approach.

Interactive Therapies

Nurse–therapists have the most difficulties with those suffering from personality disorders because clients are difficult to please, block effective communication, avoid the development of a trusting relationship, and cannot be relied upon for accurate information regarding problems or how problems arose. As noted earlier, clients with personality disorders often exhibit transference that can interfere with therapy (Lebelle, 2006).

Treatment approaches focus on restructuring the personality in age-appropriate clients, assisting clients in completing developmental levels and tasks, and setting limits for maladaptive behavior such as acting out. Most clients with a personality disorder require some combination of extended psychotherapy and medication. The key to successful treatment of clients with personality disorders is to avoid split treatment (eg,

BOX 24.3 MANAGING THE SYMPTOMS OF CLIENTS WITH PERSONALITY DISORDERS

For the client with a *disturbance in cognition,* helpful interventions may include the following:
- Reinforce reality if the client verbalizes illusions or feelings of depersonalization. Help the client select someone he or she trusts to minimize suspicious or delusional thoughts.
- Encourage the client to validate perceptions before taking action that may precipitate difficulties.
- Explore with the client present maladaptive coping mechanisms and the purpose they serve.
- Explore alternate coping mechanisms to reduce stress.
- Assist the client to develop insight regarding the purpose of nursing interventions.

If the client displays a *disturbance in affect,* try the following:
- Encourage the client to verbalize feelings of anger, hostility, worthlessness, or hopelessness.
- Give attention and support when the client expresses feelings honestly and openly.
- Encourage the client to share his or her feelings with others.
- Provide a safe environment if the client expresses suicidal ideation or exhibits self-mutilation behavior.

For the client with a *disturbance in interpersonal functioning,* possible interventions include the following:
- Explore reasons the client has difficulty establishing interpersonal relationships.
- Explore the client's self-concept and self-esteem.
- Explore the client's perception of how others view him or her.
- Provide positive feedback regarding your observations of the client's strengths.
- Encourage the client to socialize with at least one person daily.

When the client exhibits *dysfunctional behavior indicative of poor impulse control,* the following interventions may be helpful:
- State limits and behavior expected from the client.
- Enforce all limits without apologizing.
- Be direct, confronting the client when limits are not observed.
- Discuss consequences of client's failure to observe limits.
- Discuss behavior with the client in a nonjudgmental manner.

one clinician provides interactive therapy while another manages the medication), replacing it with integrated and coordinated care to avoid contradictions, discontinuities, and disagreements among all involved. If split treatment is used, the effort requires not only that the two clinicians have respect for and some basic understanding of what each is attempting to accomplish, but also that the two approaches are coordinated (Silk, 2001).

Clients with a personality disorder need to have an especially clear grasp of the often complex combination of attitudes and core beliefs that they hold. Cognitive therapists present an information-processing model to help clients understand how they incorporate data that support their belief about self while excluding or discounting data that are contrary (Beck, 1996). Dialectical behavioral therapy, a form of cognitive behavioral therapy (CBT) that focuses on coping skills so that clients learn to better control their emotions and behaviors, appears to be the most effective. Therapy sessions focus on a particular problematic

behavior or event, beginning with the chain of events leading up to it, going through alternative solutions that might have been used, and examining what kept the client from using more adaptive solutions to the problem. Dialectical behavioral therapy targets high-risk suicidal behaviors, behaviors that interfere with therapy, behaviors that interfere with quality of life, post-traumatic stress response, low-self esteem, and any goals set by the client (Linehan, 1991; Muscari, 2005). Cognitive behavioral therapy may focus on current distressing situations as well as negative childhood experiences. Group therapy is used to reinforce the client's realization that he or she is not unique and to discuss alternate ways to respond to stress. Reality therapy and intensive psychoanalysis are also used. Clients with personality disorders can learn to think about themselves in more realistic, functional ways.

Cognitive behavioral therapy has also been used with elderly clients with personality disorders (Sherman, 1999b). The purpose is not to reconfigure character (this late in life), but to relieve symptoms,

DRUG SUMMARY TABLE 24-1 Examples of Drugs Used for Personality Disorders*

GENERIC (TRADE) NAME	DAILY DOSAGE RANGE	IMPLEMENTATION
Drug Class: Antipsychotics (for paranoia, psychoses, aggression, and post-traumatic stress)		
haloperidol (Haldol)	4–16 mg	Monitor for refractory arrhythmias, abnormal BUN and WBC results, increased motor activity, EPS, TD, and NMS.
olanzapine (Zyprexa)	5–20 mg	Monitor for weight gain, EPS, TD, and NMS.
Drug Class: Anticonvulsants (for aggression, impulsivity, mood disorders, and suicidality)		
carbamazepine (Tegretol)	600–1200 mg	Administer with food to prevent GI upset; arrange for frequent liver function tests and discontinue drug if hepatic dysfunction occurs; follow protocol regarding CBC, platelet, reticulocyte, and serum iron lab work prior to initiation of drug and during drug therapy; obtain serum carbamazepine level per protocol during drug therapy; monitor for drowsiness, dizziness, GI disturbance, and skin rash.
valproate (Depakote)	500–1500 mg	Arrange for liver function, platelet count, and ammonia levels per protocol before and during drug therapy; discontinue drug if rash occurs; advise client to wear medical ID alert bracelet; monitor for bruising, jaundice, sedation, and tremor.
Drug Class: Antidepressants (for depression, anxiety, panic attacks)		
venlafaxine (Effexor)	75–375 mg	Contraindicated during pregnancy; should not be taken concurrently with MAOIs; monitor BP and reduce dose or discontinue if hypertension occurs; monitor for dreams, tremor, dizziness, somnolence, GI disturbance, and dry mouth.
Drug Class: Antianxiety Agents		
clomipramine (Anafranil)	25–300 mg	Is contraindicated during or within 14 days of MAOI therapy; administer with food; monitor for anticholinergic effects, GI disturbances, somnolence, weight gain, male sexual dysfunction, and seizures.
clonazepam (Klonopin)	0.5–20 mg	Monitor liver function and blood count in clients on long-term therapy; monitor for mild paradoxical excitement during the first 2 weeks of therapy, respiratory distress, palpitations and constipation; instruct client to avoid use of alcohol and sleep-inducing or over-the-counter drugs.

*NOTE: Various prescribing models shape the use of psychotropic agents to treat clinical symptoms of personality disorders such as psychosis, behavioral changes, depression, and anxiety.

foster interdependence, and support "healthy narcissism." Older adult clients do not tolerate confrontation or interpretation well during interactive therapy. Therapy generally has a strong psychoeducational component (Sherman, 1999a).

Family nuances are important in the treatment of clients with BPD (Johnson, 2000). Research has shown that family environment and involvement can affect the outcome of several conditions, including BPD. Family over-concern was closely related to positive outcomes, because clients interpreted family suffering as a form of caring.

Client and Family Education

Although clients frequently deny responsibility for their actions and tend to isolate themselves, after clinical symptoms are stabilized, clients are encouraged to participate in educational groups. Information may be provided regarding the impact of comorbid disorders such as anxiety or depression and how these disorders can be treated. Problem-solving groups may be offered to encourage the client to participate in role-play situations to explore positive coping skills, improve interpersonal skills, or discuss information related to

employment issues. Medication compliance, financial responsibilities, or accountability and responsibility for illegal behavior may also be addressed. Self-help or support groups that focus on anger management or substance-abuse behaviors may be provided for both the client and family members or significant others (Schultz & Videbeck, 2005; Sadock & Sadock, 2003).

EVALUATION

Evaluation of a client's progress can be difficult, given the complexity of symptoms exhibited when a client with a personality disorder enters treatment. Because of his or her ability to manipulate, resist care, distort perceptions, and transfer dependency needs to others, it may take several years to modify patterns of behavior to meet stated outcomes. Because patterns of behavior are difficult to modify or change, clients may be frequently arrested. They may require repeated hospitalizations resulting from failure to comply with treatment. Treatment of any of the described disorders tends to be long term and does not guarantee recovery. See Nursing Plan of Care 24-1, The Client With Paranoid Personality Disorder, for an example.

NURSING PLAN OF CARE 24.1

THE CLIENT WITH PARANOID PERSONALITY DISORDER

Walter, a 51-year-old president of a large accounting firm, suspected that the certified public accountant for the firm was misappropriating funds. Walter also questioned the loyalty and trustworthiness of his partners. He was reluctant to confide in the firm's attorney because he feared that the information would be used maliciously against him. He perceived attacks on his reputation by the accountant and his partners during the last corporate meeting and was quick to react angrily to their comments. Walter's partners confronted him about the change in his behavior. During the conversation it was obvious that Walter had been harboring unjustified doubts about their loyalty. They recommended that he be seen by his family physician to rule out exhaustion due to the stress of his position. Walter was seen by his family physician who ruled out any medical problems and referred him to a mental health provider for a psychiatric evaluation.

DSM–IV–TR DIAGNOSIS: Paranoid personality disorder.

ASSESSMENT: Personal strengths: Alert, oriented in all spheres; supportive business partners; supportive family physician; stable medical condition

Weaknesses: Suspicious, with unjustified doubt about partners; inability to relate to partners without displaying anger

(Continued on following page)

NURSING DIAGNOSIS: Disturbed Thought Processes related to delusional belief as evidenced by accusatory statements and questioning loyalty and trustworthiness of peers

OUTCOME: The client will recognize that others do not share his paranoid thoughts.

Planning/Implementation	Rationale
Do not validate paranoid thoughts, but introduce reality when appropriate.	Introducing and reinforcing reality may diminish delusional beliefs.
Let the client know that all feelings, ideas, and beliefs are permissible to share with nursing staff.	Reassurance may diminish the client's fears.
Encourage the client to discuss other topics such as family or hobbies.	Discussing concrete or familiar topics may redirect the client's attention to reality.

NURSING DIAGNOSIS: Defensive Coping as evidenced by repeated projection of blame and difficulty in testing perceptions against reality

OUTCOME: The client will demonstrate less defensive behavior when interacting with his peers and employees.

Planning/Implementation	Rationale
Encourage the client to verbalize his feelings.	Verbalizing feelings may help the client work through his paranoid thoughts.
Give the client positive feedback when he recognizes defensive coping behavior.	Positive feedback provides reinforcement of the client's ability to recognize defensive coping behavior and promotes acceptance of behavior.

NURSING DIAGNOSIS: Impaired Social Interaction related to alienation from others secondary to delusional thinking

OUTCOME: The client will modify behaviors that are problematic when interacting with others.

Planning/Implementation	Rationale
Role-play situations in which the client can redirect some of the anger generated by suspiciousness and doubt.	Role-playing enables the client to explore feelings and obtain feedback to develop positive behaviors.
Provide feedback for any interactions or attempts to interact with others.	Positive feedback may facilitate the development of desired behaviors.

EVALUATION: Clients such as Walter are often noncompliant with treatment due to their inability to trust others. Therefore, evaluation focuses on the progress the client makes if he or she agrees to participate in therapy. Interventions are difficult. If Walter agrees to continue in therapy, a referral to community resources (eg, occupational therapy, outpatient social clubs or groups) to build the client's socialization skills may prove to be beneficial.

KEY CONCEPTS

◆ Understanding theories of personality development is necessary to identify characteristics of healthy and unhealthy personalities.

◆ Personality disorders exist on a continuum in which symptoms may be described as mild to severe. Factors that may contribute to the development of a personality disorder have been classified as genetic, biologic, or psychoanalytic. Personality disorders are grouped according to behavioral clusters. Cluster A includes clinical symptoms of odd, eccentric behavior; Cluster B includes clinical symptoms of emotional, erratic, or dramatic behavior; and Cluster C includes clinical symptoms of anxious and fearful behavior. Cluster B personality disorders carry the highest suicide risk, similar to that of non–personality-disordered clients with major mood disorders.

◆ For the category of personality disorder, not otherwise specified, two new disorders are now listed: passive–aggressive personality disorder and depressive personality disorder.

◆ The nursing process focuses on the client's cognition, affect, interpersonal functioning, and behavior, as well as his or her ability to meet basic needs.

◆ Nursing assessment should include a detailed history of the client's childhood and adolescent behavioral patterns. Cultural diversity must be considered during the assessment process to avoid misdiagnosis of the problems associated with acculturation after immigration, or misdiagnosis as a result of the expression of habits, customs, or religious or political values professed by the client's culture of origin.

◆ Nursing interventions are directed at assistance in meeting basic needs, symptom management, and medication management, and address the diagnostic criteria of disturbance in cognition, disturbance in affect, disturbance in interpersonal functioning, and dysfunctional behavior including poor impulse control. Clients may exhibit negative responses to planned interventions.

◆ Clients with personality disorders may respond to the combination of psychotropic drugs and interactive therapies such as dialectical behavioral therapy, cognitive behavioral therapy, group, and reality therapy.

◆ Client education focuses on the impact of comorbid psychiatric disorders; problem-solving techniques; medication compliance; and participation in specific self-help or support groups. Treatment tends to be long term and does not guarantee recovery, because recidivism is high.

For additional study materials, please refer to the Student Resource CD-ROM located in the back of this textbook.

CHAPTER WORKSHEET

CRITICAL THINKING QUESTIONS

1. The theories of personality development discussed in this chapter were all developed by men. Discuss how a woman's perspective might be different.
2. Ask classmates of varying cultural backgrounds how their culture and childhood experiences have affected the development of their personality. Do they exhibit any traits of Cluster C disorders, such as obsessive–compulsive traits when studying for tests or providing care for clients? Do these traits interfere with their daily activities? If so, what interventions would you recommend?

REFLECTION

According to the chapter opening quote by the Personality Disorders Foundation, individuals with a personality disorder are among the least understood and recognized disorders in both psychiatry and general medical care; however, they are among the most common mental disorders. Do you accept this statement to be true? If so, what can be done to increase awareness of personality disorders? Explain your answers.

NCLEX-STYLE QUESTIONS

1. Which symptom would the nurse expect to assess related to anger expression in a client diagnosed with borderline personality disorder?
   a. Controlled, subtle anger
   b. Inappropriate, intense anger
   c. Inability to recognize anger
   d. Substitution of physical symptoms for anger

2. The client with a borderline personality disorder tells the nurse that he is the best nurse in the hospital until the nurse sets limits on client behavior. Then the client complains that the nurse is cruel and a "poor excuse for a person." The nurse interprets this behavior as demonstration of which of the following?

   a. Denial
   b. Rationalization
   c. Splitting
   d. Projection

3. The nurse uses which intervention for the client who expresses feelings of depersonalization as one of the manifestations of a personality disorder?

   a. Challenging feelings
   b. Identifying origin of these feelings
   c. Reinforcing reality
   d. Employing diversional activities

4. The nurse sets limits in a therapeutic manner by doing which of the following?

   a. Identifying limits in a clear manner without apologizing
   b. Negotiating limits appropriate for the individual client
   c. Providing various reasons that limits are important
   d. Substituting persuasive statements for specific limits

5. The client with a personality disorder has the nursing diagnosis of Chronic Low Self-Esteem related to feelings of worthlessness. Which outcome reflects successful intervention to increase the client's self-esteem?

   a. Client will verbally recognize that others do not see his or her belief as real.
   b. Client will demonstrate appropriate interactions with staff and peers.
   c. Client will identify accurate and realistic perception of good and bad qualities.
   d. Client will demonstrate alternate ways to deal with anxiety and frustration.

6. After teaching a group of students about personality disorders, the instructor determines that the students have understood the teaching when they identify which personality disorders as belonging to Cluster B disorders. Select all that apply.

   a. Paranoid
   b. Antisocial
   c. Borderline
   d. Histrionic
   e. Dependent
   f. Obsessive–compulsive

Selected References

American Psychiatric Association. (2000). *Diagnostic and statistical manual of mental disorders* (4th ed., text revision). Washington, DC: Author.

Beck, J. S. (1996). Cognitive therapy for personality disorders. *Psychiatric Times, 13*(2). Retrieved February 25, 2004, from http://www.psychiatrictimes.com/ p960241.html

Carpenito-Moyet, L. J. (2006). *Handbook of nursing diagnosis* (11th ed.). Philadelphia: Lippincott Williams & Wilkins.

Doskoch, P. (2001). Pharmacotherapy for borderline personality disorder. *Neuropsychiatry, 2*(9), 1, 20, 25.

Epigee.org. (2006). Borderline personality disorder. Retrieved January 5, 2006, from http://www.epigee.org/mental_health/bpd.html

Erikson, E. H. (1968). *Identity: Youth and crisis.* New York: W. W. Norton.

Evans, J. (2005). Prescribing models shape personality disorder treatment. *Clinical Psychiatry News, 33*(6), 26.

Freud, S. (1960). *The ego and the id.* (J. Strachey, Ed.; J. Riviere, Trans.). New York: W. W. Norton.

Gabbard, G. O. (1998). Treatment-resistant borderline personality disorder. *Psychiatric Annals, 28,* 561–656.

Grant, B. F., Hasin, D. S., & Stinson, F. S. (2004). Prevalence, correlates, and disability of personality disorders in the United States: Results from the national Epidemiologic Survey on Alcohol and Related Conditions. *Journal of Clinical Psychiatry, 65,* 948–958.

Johnson, K. (2000). Family nuances important in borderline personality treatment. *Clinical Psychiatry News, 27*(2), 25.

Lambert, M. T. (2003). Suicide risk and management: Focus on personality disorders. *Current Opinions in Psychiatry Online, 16*(1), 71–76.

Lebelle, L. (2006). *Personality disorders.* Retrieved January 21, 2006, from http://www.focusas.com/PersonalityDisorders.html

Lego, S. (1996). The client with borderline personality disorder. In S. Lego (Ed.), *Psychiatric nursing: A comprehensive reference* (2nd ed., pp. 234–245). Philadelphia: Lippincott-Raven.

Linehan, M. (1991). Dialectical behavioral therapy. Retrieved January 22, 2006, from http://www.palace.net/~llama/psych/dbt.html

Millon, T. (2005). *Millon clinical multiaxial inventory-III*. Minneapolis, MN: National Computer Systems, Inc.

Muscari, M. E. (2005). What therapy is recommended for borderline personality disorder in adolescents? Retrieved August 17, 2005, from http://www.medscape.com/viewarticle/508832

National Mental Health Association. (2006). Personality disorders. Retrieved January 19, 2006, from http://www.nmha.org/infoctr/factsheets/91.cfm

Paul, A. M. (2005). Am I normal? *Psychology Today, 38* (2), 54, 56, 59–63.

Personality Disorders Foundation. (2005). The impact of personality disorders. Retrieved January 12, 2005, from http://pdf.uchc.edu/impact.php

Pfohl, B., Blum, N., & Zimmerman. (1997). *Structured interview for DSM-IV personality (SIDP-IV)*. Washington, DC: American Psychiatric Publishing, Inc.

Piaget, J. (1963). *The child's conception of the world*. Ames, IA: Littlefield, Adams.

Rowe, C. J. (1989). *An outline of psychiatry* (9th ed.). Dubuque, IA: William C. Brown.

Sadock, B. J., & Sadock, V. A. (2003). *Kaplan & Sadock's synopsis of psychiatry: Behavioral sciences/clinical psychiatry* (9th ed.). Philadelphia: Lippincott Williams & Wilkins.

Schultz, J. M., & Videbeck, S. L. (2005). *Lippincott's manual of psychiatric nursing care plans* (7th ed.). Philadelphia: Lippincott Williams & Wilkins.

Sherman, C. (1999a). Cognitive therapy's reach extends to Axis II. *Clinical Psychiatry News, 26*(10), 24–25.

Sherman, C. (1999b). Elderly with personality disorders can benefit from psychotherapy. *Clinical Psychiatry News, 26*(6), 29.

Sherman, C. (2001). Meds play important role in borderline personality. *Clinical Psychiatry News, 29*(9), 17.

Silk, K. R. (2001). Split (collaborative) treatment for patients with personality disorders. *Psychiatric Annals, 31*(10), 615–623.

Straus, M. A., Sugarman, D. B., & Giles-Sims, J. (1997). Spanking by parents and subsequent antisocial behavior of children. *Archives of Pediatrics and Adolescent Medicine, 8*(151), 761–767.

Vaknin, S. (2006). Rage and anger. The common sources of personality disorders. Retrieved January 21, 2006, from http://www.geocities.com/Athens/Forum/6297/mask.html?200621

Suggested Readings

DuBose, A. P., & Linehan, M. M. (2005). Balanced therapy. How to avoid conflict and help 'borderline' patients. *Current Psychiatry, 4*(4), 13–16, 25–26.

Green, J. (2003). The client with a personality disorder. In W. K. Mohr (Ed.), *Johnson's psychiatric-mental health nursing* (5th ed., pp. 437–454). Philadelphia: Lippincott Williams & Wilkins.

Lambert, M. T. (2003). Suicide risk assessment and management: Focus on personality disorders. *Current Opinions in Psychiatry, 16*(1): 71–76.

Livesley, W. J. (2001). *Handbook of personality disorders: Theory, research, and treatment*. New York: Guilford Publications.

Maslow, A. M. (1962). *Toward a psychology of being*. Princeton, NJ: D. Van Nostrand.

Maslow, A. M. (1970). *Motivation and personality* (2nd ed.). New York: Harper & Row.

Nels, N. (2000). Being a case manager for persons with borderline personality disorder: perspectives of community mental health center clinicians. *Archives of Psychiatric Nursing, 14*(1), 12–18.

Norton, P. G. W. (2004). Personality disorders common in outpatients. *Clinical Psychiatry News, 32*(7), 23.

Pediaditakis, N. (2002). Borderline phenomena revisited: A synthesis. *Psychiatric Times, 19*(2), 37–38, 4.

Simon, C. C. (2005). The lion tamer. *Psychology Today, 38*(4), 54–60.

Stout, M. (2005). The ice people. *Psychology Today, 38*(1), 72–78.

Wettstein, R. M. (Ed.). (2000). *Treatment of offenders with mental disorders*. New York: Guilford Publications.

CHAPTER 25 / SUBSTANCE-RELATED DISORDERS

Substance abuse and addiction has serious medical and social consequences; the use of alcohol and other drugs can have an enormous impact on a person's physical, mental and emotional health. —PSYCHIATRY 24×7, 2004

LEARNING OBJECTIVES

AFTER STUDYING THIS CHAPTER, YOU SHOULD BE ABLE TO:

1. Explain the disease concept of alcoholism and the following theories of addiction: biologic, genetic, behavioral and learning, sociocultural, psychodynamic.
2. Differentiate among the following terms: *substance use, addiction, psychological dependence, tolerance*, and *physiologic dependence*.
3. Explain the dynamics of enabling and codependency.
4. Articulate the difference between alcohol dependence and alcohol abuse.
5. Recognize the more common physiologic effects of alcoholism.
6. Identify the common medical problems associated with illicit abuse of substances (drugs).
7. State the rationale for the use of substance-abuse screening tools during the initial assessment of a client with a substance-related disorder.
8. Articulate the rationale for the use of the Stages of Change Model when planning interventions for a client with a substance-related disorder.
9. Describe the treatment measures, including nursing interventions, for a client with a substance-related disorder.
10. Formulate a list of nursing interventions for a client with clinical symptoms of acute substance intoxication.
11. Develop a list of services available to clients who abuse substances.

KEY TERMS

Addiction
Addictions nursing
Addictive personality
Alcohol intoxication
Alcohol withdrawal
Aversion therapy
Behavioral dependence
Codependency
Delirium tremens
Detoxification
Drug dependence
Enabling
Habituation
Impaired nurse
Intervention
Korsakoff's psychosis
Physiologic dependence
Psychological dependence
Stages of Change Model
Substance use
Tolerance
Wernicke's encephalopathy

Substance-related disorders refers to the use and abuse of alcohol, illicit drugs, or substances such as over-the-counter (OTC) or prescription drugs. When substance use creates difficulties for the user or ceases to be entirely volitional, it becomes the concern of all the helping professions, including nursing. This chapter discusses the history of substance use and abuse; describes the terminology, epidemiology, clinical symptoms, and diagnostic characteristics of the major substance-related disorders; and focuses on the application of the nursing process as the nurse provides care for a client diagnosed with a substance-related disorder.

History of Substance Use and Abuse

Individuals have used and abused various substances to achieve desired mood states or as defense mechanisms to deal with reality. Following is a brief discussion of the limited information that is available regarding the history of the origin of substance use and abuse.

History of Drug Use and Abuse

According to a Chinese medical compendium dated from 2737 BC, the Chinese were the first to use marijuana to achieve euphoria. As early as the year 2000 BC, the Greeks used opium, and the Aztecs incorporated hallucinogens into religious rituals. During the Middle Ages (400 to 1500), witches brewed potent concoctions, and New World merchants transported opium along with slaves and rum. The use and abuse of several substances increased during the Civil War period (1861–1865), when soldiers became addicted to prescription drugs that were used to alleviate pain in the battlefield. Cocaine was introduced as a miracle drug and used in patent medicine. Heroin was also produced and sold by traveling salesmen; however, the addictive potential limited the use of these drugs by society. Marijuana was openly used until the federal government discouraged its use in 1930. The recreational use of illicit drugs resurfaced between 1950 and 1960. Cocaine, which was popular during the 1970s, became available as "crack cocaine" in the 1980s. During the 1990s, the use of heroin and smoking of marijuana regained popularity. Since that time,

several forms of illicit drugs (eg, methamphetamine, designer drugs, anabolic steroids) have become more commonplace in society than ever before. Drug use and abuse continues to be a significant public health problem despite public outcry and regulation by the U.S. Drug Enforcement Administration (DEA) (Goulding & Shank, 2005).

History of Use and Abuse of Alcohol

There was a time when the sale and consumption of alcoholic beverages was illegal in the United States. Alcohol was first introduced in the U.S. by the Puritans around 1620. The use of alcohol reflected their religious belief that drinking was a natural and normal part of life. Alcohol was also an effective analgesic, and generally enhanced the quality of life. People of both sexes and all ages typically drank beer with their meals. By 1697, distilleries were used to make rum, wine, beer, and cider.

In 1784, Benjamin Rush, a physician, argued that excessive use of alcohol caused injury to physical and psychological health. Followers of Rush formed a temperance movement in 1789 as an organized effort to encourage moderation or complete abstinence in the consumption of intoxicating liquors. Drinking had become an activity associated with masculine aggression and antisocial behavior. In fact, alcohol was blamed for many of society's problems, among them severe health issues, destitution and crime. The movement's ranks were mostly filled by women who, with their children, had endured the effects of unbridled drinking by many of the men in their lives. By 1826, the American Temperance Society was organized with a mission to educate individuals about the effects of drinking on religion and morality. Antialcohol education was introduced in the schools between 1901 and 1902. On January 16, 1920, prohibition of the sale and consumption of alcohol became a law. Speakeasies soon flourished across the country and there were underground saloons. Prohibition spawned organized crime, bootlegging, and corruption, and, by the late 1920s, prohibition became a very unpopular reality. Democrats used prohibition as an issue during the 1932 presidential campaign. In February of 1933, Congress passed the 21st amendment to repeal prohibition. Unfortunately, statistics kept by the Center for Disease Control indicate the use and abuse of alcoholism continues to have an adverse effect on society (eg, motor vehicle accidents, various medical problems, depression, suicide) (Essortment.com, 2006; Hanson, 2006).

According to the 2004 National Survey on Drug Use and Health, an annual survey of the civilian, non-institutionalized population of the United States age 12 years or older, 22.5 million Americans (or 9.4% of the population) were classified as having past-year substance dependence or abuse, about the same number as in 2002 and 2003. Alcohol- and drug-related use or abuse problems continue to contribute to enormous damage to society, and the magnitude of these costs underscores the need to find better ways to prevent and treat these disorders. The rising costs from substance-related public health issues warrant a major and continuous investment in research on prevention and treatment (Substance Abuse and Mental Health Services Administration [SAMHSA], 2005).

Overview of Substance-Related Disorders

Terminology Associated With Substance-Related Disorders

Substance use is simply the ingestion of a chemically active agent such as OTC medication, a prescribed drug, or illicit drug, alcohol, or nicotine. **Addiction** has been defined as an illness characterized by "compulsion, loss of control, and continued patterns of abuse despite perceived negative consequences; obsession with a dysfunctional habit" (American Nurses Association [ANA], Drug and Alcohol Nursing Association, & National Nurses Society on Addictions [NNSA], 1987). Addiction is a term used to define a state of chronic or recurrent drug intoxication, characterized by psychological and physical dependence as well as tolerance. **Habituation,** also referred to as **psychological dependence,** is a term used to describe a continuous or intermittent craving for a substance to avoid a dysphoric or unpleasant mood state. Habituation implies an emotional dependence on a drug or a desire or compulsion to continue taking a drug. **Tolerance** refers to the person's ability to obtain a desired effect from a specific dose of a drug. For example, as a person develops a tolerance for 10 milligrams of diazepam (Valium), she or he increases the dose to 15 or 20 milligrams to achieve the desired

effects originally experienced at the 10-milligram dose. **Physiologic dependence** refers to the physical effects resulting from the multiple episodes of substance use; it is manifested by the appearance of withdrawal symptoms after the person stops taking a specific drug. **Behavioral dependence** refers to the substance-seeking activities and pathological use patterns of the person using the substance. Behavioral dependence is often associated with social activities. For example, an individual may exhibit the behavioral dependence of smoking marijuana or using other illicit substances while watching television or attending sports activities with one's peers. **Codependency** is a term that refers to all the behavioral patterns of family members who have been significantly affected by another family member's substance use or abuse. Family members may feel the substance-using behavior of the user is voluntary and willful and that the user cares more for the substance than for them. They often experience feelings of anger, rejection, denial, failure, guilt, or depression and shift the blame for the user's behavior onto other family members. Such behavior by family members actually perpetuates the user's dependence and is referred to as **enabling** (Sadock & Sadock, 2003; Shahrokh & Hales, 2003).

In 1964, the World Health Organization (WHO) suggested substituting the term **drug dependence** for "addiction" to better describe the two concepts of dependence: behavioral dependence and physiologic dependence. In addition, the word "substance" is used in the *Diagnostic and Statistical Manual of Mental Disorders, 4th Edition, Text Revision (DSM-IV-TR)* because "drug" implies a manufactured chemical, whereas many substances associated with abuse patterns occur naturally (eg, marijuana) or are not meant for human consumption (eg, glue) (Sadock & Sadock, 2003).

According to the WHO, the words "addict" and "addiction" ignore the concept of drug abuse as a medical disorder. However, a recent literature search noted that several disciplines, including nursing and the medical profession, continue to use the word "addiction" interchangeably with "drug dependence" and "abuse."

Epidemiology of Substance-Related Disorders

Globally, alcohol consumption has increased in recent decades, with all or most of that increase in developing countries. This increase is often occurring in countries with few methods of prevention, control or treatment. The illicit use of drugs has also taken on global dimensions. There is sufficient reason to believe that unregulated excessive drug supply and consumption trends in some countries may be continuing and new problems may be developing (World Health Organization, 2006a, b).

Substance-related disorders are responsible for dysfunctional marital and family relationships, divorce, desertion, child abuse, displaced children, and impoverished families. Alcohol-related medical problems can be disabling, chronic, or fatal (Figure 25-1). Fetal alcohol syndrome is one of the leading causes of birth defects in the United States. Clients who abuse alcohol or drugs may develop comorbid conditions such as alcohol- or substance-induced mood disorders, anxiety disorders, and dementia. A discussion of the epidemiology of substance-related disorders follows.

Alcohol Use and Abuse

Agencies such as the National Institute on Drug Abuse (NIDA), National Institute on Alcohol Abuse and Alcoholism (NIAAA) and National Clearinghouse for Alcohol and Drug Information (NCADI) conduct periodic surveys on the use and abuse of alcohol in the United States. Several factors are considered during the surveys, including race and ethnicity, gender, region and urbanicity, education, and socioeconomic class (Sadock & Sadock, 2003). A summary of the most recent surveys regarding the use and abuse of alcohol follows.

NCADI and NIAAA Surveys. According to the 2003 statistics, approximately 90% of all U.S. residents have had an alcohol-containing drink at least once in their lives, and about 51% of all U.S. adults currently use alcohol. Most people engage in the reasonable and responsible use of alcohol; however, the 2003 statistics indicate that approximately 15.3 million Americans (one in every 12 adults) abuse alcohol, compared with the 5.1 million persons identified in 1990. About 30% to 56% of all adults in the United States have had at least one episode of an alcohol-related problem. Thirteen percent of men qualify for a diagnosis of current alcohol abuse or dependence, compared with 4% of women. Several million Americans engage in risky drinking patterns that result in serious alcohol-related problems such as traumatic or fatal injuries. For example, during spring break, college students who abuse alcohol have been fatally injured during falls from high places or while diving into pools from hotel balconies. Heavy

drinking patterns also result in motor vehicle accidents, burns, severe depression, suicide, or homicide (NCADI, 2003; NIAAA, 2003). See Supporting Evidence for Practice 25-1 for information about mortality and alcohol.

NIDA Survey. Fifty-three percent of the men and women surveyed in the United States reported that one or more close relatives abuse or are dependent on alcohol. Alcohol abuse is present in 3% to 15% of the elderly population, 18% of medical inpatients, and 44% of psychiatric patients. Caucasians have the highest rate of alcohol use (56%). No statistical differences are noted for race or ethnicity with the heavy use of alcohol (5.7% for whites, 6.3% for Hispanics, and 4.6% for African Americans). Approximately 70% of adults with college degrees currently are drinkers, compared with only 40% of those with less than a high school education. These statistics dispel the idea that drinking is often associated with lower educational levels. Individuals with a college education may use alcohol to reduce stress or to socialize (NIDA, 2003; Sadock & Sadock, 2003).

Abuse of alcohol also is a major health problem for older children and adolescents. Approximately 28% of high school seniors and 41% of persons in the 21- to 22-year-old age group engage in binge drinking. Heavy drinking by adolescents is associated with emotional and behavioral problems. Data show that adolescents who drink heavily also skip school, use illicit drugs, steal from others, feel sad and depressed, run away from home, and try to injure themselves or commit suicide more often than their non-drinking counterparts (*Clinical Psychiatry News*, 2000).

Illicit Drug or Substance Use and Abuse

The more commonly abused illicit drugs today are cocaine, marijuana, inhalants, and heroin. Statistics regarding illicit drug or substance use and abuse are available through various agencies including the National Survey on Drug Use and Health (NSDUH) that replaced the annual National Household Survey on Drug Abuse (NHSDA) in 2002; the NIDA; and the DEA. A summary of their latest reports follows.

NSDUH Survey. According to the NSDUH (2004) survey, more than 11.1 million people aged 12 or older (or 4.6% of the population) have used 3,4-methylenedioxymethamphetamine (MDMA; ecstasy). Between

Cardiovascular System

Cardiovascular system complications include portal hypertension, weakened heart muscle, and heart failure. Broken blood vessels in the upper cheeks close to the nose and bloodshot eyes are common.

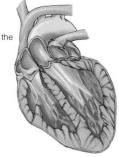

Brain

Central nervous system depression, resulting in peripheral neuropathy, interference with nerve conduction, gait changes, and nerve palsies, occurs frequently. Chronic dependence may cause dementia.

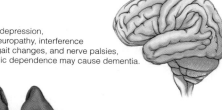

Respiratory System

Respiratory tract complications include respiratory depression and a depressed cough reflex because of the sedative effect of alcohol. The alcoholic person is susceptible to pneumonia and other respiratory infections.

Bone Marrow / Blood Cells

Anemia, an increased susceptibility to infection, and bruising and bleeding tendencies result from a decrease in red and white blood cells and abnormal bone marrow functioning.

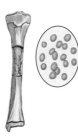

Gastrointestinal Tract

Gastrointestinal tract complications include acute gastritis, pancreatitis, hepatitis, cirrhosis of the liver, esophageal varices, hemorrhoids, and ascites. The alcoholic client usually has a poor nutritional status, including deficiencies of vitamins A, B, D, and K.

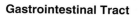

Reproduction

Reproductive system complications include prostatitis, interference with voiding, and release of sexual inhibitions. Fetal alcohol syndrome caused by maternal drinking during pregnancy results in abnormalities in the newborn such as heart defects, abnormally shaped heads and limbs, genital defects, and mental retardation.

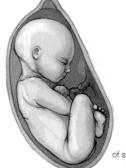

FIGURE 25.1 Effects of alcohol.

The Relationship Between Alcoholism and Mortality in White Males

PROBLEM UNDER INVESTIGATION / What is the relative risk of mortality among white male problem drinkers?

SUMMARY OF RESEARCH / Subjects were 1,853 white male problem drinkers aged 18 to 79 years who received treatment for alcohol-related problems at community mental health centers in the state of Vermont in 1991. Comparison group data were derived from the state vital records database. Researchers concluded that participation in treatment programs was highest for subjects aged 18–29 years, followed by subjects who were aged 30–49 years. Problem drinkers who were aged 18–29 years were 4.3 times as likely to die during the study compared with the general population of the same age group; problem drinkers aged 30–49 years were 2.5 times as likely to die compared with the general population of the same group; and problem drinkers over the age of 50 years were 1.5 times as likely to die than the general population of men in the same age category.

SUPPORT FOR PRACTICE / The psychiatric–mental health nurse should assess for alcohol-related problems during each visit by children, adolescents, and adults, regardless of presenting complaints. Client education should include a discussion of the risks of increased mortality when abusing alcohol.

SOURCE: Banks, S. M., Pandiani, J. A., Schacht, L. M., & Gauvin, L. M. (2000). Age and mortality among white male problem drinkers. Addiction, 95(8), 1249-1254.

2003 and 2004, the number of current users of MDMA decreased from 470,000 to 450,000 (0.2% of the population in both years). NSDUH also reported that 11.7 million people (or 4.9% of the population) used methamphetamine at least once during their lifetime. The number of current users of methamphetamine decreased from 607,000 (or 0.3% of the population) in 2003 to 583,000 (or 0.2% of the population) in 2004.

NIDA Survey. Among students surveyed by NIDA (2004), 16.6% of eighth graders (compared with 23% in 2002), 31.2% of tenth graders (compared with 41% in 2002), and 47.9% of twelfth graders (compared with 59% in 2002) reported that "club drugs" (eg, MDMA, methamphetamine, ketamine, flunitrazepam [Rohypnol], gamma-hydroxybutyrate [GHB]) were easy or very easy to obtain.

The majority of illicit substance users are white, non-Hispanic persons (74%). Men (8.5%) have a higher rate of illicit drug use than women (4.5%). The highest rates of drug abuse were found among young people ages 16 to 17 years (19.2%), compared with ages 18 to 20 years (17.3%). Only about 1% of people age 50 years and older reported using illicit drugs (NIDA, 2004).

Most illicit substance users begin to use and abuse substances when they are young. The development of addiction is rare after young adulthood. Mortality among young users is high; however, with improved medical management of various diseases, it is expected that during the coming decades, larger proportions of young-adult substance abusers will survive into old age (NIDA, 2004).

DEA Survey. According to estimates from the DEA survey, prescription medication abuse accounts for nearly 30% of the nation's drug problem. Addiction disorders affect 20% to 50% of hospitalized clients; 15% to 30% of clients in primary care settings; and as many as 50% of clients with a psychiatric illness. Moreover, approximately 72% of clients with an addiction disorder are believed to have a comorbid psychiatric diagnosis (DEA, 2006).

Hydrocodone (Vicodin, Lortab) continues to be the most widely abused prescribed medication in the U.S. Other potentially addictive medications that are not specifically regulated include carisoprodol (Soma); tramadol (Ultram); and dextromethorphan (DXM), a cough suppressant in OTC cough syrups. Attracted by easy availability, teenagers and young adults are increasingly abusing DXM, which, when taken at higher than prescribed doses, can cause euphoria and psychotic symptoms (DEA, 2006; Finn, 2004).

Approximately 80% of benzodiazepine abuse occurs in conjunction with opioids and/or alcohol. Name recognition makes trade name prescription drugs more attractive than their generic equivalents and medications in capsules are more desirable because they can be altered easily (Roscoe, 2004).

Specialty Practice: Addictions Nursing Practice

In the 1970s and 1980s, the care of clients with substance-related disorders became recognized as a unique nursing practice field. The International Nurses Society on Addictions (IntNSA) is a professional specialty organization founded in 1975 for nurses committed to the prevention, intervention, treatment, and management of addictive disorders including alcohol and other drug dependencies, nicotine dependencies, eating disorders, dual and multiple diagnosis, and process addictions such as gambling. IntNSA's mission is to advance excellence in addictions nursing practice through advocacy, collaboration, education, research and policy development (IntNSA, 2006).

In 1987, the publication *The Care of Clients With Addictions: Dimensions of Addictions Nursing Practice* described the dimensions of nursing practice associated with substance-related disorders as including the care of clients with a broad range of abuse and addiction patterns (ANA, Drug and Alcohol Nursing Association, & NNSA, 1987). **Addictions nursing** was defined as an area of specialty practice concerned with care related to dysfunctional patterns of human response that have one or more of the following key characteristics: some loss of self-control capacity, episodic or continuous maladaptive behavior or abuse of some substance, and development of dependence patterns of a physical and/or psychological nature. The addictions nurse addresses needs at every point on the health–illness continuum, uses skills from a number of nursing specialties, and collaborates with professionals in medicine, psychology, social work, and other disciplines. The recognition of addictions nursing as a distinct practice area led to the development of *Standards of Addictions Nursing Practice With Selected Diagnoses and Criteria,* published in 1988 (ANA & NNSA).

Etiology of Substance-Related Disorders

Several theories describe the onset of substance-related disorders. A brief summary of the more common theories as well as the disease concept of alcoholism follows.

Biologic Theories

The discovery that all drugs of abuse have one thing in common—namely, the stimulation of dopamine secretion—occurred in the 1980s. With scientific innovations, studies have identified the neural structures and pathways responsible for pleasure and reinforcement of behavior. For example, researchers have discovered that the brains of addicts have fewer dopamine D2 receptors in several regions of their brains than do the brains of control subjects. Addictive drugs such as cocaine, methamphetamine, heroin, and alcoholism capture these receptor sites and pathways or neural circuits and subvert normal functions (Yasgur, 2004). For instance, cocaine blocks the mechanism by which dopamine is reabsorbed into the cells that release dopamine. Amphetamines provoke the release of dopamine. Nicotine acts on a receptor for the neurotransmitter acetylcholine, possibly preventing the enzyme mono-amine oxidase from breaking up the dopamine molecule. Opiates act at receptor sites for the brain's own morphine-like substances. Sedative-hypnotics, alcohol, barbiturates, and benzodiazepines act in various parts of the brain on neurons that release γ-aminobutyric acid (GABA), which directs neurons to stop firing. Consequently, alcohol and drugs can change the way individuals feel and cause them to want to take these substances more often (Grinspoon, 1998a; Smith, 1999).

Researchers have also speculated that some individuals have a predisposition to or are at risk for addiction due to a high level of stress hormones, a deficit in dopamine function that is temporarily corrected by their drug of choice, or the presence of electrical phenomena in the brains of people at risk for alcoholism (Grinspoon, 1998b).

Genetic Theories

Separate studies of twins, adoptees, and siblings indicate that the cause of alcohol abuse has a genetic component. According to Grinspoon, "Individual differences in sensitivity to the addictive powers of drugs are almost certainly strongly influenced by genetics" (1998b, p. 1). Jellinek (1977, 1988) theorized that some individuals have a predisposition to alcoholism as a result of the "loss of control" over alcohol. His theory was supported by comparing data from studies of twins living with their biologic parents to data from studies of twins born to alcoholic parents, but separated after birth and raised by nonalcoholic foster parents. The data indicated that children born to alcoholic parents are particularly susceptible to becoming alcoholic (Goodwin, 1992, 1979). Additional studies with less conclusive data show that other types of substance-related disorders may be caused by a genetic component (Sadock & Sadock, 2003).

Behavioral and Learning Theories

Behavioral theorists believe that addiction results from the positive effect of mood alterations and reduction in feelings of fear and anxiety that one experiences using drugs or alcohol. Additionally, several types of learning are thought to be associated with compulsive self-administration of drugs.

Associative learning is exhibited during relapses experienced among clients addicted to psychostimulants. The brain is specifically designed to absorb and respond in very powerful ways to environmental cues and contexts. Nothing could be more specific, or powerful, than large doses of mind-altering drugs. The brain stores discrete patterns of information related to specific drug usage and produces context-independent sensitization of the organism to the drug or a general lethargy and unresponsiveness to the environment. The response depends on the individual's choice of substance (Medina, 2000).

Sociocultural Theories

The potential for addiction is affected by economic conditions, formal and informal social controls, cultural and ethnic traditions (eg, Asians and conservative Protestants use alcohol less frequently than do liberal Protestants and Catholics), and the companionship and approval of other drug users (Grinspoon, 1998b; Sadock & Sadock, 2003).

Additionally, a drug must be available in sufficient amounts to sustain addiction. For example, college dormitories and military bases are two social settings in which excessive and frequent drinking are often considered normal and socially expected. People risk addiction when they lack other capacities, choices, interest, or sources of attachment to something outside themselves.

Teenagers are at risk for alcohol abuse because it is the drug of choice among most adults, it is legal, and it is socially acceptable. Parents indirectly sanction the use of alcohol by drinking in front of their children and telling them that alcoholic beverages are acceptable if drunk in moderation.

Teenagers who possess more leisure time and money and experience less parental or community supervision are at risk for substance abuse, especially when they attend weekend or all-night parties. Drugs

are available "everywhere," according to grade-school children. OTC drugs, prescriptions readily obtained for insomnia, and pain-relief medication used by parents all make substance abuse easy for children and teenagers.

Peers and their values are particularly strong influences. Experimentation, curiosity, rebellion, and boredom are just a few reasons cited by adolescents when asked why they use or abuse drugs (National Criminal Justice Reference Service [NCJRS], 2004a).

Psychodynamic Theories

Although a particular **addictive personality** has not been identified, many theorists consider individuals who abuse substances to be fixed at an oral or infantile level of development. The abuser searches for immediate gratification of needs, or ways to escape tension, turning to alcohol or drugs to experience euphoria or oblivion. Characteristics frequently seen include low self-esteem, feelings of dependency, low tolerance for frustration and anxiety, antisocial behavior, and fear. Theorists are not certain whether these characteristics were present before the addictive behavior or whether the characteristics are a result of substance or alcohol abuse (Berman, 2001; Sadock & Sadock, 2003).

Other theorists believe that early childhood rejection, overprotection, or undue responsibility can cause an individual to become dependent on alcohol or drugs to cope with increased anxiety, depression, social or sexual inadequacy, increased social pressures, self-destructive behavior, or due to a desire to lower one's inhibitions (Berman, 2001).

Disease Concept of Alcoholism

The American Medical Association and the U.S. Public Health Service consider alcoholism to be a disease. Most authorities in the field of alcohol abuse base their beliefs on the pioneering work of Jellinek (1988). He surveyed 2,000 alcoholic men and classified alcoholics into five types. He also identified four progressive phases that the alcoholic experiences.

Alcohol is known to shorten an individual's life span by 12 to 15 years unless treatment is received. Like other chronic illnesses, it has certain observable symptoms. For example, tolerance occurs as the individual drinks more with less effect. Withdrawal occurs when an individual abruptly stops drinking after alcohol has become a necessity of life to maintain functioning. Finally, alcoholism can be fatal.

The same can be said for substance abuse, because both the alcoholic and the substance or drug abuser lose control over when they drink or take drugs, how much they take, and where the abuse occurs.

Clinical Symptoms and Diagnostic Characteristics of Alcohol-Related Disorders

Alcohol (eg, beer, wine, whiskey) is considered a central nervous system (CNS) depressant that causes false self-confidence, false sense of belonging, and lowering of inhibition. Figure 25-1, mentioned earlier in the chapter, depicts the potential medical problems related to the use or abuse of alcohol. Individuals who are dependent on or who abuse alcohol often exhibit impairments in judgment, orientation, memory, affect, cognition, speech, and mobility, as well as behavioral changes.

Two categories of alcohol-related disorders are included in this classification. The first, alcohol use disorders, includes alcohol dependence and alcohol abuse. The second, alcohol-induced disorders, includes 12 subtypes:

1. Alcohol intoxication
2. Alcohol withdrawal
3. Alcohol intoxication delirium
4. Alcohol withdrawal delirium
5. Alcohol-induced persisting dementia
6. Alcohol-induced persisting amnestic disorder
7. Alcohol-induced psychotic disorder
8. Alcohol-induced mood disorder
9. Alcohol-induced anxiety disorder
10. Alcohol-induced sexual dysfunction
11. Alcohol-induced sleep disorder
12. Alcohol-related disorder, not otherwise specified

Both alcohol use disorders are discussed in the sections that follow; selected alcohol-induced disorders are also discussed.

Alcohol Use Disorders

Patterns of alcohol use disorders include alcohol dependence and alcohol abuse. An understanding of these patterns is essential for psychiatric–mental health nursing practice.

Alcohol Dependence

Alcohol dependence is characterized by tolerance to alcohol or by the development of withdrawal phe-

nomena upon cessation of or reduction in intake (Shahkroh & Hales, 2003). Alcohol dependence and alcohol abuse (see discussion that follows) share features with other substance-dependence and -abuse disorders such as those associated with sedatives, hypnotics, and anxiolytics.

The essential feature of alcohol dependence is a cluster of cognitive, behavioral, and physiologic symptoms indicating that the individual continues use of the alcohol despite critical alcohol-related problems. There is a maladaptive pattern of alcohol use resulting in distress as the individual experiences a cluster of three or more of seven stated symptoms during a 12-month period:

1. Tolerance, defined as a need for markedly increased amounts of alcohol to achieve desired effect or a markedly diminished effect with continued use of the same amount of alcohol
2. Withdrawal symptoms or the continued use of alcohol to relieve or avoid withdrawal symptoms
3. Intake of alcohol in larger amounts or over a longer period of time than that which was intended
4. Persistent desire or unsuccessful efforts to cut down or control use of alcohol
5. A significant amount of time spent in activities necessary to obtain alcohol, drink alcohol, or recover from its effects
6. Social, occupational, or recreational activities given up or reduced because of drinking alcohol
7. Continued drinking of alcohol despite knowledge of having a persistent or recurrent physical or psychological problem that is likely to have been caused or exacerbated by alcohol

The *DSM-IV-TR* also lists specifiers to accompany the diagnosis. These include with physiologic dependence (evidence of tolerance or withdrawal) or without physiologic dependence (no evidence of withdrawal or tolerance).

Alcohol Abuse Disorder

The criteria for alcohol abuse disorder do not include tolerance, withdrawal, or a pattern of compulsive use. The individual exhibits one or more of the following symptoms in a 12-month period:

1. Recurrent drinking of alcohol resulting in a failure to fulfill major role obligations at work, school, or home

2. Recurrent drinking in situations in which it is physically hazardous
3. Recurrent alcohol-related legal problems
4. Continued use despite having persistent or recurrent social or interpersonal problems caused by alcoholism

Alcohol-Induced Disorders

Alcohol-induced disorders are the result of the effects of alcohol on the CNS. Clients with alcohol-induced disorders exhibit impairment of neurologic functioning such as delirium or dementia. They also may exhibit behavioral changes.

Alcohol Intoxication

Alcohol intoxication occurs after the recent ingestion of alcohol and is evidenced by behavioral changes such as decreased inhibition, impaired social or occupational functioning, fighting, or impaired judgment. The client may exhibit mood changes, increased verbalization, impaired attention span, or irritability. Other symptoms include slurred speech, disorientation, facial flushing, lack of coordination, unsteady gait, nystagmus, impaired memory, disorientation, and stupor or coma.

Alcohol Withdrawal

Clients generally experience clinical symptoms of **alcohol withdrawal** within several hours to a few days after the cessation or reduction of heavy and prolonged alcohol consumption. The client may experience symptoms such as autonomic hyperactivity; increased hand tremor; sleep disturbances, insomnia, or nightmares; nausea or vomiting; transient visual, tactile, or auditory hallucinations or illusions; delusions, psychomotor agitation; anxiety; and grand mal seizures. Increased blood pressure may occur. Elevated temperatures in excess of 100°F (37.3°C) and pulse in excess of 100 beats per minute may indicate impending alcohol withdrawal delirium.

Alcohol Withdrawal Delirium

Alcohol withdrawal delirium, also referred to as **delirium tremens,** may occur from 24 to 72 hours after the client's last drink. Elevation of vital signs accompanies restlessness, tremulousness, agitation, and hyperalertness. Any noises or quick movements are perceived as greatly exaggerated, shadows are misinterpreted, and illusions and hallucinations frequently occur. The client's speech is incoherent. Serious medical complications may occur if the client is left untreated.

Alcoholic-Induced Persisting Dementia

Individuals who experience a prolonged, chronic dependence on alcohol may develop alcoholic-induced persisting dementia. Clinical symptoms include a severe loss of intellectual ability that interferes with social or occupational functioning and impaired memory, judgment, and abstract thinking. Permanent brain damage can occur in severe cases.

Alcoholic-Induced Persisting Amnestic Disorder

Individuals who drink large amounts of alcohol over a prolonged period often have poor nutritional habits. Two CNS disorders are associated with alcoholism. The first, **Korsakoff's psychosis,** is a form of amnesia characterized by a loss of short-term memory and the inability to learn new skills. Clinical symptoms include disorientation and the use of confabulation. Degenerative changes in the thalamus occur because of a deficiency of B-complex vitamins, especially thiamine and B_{12}. The second disorder is **Wernicke's encephalopathy,** an inflammatory hemorrhagic, degenerative condition of the brain caused by a thiamine deficiency. Lesions occur in the hypothalamus, mamillary bodies, and tissues surrounding ventricles and aqueducts. Clinical symptoms include double vision, involuntary and rapid eye movements, lack of muscular coordination, and decreased mental function, which may be mild or severe.

Other Alcohol-Induced Disorders

Individuals who abuse alcohol can develop depression, anxiety, sexual dysfunction, and sleep disorders. Clinical symptoms of anxiety, depression, and sleep disorders were discussed in earlier chapters. Sexual disorders are discussed in Chapter 26.

Clinical Symptoms and Diagnostic Characteristics of Other Substance-Related Disorders

Ten classes of substances, other than alcohol, are associated with both abuse and dependence: amphetamines, caffeine, cannabis, cocaine, hallucinogens, inhalants, nicotine, opioids, phencyclidine (PCP), and the group of sedatives, hypnotics, and anxiolytics.

A diagnosis of multiple-substance or polysubstance abuse occurs when people mix drugs and alcohol. The severity of psychoactive substance dependence is classified according to the following criteria: mild, moderate, severe, in partial remission, or in full remission.

Sedative-, Hypnotic-, or Anxiolytic-Related Disorders

Substances included in the category of sedatives, hypnotics, and anxiolytics include benzodiazepines, carbamates, barbiturates, barbiturate-like hypnotics, all prescription sleeping medications, and all anxiolytic medications except the nonbenzodiazepine antianxiety agents (eg, buspirone). Ingestion of these drugs in high doses can be lethal, especially when they are mixed with alcohol.

Taken orally or intravenously, these drugs are used to relax the CNS or slow down body processes. They temporarily ease tension and induce sleep. Medically, they may be used in the treatment of hypertension, peptic ulcers, or seizures; as a relaxant before and during surgery; and as a sedative for use in mental and physical illness.

Normal effects of these drugs include a decrease in cardiac and respiratory rate, lowered blood pressure, and a mild depressant action on nerves, skeletal muscles, and the heart. Overdoses or intoxication may result in symptoms such as slurred speech, incoordination, drunken appearance, staggering gait, nystagmus, impaired memory, stupor, or coma. Other symptoms may include poor judgment, mood swings, paranoia, lack of sexual inhibition, and aggressive impulses. Medical symptoms include dry mouth, headaches, dizziness, chills, and diarrhea (American Psychiatric Association [APA], 2000; Sadock & Sadock, 2003). Street names for these drugs include "libs," "blues," "rainbows," "yellow-jackets," and "downers."

Barbiturates are the leading cause of accidental poisoning, as well as a primary method of committing suicide. Barbiturate dependency is one of the most difficult disorders to cure. Clinical symptoms of sedative, hypnotic, or anxiolytic withdrawal may include diaphoresis, increased pulse rate (greater than 100 beats per minute), hand tremors, nausea and vomiting, insomnia, transient hallucinations or illusions, psychomotor agitation, and anxiety (APA, 2000; Sadock & Sadock, 2003).

Opioid-Related Disorders

An opioid is a drug or naturally occurring substance that resembles opium or one or more of its alkaloid derivatives. *Opiates* are powerful drugs derived from the poppy plant that have been used for centuries to relieve pain. The opioid classification includes natural opioids such as morphine, semi-synthetics such as heroin, and synthetics with morphine-like action such as codeine or methadone. Medications such as pentazocine, which has both opiate agonist and antagonist effects, are also included in this classification.

Opioids are narcotic drugs that induce sleep, suppress coughing, and alleviate pain. People abuse opiates by taking them orally, inhaling them (eg, snorting or smoking), or injecting them into their veins in an attempt to help relieve withdrawal symptoms, for "kicks," or to "feel good." The user becomes passive and listless as the opioids depress the respiratory center of the brain, causing shallow respirations. The person also experiences reduced feelings of hunger, thirst, pain, and sexual desire. As the effects of the drug wear off, the user, who becomes physically and emotionally addicted by requiring increasingly larger dosages, suffers withdrawal symptoms unless another dose of the drug is taken.

Opioids, also referred to as "white stuff," "hard stuff," and "junk," are considered to be the most addictive drugs. Acute overdose or intoxication is identified by symptoms of drowsiness; slurred speech; decreased, slow respirations; constricted pupils; and a rapid, weak pulse. The client also may exhibit mood swings, psychomotor agitation or retardation, impaired judgment, or impaired social or occupational functioning (APA, 2000; Sadock & Sadock, 2003).

Opioid withdrawal symptoms begin 12 to 16 hours after the last dose and are characterized by watery eyes, rhinitis, yawning, sneezing, and diaphoresis. Other symptoms include dilated pupils, restlessness and tremors, goose bumps, irritability, loss of appetite, muscle cramps, nausea and vomiting, fever, and diarrhea. Symptoms subside in 5 to 10 days if no treatment occurs (APA, 2000; Sadock & Sadock, 2003).

Amphetamine-Related Disorders

Amphetamines or amphetamine-like substances are medically indicated for the treatment of attention-deficit–hyperactivity disorder, narcolepsy, weight reduction, and treatment-resistant depression. Amphetamines ("pep pills") are drugs that directly stimulate the CNS and create a feeling of alertness and self-confidence in the user. They are also referred to by drug abusers as "wake-ups," "speed," "eye-openers," "co-pilots," "truck drivers," "uppers," or "bennies."

These drugs are often abused by oral ingestion, injection into veins, smoking, or inhalation of large doses to obtain an exaggerated effect of the stimulating action. People also take these drugs for kicks, for thrills, or to combat boredom; to stay awake or to allow greater physical effort; or to counteract the effects of alcohol and barbiturates. Amphetamines are considered to be dangerous because they can drive a user to do things beyond his or her physical limits; they can cause mental fatigue, dizziness, and feelings of fear and confusion; and sudden withdrawal can lead to depression and suicide. The heart and circulatory system also may be damaged from the adverse effects of adrenaline overproduction due to drug abuse.

Clinical symptoms of intoxication include tachycardia or bradycardia, alterations in blood pressure, cardiac arrhythmias, respiratory depression, pupillary dilation, excitability, tremors of the hands, increased talkativeness, profuse diaphoresis, dry mouth, nausea and vomiting, weight loss, headaches, pallor, diarrhea, and unclear speech (APA, 2000; Sadock & Sadock, 2003). The abuser can develop a psychological dependence on stimulants and may experience delusions, auditory and visual hallucinations, or a drug psychosis that resembles schizophrenia. Clinical symptoms of withdrawal include dysphoria, fatigue, altered sleep patterns, increased appetite, dreams, and psychomotor agitation or retardation (APA, 2000; Sadock & Sadock, 2003).

Cocaine-Related Disorders

Cocaine is a short-acting CNS stimulant substance that is extracted from the leaves of the South American coca plant (*Erythroxylon coca*). Historically, the leaves of the plant were chewed for refreshment, and were used by peasant laborers to relieve fatigue and fight off pain or hunger. Cocaine also produces feelings of happiness, alertness, sensory awareness, and enhances one's self-esteem.

Cocaine is available as a white crystalline powder or in larger pieces referred to as "rocks." Powdered cocaine is usually sniffed, snorted, smoked in a pipe (freebasing), or injected into a vein or subcutaneous tissue.

Physical effects of cocaine intoxication include immediate dilation of the pupils and an increase or decrease in blood pressure, pulse, respirations, and body temperature. Users may also experience a loss of appetite, nausea and vomiting, weight loss, insomnia, impaired thinking, agitation, seizures, chest pain, or coma (APA, 2000; Sadock & Sadock, 2003). Long-term effects include chronic nose bleed, runny nose, chronic sore throat, exhaustion, respiratory ailments, vitamin deficiencies, dangerous weight loss, and miscarriage/birth defects.

Clients who experience cocaine withdrawal may exhibit fatigue, an increased appetite, altered sleep patterns, and behavioral changes such as agitation or psychomotor retardation. Panic attacks or cocaine psychosis may occur. Individuals with a history of cardiac disease may experience chest pain, heart attack, or heart failure. Cocaine also can cause sudden heart attack in healthy young people (APA, 2000; Sadock & Sadock, 2003).

Cannabis-Related Disorders

Marijuana is a common plant with the biologic name of *Cannabis sativa*. With the ability to act as a stimulant or depressant, it is often considered to be a mild hallucinogen with some sedative properties. As of February 2005, 12 states have legalized the use of marijuana to alleviate the symptoms of nausea and vomiting during chemotherapy, stimulate appetite in clients with HIV/AIDS, and lower ocular pressure in clients with glaucoma: Alaska, Arizona, California, Colorado, Hawaii, Maine, Montana, Nevada, Oregon, Rhode Island, Vermont, and Washington (DEA, 2006). With written certification from a physician, clients or their caregivers are able to register with a state to grow and use marijuana. The physician, client, and caregiver are all protected from arrest and prosecution.

When used illegally, marijuana is often combined with other addictive substances such as alcohol or nicotine. Most users in the 18- to 25-year-old age range are male. Many people who try marijuana go on to use it extensively, and many of these people use it in combination with other substances such as opioids, PCP, or hallucinogens (APA, 2000; Pfizer, Inc., 1996).

Persons who use marijuana usually smoke it in a pipe or as a rolled cigarette ("joint"). Individuals also may take it orally as capsules or tablets, on sugar cubes, or in food. Holders ("roach clips") are used to get the last puffs from marijuana cigarette butts when they become too short to handle with fingers. Slang names for marijuana include "pot," "herb," "grass," "weed," "smoke," and "Mary Jane."

Marijuana acts quickly, in approximately 15 minutes, after it enters the bloodstream, and its effects last approximately 2 to 4 hours. It affects a person's mood, thinking, behavior, and judgment in different ways, and in large doses it can cause hallucinations.

General physiologic symptoms of intoxication include increased appetite, lowered body temperature, depression, drowsiness, unsteady gait, inability to think clearly, excitement, reduced coordination and reflexes, and impaired judgment. Users of large amounts may experience suicidal ideation or have delusions of invulnerability, causing them to take risks.

Although marijuana is not considered to be physically addicting and no withdrawal criteria have been established, it may lead to psychological dependence, thereby retarding personality growth and adjustment to adulthood. Its use also can expose the user to those using and pushing stronger drugs (APA, 2000).

Hallucinogen- and Phencyclidine-Related Disorders

Hallucinogens and PCP are associated only with abuse because physiologic dependence has not been demonstrated. They are referred to as "mind benders" or psychedelic drugs, affecting the mind and causing changes in perception and consciousness.

Hallucinogens

Examples of hallucinogens include lysergic acid diethylamide (LSD), mescaline, dimethyltryptamine (DMT), 2,5 dimethoxy-4-methylamphetamine (STP), and psilocybin. They may be taken orally or injected.

Similar to marijuana, but stronger in the effect on the body, hallucinogens are dangerous because intoxication can lead to panic, paranoia, flashbacks, or death. Physiologic symptoms include increased pulse rate, blood pressure, and temperature; dilated pupils; tremors of hands and feet; cold, sweaty palms; flushed face or pallor; irregular respirations; and nausea. Effects on the CNS include an increased distortion of senses (visual, auditory, and tactile hallucinations), loss of the ability to separate fact from fantasy, loss of sense of time, ambivalence, and the inability to reason logically (APA, 2000; Sadock & Sadock, 2003).

Hallucinogens are quite unpredictable. One experience ("trip") with them may be good but the next one may be disastrous. The daughter of former television personality Art Linkletter leaped from her apartment in a suicidal panic brought on by LSD. Diane had an exciting career, loving family, good health, and no material worries. According to her father, no explana-tion could be found for her tragic death except the fact that she had taken LSD.

Phencyclidine (PCP)

PCP, commonly known as "angel dust," is an extremely dangerous substance. It can be taken orally or smoked. Originally used as a surgical anesthetic, PCP was found to cause extreme agitation, ataxia, stupor, hallucinations, and psychosis. Persons who experience PCP intoxication have enormous strength, experience unbelievably paranoid reactions, and literally do not know pain. They may become violent, destructive, and confused after one dose. Clinical symptoms of PCP intoxication include vomiting, seizures, tachycardia, muscle rigidity, and extremely high blood pressure (APA, 2000; Sadock & Sadock, 2003).

Inhalant-Related Disorders

Inhalants are any chemicals that give off fumes or vapors and, when inhaled, produce symptoms similar to intoxication. Commonly abused inhalants include glue, gasoline, lighter fluid, paint thinner, varnish, shellac, nail polish remover, and aerosol-packaged products. The person who inhales or sniffs such substances may experience inhalant intoxication. Clinical symptoms include unsteady gait, slurred speech, dizziness, nystagmus, tremor, blurred vision, lethargy, depressed reflexes, muscle weakness, euphoria, stupor, or coma. After such a "high," the person may experience a loss of coordination, a distorted perception of reality, and hallucinations and convulsions (APA, 2000; Sadock & Sadock, 2003). Although withdrawal-like symptoms have occurred in animals exposed to certain inhalants, no clinically meaningful withdrawal syndrome occurs in humans.

Dangers of inhaling gasoline, glue, or paint thinners include temporary blindness and damage to the lungs, brain, and liver. Immediate effects of inhalant abuse may last from a few seconds to several minutes. Chronic effects may occur at any time after inhalation of toxic products or materials. Deaths have occurred as a result of suffocation caused by placing a plastic bag, moistened cloth, or plastic container against one's face.

Caffeine- and Nicotine-Related Disorders

Caffeine is available in a variety of sources such as coffee, soda, tea, OTC analgesics and cold remedies, stimulants, and weight-loss aids. Some individuals display some aspects of dependence and exhibit tolerance, and perhaps withdrawal, when consuming large amounts of caffeine. There is evidence that caffeine intoxication can be clinically significant. Clinical symptoms of intoxication include restlessness, nervousness, excitement, insomnia, flushed face, diuresis, gastrointestinal disturbance, muscle twitching, rambling thoughts or speech, tachycardia or arrhythmia, hypertension, periods of inexhaustibility, and psychomotor agitation (APA, 2000; Sadock & Sadock, 2003).

Nicotine, the active ingredient in tobacco, is available in the form of cigarettes, cigars, chewing tobacco, and dipping tobacco. It is a stimulant that elevates one's blood pressure and increases one's heartbeat. Tar, found in the smoke, contains many carcinogens. Long-term effects of tobacco dependence include emphysema, chronic bronchitis, coronary heart disease, and a variety of cancers.

Approximately 28% of adult women and 30% of adult men smoke cigarettes for stimulation, to relax or feel better, or due to habit. Regular smokers become psychologically dependent on cigarettes and find it difficult to stop smoking. Tobacco dependence usually begins in late adolescence or by early adulthood and may result in tobacco withdrawal when the person attempts to stop smoking. Symptoms of withdrawal include a craving for tobacco, irritability, difficulty concentrating, restlessness, anxiety, headache, drowsiness, and gastrointestinal disturbances. Nicotine has been linked with respiratory problems such as emphysema, chronic bronchitis, and cancer. It can cause hypertension, cardiac disease, and low–birth-weight babies.

Designer Drugs, Club Drugs, and Anabolic Steroids

Three popular categories of illicit substances that are readily accessible to the public include designer drugs, club drugs, and anabolic steroids. To some individuals, these substances seem harmless. However, in reality, they can cause serious physical and psychological problems, even death. Some of the substances—such as anabolic steroids and methamphetamine—are included in the *DSM-IV-TR* classification of substance-related disorders, whereas others cannot be easily grouped into a specific diagnostic category (eg, GHB or "liquid ecstasy") (Sadock & Sadock, 2003).

Designer Drugs

Designer drugs are amphetamine derivatives (N-analogs) that are classified as stimulants. They are cur-

rently manufactured in clandestine laboratories ("meth labs") and then made available on the street. Instructions on how to make methamphetamine and similar drugs appear on the Internet, and the ingredients, including the common OTC decongestant, pseudoephedrine, are easy to obtain. Statistics released by the DEA revealed that authorities reported 17,170 clandestine methamphetamine laboratory incidents in 2004 compared with 327 incidents a decade ago. Methamphetamine stays in the body about 10 times longer than cocaine, making it cheaper to use, thus increasing its appeal (Herrick, 2005).

Designer drugs differ from one another in their potency, speed of onset, duration of action, and their capacity to modify mood with or without producing overt hallucinations. Described as addictive and as potent reinforcers, they are usually taken orally, sometimes snorted, but rarely injected. Because they are produced in clandestine laboratories, they are seldom pure. Thus the amount in a capsule or tablet is likely to vary considerably. Examples of designer drugs include 4-methyl-2,5-dimethoxyamphetamine (DOM, also referred to as STP), 3,4-methylenedioxyamphetamine (MDA, also referred to as "ecstasy" or "XTC"), and 4-bromo-2,5-dimethoxyhenethylamine (NEXUS).

The use of ecstasy is a global phenomenon. The prevalence of its use in the United States is increasing among young adults. Ecstasy is being used legally in Switzerland as an adjunct in psychotherapy despite the occurrence of numerous fatal intoxications. Designer drugs are notoriously dangerous when mixed with alcohol and other drugs (Drew, 1999; Valentine, 2002).

Club Drugs

The term *club drugs* applies to certain illicit substances (including some designer drugs) that are primarily synthetic and are found at nightclubs, bars, and "raves" (all-night dance parties for adolescents and young adults). Substances that are often used include, but are not limited to, ketamine (animal anesthetic), flunitrazepam (Rohypnol), burundanga (Datura), and GHB. These substances are referred to as *date rape drugs*. Commonly used *designer drugs* include MDA and MDMA, and methamphetamine (NCJRS, 2004b). Table 25-1 identifies the classification and potential adverse effects of the more common club drugs.

Anabolic Steroids

Anabolic steroids are a family of drugs that includes the natural male hormone testosterone and a group of

TABLE 25.1 Club Drugs: Classification and Potential Adverse Effects

CLUB DRUG	CLASSIFICATION	POTENTIAL ADVERSE EFFECTS
MDMA (ecstasy)	Amphetamine	Critical elevation in BP, P Severe hyperthermia Heart or kidney failure Brain damage
gamma hydroxybutyrate (GHB)	CNS depressant (date-rape drug)	Increased muscle relaxation Loss of consciousness Inability to recall information after ingesting drug
flunitrazepam (Rohypnol)	CNS depressant (date-rape drug)	Similar to GHB
ketamine	Animal anesthetic (similar to phencyclidine [PCP])	Impaired motor function Elevated BP Amnesia Respiratory depression Seizures
methamphetamine	Addictive stimulant	Dramatic CNS effects Increased energy and alertness Decreased appetite Convulsions Hyperthermia Tremors Cerebral vascular accident Cardiac arrhythmia

National Criminal Justice Reference Service. (2004b). *In the spotlight: Club drugs summary.* Retrieved February 5, 2006, from http://www.ncjrs.org/club_drugs/summary.html

many synthetic analogues of testosterone synthesized since the 1940s. They are Schedule III drugs and are subject to the same regulatory dispensing requirements as narcotics. Athletes and adolescent men abuse steroids to enhance masculine appearance; men and women abuse steroids to maximize physical development. Adverse behavioral effects as well as medical complications may result, including acne, premature balding or alopecia, jaundice, abnormal liver function tests, cerebrovascular disease, and myocardial infarction. In men, unilateral or bilateral breast enlargement and decreased testicular and prostate size may occur. In women, menstrual problems, hirsutism, and a deepened voice may occur (Riggin, 1996a; Sadock & Sadock, 2003).

Prescription Drug Abuse

Although almost all prescription drugs can be misused, the three classifications of drugs most commonly abused are opioids, CNS depressants, and stimulants. Opioids (eg, morphine, codeine, oxycodone) are generally prescribed to treat pain, relieve coughs, and treat diarrhea. CNS depressants (eg, benzodiazepines, barbiturates) are used to treat anxiety, sleep disorders, and, in higher doses, are used as anesthetics. Stimulants (eg, methylphenidate) may be prescribed to treat sleep disorders (eg, narcolepsy), attention-deficit hyperactivity disorder (ADHD), and obesity (Roscoe, 2004). (See Chapter 16 for additional information regarding these drug classifications.)

The Controlled Substance Act (DEA, 2006) categorizes addictive substances into five categories or schedules depending upon their value for medical purposes and the potential for abuse:

- Schedule I: High potential for abuse; no accepted medical use in the United States under federal law (eg, heroin, cocaine, ecstasy, LSD, marijuana)

- Schedule II: High potential for abuse; accepted medical use with severe restrictions; may lead to severe physical dependence or addiction (eg, oxycodone hydrochloride [OxyContin], oxycodone/acetaminophen [Percocet], hydromorphone [Dilaudid], morphine)
- Schedule III: Less potential for abuse than Schedules I and II; accepted medical use; abuse may lead to moderate or low physical dependence or addiction (eg, anabolic steroids, hydrocodone [Vicodin], codeine, some barbiturates)
- Schedule IV: Low potential for abuse relative to drugs listed in Schedules I, II, III; accepted medical use; abuse may lead to limited physical dependence or addiction (eg, darvon, alprazolam, diazepam, lorazepam)
- Schedule V: Low potential for abuse relative to other controlled substances; accepted medical use; abuse may lead to limited physical dependence or addiction (eg, cough syrups with codeine)

Internet Addiction Disorder

Addictions have focused mainly on highs that are produced from the use of drugs or other external forces that affect the brain's chemical responses. Researchers have brought to the public's attention that an individual can receive a similar kind of "high" from using the Internet and have identified this behavior as *Internet addiction disorder (IAD)*. For example, China's first officially licensed clinic for Internet addiction located in Beijing has admitted 12 teenagers and young adults who have left school because of Internet addiction; that is, they play games or are in chat rooms every day. Assessment of these individuals revealed clinical symptoms associated with substance-related disorders (eg, depression, anxiety, fear, panic, social isolation, sleep disturbances, tremors, paresthesia). Authorities in China have begun to shut down Internet cafes because they are considered to be eroding public morality (Ang, 2005).

IAD affects everyone involved with the "user," and, moreover, there are only few clinicians who know how to treat it. Theories explaining why people become addicted to the Internet are similar to those presented earlier in this chapter (eg, biologic, genetic, behavioral, etc.). Several research studies are being conducted to determine whether this disorder should be included as a distinct disorder in the *DSM-IV-TR* (Duran, 2003).

Impaired Nurse

Nurses, like the rest of the community, can suffer from substance abuse or dependence. Many **impaired nurses** are not aware that they have problems, and resist any offer of support or help. Others, aware of their shortcomings, go to great efforts to mask their addictions. Although the behavior of impaired nurses varies according to the substance being used, the following actions by the nurse should be considered as possible impairment behavior:

- Volunteers to work overtime frequently especially on weekends when staffing ratios are less than during the weekdays
- Leaves the floor or unit frequently or spends a considerable amount of time in the bathroom
- Is frequently involved in incidents in which clients report they haven't received relief for pain (narcotic analgesics), insomnia (sedative hypnotics), or anxiety (benzodiazepines) although documentation indicates that they have received prescribed medication
- Exhibits lapses in memory, changes in personal appearance, and appears preoccupied
- Is on duty when the inaccurate drug counts occur
- Gives questionable explanations regarding drug wastage and discrepancies in documentation

Nurses who use or abuse substances can receive help in some states from the Board of Registration in Nursing, which may offer substance-abuse rehabilitation programs. For example, in 1983 the state of Florida established the Intervention Project for Nurses (IPN). Objectives of the IPN focus on the early intervention and close monitoring of nurses who are deemed unsafe to practice; providing a program for affected nurses to be rehabilitated in a therapeutic, nonpunitive, and confidential process; and providing an opportunity for the retention of nurses. If the nurse enters a program voluntarily and successfully completes it, she or he will avoid disciplinary action and loss of license (IPN, 2001–2006). Since 1983, several state boards of nursing have developed similar programs.

THE NURSING PROCESS

ASSESSMENT

"Data collection is the necessary first step in addressing the quality of the health of the client. The data collection process must be continual, systematic, accurate, and comprehensive to enable the addictions nurse and other members of the treatment team to reach sound conclusions, plan and implement interventions, and evaluate care" (ANA & NNSA, 1988, p. 6).

Clients suffering severe, inadequately treated chronic pain can closely resemble individuals with a substance-related disorder, posing assessment, diagnostic, and nursing management challenges. The term *pseudo-addicts* has been used to characterize clients whose desperation to obtain relief may resemble drug-seeking behavior. Pseudo-addicts may have a loss of control over their medication use, seek early prescription renewals, or report that their medication was lost. Unfortunately, unresolved pain can lead to true addiction, the chronic pain client's biggest fear (Bates, 2005).

During the assessment process, which may occur in the emergency room, general hospital, psychiatric unit, or drug treatment center, questions are directed toward identifying the substance(s) used, amount and frequency of use, duration of use, and route of administration if substances other than alcohol are involved. Information regarding any prior treatment for a substance-related disorder also is important.

Assessment of the Client Who Abuses Alcohol

The assessment of a client who abuses alcohol can be frustrating as well as challenging for several reasons. The client may use defense mechanisms of denial, rationalization, and projection when confronted about his or her drinking behavior. Family members or significant others may also be in denial of the client's drinking problem. Furthermore, they may be enablers (ie, perpetuating the person's dependence on alcohol)

who share the client's addiction to alcohol (eg, co-dependency).

General Description. The nurse uses the interview process to obtain data from the client, including the client's interpretation of the drinking problem (alcoholics tend to understate drinking habits) and attitude toward control of the problem. Data regarding the client's level of sensorium, mood and affect, ability to communicate needs and follow instructions, ability to meet basic needs, and general physical condition are collected. Document whether the client is inebriated, undergoing withdrawal, dehydrated, malnourished, in any physical distress, or at risk for injury due to an unsteady gait or the presence of tremors. Also obtain information regarding available support systems at this time.

The Clinical Institute Withdrawal Assessment for Alcohol (CIWA-Ar), available at www.fpnotebook. com/psy83.htm, serves as a guide for the nurse during physical assessment of clients suspected of alcohol abuse. The assessment focuses on the client's general appearance; level of orientation (eg, date, time, place); and the presence of clinical symptoms including nausea and vomiting (none, intermittent), tremor (with arms extended or at rest), paroxysmal sweating (palms, forehead), anxiety (mild, moderate, severe), agitation (fidgets, paces), tactile dysfunction (paresthesias), auditory and visual disturbances (hallucinations), and headache (none, moderate, severe, extreme). The assessment yields an objective score of the client's potential level of withdrawal (Family Practice Notebook.com, 2005).

Behavior. Observe the client's behavior, documenting whether the client is withdrawn, argumentative, hostile, disruptive, combative, or exhibiting any behavioral symptoms due to the presence of hallucinations, illusions, or delusions. Also note whether the client has exhibited any suicidal or homicidal thoughts or behaviors in the past. Finally, ask the client about any history of driving while under the influence or any other legal charges related to the use of alcohol.

Screening Tools for Alcohol Use or Abuse. Several screening tools are frequently used during the assessment process. They include the Michigan Alcohol Screening Test (MAST) (Box 25-1) and the CAGE Screening Test for Alcoholism (Box 25-2). The Alcohol Use Disorders Identification Test (AUDIT) also may be used. The AUDIT contains ten questions about quantity

BOX 25.1   MICHIGAN ALCOHOL SCREENING TEST (MAST)

The MAST involves a list of 26 questions, each with a specific point score. A total of 5 or more points on the MAST indicates the presence of alcoholism. A total of 4 points suggests a potential problem with alcohol. A total of 3 or fewer points indicates that the individual does not have a problem with alcohol.

POINTS	QUESTIONS
(0)	1. Do you enjoy a drink now and then?
(2)	2. Do you feel you are a normal drinker?*
(2)	3. Have you ever awakened the morning after some drinking the night before and found that you could not remember a part of the evening before?
(1)	4. Does your spouse (or parents) ever worry or complain about your drinking?
(2)	5. Can you stop drinking without a struggle after one or two drinks?*
(1)	6. Do you ever feel bad about your drinking?
(2)	7. Do friends and relatives think you are a normal drinker?*
(0)	8. Do you ever try to limit your drinking to certain times of the day or to certain places?
(2)	9. Are you always able to stop drinking when you want to?*
(4)	10. Have you ever attended a meeting of Alcoholics Anonymous (AA)?†
(1)	11. Have you gotten into fights when drinking?
(2)	12. Has drinking ever created problems with you and your spouse?
(2)	13. Has your spouse (or other family member) ever gone to anyone for help about your drinking?
(2)	14. Have you ever lost friends or girl- or boyfriends because of drinking?
(2)	15. Have you ever gotten into trouble at work because of drinking?
(2)	16. Have you ever lost a job because of drinking?
(2)	17. Have you ever neglected your obligations, your family, or your work for two or more days because you were drinking?
(1)	18. Do you ever drink before noon?
(2)	19. Have you ever been told you have liver trouble? Cirrhosis?
(2)	20. Have you ever had delirium tremens (DTs), severe shaking, heard voices, or seen things that were not there after heavy drinking?
(9)	21. Have you ever gone to anyone for help about your drinking?
(4)	22. Have you ever been in a hospital because of drinking?
(0)	23. a. Have you ever been a patient in a psychiatric hospital or on a psychiatric ward of a general hospital?
(2)	b. Was drinking part of the problem that resulted in hospitalization?*
(0)	24. a. Have you ever been seen at a psychiatric or mental health clinic, or gone to any doctor, social worker, or clergyman for help with an emotional problem?
(2)	b. Was drinking part of the problem?
(2)	25. Have you ever been arrested, even for a few hours, because of drunk behavior?
(2)	26. Have you ever been arrested for drunk driving after drinking?

*Negative responses are indicative of alcoholism.
†Positive response would be diagnostic of alcoholism.
A total of 4 or more points is presumptive evidence of alcoholism, while a 5-point total would make it extremely unlikely that the individual was not alcoholic. However, a positive response to questions 10, 23 or 24 would be diagnostic; a positive response indicates alcoholism.
From Gallant, D.S. (1982). *Alcohol and drug abuse curriculum guide for psychiatric faculty* (pp. 53–54). Rockville, MD: National Institute on Alcohol Abuse and Alcoholism.

BOX 25.2 CAGE SCREENING TEST FOR ALCOHOLISM

The CAGE tool involves a list of four questions. A positive response to one question in the CAGE questionnaire indicates the individual has a potential problem with alcoholism. Two affirmative responses correctly identify 75% of persons with an alcohol problem.

1. Have you ever felt you ought to Cut down on your drinking?
2. Have people Annoyed you by criticizing your drinking?
3. Have you ever felt bad or Guilty about your drinking?
4. Have you ever had a drink first thing in the morning to steady your nerves or get rid of a hangover (Eye-opener)?

From Ewing, J.A. (1984). Detecting alcoholism: The CAGE questionnaire. *Journal of the American Medical Association, 252,* 1905–1907.

and frequency of drinking, bingeing, and drinking consequences. Because of its emphasis on drinking within the last year, this self-administered screening tool may not identify clients with previous drinking problems. Alcoholics Anonymous has also developed a 12-question quiz to identify teenagers at risk for alcohol use or abuse. Experts caution that brief screening tests may be less effective in some populations. These implications could have a significant importance, given the number of individuals who abuse alcohol (Lucas, 1998).

Diagnostic Tests. During admission, a breath analyzer reading may be performed to determine whether the client is intoxicated or in the withdrawal process. Diagnostic laboratory tests include liver function tests and mean corpuscular volume, which, when elevated, are indicators of heavy alcohol use. Other tests, such as blood alcohol level or urine screen for alcohol, may be ordered depending on the physical condition of the client or complaints verbalized during the assessment process. The Food and Drug Administration (FDA) has approved the use of a diagnostic test, the Carbohydrate-deficient Transferring Test (%CDT), for detecting alcohol abuse. Recommended use includes detection of heavy alcohol consumption, monitoring

of abstinence, and identifying relapse in clients with alcohol use disorders. The %CDT has been effective in screening clients with diseases possibly triggered by alcohol use, detecting alcohol use disorders in hospitalized clients, and in screening presurgical and trauma clients to predict alcohol withdrawal syndrome and/or postsurgical complications (Miller, Dominick, & Anton, 2005). Table 25-2 summarizes blood alcohol levels and associated findings, comparing various blood alcohol levels, the approximate amount of beverage for each level, effects of alcohol, and the amount of time it takes alcohol to leave the body (Altrocchi, 1980; Liska, 2003). A neurologic evaluation may be requested, as well as a psychiatric consultation to rule out coexisting psychiatric disorders such as depression, delirium, dementia, or anxiety.

Assessment of the Client Who Abuses Substances Other Than Alcohol

The client who abuses substances other than alcohol presents many challenges because of fear, dependency needs, feelings of insecurity, low self-esteem, the inability to cope, a low tolerance for frustration or anxiety, rebellion, or boredom. Clients who self-prescribe medication frequently do not admit readily to substance abuse. Defense mechanisms such as rationalization, projection, and repression commonly are exhibited. Therefore, obtaining a family history and information from significant others regarding the client's use of drugs are important elements of the assessment. Such information can help the nurse determine whether a client has a pseudo-addiction or a substance-related disorder (Bates, 2005).

The nurse should keep in mind that the assessment of clients with a marijuana-related disorder can be difficult because clients do not recognize that they have a problem, and abuse and associated problems commonly develop slowly. Individuals seeking treatment for cocaine addiction can be difficult to assess because they are likely to be polysubstance abusers. Also, clients with heroin addiction may require a detailed assessment that focuses primarily on detoxification (Goulding & Shank, 2005).

General Description. In addition to using the assessment format described for the client who abuses alcohol, the nurse must be able to recognize symptoms of drug overdose or drug withdrawal during the collec-

TABLE 25.2 Comparison of Blood Alcohol Levels

BLOOD ALCOHOL LEVEL (%)	APPROXIMATE AMOUNT OF BEVERAGE	EFFECTS OF ALCOHOL	TIME NEEDED FOR ALCOHOL TO LEAVE THE BODY
0.03	1 cocktail, 1 bottle beer, or 5½ oz. wine	Slight tension Euphoria Feeling of superiority	2 hr
0.06	2 cocktails, 3 bottles beer, or 11 oz. wine	Feeling of warmth and relaxation Decreased mental efficiency Loss of normal inhibitions Loss of some motor coordination	4 hr
0.09	3 cocktails, 5 bottles beer, or 16½ oz. wine	Talkative Clumsy Exaggerated behavior	6 hr
0.10	3 to 5 cocktails, 6 to 7 bottles beer, or 20 to 22 oz. wine	Legally drunk in most states Impaired motor, mental, and speech activity Decreased feelings of guilt	6 hr
0.15	5 to 7 cocktails or 26 to 27 oz. wine	Gross intoxication Slurred speech Impaired motor coordination	10 hr
0.20	8 cocktails	Angers easily Motor abilities severely impaired Blackout level Unable to recall events	At least 10 or more hr
0.30	10 cocktails	Stupor likely; possible aggressive behavior Death may occur due to deep anesthetic effect or paralysis of the respiratory center	
0.40	13 cocktails	Coma leading to death	
0.60	20 cocktails	Severely impaired breathing and heart rate Death will probably occur	

tion of data. Keep in mind that clients who abuse drugs often take multiple drugs to achieve desired effects. Each drug reacts differently and is identified in part by physical and behavioral manifestations. Therefore, focus assessment measures on obtaining baseline data and monitoring vital signs (some drugs will depress vital signs, others will cause an elevation); observing for signs of CNS depression, such as irregular respirations; recognizing signs of impending seizures or coma; assessing the client for cuts, bruises, infection, or needle tracks; assessing general nutritional status; determining the client's level of sensorium; and listening to physiologic complaints.

Behavior. Also monitor the client's behavior. Focus on the client's history of suicidal ideation or attempts; withdrawal symptoms, including hallucinations, confusion, tremors, seizures, and the like; longest drug-free period; and desire for treatment.

Screening Tools. Two frequently used assessment tools in clinical settings with individuals who have a problem with substance-related disorders include the Diagnostic Interview Schedule (DIS), which contains an alcohol dependence subscale; and the Addiction Severity Index (ASI), designed to assess alcohol and drug use as well as the medical, psychological, and legal complications of use within the family, employment, and social settings (Riggin, 1996b). Both tools can be used to assess the client who abuses substances to rule out the presence of comorbid alcohol and drug abuse. A third tool, UNCOPE, is a six-question survey to provide a simple and quick means of identifying risk for abuse or dependence of alcohol or drugs when neither is clearly identified as a problem. A copy of the survey is available at http://www.evinceassessment.com/ UNCOPE_for_web.pdf.

Diagnostic Tests. Drug screening can be done with a variety of bodily specimens including hair, urine, gastric contents, and blood. For example, cannabis may be detected in urine from 7 to 30 days after use and in blood for up to 15 weeks after use. Gastric contents have been tested in individuals suspected of ingesting drugs to smuggle them into the country. Although urine drug screening is the preferred method because it is more easily performed and more economical, hair testing can be used to determine when drug use has occurred and can usually detect results up to 90 days after use. The nurse should be aware that several products to mask controlled substances in the urine are available for purchase via the Internet (eg, Carbo Cleansing Shakes, Constant Cleanze, Herbal Pre-Cleanse, Pure Gold, Urinegative) (Colyar, 2003). Additional tests may include liver profile, electrolytes, or testing for the human immunodeficiency virus (HIV; see Chapter 34). In a crisis, data collection focuses on whatever is essential for immediate care.

Transcultural Considerations

There are wide cultural variations in attitudes toward substance consumption, patterns of use, accessibility of substances, physiologic reactions to substances, and prevalence of substance-related disorders. For example, Asians have a genetic intolerance to alcohol even when consumed in small amounts. Some cultures forbid the use of alcohol or drugs, whereas other cultures include alcoholic beverages with their meals and accept the use of various substances to achieve mood-altering effects (APA, 2000).

Substance abuse is never static. The availability of new illicit drugs, changing circumstances in our communities, and generational shifts fuel new problems. New heroin use now occurs in suburbia rather than in urban centers. Britain's rave culture is now estimated to include 500,000 people. Columbia, Puerto Rico,

Mexico, and parts of Asia are known for their drug cultures and illicit drug trafficking. Rave parties and clubs have become popular in the United States. There has been an increase in the use of ecstasy, ketamine, and "roofies" or date rape drugs imported from Mexico (Drew, 1999; NCJRS, 2004b; NIDA, 1999).

Andrews and Boyle (1999) discuss the use and abuse of alcohol by adolescents. It is noted that most teenagers have their first alcoholic drink between the ages of 12 and 15 years. Alcohol may serve as an informal rite of passage from childhood to adulthood for African American teens. Studies indicate that alcohol use among white and Native American males is relatively high compared with consumption by African American and Asian American teens. The reason for drinking cited by white, African American, and Hispanic adolescents was to relax. Indochinese youths indicated that they drink to forget.

Nurses need to be aware of these cultural variations including the social, environmental, and development trends, keeping them at the forefront when assessing the client.

NURSING DIAGNOSES

"The use of accepted diagnostic classification systems facilitates communication about the client's actual and potential health problems and response to these problems. The diagnoses identify the health needs requiring nursing interventions" (ANA & NNSA, 1988, p. 7).

Clients who use or abuse substances may have poor general health and inadequate nutrition. They are more susceptible to infections and medical complications. Sensory or perceptual alterations may occur, and there is a potential for injury resulting from impaired memory or cognition. Communication and social interaction may be impaired. Family dynamics may be dysfunctional. A dual diagnosis may exist (see Chapter 32). Examples of North American Nursing Diagnosis Association (NANDA) Nursing Diagnoses for clients with substance-related disorders are presented in the accompanying box.

OUTCOME IDENTIFICATION

Outcomes focus on providing a safe environment to prevent injury; stabilizing existing medical complications secondary to substance use or abuse; improving

EXAMPLES OF NANDA NURSING DIAGNOSES/ SUBSTANCE-RELATED DISORDERS

- Anxiety related to misperception of environmental stimuli
- Ineffective Health Maintenance related to chemical use
- Ineffective Health Maintenance related to fluid and electrolyte imbalance
- Imbalanced Nutrition: Less than Body Requirements related to chronic alcohol intake or substance abuse
- Hopelessness related to addiction
- Impaired Verbal Communication related to reluctance to talk about personal matters
- Impaired Social Interaction related to unpredictable or irresponsible behavior patterns
- Ineffective Denial related to rationalization
- Ineffective Coping related to effects of chemical use
- Deficient Knowledge regarding illness related to inadequate understanding of information presented
- Risk for Injury related to confusion
- Risk for Injury related to seizure activity
- Risk for Other-Directed Violence related to feelings of fear
- Disturbed Sleep Pattern related to withdrawal symptoms
- Spiritual Distress related to despair

EXAMPLES OF STATED OUTCOMES/ SUBSTANCE-RELATED DISORDERS

- The client will be physically safe and without injury.
- The client will establish nutritious eating patterns.
- The client will demonstrate decreased hostile or aggressive behavior.
- The client will establish a balance of rest, sleep, and activity.
- The client will verbalize increased self-esteem.
- The client will abstain from drug and alcohol use.
- The client will report decreased feelings of fear or anxiety.
- The client will express feelings openly.
- The client will identify negative effects of his or her behavior on others.
- The client will verbalize acceptance of personal responsibility for his or her behavior.
- The client will express acceptance of chemical dependence as an illness.
- The client will verbalize the need for medication compliance.
- The client will demonstrate appropriate social skills.

impaired cognition and communication; establishing nutritious eating patterns; establishing a balance of rest, sleep, and activity; establishing alternative coping skills; and resolving any personal or family issues related to the client's disorder. Examples of Stated Outcomes for clients with substance-related disorders are highlighted in the accompanying box.

PLANNING INTERVENTIONS

"The nursing plan of care documents the human response patterns that will be addressed by nursing interventions; guides each nurse to intervene in a manner congruent with client needs and goals; and provides outcome criteria for measurement of client

progress. Upon the basis of this plan, nurses can contribute effectively to formulation of the multidisciplinary treatment plan and collaborative therapeutic interventions" (ANA & NNSA, 1988, p. 8).

The treatment of a client with a substance-related disorder can be complex and must address a variety of problems. For example, is the client intoxicated or at risk for withdrawal because of abrupt cessation of alcohol or a specific drug, or has the client overdosed? Planning is similar to that used when caring for clients with eating disorders, because both client populations typically deny their illness and refuse care. Thus, planning focuses on psychobiologic, social, and pharmacologic aspects of the client's substance abuse; involves the client and family; and includes a multidisciplinary approach.

Stages of Change Model

The **Stages of Change Model**, developed by Prochaska and DiClemente (1982), is based on scien-

TABLE 25.3 Stages of Change Model Applied to Alcohol or Substance Abuse

STAGE OF CHANGE	DESCRIPTION	NURSING INTERVENTIONS
Precontemplation	Client seems unaware of problem	Ask client what he or she considers to be problematic substance abuse
Contemplation	Client is aware of problem but is not motivated to change	Offer assistance Discuss pros and cons of substance abuse Discuss possible solutions that have been effective for others
Preparation	Client is getting ready to change	Support smallest effort to change Review and recommend treatment options such as AA or NA
Determination	Client develops a plan to seek help	Offer support
Action	Client actively engages in change process and achieves abstinence	Continue to offer support Monitor efficacy of treatment
Maintenance	Client actively works to prevent relapse	Ask client to identify positive coping skills Assist with problem-solving Encourage participation in support groups
Relapse	Client returns to drinking or substance abuse	Help client identify triggers that lead to relapse Discuss strategies to prevent further relapse

tific investigation of change in humans. Their model conceptualizes change as several stages that require alterations in attitude in order to progress. They contend that it is quite normal for people to experience several trips through the stages to make lasting change because change is difficult, and it is unreasonable to expect everyone to be able to modify a habit perfectly without relapse. The stages identified by Prochaska and DiClemente include precontemplation, contemplation, preparation, determination, action, maintenance, and relapse (Table 25-3).

The model can address various substance-related disorder issues such as enabling behavior between client and family, codependency, or substance abuse. As noted earlier, relapse can occur at any time after the client agrees to treatment (Westermeyer, 2005).

IMPLEMENTATION

"Addictions nursing addresses an area of concern extending over the entire health-care continuum. Addictions nursing interventions consist of all those nursing actions that are directed toward fostering adaptive human responses to actual or potential health problems stemming from patterns of abuse or addiction" (ANA & NNSA, 1988, p. 9).

Attitudes of nursing personnel can influence the quality of care given to clients who abuse substances. Nurses may exhibit disapproval, intolerance, moralistic condemnation, anger, or disinterest. Displaying an accepting, nonjudgmental attitude or assisting clients with their activities of daily living as they exhibit manipulative, noncompliant, aggressive, or hostile behavior is difficult. Various approaches can be used to provide effective care. These include maintaining one-to-one contact, orienting the client to reality, speaking slowly and clearly in a low voice, avoiding either negative or positive judgments, and offering support if the client is willing to verbalize feelings about his or her situation.

Clients with the diagnosis of a substance-related disorder often require placement in a safe environment as the nursing staff provides assistance in meeting the client's basic needs; monitors the client's medical condition; uses interventions to stabilize the client's medical condition and behavioral problems; and assists with medication management, intervention strategies, interactive therapies, and client education.

Provision of a Safe Environment

Client safety is a priority because the client may exhibit clinical symptoms of overdose, intoxication, or withdrawal. The client also may react to substance-induced internal stimuli such as hallucinations or delusions, placing him or her at risk for injury to self or others. It may be necessary to place the hospitalized client in a room near the nurses' station or where the staff can observe the client closely. Reduce stimuli to minimize the possibility of illusions or agitation by placing the client in a partially lighted room. Chapter 31 discusses nursing interventions for clients who exhibit self-abusive or suicidal behavior.

Assistance in Meeting Basic Needs

Nursing interventions focus on providing adequate hydration and nutrition and assisting the client with personal hygiene and activities of daily living. Promoting a balance of sleep, rest, and activity and monitoring the client's elimination patterns also are important.

Stabilization of Medical Condition

Several medical problems are associated with substance abuse (Box 25-3). Seizures can occur during withdrawal from various substances. Therefore, insti-

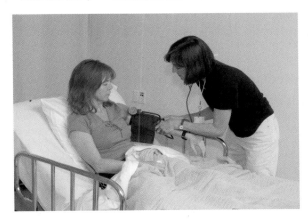

FIGURE 25.2 The nurse assessing the blood pressure of a client experiencing alcohol withdrawal.

tute seizure precautions to minimize chances of injury. Intravenous (IV) barbiturates may be required to control extreme agitation. The client is at risk for fluid and electrolyte imbalance caused by severe dehydration or malnourishment. Monitor intake and output. If the client is vomiting, IV therapy may be necessary.

Also assess vital signs frequently for changes (eg, clients who overdose on methamphetamine are at risk for hyperthermia as well as seizures) and observe for signs of impending or current delirium tremens (Figure 25-2). Because of the substance's effect on the heart, cardiac status may require monitoring. Laboratory tests may need to be repeated because of abnormal values. A computed tomography scan and electroencephalography may be ordered to rule out metabolic encephalopathy or coexisting neurologic disorders. McCabe (2001) addresses the additional emergency care of clients exhibiting clinical symptoms of alcohol withdrawal delirium and drug intoxication; detailed emergency care interventions are beyond the scope of this discussion.

Stabilization of Behavior

Clients who abuse substances are often manipulative and prone to staff-splitting. They may continue to exhibit drug-seeking behavior despite placement in a secure, controlled environment. Clients have been known to have peers bring alcoholic beverages or drugs to them during treatment. Antipsychotics may be required during an acute psychotic episode. Protocols for the use of specific psychoactive medica-

---

BOX 25.3 MEDICAL PROBLEMS ASSOCIATED WITH SUBSTANCE ABUSE

Cardiovascular: Myocardial ischemia, arrhythmias, cardiomyopathies, bacterial endocarditis, thrombophlebitis, cardiac arrest

Respiratory: Respiratory infections, pulmonary embolism, cancer

Gastrointestinal: Constipation, colitis, intestinal ischemia, hepatic dysfunction, gastroduodenal ulcer

Renal: Renal failure, rhabdomyolysis

Neurologic: Seizures, dementia, amnesia

Endocrine: Amenorrhea, adrenergic effects mimicking hyperthyroidism

Obstetric: Complications during pregnancy, birth defects

Oral: Dental caries, gingival ulceration

Other: Malnutrition, vitamin deficiencies, fluid and electrolyte imbalance, skin abscesses, cellulitis, male impotence, HIV/AIDS

tions to be used during an acute substance-induced psychotic episode must be readily available on the client's medical record.

Medication Management

"Varied individualized pharmacological treatment modalities may be needed by clients during their health maintenance, withdrawal, and recovery process. Pertinent clinical observations and judgments must be made concerning the effects of medications used with reference to the stages of this process and the nature of the abuse or addiction problem" (ANA & NNSA, 1988, p. 14).

Caution is used when prescribing medication for clients with a history of substance use or abuse. Unnecessary drugs should be avoided, and CNS stimulants are not advised because they may cause seizures. If the drug of choice is unidentifiable, the client's symptoms are treated. During delirium tremens, benzodiazepines such as lorazepam (Ativan) or diazepam (Valium) are generally administered intravenously until the client's symptoms stabilize (Sadock & Sadock, 2003). Ascorbic acid may be given to enhance excretion of the drug through acidification of the urine. Thiamine is generally prescribed because the client may exhibit a deficiency state that can affect the CNS, gastrointestinal tract, and circulatory system. Diazepam may be used to decrease anxiety, to reduce the possibility of seizures, or to provide skeletal muscle relaxation (Bernstein, 1995; Cornish, McNicholas, & O'Brien, 1995; Sadock & Sadock, 2003).

Detoxification (Detox)

Detoxification (ie, medical intervention to relieve withdrawal symptoms while clients adjust to a drug-free state) is not necessary when treating clients who abuse marijuana, amphetamines, or cocaine. *Rapid detoxification* is a term used to describe a specific type of detox that occurs under anesthesia, allowing clients to return to a productive life in a matter of days and eliminating the need to be hospitalized or participate in rehabilitation programs (Addiction Help Services, 2006).

Some substance-use disorders may require specific interventions to relive withdrawal symptoms. For example, clients who abuse hallucinogens may require 3 months of neuroleptic or antipsychotic maintenance therapy to avoid the risk of recurrent symptoms. Methadone is given to clients who abuse opioids and synthetic substances to replace their usual substance of abuse, because it decreases the severity of withdrawal. Clonidine (Catapres) is then given during the detoxification from methadone. Buprenorphine (Suboxone) and buprenorphine/ naloxone (Suboxone sublingual tablet) are opioid-agonist medications approved for treatment of opioid dependence. They provide less risk of respiratory depression, less physical dependence, and easier medical withdrawal than methadone when discontinuation is appropriate for the individual client. Abrupt discontinuation of sedatives may be fatal due to status epilepticus, hyperthermia, or possible intravascular coagulation. Long-term use of low doses of sedatives may produce discomfort when drug use is stopped, but detoxification is not generally required (Bernstein, 1995; Sadock & Sadock, 2003). Table 25-4 lists initial treatment options to counteract adverse physiologic or behavioral effects of various substances.

Disulfiram and Naltrexone Therapy (Alcohol Aversion Therapy). Substance use creates a hold on the user by operant conditioning. Each time a substance is taken, it stimulates the release of endorphins, a morphine-like action that encourages the individual to think about and seek the substance. However, learning can be reversed through extinction of the individual's desire to think about or seek the substance (Sherman, 2001).

Aversion therapy, one way of reversing the individual's desire to seek and use an illicit substance, consists of giving a drug such as emetine (an extract of the ipecac root) and then following it with alcohol. Nausea and vomiting are induced by the emetine, causing an aversion to alcohol based on the reflex association between alcohol and vomiting.

Disulfiram (Antabuse) is another drug that may be used to cause an aversion to alcohol. This drug interferes with the breakdown of alcohol, causing an accumulation of acetaldehyde, a by-product of alcohol, in the body. The person who takes disulfiram and drinks alcohol experiences severe nausea and vomiting, hypotension, headaches, rapid pulse and respirations, flushed face, and bloodshot eyes. This reaction lasts as long as there is alcohol in the blood. Persons with serious heart disease, diabetes, epilepsy, liver impairment, or mental illness should not take disulfiram.

Naltrexone (ReVia) is another drug approved for use in the treatment of alcoholism. The precise mechanism of action is unknown. However, when given with alcohol consumption ("targeted" use), it reduces

TABLE 25.4 Treatment Options for Substance Abuse

SUBSTANCE	TREATMENT OPTIONS
Heroin	Methadone, LAAM (levo-alpha-acetyl-methadol), naltrexone. Maintenance therapy may be necessary.
Narcotics	Methadone, LAAM, or switch client to a comparable drug that produces milder withdrawal symptoms, and then gradually taper off the substitute medication
Alcohol	Disulfiram to discourage use of alcohol, naltrexone (ReVia), or benzodiazepines
Hallucinogens	Diazepam, haloperidol, or talk down
Sedatives	Diazepam; detoxification should occur on an inpatient unit.
Inhalants	Haloperidol for psychotic symptoms
Amphetamines	Ammonium chloride, antipsychotics, tricyclic antidepressants, diazepam, or propranolol. Inpatient unit if client is suicidal, psychotic, or violent.
Phencyclidine	Hospitalization, because death may occur secondary to hyperpyrexia. IV medications such as benzodiazepines, haloperidol; antihypertensive drug (phentolamine), ammonium chloride, ascorbic acid, cranberry juice
Cannabis	Anxiolytic, antipsychotic, antidepressant

*There are currently no medications approved by the Food and Drug Administration (FDA) for treating addiction to cocaine, LSD, PCP, marijuana, methamphetamine, and other stimulants, inhalants, or anabolic steroids. Medications are used to treat adverse health effects of these drugs, such as seizures or psychotic reactions. Currently, a top research priority is the development of a medication useful in treating cocaine addiction.

the craving. It also helps clients to remain abstinent and interferes with the urge to drink during a relapse. It is considered to be an extremely effective therapy for alcohol addiction (eg, approximately 70% effective in reducing craving and blocking the reinforcing effects of alcohol). Clinical trials have shown that an intramuscular form of naltrexone (Vivitrol 380 mg) given monthly has proven to improve alcohol dependence treatment adherence. The estimated date of availability (ie, FDA approval) has been listed as spring or summer of 2006 (Rosenthal, 2006). The use of naltrexone is contraindicated in clients with hepatitis or liver failure and in those who have recently taken opioid drugs (Internet Alcohol Recovery Center, 2003; Sherman, 2001).

Harm avoidance is a new concept that has been embraced for alcohol treatment. Researchers believe that treatment of alcohol abuse can be effective in the absence of total abstinence. Reduced drinking may be a suitable alternative for some drinkers. Clients who relapse while taking acamprosate or naltrexone still drink a lot less, which presumably means fewer adverse consequences (Kirn, 2006).

Acamprosate (Campral), a GABA analogue approved by the FDA on July 29, 2004, is now available to reduce

discomfort (eg, restlessness, anxiety, dysphoria, insomnia) common within the first 6 months of alcohol abstinence. It does not block the high associated with alcohol consumption, diminish withdrawal symptoms, or cause alcohol aversion or unpleasant reactions. The National Institute on Alcohol Abuse and Alcoholism recently funded a study to compare the efficacy of naltrexone, acamprosate, and both agents (naltrexone/acamprosate) in combined pharmacotherapy. Preliminary safety, tolerability, and adherence results have been promising. Acamprosate is not indicated for use in children, adolescents, or the elderly (Connery & Weiss, 2005). Drug Summary Table 25-1 highlights the major drugs used for substance-related disorders.

Several research studies regarding off-label uses of drugs to reduce alcohol craving highlight advances of the harm avoidance concept. The FDA is currently reviewing the use of a long-acting injectable form of naltrexone that lasts up to 30 days. The anticonvulsants topiramate (Topamax) and gabapentin (Neurontin) target the glutamate (excitatory) and GABA (inhibitory) activity systems of the brain and are believed to relieve craving, improve impaired control, reduce withdrawal symptoms, and eliminate the desire or urge to drink. Ondansetron (Zofran), an antiemetic that affects the

DRUG SUMMARY TABLE 25-1   Substance-Related Disorders: Drugs Used for Detox

GENERIC (TRADE) NAME	DAILY DOSAGE RANGE	IMPLEMENTATION
Drug Class: Anticonvulsants		
carbamazepine (Tegretol)	600–1200 mg	Give with food to prevent GI upset; arrange for liver function tests to rule out liver dysfunction; monitor for drowsiness, dizziness, GI disturbance, and skin rash.
valproate (Depakote)	500–1500 mg	Obtain lab work regarding liver function, platelet count, and ammonia levels; discontinue drug if rash occurs; monitor for bruising, jaundice, sedation, and increased tremor if exhibiting DTs.
Drug Class: Benzodiazepines		
chlordiazepoxide (Librium)	25–300 mg	Expect parenteral form to be given initially (50–100 mg) and then orally with repeated doses not to exceed 300 mg in 24 hours; follow detox or withdrawal protocol regarding obtaining vital signs and providing a safe environment to prevent injury due to possible drowsiness, disorientation, confusion, and restlessness.
diazepam (Valium)	2–40 mg	Follow detox or withdrawal protocol and monitor vital signs; provide a safe environment to prevent injury.
Drug Class: Opioid Antagonist		
buprenorphine (Suboxone)	4–24 mg sublingual tabs	Dissolve under tongue. Do not chew. Monitor hepatic function at baseline and periodically. Follow detox protocol.
Drug Class: Central Alpha$_2$-Agonist		
clonidine (Catapres)	0.2–2.4 mg	Potentiates CNS depressants; monitor for dry mouth, dizziness, weakness, arrhythmias, hypotension, agitation, rash, myalgia, and insomnia. Follow detox protocol.
Drug Class: Antialcoholic Agents (aversion therapy)		
disulfiram (Antabuse)	500 mg	Never administer to an intoxicated client or to a client without the client's knowledge; instruct client of seriousness of disulfiram-alcohol reaction and the potential consequences of alcohol use during therapy; obtain liver function tests, CBC, and serum electrolytes before therapy and according to protocol; give single dose 12 hours after client has abstained from use of alcohol; crush tablet and mix with beverages if necessary; if a sedative effect occurs, administer next scheduled dose at h.s.; monitor for drowsiness, headache, metallic or garliclike aftertaste, and skin eruptions.

NOTE: It is beyond the scope of this text to discuss the specific protocols used during the detoxification and withdrawal phases from all substances. This table lists examples of selected adjunctive medications (anticonvulsants, benzodiazepines, opioid antagonists, central alpha$_2$-agonists, and antialcoholic agents) used during the detoxification and withdrawal phases and is not to be considered all-inclusive. For additional information regarding detox methods, see the Addiction Help Services Web site (www.addictionhelpservices.com). For information about drugs used to treat anxiety or depression associated with substance-related disorders, see Chapters 16, 19, 20, and 21.

serotonin system, has shown to be effective in individuals who develop alcoholism before the age of 25 years. Other off-label drug studies include baclofen (Lioresal), rimonabant, memantine (Namenda), and the Chinese herbal medicine kudzu (Kelly, 2005).

Pain Management of Clients With Substance-Related Disorders. Nurses face ethical decisions daily when providing safe and successful pain management to clients with, or who have a history of, a substance-related disorder. Vigilance is essential to ensure that clients don't abuse pain medication such as oxycodone hydrochloride (OxyContin), often called a miracle pain drug, while at the same time ensuring that those who need the medication have access to it. Combating abuse requires a delicate balance of getting to know a client's needs and treating the client in a way that does not cause harm. The possibility of under-treated pain is rarely explored (Nichols, 2003; Willis, 2001).

Efforts to improve pain management have created an opportunity to address the controversy surrounding the provision of pain management to clients who suffer from a comorbid substance-related disorder and are experiencing physical pain (Nichols, 2003). These clients have the right to the same quality of pain assessment and management as other clients. This right presents a challenge to the nurse who attempts to maintain a balance between providing pain relief and protecting the client from inappropriate use of prescribed pain medication (American Society of Pain Management Nurses [ASPMN], 2002).

In a position paper titled *ASPMN Position Statement: Pain Management in Patients With Addictive Disease* (2002), the ASPMN outlines basic steps for the management of pain in the following populations of clients with substance-related disorders:

- All clients with addictive disease
- Clients who are actively using alcohol or other drugs
- Clients in recovery
- Clients on methadone maintenance treatment

Information regarding these guidelines, as well as tools for assessing and treating withdrawal, information regarding the risks of unrelieved pain, treatment options for substance-related disorders, and therapeutic interventions in the event of relapse are available on the ASPMN Web site (http://www. ASPMN.org) (Nichols, 2003). Psychiatric–mental health nurses need to be aware of these guidelines to ensure adequate pain management. Skillful treatment of pain or addiction in comorbid clients will usually fail unless both conditions are addressed. The gift of sobriety combined with effective coping with pain usually leads to a life restored (Kotz, 2005).

Intervention Strategy

An **intervention,** a term used to describe an organized, deliberate confrontation of a client who uses or abuses substances, may be planned and then implemented. Although it is frequently used to encourage a person to enter treatment or rehabilitation immediately, intervention can be used once a person has entered treatment. For example, family members are aware that a loved one has exhibited several symptoms of alcoholism such as slurred speech, decreased attention span, "alcohol breath," disheveled or unkempt appearance, and numerous instances of calling out of work or avoiding other responsibilities after weekends or holidays. The nurse asks each family member to compose a testimonial letter to read aloud during the intervention. The purpose of the intervention is to help the family member recognize that a problem does exist, understand that help is available, and agree to receive help. This approach implies that a support system is available and the client is not alone during treatment. Even if an intervention succeeds, it is only the first step in treatment. The majority of individuals who enter treatment suffer at least one relapse along the road to recovery (Flora, 2005).

Interactive Therapies

"The counseling role is an inherent component of nursing practice and is used within the framework of the therapeutic relationship between nurse and client. Counseling interventions are informal or formal and include a variety of interactional modalities and strategies" (ANA & NNSA, 1988, p.16).

Several interactive therapies can be useful during the rehabilitation process. Clients with a high level of anxiety, poor coping skills, guilt feelings, and a low level of tolerance, or clients with a dual diagnosis, usually require individual or cognitive behavioral psychotherapy before participating in group or family therapy.

Individual and Cognitive Behavioral Psychotherapy. Individual psychotherapy with the nurse–therapist generally focuses on the client's pathological defense mechanisms, development of insight into behavior, and the exploration of alternate coping skills. Self-worth and self-esteem are explored. Accountability and responsibility are addressed as the nurse helps the client develop self-discipline. Cognitive behavioral therapy is considered to be the most effective treatment for methamphetamine addiction. This approach is designed to help modify the client's thinking, expectancies, and behaviors and to increase basic coping skills (Goulding & Shank, 2005).

Group Therapy. Group therapy provides the client with an opportunity to identify with peers and respond to confrontation about ineffective coping or dysfunctional behavior. The client has an opportunity to improve communication skills as he or she receives emotional support from the group. Feelings of hopelessness, discouragement, and demoralization are shared with peers. The importance of establishing social skills and developing interpersonal relationships in a drug-free environment is stressed (Riggin, 1996a, 1996b; Thurston, 1997; Sadock & Sadock, 2003).

Family Therapy. Family therapy, effective if the family members are supportive of the client and willing to participate, provides an opportunity for the client and family members to share personal feelings, to rebuild relationships, and to reestablish healthy roles in the family. Helping the family to gain knowledge about alcoholism and put that knowledge into effect may also occur during family therapy, because problem-solving guidance and direction are available.

The concept of codependency is usually addressed in family or marital therapy. The codependent becomes so involved with the family member's drinking problem that the codependent's needs and desires are ignored. As a result, the codependent may allow abusive behavior to continue even when it is dangerous. Codependent behavior impedes recovery.

Craft Reinforcement and Family Training Program. Community Reinforcement and Family Training (CRAFT) is a new program in Albuquerque, New Mexico, that trains a spouse or other family members on how to deal with the addicted client. It helps family members develop skills aimed at promoting sobriety in the loved ones by teaching them how to change their own behavior. Three major goals of the CRAFT program are to reduce the loved one's drinking, engage the person into treatment, and improve the functioning of the concerned significant other. The program received funding from the National Institute on Drug Abuse for a demonstration project targeting treatment-resistant drug abusers. After spouses and relatives underwent the CRAFT program, 74% of the drug abusers entered treatment (Little, 2005).

Client Education

Client education can be provided by the nurse in several ways depending on the client's level of motivation, reading ability, educational background, willingness to participate in group discussions, and availability of a family support system. Some of the methods used to educate clients who have a substance-related disorder are highlighted in the following sections.

Smoking-Cessation Program

Nicotine replacement therapy (NRT) and behavior modification (discussed in Chapter 12) are approaches commonly used to assist motivated clients to stop smoking. Nicotine replacement therapy involves the use of a stop-smoking aid such as a transdermal patch, inhaler, nasal spray, lozenge, or chewing gum. Sustained-release tablets such as bupropion hydrochloride (Zyban) have also been used, but the drug is contraindicated in individuals with seizure disorders or eating disorders. For clients in whom first-line agents are ineffective, recommended second-line monotherapies include the antihypertensive clonidine and the tricyclic antidepressant nortriptyline. However, neither of these agents is approved for smoking cessation. Researchers are investigating the simultaneous use of more than one NRT on an individualized basis (Mitchell & Parish, 2005).

Smoking cessation counseling may range in intensity from brief advice provided by a nurse, to a more formalized, intensive counseling program and follow up on an individual or group basis. The U.S. Public Health Service Report published in 2000 discusses key components of comprehensive counseling for tobacco cessation. The guidelines address the "5 A's" or Key Components of Structured Tobacco Cessation Counseling Intervention and the "5 R's" or Ways to Promote Motivation in Patients Not Ready to Quit (Anthenelli, 2005). These guidelines are available at http://www.ahcpr.gov/path/tobacco.htm.

Ruppert (1999) lists several behavioral modification tips to help ex-smokers stay tobacco free. They include behaviors such as:

- Maintaining a routine schedule
- Avoiding the substitution of food for tobacco
- Avoiding the practice of lingering after a meal

- Drinking plenty of water
- Practicing deep breathing and relaxation exercises
- Exercising or doing labor-intensive tasks such as gardening or housekeeping to divert attention from smoking
- Replacing items that have been associated with smoking or that may be saturated with nicotine

Support and Self-Help Groups. *"Self-help groups have proven to be of therapeutic value for clients with problems of abuse and addiction. Self-help groups teach new ways of thinking, support constructive behavior change, and provide motivation and social support for members"* (ANA & NNSA, 1988, p. 13).

Several types of support and self-help groups are available for clients who are motivated for treatment:

- Alcoholics Anonymous (AA) (founded in 1935 by a surgeon and a stockbroker who were unable to obtain help for their alcoholism): A voluntary, nonprofessional, nondenominational fellowship of alcoholics who help themselves and each other recover from the illness of alcoholism by following 12 steps (Box 25-4); educational materials, including videos, pamphlets, and books, available online through AA's Web site
- Al-Anon: A fellowship of spouses, relatives, and friends
- Alateen and Adult Children of Alcoholics (ACOA): Components of Al-Anon
- Narcotics Anonymous (NA): Program for recovering addicts who have abused any mood-altering substances; format for NA similar to that of AA
- Cocaine Anonymous (CA): Available for individuals who prefer the support of peers who abused cocaine
- Mentally Ill Chemical Abusers (MICA): Group available for individuals with a dual diagnosis
- Co-Dependents Anonymous (CoDA): Fellowship of men and women whose common problem is an inability to maintain functional relationships; relies on the wisdom, knowledge, 12 steps, and 12 traditions of AA

In addition, there are nationally known treatment centers including the Betty Ford Treatment Center in Palm Desert, California; the Hanley-Hazelden Center at St. Mary's in Minneapolis, Minnesota; and the Phoenix House in New York, New York.

Moreover, a variety of resources can be obtained from NIAAA and National Institute on Aging (NIA). The National Council on Alcoholism and Drug Depend-

---

BOX 25.4   TWELVE STEPS OF ALCOHOLICS ANONYMOUS

1. We admitted we were powerless over alcohol, that our lives had become unmanageable.
2. Came to believe that a Power greater than ourselves could restore us to sanity.
3. Made a decision to turn our will and our lives over to the care of God as we understood Him.
4. Made a searching and fearless moral inventory of ourselves.
5. Admitted to God, to ourselves, and to another human being the exact nature of our wrongs.
6. Were entirely ready to have God remove all these defects of character.
7. Humbly asked Him to remove our shortcomings
8. Made a list of all persons we had harmed, and became willing to make amends to them all.
9. Made direct amends to such people wherever possible, except when to do so would injure them or others.
10. Continued to take personal inventory, and when we were wrong, promptly admitted it.
11. Sought through prayer and meditation to improve our conscious contact with God as we understood Him, praying only for knowledge of His will for us and the power to carry that out.
12. Having had a spiritual awakening as the result of these steps, we tried to carry this message to alcoholics and to practice these principles in all our affairs.

The Twelve Steps are reprinted with permission of Alcoholics Anonymous World Services, Inc. (A.A.W.S.). Permission to reprint the Twelve Steps does not mean that A.A.W.S. has reviewed or approved the contents of this publication, or that A.A.W.S. necessarily agrees with the views expressed herein. AA is a program of recovery from alcoholism only—use of the Twelve Steps in connection with programs and activities which are patterned after AA, but which address other problems, or in any other non-AA context, does not imply otherwise.

---

ence, Inc., can refer anyone to treatment services in local areas.

EVALUATION

"The nursing process is a dynamic activity that incorporates alternative strategies at every stage of

the process, based on ongoing and systematic evaluation of client assessment data" (ANA & NNSA, 1988, p. 17).

The nurse evaluates the response of the client to the interventions and revises the nursing diagnoses, interventions, and treatment plan accordingly. Data are obtained from multiple sources, such as the staff, documentation, the client, and his or her family or significant others. The ultimate outcome is complete freedom from drug use and abuse. However, the potential for relapse is ever-present.

Continuum of care is difficult and costly. Although some professionals have suggested that problem drinkers can return to controlled drinking, many experts feel that abstinence should be the ultimate goal because relapse can occur at any time. It is not unusual for a client to give a history of several attempts to achieve sobriety or to be "clean" of drugs. Such individuals believe that they can drink or do drugs socially. Examples of services available to clients who relapse include:

- 28-day inpatient program
- Short-term residential rehabilitation for 3 months
- Long-term therapeutic community programs for 6 to 18 months
- Day-treatment centers
- Re-entry programs
- Outpatient or aftercare programs

Halfway houses provide group living in a structured environment for recovering alcoholic clients who need a "home away from home" or who have no home. Comprehensive industrial programs for alcoholic employees have been developed in an effort to save corporations an estimated $10 billion per year. Employee assistance programs, such as in-house counseling and AA programs, have been developed. Hospitals and mental health centers also provide support groups. See Nursing Plan of Care 25-1: The Client With Alcohol Dependence.

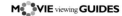 M VIE viewing GUIDES

NURSING PLAN OF CARE 25.1

THE CLIENT WITH ALCOHOL DEPENDENCE

Alan, a 54-year-old accountant, was seen by his attending physician for a yearly physical examination required by his company. During the evaluation, Alan informed the physician that he drank a six-pack or two of beer nightly to relax after a stressful day at work. He further stated that he had been drinking on and off since his early 20s, but was always able to handle his drinking. He denied having any problems with his wife or children. He also denied being depressed or anxious.

When asked whether he considered himself to be an alcoholic, Alan stated he was a "social drinker" and could quit drinking anytime: however, he could not state when he last abstained from drinking.

Alan's physician informed him that he was anemic and that his weight was below the ideal body weight range for his height. He recommended that Alan be seen for an evaluation regarding the possibility of alcoholism before he developed any medical complications secondary to alcoholism.

DSM-IV-TR DIAGNOSIS: Alcohol dependence

ASSESSMENT: Personal strengths: Good health except for anemia and being underweight, married with children, accountant

Weaknesses: Denial of a drinking problem, weight loss below ideal body weight, anemic, inadequate coping skills

NURSING DIAGNOSIS: Imbalanced Nutrition: Less than Body Requirements due to effects of alcohol.

OUTCOME: Client will increase nutritional and caloric intake.

Planning/Implementation	Rationale
Determine daily caloric requirements that are realistic and adequate.	The client's physical health is a priority Many physical problems besides anemia and weight loss may develop as a result of imbalanced nutrition.
Explain the importance of adequate nutrition.	The client may lack knowledge about the physiologic effects of alcohol (eg, weight loss, anemia).
Arrange dietary consultation with input by the client.	The client needs to develop adequate eating habits to meet minimum daily caloric requirements.

NURSING DIAGNOSIS: Ineffective Coping identified by the statement that he drinks to relieve stress

OUTCOME: Client will identify alternate methods of coping with stress.

Planning/Implementation	Rationale
Encourage client to identify stressful situations at work.	The client may need to learn to recognize the cause of his stress and develop stress management techniques.
Explore relationships with employer, wife, and children	The client can learn to express feelings and deal with emotions without using alcohol.

NURSING DIAGNOSIS: Ineffective Denial about alcohol dependence as evidenced by minimizing the seriousness of his drinking history and stating that he could quit drinking anytime

OUTCOME: Client will develop an understanding that alcohol use is an ineffective coping mechanism that can result in physical damage.

Planning/Implementation	Rationale
Discuss evidence of physical change.	Client may be unaware of the deleterious effects of alcohol.
Acquire commitment to keep a diary of alcohol use.	Client may be able to determine his pattern of drinking and recognize it as an ineffective method of coping with stress.
Provide self-help manuals and information about groups for client and his family.	The client is dealing with feelings and behaviors that have been accumulating for years.
	Resolving these issues and making personal changes is facilitated by ongoing support of his family and others in similar situations.

EVALUATION: Evaluation focuses on the client's understanding of the physical damage of alcohol abuse that he has experienced (anemia and low body weight), the potential for additional damage in other aspects of his life, and the need to develop effective coping skills.

KEY CONCEPTS

◆   According to the 2003 statistics, about 51% of all U.S. adults currently use alcohol. Approximately 15.3 million Americans (one in every 12 adults) abuse alcohol, compared with the 5.1 million persons identified in 1990.

◆   Data from major surveys painted a mixed picture of the nation's drug-use problems between 2002 and 2004. The use of ecstasy and methamphetamine declined since 2002. "Club drugs" remain easy to obtain and prescription medication abuse accounts for nearly 30% of the nations' drug problem. The highest rates of drug abuse were found among young people ages 16 to 17 years.

◆   In 1964, the World Health Organization recommended using the term "drug dependence" instead of "addiction" to describe the two concepts of dependence: behavioral dependence and physiologic dependence. Addiction is a term used to define a state of chronic or recurrent drug intoxication characterized by psychological and physical dependence as well as tolerance. Tolerance is a term used to describe a person's ability to obtain the desired effect from a specific dose of a drug or alcohol.

◆   Physiologic effects of alcohol are numerous and affect systems such as the gastrointestinal tract, cardiovascular system, respiratory tract, reproductive system, and central nervous system.

◆   Biologic theories of addiction state that all drugs of abuse affect dopamine secretion and subvert normal functions of neural structures and pathways. Some researchers have also speculated that individuals have a predisposition to or are at risk for addiction because of having fewer D2 dopamine receptors; interference with enzyme action on dopamine molecules; a high level of stress hormones; a deficit in dopamine function that is temporarily corrected by their drug of choice; or electrical phenomena in the brains of people at risk for alcoholism.

◆   Studies of twins, adoptees, and siblings indicate that the cause of alcohol abuse has a genetic component.

◆   Behavior and learning theories, sociocultural theories, and psychodynamic theories have also been described by theorists in an attempt to understand the etiology of substance dependence and abuse. In addition, the disease concept of alcoholism has been accepted by the medical profession.

◆   Alcohol-related disorders include two categories: alcohol use disorders, including alcohol dependence and alcohol abuse; and alcohol-induced disorders, including intoxication, withdrawal, delirium, dementia, amnestic disorder, psychotic disorder, mood, anxiety, sexual dysfunction, and sleep disorders.

◆   Ten classes of substances, other than alcohol, are associated with both abuse and dependence: amphetamines, caffeine, cannabis, cocaine, hallucinogens, inhalants, nicotine, opioids, phencyclidine (PCP), and the group of sedatives, hypnotics, and anxiolytics.

◆   Designer drugs, club drugs (also referred to as date rape drugs), and anabolic steroids are three popular categories of illicit substances readily accessible to the public.

◆   Research studies are being conducted to determine whether the clinical symptoms (eg, "high" similar to substance abuse) experienced by individuals who are addicted to the use of the Internet meet the criteria for the proposed diagnosis of Internet Addiction Disorder.

◆   Several assessment tools are available for evaluating alcohol abuse. They include the MAST, CAGE, and AUDIT, and a 12-question quiz designed to identify teens with drinking problems. The Clinical Institute Withdrawal Assessment for Alcohol serves as a guide when determining whether a client is intoxicated or at risk for withdrawal from alcohol abuse. The DIS and ASI are used to assess both alcohol and drug abuse. Because of the possibility of complex medical problems secondary to substance abuse, a complete medical evaluation includes urine and blood alcohol or drug screen, laboratory tests, and neurologic evaluation. A new diagnostic tool for alcoholism, the Carbohydrate-deficient Transferring Test, is now available. Additional tests are completed when indicated.

◆   Nurses are not immune to the development of a substance-related disorder. Several states have adopted programs for impaired nurses to provide early intervention, rehabilitation, and possible retention in the nursing profession without fear of disciplinary action or loss of license.

◆   Nursing diagnoses identify the client's health needs requiring interventions, such as poor general health, inadequate nutrition, infections, medical complications, and sensory or perceptual alterations. Communication, social interactions, and family dynamics are also addressed.

◆ Nursing interventions include providing assistance in meeting basic needs, creating a safe environment, stabilizing medical condition, stabilizing behavior, medication management, providing interactive therapies, and providing client education.

◆ Relapse can occur at any time during treatment. The nurse assists the client in planning continuum of care.

For additional study materials, please refer to the Student Resource CD-ROM located in the back of this textbook.

CHAPTER WORKSHEET

CRITICAL THINKING QUESTIONS

1. Prepare a genogram of a client with alcohol abuse and his or her family. What patterns do you find? What conclusions can you make about alcoholism as a disease?
2. Attend an Alcoholics Anonymous, Al-Anon, or Alateen meeting in your community. What kinds of appropriate and inappropriate coping skills did you see? What kinds of group tasks did you observe?
3. Professional nurses are not exempt from substance abuse; in fact, many communities have support groups for recovering nurses. Research the available services for impaired nurses at your hospital and in the community. Explore the behaviors and personality traits of the impaired nurse. What assessment parameters might assist the profession to quickly identify and help these nurses?
4. One needs only to turn on a television or read a newspaper to realize that drug abuse is a major social, economic, and political problem in this country. What actions might a community mental health nurse take to create awareness among children in his or her community? What actions might a hospital-based nurse take?

REFLECTION

Reflect on the chapter opening quote. Compare and contrast the serious medical and social conse-quences of alcohol abuse to drug abuse. Which abuse do you think is more detrimental to a client's quality of life? Why? Which abuse do you think is more detrimental to a client's family? Explain your answers.

NCLEX-STYLE QUESTIONS

1. The nurse understands that the biochemical theory of addiction is based on research establishing that all drugs of abuse have one thing in common, that is, the stimulation of which neurotransmitter?
   a. Acetylcholine
   b. Dopamine
   c. Norepinephrine
   d. Serotonin

2. The nurse teaches a client who has a *DSM-IV-TR* diagnosis of alcohol abuse about the physical consequences of continued abuse, including the central nervous system disorders of Korsakoff's psychosis and Wernicke's encephalopathy. The nurse emphasizes that alcohol and deficiency of which vitamin are associated with these disorders?
   a. Vitamin C
   b. Vitamin A
   c. Niacin
   d. Thiamine

3. The nurse identifies which substance commonly abused as the most common cause of sudden heart attack in healthy young people?
   a. Alcohol
   b. Cocaine
   c. Marijuana
   d. Steroids

4. The nurse and the family of a client participate in a planned intervention for the client with an alcohol problem. Which statement best explains the rationale for this technique?
   a. Assists the family to identify client's problems
   b. Confronts the client's denial of the problem
   c. Prepares the client for a treatment program
   d. Teaches the client about Alcoholics Anonymous

5. A client is admitted to an inpatient unit for alcohol detoxification. The nurse plans to protect the client from injury resulting from which of the following complications?
   a. Anxiety
   b. Tremors
   c. Seizures
   d. Headaches

6. When describing the Alcoholics Anonymous program to a client, the nurse identifies some of the 12 steps involved. Place the steps below in their proper sequence from first to last.
   a. Making direct amends to persons
   b. Experiencing a spiritual awakening
   c. Admission of powerlessness over alcohol
   d. Belief in a power greater than one's self
   e. Admission of wrongs to self and others
   f. Taking a searching and fearless moral self-inventory

Selected References

Addiction Help Services. (2006). Detox methods. Retrieved February 12, 2006, from http://www.addictionhelpservices.com

Altrocchi, J. (1980). *Abnormal behavior.* New York: Harcourt Brace Jovanovich.

American Nurses Association, Drug and Alcohol Nursing Association, & National Nurses Society on Addictions. (1987). *The care of clients with addictions: Dimensions of nursing practice.* Kansas City, MO: American Nurses Association.

American Nurses Association, & National Nurses Society on Addictions. (1988). *Standards of addictions nursing practice with selected diagnoses and criteria.* Washington, DC: American Nurses Publishing.

American Psychiatric Association. (2000). *Diagnostic and statistical manual of mental disorders* (4th ed., text revision). Washington, DC: Author.

American Society of Pain Management Nurses. (2002). ASPMN position statement: Pain management in patients with addictive disease. Retrieved February 5, 2006, from http://www.aspmn.org/organization/position_papers.htm

Andrews, M. M., & Boyle, J. S. (1999). *Transcultural concepts in nursing care* (3rd ed.). Philadelphia: Lippincott Williams & Wilkins.

Ang, Audra. (2005, July 3). China clinic treats Net addiction. *Orlando Sentinel,* p. A4.

Anthenelli, R. M. (2005). How—and why—to help psychiatric patients stop smoking. *Current Psychiatry, 4*(1), 77-78, 82, 85-87.

Banks, S. M., Pandiani, J. A., Schacht, L. M., & Gauvin, L. M. (2000). Age and mortality among white male problem drinkers. *Addiction, 95*(8), 1249-1254.

Bates, JB. (2005). Watch for the hallmarks of "pseudoaddiction." *Clinical Psychiatry News, 33*(9), 55.

Berman, C. W. (2001). Alcohol addiction: A case history. *CNS News, 3*(5), 4.

Bernstein, J. G. (1995). *Handbook of drug therapy in psychiatry* (2nd ed.). Littleton, CT: PSG Publishing.

Clinical Psychiatry News. (2000, May). *28*(5), 37.

Colyar, M. R. (2003). Testing for drugs of abuse. *ADVANCE for Nurse Practitioners, 11*(9), 30-31.

Connery, H. S. M., & Weiss, R. D. (2005). Acamprosate: For discomfort of early alcohol abstinence. *Current Psychiatry, 4*(2), 90-91, 95-96.

Cornish, J. W., McNicholas, L. F., & O'Brien, C. P. (1995). Treatment of substance-related disorders. In A. F. Schatzberg & C. B. Nemeroff (Eds.), *Textbook of psychopharmacology* (pp. 707-724). Washington, DC: American Psychiatric Press.

Drew, D. C. (1999). Drugs of abuse: Designer drugs. Retrieved May 23, 2003, from http://www.drugfreeworkplace.com/drugsofabuse/designer.htm

Drug Enforcement Administration. (2006). Controlled Substance Schedules I-V. Retrieved February 7, 2006, from http://www.deadiversion.usdoj.gov/drugs.html

Duran, M. G. (2003). Internet addiction disorder. Retrieved February 5, 2006, from http://allpsych.com/journal/internetaddiction.html

Essortment.com. (2006). Prohibition in America. Retrieved February 5, 2006, from http://inin.essortment.com/prohibitionamer_refo.htm

Ewing, J. A. (1984). Detecting alcoholism: The CAGE questionnaire. *Journal of the American Medical Association, 252,* 1905-1907.

Family Practice Notebook.com. (2005). Clinical Institute Withdrawal Assessment for Alcohol (CIWA-Ar). Retrieved July 29, 2005, from http://www.fpnotebook.com/PSY83.htm

Finn, R. (2004). Young people increasingly abuse DXM. *Clinical Psychiatry News, 32*(5), 10.

Flora, C. (2005). Tough love. *Psychology Today, 38*(6), 40-41.

Gallant, D. S. (1982). *Alcohol and drug abuse curriculum guide for psychiatric faculty* (pp. 53-63). Rockville, MD: National Institute on Alcohol Abuse and Alcoholism.

Goodwin, D. W. (1979). Alcoholism and heredity. *Archives of General Psychiatry, 36*(1), 57-61.

Goodwin, D. W. (1992). *Is alcoholism hereditary?* New York: Ballantine Books.

Goulding, P. M., & Shank, S. L. (2005). Substance abuse. In *Catalog 27 JLS, Florida nurses CE hours* (pp. 26-52). Lakeway, TX: National Center of Continuing Education, Inc.

Grinspoon, L. (Ed.). (1998a). Addiction and the brain—Part I. *The Harvard Mental Health Letter, 15*(6), 1-3.

Grinspoon, L. (Ed.). (1998b). Addiction and the brain—Part II. *The Harvard Mental Health Letter, 15*(7), 1-3.

Hanson, D. J. (2006). National prohibition of alcohol in the U.S. Retrieved February 5, 2006, from http://www2.potsdam.edu/hansondj/Controversies/1091124904.html

Herrick, T. (2005). The meth epidemic: Ravaging communities, straining health care resources. *Clinician News, 9*(10), 1, 21.

International Nurses Society on Addiction. (2006). Mission statement. Retrieved February 5, 2006, from http://www.intnsa.org/about.htm

Internet Alcohol Recovery Center. (2003). Naltrexone: Frequently asked questions. Retrieved December 13, 2003, from http://www.uphs.upenn.edu/recovery/

Intervention Project for Nurses. (2001–2006). Retrieved February 4, 2006, from http://www.ipnfl.org/history.html

Jellinek, E. M. (1977). Phases of alcohol addiction. *Quarterly Journal of Studies on Alcohol, 38,* 114–130.

Jellinek, E. M. (1988). *The disease concept of alcoholism.* New Haven, CT: Alcohol Research Documentation, Inc.

Kelly, J. (2005). New medications for alcoholism enter clinical trials. *Neuropsychiatry Reviews, 6*(9), 1, 16, 20.

Kirn, T. F. (2006). New paradigm embraced for alcohol treatment. *Clinical Psychiatry News, 34*(1), 1, 47.

Kotz, M. (2005). Comorbid addiction and chronic pain. *Clinical Psychiatry News, 33*(10), 17.

Liska, K. (2003). *Drugs and the human body: With implications for society* (7th ed.). New York: Prentice-Hall.

Little, L. (2005). Program uses families to address addiction. *Clinical Psychiatry News, 33*(11), 53.

Lucas, B. D. (1998). Recognizing and treating patients with drinking problems. *Patient Care Nurse Practitioner*, (12), 35–42.

McCabe, Donna. (2001). Emergent conditions. In S. M. Netting (Ed.), *Lippincott manual of nursing practice* (7th ed., pp. 1090–1092). Philadelphia: Lippincott Williams & Wilkins.

Medina, J. (2000). The biology of human addiction, Part I. *Psychiatric Times, 17*(8), 19–21.

Miller, P. M., Dominick, C., & Anton, R. F. (2005). Carbohydrate-deficient transferring test: A tool for detecting alcohol abuse. *Current Psychiatry, 4*(6), 80–82, 87.

Mitchell, A. E., & Parish, T. G. (2005). Using combination therapy for smoking cessation. *Clinician Reviews, 15*(5), 40–45.

National Clearinghouse for Alcohol and Drug Information. (2003). Quick facts. Retrieved February 5, 2006, from http://www.health.org/

National Criminal Justice Reference Service. (2004a). Club drugs: Facts and figures. Retrieved February 5, 2006, from http://www.ncjrs.gov/spotlight/club_drugs/facts.html

National Criminal Justice Reference Service. (2004b). In the spotlight: Club drugs summary. Retrieved February 5, 2005, from http://www.ncjrs.gov/spotlight/club_drugs/summary.html

National Institute on Alcohol Abuse and Alcoholism. (2003). Quick facts. Retrieved May 28, 2003, from http://www.niaaa.nih.gov/databases/qf.htm

National Institute on Drug Abuse. (1999). Drug abuse and addiction research: The sixth triennial report to Congress. Retrieved December 13, 2003, from http://www.drugabuse.gov/STRC/STRCindex.html

National Institute on Drug Abuse. (2004). Trends and statistics. Retrieved February 5, 2006, from http://www.nida.nih.gov/drugpages/stats.html

National Survey on Drug Use and Health. (2004). Club drugs—Facts and figures. Retrieved February 5, 2006, from http://www.ncjrs.gov/spotlight/club_drugs/facts.htm

Nichols, R. (2003). Pain control: Pain management in patients with addictive disease. *American Journal of Nursing, 103*(3), 87–90.

Pfizer, Inc. (1996, March/April). Understanding psychiatric disorders: What is substance abuse? *Clinical Advances in the Treatment of Psychiatric Disorders.*

Prochaska, J. O., & DiClemente, C. C. (1982). Transtheoretical therapy: Toward a more integrative model of change. *Psychotherapy: Theory, Research, and Practice, 19,* 276–288.

Psychiatry 24×7. (2004). Substance abuse. Retrieved October 24, 2004, from http://www.psychiatry24×7.com

Riggin, O. Z. (1996a). The client who is abusing substances other than alcohol. In S. Lego (Ed.), *Psychiatric nursing: A comprehensive reference* (2nd ed., pp. 264–274). Philadelphia: Lippincott-Raven.

Riggin, O. Z. (1996b). The client who is addicted to alcohol. In S. Lego (Ed.), *Psychiatric nursing: A comprehensive reference* (2nd ed., pp. 253–263). Philadelphia: Lippincott-Raven.

Roscoe, M. S. (2004). The drug-seeking patient: Undertreated pain or underhanded motives? *Clinician Reviews, 14*(2), 51–58.

Rosenthal, R. N. (2006). Intramuscular naltrexone: Targeting adherence in alcohol dependency treatment. *Current Psychiatry, 5*(3), 106–108, 111.

Ruppert, R. A. (1999). The last smoke. *American Journal of Nursing, 99*(11), 26–32.

Sadock, B. J., & Sadock, V. A. (2003). *Kaplan & Sadock's synopsis of psychiatry: Behavioral sciences/clinical psychiatry* (9th ed.). Philadelphia: Lippincott Williams & Wilkins.

Shahrokh, N., & Hales, R. E. (Eds.) (2003). *American psychiatric glossary* (8th ed.). Washington, DC: American Psychiatric Press.

Sherman, C. (2001). "Targeted" naltrexone: Last call for alcohol. *Clinical Psychiatry News, 29*(11), 27.

Smith, J. (1999). Alcoholism and free will. *Psychiatric Times, 16*(4), 59–62.

Substance Abuse and Mental Health Services Administration. (2005). Statistics and data. Retrieved January 13, 2005, from http://www.samhsa.gov/index.aspx

Thurston, B. A. (1997). Substance abuse and dependency. In B. S. Johnson (Ed.), *Psychiatric–mental health nursing: Adaptation and growth* (4th ed., pp. 653–694). Philadelphia: Lippincott-Raven.

Valentine, G. (2002). Addiction: MDMA and ecstasy. *Psychiatric Times, 19*(2), 46–49.

Westermeyer, R. (2005). A user-friendly model of change. Retrieved January 23, 2005, from http://www.habitsmart.com/motivate.htm

Willis, M. (2001). OxyContin: A drug with a reputation. *ADVANCE for Nurses, 2*(23), 23–24, 35.

World Health Organization. (2006a). Alcohol. Retrieved February 4, 2006, from http://www.who.int/substance_abuse/facts/alcohol/en/print.html

World Health Organization. (2006b). Other dependence-producing drugs. Retrieved February 4, 2006, from http://www.who.int/substance_abuse/facts/oghers/ en/print.html

Yasgur, B. S. (2004). The neurologic roots of addiction. *NeuroPsychiatry Reviews, 5*(5), 1, 18, 20.

Suggested Readings

Banks, S. M., Pandiani, J. A., Schacht, L. M., & Gauvin, L. M. (2000). Age and mortality among white male problem drinkers. *Addiction, 95*(8), 1249-1254.

Carpenito-Moyet, L. J. (2006). *Handbook of nursing diagnosis* (11th ed.). Philadelphia: Lippincott Williams & Wilkins.

Colyar, M. R., & Call-Schmidt, T. (2005). Through the haze: Reaching out to patients with drug and alcohol addiction. *ADVANCE for Nurse Practitioners, 13*(9), 49-54.

Community Epidemiology Work Group. (2000, June). *Epidemiologic trends in drug abuse: Advance report.* Bethesda, MD: National Institute on Drug Abuse.

Connery, H. S., McHugh, R. K., & Greenfield, S. F. (2005). Does AA work? That's (in part) up to you. *Current Psychiatry, 4*(5), 56, 59-61, 65-67.

Fink, P. J. (2005). Helping elderly drug abusers. *Clinical Psychiatry News, 33*(3), 15.

Graham, J. (2000). Rock bottom: Recognizing alcoholism in your patients. *ADVANCE for Nurse Practitioners, 8*(9), 34-35, 37-38.

Henderson-Martin, B. (2000). No more surprises: Screening patients for alcohol abuse. *American Journal of Nursing, 100*(9), 27-32.

Kaplan, A. (2001). Trying to solve the prescription drug abuse equation. *Psychiatric Times, 18*(2), 1, 3, 7.

Jancin, B. (2005). Smoking cessation: Physicians urged to lead. *Clinical Psychiatry News, 33*(2), 43.

Latimer, G. S. (2005). Alcohol screening in the ED. *ADVANCE for Nurses, 6*(20), 23-25.

Luggen, A. S. (2006). Alcohol and the older adult. *ADVANCE for Nurse Practitioners, 14*(1), 47-52.

Melick-Shield, J., Barloon, D., & Liesveld, J. (2005). Dependence risk with chronic dextromethorphan abuse. *Current Psychiatry, 4*(2), 13-16, 22-23.

Schultz, J. M., & Videbeck, S. L. (2005). *Lippincott's manual of psychiatric nursing care plans* (7th ed.). Philadelphia: Lippincott Williams & Wilkins.

Valente, S. M. (2000). Cocaine abuse in primary care. *American Journal for Nurse Practitioners, 4*(4), 7-16.

Washington, O. G. M., & Moxley, D. P. (2004). Using scrapbooks and portfolios in group work with women who are chemically dependent. *Journal of Psychosocial Nursing and Mental Health Services, 42*(6).

CHAPTER 26 / SEXUALITY AND SEXUAL DISORDERS

*Sexuality is determined by anatomy, physiology, psychology, the culture in which
one lives, one's relationship with others and developmental experiences throughout
the life cycle. It includes the perception of being male or female and all those thoughts,
feelings, and behaviors connected with sexual gratification and reproduction,
including the attraction of one person to another.* —SADOCK & SADOCK, 2003

*The concept of sexual identity involves a sense of masculinity and femininity that is
derived not only from biological sex drives but also from the individual's perception
of his or her sexual being. This perception is partially based on experiences and
interests and the attitudes of society, the culture, family, and friends.* —HAFFNER, 1994

AFTER STUDYING THIS CHAPTER, YOU SHOULD BE ABLE TO:

1. Differentiate among the terms *sex, sexual acts,* and *sexuality.*
2. Describe the theories of gender identity development.
3. Differentiate between the terms *gender identity* and *sexual identity.*
4. Articulate the attitudes and behaviors of sexuality exhibited by individuals at various developmental stages: infancy and childhood, preadolescence and adolescence, and adulthood.
5. Identify factors that contribute to sexual aggression in children and adolescents.
6. Describe the phases of the human sexual response cycle.
7. Relate the dynamics of female and male sexual dysfunctions.
8. Describe masochistic and sadistic behavior.
9. Explain the consequences of sexual addiction.
10. Analyze the barriers to taking a sexual history.
11. Articulate the importance of addressing transcultural considerations when conducting a sexual history.
12. Discuss the various pharmacologic approaches used to treat female and male clients with clinical symptoms of a sexual disorder.
13. Formulate a list of nursing interventions for a female client with clinical symptoms of a sexual disorder.

LEARNING OBJECTIVES

KEY TERMS

Ambiguous genitalia
Chromosomes
Gender identity
Hermaphrodism
Homosexuality
Klinefelter's syndrome
Male pseudohermaphro-
  dites
Masochistic behavior
Paraphilia
Sadistic behavior
Sex
Sexual acts
Sexual addiction
Sexual behavior
Sexual dysfunction
  disorder
Sexual identity
Sexuality
Sexual orientation
Sexual response
Transgender
Transsexual
Transvestite
Turner's syndrome

The terms *sex, sexual acts,* and *sexuality* are often used interchangeably. Trieschmann (1975), though, believes the terms should be differentiated. **Sex** is described as one of four primary drives that also include thirst, hunger, and avoidance of pain. **Sexual acts** occur when behaviors involve the genitalia and erogenous zones. **Sexuality** is the result of biologic, psychological, social, and experiential factors that mold an individual's sexual development, self-concept, body image, and behavior. Sexuality depends on four interrelated psychosexual factors. They include:

- **Sexual identity:** Whether one is male or female based on biologic sexual characteristics
- **Gender identity:** How one views one's gender as masculine or feminine; socially derived from experiences with the family, friends, and society
- **Sexual orientation:** How one views one's self in terms of being emotionally, romantically, sexually, or affectionately attracted to an individual of a particular gender
- **Sexual behavior:** How one responds to sexual impulses and desires

Sexuality is associated with attractiveness, sensuality, pleasure, intimacy, trust, communication, love and affection, affirmations of one's gender identity, and reverence for life (Krozy, 1998; Sadock & Sadock, 2003). It partially defines our role in society and influences our feelings. It can be expressed verbally while talking to a significant other; it can be communicated in written forms such as letters, poetry, or songs; and it can be expressed artistically. Behavioral expressions of sexuality include actions such as looking, touching, handholding, and kissing. Sexuality can be expressed in various ways during the development of an intimate interpersonal relationship.

Sexuality can be influenced by cultural or ethnic factors, religious views, health status, physical attributes, age, environment, or personal choice as a result of one's personality development. The term *normal sexual behavior* refers to a sexual act that is acceptable in our society, occurs between consenting adults, lacks any type of force, and is performed in a private setting in the absence of unwilling observers. Any act that does not meet the criteria set forth in this definition is referred to as *abnormal sexual behavior.*

Nurses come into contact with a variety of client concerns regarding sexual identity or activity (Box 26-1). Sexuality influences how we view ourselves and how we relate to others. It has become an integral part of the nursing process in planning holistic health care. Nurses who are uncomfortable with or confused about their own sexuality may have difficulty discussing sexual issues with clients. Sexual concerns may conflict with the religious beliefs of both clients and staff members. Having respect for the client, examining your own feelings, and maintaining a nonjudgmental attitude are the standards for working with clients in any aspect of human sexuality (Schultz & Videbeck, 2005).

This chapter focuses on theories related to the development of gender identity disorders, the development of sexuality, the human sexual response cycle, and the clinical symptoms and diagnostic characteristics of sexual disorders. Using the nursing process

---

BOX 26.1 | **SEXUALITY: EXAMPLES OF CLIENTS' CONCERNS**

- A mastectomy client verbalizes that her husband no longer finds her sexually attractive.
- A cardiac client expresses fear of resuming sexual activity.
- A colostomy client fears rejection due to change in body image and stoma odors.
- A teenager discloses that he is gay and expresses fear of contracting AIDS.
- A paraplegic client asks his attending practitioner about alternate sexual activity.
- A chemotherapy client requests privacy during visits by a significant other.
- Elderly clients of the opposite sex ask permission to share a room in the nursing home.
- A middle-aged client makes sexual advances while being bathed and attempts to expose his genitals to the nurse.
- A young male client asks a nurse for her address and telephone number.
- A teenaged client tells a male nurse that she thinks she has a sexually transmitted disease.

approach, the chapter describes the care necessary for clients with sexual disorders.

Overview of Gender Identity and Sexual Orientation

Identity is the core of human existence. This reality manifests itself in the human as an evolutional focal point. No other species contemplates its very nature. Understanding gender identity encompasses knowledge about sexual development, interpersonal relationships, affection, intimacy, body image, and gender roles. Almost no information is available about the prevalence of gender identity disorders. Most estimates are based on the number of individuals seeking sexual reassignment surgery (sex-change surgery) (Sadock & Sadock, 2003). The following is a discussion of terminology as it relates to gender identity and sexual orientation and a discussion of the etiology of gender identity development.

Terminology

Sexual identity is the pattern of a person's biologic sexual characteristics including chromosomes, external genitalia, internal genitalia, hormonal composition, gonads, and secondary sex characteristics. *Gender identity* is a person's sense of maleness or femaleness (Sadock & Sadock, 2003). Boys with gender identity disorders are at odds with their body image. They rigidly insist that their male sex organs are disgusting or that they will disappear as they grow up. They elicit a variety of social reactions as they reject their own anatomy and demand that others accept their feminine names and female identity (Rekers & Kilgus, 2001). Girls with gender identity disorders have male companions and an avid interest in sports and rough-and-tough play. They show no interest in dolls or playing house (unless they play the male role). They may refuse to urinate in a sitting position, claim that they have or will develop a penis, do not want to develop breasts or experience menses, and state that they will grow up to be a man (Sadock & Sadock, 2003).

Sexual orientation refers to the object of an individual's sexual impulses. Although normal gender identity may be established at an early age, such as 2 to 3 years, sexual orientation may develop in conflicting or opposite ways as the child progresses through different developmental stages. Sexual orientation may be *heterosexual* (opposite sex), *homosexual* (same

sex), or *bisexual* (both sexes). A conflict between gender identity and sexual orientation may precipitate a gender identity disorder in which the individual has a persistent desire to be, or believes that one is, of the opposite sex and experiences extreme discomfort with one's assigned sex and gender role (Sadock & Sadock, 2003).

The term **transgender** is an umbrella term used to describe **transsexuals** (individuals whose sexual identities are entirely with the opposite sex), **transvestites** (persons who derive sexual pleasure from dressing or masquerading in the clothing of the opposite sex; commonly called "cross-dressers"), and hermaphrodites. A transgender person is someone whose gender identity doesn't coincide with birth gender and the individual can be bisexual, homosexual, or heterosexual (WordReference.com English Dictionary, 2006).

Etiology of Gender Identity Development

The etiology of gender identity is likely biologically determined and secondarily affected by environment. Maintaining skepticism of assumptions and proclamations of etiology is important even while indulging our scientific faith. Look to the longitudinal outcomes of gender identity studies. Gender is anatomic, physiologic, psychosocial, and psychosexual (Reiner, 1997).

Genetic and Biologic Theories

Chromosomes are the carriers of genetic programming information. The male's sperm cell determines the sex of the embryo at conception by adding either an X or a Y chromosome to the X chromosome of the ovum. An X and Y chromosome combination (XY) results in a male fetus; two X chromosomes (XX) result in a female fetus. **Klinefelter's syndrome,** seen in males, occurs as the result of an XXY chromosome grouping (an extra X chromosome). The male appears normal until adolescence, when low levels of testosterone result in small testes, infertility, and a low level of sexual interest. **Turner's syndrome,** seen in females, occurs as the result of a missing sex chromosome (XO grouping instead of XX combination). The female appears short in stature and lacks functioning gonads. During puberty, breasts do not develop and menstruation does not occur. XYY syndrome, seen in males, contributes to a slightly taller stature, low sperm count, and abnormalities of the seminiferous tubules.

The search for a gene related to male **homosexuality,** defined as a primary erotic attraction to others of the same sex, has focused on a genetic link between an unknown gene on the human X chromosome and male homosexual behavior (Xq28 marker). Initially, it was thought that this gene or its mutation appeared to influence development of homosexual traits. However, findings revealed a confusing picture as it became evident that more data are needed from much larger samples before any conclusions can be drawn (Medina, 1999).

The work of Imperato-McGinley proposed that gender identity continually evolves under the influence of androgens despite contrary social forces (Baker, 1999). Individuals with an inherited deficiency of the enzyme 5 x-reductase are born with male genes and male internal organs but lack external male genitalia. Referred to as **male pseudohermaphrodites,** such individuals are declared female at birth and raised as girls. During puberty, they experience a surge in testosterone and gender confusion as they develop emotions and physical signs of masculinization.

Hormonal imbalances may result in a genetic girl or boy developing **ambiguous genitalia** (a penis and a small vaginal opening). True **hermaphrodism** or hermaphroditism is a rare occurrence characterized by the presence of testicular tissue containing seminiferous tubules and spermatozoa, and ovarian tissue containing follicles, in the same person (Sadock & Sadock, 2003). Attempts to explain other abnormalities that can occur biologically or genetically have been made. It is believed that subtle chemical imbalances affecting the central nervous system are also involved in forming one's gender identity (Rippel, 2003).

Psychosocial Theories

Sigmund Freud (1960) theorized that gender identity problems result within the oedipal triangle when conflict is fueled by both real family events and fantasies. Whatever interferes with a child loving a parent of the opposite sex and identifying with the same-sex parent interferes with normal gender identity. For example, the quality of mother–child relationship in the first years of life affects the development of gender identity because mothers normally facilitate their children's awareness of and pride in their gender. Devaluing, hostile mothering can result in gender identity problems. The father's role is equally important during the early years, because his presence generally helps the separation–individuation process. Without a father, the mother and child may remain overly close, and the child may not have the opportunity to develop a sense of maleness or femaleness, or distinguish between the roles of males and females. The father represents future love objects for girls and a model of male identification for boys (Sadock & Sadock, 2003).

According to Zucker, head of the Child and Adolescent Gender Identity Clinic at Clarke Institute of Psychiatry in Toronto, Canada, research in the 1950s showed that among children with physical intersex conditions (ie, both male and female sexual characteristics), sexual assignment and rearing was a better predictor of gender identity than chromosomal, gonadal, and other physical variables (Baker, 1999). Little evidence exists that frank parent-initiated cross-gender rearing attitudes caused gender identity disorder (eg, dressing a girl in boy's clothing or enrolling a girl in sports with boys). Most often, parents just tolerate signs of cross-gender behavior.

Recent theories explore the impact of gender, race, and ethnicity on gender identity. Gender identity, considered to evolve over time, is thought to be shaped by attitudes, values, beliefs, sex roles, religious values, family and ethnic communities, and degree of acculturation. Ryan, Futterman, and Stine (1998) discuss the psychosocial aspects of gender identity development, including the average age of "coming out" (self-identification as lesbian, gay, or same sex and sharing one's sexual identity with others). They reported that this age has dropped from the early twenties to age 16 years.

Clinical Symptoms and Diagnostic Characteristics of Gender Identity Disorders

The features of gender identity disorders are twofold. The *Diagnostic and Statistical Manual of Mental*

Disorders, 4th Edition, Text Revision (DSM-IV-TR) states that there must be evidence of a strong and persistent cross-gender identification in which one expresses the desire to be, or the insistence to be, of the opposite sex (American Psychiatric Association, 2000). The individual also experiences persistent discomfort about his or her assigned sex or feels inappropriate in the role of the assigned sex. Impairment occurs in social, occupational, or other important areas of functioning. For example, boys, who outnumber girls more than six to one in diagnosed cases of gender identity disorder, identify with girls or women and are preoccupied with traditionally feminine activities (Zucker, Bradley, & Sanikhani, 1997).

Girls with gender identity disorders display intense negative reactions when parents attempt to feminize them. They polarize to male attire and activities and prefer to associate with boy playmates. Adult men and women who are preoccupied with their wish to live as the opposite sex may act on their desires by adopting behavior, dress, and mannerisms of the opposite sex. Cross-dressing, hormonal treatments, or sex reassignment in the presence of genital ambiguity may be attempted to pass convincingly as the other sex. European statistics cited in the *DSM-IV-TR* indicate that approximately 1 per 30,000 adult men and 1 per 100,000 adult women seek sex-reassignment surgery. No statistics are available for the United States.

Overview of Sexual Disorders

Sexuality is an important aspect of intimate relationships. The presence or absence of sexual intimacy is a powerful indicator of the health of a couple's relationship. For many individuals, sexuality is an important part of self-esteem. Men and women both may pride themselves on their fertility, their capacity for sexual activity, or their attractiveness to sexual partners. Sexual problems and incompatibilities have a negative impact on how partners feel about themselves and each other. The impairment of sexual function or presence of sexual disorders can make it difficult for partners to enjoy satisfying sex.

Sexual disorders are generally classified as sexual dysfunctions, paraphilias, and sexual addiction. Few systematic epidemiologic data are available regarding the prevalence of various sexual disorders. The most recent comprehensive survey to date focused on a representative sample of the U.S. population between the ages of 18 and 59 years (Gender Identity Research and Education Society, 2003). Table 26-1 compares the

TABLE 26.1 Comparison of Sexual Dysfunctions Between Men and Women

SEXUAL DYSFUNCTION	MEN	WOMEN
Dyspareunia	3%	15%
Incomplete orgasm	10%	25%
Hypoactive sexual desire	10%	33%
Premature ejaculation	27%	n/a
Premature arousal	n/a	20%

SOURCE: Gender Identity Research and Education Society (GIRES). (2003). Epidemiological data. Retrieved August 31, 2003, from http://www.glres.org.uk/text_assets/etiology_definition.pdf

frequency of various sexual dysfunctions between men and women.

Two major factors that influence sexual performance are the presence or absence of normal sexuality (ie, feelings of desire and pleasure to engage in the sexual act) and the presence or absence of an adequate sexual response cycle. A discussion of these two factors follows.

Development of Sexuality

Family is the most important first source of learning about issues of sexuality. Parental attitudes and behaviors begin to shape feelings about male and female gender identity. Developmentally appropriate communication about sex should begin at home with young children and continue through adolescence.

Infancy and Childhood

Infants up to 12 months of age explore their genitalia. Toddlers (ages 1–3 years) master bodily functions and develop a solid core of gender identity. For example, a toddler may experience pleasure from touching his or her genitalia and learns to differentiate between sexual and excretory organs. The toddler also is capable of learning proper terminology regarding body parts, decreasing the likelihood of confusion in the future. Between the ages of 3 and 6 years, the preschooler identifies with the same sex, may ask questions about the origin of babies, and may ask about the anatomic differences between sexes. These are considered to be normal behaviors for children in this age group.

As children interact with other children, they may obtain inaccurate information that could affect the development of healthy sexuality. Parents may consider their children to be asexual beings and avoid discussing or clarifying information related to sexuality because they feel their children may become preoccupied with sex. They also may feel threatened by their child's natural sexual curiosity and respond with hostility or punishment (Finan, 1997; Krozy, 1998). Guidelines are available for parents who wish to deal with sexuality issues from infancy through preschool (Finan, 1997). A sexuality values scale is also available to help clinicians evaluate parental knowledge about sexuality.

Sexual Aggression in Children. One issue associated with sexuality is sexual aggression, which has been linked to general aggression in children between the ages of 5 or 6 years up until puberty (the latency stage). These children describe a history of neglect and physical abuse; a dysfunctional relationship with parents who quarrel or abuse alcohol; physical or sexual aggression against their mother or siblings by their father or another male figure; confrontation with adult sexuality at an early age; or exposure to distorted or deviant sexuality such as pornography. They often name anger, family problems, and boredom as triggers for sexually aggressive behavior, which includes forcing other children to engage in fondling, oral sex, or intercourse. They are unable to handle stress and have poor impulse control, problem-solving abilities, and social skills. They have internalized adults' reactions to their aggressiveness to the extent that they see themselves as perverts. Approximately two thirds of young abusers see sexuality not as an expression of love and affection, but rather as a way of hurting, humiliating, and punishing others.

Although child and youth offenders generally are male in the cases known to date, more cases of sexual exploitation by girls committing acts of sexualized violence against younger/weaker children and young people are becoming known (Moon, 2001; Theme Paper, Young Offenders and Prevention, 2003).

Preadolescence and Adolescence

During preadolescence and adolescence (ages 12–18 years), children experience sexual feelings, exhibit a level of sexual interest, and undergo sexual body changes as they develop interpersonal relationships. Various issues such as menses, nocturnal emissions, masturbation, sexual activity, and sex education are explored. During this time, peer pressure promotes sexually active behavior, and teens may declare an interest in or experiment with alternative sexual lifestyles.

Sexual Aggression in Adolescents. Professional recognition of adolescent aggression and sex crimes has been hampered by the long-standing myth that adolescents are merely experimenting with their sexuality (Hornor, 2003). The etiology of sexually aggressive, exploitive, or threatening behavior in adolescents is similar to that cited in childhood aggression. This includes the presence of psychological problems, history of a dysfunctional family relationship, social awkwardness, history of violence or sexual abuse, and the development of a paraphilia which generally begins in adolescence (See Clinical Symptoms and Diagnostic Characteristics of Sexual Disorders). Nearly 50% of adult sexual offenders report that they committed their first sexual offense before age 18. The younger the age when aggressive behaviors first occur, the greater the likelihood that such behavior will recur (Hornor, 2003). Chapter 33 addresses the issue of sexual abuse.

Adulthood

Preadolescent and adolescent behaviors may continue during young adulthood (ages 19–40 years) as individuals attempt to establish mature relationships with peers. Decisions are made regarding career, marriage, and lifestyle. Young adults may lack knowledge about relationships with significant others, contraceptive measures, sexual trends, sexually transmitted diseases, and alternative lifestyles (Krozy, 1998).

Sexual patterns established during early adulthood are the best predictors of sexual expression in midlife and beyond. However, expressions of sexuality may vary as the individual continues to work through the developmental stages of middle adulthood (ages 41–64 years) and late adulthood or maturity (65 years to death) (Baxer, 2001). Although physiologic changes occur and chronic illnesses may begin, interest in sexual activity among the elderly may continue, or in some instances, increase rather than decrease. Frequency of sex acts may decline, but the quality need not change. Companionship and physical activities such as touching, hugging, and handholding may replace the individual's earlier expectations of intimacy. The ability to interact intellectually with people who share similar interests and experiences and the supportive love that grows between human beings (whether romantic or platonic) are equally, and in some instances, more important than physical intimacy (Youngkin, 2004).

Krozy (1998) discusses the role of sexuality as a human force throughout life. Individuals generally value intimacy over isolation and express a need for closeness with another person during a terminal illness. Members of the nursing profession or hospice staff often meet this need when individuals are hospitalized, relocated to a long-term care facility, or cared for at home. Family members may be concerned, surprised, or embarrassed as a family member or partner expresses an interest in continuing a sexual relationship with his or her husband, wife, or significant other. Nurses should encourage the client and family to discuss sexual issues and needs.

Human Sexual Response Cycle

Sexual response is a psychophysiologic experience. Psychosexual development, psychological attitudes about sexuality, and attitudes toward one's sexual partner are directly involved with and affect the physiology of the human sexual response. The human sexual response cycle is commonly divided into four phases: desire, excitement, orgasm, and resolution.

Desire

Sexual desire is described as the ability, interest, or willingness to receive sexual stimulation. This phase involves activation of the inhibitory and excitatory functions of the brain by neurotransmitters in the limbic system. Desire appears to be controlled by the individual's perception of the environment, personal preferences, attractions to other people, and the absence of inhibitions. Desire may be inhibited by the presence of fear, anxiety, discomfort, other basic needs such as hunger, or an intense emotion such as anger (Byers & Esparza, 1997; Krozy, 1998).

Excitement

Sexual excitement or arousal occurs as the result of psychological stimulation (eg, fantasizing during the desire phase, foreplay involving erogenous zones, or watching sexually explicit movies). Foreplay involves petting and fondling of erogenous zones, areas of the body that are particularly sensitive to erotic stimulation. During this phase, females generally experience vaginal lubrication, pelvic congestion, clitoral swelling, and nipple erection. Males experience stiffening and

an increase in the length and width of the glans penis. Testes increase in size and elevate. For both sexes, vital signs increase, motor restlessness occurs, and a fine rash or "sex flush" may appear over the chest and abdomen (Byers & Esparza, 1997; Krozy, 1998).

Orgasm

The third phase of sexual response, orgasm, was formerly termed *climax*. During this phase, women experience several strong, rhythmic contractions of the vagina, which are followed by spastic contractions. The vagina enlarges, the uterus contracts irregularly, generalized muscle spasm and loss of voluntary muscle control occurs, and vital signs and the sex flush peak. Men experience emission and ejaculation of seminal fluid. Ejaculatory contractions involve the entire length of the penis. They are initially expulsive, followed by several contractions of less intensity. Some women are capable of experiencing multiple orgasms. Men generally experience a refractory period following orgasm and before resolution (Byers & Esparza, 1997; Krozy, 1998).

Resolution

Resolution is the final phase of the sexual response cycle. The organs and body systems gradually return to the unaroused state. Vital signs return to normal. The sex flush disappears. Relaxation and satisfaction are felt.

Clinical Symptoms and Diagnostic Characteristics of Sexual Disorders

Sexual disorders are categorized as sexual dysfunction disorders or paraphilias. **Sexual dysfunction disorders** involve an impairment of the sexual physiologic response. **Paraphilias** refer to disorders involving recurrent intense sexual urges and sexually arousing fantasies generally involving nonhuman objects. The major sexual dysfunctions and paraphilias are highlighted here.

Sexual Dysfunctions

Sexual dysfunction disorders involve a disturbance in the processes that characterize the sexual response cycle, or the presence of pain during sexual intercourse. Specific subtypes indicate the underlying etiology and context of the disorder. For example, the dysfunction may be the result of inhibitions, psychological factors such as depression or anxiety, impaired communication between partners, or certain types of stimulation. It may occur at the onset of sexual functioning, or it may develop after a period of normal functioning.

The psychologically induced inability to perform sexually also may result in one of the following *DSM-IV-TR* subtypes of sexual dysfunctions. For example, a female whose first sexual act caused a vaginal tear may be afraid to engage in sex with her significant other.

Sexual Desire Disorders

Two sexual desire disorders are identified: hypoactive sexual desire disorder and sexual aversion disorder. The diagnosis of hypoactive sexual desire disorder is used only if the lack of desire causes distress to the client or the client's partner. Factors such as age, health, frequency of sexual desire (diminished libido), and lifestyle are considered when one is interviewing the person seeking help. The diagnosis of sexual aversion disorder is used if anxiety, fear, or disgust occurs when an individual is confronted with a sexual opportunity.

Sexual Arousal Disorders

In female sexual arousal disorder, the woman may experience little or no subjective sense of sexual arousal. Physiologic studies of sexual dysfunctions indicate that a hormonal pattern may contribute to responsiveness in women who have excitement-phase dysfunction. Alterations in testosterone, estrogen, prolactin, and thyroxin levels, as well as medications with antihistaminic or anticholinergic properties, have also been implicated in female sexual arousal disorder (Sadock & Sadock, 2003).

In males, sexual arousal disorder, also termed *male erectile disorder* or more commonly *erectile dysfunction* (ED), refers to the inability to attain or maintain an erection adequate for sexual activity. The causes may be organic or psychological, or a combination of both. Risk factors include cardiovascular disease, cigarette smoking, and diabetes mellitus. Neurologic disorders associated with ED include spinal cord injury, multiple sclerosis, cerebral vascular accident, Parkinsonism, and multisystem atrophy (Shy-Drager syndrome). Numerous prescription and over-the-counter medications may contribute to ED, possibly affecting the neurovascular

events that lead to an erection directly or indirectly, by reducing libido (Gray, 2001).

Orgasmic Disorders

The diagnoses of female orgasmic disorder and male orgasmic disorder are used to describe recurrent, persistent inhibited orgasm after an adequate phase of sexual excitement in the absence of any organic cause.

Numerous psychological factors are associated with female orgasmic disorder. These factors include fears of rejection, impregnation, or damage to the vagina; hostility toward men; and guilt feelings related to sexual desires and impulses.

Male orgasmic disorders may include premature ejaculation (ie, ejaculation occurring before the person wishes, due to the absence of reasonable voluntary control during the sexual act) and retarded ejaculation or inhibited ejaculation (ie, ejaculation occurring during coitus with great difficulty, if at all) (Sadock & Sadock, 2003).

Sexual Pain Disorders

Sexual pain disorders typically include dyspareunia and vaginismus. The diagnosis of dyspareunia is used to describe recurrent, persistent genital pain in the female or male that occurs during or after intercourse and is not due to a general medical condition. Approximately 30% of all surgical procedures on the female genitalia are estimated to cause temporary dyspareunia. Dyspareunia in men is uncommon and is usually associated with Peyronie's disease, the presence of sclerotic plaques on the penis that causes penile curvature (Sadock & Sadock, 2003).

In vaginismus, spasms of the musculature of the outer third of the vagina are recurrent, persistent, and involuntary, thus interfering with the sexual act. A female engaging in sex for the first time, a victim of rape, or a woman who has had a strict religious upbringing in which sex is associated with sin may experience vaginismus (Sadock & Sadock, 2003).

Sexual Dysfunction Due to a General Medical Condition

This disorder is distinguished from the previous disorders by the presence of clinically significant sexual dysfunction that is due to the direct physiologic effects of a general medical condition. Marked distress or interpersonal difficulty occurs during sexual activity. The subtypes of this disorder include:

- Male or female hypoactive sexual desire disorder due to... (indicate the general medical condition)
- Male erectile disorder due to...
- Male or female dyspareunia due to...
- Other male or female sexual dysfunction due to...

Some common physical disorders could cause difficulty with sexual activity. These include chronic pain syndrome, arteriosclerosis, diabetes, liver disease, hypertension, thyroid disorder, and sexually transmitted diseases. Sexual dysfunction may also occur as a result of treatments used to manage a general medical condition, such as radiation therapy, nerve blocks, or surgical procedures that physically alter the central nervous system (Paice, 2003).

Medication or substances can diminish libido or inhibit sexual function by causing changes in the blood flow or the nervous system. Examples of substances that interfere with sexual activity have been identified as alcohol, antihypertensive drugs, chemotherapeutic agents, cortisone, hormonal therapy used to treat cancer, narcotic analgesics such as morphine and codeine, antihistamines, anticonvulsants, antipsychotics, SSRIs, sedatives, and recreational drugs (Jensen, Lewis, & Jones, 2004; Paice, 2003). The presence of these conditions needs to be investigated before a diagnosis of sexual dysfunction is made.

Paraphilias

The term *paraphilia* did not enter the *DSM* until 1980. Since that time, it has come to mean different things to different individuals. Often, people confuse the term with *pedophile* (sexual activity with a prepubescent child usually of the same sex). It is important that these terms are used correctly when describing client behavior because this is arguably the most disparaging label society can currently attach to a human being (Frieden, 2005). See Chapter 33 regarding abuse and violence.

The *DSM-IV-TR* describes paraphilias as disorders in which unusual or bizarre sexual imagery or acts are enacted to achieve sexual excitement. These fantasies, urges, or behaviors generally involve nonhuman objects, the suffering and humiliation of oneself or another person, or children or other nonconsenting persons. An example of a paraphilia is sexual sadism, in which an individual achieves sexual excitement from the psychological or physical suffering of another. Sadism can involve the infliction of pain with materials such as leather straps, handcuffs, and whips.

Sexual masochism involves the act of being injured, bound, humiliated, or otherwise made to suffer.

Mental health professionals generally do not see clients with paraphilias unless their behavior creates a conflict with society. Nonconsenting partners may report such activity to legal authorities. Concerned neighbors may suspect that children are the object of sadistic sexual behavior and inform the police or the child welfare bureau of such abuse. Voyeurism, exhibitionism, and pedophilia are three subclassifications of behavior that often result in arrest and incarceration. A description of paraphilias is included in Box 26-2.

Characteristics of Paraphiliacs

A person may experience more than one paraphiliac disorder at the same time, or may exhibit clinical symptoms of other mental disorders such as a personality disorder or schizophrenia. Characteristics or associated features of persons who are classified as paraphiliacs include:

- Emotional immaturity (seen in the pedophile or "peeping Tom" who is unable to engage in a mature sexual relationship because of feelings of inadequacy)
- Fear of a sexual relationship that could result in rejection
- Shyness (seen in the voyeur who views others from a distance)
- The need to prove masculinity, demonstrated by the exhibitionist
- The need to inflict pain on another to achieve sexual satisfaction (seen in **sadistic behavior**)
- The need to endure pain to achieve sexual satisfaction (seen in **masochistic behavior**)
- Low or poor-self concept
- Depression

Not all of the characteristics listed are present in each paraphiliac. The way a paraphiliac expresses himself or herself sexually affords a clue to the paraphiliac's self-concept. For example, the fetishist who has a very low self-concept chooses inanimate objects to satisfy sexual needs, and therefore does not have to fear rejection by a partner.

Sexual Addiction

Although sexual addiction is not a *DSM-IV-TR* diagnosis, it is presented here because individuals who are

BOX 26.2 PARAPHILIAS

Bestiality or Zoophilia: Sexual contact with animals serves as a preferred method to produce sexual excitement. It is rarely seen.

Exhibitionism: An adult male obtains sexual gratification from repeatedly exposing his genitals to unsuspecting strangers, usually women and children who are involuntary observers. He has a strong need to demonstrate masculinity and potency.

Fetishism: Sexual contact with inanimate articles (fetishes) results in sexual gratification. Most often it is a piece of clothing or footwear. Parts of the body may also take on fetishistic significance. Its occurrence is almost exclusive to men who fear rejection by members of the opposite sex.

Frotteurism: Sexual excitement is achieved by touching and rubbing against a nonconsenting person.

Sexual Masochism: Sexual pleasure occurs while one is experiencing emotional or physical pain. The willing recipient of erotic whipping is considered to be masochistic.

Necrophilia: Sexual arousal occurs while the person is using corpses to meet sexual needs.

Pedophilia: The use of prepubertal children is needed to achieve sexual gratification. Pedophilia can be an actual sexual act or a fantasy.

Sexual Sadism: Sexual gratification is experienced while the person inflicts physical or emotional pain on others. Severe forms of this behavior may be present in schizophrenia.

Telephone Scatologia: Sexual gratification is achieved by telephoning someone and making lewd or obscene remarks.

Transvestic Fetishism: A heterosexual male achieves sexual gratification through wearing the clothing of a woman (cross-dressing). It is a learned response due to encouragement by family members. As a child, the person was considered more attractive when dressed up as a girl.

Voyeurism: The achievement of sexual pleasure by looking at unsuspecting persons who are naked, undressing, or engaged in sexual activity. Individuals engaging in voyeurism are commonly called "Peeping Toms."

---

addicted to sex often develop clinical symptoms of sexual disorders.

Sexual addiction, first described by Dr. Patrick Carnes in his book, *Out of the Shadows: Understanding Sexual Addiction* (2001), is defined as engaging in obsessive–compulsive sexual behavior that causes severe stress to addicted individuals and their families. Sexual addicts make sex a more important priority than family, friends, work, and values. Sex becomes the source of nurturing and trust, and addicts are willing to sacrifice what they cherish most to preserve their behavior. Approximately 6% to 8% of the population is affected by sexual addiction (Klein, 2003).

Sexual addicts have admitted that their unhealthy use of sex began with an addiction to masturbation, paraphilia, pornography, or a heterosexual or homosexual behavior. Sexual addiction also includes prostitution, exhibitionism, voyeurism, indecent phone calls, child molestation, incest, rape, and violence. (See Chapter 33 regarding abuse and violence.) Addiction to cybersex is a new but growing disorder that often goes undiagnosed. The explosive growth of the Internet has provided a new outlet for individuals with sexual compulsions. For some, the computer has become the primary focus of their sexual or romantic life. Children (middle school–aged boys in particular) are becoming addicted to sex on the Internet in numbers that would startle most clinicians and parents. It provides the three A's of affordability, accessibility, and anonymity. Signals that a client is addicted to sex online may be missed because clinicians may be unaware of the breadth and variety of sexual activities available on the Internet (Jancin, 2005; Macready, 2001). Addicts experience powerlessness over a compulsive behavior that has made their lives unmanageable. They may feel out of control; experience tremendous shame, pain, and self-loathing; and try to stop, yet repeatedly fail to do so. The unmanageability of addicts' lives is seen in the consequences they suffer: school absenteeism or difficulty with school work, loss of relationships, difficulties with work, arrests, financial troubles, a loss of interest in things not sexual, low self-esteem, and despair. Many sexual addicts have a dual diagnosis including substance abuse or depression.

THE NURSING PROCESS

ASSESSMENT

"In a perfect world, health care providers would be both trained and proficient in all areas of care. In reality, sexual health is often the exception" (Warner, Rowe, & Whipple, 1999, p. 34).

This statement was made regarding the lack of emphasis placed on including a sexual history as part of the assessment phase of the nursing process.

Katz (2005) lists several reasons that the subject of sex may not be addressed by nurses during the assessment process. For example, nurses may be embarrassed, may not believe that sexuality is part of a presenting problem, may feel that discussing sex is an invasion of a client's privacy, or may feel inadequately equipped to provide appropriate nursing interventions. Fear of legal ramifications may also play a role, particularly when the nurse and client are of opposite sexes. Guidelines to obtaining a sexual history are included in the following section.

Sexual History

Obtaining a sexual history in a nonthreatening, quiet, and private environment is essential. Too often, the discomfort of both the nurse and the client interferes with communication during this time. By focusing on the universal aspects of human sexuality, including the need for acceptance, personal bias can be overcome and compassionate interaction with clients can occur (Bresolin, 2001).

During the assessment, ask the client's permission to discuss his or her "sex life," emphasizing that all client information provided is confidential. Be professional when approaching the subject about sexuality and provide support without appearing judgmental. Keep in mind the client's educational level and familiarity with terminology. Use simple words and phrases when asking questions to avoid any misunderstanding or confusion.

Gather data regarding the client's earliest sexual behavior and experiences, attitude about sex, and gender identity. Present questions in order of least sensitive to most sensitive material. Be sure to word the questions in a closed-ended style to elicit a specific response. Examples of questions may include "Are you married?" or "Are you living with a partner?" Allow the information revealed to guide the discussion.

Explore the client's role in sexual relationships, both past and present. Also obtain information about the client's perception of any sexual issues in the relationships. Be especially sensitive with questions regarding the history of any sexual trauma. Also explore any history of depression, anxiety, and substance abuse and legal problems, and pay particular attention to any cultural and religious influences affecting the client's sexuality (Byers & Esparza, 1997; Warner et al., 1999).

As the assessment progresses, determine whether additional data, including a history and physical, genital or pelvic examination, and laboratory tests, are indicated; whether the client is willing to involve a family member or significant other in the collection of data; whether the client would benefit from a referral to a support group; or whether the client and spouse or significant other would benefit from a referral to a knowledgeable family or sex therapist who understands the dynamics of sexual problems. Box 26-3 describes the basic principles of a sexual assessment. Chapter 9 also discusses assessment of sexuality.

Barriers to Taking a Sexual History. Because of the sensitive nature of the subject, obtaining a sexual history can be problematic for the client and nurse. Several

---

BOX 26.3 BASIC PRINCIPLES FOR PERFORMING A SEXUAL ASSESSMENT

- Be comfortable and at ease with the client.
- Present an open and accepting attitude.
- Be empathetic.
- Avoid personal values and biases during the interview.
- Ensure a thorough knowledge base.
- Establish familiar terminology with the client.
- Encourage the client to verbalize any sexual concerns or emotions.
- Support the expression of feelings and validate them.
- Ask specific, open-ended questions.
- Approach emotional or more sensitive questions gradually.
- Progress from how information was learned, to attitudes, then behaviors.
- State that certain sexual behaviors are common before asking questions about them.

issues can create barriers to obtaining the necessary information. Common barriers to taking a client's sexual history include failure to view the client's sexual history as relevant to the plan of care; inadequate training of the health care professional; embarrassment on the part of the health care professional; fear of offending the client by asking personal questions; and the perception by the health care provider that any sexual concern of the client will be overly complex and time consuming for the provider to assess, much less manage (Postlethwaite, Stump, Bielan, & Rudy, 2001).

Another barrier that could interfere with assessment involves legal issues. Providers may be uncertain about state laws regarding a minor's consent to treatment or may feel uncomfortable in supporting an adolescent's decisions that may conflict with a parent's wishes. For lesbian and gay youth who haven't informed their parents of their sexual preference, fear that their confidentiality may not be protected can be a significant barrier to care (Ryan et al., 1998). One or all of these barriers could result in an incomplete sexual health assessment of clients seen in private practice, a general hospital setting, an inpatient psychiatric unit, and a long-term care facility.

Following are some examples for the reader to determine which, if any, of the common barriers could interfere with the assessment process:

1. Clients seen in private practice may complain of hypoactive sexual desire due to a medical condition or decreased libido or impotence due to new medication, or may ask the practitioner for advice regarding sex-reassignment surgery. Transference may occur, because the client believes he or she is in love with the therapist.
2. Sexual acting-out may occur in the general hospital as the client attempts to test his or her sexuality because of loss of independence, low self-esteem, loss of a body part, loneliness, fear, anxiety, or loss of control. Behavior frequently seen includes flirting, deliberately exposing the genital area, dressing in seductive attire, touching the caregiver inappropriately, using profanity, or making provocative comments. Some clients use a shock approach by blatantly discussing promiscuous sexual activity or telling jokes that center on sexual contact.
3. Issues regarding sexuality may occur on an inpatient psychiatric unit. For example, clients may engage in sexually explicit conversation, make sexual advances toward staff or peers of the same

or opposite sex, or openly masturbate on the unit. Clients who are confused or delirious may undress or urinate in public. A teenager, admitted because of a suicide attempt, may be struggling with an emerging sexual identity. Family members express embarrassment to the staff because their loved one is exhibiting impulsive, uninhibited behavior.

4. Restricting the emotional and sexual desires of long-term care clients can result in a loss of their will to live. It is also a violation of their rights. Spouses may ask to take their wife or husband home for a few hours or on an overnight leave of absence. Clients with dementia may be sexually attracted to other residents and exhibit overt sexual behavior. A referral may be made to a mental health provider to assess how competent the client is to engage in an intimate relationship, considering the client's sexual needs and protecting the rights of both competent and incompetent clients.

Assessment of Children and Adolescents

Assessing children and adolescents requires sensitivity. A cultural consensus still remains concerning certain sex-role distinctions that children are expected to master in early development. For example, in our society, only females wear lipstick or dresses in public. If a boy wears a dress and lipstick to school, adults react with disapproval and peers react with ridicule (Rekers & Kilgus, 2001).

Children and adolescents who have concerns about body image, sexual identity, or attraction to the same sex, or who verbalize sexual fantasies, may experience distress and exhibit severe adjustment problems or sexually aggressive behavior that warrants a psychosocial assessment.

If cross-gender behavior is observed in a child or adolescent over a 6-month period, a careful assessment should be made regarding the significance of the behavior to the child or adolescent. The cluster of behaviors requires assessment because the ratio of masculine to feminine behaviors, rather than the exact number of cross-gender behaviors, is diagnostically significant (ie, the pattern of behavior and frequency of mannerisms and gestures are compared with normative data on boys and girls of the same age group) (Rekers & Kilgus, 1995; Zucker et al., 1997).

Children younger than 8 years often are open to answering questions truthfully about sexual behavior, including sexual fantasies or their attraction to peers of the same sex. Older children and adolescents are more aware of the social significance of their behavior and may conceal their true interests. Lesbian and gay youth who report significant stress associated with school and related activities need assessment for evidence of alcohol abuse, depression, and suicidal ideation. Clinical psychological testing may be necessary to obtain additional data during the assessment process (Rekers & Kilgus, 1998; Ryan et al., 1998; Zucker et al., 1997).

Transcultural Considerations

A client's ethnic, cultural, religious, and social background influences sexual attitude, desire, and expectations. Andrews and Boyle (2003) comment about cultural norms related to appropriate male–female and same-sex relationships. Failure to adhere to cultural codes is considered to be a serious transgression. For example, in some cultures, the sexual desires of the woman are not considered relevant; fertility is the primary function of the woman. Also, what is considered deviant sexual behavior in one cultural setting may be an acceptable practice in another culture. Furthermore, a client may experience conflict or disagreement between the messages learned from the social/cultural group in which client grew up and the current social/cultural group in which the client lives. Therefore, be as familiar as possible with the customs of each client's culture.

NURSING DIAGNOSES

The diagnoses of Ineffective Sexuality Patterns and Sexual Dysfunction are difficult to differentiate. Ineffective Sexuality Patterns is a broad diagnosis of which sexual dysfunction can be one part. Defining characteristics of Ineffective Sexuality Patterns include the presence of actual or anticipated negative changes in sexual functioning or sexual identity. Other characteristics that may be present include the expression of concern about sexual functioning or sexual identity; inappropriate sexual verbal or nonverbal behavior; or changes in primary and/or secondary sexual characteristics. (Carpenito-Moyet, 2006).

The nursing diagnosis of Sexual Dysfunction may be more appropriately used by a nurse with advanced

---

EXAMPLES OF NANDA NURSING DIAGNOSES/ SEXUALITY DISORDERS

- Ineffective Sexuality Patterns related to ineffective role models
- Ineffective Sexuality Patterns related to negative sexual teaching
- Ineffective Sexuality Patterns related to absence of sexual teaching
- Ineffective Sexuality Patterns related to values conflict
- Sexual Dysfunction related to limited sexual performance with an impotent partner
- Sexual Dysfunction related to lack of fulfillment due to dyspareunia
- Rape-Trauma Syndrome related to fear of sexual intercourse due to distrust of men
- Rape-Trauma Syndrome related to fear of intimidation by a sexually abusive husband

---

preparation in sex therapy when a client experiences or is at risk of experiencing a change in sexual function that is viewed as unrewarding or inadequate. Defining characteristics include the client's verbalization of a problem with sexual function or report of a limitation on sexual performance imposed by disease or therapy (Carpenito-Moyet, 2006).

The nursing diagnosis of Rape-Trauma Syndrome is used when a client experiences a forced, violent sexual assault against his or her will and without his or her consent. The trauma syndrome develops as a result of the attack or attempted attack. Defining characteristics include a report or evidence of sexual assault (Carpenito-Moyet, 2006) (see Chapter 33). See the accompanying box for Examples of North American Nursing Diagnosis Association (NANDA) Nursing Diagnoses related to sexuality disorders. Other nursing diagnoses that may be used when implementing care for clients with sexual problems or concerns include Chronic Low Self-Esteem, Disturbed Body Image, Anxiety, Fear, Hopelessness, Social Isolation, and Spiritual Distress.

New diagnostic labels regarding women's sexual problems have become increasing prevalent and are currently used by medicine centers that specialize in sexual dysfunction, Web sites, continuing education symposia, and professional organizations (Medscape

Today, 2004). Nurses who obtain sexual histories should familiarize themselves with the following diagnoses although the true prevalence has not been established:

- Female androgen-deficiency syndrome
- Psychotropic-induced sexual dysfunction
- Sexual problems due to sociocultural, political, or economic factors
- Sexual problems related to partner and relationship
- Sexual problems related to psychological factors
- Sexual problems related to medical factors

OUTCOME IDENTIFICATION

Outcomes related to gender identity and sexual functioning cannot be developed without input from the client because they are too personal (Krozy, 1998). Examples of Stated Outcomes are presented in the accompanying box.

PLANNING INTERVENTIONS

The ideal approach to planning treatment of sexual problems is utilization of an integrated sexual health team model involving nurses, sex counselors, medical social workers, and sexuality educators. Familiarity with sexual abuse and domestic violence screening is essential (Medscape Medical News, 2004). Planning focuses on the individual client's specific problems or complaints and respects the client's age, sex, and cultural and religious preferences. The nurse assumes the role of client advocate to ensure the promotion of gender identity and sexual health in the plan of care. Involvement of a spouse, significant other, or family may be necessary.

Normal sexual function requires an intact endocrine system, vascular system, central nervous system, and autonomic and peripheral nervous systems. Generally, a comprehensive medical examination, including a review of medications, is planned to validate the presence of a gender identity disorder or determine the cause of sexual dysfunction.

Negative attitudes about homosexuality, myths, and misperceptions are internalized from early childhood. Children and adolescents may require assistance in learning to manage a stigmatized identity, discrimination, rejection, loss of critical relationships, and ejection from their homes. Lesbian and gay youth may have misperceptions about their physiology, health needs, and health risks. They may have questions about

> **EXAMPLES OF STATED OUTCOMES/**
> **SEXUAL DISORDERS**
>
> - The client will verbalize feelings that lead to sexually aggressive behavior.
> - The client will modify behavior to reduce stressors.
> - The client will identify limitations on sexual activity caused by health problem.
> - The client will share concerns regarding sexual function.
> - The client will identify stressors affecting sexual function.
> - The client will report a desire to resume sexual activity.
> - The client will describe improved body image following reconstructive breast surgery.
> - The client will verbalize satisfaction with sex role.
> - The client will discuss sexual concerns with his or her sexual partner.
> - The client will verbalize understanding of the relationship between adverse effects of drug therapy and sexual dysfunction.

parenting and the risk of sexually transmitted diseases. Finally, they may lack knowledge of support services that can reduce social isolation, provide accurate information, and connect them with positive role models (Ryan et al., 1998).

Interventions are planned to meet the client's basic human needs, provide structured and protective care, and explore methods to re-channel sexually unacceptable behavior. Counseling may be necessary if the client has experienced a recent life change (eg, illness, divorce, death of a spouse, or a second marriage) or traumatic event that has had an impact on the client's sexuality. The client works with the nurse to determine which interactive therapies may be beneficial during the implementation of care.

IMPLEMENTATION

Interventions are individualized based on the client's concerns about sexual identity, gender identity, identified sexual disorder, causative factors, and clinical symptoms. The nurse also considers the client's needs, nursing diagnosis or diagnoses, problem severity, and the nurse's own competence (Krozy, 1998). Knowledge of psychosexual development is imperative. Ensuring the client's rights also is important. Jacobson (1974) describes a bill of rights to guarantee sexual freedom and promote sexual health. These rights include the client's right to express his or her sexuality, to become the person he or she desires to be, and to select a partner of choice, regardless of the partner's gender identity.

Nurses must examine feelings about their own sexuality before they are able to provide care for clients who present with issues related to sexuality. Feelings of disgust, contempt, anger, or fear need to be identified and explored so that they do not interfere with the development of a therapeutic relationship. If the nurse is unable to be objective while providing care for a specific client, the nurse should relinquish responsibility to another member of the health care team.

Assistance in Meeting Basic Needs

Adequate rest, exercise, and nutrition, and good general physical health, promote sexual health. Clients with health problems or who are elderly are assisted in identifying barriers that interfere with sexual functioning (eg, pain, impaired mobility, or adverse effects of medication). Techniques are taught to reduce oxygen consumption and cardiac workload and reduce or eliminate pain during sexual activity.

Provision of a Safe Environment

Client safety is a priority. Clients with impulsive, unpredictable sexual behavior can pose a threat to the safety of others as well as to themselves. The client who has a gender identity conflict may become severely depressed, develop a substance-abuse disorder, exhibit violent behavior toward others, or be victimized by family members.

Children who are sexually aggressive may victimize other children. Clients with paraphilias can be aggressive as they participate in masochistic or sadistic behavior. Some paraphiliacs are disturbed by their thoughts and behaviors and seek help; some are mandated by the courts to seek therapy; and others do not experience any conflict and do not seek therapy.

Environmental manipulation has proven effective in relieving anxiety and altering the undesirable behavior of children who are sexually aggressive, paraphiliacs, and sex offenders. Incarceration may be imposed legally to protect the public, especially children, from being victimized by sex offenders (ie, pedophiles, prostitutes, and other paraphiliacs). The incarcerated client may then be interviewed and accepted into a special program to provide treatment for the specific sexual disorder or problem (see Chapter 35).

The client with a sexual addiction may wish to stop his or her destructive behavior, but fear of consequences keeps many from seeking help. The addict often experiences extreme despair over constant failure to control obsessive behavior. This despair may lead them to contemplate or attempt suicide.

Research reveals that many young people who are gay face abuse from family members after they disclose their sexual orientation (Worcester, 1999). Lesbians are most likely to be attacked by mothers, and gay men are most likely to be attacked by brothers. Such individuals have been known to make suicidal threats, which resulted in involuntary admission to a psychiatric facility. See Supporting Evidence for Practice 26-1.

Medication Management

Various pharmacologic approaches are used to treat clients with sexual disorders. Nurses need to be knowledgeable about and familiar with their application and potential adverse effects. Following is a brief discussion of medication management of female and male sexual disorders.

Female Sexual Disorders. Hormone-replacement therapy is used to reduce dyspareunia in female clients. Such therapy may be given orally, parenterally, or transdermally.

Avlimil is a homeopathic remedy manufactured by Berkeley Premium Nutraceticals in Cincinnati, Ohio. It is used for treatment of female sexual dysfunction. Avlimil is a nonsynthetic, nonhormonal composite of 11 herbs that promotes blood flow and muscle relaxation to achieve an improved sexual response. Examples of drugs that may interact adversely with Avlimil include anticoagulants, antidiabetics, antihypertensives, antiplatelets, contraceptives, estrogens, and drugs that are cytochrome P-450 (CYP) 3A4 and CYP2BC substrates (Aschenbrenner, 2004). Other homeopathic remedies such as aromatherapy, massage therapy, and therapeutic touch are used to reduce pain, depression, or anxiety and promote sexual health.

Studies regarding the treatment of female sexual arousal disorder have focused on the use of the topical phosphodiesterase type-5 inhibitor alprostadil (MUSE); subcutaneous dopamine agonist, apomorphine (Apokyn); and a clitoral vacuum pump. A vali-

SUPPORTING EVIDENCE FOR PRACTICE 26.1
The Relationship Between Suicide Risk and Sexual Orientation

PROBLEM UNDER INVESTIGATION / What is the suicide risk among bisexual/homosexual and heterosexual students?

RESEARCH SUMMARY / The study consisted of 152 female and 184 male bisexual and homosexual groups. Data were obtained from the Adolescent Health Survey to identify the sexual preference of the subjects. Suicide risk was identified from questions that were asked about previous attempts, current suicide thoughts, and suicide plans. Results indicated that 90% of the subjects answered the questions regarding suicide and that bisexual/homosexual males (84%) were less likely to complete these questions when compared with their heterosexual counterparts (91%). Economic status was higher among the heterosexual males (69%) compared with their bisexual/homosexual counterparts (56%).

Results also indicated that there were more white heterosexual females (86%) compared with bisexual/homosexual females (73%). Suicidal intent was significantly associated with male bisexual/homosexual orientation as was previous suicide attempt. Suicidal ideation was not proven to be significant among males and none of the suicidal variables were associated with bisexuality/homosexuality in females.

SUPPORT FOR PRACTICE / Psychiatric–mental health nurses working with teens need to be aware of the findings that males whose sexual preference is that of bisexuality or homosexuality are at risk for attempted suicide. In addition, assessment needs to focus on other factors that may also play a role in suicidal behavior, such as self-identification of homosexuality at a young age, substance abuse, interpersonal conflict, nondisclosure, or family dysfunction.

SOURCE: Remafedi, G., French, S., Story, M., Resnick, S. C., & Blum, R. (1998). The relationship between suicide risk and sexual orientation: Results of a population-based study. American Journal of Public Health, 88(1), 57–60.

dated questionnaire during the studies demonstrated significant benefit in sensation, lubrication, orgasm, and sexual satisfaction (Medscape Medical News, 2004, 2006).

Male Sexual Disorders. ED has been reported to improve significantly with the use of a phosphodiesterase type-5 inhibitor, sildenafil citrate (Viagra). However, the drug is limited in its use. For example, there is potential cardiac risk for clients with preexisting cardiovascular disease. Also, clients have reported prolonged erection lasting longer than 4 hours and priapism (painful erections more than 6 hours in duration). If priapism is not treated immediately, penile tissue damage and permanent loss of potency could result.

Vardenafil (Levitra), tadalafil (Cialis), and transurethral alprostadil (MUSE) are also phosphodiesterase type-5 inhibitors used in the treatment of ED. Clients taking sildenafil or tadalafil should not drink grapefruit juice because the juice inhibits metabolic enzyme activity with possibly fatal consequences (Karch, 2004).

Other medications used in the treatment of male sexual disorders include the injectable agent phentolamine (Vasomax), an alpha-adrenergic receptor blocker; injectable alprostadil (Caverjest), a prostaglandin; and the sublingual dopaminergic agent apomorphine (Spontane); (Google Directory Health Pharmacy, 2006; Sadock & Sadock, 2003). Drug injection therapy, including mixtures of phentolamine, papaverine, prostin, and/or atropine injected directly into the corpora cavernosa prior to intercourse, is effective in clients with ED regardless of the cause.

Hormone therapy may be effective in men with low testosterone levels. Hormonal therapy, however, may suppress natural hormone production and increase the risk of prostate cancer or hypertrophy. Hormone therapy with progestins such as medroxyprogesterone acetate, as well as antianxiety agents and selective serotonin reuptake inhibitors (SSRIs), is also used as adjunctive therapy to reduce libido in clients with sexual addiction and paraphilias, and other sex offenders (Drug Summary Table 26-1: Selected Drugs Used for Male Sexual Disorders).

DRUG SUMMARY TABLE 26-1 — Selected Drugs Used for Male Sexual Disorders

GENERIC (TRADE) NAME	DAILY DOSAGE RANGE	IMPLEMENTATION
Drug Class: Dopaminergic Agents (to improve sexual response)		
levodopa (Larodopa)	0.5–8 g	Give in divided doses (two or more doses with food if GI upset occurs); observe for development of suicidal tendencies; monitor hepatic, renal, hematopoietic, and CV function; instruct client not to take multivitamin preparations with pyridoxine because they may prevent therapeutic effects of drug; instruct client to report vertigo, syncope, abnormal facial or body movements, irregular heartbeat or palpitations, difficulty with urination, and severe or persistent nausea or vomiting.
Drug Class: Impotence Agents (to treat decreased libido and response-cycle dysfunction)		
sildenafil citrate (Viagra)	25–100 mg	Instruct client that drug is usually taken 1 hr before anticipated sexual activity, but it may be taken 30 min to 4 hr before sexual activity; limit use to once per day; instruct client to avoid use of nitrates because serious side effects and death can occur; monitor for headache, dizziness, rash, flushing, palpitations, and painful urination.
Drug Class: Antidepressants (to treat decreased libido and orgasm dysfunction)		
bupropion (Wellbutrin)	200–450 mg	Ask client whether he is taking levodopa, an MAOI, or using alcohol because there is a risk for adverse drug–drug interactions including seizures due to lowering of seizure threshold; give t.i.d. with no dose >150 mg; monitor for dizziness, lack of coordination, tremors, dry mouth, headache, GI disturbances, insomnia, tachycardia, and weight loss.
Drug Class: SSRIs (treatment of premature ejaculation or hyperarousal disorder)		
paroxetine (Paxil)	10–50 mg	Contraindicated during or within 14 days of MAOI therapy; administer in the morning; use cautiously in the presence of renal or hepatic impairment; discuss rationale for use with client who has a sexual hyperarousal disorder; monitor for drowsiness, tremor, somnolence, and GI disturbances; instruct client to report any genitourinary symptoms.

Assistance With Medical Management

The nurse's role in medical management varies depending on the setting in which the client is assessed and treated. For example:

- Is the client being seen in the office primarily for the treatment of impotence secondary to muscular dystrophy?
- Is a referral made because a primary care physician suspects alcoholism in a client who is infertile?

- Does a hospitalized client verbalize concerns about sexuality after a mastectomy?
- Does a hospitalized client exhibit impulsive, sexual acting-out behavior postoperatively?
- Has a client been admitted for a penile implant?
- Has the client experienced a decrease in sexual desire since being placed on lithium?

Comorbidity of sexual dysfunction with depression, anxiety, and alcohol abuse is high. As mentioned earlier, surgical procedures such as cystectomy or arterial vascular surgery as well as medical conditions such as diabetes, multiple sclerosis, renal failure, cardiovascular disease, and peripheral neuropathy can lead to ED (Sadock & Sadock, 2003). Nurses need to be aware of these possible underlying conditions and comorbidities to be better equipped to address the client's concerns.

Nursing responsibilities include being aware of the processes and techniques of mechanical treatment approaches, such as the vacuum pump or penile prosthetic devices that can improve clients' sexual functioning, and knowledgeable of performing appropriate care and procedures when these approaches are used. Interventions also may include explaining the dynamics of sexual response and facilitating sexual communication between partners. Be aware of your own limitations and anticipate the need for referrals to formally trained, certified sex therapists as needed (Krozy, 1998; Sadock & Sadock, 2003).

Interactive Therapies

"The true meaning, and indeed, the deep pleasure associated with sexuality cannot be found in a pill... Exploring the deeper aspects of sexuality is an opportunity and a challenge" (Tamerin, 1998, p. 56).

Various interactive therapies are available to clients. The nurse and client discuss which, if any, of the interactive therapies would be therapeutic: individual, marital or couple, family, sex, group, or behavioral therapy.

Most individuals with a gender identity disorder have fixed ideas and values and are unwilling to change. They may participate in psychotherapy to address issues such as depression or anxiety or how to deal with their disorder, not alter it. Therapy is also used to explore issues related to sex-reassignment surgery (Sadock & Sadock, 2003).

One exciting new program combining many different types of therapy, The INTEGRIS Sexual Trauma and Abuse Recovery (STAR) program in Oklahoma City,

Oklahoma, combines various interactive therapies (eg, individual, group, family, behavior) to address children's sexually abusive behavioral problems. Almost one third of children who are sexually abused and do not receive treatment act out their abuse by behaving in inappropriately sexual ways with others or hurting themselves due to their emotional trauma. Children learn "Sexual Behavior Rules" and coping skills such as the "Turtle Technique," a method used to teach children to control their impulses and anger by helping them stop and think through the consequences of their behavior and make good choices. Treatment also includes individual therapy, family therapy, recreational therapy, social skills training, self-esteem development, anger management, stress management, and expressive groups. Groups also address inappropriate sexual behavior and how to maintain appropriate boundaries with others (INTEGRIS Health Essentials, 2006).

Individual Psychotherapy. Individual therapy is recommended for clients who have had a recent life change, such as illness, loss, divorce, surgery, and any factors resulting in change in self-esteem or body image. A common cause of the cessation of sexual activity is the loss of a partner. Sexual self-confidence may be lost along with the familiar partner, and new relationships may seem threatening. Individuals who have experienced a life-threatening illness may fear that sexual behavior will result in further debilitation. Conformity to cultural taboos about sexuality and aging may play an important part in impotence.

Although the majority of ED is physiologically based, it may be secondary to lack of practice, unfamiliarity with a new partner, guilt feelings, or performance anxiety. Encourage clients to seek counseling for themselves and their partners if they are involved in a relationship. Interviewing the partner allows the nurse–therapist to assess relationship strengths and weaknesses and incorporate interventions during therapy.

Marital or Couple Therapy. Marital or couple therapy or counseling can be used to clarify, discuss, and work through problems such as feelings of sexual inadequacy, infidelity, or incompatibility. It can be effective in resolving conflicts, especially if the couple has a difference in opinion regarding what is normal sexual behavior. For example, disclosure, the self-reporting of marital or partner infidelity during therapy, has been viewed as a positive way to end an extramarital relationship or a secret life, establish hope for the future, and experience the healing value of honesty. The partner or spouse is encouraged to reflect and respond to the disclosure and decide whether he or she accepts the disclosure as a step toward healing the couple or marital relationship (Levin, 1999).

Family Therapy. As adolescents and young adults struggle with emerging sexual identity, parents and families go through a parallel coming-out process and are affected by the stigma associated with being gay or lesbian. Family therapy or a referral to Parents, Families, and Friends of Lesbians and Gays (PFFLAG), a national organization that provides education, information, and support, helps parents learn to cope with and ultimately accept their adolescent's gender identity (Ryan et al., 1998).

Parents may bring children with cross-gender behavior patterns to therapy in an attempt to instill culturally acceptable behavior patterns in the child. For example, adults or peers role-model masculine or feminine behavior (Sadock & Sadock, 2003).

Sex Therapy. Individuals who are trained and certified generally provide sex therapy. The way in which sexual material is experienced and expressed during therapy depends on the gender and age of the client or couple, and to some extent, of the therapist or co-therapists as seen in dual-sex therapy. Specific techniques and exercises to reduce physiologic problems may be explored. Hypnotherapy may be employed to remove anxiety-producing symptoms and to develop alternative means to deal with fears during sexual encounters. Sensitivity to gender aspects of human sexuality facilitates all aspects of the psychotherapeutic process (Friedman & Downey, 2000; Sadock & Sadock, 2003).

Group Therapy. The purpose of group therapy is to examine intrapsychic and interpersonal problems in clients with sexual or gender identity disorders. Group therapy provides a strong support system for children and adolescents as well as for adults who feel ashamed, anxious, or guilty about a particular sexual problem. It provides a useful forum in which to discuss sexual myths; correct misconceptions; and provide accurate information about sexual anatomy, physiology, and various behaviors (Sadock & Sadock, 2003).

Behavioral Therapy. Behavioral therapy interventions have been found to be effective in the treatment of emergent transvestite-like behavior in male adolescents (Rekers & Kilgus, 2001). Systematic desensitiza-

tion is utilized to minimize anxiety-producing situations in clients who experience sexual fantasies. Assertiveness training is helpful in teaching clients to express sexual needs openly and without fear (Sadock & Sadock, 2003).

Support Groups

A variety of organizations offer support groups regarding issues of sexuality and sexual health. Information can be accessed through local community mental health centers, local hospitals, libraries, the National Institutes of Health, and various Web sites. Examples include Reach to Recovery for clients who have had a mastectomy; United Ostomy Association, Inc., for clients who have had surgery such as ileal conduits or colostomies; the Endometriosis Association for clients who experience infertility; Sex Addicts Anonymous, a spiritual program based on the principles and traditions of Alcoholics Anonymous; the PFFLAG program mentioned earlier in this chapter; ED research groups supported by pharmaceutical companies; Impotency Anonymous; support groups for clients who are HIV-positive or have been diagnosed with AIDS and have a history of sexual addiction, sexual dysfunction, or gender identity disorder; and the National Youth Advocacy Coalition.

Client Education

Because human sexuality encompasses so many facets of a person's life, nurses who are educated about psychophysiologic changes in sexual response are able to assist clients in maintaining sexual health through their lifespan (Baxer, 2001). Recognize each client's particular cultural, physiologic, and psychological circumstances when teaching clients. Adapt client teaching by keeping an open mind and nonjudgmental attitude about human sexual expression.

Education can begin with an explanation of normal sexual response (Masters & Johnson, 1966). Be aware of variability among individuals with respect to normal sexuality, stressing this variation with clients. Educating the client and partner about the natural changes in sexual function with aging can dispel some fear and anxiety. Education also may include information about various medications, recreational drugs (see Chapter 25), psychoactive drugs (see Chapter 16), and medical conditions (such as chronic pain syndrome, respiratory problems, or cardiac disease) that can interfere with normal sexual response cycle.

EVALUATION

The evaluation of nursing interventions for clients with issues or concerns related to their gender identity or sexuality is important because outcomes are based on the client's expectations. Clients with sexual dysfunction generally expect an improvement to occur. Partner satisfaction, also a concern, is a part of this evaluation, if possible. The nurse evaluates the response of the individual with a gender identity disorder to medication if treatment for anxiety or depression was implemented. In addition, the client's ability to cope with issues related to his or her gender identity disorder also is determined.

As noted earlier in the chapter, not all paraphiliacs want or receive treatment. Those who do generally participate in individual or group therapy to explore feelings of sexuality, anxiety, depression, and frustration. Behavioral therapy focuses on altering or managing unacceptable or undesirable behaviors. Thus, outcomes are evaluated based on resolution or change in these unacceptable or undesirable behaviors.

Clients who exhibit clinical symptoms of sexual addiction may have difficulty resolving social, marital, and professional issues. Fear of consequences may keep them from continuing with treatment. Recidivism for paraphiliacs and sex addicts is high.

For example, the nurse and client would discuss whether the client's clinical symptoms, such as pain, frustration, anxiety performance, depression, or anxiety, have improved. They would also discuss whether the client accepted or tried suggested interventions and how effective these actions were.

Evaluation focuses on whether the expectations of the client are realistic and whether the client feels a need to continue with supportive therapy. Some clients may not want to change their behavior or are not ready to change. Partners may be resistant to new suggestions. Evaluation may indicate that the need for a referral to another therapist with a perspective more consistent with the client's, or to a clinician with more experience, would benefit the client. See Nursing Plan of Care 26-1: The Client Experiencing Hypoactive Sexual Desire Disorder.

NURSING PLAN OF CARE 26.1

THE CLIENT EXPERIENCING HYPOACTIVE SEXUAL DESIRE DISORDER

Jim, a 36-year-old executive, was admitted to the ICU with the diagnosis of myocardial infarction. The father of two children, Jim confided in the nurse that he is afraid to resume his duties as husband and father. He also stated that he is afraid to play golf, even though the attending physician assured him he would eventually be able to lead a normal life if he adhered to the doctor's orders. After a visit by his wife, Jim appeared withdrawn and apprehensive. As the nurse made evening rounds, Jim complained of chest pain and stated that he thought his doctor was sending him home too early. Later that evening, Jim's wife called the nurses' station and asked to talk to the head nurse. She expressed concern over her husband's withdrawal, lack of interest in visiting with her, and fear of going home.

DSM-IV-TR DIAGNOSIS: Hypoactive sexual desire disorder due to myocardial infarction

ASSESSMENT: Personal strengths: Married with children, supportive wife who has verbalized her concerns about her husband's behavior, able to verbalize his feelings

Weaknesses: Withdrawn, apprehensive, fearful of resuming normal daily activities

NURSING DIAGNOSIS: Ineffective Sexuality Patterns related to biochemical effects on energy and libido secondary to myocardial infarction

OUTCOME: The client will identify limitations on sexual activity caused by recent myocardial infarction.

Planning/Implementation	Rationale
Explain the effects of cardiovascular disease and medications on sexual functioning.	The client may have misconceptions about the effects of cardiovascular disease and medications on his sexual functioning.
If the client agrees, include his wife in the development of his treatment plan.	The client's wife verbalized a concern about the change in his behavior. Giving the wife specific information will help clarify expectations of the client and his wife.

NURSING DIAGNOSIS: Ineffective Coping as evidenced by withdrawal, lack of interest, and expression of fear of resuming normal daily activities

OUTCOME: The client will verbalize a decrease in fear regarding the resumption of activities of daily living.

Planning/Implementation	Rationale
Encourage client to verbalize feelings.	Identifying and verbalizing feelings is a necessary initial step toward resolving fears and developing effective coping skills.
Reassure client that the concerns he has are not unusual.	The client may have difficulty expressing concerns directly. Reassurance may decrease the client's fears.
Explore successful past and present coping skills.	The client can build on his previous or present successful coping skills to deal with his current situation.
Establish a schedule, with client's input, to gradually resume activities of daily living.	The client can gain confidence as he gradually resumes activities of daily living. Establishing a schedule allows the client to pace himself and verbalize concerns about specific activities when necessary.

EVALUATION: Evaluation focuses on the client's understanding of the recovery process after myocardial infarction, the development of positive coping skills, and an improvement in his sexual functioning.

KEY CONCEPTS

◆ The terms *sex*, *sexual acts*, and *sexuality* are often used interchangeably; however, there is a distinction to be made. Sex is a primary drive; sexual acts occur when behaviors involve the genitalia and erogenous zones; and sexuality is the result of an individual's biopsychosocial and experiential factors that mold an individual's sexual development, self-concept, body image, and behavior.

◆ Sexuality consists of four interrelated psychosexual factors: sexual identity, gender identity, sexual orientation, and sexual behavior.

◆ Sexual identity is the pattern of a person's biologic sexual characteristics.

◆ Gender identity is a person's sense of maleness or femaleness and is believed to be determined primarily by chromosomes and hormones and secondarily affected by one's environment.

◆ Sexuality develops over time and is subject to change as one experiences the stages of infancy and childhood, preadolescence and adolescence, and the different phases of adulthood.

◆ Latency-age children and adolescents who have problems with general aggressiveness may, as a result of anger, boredom, dysfunctional family relationships, social awkwardness, or history of violence or abuse, exhibit sexual aggression toward peers.

◆ The human sexual response cycle includes four phases: desire, excitement, orgasm, and resolution.

◆ Psychological factors, medication, substances, or physical disorders can precipitate a sexual dysfunction disorder in both male and female clients.

◆ Individuals who participate in unusual or bizarre sexual acts to achieve sexual excitement are referred to as paraphiliacs. They are generally not seen by mental health professionals unless their behavior creates a conflict with society.

◆ Sexual addiction is characterized by the participation in obsessive–compulsive sexual behavior that causes stress to addicted individuals and their families. Children as well as adults experience symptoms of sexual addiction. The consequences of such behavior include school absenteeism or difficulties in school, difficulties with work, financial problems, loss of relationships with significant others, divorce, arrests, low self-esteem, and despair. Many sexual addicts have a dual diagnosis including substance abuse or depression.

◆ Several common barriers to taking a sexual history have been identified. They include not considering the client's sexual history as relevant to the plan of care, inadequate training of the health care professional, embarrassment on the part of the health care professional, fear of offending the client by asking personal questions, and the perception by the health care provider that any sexual concern of the client will be overly complex and time consuming for the provider to assess, much less manage.

◆ Planning focuses on the individual client's specific problems or complaints and respects the client's age, sex, and cultural and religious preferences. The nurse assumes the role of client advocate to ensure the promotion of gender identity and sexual health in the plan of care.

◆ Interventions are individualized on the basis of the client's concerns about sexual identity, gender

identity, identified sexual disorder, causative factors, and clinical symptoms.

◆ Although the plan of care is developed with the client's input, the competence of the nurse has an effect on the outcomes. If the nurse is unable to be objective while providing care for a specific client, the nurse should relinquish responsibility to another member of the health care team.

◆ Evaluation focuses on whether the client's expectations are realistic and whether the client feels a need to continue with supportive therapy. The nurse may decide that a referral to another therapist or clinician would be in the best interest of the client.

For additional study materials, please refer to the Student Resource CD-ROM located in the back of this textbook.

CHAPTER WORKSHEET

CRITICAL THINKING QUESTIONS

1. Team up with a classmate and interview each other concerning personal sexual history.
2. After the interviews, discuss when you considered not telling the truth, when you became embarrassed, and what thoughts and feelings you experienced when evaluating how to answer each question. Could the interviewer tell when these feelings were occurring?
3. If you and your classmate, who know each other, felt embarrassed, how might a new client feel? How might you make the client more comfortable? How would you adjust the interview for a client your own age? For a client your father's age?
4. Prepare a presentation on the anatomy and physiology of human sexual response. What did you learn? How will this information help you understand clients with sexual dysfunction?

REFLECTION

Review the chapter opening quote about the development of sexuality by Sadock and Sadock. In some Middle Eastern countries, women are not allowed to show their faces in public, wear Western-style clothes, or drive a car. What influence do you think these cultural practices might have on the development of a woman's sexual identity? What impact would these cultural practices have on a female American citizen working in such a country? Explain your answers.

NCLEX-STYLE QUESTIONS

1. A female client suffering from an anxiety disorder tells the nurse that she was diagnosed with Turner's syndrome in adolescence. The nurse understands that which of the following is true with this disorder?
   a. An extra X chromosome is present.
   b. The client will be unable to bear children.
   c. The client has an extra Y chromosome.
   d. Early menopause will occur.

2. When performing a sexual assessment, which of the following should the nurse do? Select all that apply.
   a. Ask questions requiring a yes-or-no response
   b. Gradually introduce more sensitive questions
   c. Demonstrate an open and accepting attitude
   d. Provide personal views and input
   e. Investigate behaviors first, then client's attitudes
   f. Use terminology that the client is familiar with

3. The parents of a 4-year-old boy verbalize concern to the pediatric clinic nurse that their son is already asking questions about the anatomic differences between the sexes. The nurse responds to the parents' concern on the basis of which of the following?
   a. Children with a history of sexual abuse are preoccupied with sexual issues.
   b. Curiosity about sexual identity is normal in preschool children.
   c. Interest in sexuality is generally latent in preschool children.
   d. Preschool children are too young to be instructed about sexuality.

4. A 40-year-old male client, paralyzed from the waist down as a result of a car accident, is in a drug and alcohol rehabilitation unit for treatment of substance abuse. The client frequently exposes himself to female staff. Which response by the nurse would be most appropriate?
   a. Ignoring the client's behavior, realizing that the client has low self-esteem
   b. Informing client that behavior is unacceptable, knowing limit-setting is appropriate
   c. Holding a community meeting in which unit-appropriate behavior is discussed
   d. Requesting that the client's physician speak with the client about this behavior

5. A 36-year-old female client with a depressive disorder reports loss of interest in sexual activity during the nurse–client interview. Questions focusing on which factor would be most appropriate for the nurse to ask to identify a possible contributor to this problem?
   a. Early age of onset of puberty
   b. Medications taken by the client
   c. Difficulty with childbirth
   d. High dietary intake of fats

6. Which area represents the most significant barrier to the taking of a sexual history by the nurse?
   a. Client discomfort and embarrassment
   b. Concerns about privacy
   c. Inadequate time for discussion
   d. Nurse's discomfort and embarrassment

Selected References

American Psychiatric Association. (2000). *Diagnostic and statistical manual of mental disorders* (4th ed., text revision). Washington, DC: Author.

Andrews, M. M., & Boyle, J. S. (2003). *Transcultural concepts in nursing care* (4th ed.). Philadelphia: Lippincott Williams & Wilkins.

Aschenbrenner, D. S. (2004). Avlimil taken for female sexual dysfunction. *American Journal of Nursing, 104*(10), 27, 29, 31.

Baker, B. (1999). Gender identity can keep shifting. *Clinical Psychiatry News, 27*(5), 30.

Baxer, P. M. (2001). Midlife changes in sexual response. *ADVANCE for Nurse Practitioners, 9*(3), 67–70.

Bresolin, J. (2001). Connecting with gay patients. *ADVANCE for Nurse Practitioners, 9*(2), 114.

Byers, S. E., & Esparza, D. (1997). Sexuality and sexual concerns. In B. S. Johnson (Ed.), *Psychiatric-mental health nursing: Adaptation and growth* (4th ed., pp. 171-197). Philadelphia: Lippincott-Raven.

Carnes, P. J. (2001). *Out of the shadows: Understanding sexual addiction.* Golden Valley, MN: CompCare.

Carpenito-Moyet, L. J. (2006). *Handbook of nursing diagnosis* (11th ed.). Philadelphia: Lippincott Williams & Wilkins.

Finan, S. L. (1997). Promoting healthy sexuality: Guidelines for infancy through preschool. *Nurse Practitioner, 22*(10), 70-100.

Freud, S. (1960). *The ego and the id* (J. Strachey, Ed., & J. Rivere, Trans). New York: W. W. Norton.

Frieden, J. (2005). Debate continues over categorizing paraphilias. *Clinical Psychiatry News, 33*(2), 53.

Friedman, R. C., & Downey, J. I. (2000). Discussing sex in the psychotherapeutic relationship. *Psychiatric Times, 17*(7), 57-60.

Gender Identity Research and Education Society. (2003). Epidemiological data. Retrieved August 29, 2003, from http://www.gires.org.uk/text_assets/etiology_definition.pdf

Google Directory Health Pharmacy. (2006). Drugs and medications. Retrieved February 16, 2006, from http://directory.google.com/Top/Health/Pharmacy/drugs_and_medications/

Gray, M. (2001). The etiology of erectile dysfunction. *Therapeutic Spotlight, 12,* 9-14.

Haffner, D. (1994). Sexuality and aging: The family physician's role as an educator. *Geriatrics,* (9).

Hornor, G. (2003). Adolescent sexual offenders: A challenge for primary care NPs. *American Journal for Nurse Practitioners, 7*(9), 37-38, 41-42, 44-45.

INTEGRIS Health Essentials.com. (2006). The STAR program: Sexual trauma and abuse recovery. Retrieved February 17, 2006, from http://www.integris-health.com/newsletter/fall2004/story14.html

Jacobson, L. (1974). Illness and human sexuality. *Nursing Outlook,* (1).

Jancin, B. (2005). Addiction to cybersex called pervasive. *Clinical Psychiatry News, 33*(6) 32.

Jensen, P. K., Lewis, J., & Jones, K. B. (2004). Improving erectile dysfunction: Incorporating new guidelines into clinical practice. *ADVANCE for Nurse Practitioners, 12*(27), 40-50.

Karch, A. (2004). The grapefruit challenge. *American Journal of Nursing, 104*(12), 33.

Katz, A. (2005). Sexually speaking: Do ask, do tell. *American Journal of Nursing, 105*(7), 66-68.

Klein, M. (2003). Epidemiology of sexual addiction. Retrieved August 31, 2003, from http://www.sexed.org/arch/arch08.html

Krozy, R. A. (1998). Sexual disorders. In M. A. Boyd & M. A. Nihart (Eds.), *Psychiatric nursing: Contemporary practice* (pp. 800-836). Philadelphia: Lippincott Williams & Wilkins.

Levin, A. (1999). Disclosure by sex addicts doesn't prevent relapse. *Clinical Psychiatry News, 27*(10) 26.

Macready, N. (2001). Online sexual addiction often missed by therapists. *Clinical Psychiatry News, 29*(6), 18.

Masters, W., & Johnson, V. (1966). *Human sexual response.* Philadelphia: Lippincott Williams & Wilkins.

Medina, J. (1999). Genes and human sexuality. *Psychiatric Times, 16*(8), 16-17.

Medscape Medical News. (2004). Daily apomorphine may be useful for women with sexual arousal disorder. Retrieved May 31, 2004, from http://www.medscape.com/viewarticle/478481_print

Medscape Medical News. (2006). New approaches to female sexual arousal disorder. Retrieved February 18, 2006, from http://www.medscape.com/viewarticle/ 434478_print

Medscape Today. (2004). Women's sexual problems: A guide to integrating the "New View" approach. Retrieved October 14, 2004, from http://www.medscape.com/viewarticle/4892000_4

Moon, M. A. (2001). Addressing sexual aggression in children. *Clinical Psychiatry News, 29*(11), 45.

Paice, J. (2003). Sexuality and chronic pain. *American Journal of Nursing, 103*(1), 87-89.

Postlethwaite, D., Stump, S., Bielan, B., & Rudy, S. J. (2001, Spring). Sexual history and counseling for patients on teratogenic drugs. *American Journal for Nurse Practitioners, Special Supplement,* 14-18.

Reiner, W. G. (Ed.). (1997). To be male or female—that is the question. *Archives of Pediatric Adolescent Medicine, 151,* 224-225.

Rekers, G. A., & Kilgus, M. D. (1995). Differential diagnosis and rationale for treatment of gender identity disorders and transvestism. In G. A. Rekers (Ed.), *Handbook of child and adolescent sexual problems.* New York: Lexington Books.

Rekers, G. A., & Kilgus, M. D. (1998). Diagnosis and treatment of gender identity disorders in children and adolescents. In L. Vande-Creek, S. Knapp, & T. L. Jackson (Eds.), *Innovations in clinical practice: A sourcebook* (Vol. 15). Sarasota, FL: Professional Resource Press.

Rekers, G. A., & Kilgus, M. D. (2001). Early identification and treatment of gender identity disorder. *Psychiatric Times, 18*(12), 44-47.

Remafedi, G., French, S., Story, M., Resnick, S. C., & Blum, R. (1998). The relationship between suicide risk and sexual orientation: Results of a population-based study. *American Journal of Public Health, 88*(1), 57-60.

Rippel, A. C. (2003, March 24). Transgenders seek equality in eyes of law. *Orlando Sentinel,* B1-B2.

Ryan, C., Futterman, D., & Stine, K. (1998). Helping our hidden youth. *American Journal of Nursing, 98*(12), 37-41.

Sadock, B. J., & Sadock, V. A. (2003). *Kaplan & Sadock's synopsis of psychiatry: Behavioral sciences/clinical psychiatry* (9th ed.). Philadelphia: Lippincott Williams & Wilkins.

Schultz, J. M., & Videbeck, S. L. (2005). *Lippincott's manual of psychiatric nursing care plans* (7th ed.). Philadelphia: Lippincott Williams & Wilkins.

Tamerin, J. S. (1998). Viagra and the essence of male sexuality. *Psychiatric Times, 15*(12), 56.

Theme Paper, Young Offenders and Prevention. (2003). Retrieved May 28, 2003, from http://www.childhood.com/de/text_p711.html

Trieschmann, R. B. (1975). Sex, sex acts, and sexuality. *Archives of Physical Medicine and Rehabilitation, 56,* 8–9.

Warner, P. H., Rowe, T., & Whipple, B. (1999). Shedding light on the sexual history. American *Journal of Nursing, 99*(6), 34–41.

WordReference.com English Dictionary. (2006). Definition of transsexual. Retrieved May 3, 2006, from http://www.wordreference.com/definition/transsexual

Worcester, S. (1999). Revealing homosexuality puts youths at risk of family abuse. *Clinical Psychiatry News, 27*(1), 26.

Youngkin, E. Q. (2004). The myths and truths of mature intimacy: Guidance for nurse practitioners. *ADVANCE for Nurse Practitioners, 12*(9), 45–48.

Zucker, K. J., Bradley, S. J., & Sanikhani, M. (1997). Sex differences in referral rates of children with gender identity disorder: Some hypotheses. *Journal of Abnormal Child Psychology, 25*(3), 217–227.

Suggested Readings

Barden, C. (2004). Lesbian and gay youths at risk. *American Journal of Nursing, 104*(10), 13.

Finn, R. (2004). It's important to take sexual history in diabetics. *Clinical Psychiatry News, 32*(5), 99.

Katz, A. (2005). Sexually speaking: Do ask, do tell. *American Journal of Nursing, 105*(7), 66–68.

Kellog-Spadt, S. (2004). Valuable resources for female sexual dysfunction. *American Journal for Nurse Practitioners, 8*(9), 75–76.

Kellog-Spadt, S. (2005). Erectile dysfunction: What your patients should know. *American Journal for Nurse Practitioners, 9*(9), 62–63.

Kellog-Spadt, S., & Pillai-Friedman, S. (2005). Women, sexuality, and aging. *American Journal for Nurse Practitioners, 9*(5), 27–28.

Krassner, D., Hierholzer, R., & Battista, M. (2005). Nothing more than feelings? *Current Psychiatry, 4*(7), 77–78, 83–87.

Masters, W., & Johnson, V. (1970). *Human sexual inadequacy.* Boston: Little, Brown.

Medscape Today. (2004). Taking a sexual history using guidelines from a new view. Retrieved October 14, 2004, from http://www.medscape.com/viewarticle/ 489200_9

Rollet, J. (2005). The quest for a little pink pill: Female sexual dysfunction finally attracting attention. *ADVANCE for Nurse Practitioners, 13*(6), 51–54.

Schultz, J. M., & Videbeck, S. D. (2005). *Lippincott's manual of psychiatric nursing care plans* (7th ed.). Philadelphia: Lippincott Williams & Wilkins.

Sexuality Information and Education Council of the United States. (2003). Sexuality education. Retrieved May 26, 2003, from http://www.siecus.org/school/sex_ed/sex_ed0000.html

Sherman, C. (2004). Treating sexual dysfunction. *Clinical Psychiatry News, 32*(12), 26.

CHAPTER 27 / COGNITIVE DISORDERS

In older people, the development of delirium or acute confusion...has been associated with increased lengths of hospital stay, the need for chemical and physical restraints, readmission, and increased mortality. —WAKEFIELD, 2002

The death of the mind is the worst death imaginable, and for millions of Americans the slow death...creates a world of pain and suffering. The number of affected individuals signal[s] the profound magnitude of the public health challenges to our society. —COHEN, 1995

Time is the most precious gift in our possession, for it is the most irrevocable. —DIETRICH BONHOEFFER (1906–1945)

LEARNING OBJECTIVES

AFTER STUDYING THIS CHAPTER, YOU SHOULD BE ABLE TO:

1. Discuss the changes that occur in the aging brain.
2. Describe the four distinct, yet mutually interacting, memory systems identified by Heindel and Salloway.
3. Discuss the latest research findings related to the etiology of dementia of the Alzheimer's type.
4. Compare and contrast the etiology of vascular dementia and dementia with Lewy bodies.
5. Distinguish the clinical symptoms of delirium, dementia, and amnestic disorders.
6. Describe the onset and course of dementia from early to terminal stages.
7. Explain the rationale for use of the Wong-Baker Faces Rating Scale, NEECHAM Confusion Scale, and Agitated Behavior in Dementia Scale when assessing clients with cognitive disorders.
8. Articulate the importance of identifying a client's cultural and educational background during the assessment process.
9. Describe the elements of a comprehensive history and physical examination for a client who exhibits clinical symptoms of dementia of the Alzheimer's type.
10. Formulate nursing interventions for a client with the diagnosis of delirium who exhibits agitated and aggressive behavior.
11. Develop an educational program to use with family members of clients with the diagnosis of dementia.

KEY TERMS

Agnosia
Anterograde amnesia
Aphasia
Apraxia
Asterixis
Binswanger's disease
Cognition
Cognitive disorder
Confabulation
Delirium
Dementia
Dementia with Lewy bodies
Disturbances in executive functioning
Dysgraphia
Dysnomia
Perseveration
Retrograde amnesia
Sundown syndrome

Cognition refers to the mental processes of comprehension, judgment, memory, and reasoning in contrast to emotional and volitional (willful or free-will) processes (Shahrokh & Hales, 2003). A **cognitive disorder** occurs when there is a clinically significant deficit in cognition from a previous level of functioning. Although cognitive disorders are the most prevalent psychiatric disorders occurring in later life, they can occur at any time. At least 70 known cognitive disorders are caused by intracranial or primary diseases of the central nervous system (eg, epilepsy, brain trauma, infection) and extracranial diseases or diseases of other organ systems (eg, drug intoxication, poisons, systemic infections). Cognitive impairment ranges from irreversible to fully reversible, depending on the contributing factor. One half of the beds in community long-term care facilities contain clients with the diagnosis of dementia. Other cognitive disorders, such as delirium and amnestic disorders, also consume large amounts of public health resources. As the United States population increases and ages, more older adults will be diagnosed with cognitive deficits such as delirium, dementia, or amnesia (Peskind & Raskind, 1996; Sadock & Sadock, 2003).

In the hospital setting, delirium is a frequent problem. In the primary care setting, dementia has become a common ailment. In some cases, Alzheimer's disease (AD) is diagnosed prematurely and incorrectly. Amnesia may occur at any age, depending on the primary pathological process (eg, traumatic brain injury, stroke, exposure to toxic substances).

This chapter discusses the major cognitive disorders and their subtypes, when applicable, as identified by the *Diagnostic and Statistical Manual of Mental Disorders, 4th Edition, Text Revision (DSM-IV-TR)* (American Psychiatric Association [APA], 2000). Cognitive disorders secondary to substance-related disorders are included in the classifications but are discussed fully in Chapters 25 and 32. According to criteria established by the *DSM-IV-TR*, the differential diagnosis of each disorder is based on the type of onset and course of symptoms. Mental processes, speech, behavior, and level of consciousness, as well as presumed or established etiology, are considered in determining a diagnosis (APA, 2000).

History of Dementia

Dementia was first described in a book about mental illness in 1838. In 1894, Dr. Alois Alzheimer, a German neuropathologist who had a particular interest in "nervous disorders," described changes in the brain caused by vascular disease (now known as vascular dementia). In 1901, he treated a middle-aged woman who had exhibited clinical symptoms of memory loss, disorientation, "peculiar behavior," anxiety, and hallucinations. When the woman died in 1906 as a result of multiple causes, including pneumonia and nephritis, Dr. Alzheimer was unable to classify the disease into any existing category. A postmortem examination of the brain revealed microscopic and macroscopic lesions and distortions, including neuritic plaques and neurofibrillary tangles. The woman's neurologic changes were identified as AD (dementia of the Alzheimer's type [DAT]) (E-MentalHealth.com, 2005; Needham, 2006).

The clinical symptoms of dementia were attributed to the aging process until the 1970s when researchers determined that dementia was caused by several factors such as organic change, disease process, or neurochemical deficiency within the brain. This discovery enabled researchers to develop a classification of the various types of dementia now included in the *DSM-IV-TR*.

Cognitive Function

The brain integrates, regulates, initiates, and controls functions in the entire body. The processes of thinking, remembering, and learning occur in different areas of the brain. For example, the frontal lobe organizes and classifies information; the parietal lobe processes sensory input; the temporal lobe synthesizes auditory, visual and somatic input into thought and memory; and the occipital lobe controls visual information that is received and processed through the retina (Needham, 2006).

Research has been done to determine the effects of aging on the brain and cognitive function. Figure 27-1 illustrates the major areas of the brain involved in cognitive functions. Some findings include the following:

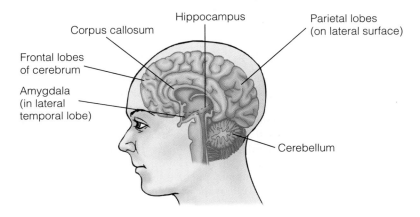

Corpus callosum — Frontal lobes of cerebrum — Amygdala (in lateral temporal lobe) — Hippocampus — Parietal lobes (on lateral surface) — Cerebellum

Different parts of the brain have different functions

- The frontal lobes of the cerebrum allow us to solve problems, plan ahead, understand the behavior of others, and restrain our impulses.

- The corpus callosum passes information from one side of the brain to the other.

- The parietal areas control hearing, speech, and language.

- The amygdala directs our emotional responses.

- The hippocampus makes it possible to recall recent experiences and new information.

- The cerebellum regulates balance, body movements, coordination, and the muscles used in speaking.

FIGURE 27.1 Areas of cognitive function within the brain.

- The normal human brain weighs approximately 1,350 grams and declines approximately 7% to 8% in weight as one ages.
- Cell loss is not uniform because the frontal lobes degenerate at a faster rate than the other lobes.
- Gray matter is lost at a greater rate initially, but white matter loss disproportionately increases as one ages.
- Ventricular size increases with age.
- Approximately 50% of aging individuals experience atherosclerosis in cerebral vessels.
- Changes in neurotransmitter function occur, such as alterations in neurotransmitter concentration, receptor density, and functional activity (Salloway, 1999).

Results also demonstrate that intellect peaks at age 30 years, plateaus at ages 50 to 60 years, and then slowly declines until the age of 70 years. Decline of intellect accelerates as one's age nears 80 years (Salloway, 1999).

According to neuropsychological investigative studies of brain-injured clients by Heindel and Salloway (1999), results demonstrate convincingly that memory is not a single homogeneous entity. Rather it is composed of four distinct, yet mutually interacting, memory systems: working memory, episodic memory, semantic memory, and procedural memory. Figure 27-2 illustrates the different memory systems and their locations, including examples of the specific types of memory impairment. Understanding these systems provides a powerful clinical tool for assessing cognitive disorders in clients.

Etiology of Cognitive Disorders

Studies regarding the etiology of delirium and amnestic disorders have focused almost exclusively on biologic factors. Various theories have been proposed to

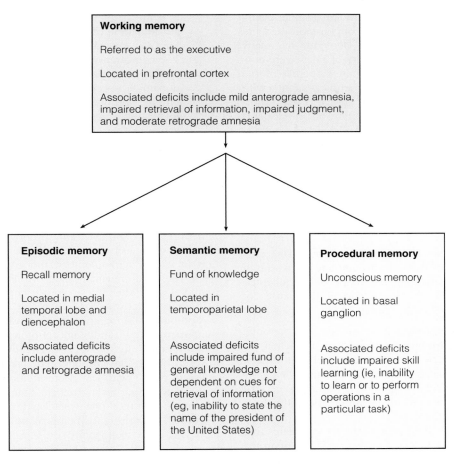

FIGURE 27.2 Memory systems and associated deficits.

suggest the etiology of dementia, diseases associated with dementia, and amnestic disorders.

Etiology of Delirium

Delirium is defined as a transient cognitive disorder, usually acute or subacute in onset, presenting as a reversible global dysfunction in cerebral metabolism. It is usually caused by disturbance of brain pathology by a medical disorder or an ingested substance. Delirium is considered a syndrome (ie, a group of signs and symptoms that cluster together), not a disease, that has many causes.

The three major causes are central nervous system diseases (eg, epilepsy, meningitis, encephalitis), systemic illnesses (eg, heart failure or pulmonary insufficiency), and either drug intoxication or withdrawal from pharmacologic or toxic agents. For example, any drug taken by a client has the potential to precipitate delirium secondary to adverse effects.

Other causes of delirium include endocrine or metabolic disorders (eg, hypoadrenocorticism or hypercalcemia) and deficiency diseases (eg, thiamine, nicotinic acid, folic acid). In addition, systemic infections, electrolyte imbalance, postoperative states, and traumatic injury to the head or body also are associated with causing delirium (APA, 2000; Peskind & Raskind, 1996; Sadock & Sadock, 2003).

Etiology of Dementia

Dementia refers to a syndrome of global or diffuse brain dysfunction characterized by a gradual, progressive, chronic deterioration of intellectual function. The persistent and stable nature of the impairment distinguishes it from the altered levels of consciousness and fluctuating deficits of delirium. Dementia has many causes. Until recently, the majority of cases were considered to be of two main types: dementia of the Alzheimer's type and vascular dementia. Dementia with Lewy bodies (DLB) is a form of dementia that shares characteristics of both DAT and Parkinson's disease. It is now thought to account for 10% to 15% of all dementia cases in older people. Furthermore, up to 40% of clients with DAT also have concomitant DLB (DLB-DAT) (Peskind & Raskind, 1996; Sadock & Sadock, 2003; Newsline, 2004; Alzheimer's Society, 2006).

Etiology of Dementia of the Alzheimer's Type (DAT)

The search for the causes and treatment of DAT continues. Several theories exist. A complete discussion of these theories is beyond the scope of this chapter. However, current theories regarding the causes of dementia are cited below and include:

1. The apolipoprotein theory focuses on the build up of apolipoprotein deposits or plaques in the brain. Genetic screening, based on this theory, is now available to determine an individual's apolipoprotein E genotype, revealing genetic risk information to asymptomatic individuals (Wachter, 2006).
2. The beta-amyloid protein theory postulates that symptoms of DAT are the result of neuronal degeneration due to the neurotoxic properties of these proteins (Peskind & Raskind, 1996; Medina, 2001; Sadock & Sadock, 2003).
3. The genetic theory, which proposes a genetic link to DAT, which focuses on three genes on three separate chromosomes (1, 14, and 21).
4. The immune system theory suggests that DAT is the result of immune system malfunctions.
5. The oxidation theory states that the buildup of damage from oxidative processes in neurons results in the loss of various body functions.
6. The virus and bacteria theory proposes that DAT may be caused by a viral- or bacterial-induced condition secondary to the breakdown of the immune system (eg, herpes virus).
7. The nutritional theory postulates that poor nutrition and lack of mental stimulation during childhood may predispose one to DAT later in life.

8. The metal deposit theory speculates that an accumulation of aluminum ions replacing iron ions may contribute to existing dementia.
9. The neurotransmitter theory hypothesizes that DAT is caused by a decrease in acetylcholine, dopamine, norepinephrine, or serotonin levels, limiting neuronal activity. A second theory postulates that excessive stimulation of glutamate damages neurons.
10. The membrane phospholipid metabolism theory proposes that DAT is caused by an abnormality in metabolism that causes neuronal cell membranes to be less fluid or more rigid than normal.

Researchers continue to work diligently to determine the cause of DAT and proposed treatments. Neuroimaging has been used in the diagnostic evaluation of clients with memory and cognitive impairment. The predominant finding of bilateral posterior temporal and parietal perfusion defects is thought to be highly predictive of DAT.

Computed tomography (CT), positron emission tomography (PET), and single photon emission computed tomography (SPECT) scans show atrophy and lowered blood flow and energy consumption in the brains of clients with DAT. Deterioration appears first in the superior parietal cortex, the temporal lobes, and the hippocampus. In late stages, atrophy is severe (Figure 27-3). At present, brain imaging can distinguish early DAT fairly well from depression but not always from other brain diseases. Microscopic findings (postmortem) show senile plaques, neurofibrillary tangles, neuronal loss, synaptic loss, and granulovascular degeneration of neurons (Holman & Devous, 1992; Sadock & Sadock, 2003).

Etiology of Dementia With Lewy Bodies (DLB)

DLB is difficult to clinically differentiate from DAT. Both dementias indicate cognitive decline inappropriate to age that interferes with normal tasks of daily living.

Research studies have found that **dementia with Lewy bodies** (DLB) is caused by neurohistologic changes (spherical protein deposits in nerve cells) in the cerebral cortex and other areas of the brain. Their presence in the brain disrupts the brain's normal functioning, interrupting the action of important chemical messengers, including acetylcholine and dopamine. When lesions collect in the substantia nigra of the

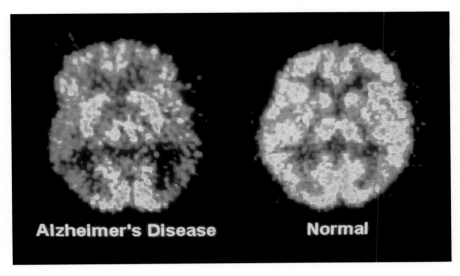

Alzheimer's Disease   Normal

FIGURE 27.3   Positron emission tomography scan comparing a control client subject and a client with dementia of the Alzheimer's type. (Courtesy of Monte S. Buchsbaum, MD. The Mount Sinai Medical Center and School of Medicine, New York, NY.)

brain stem, they cause Parkinson's disease. Researchers have found that Lewy bodies never form in normal brains (Newsline, 2004; Sylvester, 2004).

Etiology of Vascular Dementia

Vascular dementia is thought to result from infarction of small- and medium-sized cerebral vessels causing parenchymal lesions to occur over wide areas of the brain. Plaques or thromboemboli from distant organs such as heart valves are presumed to be the cause of the infarction. **Binswanger's disease** is a type of vascular dementia that is characterized by the presence of many small infarctions affecting the white matter of the brain that spare the cortical regions (Peskind & Raskind, 1996; Sadock & Sadock, 2003).

Etiology of Diseases Associated with Dementia

Several diseases are often associated with dementia (APA, 2000; Busse & Blazer, 1996; Sadock & Sadock, 2003). They include:

- Familial multiple system taupathy (eg, a buildup of tau protein in the neurons and glial cells) occurring in individuals in their forties or fifties; thought to be carried on chromosome 17 and shares some brain abnormalities with DAT; often referred to as *presenile dementia.*
- Pick's disease, progressive disorder of middle and late life characterized by atrophy and microscopic changes of the frontotemporal regions; difficult to differentiate from DAT.
- Parkinson's disease due to the presence of neurohistologic lesions in the basal ganglia; associated impairment of cognitive abilities; commonly associated with dementia.

Etiology of Amnestic Disorders

Amnestic disorders are described as the acquired impaired ability to learn and recall new information or to recall previously learned information. The etiology of an amnestic disorder is usually damage to diencephalic and medial temporal lobe structures, important in memory functions (Peskind & Raskind, 1996). The causes of amnestic disorders may be many, and are typically classified as medical conditions such as thiamine deficiency and hypoglycemia; primary brain conditions such as head trauma; and substance-related disorders such as those involving alcohol and neurotoxins (APA, 2000; Sadock & Sadock, 2003). Alcohol-induced persisting amnestic disorder is discussed in Chapter 25, Substance-Related Disorders.

Clinical Symptoms and Diagnostic Characteristics of Cognitive Disorders

Differentiating delirium from dementia or depression is challenging. It would be easier if a client developed only one syndrome at a time. Unfortunately, this is not always the case, because clients can actually suffer from all three syndromes at once. Many of the clinical symptoms overlap, requiring a thorough investigation during the assessment process (Table 27-1).

The diagnostic characteristics of cognitive disorders described here help to clarify difference among delirium, dementia, and depression. Although depression was discussed in detail in Chapter 21, reference is made to depression in this chapter to compare and contrast clinical symptoms with those of delirium and dementia.

TABLE 27.1 Comparison of Dementia, Delirium, and Depression

	DEMENTIA	DELIRIUM	DEPRESSION
Symptoms			
Judgment	Impaired	May be impaired	May seem impaired
Mood	Fluctuates Apathetic	Fluctuates	Labile Apathetic
Memory	Recent and remote are impaired	Recent and remote are impaired	May seem impaired; selective
Cognition	Disordered reasoning	Disordered reasoning	"I don't know" responses
Orientation	Disoriented	Disorientation fluctuates	Selective disorientation with "It doesn't matter" responses
Thoughts	Confused Suspicious Paranoid	Confused Suspicious	Low self-concept Negativistic, hopeless Death related Possible delusions
Perception	No change	Misinterpretations Visual hallucinations	Delusions and hallucinations may occur in severe cases
Consciousness	Normal	Clouded	Normal
Speech	Sparse Repetitive	Sparse or fluent Incoherent	Fluent or retarded (slow response) Soft-spoken, selectively mute
Behavior	Agitation Wanders Disturbed sleep–wake cycle	Agitation May wander Disturbed sleep–wake cycle	Changes in appetite Complains of fatigue Insomnia or sleeps often
Mental status	Poor testing Progressively worsens Inappropriate answers	Poor testing Improves when medically stable Improves with treatment	Inconsistently poor performance "I don't know" answers
Activities of daily living	Deteriorate as dementia progresses	Usually remain stable unless medically unstable	May deteriorate with major depression due to apathy
Prognosis	No return to premorbid function, chronic, depends on cause as is generally insidious in onset	Return to premorbid function if cause is correctable and is corrected in time. Generally acute onset, often at twilight	Risk of injury or suicide. Return to premorbid function on recovery Usually requires treatment Coincides with major life changes

Delirium

Delirium is one of the most common and, by far, one of the most life-threatening psychiatric illnesses. Several terms may be used to identify delirium, including *ICU* (intensive care unit) *psychosis, encephalopathy, acute brain failure,* and *acute confusional state.*

Clinical symptoms include a rapid onset with symptoms varying sharply in a short period. Judgment may be impaired. Affect or mood fluctuates. Memory of recent events is impaired. Disorientation to person and place usually occurs. **Dysnomia,** the inability to name objects, and **dysgraphia,** the impaired ability to write, may occur. Speech may be incoherent, sparse, or fluent. Perceptual disturbances may include misinterpretations, illusions, or hallucinations. Thought processes appear confused, with possible delusional content.

Behavior exhibited may include agitation, restlessness, wandering, and disturbance in sleep–wake cycle. **Asterixis,** an abnormal movement in which the client exhibits a peculiar flapping movement of hyperextended hands, is seen in various delirious states. Hypoactive symptoms, such as lethargy and reduced psychomotor activity, are common but less frequently identified.

Although the client may perform poorly on mental status examinations, cognitive ability generally improves when the client recovers, unless the delirium is superimposed on moderate to severe dementia. The prognosis includes a return to premorbid function if the cause is corrected in time.

High-risk populations include the following individuals: those who take numerous medications that may interact and cause adverse reactions; persons who undergo age-related physiologic changes that reduce cerebral reserve capacity and limit the ability to tolerate stressors; individuals with inefficient homeostatic and immune mechanisms; persons with impaired hepatic function or reduced renal excretion; and those who are drug dependent (Branski, 1998; Radovich, 1999).

The incidence of delirium in hospitalized individuals older than 65 years is approximately 10% to 15% at the time of admission; another 10% to 40% may develop delirium while in the hospital. Approximately 40% to 50% of clients recovering from surgery for a hip fracture exhibit clinical symptoms of delirium. The highest rate is exhibited by clients after cardiotomy. Additionally, delirium is seen frequently in individuals who relocate from the hospital to rehabilitation centers or long-term care facilities, especially when the length of hospital stay is less than 3 or 4 days and the client has not fully responded to medical or nursing interventions (APA, 2000; Peskind & Raskind, 1996; Sadock & Sadock, 2003).

Delirium Due to a General Medical Condition

The diagnosis Delirium Due to a General Medical Condition is given when findings indicate that the cognitive disturbance is the direct physiologic consequence of a general medical condition such as a urinary tract infection (see Clinical Example 27-1), respiratory tract infection, septicemia, or end-stage renal disease.

Certain focal lesions of the right parietal lobe and occipital lobe also may cause delirium. Other causes include metabolic disorders, fluid or electrolyte imbalances, hepatic disease, thiamine deficiency, postoperative states, hypertensive encephalopathy, and sequelae of head injury (APA, 2000; Peskind & Raskind, 1996).

Substance-Induced Delirium

Clinical symptoms of substance-induced delirium occur within minutes to hours after taking relatively

---

CLINICAL EXAMPLE 27.1

THE CLIENT WITH DELIRIUM DUE TO A URINARY TRACT INFECTION

LS, a 65-year-old retired mechanic, had just been transferred to a rehabilitation center from a local hospital after surgical repair of a fractured hip. During hospitalization, he had an indwelling Foley catheter in place. The catheter was removed 2 days after surgery. On the fifth postoperative day, LS began to exhibit agitation and complained of seeing animals in his room. He also expressed a concern that someone was going to hurt him. He was oriented to person only. At night, LS attempted to crawl out of bed over the side rails. During the day, he appeared to be aware of his surroundings and was able to make his needs known. He had no recall of the episodic confusion or disorientation he exhibited. The result of a urinalysis with culture and sensitivity revealed a urinary tract infection due to *Escherichia coli*. LS was exhibiting clinical symptoms of delirium that resolved after a 10-day course of treatment with Bactrim.

high doses of certain drugs. The delirium resolves as the substance is discontinued or eliminated from the body. Substances and medications reported to cause delirium include anesthetics, analgesics, antihistamines, anticonvulsants, anti-asthmatic agents, antiparkinsonism drugs, corticosteroids, and muscle relaxants. Antibiotics and nonsteroidal anti-inflammatory agents also have been identified as causes of delirium in the elderly (Sadock & Sadock, 2003).

Delirium Due to Multiple Etiologies

This diagnosis is used to alert clinicians to the common situation in which the delirium has more than one etiology. For example, a 55-year-old male who undergoes coronary artery bypass surgery may exhibit clinical symptoms of delirium secondary to anesthesia, pain medication, antibiotics, and environmental stimuli secondary to high-tech equipment in the recovery room.

Delirium, Not Otherwise Specified

This diagnosis refers to delirium that does not meet criteria for any specific type of delirium. There is insufficient evidence to establish a specific etiology.

Dementia

Dementia is characterized by impaired judgment, orientation, memory, attention, and cognition (JOMAC), which are affected either by a pattern of simple, gradual deterioration or by rapid, complicated deterioration. Impaired judgment, or the inability to make reasonable decisions, is one of the earliest signs of dementia. It may occur during business dealings or social functions; for example, the person engages in a reckless business venture or displays a disregard for conventional rules of social conduct.

Disorientation to person, place, and time is one of the most common signs of brain dysfunction. An individual becomes more disoriented as the impairment becomes more extensive. A person with minimal impairment may misjudge the date by weeks or months. Moderate impairment generally involves confusion about geographic location such as city or state as well as time, whereas severe impairment is demonstrated by disorientation with respect to time, place, and person. Short-term memory, attention, and concentration deficits are observable in this disorder because the person loses his or her train of thought, forgets what was said just a few minutes earlier, and may be unable

to repeat the information just communicated (Peskind & Raskind, 1996; Sadock & Sadock, 2003).

Other characteristics or associated features include confabulation, perseveration, concrete thinking, and emotional lability. **Confabulation** is the filling in of memory gaps with false but sometimes plausible content to conceal the memory deficit. **Perseveration** is the inappropriate continuation or repetition of a behavior such as giving the same details over and over even when told one is doing so. Abstraction skills are impaired; therefore, the person tends to think in concrete terms. The tendency to manifest rapid, inappropriate, exaggerated mood swings often occurs, and marked anxiety or depression may be seen in mild cases.

Personality changes are often seen in clients with dementia. The normally active person may become withdrawn and apathetic when social involvement narrows.

Psychotic or behavioral disturbances such as agitation, wandering, hallucinations, delusions, suspiciousness, reversal of sleep–wake pattern, inappropriate sexual behavior, hostility, aggressiveness, and combativeness may occur.

Clients with dementia often seem to exhibit increased confusion, restlessness, agitation, wandering, or combative behavior in the late afternoon and evening hours. This phenomenon, referred to as the **sundown syndrome,** may be due to a misinterpretation of the environment, lower tolerance for stress at the end of the day, or overstimulation due to increased environmental activity later in the day. Clients may also exhibit a reversal in their sleep pattern, sleeping during the day and staying awake during the night (APA, 2000; Peskind & Raskind, 1996; Sadock & Sadock, 2003).

The *DSM-IV-TR* lists 12 subtypes of dementia:

1. Dementia of the Alzheimer's type
2. Vascular dementia
3. Dementia due to human immunodeficiency virus (HIV) disease
4. Dementia due to head trauma
5. Dementia due to Parkinson's disease
6. Dementia due to Huntington's disease
7. Dementia due to Pick's disease
8. Dementia due to Creutzfeldt-Jakob disease
9. Dementia due to other general medical conditions
10. Substance-induced persisting dementia
11. Dementia due to multiple etiologies
12. Dementia, not otherwise specified

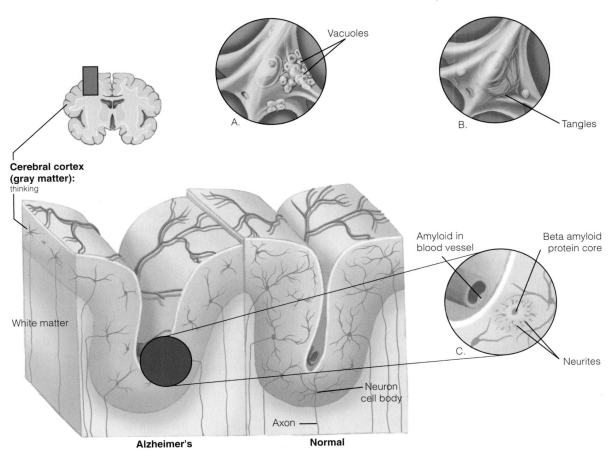

FIGURE 27.4 Pathophysiologic changes associated with DAT: (**A**) granulovascular degeneration; (**B**) neurofibrillary tangles; and (**C**) amyloid plaques as physical changes in the cortex.

Clinical symptoms of DAT, DLB, and vascular dementia are discussed because these disorders constitute the majority of all dementias. Definitions of Parkinson's disease, Huntington's disease, Pick's disease, and Creutzfeldt-Jakob disease appear in the glossary in the back-of-book CD.

Dementia of the Alzheimer's Type

AD is considered the fourth most common cause of death for people older than 65 years in the United States. It is not a natural course of aging. Rather, it is a silent epidemic characterized by the development of multiple cognitive deficits including memory impairment, **aphasia** (language disturbance), **apraxia** (impaired ability to carry out motor activities despite motor function), **agnosia** (failure to recognize or identify objects despite intact sensory function), and **disturbances in executive functioning** (eg, planning, organizing). Figure 27-4 depicts some of the pathophysiologic changes that are believed to occur with DAT.

The course is characterized by gradual onset. The client is aware of the loss of mental abilities as they occur. The diagnosis is coded or labeled based on when and what symptoms appear. If clinical symptoms appear before age 65 years, the diagnosis is coded as *DAT with early onset;* after age 65, the coding *with late onset* is used. Additional coding indicates *with delir-*

ium, with delusions, with depressed mood, or *uncomplicated.* The *DSM-IV-TR* also may include the phrase "specify if." This "specifier" enables the clinician to select additional information from the criteria, such as *with behavioral disturbance,* during the collection of data. Although the specifier is not coded, it can be used to indicate clinically significant behavior such as wandering, throwing items, or combativeness (APA, 2000). As the dementia progresses, personality changes, paranoia, stooping gait, loss of voluntary functions, seizures, and violent behavior may occur. Death can result from neglect, malnutrition, dehydration, incorrect diagnosis, inappropriate treatment, or suicide.

Risk factors associated with the occurrence of AD include advanced age, female gender, head trauma, low educational level, and family history of Down syndrome (Cummings, 1995).

Stages of Dementia of the Alzheimer's Type. Attempts to describe the progression of DAT have resulted in two frequently used classification systems. The first system groups clinical symptoms into four progressive stages. Stage 1 (also referred to as *mild* or *early* stage*)* may last for as long as 2 years. The individual attempts to compensate for memory deficits and difficulty with word recall. Stage 2 (also referred to as *moderate* or *middle* stage) is a progressive stage in which the individual requires cuing and prompting as clinical symptoms continue to intensify and interfere with activities of daily living (ADLs). Stage 2 generally lasts 2 to 5 years. During Stage 3 (also referred to as *severe* or *late* stage), expressive and receptive language is quite limited and gross motor skills are impaired. The length of Stage 3 varies from 2 to 5 years. During Stage 4 (also referred to as *terminal* stage), the individual is unable to communicate, has no recognition of self or others, and is totally dependent upon caregivers. This stage may last from 5 to 10 years (Williams, 1986; Blazer, 1996; Cummings, 2001; Needham, 2006).

The second system describes seven stages of AD according to functional consequences (Reisberg, 1986). For example, stage 3 lists functional manifestations of normal aging such as forgetting names and the location of objects and exhibiting decreased ability to recall appointments. In comparison, stage 7 lists functional manifestations such as progressive loss of all verbal and psychomotor abilities, at which point the individual eventually requires total assistance in all activities. The duration of stage 7 is usually 12 to 18 months before death occurs. See Clinical Example 27-2, The Client With Dementia of the Alzheimer's Type, Stage 6.

CLINICAL EXAMPLE 27.2

THE CLIENT WITH DEMENTIA OF THE ALZHEIMER'S TYPE, STAGE 6

MM, an 80-year-old female client, was admitted to the special care unit of a long-term care facility because her family is no longer able to meet her needs. During the assessment process, MM scored 8 of 30 points on the Mini-Mental State Exam. Deficits were noted in the area of orientation, recall, inability to spell "world" backwards, inability to write a complete sentence, and the inability to copy a diagram. MM also had difficulty performing activities of daily living while residing at home. She had become incontinent of bowel and bladder and was resistant to care provided by her family. MM had wandered outside at night and was returned home by the police. During the interview process, MM used confabulation during responses to questions about her husband, family, and past employment as an executive secretary. After the completion of a dementia workup, the diagnosis of Dementia of the Alzheimer's Type, Late Onset, Stage 6, was noted.

Knowledge of both classification systems is important when providing care for individuals with the diagnosis of AD.

Dementia with Lewy Bodies

DLB is a cognitive disorder that progresses at about the same rate as DAT. Individuals with DLB will typically have some of the clinical symptoms of DAT (eg, memory loss, spatial disorientation, communication difficulties) and Parkinson's disease (eg, slowness, muscle stiffness, trembling of the limb, shuffle gait, loss of facial expression). Persons with DLB find that their cognitive abilities decline early, but significant memory impairment may not become evident until later stages of the disease. Clinical symptoms also include fluctuating cognition; motor deficits such as falls or "funny turns"; detailed and convincing visual hallucinations often of people and animals; falling asleep very easily by day; and restless, disturbed nights with confusion, nightmares, and hallucinations (Alzheimer's Society, 2006). The *DSM-IV-TR* classification of DLB is listed under Dementia Due to Other Medical Conditions.

Vascular Dementia

Vascular dementia, formerly known as *multi-infarct dementia,* is also a common cognitive disorder. It is more common in males than in females. The onset of vascular dementia is usually earlier than that of DAT. Onset is generally abrupt, with fluctuating, rapid changes in memory and other cognitive impairment. Apathy, unsteady gait, weakness, dizziness, and sensory loss generally occur. Clients with vascular dementia often exhibit the same clinical symptoms seen in DAT: aphasia, apraxia, agnosia, and disturbances in executive functioning. Medical conditions associated with the development of vascular dementia include long-standing arterial hypertension, valvular heart disease, cerebrovascular disease, and extracellular vascular disease that may precipitate cerebral emboli. Risk factors also include diabetes mellitus, cardiac arrhythmias, smoking, hypercholesterolemia, and genetics (APA, 2000; Peskind & Raskind, 1996; Sadock & Sadock, 2003).

Vascular dementia may be classified into subtypes due to the presence of large vessel disease, lacunar infarct, strategic infarct, microvascular disease such as Binswanger's disease, small vessel disease, and hypoxic conditions.

The *DSM-IV-TR* diagnosis of vascular dementia is used when focal neurologic signs and symptoms or laboratory evidence indicative of cerebrovascular disease are judged to be etiologically related to the disturbance. The focal neurologic signs and symptoms include exaggeration of deep tendon reflexes, extensor plantar response, pseudobulbar palsy, gait abnormalities, or weakness of an extremity. Computed tomography scan usually reveals multiple infarcts involving cortex and underlying white matter. Anxiety, depression, delirium, delusions, socially inappropriate behavior, lack of inhibition, and increased agitation related to environmental stimulation may occur (APA, 2000). See Clinical Example 27-3.

Dementia Due to Other General Medical Conditions

This classification is used to diagnose dementia due to general medical conditions (eg, HIV, traumatic brain injury, and Parkinson's disease); endocrine, nutritional, and infectious conditions; structural lesions of the brain; and renal or hepatic dysfunction.

Identifying the specific type of dementia is important because treatment guidelines have been developed for the different types of dementia. For example,

---

CLINICAL EXAMPLE 27.3

THE CLIENT WITH VASCULAR DEMENTIA

BW, a 49-year-old male, was admitted to the subacute unit of a rehabilitation center. Upon admission, he presented with expressive aphasia, left-sided hemiparesis, and had an indwelling catheter in place. His wife of 20 years accompanied him. She provided information regarding his recent hospitalization and current plan of care. According to the client's wife, BW had experienced his first stroke at the age of 48 years. His recovery was uneventful; however, she noted that BW had difficulty expressing himself and would become frustrated because he was unable to recall previously learned information. At that time, he also exhibited apraxia, the inability to carry out motor activities despite intact motor function. Approximately 8 months ago, BW had another stroke that left him with his current symptoms. During his course of rehabilitation, BW was able to speak but continued to exhibit some expressive aphasia. He was oriented to person and knew that he was not at home, but could not state where he was. He was unable to state the date. Before discharge, a follow-up neurologic evaluation was conducted. BW was able to complete a modified Mini-Mental State Exam. The results indicated the presence of vascular dementia.

---

as noted earlier, persons with DAT may also have DLB. Conversely, individuals with DLB may be misdiagnosed as having DAT. Often individuals with DLB have extreme adverse reactions (eg, stiff, rigid movements or immobility) to drugs commonly used to treat behavioral problems associated with dementia. These adverse reactions can be serious and could jeopardize the person's health.

Amnestic Disorders

Individuals with amnesia experience impairment in their ability to recall information or past events. Clients with **anterograde amnesia** are unable to recall events of long ago but have normal recall of recent events. **Retrograde amnesia** refers to the loss of memory of events occurring before a particular time in a person's life. (The terms *working*, *episodic*, *semantic*, and *procedural* memory are described in Figure 27-2.) An understanding of these different memory systems and their location in the human brain enables the clinician to effectively evaluate the client's memory functioning and area of pathology.

The *DSM-IV-TR* describes three subtypes of amnestic disorders: amnestic disorder due to a general medical condition; substance-induced persisting amnestic disorder; and amnestic disorder, not otherwise specified (NOS). See the accompanying Clinical Symptoms and Diagnostic Characteristics box for amnestic disorder due to a general medical condition.

Substance-induced persisting amnestic disorder can occur in association with alcohol, sedatives, hypnotics, anxiolytics, and other or unknown substances. The diagnostic characteristics are the same as those listed for amnestic disorder due to a general medical condition. If there is insufficient evidence to establish a specific cause for amnesia, the diagnosis of amnestic disorder, NOS, is used.

Cognitive Disorder, Not Otherwise Specified

This category is for disorders—characterized by cognitive dysfunction presumed to be caused by the direct physiologic effect of a general medical condition or substance use—that do not meet the criteria for any of the specific deliriums, dementias, or amnestic disorders already described in this classification. Examples include postconcussion disorder following head trauma or a mild neurocognitive disorder due to central nervous system pathology (APA, 2000). Box 27.1 summarizes behavior caused by central nervous system pathology.

CLINICAL SYMPTOMS AND DIAGNOSTIC CHARACTERISTICS /
AMNESTIC DISORDER DUE TO A GENERAL MEDICAL CONDITION

CLINICAL SYMPTOMS

- Impaired ability to learn new information
- Inability to recall previously learned information or past events
- Possible confusion and disorientation prior to development of memory deficit

DIAGNOSTIC CHARACTERISTICS

- Evidence of memory impairment: memory significantly decreased from usual level; considered transient if impairment lasting for 1 month or less, considered chronic if impairment occurring longer than 1 month
- Memory impairment not solely limited to periods of delirium or dementia
- Demonstration of significant problems with social or occupational functioning
- History, physical examination, and laboratory findings indicative of medical condition underlying the memory impairment

---

BOX 27.1 BEHAVIOR DUE TO CENTRAL NERVOUS SYSTEM PATHOLOGY

FRONTAL LOBE:

Lack of attention tenacity or persistence

Loss of emotional control, rage, violent behavior

Changes in mood and personality, uncharacteristic behavior

Expressive aphasia or dysphasia

PARIETAL LOBE:

Neglect or inattention to left half of space, resulting in possible self-injury or unintentional contact with others that could be viewed as aggressive behavior

TEMPORAL LOBE:

Inability to store or retrieve information

Inability to comprehend speech due to loss of hearing or receptive aphasia

OCCIPITAL LOBE:

Visual disturbances such as agnosia or the inability to recognize by sight

LIMBIC LOBE:

Inability to feed self

Decrease in socialization

Lack of emotional expression or apathy

Inability to learn or store information

THE NURSING PROCESS

ASSESSMENT

The single most important piece of information when assessing a client with cognitive impairment is a careful history from the client's family or another reliable observer. To identify a cognitively impaired client's baseline mental status and the characteristics of any change is crucial (Henry, 2002).

Assessment focuses on the client's ability to meet basic needs, appearance, severity and duration of cognitive impairment, and behavioral manifestations, including any associated clinical symptoms to determine the presence of delirium, dementia, or amnestic disorder. Judgment, orientation, memory, affect, and cognition (JOMAC) are key areas to assess. Also note the client's intellectual ability, both past and present, and document the following assessment data.

Ability to Meet Basic Needs

Clients with impaired cognition, such as those with dementia, may exhibit a slow, progressive decline in their ability to perform ADLs that goes unnoticed over a period of time. Conversely, clients with clinical symptoms of delirium or amnestic disorder exhibit an acute change in their ability to meet basic needs. Examples of questions that can be used to collect data include the following:

- Does the client live alone? If not, where does the client reside? With whom? Has the client relocated recently? If so, why?
- Is the client able to provide self-care? If not, who assists the client? Does the client require supervision or minimal prompting to complete ADLs?
- Does the client have impaired hearing or vision that interferes with his/her ability to follow directions to meet basic needs?

Appearance, Mood, and Affect

Changes in appearance, mood, and affect may go unnoticed unless a client with cognitive impairment has a support system or is brought to the attention of a health care provider because of a medical or psychiatric emergency. The following questions may be helpful in collecting data in this area:

- Does the client appear tense, anxious, depressed, or frightened?

- Is the client dressed appropriately?
- Does the client present with disturbances in gait, balance, or movements?
- Does the client present with any signs of physical abuse or self-sustained injuries?
- Do the client's height and weight appear to be within normal limits?

Cognitive Abilities

Assess judgment, orientation, memory and cognitive abilities. Focus on clinical symptoms of memory loss, confusion, rambling speech, or a change in personality. If any of the symptoms are noted, use the following questions to collect more information:

- How and when did the symptoms first occur? Do they fluctuate frequently?
- Does the client require cues or prompting to complete tasks?
- Does the client use confabulation, negativistic behavior, perseveration, projection, or rationalization, or feign deafness for lack of appropriate responses?

Delirium should be considered any time there is an acute change in mental status or cognitive abilities.

Behavioral Manifestations

Assessment of behavioral manifestations takes into account the complexity of a client's medical, psychiatric, social, and environmental conditions. During the assessment, focus attention on data obtained from the following questions:

- Is the client restless, pacing, groaning, withdrawn, or exhibiting loss of mobility? Such behaviors are the most common signals of pain in clients who can't provide rational information on a verbal basis.

- Does the client exhibit behavioral disturbances such as sleep–wake pattern disturbance, agitation, anxiety, irritability, or a change in appetite? Common problems that contribute to such behavior, but often go undiagnosed, include sensory impairment, constipation, gastroesophageal reflux disease, poor dentition, and pain.
- Does the client take any medication such as anticholinergic agents, histamine-blocking agents, analgesics, sedative–hypnotics, or cardiovascular drugs that can produce adverse effects? Also ascertain whether the client takes over-the-counter medications, medications prescribed for someone else, eye drops, eardrops, topical medications, and herbal and vitamin preparations.
- Does the client have any medical conditions that are currently being treated by an attending physician or that the client has refused to have treated?
- Has the client been exposed to any chemical toxins?
- Does the client have a history of getting lost in familiar territory, inappropriate behavior, disinhibition, suspiciousness, delusions, or hallucinations? If so, who is involved? Where and when does the behavior occur? What is the duration and frequency of the behavior? What occurs prior to (antecedents) and after the behavior (consequences)? Sensory impairments are often the cause of such behavior in older adults.
- Is the client's behavior affected by any specific environmental changes or stimuli (eg, temperature, noise levels, or the presence of strangers)?
- Does the client drink alcohol or use any addictive or chemical substances?
- Has the client ever been evaluated and treated for a psychiatric disorder? If so, when and where?

Assessment Tools

Several assessment tools are available to assess a client's mental status or cognitive abilities (eg, orientation, concentration, memory), instrumental functionality (eg, ability to perform ADLs), neurologic or motor functioning (eg, gait, reflex changes), and behavioral symptoms (eg, agitation, mood, wandering). A few assessment tools also use caregiver input to assess the client's status. Examples of the assessment tools used include:

- MMSE (Mini-Mental Status Exam)
- ADAS-Cog (AD Assessment Scale-Cognitive Subscale)
- Clock Drawing Test (cognition)
- Delirium Scale

- IADL Scale (Instrumental Activities of Daily Living Scale)
- Functional Assessment Staging Test (FAST) Scale (Table 27-2)
- Short Geriatric Depression Scale
- Behavioral Syndromes Scale for Dementia
- NPI-Q (Neuropsychiatric Inventory Questionnaire) (behaviors)
- Algase Wandering Scale (AWS)
- Caregiver Dementia Screener
- Caregiver Strain Index
- Caregiver's Burden Scale (CBS)

The Wong-Baker Faces Rating Scale may be useful in determining the presence or absence of pain in clients who are not able to communicate their needs.

The NEECHAM Confusion Scale may be used to assess clients who may exhibit signs and symptoms of confusion in a variety of ways and differently with each episode (Allen, 1999). This scale, a nine-item checklist that then can be used during routine care, assesses the client's behavior and physiologic control, including vital sign stability, urinary continence, and oxygen saturation levels, as well as the client's ability to process information.

The Agitated Behavior in Dementia Scale is used to assess behaviors that represent verbal and physical agitation. A 4-point scale is used to rate the hourly, daily, or weekly frequency of occurrence for each of the 16 identified behaviors commonly exhibited by individuals with dementia. Care-giver reaction is also rated on a 5-point scale to indicate "not at all" to "extremely." Effective behavioral interventions can be planned based on the results of this assessment scale (Smith & Buckwalter, 2005).

Expect to obtain a comprehensive history and physical examination, including a variety of tests, to aid in determining the type of cognitive disorder present and whether a mood disorder exists (Box 27-2). A medication history also is conducted. Clients may be referred to a memory clinic for a complete neurologic workup, including assessment of sensory function, to rule out pathological changes. Neuroimaging techniques such as the magnetic resonance imaging (MRI), SPECT, PET, and CT are being utilized to help in the assessment by identifying structural changes that could produce cognitive disorders. If the assessment does not clearly confirm the presence of a cognitive disorder such as dementia or delirium, the assessment should be repeated in 6 months to determine whether a progression in the clinical symptoms has occurred.

TABLE 27.2 Functional Assessment Staging Test (FAST) Scale

The Functional Assessment Staging Test (FAST) Scale evaluates the progression of functional decline in clients with uncomplicated dementia of the Alzheimer's type (DAT). It describes in detail the entire course of DAT, including both the well-documented early stages of the disease and the less well-documented late stages. The first two stages address characteristics of a normal aging adult. During the third stage the client exhibits clinical symptoms related to impaired memory (eg, forgetting important appointments for the first time). The average duration of the third stage is 7 years (Reisberg, 1986). Following is a summary of stages four through seven, including characteristics, clinical diagnosis, and average duration of each stage.

STAGE	CHARACTERISTICS	DIAGNOSIS	DURATION
4	The client has difficulty completing complex tasks related to finances and shopping.	Mild DAT	2 years
5	The client has difficulty with independent community functioning and choosing proper clothing.	Moderate DAT	$1\frac{1}{2}$ years
6	During this stage, the client requires assistance with dressing, bathing, and toileting. Urinary and fecal incontinence develop at the end of this stage. Stage 6 consists of five substages to show the progression of this disease.	Moderately severe DAT	Approximately 5 months to 2 years
7	During this stage the client progressively loses the ability to speak, ambulate, sit up, smile, and hold up one's head. Stage 7 consists of six substages to show the progression of this disease.	Severe DAT	Approximately 12 months to 18 months

Also assess the client's social support to determine which resources are needed and whether they are available. Family members may also benefit from support group programs or reading or viewing educational material about cognitive impairment.

Transcultural Considerations

Always consider the client's cultural and educational background when evaluating his or her cognitive capacity. Individuals from various backgrounds may have difficulty answering questions in certain tests because they are unfamiliar with the general knowledge of other cultures or their culture does not place an emphasis on information such as date of birth, state capitals, names of presidents, and so forth. The prevalence of different causes of dementia varies across cultural groups; for example, dementia secondary to nutritional deficiency or infections may occur with more frequency in countries where poverty is prevalent. Strickland, Longobardi, and Gray (1999) cite several studies regarding the prevalence of dementia in minority elderly. According to their literature research

of various studies, cognitive impairment was more prevalent in chronically ill African Americans than in the white population after hospital discharge; vascular dementia and dementia due to chronic alcohol use were higher among African Americans than in the white population; and mixed or vascular dementia was found to be more common among Mexican American nursing home residents than among comparable white residents.

Language and ability to comprehend it also may affect assessment. If the client speaks a different language or has difficulty with the English language, enlist the aid of an interpreter. Then when interviewing a client who needs an interpreter, make sure that the interpreter does not provide additional information or elaborate on the client's responses.

NURSING DIAGNOSES

The goals of the diagnostic process are to make a specific diagnosis to avoid implementing the wrong nursing interventions as a result of misdiagnosis; identify

BOX 27.2 COMPREHENSIVE ASSESSMENT OF IMPAIRED COGNITION AND BEHAVIORAL MANIFESTATIONS

HISTORY

Will likely require interview with close family or friend

Data regarding birth, developmental stages, medical history, medication, time of onset of clinical symptoms, rate of progression, and any family history of dementia

PHYSICAL EXAMINATION

Mental status evaluation: Obtain information regarding any past psychiatric treatments.

General physical and neurologic examination including pain assessment (client may not be able to self-report pain). Observe for behaviors associated with pain such as crying or moaning, rubbing or guarding, frowning or grimacing. Assess the client during activity whenever possible because pain may be more evident during ambulation or repositioning.

STUDIES

Complete blood count

Sedimentation rate

Chemistry panel (electrolytes, calcium, albumin, BUN, creatinine, transaminase, blood sugar)

Thyroid function tests

VDRI or RPR

Urine Alzheim Alert TM Test (a noninvasive urinary test that measures neural thread protein and is elevated in DAT)

Urinalysis

Serum B_{12} and folate levels

Human immunodeficiency virus (HIV), if permission is granted

IMAGING

Chest x-ray

Head computed tomography (CT) scan

Electrocardiogram (ECG)

ADDITIONAL STUDIES (IF INDICATED)

Electroencephalogram (EEG)

Neuropsychiatric testing

Head magnetic resonance imaging (MRI) if vascular dementia suspected

Lumbar puncture (LP)

Drug and alcohol toxicology

Heavy metal screen

---

any existence of a comorbid medical condition or psychiatric disorder; avoid labeling a person with a diagnosis of dementia or DAT when it does not exist; identify the practical and psychosocial needs of the client, the family, and the primary caregivers; and to plan for the future (Needham, 2006).

Early diagnosis of a cognitive disorder such as dementia is important because it provides time for decision-making. For example, it may allow a client to participate as a candidate for one of the Food and Drug Administration (FDA)–approved drugs that may slow the progression of some symptoms and delay the need for long-term care placement. Additionally, the client can have time to complete advance directives, making his or her wishes for future care known. Moreover, family members may have more time to adjust to the needs of the client and consider home-based care as the clinical symptoms progress (Douris, 2003).

Six basic commonalities link delirium, dementia, and amnestic disorders: impaired cognition, alteration in thought processes, impaired communication, behavioral disturbances, self-care deficits, and impaired socialization. In addition, a comorbid medical condition may exist. These commonalities are considered during the formulation of the nursing diagnoses.

See the accompanying Examples of North American Nursing Diagnosis Association (NANDA) Nursing Diagnoses box for examples of nursing diagnoses for clients with cognitive disorders.

OUTCOME IDENTIFICATION

Stating outcomes for clients with cognitive disorders can be challenging because of the variety of identified problems. Generally, outcomes for clients with cognitive disorders include the elimination of organic etiol-

EXAMPLES OF NANDA NURSING DIAGNOSES/ COGNITIVE DISORDERS
• Interrupted Family Processes related to shift in family roles • Ineffective Role Performance related to loss of previous capabilities • Disturbed Thought Processes related to hallucinations and delusions • Hopelessness related to progressive nature of Alzheimer's disease • Impaired Social Interaction related to attention deficits • Ineffective Coping related to memory deficits • Risk for Injury related to impulsive behavior • Risk for Injury related to poor judgment • Situational Low Self-Esteem related to loss of previous capabilities • Social Isolation related to irritability • Social Isolation related to bizarre behavior

EXAMPLES OF STATED OUTCOMES/ COGNITIVE DISORDERS
• The client will verbalize decreased frequency of delusions and hallucinations. • The client will demonstrate decreased agitation. • The client will be free of injury. • The client will not harm others or destroy property. • The client will verbalize feelings of powerlessness or hopelessness. • The client will develop alternate communication skills. • The client will verbalize increased feelings of self-worth. • The client will demonstrate decreased socially inappropriate behavior. • The client will identify life areas that require alterations due to illness. • The client will verbalize beginning of the grieving process related to loss of mobility. • The client will live in the least restrictive environment that is safe.

ogy, if possible; the prevention of acceleration of symptoms; and the preservation of the client's dignity (Detwiler, 2003).

When developing outcomes, consider the client's present physical and emotional status, any behavioral disturbances the client manifests, the environment in which he or she lives, the client's level of independent functioning and ability to socialize, and the availability of a support system. Also keep in mind the client's degree of insight into his or her diagnosis, verbalized expectations, and capabilities to meet stated outcomes. The clinical prognosis for cognitive disorders may be reversible (eg, delirium secondary to anesthesia), treatable but not reversible (eg, prevention of further ischemia in cardiovascular disease), or progressive (eg, DAT). See the accompanying Examples of Stated Outcomes box.

PLANNING INTERVENTIONS

Nursing interventions planned for a client with a cognitive disorder often vary depending on the client's diagnosis of delirium, dementia, or amnestic disorder. However, the focus is on maintaining the client's contact with reality, reducing agitation, preventing injury, promoting adequate nutritional and fluid intake, pro-

moting adequate sleep and rest, treating any underlying causes, encouraging expression of feelings, and stimulating the memory through various activities. Attempts to maximize remaining learning potential are important while making the client feel comfortable both physically and emotionally.

Meeting basic needs becomes increasingly demanding as physical deterioration occurs. Gradually introduce new devices or material to provide self-care simply. Ensure that the environment allows the client the opportunity to adapt to impairments by doing things in less-complex ways than in the past, thus promoting an optimal level of independence.

Planning also focuses on decreasing socially inappropriate behavior, encouraging satisfactory social relationships, and assisting the client to live in as nonrestrictive an environment as possible.

IMPLEMENTATION

Working with clients with cognitive impairment frequently results in health care personnel being confronted with their own human limitations, especially when deficits are irreversible and become progressively worse over time. Repeating oneself constantly, knowing that the client is unable to recall information or will soon forget, is frustrating. Emotional reactions are possible when faced with the inability to control inevitable deterioration in some clients. Feelings of helplessness, impatience, anger, disgust, overprotectiveness, chronic helpfulness, or "burnout" may result (Husseini, 1996).

Establishment of a Safe Environment

Clients with cognitive disorders require an environment that will promote health and safety and maximize independence (Needham, 2006). A calm, direct, supportive approach with a predictable schedule is necessary when providing care for clients who are forgetful, disoriented, confused, or frightened, or who exhibit alterations in perception. The Alzheimer's Disease Research Center at the University of California at San Diego suggests implementing three standards when creating a safe environment for a client with DAT or cognitive disorders such as delirium: think prevention, change the environment rather than the behavior, and minimize danger to maximize independence (Johnson, 2002).

Reorient client to the environment frequently. Have familiar or personal objects available to create a safe, comfortable atmosphere and to add meaning to the surroundings. Encourage the use of eye glasses and hearing aides when appropriate to improve sensory input. Provide way-finding cues. Assess safety of lighting, flooring, and furniture. Remove any items from the environment that are safety hazards or potentially harmful. Although the goal of a restraint-free environment is considered to be the gold standard of care for clients with cognitive disorders, the emergency use of physical or chemical restraints may be necessary to safeguard against injury when clients who are placed in unfamiliar surroundings or require hospitalization exhibit combative or assaultive behavior or are at risk for self-injury. It is beneficial to have a discussion with the family or health care surrogate of a client regarding the limited use of restraints (Branski, 1998; Foreman & Zane, 1996; Needham, 2006; Wheldon, 2005).

Furthermore, encourage the family of clients who have been diagnosed with DAT and have a tendency to wander to register the client in the Alzheimer's Association's Safe Return program.

Assistance in Meeting Basic Needs

If a comorbid medical condition exists, be sure to provide routine care such as monitoring vital signs, assessing level of consciousness, and meeting physiologic needs. Unmet needs can cause a client with a cognitive disorder to become agitated and anxious. The client may be unaware of the source of discomfort or be unable to respond to the cues resulting from unmet needs (Needham, 2006). In addition, assist with ADLs as necessary. Branski (1998) discusses providing assistance with some or all ADLs, such as bathing, eating, dressing, and toileting. Provide a balance of rest and activity because excessive activity may lead to fatigue and can present as acute confusion. Inadequate activity and stimulation may lead to apathy and little desire to attend to information. Also promote restorative care, including that of range of motion or ambulation when appropriate. Finally, remember that clients with delirium might be unaware of deficits or limitations.

Stabilization of Behavior

Approximately 90% of clients with dementia may exhibit measurable behavioral disturbances, and one half to one third of all clients with the diagnosis of cognitive disorder are overtly aggressive (Rawlings & Verma, 2001). Agitation tends to increase with the severity of cognitive impairment and may predict the need for early institutionalization.

Behavioral manifestations (eg, agitation, aggressiveness, combativeness, pacing, wandering, yelling, hoarding, lack of sexual inhibition, impulsivity) may be caused by the client's inability to verbalize distress in socially appropriate ways. Common forms of distress that often go undetected in older clients with cognitive disorders include constipation, infection (eg, urinary tract infection), and pain (eg, arthritis). Other causes of behavioral manifestations include personality changes, internal stimuli such as anxiety or agitated depression, delusions, hallucinations, environmental stimuli (eg, excessive heat, noise, light or humidity), or any number of sources too numerous to list (Rawlings & Verma, 2001).

Nursing research identified causes of behavioral manifestations exhibited by cognitively impaired clients (eg, hitting, kicking, pinching, biting) during bathing. Although most nurses have a desire to deal compassionately with clients, they need to be aware of situations that could evoke disturbances in behavior by clients during the delivery of care. Examples of situations that could evoke unexpected behavioral disturbances include failure to prepare a client for a task or treatment; unexpected touch; hurried pace when assisting a client; addressing a client in an irritated voice or manner; confrontational communication; invalidation of the client's feelings; and the presence of multiple caregivers (Somboontanont, Sloane, Floyd, Holditch-David, Hogue, & Mitchell, 2004). Before establishing interventions to stabilize behavioral manifestations of clients, determine whether the safety of the client or other individuals is at risk because of the behavior and whether the problem is truly a client problem or a staff problem (Needham, 2006).

Behavioral Intervention Techniques and Programs

Redirection is a form of behavioral intervention that uses distraction techniques. The client's memory deficits and short attention spans help to ensure the success of distraction. If used correctly, redirection avoids confrontation and the risk of catastrophic reactions.

Stimulated response therapy (SRT) is a form of behavioral intervention that uses audiotapes composed of a family member's voice in a telephone conversation with blank spaces that correspond to the client's side of the conversation. During the conversation, the family member reminisces about cherished and loved experiences of the person's life (Needham, 2006).

Several programs have been developed to minimize behavioral problems including the consequences seen in clients with DAT (Moyer, 1995). These programs include using creative reality by entering the world of the client, using validation rather than reality orientation, using low-stimulation activities, focusing on former lifestyle and current capabilities, and providing for physical activities appropriate to the client's age and physical capabilities. Music also has been shown to be an effective intervention to minimize behavioral manifestations (see Supporting Evidence for Practice 27-1).

Many hospitals, rehabilitation centers, and long-term care facilities take pride in having "restraint-free" environments. If a client is at risk for injury and needs to be restrained, some facilities have committees that review the client's behavior to determine the least restrictive device to be used. Also, family members or companion sitters are considered an alternate measure to the use of restraints (Branski, 1998).

Outreach Programs

Several outreach programs are available for clients with behavioral problems related to dementia. The Mayo Clinic Internal Medicine outreach program in

---

SUPPORTING EVIDENCE FOR PRACTICE 27.1

The Use of Music to Decrease Aggressive Behavior in Clients With the Diagnosis of Dementia

PROBLEM UNDER INVESTIGATION / How does playing music affect aggressive behaviors among institutionalized elders with dementia?

SUMMARY OF RESEARCH / The study included 18 elders (14 women) between the ages of 55 and 95 years. Scores on the Mini-Mental State Examination (MMSE) ranged from 1 to 22, with only three subjects scoring above 15. Three subjects were untestable. Data were collected during ten observation periods in which subjects were randomly assigned to an intervention (favorite music was played during bath) or to the control (no music was played). Conditions were then reversed for the subjects. Researchers concluded that the total number of aggressive behaviors

(eg, biting, kicking, spitting, and yelling) was significantly lower when music was played. Caregivers noted improved mood, smiling, clapping, and dancing during music interventions.

SUPPORT FOR PRACTICE / Psychiatric–mental health nurses should consider music as a form of non-pharmacologic therapeutic intervention when providing care for older adult clients who exhibit agitation or aggressive behaviors. Additional research is suggested to study the type of music that decreases agitation, and the impact of music on caregivers.

SOURCE: Clark, M. E., Lipe, A. W., & Bilbrey, M. (1998). Use of music to decrease aggressive behaviors in people with dementia. Journal of Gerontological Nursing, 24(7), 10–17.

Rochester, Minnesota, provides a multidisciplinary team approach to the behavioral manifestations of clients with dementia (Allen, 1999). This program is called the Dementia-Behavioral Assessment and Response Team (D-BART). The target population of D-BART includes clients whose behavior puts them at risk for increased use of physical or pharmacologic restraints, potential abuse of self or others, compromised safety, dismissal from a facility, or institutionalization; or clients whose behavior puts their caregivers at risk for extreme physical and psychological stress. The team consists of geriatric health specialists, including a geriatric nurse practitioner, who meet with caregivers and families in a client's home or care facility. The team's goal is to educate caregivers about the disease process and its impact on behavior and to develop an individualized plan of care to reduce or eliminate problem behaviors.

A Home-Based Primary Care program (HBPC) operated by 70 Veterans' Administration centers throughout the country also has been described (Douris, 2003). The goal of this outreach program is to improve the care of veterans with dementia. A multidisciplinary team visits homebound veterans and provides services such as pain assessment of cognitively impaired veterans; client education about advance directives and community resources; and assessment of caregiver stress. Palliative care and end-of-life care are also provided in the home if requested.

Medication Management

Although there are no specific medications to cure cognitive disorders such as DAT and related disorders, pharmacologic interventions can be considered in addition to social, environmental, and behavioral management approaches. Medication may be required to treat comorbid medical conditions such as CVA or Parkinson's disease or manage clinical symptoms of dementia, delirium, or a comorbid psychiatric disorder. For example, atypical antipsychotics may be used to alleviate agitation or anxiety secondary to hallucinations or delusions when behavioral interventions are ineffective. Preliminary evidence suggests that atypicals are also safe and effective in treating delirium if low to modest dosages are used.

The anticonvulsant gabapentin (Neurontin) has proven to be safe and effective in controlling agitation and combativeness in cognitive disorders. It has no significant drug interactions, is only 3% plasma bound, and is not appreciably metabolized. Should treatment with gabapentin prove ineffective or poorly tolerated, a reasonable second-line choice is divalproex (Depakote), although it requires periodic blood level be measured and venipunctures for easily agitated clients need to be kept at a minimum (Smith, 2005).

Antidepressants may be prescribed for a comorbid mood disorder or as a hypnotic in clients with delirium. Although benzodiazepines are frequently used to treat clinical symptoms of anxiety and agitated depression, they appear ineffective and generally play only an adjunctive role in treating delirium. An exception is in the treatment of delirium induced by acute alcohol or benzodiazepine withdrawal. General anesthetics, narcotics, and cholinomimetics may also help manage hyperactive delirious clients. Caution must be taken to avoid over-sedation and adverse reactions that can occur during drug–drug interactions (O'Connor, 2005).

Evidence regarding the use of alternative therapies such as nonsteroidal anti-inflammatory drugs (NSAIDS), ginkgo biloba, B vitamins, statins, tocopherol (Vitamin E), and estrogen in the treatment of dementia is weak. Although antihypertensive treatment reduces the development of stroke and vascular dementia, the evidence is limited that similar treatment of people with mild to moderate dementia delays disease progression (Needham, 2006; U.S. Preventive Services Task Force, 2003).

Medicating clients may prove to be challenging due to several factors. Clients may:

- Be unable to comprehend the need for a medication
- Be unable to identify self due to impaired cognition and communication
- Resist taking medication because of impaired thoughts such as delusions or paranoid thoughts
- Exhibit fluctuations in cognition, mood, and behavior
- Exhibit behavioral manifestations similar to adverse effects of prescribed medication

Recent advances in the treatment of dementia, specifically DAT, have resulted in several pharmacologic approaches to slow the progression of the disease and to stabilize clinical symptoms. Cholinesterase inhibitors are agents thought to improve memory and goal-directed thought processes by reducing inactivation of acetylcholine and potentiating cholinergic transmission. As a result, the concentration of acetylcholinesterase is increased in the cerebral cortex (Sadock & Sadock, 2003). Cholinesterase inhibitors include donepezil (Aricept), rivastigmine (Exelon), tacrine (Cognex), and galantamine (Razadyne). Galantamine has been proven safe and effective for improving behavior and global function in clients with DLB (Zoler, 2004).

Memantine (Namenda), an N-methyl-D-aspartate (NMDA) antagonist, has been approved for the treatment of moderate-to-severe DAT. It can be used alone or in combination with donepezil and has been shown to slow the decline in mental function in clients with more advanced dementia. Memantine is generally safe and effective, with a low potential for drug interactions, even when combined with a cholinesterase inhibitor (Peskind, Tangalos, & Grossberg, 2005). These drugs are highlighted in Drug Summary Table 27-1.

Client and Family Education

The diagnosis of a cognitive disorder can have devastating consequences for clients and their families. After a client has been diagnosed, be sure that the client and family are informed about the disease and the progression of clinical symptoms. Also inform families about the availability of community-based programs (Andrews & Andrews, 2003).

The D-BART outreach program mentioned earlier in this chapter is an example of a program designed to educate clients, family members, and caregivers about the disease process and the management of clinical symptoms of cognitive disorders. Other sources of educational information include community support

DRUG SUMMARY TABLE 27-1   Drugs Used for Cognitive Disorders

GENERIC (TRADE) NAME	DAILY DOSAGE RANGE	IMPLEMENTATION
Drug Class: Cholinesterase Inhibitors*		
donepezil (Aricept)	5–10 mg	Give once daily in A.M. or h.s.; provide small, frequent meals if GI disturbance occurs; monitor for bradycardia, insomnia, fatigue, GI disturbances, muscle cramps, skin rash, jaundice, and changes in color of urine or stool; use with caution in clients with peptic ulcer disease.
galantamine (Razadyne) (also available in extended-release form)	8–24 mg	Give with AM and PM meals; monitor for bradycardia, GI disturbance, syncope, and weight loss. XR form is given once daily after a meal.
rivastigmine (Exelon)	3–12 mg	Give in AM and PM with meals; monitor for GI disturbance, fatigue, headache, and malaise, weight loss.
tacrine (Cognex)	40–160 mg	Give q.i.d. in divided doses on an empty stomach unless severe GI disturbance occurs; arrange for regular transaminase level determination before and during therapy; monitor for symptoms of impaired hepatic function, syncope, and bleeding; give with vitamin E 1000 IU b.i.d. if ordered.
Drug Class: N-methyl-D-aspartate (NMDA) receptor antagonist		
memantine (Namenda)	5–20 mg	FDA approved for use in moderate-to-severe AD. Use caution with other NMDA antagonists; may affect or be affected by renally excreted drugs; monitor for dizziness, headache, hypertension, pain, GI upset, somnolence, hallucinations, and dyspnea.

*Cholinesterase inhibitors are the drug of choice to improve memory and thought process in clients with the diagnosis of a cognitive disorder.

groups sponsored by the Alzheimer's Disease and Education Referral Center, free community programs for the public, continuing educational programs for nursing and medical professionals provided by drug companies, and the Internet.

Continuum of Care

According to the findings of research comparing end-of-life care between clients with advanced dementia and clients with terminal cancer, clients with advanced dementia are not always recognized as having a terminal condition and do not receive adequate palliative care in the final stage of the illness. Distressing signs and symptoms are not recognized or managed adequately. Lacking advance directives that limit aggressive care, many clients with advanced dementia undergo painful, unnecessary interventions including the insertion of feeding tubes in the final weeks before death. Clients with advanced dementia are eight times less likely to have a Do Not Resuscitate order than other clients (Moon, 2004).

Continuum of care is vital if clients with cognitive disorders are to experience a good quality of life. Although delirium is considered a reversible process, the client could experience recurrent symptoms due to the progression of a chronic medical problem; drug–drug interactions; or other physiologic changes such as fluid and electrolyte imbalance when using diuretics. Clients with dementia may exhibit stabilization of clinical symptoms, a slow progression of the illness, or clinical symptoms of end-stage DAT or a related disorder. Clients with amnestic disorders may never regain full functioning of their memory and may require continued supervision of ADLs.

The client's physical and psychosocial changes and the availability of caregivers determine the setting in which continuum of care will occur. Nearly 4 million U.S. residents have DAT, and approximately 70% of these people live at home, with the majority of care being provided by friends and family. To assist families in caring for clients, several resources are available, such as the Administration on Aging, Alzheimer's Association, Family Caregiver Alliance Resource Center, and the National Council on Aging (Johnson, 2002). These resources also help family members locate providers of continuum-of-care services such as adult day care centers, assisted-living facilities, and long-term care facilities that have special units for clients with dementia, as well as respite care centers.

Every year about 540,000 terminally ill Americans enter hospice programs to receive a wide array of supportive care for themselves and their families. Hospice care is available to clients with cognitive disorders, including DAT. Hospice workers provide medical support; assist clients and family members with emotional support including life closure, grief counseling, and spiritual counseling; and may provide art, touch, and music therapy when the need is identified. Follow-up contact and bereavement counseling continue if family members indicate a need or desire. Although care can be delivered in a variety of settings, it is usually given in the home setting at no out-of-pocket expense. Medicare and most insurance companies have established guidelines for certification of hospice care (Knowlton, 2000a; Knowlton, 2000b).

Future Research

Several research studies regarding the etiology and treatment of cognitive disorders are being conducted by the National Institute of Health, National Institute of Mental Health, and independent groups. The studies are focusing on:

- The short-term and long-term efficacy of donepezil and cognitive training to improve memory in elderly adults not affected by dementia
- The effects of nonsteroidal anti-inflammatory drugs in the delay of cognitive decline in older adults with age-associated memory impairment
- Alzhemed, an investigational drug that appears to prevent formation of amyloid fibrils in the brain
- Use of a low-flow cerebrospinal fluid shunt to increase the clearance of beta amyloid deposition from the brain to improve cognitive stability
- Passive immunization by vaccine to develop antibodies that target the beta amyloid peptide in the brain to prevent DAT

EVALUATION

Because the client with a cognitive disorder generally exhibits a fluctuation in physical and psychosocial functioning, evaluation is an ongoing process. Input is obtained from caregivers and family members. Success may be measured in terms of quality of life as achieved by slowing down the disease process, rather than by reversing, stopping, or curing medical or psychosocial problems. See Nursing Plan of Care 27-1 for an example.

M●VIE viewing GUIDES

NURSING PLAN OF CARE 27.1

THE CLIENT WITH DELIRIUM

Mike, a 35-year-old real estate broker, was admitted to the emergency room for evaluation of a possible fractured right arm following a rollerblading accident. He was then admitted to the hospital for surgical intervention. The evening of surgery, Mike was given pain medication. A few hours later he was found to be confused and began talking incoherently. His level of consciousness changed as he was no longer oriented to place and time. He thought that he was trapped on a boat and kept asking the staff for assistance to find the bathroom. The following day, a neurologic evaluation was requested. Mike was diagnosed as exhibiting clinical symptoms of delirium due to pain medication, anesthesia, and changes in his environment.

DSM–IV–TR DIAGNOSIS: Delirium due to multiple etiologies

ASSESSMENT: Personal strengths: Employed as a real estate broker, good physical health except for fractured arm.

   Weaknesses: Disoriented, confused, incoherent speech, impaired mobility.

NURSING DIAGNOSIS: Disturbed Thought Processes related to side effects of anesthesia pain medication, and changes in his environment as evidenced by disorientation and confusion.

OUTCOME: The client will demonstrate decreased confusion and disorientation.

Planning/Implementation	Rationale
Assess the client's level of functioning daily or more frequently if necessary.	Clients with delirium exhibit fluctuating capabilities until the delirium clears.
Provide factual information to minimize the client's confusion and disorientation.	The client will become aware that his perceptions are not real to others.
Refer to the day, date, and time when providing care.	Reminders help to re-orient the client.

NURSING DIAGNOSIS: Impaired Verbal Communication secondary to delirium as evidenced by incoherent speech

OUTCOME: The client will demonstrate appropriate responses to questions

Planning/Implementation	Rationale
Talk distinctly and clearly, facing the client.	This approach minimizes the possibility of environmental distraction during interactions with the client.
Ask the client to clarify any responses that are vague.	Clarification can prevent a misunderstanding of responses.

(Continued on following page)

NURSING DIAGNOSIS: Risk for Injury related to disorientation and confusion

OUTCOME: The client will be free of injury.

Planning/Implementation	Rationale
Utilize the least restrictive devices if necessary to prevent injury.	Restrictive devices may be necessary until the client's cognitive impairment clears.
Provide adequate lighting.	Adequate lighting minimizes the client's misperception of the environment and risk for injury.

NURSING DIAGNOSIS: Self-Care Deficit related to fracture

OUTCOME: The client will demonstrate an increased ability to perform ADLs.

Planning/Implementation	Rationale
Evaluate client's ability to perform self-care.	Independence is important but safety is a priority.
Allow the client ample time to perform each task related to ADLs.	Rushing the client may frustrate him.
Assist the client daily as needed to maintain daily functions and complete ADLs.	The client will develop a sense of dignity and well-being as his cognitive abilities improve and he can resume his previous level of independence.

EVALUATION: Prior to discharge from the hospital, assess client's level of consciousness to determine if the delirium has resolved. Review client's understanding of post-operative orders and discharge plan of care. Explore client's understanding of adverse response to the specific pain medication administered in the hospital and the importance of including the information in any future physical examinations or medical consultations.

KEY CONCEPTS

◆ Delirium, dementia, and amnestic disorders are classified as cognitive disorders in which impairment of mental processes, speech, behavior, and level of consciousness occurs. The impairment may be reversible, partially reversible, or irreversible, depending on the cause of the impairment.

◆ Research has shown that as the brain ages, the potential for cognitive impairment exists.

◆ Neuropsychological investigative studies of brain-damaged clients have concluded that four distinct memory systems exist: working, episodic, semantic, and procedural.

◆ Several theories have been established regarding the development of dementia of the Alzheimer's type (DAT), including genetic, immune system, oxidation,

virus and bacteria, nutritional, metal deposit, neurotransmitter, membrane phospholipid metabolism, and beta-amyloid protein. Researchers continue to investigate potential causes of DAT and proposed treatments.

◆ Clinical symptoms of more than one cognitive disorder may occur at the same time, which can be challenging to the assessment process.

◆ Delirium, considered to be one of the most life-threatening acute psychiatric illnesses, is a syndrome that presents as a reversible global dysfunction in cerebral metabolism. Three major causes of delirium are central nervous system diseases, systemic illnesses, and either drug intoxication or withdrawal from pharmacologic or toxic agents. Prognosis is good if the cause is corrected in time.

◆ Dementia is a syndrome of global or diffuse brain dysfunction that is characterized by a gradual, progressive, chronic deterioration of intellectual function. Twelve subtypes of dementia have been identified. DAT and vascular dementia are the most frequently diagnosed types, constituting approximately 75% of all dementias.

◆ DAT, vascular dementia, and dementia with Lewy bodies (DLB) constitute the majority of all dementias.

◆ Diseases commonly associated with dementia include familial multiple system taupathy, Pick's disease, and Parkinson's disease.

◆ Amnestic disorders are the acquired impaired inability to recall information or past events usually due to damage to the diencephalic and medial temporal lobe structures of the brain. The terms *anterograde* and *retrograde* amnesia are used to discuss the type of amnesia one experiences.

◆ Input by a client's family member or another reliable observer is important when assessing a client with a cognitive impairment. A comprehensive history and physical examination is necessary to determine the type of cognitive disorder present and whether a mood disorder exists.

◆ The basic commonalities that link delirium, dementia, and amnestic disorders include self-care deficits; alteration in appearance, mood, and affect; cognitive impairment, including alteration in thought processes and the inability to communicate needs; and behavioral manifestations. Impaired socialization often occurs because of a decline in the client's cognitive abilities and the presence of behavioral manifestations.

◆ Several assessment tools are available to assess a client's mental status or cognitive abilities, instrumental functionality (eg, ability to perform ADLs), neurologic or motor functioning, and behavioral symptoms.

◆ Although there are no specific medications to cure cognitive disorders such as DAT and related disorders, pharmacologic interventions can be considered in addition to social, environmental, and behavioral management approaches.

◆ Continuum of care is based on the client's needs and his or her ability to experience quality of life. The setting is determined by the client's physical and psychosocial changes and the availability of caregivers.

◆ Several research studies regarding the etiology and treatment of cognitive disorders are currently being conducted by the National Institutes of Health, the National Institute of Mental Health, and independent groups.

◆ Evaluation of clients with a cognitive disorder is an ongoing process because of fluctuating physical and psychosocial functioning.

For additional study materials, please refer to the Student Resource CD-ROM located in the back of this textbook.

 ## CHAPTER WORKSHEET

CRITICAL THINKING QUESTIONS

1. Attend a local support group for families of people with Alzheimer's disease. What did you observe? What techniques did the group leader employ? What role can nursing play to help these families?

2. Your 35-year-old client, who underwent surgery today, appears disoriented and confused during a dressing change. He was alert and oriented prior to surgery. He can't remember his name or where he is. What data do you need to collect? What nursing diagnoses would you consider? What nursing interventions would you provide to minimize the occurrence of such symptoms in clients who undergo surgery in the future?

3. Observe a client with early-stage Alzheimer's disease and a client with late-stage Alzheimer's disease. What similarities and differences do you observe? How does nursing care differ for these two clients?

REFLECTION

Reflect on the chapter opening quote by Wakefield. Articulate the rationale for increased length of hospital stay, the need for chemical and physical restraints, readmission, and increased mortality in older clients who exhibit clinical symptoms of delirium or acute confusion. What nursing interventions could you provide to older clients who exhibit clinical symptoms of delirium or acute confusion after relocation to a rehabilitation unit?

NCLEX-STYLE QUESTIONS

1. Assessment of an 84-year-old client admitted to the medical–surgical unit for treatment of renal insufficiency reveals disorientation to time and place after dark. The nurse interprets this finding as which of the following?
   a. Amnesia
   b. Degeneration
   c. Perseveration
   d. Sundown syndrome

2. The family of a client with Alzheimer's disease questions the nurse about what to expect as the disease progresses. The nurse bases the answer on which fact associated with this disorder?
   a. Improvement depends on what medications are used for treatment.
   b. Improvement can occur when underlying medical problems are treated.
   c. The disorder occurs in a chronic, progressive manner over time.
   d. The disorder typically involves periods of remission and exacerbation.

3. Which nursing intervention would be most appropriate for the client with dementia who is upset and agitated?
   a. Decreasing environmental stimuli while remaining with client
   b. Firmly telling the client that the behavior is not acceptable
   c. Offering to provide medication that will have a calming effect
   d. Questioning the client about the cause of the problem

4. Which assessment question would be most useful when questioning the family to differentiate delirium from dementia in a client admitted to the hospital after experiencing increased confusion at home?
   a. How long have you noticed the confusion in your family member?
   b. Has there been a history of dementia in your family?
   c. Do you think something happened that was upsetting to your family member?
   d. Does your family member live alone or with someone?

5. Which outcome would the nurse determine as most realistic for a client in the late stages of Alzheimer's disease?
   a. The client will verbalize increased feelings of self-worth.
   b. The client will identify life areas that require alterations due to illness.
   c. The client will maintain reality orientation.
   d. The client will remain safe in the least restrictive environment.

6. A client with DAT is to receive pharmacologic therapy with a cholinesterase inhibitor. Which of the following agents might be prescribed? Select all that apply.
   a. Donepezil (Aricept)
   b. Rivastigmine (Exelon)
   c. Tacrine (Cognex)
   d. Memantine (Namenda)
   e. Galantamine (Razadyne)

Selected References

Allen, L. A. (1999). Treating agitation without drugs. *American Journal of Nursing, 99*(4), 36–40.

Alzheimer's Society. (2006). Facts about dementia. What is dementia with Lewy bodies (DLB)? Retrieved February 23, 2006, from http://www.alzheimers.org

American Psychiatric Association. (2000). *Diagnostic and statistical manual of mental disorders* (4th ed., text revision). Washington, DC: Author.

Andrews, J. C., & Andrews, N. C. (2003). Counseling Alzheimer's patients and their families. *Clinician Reviews, 3*(4), 56–62.

Blazer, D. G. (1996). The psychiatric interview of the geriatric patient. In E. W. Busse and D. G. Blazer (Eds.), *Textbook of geriatric psychiatry* (2nd ed., pp. 175–189). Washington, DC: American Psychiatric Press.

Branski, S. H. (1998). Delirium in hospitalized geriatric patients. *American Journal of Nursing, 98*(4), 16d–16l.

Busse, E. W., & Blazer, D. G. (1996). *Textbook of geriatric psychiatry* (2nd ed.). Washington, DC: American Psychiatric Press.

Clark, M. E., Lipe, A. W., & Bilbrey, M. (1998). Use of music to decrease aggressive behaviors in people with dementia. *Journal of Gerontological Nursing, 24*(7), 10–17.

Cohen, D. (1995). Preface. In R. E. Cairl (Ed.), *Somebody tell me who I am*. St. Petersburg, FL: Caremor Publications.

Cummings, J. (1995). Alzheimer's disease: A look at disease characteristics and etiology. *Current Approaches to Dementia, 1*(11), 5–6.

Cummings, J. (2001). New practice parameters for dementia. *Psychiatric Times, 18*(10), 45.

Detwiler, C. (2003). The client with a cognitive disorder. In W. K. Mohr (Ed.), *Johnson's psychiatric-mental health nursing*

(5th ed., pp. 607-640). Philadelphia: Lippincott Williams & Wilkins.

Douris, K. R. (2003). Home-based primary care for dementia. *ADVANCE for Nurse Practitioners, 11*(1), 50-52.

E-MentalHealth.com. (2005). History of Alzheimer's disease. Retrieved July 2, 2005, from http://www.emental-health.com/alzh_history.htm

Foreman, M. D., & Zane, D. (1996). Nursing strategies for acute confusion in elders. *American Journal of Nursing, 96*(4), 44-52.

Heindel, W. C., & Salloway, S. (1999). Memory systems in the human brain. *Psychiatric Times, 16*(6), 19-21.

Henry, M. (2002). Descending into delirium. *American Journal of Nursing, 102*(3), 49-56.

Holman, L., & Devous, M. D. (1992). Functional brain SPECT: The emergence of a powerful clinic method. *Journal of Nuclear Medicine, 33*(10), 1888-1904.

Husseini, M. B. (1996). The client who has dementia. In S. Lego (Ed.), *Psychiatric nursing: A comprehensive reference* (2nd ed., pp. 285-290). Philadelphia: Lippincott-Raven.

Johnson, C. (2002). Ensuring home safety for your Alzheimer's patients. *ADVANCE for Nurse Practitioners, 10*(7), 65.

Knowlton, L. (2000a). Delivering hospice care to Alzheimer's patients. *Psychiatric Times, 17*(7), 1, 5-6.

Knowlton, L. (2000b). Hospice and Alzheimer's disease. *Geriatric Times, 1*(4), 29-30.

Medina, J. (2001). Yet another gene for Alzheimer's disease. *Geriatric Times, 2*(5), 15, 18.

Moon, M. A. (2004). Dementia patients get feeding tubes instead of palliation. *Clinical Psychiatry News, 32*(4), 65.

Moyer, D. M. (1995). Dementia care: The nurse practitioner's role. *ADVANCE for Nurse Practitioners, 3.*

Needham, J. (2006). Alzheimer's disease. *CME Resource: Continuing Education for Florida Nurses, 2006* (pp. 69-122). Irvine, CA: Continuing Medical Education, Inc.

Newsline. (2004). Don't mistake Alzheimer's for this dementia. *Clinical Advisor, 7*(3), 12.

O'Connor, M. K. (2005). Delirium: Apply the "4 Ps" for comprehensive treatment. *Current Psychiatry, 4*(1), 53-54, 60-62, 68-70.

Peskind, E. R., & Raskind, M. A. (1996). Cognitive disorders. In E. W. Busse & D. G. Blazer (Eds.), *Textbook of geriatric psychiatry* (2nd ed., pp. 213-234). Washington, DC: American Psychiatric Press.

Peskind, E. R., Tangalos, E. G., & Grossberg, G. T. (2005). A case-based approach to Alzheimer's disease. *Clinical Advisor, 8*(6), 32, 35-36, 39-40, 42, 46.

Radovich, C. (1999, November 11-14). *The three D's: Dementia, depression and delirium.* Paper presented at the 12th Annual United States Psychiatric & Mental Health Congress, Atlanta, GA.

Rawlings, J. N., & Verma, S. (2001). Guidelines for management of behavioral disturbances. *Geriatric Times, 2*(4), 28-31.

Reisberg, B. (1986). Dementia: A systematic approach to identifying reversible causes. *Geriatrics, 41*(4), 30-46.

Sadock, B. J., & Sadock, V. A. (2003). *Kaplan & Sadock's synopsis of psychiatry: Behavioral sciences/clinical psychiatry* (9th ed.). Philadelphia: Lippincott Williams & Wilkins.

Salloway, S. (1999, November 11-14). *The aging brain.* Paper presented at the 12th Annual United States Psychiatric & Mental Health Congress, Atlanta, GA.

Shahrokh, N., & Hales, R. E. (Eds.) (2003). *American psychiatric glossary* (8th ed.). Washington, DC: American Psychiatric Press.

Smith, M., & Buckwalter, K. (2005). Behaviors associated with dementia. *American Journal of Nursing, 105*(7), 40-53.

Smith, M. N. (2005). Tips for controlling agitation and combativeness in dementia. *Neuropsychiatry Reviews, 4*(4), 14.

Somboontanont, W., Sloane, P. D., Floyd, F. J., Holditch-David, D., Hogue, C. C., & Mitchell, C. M. (2004). Assaultive behavior in Alzheimer's disease: Identifying immediate antecedents during bathing. *Journal of Gerontological Nursing, 30*(9), 22-29.

Strickland, T. L., Longobardi, P., & Gray, G. E. (1999). Dementia in minority elderly. *Clinical Geriatrics, 7*(11), 83-92.

Sylvester, B. (2004). Key clues differentiate Alzheimer's from Lewy body dementia. *Clinical Psychiatry News, 32*(3), 54.

U. S. Preventive Services Task Force. (2003). Screening for dementia: Recommendations and rationale. *American Journal of Nursing, 103*(9), 87, 89, 91, 93, 95.

Wachter, K. (2006). Genetic screening for AD appears beneficial. *Clinical Psychiatry News, 34*(2), 28.

Wakefield, B. J. (2002). Acute confusion in the elderly. *Clinical Nursing Research, 11*(2), 153-172.

Wheldon, M. (2005). Untangling the confusion: Alzheimer's management today. *ADVANCE for Nurse Practitioners, 13*(5), 47-48, 50, 52.

Williams, L. (1986). Alzheimer's: The need for caring. *Journal of Gerontological Nursing, (2).*

Zoler, M. L. (2004). Galantamine shows safety and efficacy as tx for dementia with Lewy bodies. *Clinical Psychiatry News, 32*(10), 49.

Suggested Readings

Annerstedt, L., Elmstahl, S., Ingvad, B., & Samuelson, S. M. (2000). Family caregiving in dementia—An analysis of the caregiver's burden and the breaking point when home care becomes inadequate. *Scandinavian Journal of Public Health, 28*(1), 23-31.

Brandt, D., & Jacobson, J. (2005). Dementia: How well do drugs treat neuropsychiatric symptoms? *American Journal of Nursing, 105*(5), 20.

Byrd, L. (2003). Terminal dementia in the elderly. *ADVANCE for Nurse Practitioners, 11*(9), 65-68, 72.

Carpenito-Moyet, L. J. (2006). *Handbook of nursing diagnosis* (11th ed.). Philadelphia: Lippincott Williams & Wilkins.

Cheng, G. S. (2000). Following the trail left by Alzheimer's biologic markers. *Clinical Psychiatry News, 28*(1), 1-2.

Cummings, J. L. (2000). Advances in Alzheimer's disease research: Implications for new treatments. *Psychiatric Times, 17*(1), 61-62.

Doskoch, P. (2000). Treating behavioral disturbances in Alzheimer's disease: What works. *NeuroPsychiatry, 1*(5), 18–20.

Evans, J. (2005). Study is shedding light on predementia criteria. *Clinical Psychiatry News, 33*(11), 48.

Fick, D., & Foreman, M. (2000). Consequences of not recognizing delirium superimposed on dementia in hospitalized elderly individuals. *Journal of Gerontological Nursing, 26*(1), 30–40.

Fitzsimmons, S. (2004). Recreation therapy for dementia-related behaviors. *ADVANCE for Nurse Practitioners, 12*(9), 38–42, 86.

Grossberg, G. T. (2000). The current era of anti-dementia compounds. *Clinical Geriatrics, 8*(11), 28–31.

Hashmi, F. H., Drady, A. I., Qayum, F., & Grossberg, G. T. (2000). Sexually disinhibited behavior in the cognitively impaired elderly. *Clinical Geriatrics, 8*(11), 61–68.

Henry, M. (2002). Descending into delirium. *American Journal of Nursing, 102*(3), 49–56.

Higgins, E. S. (2006). Can a vaccine prevent Alzheimer's disease? *Clinical Psychiatry, 5*(2), 28, 30.

Kamat, S. M., Grossberg, G. T., & LeFevre, P. M. (2005). Which cholinesterase inhibitor for early dementia? *Current Psychiatry, 4*(11), 55–58, 61–62, 67–68.

Karch, A. M. (2005). A cognitive conundrum: What is causing changes in cognition for this older adult? *American Journal of Nursing, 105*(10), 33, 35.

Kelly, P. A., & Carney, E. A. (2005). Managing dementia: Risks of using vs. not using atypical antipsychotics. *Current Psychiatry, 4*(8), 14–16, 22–24, 27–28.

Luggin, A. S. (2003). You must remember this: An overview of memory loss. *ADVANCE for Nurse Practitioners, 11*(12), 53–60.

Rasin, J., & Barrick, A. L. (2004). Bathing patients with dementia: Concentrating on the patient's needs rather than merely the task. *American Journal of Nursing, 104*(3), 30–32, 34.

Simard, M., van Reekum, R., & Suvajac, B. (2000). Improving cognition, behavior, and function, and slowing disease progression of Alzheimer's disease. *Clinical Geriatrics, 8*(11), 32–58.

Sullivan, M. T. (2004). Caregiver strain index. *Dermatological Nursing, 16*(4), 385–386.

Terry, B. R. (2004). Is wandering reversible? *ADVANCE for Nurse Practitioners, 5*(25), 20–21.

Tuschner, J. (2004). Doctor, patient, family: The synchronized Alzheimer's/dementia team. *Central Florida M.D. News, 6*(5), 22.

Wilner, A. (2002a). Alzheimer's-related delusions may be predictable. *CNS News, 4*(1), 31.

Wilner, A. (2002b). Alzheimer's severity dictates behavior patterns. *CNS News, 4*(1), 27.

Wright, S. W. (2000). Delirium in the elderly: Recognition and management issues. *ADVANCE for Nurse Practitioners, 8*(4), 71–74.

Zoler, M. L. (2004). Alzhemed may stabilize cognitive function. *Clinical Psychiatry News, 32*(9), 55.

CHAPTER 28 / DELUSIONAL AND SHARED PSYCHOTIC DISORDERS

Delusional disorder is relatively uncommon in clinical settings, with most studies suggesting that the disorder accounts for 1% to 2% of admissions to inpatient mental health facilities. The annual incidence is one to three new cases per 100,000 persons. —AMERICAN PSYCHIATRIC ASSOCIATION, 2000

LEARNING OBJECTIVES

AFTER STUDYING THIS CHAPTER, YOU SHOULD BE ABLE TO:

1. Discuss five risk factors related to the development of delusional disorders.
2. Identify the clinical symptoms of delusional disorders.
3. Articulate the predominant theme of each of the following subtypes of delusional disorders: persecutory, conjugal (jealous), erotomanic, grandiose, and somatic.
4. Differentiate between delusional disorder and shared psychotic disorder.
5. Explain the importance of identifying the specific cultural and religious background of a client diagnosed with a delusional disorder.
6. Articulate the rationale for the use of atypical antipsychotics and anticonvulsants in the treatment of delusional and shared psychotic disorders.
7. Explain why individual psychotherapy is considered to be more effective than other interactive therapies in the treatment of delusional and shared psychotic disorders.
8. State nursing interventions for the following nursing diagnosis related to delusional disorder: Disturbed Thought Processes related to delusions of persecution as evidenced by statement that drinking water is poisoned.

KEY TERMS

Conjugal paranoia
Content-specific delusions (CSDs)
Delusion
Erotomanic delusions
Folie à deux
Grandiose delusions
Ideas of reference
Nonbizarre delusions
Paradoxical conduct
Paranoid
Persecutory delusions
Somatic delusions

Delusion is a term used to describe a false belief based on an incorrect inference about external reality that is firmly sustained despite clear evidence to the contrary. Conversely, the term **paranoid** is used to describe a wide range of behaviors, ranging from aloof, suspicious, and nonpsychotic behaviors (Chapter 24, paranoid personality disorder) to well-systematized and psychotic symptoms (Chapter 22, paranoid type of schizophrenia) (Shahrokh & Hales, 2003).

The *Diagnostic and Statistical Manual of Mental Disorders, 4th Edition, Text Revision (DSM-IV-TR)* lists several disorders in which the clinical symptom of delusional thoughts may occur. They include dementia, alcohol-induced psychotic disorder, substance-induced psychotic disorder, schizophrenia, psychotic disorder due to a medical condition, mood disorder, paranoid personality disorder, delusional disorder, and shared psychotic disorder. This chapter focuses on delusional disorder and shared psychotic disorder; the remaining disorders are addressed elsewhere in the text.

History of Delusional and Shared Psychotic Disorders

History of the first identification of delusional disorder is hampered by its relative rareness, the variety of theories regarding its etiology, and changing definitions in recent history. Freud believed that delusions were part of a healing process. In 1896, he described projection as the main defense mechanism in paranoia (now referred to as delusional disorder). He also theorized that individuals with paranoia (delusional disorder) utilized the defense mechanisms of denial and projection to defend against unconscious homosexual tendencies. Although careful studies of clients with delusions have been unable to corroborate Freud's theories regarding the dynamics of homosexual tendencies, his major contribution was to demonstrate the role of projection in the formation of delusional disorders (Sadock & Sadock, 2003).

Shared psychotic disorder, also referred to as *shared paranoid disorder, induced psychotic disorder,* and *double insanity,* was first described in 1651 in a case of phantom pregnancy associated with two sisters. In 1877, the term **folie à deux** (which refers to two individuals who have a close relationship and shared delusions) was used in a classic report by Lasegue and Falret. Almost a century later (1942), a classification

of four subtypes of folie à deux was published by Gralnick: *folie imposèe* (delusions of a person with psychosis are transferred to a person who is mentally sound); *folie simultanèe* (simultaneous appearance of an identical psychosis occurs in two individuals who are intimately associated and morbidly predisposed); *folie communiquèe* (the recipient develops psychosis after a long period of resistance and maintains the symptoms even after separation); and *folie induite* (new delusions are adopted by an individual with psychosis who is under the influence of another individual with psychosis). A literature review by Sharon, Sharon, Eliyahu, and Shteynman (2006) revealed the existence of several complex cases of shared psychotic disorders (husband/wife, mother/daughter, twins). Their article sheds light on the seriousness of the disorder, complications associated with the disorder, and the need for treatment.

Etiology of Delusional Disorders

Although the cause of delusional disorders is unknown, several predisposing factors have been identified. These include risk factors such as:

- Relocation due to immigration or emigration
- Social isolation
- Sensory impairments such as deafness or blindness
- Severe stress
- Low socioeconomic status in which the person may experience feelings of discrimination or powerlessness
- Personality features such as low self-esteem or unusual interpersonal sensitivity
- Trust–fear conflicts

Research has demonstrated that delusions can also result from an identifiable neurologic disease, primarily those diseases that affect the limbic system and the basal ganglia. Clients with a neurologic condition may have intact cerebral cortical functioning, but exhibit complex delusions that are referred to as **content-specific delusions (CSDs)** to distinguish them from the delusions exhibited in psychiatric disorders such as paranoid schizophrenia. Content-specific delusions are also associated with focal lesions of the frontal lobe or right hemisphere of the brain (Sadock & Sadock, 2003).

Information about the familial pattern of delusional disorders is conflicting. Some studies have found that delusional disorders are more common among relatives of individuals with schizophrenia than would be expected by chance. Other studies have found no familial relationship between delusional disorders and schizophrenia (American Psychiatric Association [APA], 2000).

Clinical Symptoms and Diagnostic Characteristics

Although often difficult to differentiate from paranoid schizophrenia, the delusions in delusional disorder are characteristically systematized (an ordered grouping of sustained false beliefs) and nonbizarre. **Nonbizarre delusions** involve situations that could occur in real life, usually involving phenomena that, although not real, are possible (Sadock & Sadock, 2003).

Although nonbizarre delusions can occur at a younger age, the typical age of onset is usually middle or late adult life. Clients with nonbizarre delusions usually verbalize extreme suspiciousness, jealousy, and distrust, and are generally convinced that others intend to do them harm. They may complain about various injustices, and frequently instigate legal actions as they verbalize resentment, anger, and grandiose ideas. Social and marital functioning are often impaired, although the client preserves daily, intellectual, and occupational functioning.

Other clinical symptoms may include social isolation, seclusiveness, or eccentric behavior. Anxiety or depression may occur as the client attempts to cope with delusional thoughts. Clients rarely seek treatment. Usually clients are brought to the attention of mental health professionals by friends, relatives, or associates who are concerned about their behavior.

Clients with delusional disorders also may experience CSDs, occurring at any time. CSDs are not categorized in the *DSM-IV-TR*. Clients with CSDs are usually described as forthcoming and cooperative. They insist that their delusions are true, but also admit to puzzlement or bemusement regarding aspects of the delusion. They are more likely to confabulate explanations for their delusions rather than become defensive and hostile (Malloy & Salloway, 1999). Types of CSDs include delusions of place, delusions of person, sexual delusions, and somatic delusions.

According to *DSM-IV-TR* criteria, delusional disorder is differentiated from schizophrenia in that clients with delusional disorder do not have prominent or sustained hallucinations associated with schizophrenia. However, clients may verbalize the presence of tactile, olfactory, or auditory hallucinations consistent with their delusions. Delusions, as noted earlier, are not bizarre, but rather could conceivably occur in real life (eg, client believes he or she is being poisoned or that someone has tampered with the brakes in his or her car). The delusions are not due to any other mental disorder such as schizophrenia, and are not the direct physiologic effects of a substance or the direct result of a general medical condition.

Clients with delusional disorder have no insight into their condition. They refuse to acknowledge negative feelings, thoughts, motives, or behaviors in themselves and project such feelings onto others by blaming others for their problems. They also spend much time confirming suspicions and defending themselves against imagined persecution. Such self-centered thoughts, in which everything is taken personally, are called **ideas of reference.**

The *DSM-IV-TR* identifies five subtypes of delusional disorder: persecutory, conjugal or jealous, erotomanic, grandiose, and somatic. In all subtypes, mood changes, including irritability, anger, depression, and violence, may occur. Legal difficulties also may arise. Clients may be subjected to unnecessary medical tests and procedures. Social, marital, or work problems are common. However, cognitive disorganization or emotional deterioration usually does not occur. The type of delusional disorder with which a client is diagnosed is based on the predominant delusional theme, because cases with more than one theme are frequent. See Clinical Example 28-1.

Persecutory Subtype

Clients who exhibit **persecutory delusions** believe they are being conspired against, spied on, poisoned or drugged, cheated, harassed, maliciously maligned, or obstructed in some way. No other psychopathology is present. Deterioration in personality or in most areas of functioning is absent (Sadock & Sadock, 2003). Compton (2003) discusses the increasing prevalence of controlling, broadcasting, and persecutory delusions in clients with delusional disorders as a result of the use of computers, the Internet, and Internet technology. Individuals with no real familiarity with the Internet may just as readily incorporate computer-associated themes in delusional thought patterns as those individuals who utilize such technology on a regular basis.

THE CLIENT WITH DELUSIONAL DISORDER, PERSECUTORY TYPE

MS, a 45-year-old Cuban man who recently moved to Florida with his family, suddenly becomes suspicious that Fidel Castro is "out to get him." He barricades the windows and doors of his home, has his telephone number unlisted, and warns his family to be careful whenever they leave the house. Although he displays this delusion of persecution and exhibits hypervigilance, he is able to function with minimal impairment. When questioned, his wife states that he has felt guilty about leaving his parents behind in Cuba.

Working with such a client could be extremely difficult because his delusional system may have an element of truth in it. People who have emigrated to the United States from Cuba and other countries have related stories of persecution for crimes they did not commit, whereas others have fled to avoid persecution for crimes committed. Living in such an environment could predispose someone to the development of a highly suspicious thought process.

Conjugal (Jealous) Subtype

The client who is convinced that his or her mate or significant other is unfaithful exhibits clinical symptoms of **conjugal paranoia** or *delusional jealousy*. This delusion may occur suddenly and usually affects men with no prior psychiatric illness. The delusion may diminish only upon separation, divorce, or death of the spouse or significant other.

Erotomanic Subtype

An individual, usually an unmarried woman, exhibiting clinical symptoms of **erotomanic delusions** believes a person of elevated social status loves her. The delusion, which can occur suddenly, is usually of romantic or spiritual love rather than sexual love. The delusional phenomenon **paradoxical conduct** occurs as the client interprets all denials of love, no matter how clear, as secret affirmations. Individuals such as movie stars or prominent television personalities have been victimized by such persons, who write letters, stalk the individuals, send gifts, or attempt to visit them.

Grandiose Subtype

Grandiose delusions, also referred to as *megalomania,* are present when the client believes he or she possesses unrecognized talent or insight, or has made an important discovery. Less commonly, the client may have the delusion of being a prominent person or of being involved in a special relationship with a prominent person (eg, secretary to the Queen of England). Grandiose delusions may involve religious content, such as the client believing he is a messenger of God (APA, 2000).

Somatic Subtype

The client with delusional disorder, somatic subtype demonstrates a preoccupation with the body by verbalizing unusual **somatic delusions.** For example, clients may complain of disfigured or nonfunctioning body parts, or believe that they are infested with insects or bugs (*delusional parasitosis*), or have a serious illness. These delusions are fixed, unarguable, and presented intensely, because the client is convinced that the condition exists. A substantial suicide risk exists because some clients believe death is imminent (Sadock & Sadock, 2003).

Etiology of Shared Psychotic Disorder

As noted earlier in this chapter, shared psychotic disorder, or folie à deux, involves two individuals who have a close relationship and share the same delusion. This occurrence is attributed to the strong influence of the more dominant (primary case or inducer) person over the submissive (secondary case) individual. Traditional views believed this disorder was seen more frequently in women who were isolated by language, culture, or geography; however, literature analysis revealed that females and males are affected equally. Such persons are often related by blood or marriage and have lived together for an extended period of time. The incidence in married or common-law couples is equal to that in siblings. Contributing factors include low intelligence, sensory impairment, cerebrovascular disease, and alcohol abuse. Age used to be considered a contributing factor (ie, submissive individual was younger than the dominant person); however, recent views have shown that the submissive individual has an equal chance of being either younger or older than the dominant individual. This disorder has been diagnosed in twins and in individuals, both of whom had a chronic psychotic disorder. This disorder also has occurred in a group of individuals or in families in which the parent is the primary case (inducer) (Sadock & Sadock, 2003; Sharon et al., 2006).

Clinical Symptoms and Diagnostic Characteristics

In shared psychotic disorder, delusions may be bizarre or nonbizarre. The dominant individual (primary case or inducer) usually has a chronic psychotic disorder with prominent delusions that the submissive individual (secondary case) begins to believe. The submissive individual is usually healthy, but frequently less intelligent, more gullible, more passive, or more lacking in self-esteem than the dominant individual (Sadock & Sadock, 2003). See Clinical Example 28-2.

According to the *DSM-IV-TR*, an individual adopts a delusion from another individual (who already has an

---

CLINICAL EXAMPLE 28.2

THE CLIENTS WITH SHARED PSYCHOTIC DISORDER

Mr. and Mrs. G were brought to the local psychiatric receiving facility by the country sheriff. Neighbors had reported both individuals were observed boarding up their windows, chasing people off the sidewalk in front of their house, and accusing people of spying on them. Garbage was piled in the driveway, attracting rodents and stray cats. Mail was left uncollected in their mailbox.

During the interview, it was noted that the wife agreed with the bizarre story that the husband related. He described delusions of persecution in which he believed aliens were spying on them. They had moved several times because they feared for their safety. When interviewed separately, they gave identical stories. It was determined that the husband was the inducer.

SELF-AWARENESS PROMPT

Reflect on your comfort level in the presence of clients who verbalize suspiciousness, ideas of reference, jealousy, somatic complaints, or erotomanic thoughts. Which of these behaviors are uncomfortable for you? What feelings or thoughts do you experience? What can you do to increase your comfort level and provide therapeutic care to clients diagnosed with delusional disorders?

established delusion) with whom he or she has a close relationship. The delusional content of both persons is shared. In addition, neither person has been diagnosed with a psychotic or mood disorder with psychosis to account for the delusion. Moreover, the effects of substance use or of a medical condition are not the underlying reason for the development of the delusion.

THE NURSING PROCESS

ASSESSMENT

Assessment of clients with delusional disorders or shared psychotic disorder is challenging because the clients typically deny any pathology. This challenge is further compounded by the presence of suspiciousness or ideas of reference, their inability to trust others, and their resistance to therapy.

History and Physical Examination

Observe the client for specific behaviors. For example, clients with persecutory delusions may exhibit erratic, impulsive, or socially inappropriate behavior; illogical thinking; poor judgment; agitation; or extreme, intense feelings such as suicidal ideation; or they may exhibit violence against those persons they believe to be threatening or harmful to them. Further, the client is generally threatened by any close or personal contact, such as a physical examination, that may occur during the assessment process.

If the client refuses a physical examination, the nurse may elect to reschedule the examination when a trusted family member or significant other is present to provide support to the client. Conversely, if a medical emergency exists, and the client refuses to be examined, it may be necessary to medicate the client to stabilize the clinical symptoms before performing the examination.

Investigate if the client exhibits tactile, olfactory, or auditory hallucinations. Are there any sensory handicaps that could contribute to the presence of delusional thoughts? Such handicaps can interfere with the ability to test reality. For example, elderly persons with impaired vision or hearing may develop ideas of reference. It is not uncommon for alert and oriented elderly clients who have delegated power of attorney to others to verbalize that there is a conspiracy to take their money or personal property.

Also assess for the presence or absence of clinical symptoms of depression (eg, low self-esteem, suicidal ideation), anxiety, and behavioral disturbances, which may be indicative of the diagnosis of mood disorder with psychotic features rather than a delusional disorder. Social and marital functioning is more likely to be impaired in a client with a delusional disorder.

Transcultural Considerations

The client's cultural and religious background must be considered while collecting data from the client, support person, or family member. For example, individuals relocating from countries such as Cuba or Yugoslavia may exhibit what appear to be ideas of reference or delusions of persecution. Family members, though, may describe the client as "normal" most of the time and substantiate the validity of a client's concerns, thus negating the diagnosis of delusional disorder.

Be aware that the content of delusions varies in different cultures and subcultures, and reflects cultural patterns. Also, the distribution of the shared psychotic disorder relationships in Western countries differs from those indicated by Japanese data. In Japan, cases of shared psychotic disorder usually involve a mother–child or spousal relationship. Also in Japan, contrary to Western countries, the dominant individual is often younger than the submissive individual. The conclusion has been made that close association contributes more to the development of shared psychotic disorder than age (Sharon et al., 2006).

Delusions may be primarily psychological, religious or spiritual, moral or social, naturalistic or supernatural, or physical or medical (Andrews & Boyle, 2003). Also, some cultures have widely held and culturally sanctioned beliefs that might be considered delusional in other cultures.

NURSING DIAGNOSES

After data have been collected, the nursing diagnoses are stated. Examples of nursing diagnoses related to clients exhibiting clinical symptoms of delusional and shared psychotic disorders are listed in the accompanying box.

OUTCOME IDENTIFICATION

The statement of outcomes depends on the severity of the disorder and the ability of the client to function

---

EXAMPLES OF NANDA NURSING DIAGNOSES/ DELUSIONAL AND SHARED PSYCHOTIC DISORDERS

- Disturbed Thought Processes related to erotomanic delusions (idealized romantic love with employer) as evidenced by efforts to contact object of delusion through phone calls, letters, and visits
- Disturbed Sensory Perception (olfactory) related to somatic delusion as evidenced by statement that one's skin is emitting a foul odor
- Social Isolation related to persecutory delusions (fear of being kidnapped) as evidenced by withdrawal and uncommunicativeness
- Risk for Other-Directed Violence related to delusional thoughts and hallucinatory commands as evidenced by overt aggressive acts toward employees
- Defensive Coping related to delusional jealousy as evidenced by accusatory statements about spouse's fidelity
- Fear related to persecutory delusions as evidenced by thinking not based in reality
- Impaired Social Interaction related to grandiose delusions as evidenced by inappropriate responses
- Noncompliance with medication regimen related to delusions of persecution as evidenced by failure to adhere to medication schedule

---

EXAMPLES OF STATED OUTCOMES/ DELUSIONAL AND SHARED PSYCHOTIC DISORDERS

- The client will experience control of behavior with assistance from others.
- The client will exhibit a decreased number of violent responses.
- The client will describe the causes of violent responses.
- The client will identify situations that evoke anxiety.
- The client will describe problems to relating to others.
- The client will identify alternatives to present coping patterns.
- The client will describe possible preventive measures of violent behavior.
- The client will express delusional thoughts less frequently.
- The client will differentiate between reality and fantasy.

---

outside the hospital setting. For example, persecutory delusional disorder, the most common subtype, may be a chronic disorder, or the client may exhibit full periods of remission followed by relapses. The jealous subtype, considered to be more common in men, may have a better prognosis than the persecutory type.

Stated outcomes focus on several factors, including the client's ability to:

- Identify situations that contribute to delusional thoughts
- Identify problems in relating with others
- Minimize delusional material
- Differentiate between fantasy and reality
- Utilize interventions to stabilize mood and behavior

See the accompanying box for examples of stated outcomes.

PLANNING INTERVENTIONS

In the past, delusional disorder was generally regarded as resistant to treatment; however, in recent years the outlook has become less pessimistic. The goals of treatment are to establish the diagnosis, to decide on appropriate interventions, and to manage complications (Sadock & Sadock, 2003).

Intervention may occur in a private-practice setting or in a mental health clinic, where symptoms can be alleviated to the degree that is essential for continued employment and community living. If feelings of persecution persist and the tendency toward impulsive, suicidal, or destructive behavior presents a problem to the client, family, or community, hospitalization may be required to determine the cause—such as a nonpsychiatric medical condition—for the delusional symptoms. Hospitalization may also be necessary to stabilize the client's social and occupational relationships.

Clients with the diagnosis of shared psychotic disorder are seen individually and placed on separate units if hospitalized to avoid contact with each other. In general, the healthier of the two clients will give up the delusional belief. The sicker of the two clients will maintain the fixed false belief (Sadock & Sadock, 2003).

Clients exhibiting paranoia may arouse feelings in the nurse of being attacked, assaulted, or belittled. The nurse also may feel frustrated because the client blames the nurse or others for his or her difficulties. Be aware that delusions protect clients from recognizing or coping with feelings that are often the opposite of those represented by the delusion; result from overwhelming anxiety; represent an exaggerated picture of what the person believes; and often result in the use of defenses such as projection or intellectualization. Plan effective interventions by keeping in mind five nonproductive reactions to delusional clients:

1. Becoming anxious and avoiding the client
2. Reinforcing delusions by actually believing the client
3. Attempting to prove that the client is mistaken by presenting a logical argument
4. Setting unrealistic goals that lead to disappointment, frustration, or anger
5. Being inconsistent with nursing interventions (Barile, 1984)

IMPLEMENTATION

Caring for clients with delusional disorders and shared psychotic disorder focuses on assisting the client in the activities of daily living; providing a safe environment to observe for suicidal ideation; stabilizing behavior such as hostility and aggression; establishing rapport; enhancing self-esteem; and decreasing fears,

BOX 28.1 NURSING INTERVENTIONS FOR DELUSIONAL AND SHARED PSYCHOTIC DISORDERS

- Assure the client that he or she is in a safe environment.
- Utilize listening and acceptance to establish a trusting relationship.
- Identify irrational thoughts and investigate whether there is a precipitating stressor that triggered the delusion.
- Encourage the client to discuss the logic or reasoning behind the delusion.
- If the client asks you if you believe the delusion, inform the client that you do not share the perception or delusional belief.
- Acknowledge the plausible elements of the delusion.
- Identify the purpose or needs the delusion serves.
- If possible, meet the needs the delusion fulfills (ie, dependence, low self-esteem).
- Identify ways to help the client control thoughts, such as distracting oneself from thinking the same thought repeatedly; using thought-switching techniques; identifying signs, such as staring, that indicate thoughts are becoming disorganized; and anticipating new situations that may increase anxiety or enhance delusional thoughts.

suspicions, ideas of reference, and delusions. Box 28-1 lists some examples of nursing interventions for delusional and shared psychotic disorders.

Assistance in Meeting Basic Needs

Clients with clinical symptoms of a delusional or shared psychotic disorder may neglect activities of daily living. The more severe the clinical symptoms are, the more difficult it may be to assist the client in meeting basic needs such as adequate food and fluid intake, adequate sleep, bathing, grooming, personal hygiene, and the selection of appropriate attire. For example, the client may avoid eating because of fear of food being poisoned or fear that a medical problem exists that interferes with eating. It may be necessary to discuss food preferences with family members or have food prepared by a specific family member. The client may agree

to eat canned food or choose to select specific food to be served at mealtime. Establishing rapport can be challenging when a client exhibits fears, suspicions, ideas of reference, and delusions. When a trusting relationship develops with health care providers, more routine procedures may be introduced.

A disturbance in the client's sleep pattern may occur as a result of fear of being harmed while sleeping. Allowing the client to choose a place and time he or she feels comfortable with may promote sleep. Sedatives may be needed initially.

Personal hygiene may be neglected due to a deterioration in functional ability or delusions of persecution. A daily schedule developed with input from the client may encourage compliance with bathing, grooming, and dressing.

Medication Management

If the client is extremely belligerent, agitated, suicidal, or exhibiting violent behavior, injectable or depot antipsychotics such as haloperidol (Haldol) are very effective in controlling feelings of distress. Medication management has been effective in the treatment of anxiety, depression, and somatic delusions. Most clinicians consider psychotropic drugs, including the atypical antipsychotics and newer-generation anticonvulsants, to be the treatment of choice for delusional and shared psychotic disorders. Examples of psychotropic drugs considered to be effective in the treatment of delusional disorders include ziprasidone (Geodon), tiagabine (Gabitril), pimozide (Orap), lithium (Lithobid), carbamazepine (Tegretol), oxcarbazepine (Trileptal), and valproate (Depakote). The new standard of treatment for shared psychotic disorders includes the use of three agents: aripiprazole (Abilify), olanzapine/fluoxetine (Symbyax), and quetiapine (Seroquel). The anticonvulsant, oxcarbazepine, is also very effective in the treatment of shared psychotic disorders as a main agent or as an adjunctive agent clinically (Sadock & Sadock, 2003; Sharon et al., 2006). Drug Summary Table 28-1 highlights selected antipsychotic agents used for delusional and shared psychotic disorders. Also see Chapter 16 for a more complete discussion of these medications.

Unfortunately, clients may incorporate the administration of drugs into their delusional system, possibly refusing to take medication if rapport has not been established between client and nurse or clinician. Allowing the client to open pre-packaged unit-dose

DRUG SUMMARY TABLE 28-1 ☐ Selected Antipsychotic Drugs Used for Delusional and Shared Psychotic Disorders

GENERIC (TRADE) NAME	DAILY DOSAGE RANGE	IMPLEMENTATION
aripiprazole (Abilify)	5–60 mg	Monitor for GI upset; drug–drug interactions may occur with anticholinergics; avoid alcohol; monitor for adverse effects.*
pimozide (Orap)	1–10 mg	Monitor ECG for prolonged Q-T intervals, severe cardiac complications, and major motor seizures.
quetiapine (Seroquel)	25–800 mg	Administer small quantity to any client with suicidal ideation; monitor for adverse effects.*
ziprasidone (Geodon)	20–160 mg	Monitor ECG for Q-T changes; monitor for adverse effects.*

NOTE: If the client does not respond adequately to the prescribed antipsychotic, adjunctive medication such as lithium (Eskalith) or an anticonvulsant (eg, oxcarbamazepine [Trileptal] or valproate [Depakene]) may be warranted. Refer to Chapter 16, Psychopharmacology, for additional information.

*Adverse effects: Agranulocytosis, changes in blood sugar and lipid serum levels, constipation, dehydration in the elderly, dry mouth, movement disorders (eg, extrapyramidal symptoms [EPS], tardive dyskinesia [TD], and neuroleptic malignant syndrome [NMS]), orthostatic hypotension, seizures, sexual dysfunction, and somnolence.

medications and identifying the times of administration for each medication helps to increase the client's participation in his or her care and may encourage compliance.

Interactive Therapies

After behavior and mood are stabilized and psychotherapeutic intervention begins, be honest and straightforward while focusing on the client's emotional response to the environment. Be sure to convey to the client interest in the client's welfare even without agreeing with any of the delusions.

Individual therapy, which is considered to be more effective than other forms of psychotherapy, generally focuses on improving self-esteem and social interactions and developing positive coping skills and problem-solving skills. Although cognitive-behavioral therapy may help some clients with delusional disorders, insight-oriented, problem-oriented, and group therapies can be ineffective because confronting delusions directly may increase agitation. Conjoint therapy (a form of marital therapy in which the therapist sees both clients together in sessions) has proven effective in some cases of shared psychotic disorders. Somatic therapy and alternative therapies generally are not used to treat delusional or shared psychotic disorders because the mark of successful treatment usually depends on a satisfactory social adjustment rather than a reduction or suppression of the client's delusions (Sadock & Sadock, 2003).

Client Education

Client education can be effective if the client has developed trust in the nursing staff and is able to focus on reality. Inform the client about the rationale for the use of any prescribed medication and instruct him or her to inform the health care provider of any adverse effects. As noted previously, some clients incorporate the use of medication into their delusional system and refuse to take medication. With the assistance of the client, develop a chart or schedule that lists the prescribed medication and times of administration. This approach will educate the client about the need to follow a schedule to maintain a therapeutic blood level of medication and stabilize clinical symptoms.

Have the client identify a contact person, such as a nurse or family member, who will be able to provide immediate feedback and validate perceptions before taking any actions that may precipitate problems.

Instruct the client to notify the contact person of any significant changes in mood or affect to avoid the recurrence of any comorbid anxiety or depression.

EVALUATION

The purpose of evaluation is to compare the client's current mental and behavioral status with the identified outcomes. This phase of the nursing process may be difficult to complete because it is common for clients to discontinue treatment abruptly. As stated earlier in the chapter, clients with delusional or shared

psychotic disorders do not normally seek help independently because of their inability to establish trust.

Because social and marital functioning are more likely to be impaired than are intellectual and occupational functioning, the mark of successful treatment is satisfactory social adjustment rather than the abatement of delusions. Long-term management of clients who are compliant generally consists of the administration of low-dosage antipsychotic or neuroleptic drugs and supportive individual psychotherapy. Nursing Plan of Care 28-1 provides an example of nursing care for the client with a diagnosis of delusional disorder, persecutory type.

NURSING PLAN OF CARE 28.1

THE CLIENT WITH DELUSIONAL DISORDER, PERSECUTORY TYPE

Robert, 65-year-old Polish immigrant, was brought to the mental health center by his wife, who verbalized concern about her husband's behavioral changes within the last 2 months. According to Robert's wife, he had become seclusive. He refused to accompany her to the grocery store and would not allow her to answer the telephone. He believed that the police were going to arrest him because he was Polish.

Robert and his wife relocated to the United States approximately 40 years ago. During that time, he was gainfully employed as a press operator in a steel mill. They had no children and seldom socialized with their neighbors. Robert recently retired and completed odd jobs for his former employer until his delusional thoughts began to interfere with his part-time work.

Robert presented as an alert, physically healthy individual who was oriented in all spheres. Eye contact was minimal and he was hypervigilant. His responses were guarded. He did not exhibit any violent behavior. His wife stated that he did not appear to exhibit any clinical symptoms of depression. He did not drink alcohol, and he quit smoking several years ago.

DSM-IV-TR DIAGNOSIS: Delusional disorder, persecutory type

ASSESSMENT: Personal strengths: Alert, oriented in all spheres; independently capable of caring for self; supportive wife; nonviolent behavior; physically healthy

Weaknesses: Delusional thoughts, persecutory type; limited socialization

---

NURSING DIAGNOSIS: Disturbed Thought Processes related to misperception of external stimuli resulting in delusions of persecution

OUTCOME: The client will verbalize feelings and report persecutory thoughts as they occur.

Planning/Implementation	Rationale
Encourage verbalization of feelings and thoughts.	The client will identify with the nurse as someone who will not censure his feelings or thoughts, even if they are unusual or bizarre.
Explore feelings of fear and suspicious thoughts.	The client has a nonthreatening outlet if he is able to discuss his fears and suspicions with the nurse.
Do not argue or attempt to correct distortions.	The client believes the persecutory thoughts to be true and cannot be convinced otherwise. Arguing or attempting to correct distortions will damage the therapeutic relationship.

NURSING DIAGNOSIS: Ineffective Individual Coping related to misperception of external stimuli and inadequate coping skills

OUTCOME: The client will develop positive coping skills to minimize disturbed thought processes related to misperception of the external stimuli.

Planning/Implementation	Rationale
Investigate whether there is a precipitating stressor.	If the client can identify the relationship between his delusions and life events that triggered the delusional thoughts, he may be able to make behavioral changes and develop more positive coping skills.
Explore alternative coping measures and problem-solving skills to minimize or avoid further problems at work or a t home.	If the client is willing to explore alternative coping measures and problem-solving skills, behavioral changes may occur without focusing on the validity of the delusions.

NURSING DIAGNOSIS: Impaired Social Interaction related to delusions of persecution

OUTCOME: The client will explore the impact of delusions on his socialization.

Planning/Implementation	Rationale
Involve wife in treatment to discuss the changes that have occurred in their socialization with others.	If the client can discuss his concerns with his wife and receive immediate feedback, he is more likely to understand the impact of his delusions on others.
Educate client's wife about the delusional process and therapeutic responses (ie, do not argue or attempt to disprove the delusion).	The client's wife can provide feedback to assist the client in changing behaviors to improve social interactions.

EVALUATION: Prior to termination of individual therapy, client will discuss his progress during treatment. Client and wife will verbalize an understanding of the plan of care. Follow-up visit is to be scheduled in 1 month. Wife will return with client to provide supportive data regarding client's progress.

KEY CONCEPTS

◆ Delusional disorders, generally characterized by extreme suspiciousness, jealousy, and distrust, are relatively uncommon in the psychiatric clinical setting.

◆ Delusional disorders focus on situations that could conceivably occur in real life, and they generally interfere with social and marital functioning. There are five subtypes of delusional disorder: persecutory, conjugal or jealous, erotomanic, grandiose, and somatic.

◆ Shared psychotic disorder occurs when two individuals who have a close relationship share the same delusion. The individual who has a psychotic disorder with prominent delusions is referred to as dominant (primary case or inducer). The individual who is usually passive and initially healthy, but begins to believe the inducer, is referred to as submissive (secondary case).

◆ Be aware that the content of delusions varies in different cultures and subcultures, and reflects cultural patterns. Also, some cultures have widely held and culturally sanctioned beliefs that might be considered delusional in other cultures.

◆ Implementing the nursing process is challenging because clients with delusional or shared psychotic disorders generally deny the presence of any pathology, are distrustful of others, and are resistant to therapy.

◆ Intervention generally occurs on an outpatient basis, unless the client exhibits violent behavior secondary to persecutory delusions or verbalizes suicidal ideation secondary to somatic delusions or major depression. Hospitalization may be necessary to determine whether a nonpsychiatric medical condition is causing the delusions; to stabilize behavior; and to provide interventions to improve social or occupational relationships.

◆ Clients with the diagnosis of shared psychotic disorder are separated and seen individually to avoid contact. The healthier of the two will generally give up the delusion, whereas the sicker of the two will maintain the false fixed belief.

◆ Nursing interventions focus on establishing rapport; enhancing self-esteem; decreasing fears and suspicion; decreasing hostility, aggression, ideas of reference, and delusions; observing for suicidal ideation; and assisting the client in the activities of daily living.

◆ Injectable antipsychotic medication may be required to control violent behavior before the implementation of nursing interventions. If the client(s) agree, atypical antipsychotics and/or newer generation anticonvulsants may be used to stabilize clinical symptoms of delusional disorders and shared psychotic disorders.

◆ Individual psychotherapy is the treatment of choice because clients with delusional thoughts do not respond well to insight-oriented, problem-oriented, or group therapy in which delusions are confronted by peers or therapists. Conjoint therapy has proven effective for couples with shared psychotic disorder.

◆ Long-term management may be required because clients may exhibit periods of remission followed by relapses or may have a chronic delusional disorder.

For additional study materials, please refer to the Student Resource CD-ROM located in the back of this textbook.

CHAPTER WORKSHEET

CRITICAL THINKING QUESTIONS

1. Newspapers and television programs frequently report on celebrities being stalked by fans. Select a recent or current story. Using what you have learned about delusional disorders, analyze the stalker's behavior. What conclusions can you draw from this situation?

2. As mentioned in the chapter, delusional disorders can occur in recent immigrants. Identify the immigrant population closest to where you live. Contact the community health department that services this population. What questions would you ask a community health nurse to determine whether any of the immigrants show symptoms of delusional disorders?

REFLECTION

According to the chapter opening quote, delusional disorder is considered to be relatively uncommon.

Given the numerous precipitating factors that are believed to cause delusional disorders, explain why you believe the frequency of occurrence is only 1% to 2% of admissions to inpatient mental health facilities. What questions could you ask a client during the assessment process to determine whether the client is at risk for the development of a delusional disorder? Explain the rationale for your questions.

NCLEX-STYLE QUESTIONS

1. The nurse interacting with a client with a delusional disorder understands that which defense mechanism underlies this disorder?
   a. Projection
   b. Regression
   c. Suppression
   d. Sublimation

2. Which intervention would be the priority for a client exhibiting delusions of persecution?
   a. Establishing trust
   b. Encouraging activities
   c. Presenting reality
   d. Reducing anxiety

3. A 51-year-old female client tells you she believes a popular male vocalist is in love with her and wants her to live with him. She is exhibiting clinical symptoms of which subtype of delusional disorder?
   a. Jealous
   b. Conjugal
   c. Erotomanic
   d. Grandiose

4. The nurse anticipates which problem when completing an admission assessment for a client with a delusional disorder?
   a. Client assuming unusual body postures
   b. Client exhibiting bizarre behaviors such as grimacing and giggling
   c. Client feeling threatened by any personal contact such as a physical examination
   d. Client remaining mute and refusing to answer any questions

5. Clients with a delusional disorder may require which type of medication to stabilize aggressive behavioral disturbances?
   a. Antidepressants
   b. Depot antipsychotics
   c. Sedative–hypnotics
   d. Antiparkinsonism agents

6. The nurse is assessing a client with a delusional disorder for possible risk factors for the disorder. Which of the following would the nurse identify as increasing the client's risk for delusional disorder? Select all that apply.
   a. Social isolation
   b. Low to moderate stress
   c. Feelings of discrimination
   d. Low self-esteem
   e. Conflicts involving trust and fear

Selected References

American Psychiatric Association. (2000). *Diagnostic and statistical manual of mental disorders* (4th ed., text revision). Washington, DC: Author.

Andrews, M. M., & Boyle, J. S. (2003). *Transcultural concepts in nursing care* (4th ed.). Philadelphia: Lippincott Williams & Wilkins.

Barile, L. (1984). The client who is delusional. In S. Lego (Ed.), *The American handbook of psychiatric nursing* (pp. 450–454). Philadelphia: J. B. Lippincott.

Compton, M. T. (2003). Internet delusions. *Southern Medical Journal, 96*(1), 61–63.

Malloy, P. F., & Salloway, S. (1999). The neurological basis of content-specific delusions. Psychiatric Times, *16*(10), 25–29.

Sadock, B. J., & Sadock, V. A. (2003). *Kaplan & Sadock's synopsis of psychiatry: Behavioral sciences/clinical psychiatry* (9th ed.). Philadelphia: Lippincott Williams & Wilkins.

Shahrokh, N., & Hales, R. (Eds.) (2003). *American psychiatric glossary,* (8th ed.). Washington, DC: American Psychiatric Press.

Sharon, I., Sharon, R., Eliyahu, Y., & Shteynman, S. (2006). Shared psychotic disorder. Retrieved February 28, 2006, from http://www.emedicine.com/med/topic3352.htm

Suggested Readings

Carpenito-Moyet, L. J. (2006). *Handbook of nursing diagnosis* (11th ed.). Philadelphia: Lippincott Williams & Wilkins.

Cervini, P., Newman, D., Dorian, P., Edwards, J., Greene, M., & Bhalerao, S. (2003). Folie à deux: An old diagnosis with a new technology. *Canadian Journal of Cardiology, 19*(13), 1539-40.

Mohr, W. K. (2003). *Johnson's psychiatric-mental health nursing: Adaptation and growth* (5th ed.). Philadelphia: Lippincott Williams & Wilkins.

Reif, A., & Pfuhlmann, B. (2004). Folie à deux versus genetically driven delusional disorder: Case reports and nosological considerations. *Comprehensive Psychiatry, 45*(2), 155-60.

Schanda, H. (2000). Paranoia and dysphoria: Historical developments, current concepts. *Psychopathology, 33,* 204.

Schultz, J. M., & Videbeck, S. D. (2005). *Lippincott's manual of psychiatric nursing care plans* (7th ed.). Philadelphia: Lippincott Williams & Wilkins.

Wenning, M. T., Davy, L. E., Catalano, G., & Catalano, M. C. (2003). Atypical antipsychotics in the treatment of delusional parasitosis. *Annals of Clinical Psychiatry, 15*(3-4), 233-239.

CHAPTER 29 / INFANT, CHILD, AND ADOLESCENT CLIENTS

UNITY

I dreamed I stood in a studio and watched two sculptors there. The clay they used was a young child's mind and they fashioned it with care. One was a teacher; the tools she used were books and music and art. One a parent with a guiding hand and gentle loving heart. Day after day the teacher toiled with touch that was deft and sure, while the parent labored by the side and polished and smoothed it o'er. And when at last their task was done, they were proud of what they had wrought. For the things they had molded into the child could neither be sold nor bought. And each agreed they would have failed if they had worked alone, for behind the parent stood the school and behind the teacher, the home. —AUTHOR UNKNOWN

LEARNING OBJECTIVES

AFTER STUDYING THIS CHAPTER, YOU SHOULD BE ABLE TO:

1. Explain the limitations involving the study of the genetics of behavioral disorders in children.
2. Articulate the relationship between the psychosocial process of attachment and child development.
3. Identify the seven groups of children considered to be at high risk for mental health disorders
4. Differentiate the four types of mental retardation.
5. Distinguish attention-deficit hyperactivity disorder from conduct disorder.
6. Articulate the etiology and clinical symptoms of attention-deficit hyperactivity disorder in adults.
7. Distinguish autistic disorder from Asperger's disorder and Rett's disorder.
8. Compare and contrast clinical symptoms of oppositional defiant disorder and conduct disorder.
9. Develop an assessment tool for childhood and adolescent depression.
10. Propose at least three nursing interventions for each of the following clients:
    - a 15-year-old girl with conduct disorder
    - a 12-year-old boy with clinical symptoms of depression
    - a 7-year-old boy with attention-deficit hyperactivity disorder
    - a 4-year-old girl with autistic behavior
    - a 3-year-old girl with separation anxiety disorder
    - a 9-year-old boy with childhood psychosis
11. Formulate a list of pharmacologic agents approved for use in the treatment of children and adolescents.

KEY TERMS

Asperger's disorder
Attachment theory
Attention-deficit hyperactivity disorder
Autistic disorder
Conduct disorder
Encopresis
Enuresis
Mental retardation
Oppositional defiant disorder
Rett's disorder
Scapegoat
Tic
Tourette's syndrome

Psychiatric care for children continues to be a growing crisis in America. Since the inception of child and adolescent training programs, there has been a shortage of child and adolescent psychiatrists. In 1993, the American Medical Association predicted that the number of youths needing psychiatric services would continue to increase and that the supply of child and adolescent psychiatrists would not keep up with the demand. This prediction has come true. Currently there is a severe shortage of child and adolescent psychiatrists to service the growing needs of this population. For example, attention-deficit hyperactivity disorder (ADHD), one of the most common mental disorders in children and adolescents, affects an estimated 4.1% of youth's ages 9 to 17 years in a 6-month period. Autism affects an estimated 1 to 2 cases per 1,000 individuals. The prevalence of oppositional defiant disorder and conduct disorders among school-aged children is approximately 2% to 16%. Over 5 million youths, by the age of 16 years, have met the diagnostic criteria for substance use disorder. Furthermore, approximately 103,000 short-term psychiatric hospitalizations (of less than 30 days) of youths under age 15 occur yearly (National Institute of Mental Health, 2005). Table 29-1 lists the most current statistics regarding the prevalence of mental or addictive disorders exhibited by children and adolescents. Table 29-2 compares the prevalence of critical mental health related problems between adolescent males and females.

In 2000, the Surgeon General's report on children's mental health, *National Action Agenda for Children's Mental Health,* drew attention to the crisis in children's mental health services. The agenda reflects the culmination of several activities and incorporates recommendations from federal agencies, clinicians, professional and advocacy organizations, and other mental health advocates (Imperio, 2001). The report listed eight goals to improve mental health services to children. Summarized, they include:

- Promoting public awareness of and reducing stigma associated with children's mental health issues
- Developing, disseminating, and implementing scientifically proven prevention and treatment services in the field of children's mental health
- Improving the assessment and recognition of mental health needs in children
- Eliminating racial/ethnic and socioeconomic barriers to mental health care
- Improving the infrastructure for children's mental health services
- Increasing access to and coordination of quality mental health care services
- Training providers (eg, family practitioners or primary care physicians) to recognize and manage mental health issues, and educating mental health providers in scientifically proven prevention and treatment services
- Monitoring access to and coordination of quality mental health care services

Diagnosing childhood and adolescent psychiatric disorders is not an easy task. The etiology of mental health and psychiatric disorders is multifactorial; that is, there is no single cause. Several risk factors (eg, overprotective or controlling parents, behavior problems in the toddler or preschool period, lack of resilience, and gay or bisexual orientation) have been identified as placing children and teens at risk for mental health disorders. In addition to the shortage of child and adolescent psychiatrists noted earlier, the problem of diagnosing and treating young clients is further compounded by the scarcity of trained clinicians such as psychiatric–mental health clinical nurse specialists,

TABLE 29.1 Prevalence of Mental or Addictive Disorders in Children and Adolescents Ages 9 to 17 Years

TYPE OF DISORDER	PERCENTAGE*
Anxiety disorders	13.0
Disruptive disorders	10.3
Mood disorders	6.2
Substance use disorders	2.0
Any disorder	20.9

*Prevalence for 6-month period in 1999.

SOURCE: U.S. Department of Health and Human Services. (1999). *Mental health: A Report of the Surgeon General.* Rockville, MD: DHHS, Substance Abuse and Mental Health Services Administration, Center for Mental Health Services, NIH, NIMH.

TABLE 29.2 Prevalence of Critical Adolescent Mental Health–Related Problems

PROBLEM	MALES	FEMALES
Disabling sadness, unhappiness, or depression	33%	34%
Suicide attempts requiring medical attention	2.1%	3.1%
Drinking and driving	17.0%	9.5%
Alcohol consumption (prior to age 13 years)	24.0%	34.0%
Physical fights	43.0%	33%
Carrying a weapon at school	10.0%	3.0%
Chlamydia trachomatis	15.7%	12.2%

SOURCE: Elster, A. B., & Marcell, A. V. (2003). Health care of adolescent males: Overview, rationale, and recommendations. *Adolescent Medicine: State of the Art Professional Reviews, 14*(3), 525–540.

advanced nurse practitioners, clinical child psychologists, and social workers. Inadequate screening and referral is a major contributing factor to misdiagnosis, leaving approximately 70% of affected children and teens without proper diagnosis and treatment (Kaplan, 2000; Sadock & Sadock, 2003).

This chapter focuses on etiology of disorders of infancy, childhood, and adolescence, which usually occur as a result of complex reactions during one's early developmental stages. The clinical symptoms and diagnostic characteristics are also presented. Using the nursing process, care of children and adolescents is discussed. (See Chapter 24 for information regarding developmental theories.)

History of Child and Adolescent Psychiatry

Most historians of child and adolescent psychiatry trace its beginning in the United States to the year 1899, when Illinois established the nation's first juvenile court in Chicago. In 1909, a group of influential, socially concerned women, who wanted to understand the origin, prevention, and treatment of behavior that contributed to juvenile delinquency, created the Juvenile Psychopathic Institute. They hired William Healy, a neurologist, to be the program director. He

formed teams composed of a psychologist, neuropsychiatrist, and social worker to study brain functioning and intelligence quotient (IQ) of clients with behavioral disturbances. Although research was a primary goal, the institute's board of directors also expected the teams to focus attention on the social factors, attitudes, and motivations of juveniles (Schowalter, 2006).

Around 1911, the noted Swiss psychiatrist Eugene Bleuler, who was also studying behavior, introduced the term autism to describe an individual's exclusion of the outside world and virtual withdrawal from social life. Shortly thereafter, in 1922, behavioral symptoms now associated with ADHD were documented and given a diagnosis of "Post-Encephalitic Behavior Disorder." The first edition of *Child Psychiatry*, published by an American physician, Leo Kanner, in 1935 was very influential in the field of psychiatry. In 1943, Kanner published a paper in which he described autistic behavior as a specific childhood mental health disorder. The following year, Hans Asperger of Vienna, Austria, published a paper in which he described a similar condition that later became known as Asperger's syndrome. These landmark papers featured the first theoretical attempts to explain such complex disorders (About.com, 2006; National Alliance for Autism Research, 2006; Schowalter, 2006).

During the 1940s, World War II also played an important part in the research of child and adolescent psychiatry. Background histories about soldiers who had behavior problems as children or adolescents and were prematurely discharged, disciplined, wounded, or killed in action were researched. The findings provided important statistical information about the etiology of childhood and adolescent mental illness. The movement toward subspecialization in the field of child and adolescent psychiatry accelerated in 1943 when the American Psychiatric Association (APA) converted its section on *Mental Deficiency* to the *Section of Child Psychiatry* (Schowalter, 2006).

The American Academy of Child Psychiatry was founded in 1953. In 1983, the academy published *Child Psychiatry: A Plan for the Coming Decades*. Recommendations were made to focus on the understanding and treatment of mental illnesses in children. In 1986, the academy expanded its name to American Academy of Child and Adolescent Psychiatry. The academy continues to conduct research in an attempt to improve understanding of developmental psychopathology of children and adolescents with mental illnesses.

Etiology

Several theories (eg, genetic, biologic) have been proposed for the different psychiatric–mental health disorders affecting infants, children, and adolescents. In addition, attachment theory and psychosocial and environmental risk factors pertaining to the development of disorders of infants, children, and adolescents have been discussed in the literature.

Theories

The more common psychiatric–mental health disorders occurring in infants, children, and adolescents include mental retardation, pervasive developmental disorder, ADHD, childhood psychosis, anxiety disorders, depression, and disruptive behavior. The theories underlying the causes of these disorders are presented here.

Mental Retardation

Mental retardation is a term used to describe individuals who exhibit subaverage intelligence, as measured by a standardized IQ test, and deficits in adaptive functions (eg, activities of daily living). The etiologic factors associated with the development of mental retardation have been identified as genetic (eg, chromosomal and inherited conditions), developmental (eg, prenatal exposure to toxins and infections), and acquired syndromes (eg, perinatal trauma and sociocultural factors). For example, although Down syndrome (also known as trisomy 21) is a general medical condition, it is a form of mental retardation caused by the chromosomal abnormality. Phenylketonuria is a genetic, metabolic disorder characterized by the inability to convert phenylalanine to tyrosine. Abnormal accumulation of chemicals interferes with brain development and, if untreated, can result in mental retardation. Mental retardation has also occurred when fetuses were exposed to radiation, syphilis, oxygen deprivation, poor maternal nutrition, alcohol, or drugs in utero.

In approximately two thirds of all individuals with mental retardation, the probable cause can be identified. It is not unusual for a comorbid mental disorder to be present (Sadock & Sadock, 2003).

Pervasive Developmental Disorders

Pervasive developmental disorders (also called *autism spectrum disorders*) are characterized by severe deficits and impairment in reciprocal social interaction and communication, and include the presence of stereotyped behavior, interests, and activities. Genetic or biologic theories of Rett's disorder, autistic disorder, and Asperger's disorder are presented.

Rett's Disorder. **Rett's disorder** is an X-linked, progressive neurodevelopmental disorder. Although it was once thought to only occur in girls, there are now several case reports with boys. The gene for this disorder has been found (Baker, 2000). For families who have an identified mutation in the gene, genetic testing may be considered for prenatal diagnosis. That is, for those families who have a child with Rett's disorder or someone in the family with Rett's disorder and the identified gene, genetic testing will be done to help with a possible prenatal diagnosis.

Autistic Disorder. **Autistic disorder** refers to a disorder of development consisting of gross and sustained impairment in social interaction and communication accompanied by restricted and stereotypical patterns of behavior. On the basis of recent genetic analyses, behavioral and brain chemistry studies, and imaging analyses of autistic children, approximately 70% of idiopathic autism cases appear to be an inherited form of an affective disorder (Sadock & Sadock, 2003).

Researchers have hypothesized that there are two distinct forms of autistic disorder. The first type is caused by bilateral brain damage early in life. The second type, which is a more common form, is not associated with brain damage, neurologic findings, or biologic markers. Children with the more common form exhibit very low levels of serotonin on the left side of the brain in the area responsible for language. Symptoms of autism are thought to occur when serotonin levels in the left hemisphere of the brain do not reach a critical level in early childhood (APA, 2000; Sadock & Sadock, 2003). According to recent research, concrete evidence proves that several mutations within the serotonin transporter (SERT) gene, which regulates serotonin levels, constitute a risk factor in autism (Neuropsychiatry Reviews, 2005).

Recent research, based on the premise that not being able to detect autism until a child is close to the age of 3 years eliminates a valuable window of treatment opportunity, is focusing on hematologic changes (ie, unique immune responses) of children ages 2 to 5 years with autism. This study is ongoing. In another study, researchers have isolated the regions of an autism gene on chromosomes 7 and 21. These regions are linked to susceptibility of a type of autism characterized by developmental regression, the loss of previously acquired sociocommunicative skills (Spittler, 2005).

Smith-Lemli-Opitz syndrome (SLOS), a genetic disorder that often presents as a "mild case of autism," is included in the classification of pervasive developmental disorders. It is caused by a defect in the cholesterol metabolic pathway and may exist alone or as a comorbid condition in children with autism. Research has shown that some autistic children with SLOS benefit from cholesterol treatment, which lessens behavioral symptoms associated with autism (Little, 2005).

Asperger's Disorder. Although the cause of **Asperger's disorder**—a disorder similar to autism characterized by impaired behavior and social interaction but with no impairment in communication—is unknown, family studies suggest a possible relationship to autistic disorder. The similarities between the two disorders support the presence of genetic, metabolic, infectious, and perinatal contributing factors. Although definitive data regarding the prevalence of Asperger's disorder are lacking, the disorder appears to be diagnosed much more frequently in males (at least five times more) than in females (APA, 2000; Sadock & Sadock, 2003).

Attention-Deficit Hyperactivity Disorder

Attention-deficit hyperactivity disorder (ADHD), one of the best-researched disorders in medicine, is characterized by prominent symptoms of inattention and/or hyperactivity–impulsivity. Although overall data on the validity of its existence are far more compelling than for most mental disorders, a major limitation in the study of the genetics of such disorders in children has been the overlap of one or more syndromes such as anxiety, depression, or conduct disorder. The rate of overlap is greatly increased with ADHD.

Given that any child has a 10% possibility of being diagnosed with ADHD, overlap with other syndromes can occur merely by chance (Baren, 2000; Flick, 2002; Myers, Eisenhauer, & Ryan, 2003).

ADHD is a heterogeneous behavioral disorder with multiple etiologies. The symptoms have been attributed to neuromaturational delay, catecholamine deficits, altered glucose metabolism in the brain, and frontal lobe dysfunction. For example, genetic influences such as rare mutations in the human thyroid receptor gene on chromosome 3, dopamine transporter gene on chromosome 5, and D4 receptor gene

on chromosome 11 have been identified in studies of twins and families (Biederman, 1999). Additionally, severe central nervous system infections such as Reye's syndrome and meningitis; perinatal insults such as substance abuse during pregnancy, poor maternal nutrition, premature labor, and anoxia; and brain injuries during or after birth are also considered to be causes of ADHD (Baren, 2000).

ADHD in Adults. Until the 1970s, it was believed that ADHD was strictly a childhood disorder, and that children outgrew it in adolescence. Recent research supports the diagnostic continuity of ADHD throughout the life cycle. Estimates suggest that ADHD affects approximately 5% of adults (or about 8 million American adults). Although the hyperactivity component may diminish, the attention and impulsive aspects can persist into adulthood. To be diagnosed with ADHD, an adult must have a childhood onset on clinical symptoms that are persistent during adulthood. According to a 10-year follow-up study of male subjects with ADHD, the chance of boys retaining ADHD into manhood was 56% (McDonnell & Dougherty, 2005; Waite, 2004; Zoler, 2004).

Childhood Psychosis

Although there is clearly a genetic component, genetic predisposition alone does not explain the development of childhood schizophrenia. Early-onset schizophrenia and schizophrenia-like disorders (such as schizoaffective, schizoid personality, and schizophreniform disorders) are due to neuropathology, which includes neurostructural changes, neurochemical influences, and changes in brain metabolism. Intrauterine stress, neuropsychological abnormalities, communication style, life events, and stress are important etiologic factors as well.

More than 50% of adults with bipolar disorder experience the onset in childhood or adolescence. Biologic contributions include genetic factors, neuropathology, and neurotransmitter abnormalities (Hendren, 1997). Box 29-1 summarizes possible causes of psychosis in childhood. Chapters 21 and 22 provide additional information regarding theories related to the development of bipolar disorder and schizophrenia.

Mood Disorders

Although the cause of childhood mood disorders, such as depression or bipolar disorder, is unknown, the evi-

BOX 29.1 POSSIBLE CAUSES OF PSYCHOSIS IN CHILDHOOD

METABOLIC AND INFECTIOUS CAUSES	NEUROLOGIC CAUSES	DRUG-INDUCED CAUSES
Adrenal cortical hypofunction	Head trauma	Prescription drugs, stimulants, corticosteroids, anticholinergics
Thyroid and parathyroid disease	Multiple sclerosis	Drug interactions
Porphyria	Seizure disorder	Nonprescription drugs, cocaine, phencyclidine (PCP), hallucinogens, solvents
Endocrinopathies	Brain tumor	
Wilson's disease	Congenital malformations	Heavy metals
Encephalitis, meningitis, AIDS	Huntington's disease	
	Neurosyphilis	

dence is strongest for a transaction between biologic, personality, and environmental factors. Biologic factors include genetic heritability, dysregulation of central serotonergic or noradrenergic systems, hypothalamic–pituitary–adrenal (HPA) axis dysfunction, and the influence of prepubertal sex hormones (Jeffrey, Sava Bianca, & Winters, 2005). Recent studies of pediatric clients also point to a possible neurobiologic marker (eg, reduced glutamatergic concentrations in the anterior cingulated cortex) in the pathogenesis of major depressive disorders as well as obsessive–compulsive disorder. Future studies are warranted and necessary because alterations in glutamatergic concentrations can be reversed with effective treatment (Romano, 2004). Studies of adults with depression point to a genetic predisposition and environmental influence. The children of depressed parents are three times more likely to develop a mood disorder than their peers with unaffected parents. Possible risk factors include a history of abuse, neglect, trauma, or loss of significant other. Although divorce and the loss of a loved one can place a child at risk, these factors do not necessarily trigger the onset of depression. Learning disabilities may also contribute to childhood depression (National Institute of Mental Health, 2003). Chapter 21 provides additional information regarding the development of mood disorders in children and adolescents.

Anxiety Disorders

Children and teens experience stress and anxiety in their lives, just as adults do. Kids Health Kids Poll, a survey of 875 children conducted from May 10 to June 7, 2005, identified the top ten triggers of stress in children ages 9 to 13 years. Identified triggers included grades/school/homework (36%), family (32%), friends/

teasing/gossip (21%), siblings (20%), mean/annoying people (20%), parents (14%), yelling/loud noise (9%), fighting (9%), sports (8%), and lack of autonomy (7%) (Foley & Keller, 2006). Although events such as starting school, moving, or the loss of a parent precipitate stress, a specific stressor need not be the precursor to the development of an anxiety disorder. As a group, anxiety disorders affect 20% of youth up to age 18 years; however, clinical symptoms are generally evident around the age of 11 years (Bryant & Cheng, 2005). The most common diagnoses include separation anxiety disorder, social phobia, school phobia, panic disorder in adolescents, and generalized anxiety disorder.

Insufficient data exist regarding the etiology of anxiety disorders in very young children. Studies do not prove whether anxiety is the result of biologic or environmental factors or both (Anxiety Disorders Association of America, 2003). Psychosocial risk factors, including attachment theory, are discussed in the next section. Chapters 19 and 20 provide additional information regarding theories related to the development of anxiety disorders.

Disruptive Behavior Disorder: Conduct Disorder

Conduct disorder is classified as a disruptive behavior disorder that is characterized by a pattern of behavior that violates the basic rights of others or major age-appropriate norms or rules (APA, 2000). No single factor can account for the etiology of conduct disorder. Rather many risk factors are considered to contribute to development of this disorder including parental and family, sociocultural, psychological, and school-related factors (Perepletchikova & Kazdin, 2005; Sadock & Sadock, 2003). Psychosocial risk factors, including attachment theory, are discussed in the next section.

Neurobiologic theories state that conduct disorders may be a result of decreased noradrenergic functioning or high serotonin blood levels. Medical and metabolic explanations given for the development of a conduct disorder include encephalopathy, phenylketonuria, lead poisoning, hyperthyroidism, fragile X syndrome, Lesch-Nyhan syndrome, Tourette's syndrome, brain tumors, or head trauma. Some teenagers with conduct disorder have been found to be exposed to cocaine in utero. The most salient contributor to their behavior lies in the brain, in which abnormalities and atrophy can be confirmed by magnetic resonance imaging and electroencephalogram (Bates, 1999; Sadock & Sadock, 2003).

Attachment Theory

John Bowlby, a British psychoanalyst (1907–1990), formulated a theory about the psychological concept of attachment. His **Attachment theory** states that normal attachment in infancy is crucial to a person's healthy development. He differentiates attachment from bonding. *Attachment*, according to Bowlby, occurs when there is a warm, intimate and continuous relationship with the mother in which both the infant and mother find satisfaction and enjoyment. Attachment is also referred to as the emotional tone between children and their caregivers and is evidenced by the child's clinging to the caregiver. *Bonding* occurs during skin-to-skin contact between a mother and infant or when other types of contact, such as voice and eye contact occur (Sadock & Sadock, 2003; Wikipedia.org, 2006.).

Charles Zeanah, professor of psychiatry and neurology at Tulane University Medical School, New Orleans, believes the quality of early attachments is a good predictor of later social adaptation. Children who have difficulty with attachment often exhibit anxiety and aggressive behavior and are more likely to have difficult relationships with parents, peers, and teachers. Attachment problems often overlap with other diagnoses including autism, conduct disorders, and depression. Separation anxiety disorder, avoidant personality disorder, depressive disorders, and borderline intelligence have also been traced to negative attachment experiences (Sadock & Sadock, 2003; Sullivan, 2004).

A meta-analysis of attachment studies indicates that about 15% of children in a general population sample exhibit disorganized attachment. The percentage is much higher, however, in a high-risk sample where there is poverty, neglect, or abuse. In those samples, up to 82% of children may exhibit disorganized attachment (Sullivan, 2004).

Psychosocial Risk Factors

Seven specific groups of children, many of whom experienced maternal or caregiver deprivation (detachment), are considered to be at high risk for psychiatric–mental disorders. The summary that follows reflects the risk factors identified by the United States Congress, Office of Technology Assessment (USCOTA; 1986).

Children in Families With Conflict or Divorce

Scapegoat is a term used to describe the role within a family of a person who receives the angry, hostile, frustrated, or ambivalent emotions experienced by various family members. The scapegoat, usually a child, is singled out by family members who project their feelings onto this person. As a result, the child may resort to acting-out behavior in an attempt to cope, decrease anxiety, receive love and attention, or preserve self-esteem.

Placing too much responsibility on a child, making him or her a "little adult" in the absence of an adult partner, creates an abnormal family role that can also lead to a behavior disorder. Such a child might be expected to baby-sit siblings, help with adult tasks, or even fulfill the role of the absent adult. The child does not have the opportunity to progress through the normal stages of growth and development. Children of divorce may exhibit low self-esteem and ineffective coping skills and lack social support.

Children Who Experience Poverty

Children who live in poverty are generally denied access to health care, child care, nutrition, adequate housing, and school and play environments. Social isolation occurs. Family functioning is compromised because parents in poverty live under chronic stress, which exposes children to other risk factors (eg, crime or illicit drug use or abuse) for psychiatric–mental health disorders.

Children of Minority Ethnic Status

According to 1990 statistics from the National Center for Children in Poverty, children ages 18 years and younger from culturally diverse groups constituted approximately one third of the U.S. and Canadian populations (Li & Bennett, 1994). These children lived in families in which there was racial, ethnic, and/or religious diversity. Nearly 50% of African American children and more than 40% of young Hispanic children live in poverty. These children experience adverse effects related to their ethnicity because of poverty and racism. Learning disabilities, deteriorating grades, and lack of developmental assets such as self-esteem and coping skills often place these children at risk (Andrews & Boyle, 2003).

Children Who Are Abused

Child abuse, which can be physical, emotional, or sexual, places children at risk for emotional and behavioral disorders possibly resulting in death. Clinicians who routinely provided care for children saw an average of four to six victims of abuse and neglect each year (United States Department of Health and Human Services [USDHHS], 1999). It is estimated that more than 2.4 million cases of suspected child abuse and neglect are reported yearly to state child protective agencies in the United States. Estimates of abuse continue to rise yearly.

Child abuse can occur in the home, where the abusers are parents or parent substitutes; in institutional settings, such as daycare centers, child-care agencies, schools, welfare departments, correctional settings, and residential centers; and in society, which allows children to live in poverty or be denied the basic necessities of life. (Chapter 33 discusses child abuse in more detail.)

Children of Substance-Abusing and Mentally Ill Parents

The terms *crack babies* and *fetal alcohol syndrome* are used to describe the effects of maternal crack addiction and alcoholism on children. Children exposed to substance abuse in utero or to substances at any early age may experience altered physical development, decreased intellectual ability, behavior or conduct disorders, substance abuse, depression, suicide, and criminality (Johnson, 1997).

Children who live with substance-abusing or mentally ill parents also are at risk for parental abuse and the development of a psychiatric–mental health disorder if they remain in a dysfunctional family unit. Children of mentally ill parents are often neglected because of lack of bonding with parents after birth,

and separation or detachment from the ill parent who is unable to function as a positive role model.

Children of Teenaged Parents

Teenage pregnancy is often the result of impulsive sexual behavior without any thought given to the consequences (USCOTA, 1986). In addition, the sexual act may occur while the teenager is under the influence of alcohol or other substances, placing the teenager and infant at risk for a sexually transmitted disease or acquired immunodeficiency syndrome (AIDS). Infants born to teenage mothers are likely to be premature and to present with health problems. The parenting skills of teenagers to deal with stressors of family life are generally lacking. As a result, the child is at risk for developmental disorders, behavior or conduct disorders, and emotional problems.

Children With Chronic Illness or Disability

Just as adults may develop psychiatric–mental health problems secondary to a chronic medical condition or disability, children are also at risk. For example, a child with a physical handicap due to a neuromuscular disorder is at risk for the development of an emotional or behavioral problem. A child taking medication to control asthma symptoms is at risk for the development of anxiety due to adverse effects of medication, or may exhibit behavior similar to conduct disorder due to low self-esteem or a disturbance in self-concept. Children of parents with a chronic illness or disability are also at risk for the development of psychiatric–mental health disorders. They may be subjected to unrealistic expectations (eg, serving as caretakers for the disabled parent) or they may be verbally or emotionally abused by a parent who is unable to cope with his or her medical condition.

Environmental Risk Factors

Two environmental factors that place children at risk for the development of psychiatric–mental health disorders include public schools and the community, also referred to as "neighborhood" or the inner city.

Public Schools

According to a public school education survey conducted in 1999, the National Public Radio (NPR)/

Kaiser/Kennedy School Poll, parents think the nation's public schools have six major problems: the presence of undisciplined and disruptive students, lack of parental involvement, overcrowded classrooms, violence and lack of school safety, students' use of alcohol and drugs, and inequality in funding among school districts. All of these factors can influence the development of psychiatric–mental health disorders in children and adolescents (NPR online, 2003).

Behavioral Approaches. The public school setting is becoming an entry point of contact for behavioral health services in an attempt to prevent and reduce environmental factors that place children and youth at risk for the development of a psychiatric–mental health disorder. Partnerships between psychiatric–mental health clinical nurse specialists in the public-school setting and primary-care nurse practitioners can provide comprehensive services of early identification and timely intervention. When mental health services are provided within the school system, accessibility and efficiency of interventions increase, fragmentation decreases, and there is no unnecessary stigma that often surrounds referrals for mental health treatment (Hales, Karshmer, Monter-Sandoval et al., 2003).

Promotion of Positive Behaviors. The poem at the beginning of this chapter addresses the role of a positive parent–teacher relationship in child development. Barker (1995) lists the characteristics of a school environment that minimize risk factors and influence the development of normal, positive behavior in children and adolescents. The characteristics are summarized as follows:

- Integration of the intellectually able and less able children provides for a well-balanced classroom, encouraging normal growth and development.
- Acknowledgment and praise by teachers promotes the development of a positive self-concept.
- Encouragement of participation in running the school fosters responsibility.
- Moderate emphasis on academic achievement permits the child to participate in a variety of activities and to develop a well-rounded personality.
- Good role-modeling by teachers promotes positive behavior in children.
- A comfortable, pleasant, and attractive environment is conducive to the development of mentally healthy persons.

Neighborhoods

Neighborhoods can also influence the development of behavior disorders. Poor socioeconomic conditions in crowded inner cities produce higher rates of childhood psychiatric–mental health disorders than are seen in suburban areas. Delinquency, substance abuse, childhood depression, and antisocial personality are just a few examples of disorders prevalent in such neighborhoods.

Clinical Symptoms and Diagnostic Characteristics

Disorders usually evident in infancy, childhood, or adolescence have been classified by the *Diagnostic and Statistical Manual of Mental Disorders, 4th Edition, Text Revision (DSM-IV-TR)* (APA, 2000). These disorders are as follows:

1. Mental retardation
2. Learning disorders related to reading, mathematics, and writing
3. Motor skills disorder related to coordination
4. Communication disorders
5. Pervasive developmental disorders
6. Attention-deficit and disruptive behavior disorders
7. Feeding and eating disorders
8. Tic disorders
9. Elimination disorders
10. Other disorders of infancy, childhood, and adolescence, such as excessive anxiety, selective mutism, or repetitive nonfunctional motor behavior

Several disorders such as personality disorders, dual diagnosis disorders, psychotic disorders, and substance-related disorders that are discussed in this text may be diagnosed in children or adolescents. Age-specific features have been included in each chapter. Specific content regarding eating disorders, adolescent suicide, and child abuse is discussed in separate chapters.

Many texts present an excellent summary of psychological development, focusing on the developmental stage, motor and physical development, language or communication, cognitive behavior, interpersonal behavior, developmental crisis, and the most frequent disturbing behaviors in that particular developmental stage. The reader is referred to such texts on growth and development for additional information because it is important in the assessment and treatment of disorders affecting infants, children, and adolescents.

Mental Retardation

The last two decades have seen enormous changes in services for children with learning and developmental difficulties such as mental retardation, who are referred to by the general public as "mentally or developmentally challenged." Although onset occurs before the age of 18 years, the incidence is difficult to calculate because mental retardation sometimes goes unrecognized until middle childhood. Its prevalence rate has been estimated at approximately 1% of the population, with the highest incidence in school-age children

peaking at ages 10 to 14 years. It occurs about $1\frac{1}{2}$ times more frequently among men than among women. The trend toward deinstitutionalization has made family and community support a central issue (Sadock & Sadock, 2003).

Mental retardation is described in the *DSM-IV-TR* as the presence of subaverage general intellectual functioning (an IQ of approximately 70 or below) associated with or resulting in impairments in adaptive behavior. Table 29-3 lists the subtypes and associated severity of mental retardation. Clients with mental impairment experience or exhibit significant limitations in at least two of the following skill areas: communication, self-care, home living, social/interpersonal skills, use of community resources, self-direction, functional academic skills, work, leisure, health, and safety.

TABLE 29.3 Severity of Mental Retardation

Subtype	IQ Level	Deficits	Comments
Mild	50 to 70	None in early childhood Difficulty adapting to school Sixth-grade level by late teens May need assistance when experiencing social or economic stress	85% of all persons with mental retardation Can achieve social and vocational skills for minimum self-support "Educable"—can acquire academic skills up to approximately sixth-grade level
Moderate	35 to 55	Poor awareness of needs of others Usually no progression beyond second-grade level Need moderate supervision due to self-care deficit Require supervision and guidance under mild social or economic stress	10% of all persons with mental retardation May profit from vocational training Can function in sheltered workshops as unskilled or semiskilled persons "Trainable"
Severe	20 to 40	Poor motor development and minimal speech Unable to learn academic skills but may learn to talk and be trained in elementary hygiene skills or activities of daily living Require complete supervision in a controlled environment	3% to 4% of all persons with mental retardation May learn to perform simple work tasks
Profound	Below 20 or 25	Minimal capacity for sensorimotor functioning Require total nursing care and highly structured environment with supervision due to self-care deficit	1% to 2% of all persons with mental retardation May learn some productive skills "Custodial"

THE CLIENT WITH SEVERE MENTAL RETARDATION

MW, 18 years old, was born by a normal spontaneous vaginal delivery without any complications. Two months after birth, MW developed a temperature of 105°F and had a grand mal seizure. He was admitted to the neonatal intensive care unit with the diagnosis of fever of undetermined origin (FUO). Diagnostic tests revealed the presence of encephalitis. MW recovered, but his parents were cautioned about the possibility of central nervous system damage because of the severity of his illness. During early childhood, ages 1 to 5 years, MW was able to communicate with his parents to some extent but exhibited poor motor-skill development. He was unable to learn basic skills such as reading, writing, and arithmetic, and it became evident that he needed supervision in a controlled environment. Testing revealed MW's IQ to be that of a person with severe retardation or mental impairment. At age 18 years, he continues to live at home with very supportive parents who have been able to teach him some self-care activities. He relates well to a pet cat, helps his mother with simple household chores, and helps his father with gardening and lawn care.

Associated features of mental retardation include irritability, aggressiveness, temper tantrums, stereotyped repetitive movements, nail biting, and stuttering. See Clinical Example 29-1.

Pervasive Developmental Disorders

Five disorders are classified as pervasive developmental disorders: autistic disorder; Rett's disorder; childhood disintegrative disorder; Asperger's disorder (also referred to as Asperger's syndrome); and pervasive developmental disorder, not otherwise specified. Between 70% and 85% of individuals with the diagnosis of developmental disability referred for psychiatric consultation have one or more untreated or undiagnosed medical problems influencing their behavior. Between 60% and 100% have experienced trauma, usually repeated incidents of abuse (Ryan & Sunada, 1997;

Sobsey, 1997). A summary of autistic disorder and Asperger's disorder follows.

Autistic Disorder

According to statistics provided by the Autism Society of America in 2002, an estimated 500,000 to 1.5 million individuals in the United States have the diagnosis of autistic disorder or some form of pervasive developmental disorder. The incidence of autism is one or two of 1,000 live births. The onset of the disorder is generally noted before the age of 3 years. However, in some cases, it is not detected until a child is much older. In addition, it is estimated that children having autistic-like behavior number 15 to 20 of 10,000. These statistics have increased during the last 5 years.

Autism is four to five times more likely to affect males than females. However, girls with autistic disorder are more likely to have more severe mental retardation. Autistic disorder knows no racial, ethnic, or social boundaries. It is incurable and is considered a life-long disability (Johnson & Dorman, 1998; Sadock & Sadock, 2003).

Sometimes referred to as *early infantile autism, childhood autism,* or *Kanner's autism,* this disorder is characterized by qualitative impairments in social interaction and communication, and restricted repetitive and stereotyped patterns of behavior, interest, and activities. Before the age of 3 years, the child exhibits delays or abnormal functioning in social action, language as used in social communication, or symbolic or imaginative play.

Specifically, autistic children have an inability to establish a meaningful relationship because of their lack of responsiveness to others. They do not display an interest in or need for cuddling, touching, or hugging. They ignore people as if they were inanimate objects or not present in the environment.

Children with autistic disorder also possess gross deficits in language development, including mutism, echolalia, and the inability to name objects. Language deficits may also consist of pronominal reversal, or the use of the pronoun "you" when "I" should be used, and immature grammar.

Other symptoms include withdrawal, which may be mistaken for deafness; obsessive ritualistic behavior, such as rocking and spinning; obsessive attachments to particular objects, even mechanical objects; and anxiety or fear associated with harmless objects. The child may exhibit an obsessive desire for sameness; that is, he or she becomes resistant to change and is severely distressed if environmental change occurs.

Overactivity, distractibility, poor concentration, sudden unprovoked anger or fear, or aggressive outbursts also may occur. Autistic children do not experience delusions, hallucinations, incoherence, or looseness of association.

Intellectual functioning varies, because children who are autistic may function at a normal, high, or retarded level. Approximately 50% of autistic children have an IQ below 50 (APA, 2000). Memory may be exceptional, as observed in the behavior of an autistic child who plays several pieces of complicated classical music on the piano. See Clinical Example 29-2.

Asperger's Disorder

Asperger's disorder, incorporated into the *DSM-IV* in 1994, has been widely recognized as part of the mild end of the autistic spectrum. More commonly seen in boys, the typical child with this syndrome lives in the real world on his or her terms, has normal or higher intelligence, exhibits pedantic speech (overemphasis on detail when speaking) by age 5 years, is clumsy, has poor handwriting, and exhibits autistic-type behavior such as hand flapping or pacing when excited or upset.

Verbal functioning is essentially normal, but range of interests is highly circumscribed and social deficits are striking. The child is unable to develop peer relationships, lacks the ability to exhibit social or emotional reciprocity (ie, is unable to respond emotionally to others), and displays an impaired ability to express pleasure in other persons' happiness (APA, 2000; Sadock & Sadock, 2003).

Verbal IQ is higher than performance IQ. Developmental delay may not be apparent until preschool or school age when social deficits become apparent. Certain psychiatric disorders occur with unusual frequency in children with Asperger's disorder, including bipolar disorder, ADHD, obsessive–compulsive disorder, and Tourette's syndrome (Reed, 2001; Sherman, 2000).

Attention-Deficit and Disruptive Behavior Disorders

This category includes the diagnoses of ADHD and disruptive behavior disorders (childhood-onset type and adolescent-onset type) that manifest themselves in home, academic, or social environments. A summary of each follows.

Attention-Deficit Hyperactivity Disorder

Approximately 3% to 7% of prepubertal elementary school children have ADHD, and at least 25% of those children have a parent who also has ADHD. It is not unusual for the proper diagnosis in a child to lead to identification of ADHD or another psychiatric diagnosis in a parent and/or siblings. ADHD is more prevalent in boys, with a ratio ranging from 2 to 1 to as much as 9 to 1 (Glod, 2001; Myers et al., 2003; Sadock & Sadock, 2003).

Characteristics of ADHD include a short attention span, impulsivity, and distractibility. See the accompanying Clinical Symptoms and Diagnostic Characteristics box.

Although manifestations of symptoms are typically present before age 3 years and may cause life-long dysfunction, delayed or missed diagnoses are not unusual. ADHD appears to have many associated comorbid disorders including learning disability, depression, oppo-

---

CLINICAL EXAMPLE 29.2

THE CLIENT WITH AUTISTIC DISORDER

TJ, age 16 years, was diagnosed with autistic disorder at age 2 years. He lives at home with his parents and attends a school for developmentally disabled children. His ability to communicate verbally is restricted to making guttural sounds at times. TJ requires constant supervision because of behavior such as head banging and biting himself. Custodial care is also necessary to feed and toilet TJ. He has occasional outbursts in which he hits others and attempts to bite them. TJ responds to music, which seems to have a soothing effect on him and he will stand on the basketball court for hours shooting baskets. Although he appears to be in his own world, TJ will unexpectedly respond to the voice of his classroom teacher by looking directly at her and nodding his head or making guttural sounds. His parents report that his conduct at home fluctuates from manageable behavior to hostile, aggressive outbursts, at which time he needs to be medicated to stabilize his behavior.

CLINICAL SYMPTOMS AND DIAGNOSTIC CHARACTERISTICS / ADHD

CLINICAL SYMPTOMS

Lasting at least 6 months and occurring before the age of 7 years:
- Stubbornness
- Negativism
- Temper tantrums
- Obstinacy
- Inability to tolerate frustration
- Deficit in judgment
- Poor self-image
- Aggressiveness

DIAGNOSTIC CHARACTERISTICS

- Inattention
  - Failure to complete a task, pay attention, or listen
  - Distractibility
  - Inability to concentrate
  - Difficulty participating in activities for a period of time
- Hyperactivity
  - Fidgeting
  - Inability to sit still
  - Running, climbing, or moving during sleep
  - Behavior indicating being in "high gear"
- Impulsivity
  - Failure to think before acting
  - Frequent shifting from one activity to another (poor attention span)
  - Inability to organize work
  - Frequent disrupting of class or groups

CLINICAL EXAMPLE 29.3

THE CLIENT WITH ATTENTION-DEFICIT HYPERACTIVITY DISORDER

BS, age 6, diagnosed as having attention-deficit hyperactivity disorder, was interviewed by a clinical psychologist in the presence of several student nurses. When BS first entered the room, he jumped up and down several times, giggled nervously, and then said "I'm sorry." The psychologist asked BS to sit still as he attempted to time the child's ability to remain immobile for a period of time. One minute seemed an eternity to BS, who insisted time was up in 15 seconds. When asked to draw a picture of the psychologist, BS was unable to sit still long enough to complete the drawing. He ran about the room investigating electrical outlets and various pieces of equipment. After he knocked over a table lamp, BS repeatedly stated that he was sorry. When the psychologist asked him to participate in a ring-toss game, he stated, "You go first, I always go last." He was unable to stand still as he awaited his turn. The student nurses who observed BS's behavior stated they were exhausted after 30 minutes. "How do his parents keep up with him 24 hours a day?" "Does he ever unwind?" "Does he always break things?" and "Why does he say that he is sorry so often?" were a few of the comments by the students. One student questioned how his behavior would affect other children when he played with them. Another student wanted to know how long BS would remain hyperactive. Postclinical conference discussion focused on assessment of BS's behavior and the development of a nursing plan of care.

sitional defiant disorder, Tourette's syndrome, general anxiety, conduct disorder, and bipolar disorder. Diagnosis is usually not made until the child enters school, when academic and social functioning may be impaired (Flick, 2002; Sadock & Sadock, 2003). See Clinical Example 29-3.

ADHD in Adults

As noted earlier, the impact of clinical symptoms of ADHD continue into adulthood for many people. Clinical symptoms frequently manifest as difficulty in reading, thinking critically, regulating performance, dealing with unfamiliar events, multitasking, and working as a member of a team, all relevant in the workplace (AdultADD.com, 2006; Moore, 2005).

Disruptive Behavior Disorders

Disruptive behavior disorders are subcategorized as oppositional defiant disorder and conduct disorder. Children with these disorders are impaired by the frequency and severity of their disruptive behaviors (Sadock & Sadock, 2003).

Oppositional Defiant Disorder (ODD). **Oppositional defiant disorder** (ODD) refers to a recurring pattern of negativistic and hostile behavior in a child or adolescent. According to epidemiologic studies in nonclinical populations, ODD was identified in 16% to 22% of school-age children. The actual diagnostic rate for this disorder ranges from 2% to 6%. Although it can occur as early as 3 years of age, ODD is generally diagnosed in children by 8 years of age or no later than adolescence and is more prevalent in boys than in girls, especially before puberty (APA, 2000: Sadock & Sadock, 2003; Perepletchikova & Kazdin, 2005).

Children experience normal oppositional behavior between the ages of 18 and 24 months. Pathology begins when this developmental phase persists abnormally and the child is unable to develop skills such as flexibility, adaptability, and frustration tolerance. Authority figures overreact, and as a result of this conflict, the child exhibits negativistic, hostile, and defiant behavior. Specific behaviors include loss of temper, anger, resentment, and vindictiveness. Children with ODD also argue frequently with adults, deliberately annoy others, blame others for their mistakes or misbehavior, and are easily annoyed (APA, 2000: Sadock & Sadock, 2003).

Conduct Disorders. Conduct disorder refers to disruptive behavior by a child or adolescent characterized by persistent and repetitive violation of the rights of others. Studies indicate that conduct disorders are the largest single group of psychiatric illnesses in adolescents. Conduct disorders affect approximately 6% to 16% of boys and 2% to 9% of girls younger than age 18 years. Conduct disorders usually occur just before, during, or immediately after puberty. Causes of such behavior may include:

- A poor parent–child interpersonal relationship
- Lack of a father figure
- Parental rejection
- Lack of a secure, permanent family group, as experienced by orphans or foster children during institutional living
- Failure to bond during infancy
- Incompatibility of the child's and parents' temperaments
- Inconsistency in setting limits and disciplining a child by parents or authority figures
- Large family size
- Association with children of a lower socioeconomic class, including exposure to "delinquent groups"

Interpersonal behavior during puberty includes developing peer relationships, participating in activities outside the family, lessening family ties, and exhibiting independence. If the child does not successfully complete the developmental stages of industry versus inferiority (age 6 years to puberty) and identity versus role confusion (puberty and adolescence) as described by Erikson (1964), the child may develop a sense of inferiority, may experience difficulty learning and working, and may fail to develop a sense of identity.

Symptoms may develop first within the family unit when the child attempts to cope with anxiety or resolve an inner conflict. Involvement in adolescent gangs also may precipitate the onset of antisocial behavior. In either case, interpersonal relationships within the family are usually unstable or poor. See the accompanying Clinical Symptoms and Diagnostic Characteristics box.

Tic Disorders

A **tic** is a rapid, largely involuntary movement or noise. Although the etiology of tics is unknown, possible causes include stress, tension, brain damage, or a decreased production of the neurotransmitters serotonin and dopamine.

CLINICAL SYMPTOMS AND DIAGNOSTIC CHARACTERISTICS /
CONDUCT DISORDER

CLINICAL SYMPTOMS

Demonstrated in an individual under the age of 18 years; three or more symptoms exhibited within the last 12 months or one symptom exhibited within the last 6 months:
- Aggressive behavior toward persons and animals
- Property destruction
- Deceitfulness and theft
- Significantly serious violations of rules

DIAGNOSTIC CHARACTERISTICS

- Violation of another's basic rights or age-appropriate norms or rules of society
- Significantly impaired functioning in the social, academic, or occupational setting due to behavior

Tics are divided into two types: motor tics, involving the rapid movement of a muscle; and vocal tics, which can range from simple throat clearing to more complex vocalizations involving words or phrases. Tics are relatively common in childhood (with onset of motor tics by the age of 7 years and vocal tics by the age of 11 years), with 5% to 24% of school-age children reporting past or present tics. Usually, tics are mild and last less than 1 year, generally referred to as *transient tic disorder. Chronic tic disorder* refers to the presence of either motor tics or vocal tics, but not both. The tics occur many times a day, nearly every day for more than 1 year. Some individuals with tic disorders can suppress the tics for minutes or hours, but young children either are not cognizant of their tics or experience their tics as insuppressible. The frequency of involuntary movement or noise may be reduced during sleep, relaxation, or absorption in an activity. This disorder occurs before age 18 years (APA, 2000; Sadock & Sadock, 2003).

Tourette's syndrome, or Gilles de la Tourette's syndrome, is described as a combination of motor tics and involuntary vocal and verbal utterances that often are obscene (coprolalia). Repeating one's own sounds or words (palilalia); repeating the last-heard sound, word, or phrase (echolalia); and imitating someone else's movements (echokinesis) may be present. The tics occur many times a day nearly every day, or intermittently for more than 1 year. The onset of this disorder is before age 18 years and it can persist for a lifetime.

Several studies have addressed the comorbidity of Tourette's syndrome, obsessive–compulsive disorder, and ADHD. Findings indicate that approximately 50% of clients diagnosed with Tourette's syndrome have obsessions and compulsions (obsessive–compulsive disorder) and clinical symptoms of ADHD. Conversely, findings support that 30% to 40% of children with the diagnosis of ADHD also have clinical symptoms of Tourette's syndrome (APA, 2000; Jetmalani, 2005).

Elimination Disorders

Elimination disorders include enuresis and encopresis. **Enuresis** is the repeated urination, day or night, into bed or clothes. The presence of clinically significant distress or impairment in social, academic, occupational, or other important areas of functioning is considered when using the diagnosis of enuresis, which usually begins by age 5 years.

Primary or functional nocturnal enuresis affects approximately 5 to 7 million children older than 5 years and is a common presentation in the primary care setting. Enuresis may be caused by physiologic factors such as decreased arousal from sleep in response to a full bladder; small functional bladder capacity; food sensitivities; or high nocturnal urine production. Psychological factors include anxiety, regression, adjustment reaction, or psychosis (Mercer, 2003; Sadock & Sadock, 2003).

Encopresis, or fecal soiling, is the passage of feces in inappropriate places or settings. The behavior may be involuntary, resulting from inadequate or lack of appropriate toilet training secondary to inefficient or ineffective sphincter control, or it may be intentional as a result of anger, anxiety, fear, or a combination of psychological factors. Bowel control is established in 95% of children in Western cultures by the age of 4 years and in 99% by the age of 5 years. After the age of 4 years, encopresis is three to four times more common in boys than in girls (Sadock & Sadock, 2003).

A child must experience encopresis at least once a month for 3 months before the diagnosis is given. Age of onset is at least 4 years or the equivalent developmental level. In the absence of a physical disorder, the main causative factor is said to be a dysfunctional relationship between the child and parents, usually the mother. The child may be poorly cared for, under stress, immature, experiencing increased anxiety or regression, or mentally retarded (APA, 2000).

Other Disorders

Other disorders diagnosed in children prior to the age of 18 years include separation anxiety disorder, mood disorders, and adjustment disorders.

Separation Anxiety Disorder

Anxiety among young people has increased measurably and significantly in recent decades according to two meta-analyses reported by Zolot and Sofer (2001). The first meta-analyses involved 170 studies of self-reported anxiety measures collected from college students between 1952 and 1993. Researchers determined that every measure of anxiety increased steadily and substantially from 1952 to 1993. The second meta-analyses analyzed 99 studies of American schoolchildren who completed an anxiety measure between 1954 and 1981. Results of self-reported anxiety paralleled those of the college students (Zolot & Sofer, 2001).

Separation anxiety disorder may begin quite early in life with increasing identification as the child begins school or it may develop after some life stressor, such as the terrorist attack on the World Trade Center and Pentagon on September 11, 2001. Onset may be as early as preschool age and may occur at any time before age 18 years. There may be periods of exacerbation and remission.

Separation anxiety disorder is characterized by excessive anxiety that is severe and persistent when the child is separated from the parent (usually the mother), a significant other, the home, or familiar surroundings. As the child grows older, he or she may refuse to travel independently from home, spend the night at a friend's house, attend camp, or go to school (school phobia). Psychophysiologic symptoms, such as headache, nausea, vomiting, and stomachache, are seen frequently when the child anticipates separation or when it actually occurs. The child may show a reluctance or refusal to go to sleep at night or stay alone in the home, possibly withdrawing socially. The child may become housebound or incapacitated in the severe form of separation anxiety disorder, due to the presence of morbid fears of illness, injury, danger, or death. Before a diagnosis is made, the symptoms must have been present for at least 4 weeks. See Clinical Example 29-4. See Chapters 19 and 20 for additional information on anxiety.

Mood Disorders

The idea that children can develop conditions that are the same as the depressive disorders of adults has been controversial. However, children and adolescents have exhibited clinical symptoms of dysthymic disorder, major depressive disorder, and bipolar disorder. The use of symptom-oriented, personal interviews with children has led to widespread recognition that disorders resembling adult depression can and do occur in childhood. The *DSM-IV-TR* criteria for prepubertal, adolescent, and adult depression are identical.

Epidemiologic surveys indicate the prevalence of depressive disorders among children to be approximately 5% and range between 10% and 20% for adolescents. The gender ratio is approximately equal before puberty. This changes to a 2:1 female-to-male ratio when approaching adulthood. Depression is a major factor for suicide, the third leading cause of death among teens, and represents approximately 12% of the mortality rate in this age group (Melnyk &

> **CLINICAL EXAMPLE 29.4**
>
> ### THE CLIENT WITH SEPARATION ANXIETY DISORDER
>
> CW, 5 years old, began to complain of a stomachache each morning as her mother prepared to go to work. The complaint had persisted for approximately a week when CW began to wander into her parents' bedroom each night after she had gone to bed. During the day, the babysitter noticed that CW would follow her from room to room and refuse to play outside. The babysitter brought CW's behavior to the attention of her parents, who decided to consult the pediatrician. A diagnosis of separation anxiety disorder was made. Fortunately, CW's behavior was identified early in its development, and she responded well to the pediatrician's suggestions for managing her anxiety.

Moldenbauer, 1999). Supporting Evidence for Practice 29-1 highlights a study addressing adolescents and self-esteem, and possible risk for self-destructive acts.

The diagnostic characteristics of depression in children and adolescents are the same as those for adults (see Chapter 21). However, the clinical symptoms vary based on age. See the accompanying Clinical Symptoms and Diagnostic Characteristics box.

Adolescence is often a period of complicated and demanding conflicts. Teens undergo physical, emotional, psychological, and social changes. They are vulnerable to being overwhelmed by the many changes and pressures during this critical time. The high rate of depression and suicide among young people has prompted researchers to identify those factors relevant to adolescent depression.

Adjustment Disorders

An adjustment disorder is differentiated from other disorders in that the maladaptive reaction is in response to an identifiable, stress-producing event or situation and is not the result of or part of a mental disorder. The reaction usually occurs within 3 months after the onset of the stressor, manifests itself as impaired social or occupational functioning, and is exaggerated beyond the

SUPPORTING EVIDENCE FOR PRACTICE 29.1
The Relationship Between Self-Esteem and Lifestyle Choices by Adolescents

PROBLEM UNDER INVESTIGATION / What effect does self-esteem have on adolescent coping strategies and behavioral choices?

SUMMARY OF THE RESEARCH / The study consisted of 1,237 adolescent subjects between the ages of 11 and 18 years in a rural school district who were given the Miller Self-Esteem Questionnaire. Sixty percent of the sample were female and 46% were African American.

More than 33% did not have a father in the home, and 12% received food stamps. The average self-esteem score among the subjects was 3.0 (slightly above average) on a 4.0 scale. African American students scored higher than white students. Although the overall score did not differ between boys and girls, girls scored higher

in the areas of acceptance, popularity, and self-worth. Boys showed a higher sense of victimization and manipulation.

SUPPORT FOR PRACTICE / Psychiatric–mental health nurses who work with adolescents should consider racial and gender differences when exploring adolescent self-esteem. Positive self-esteem influences lifestyle choices and helps promote participation in various activities, whereas low self-esteem can impair school performance and lead to negative behavior including self-destructive acts.

SOURCE: Hendricks, C. S., Tavakoli, A., Hendricks, D. L., et al. (2001). *Self-esteem matters: Racial and gender differences among rural southern adolescents.* Journal of National Black Nurses Association, 12, *15–22.*

---

normal reaction to an identified stressor. Remission of the reaction usually occurs within 6 months as the stressor diminishes or disappears.

The *DSM-IV-TR* lists six subtypes of adjustment disorders based on the behavioral manifestations:

1. With depressed mood
2. With anxiety
3. With mixed anxiety and depressed mood
4. With disturbance of conduct
5. With mixed disturbance of emotions and conduct
6. Unspecified

The specifiers *acute* (less than 6 months) and *chronic* (6 months or longer) are used to indicate the persistence of symptoms. The criteria listed apply to children, adolescents, and adults.

Stress-Producing Events or Situations. Types of stressors considered include natural or man-made disasters; unwanted pregnancy; physical illness or injury; developmental stressors (eg, puberty, adolescence, or menopause); legal difficulties (eg, being arrested or incarcerated); financial problems; living circumstances (eg, change in residence or immigration); occupational changes (eg, unemployment or retirement); conjugal stressors (eg, separation or death of a spouse); par-

enting (eg, becoming a parent); and interpersonal problems (eg, relating to one's friends, neighbors, or associates). A review of Erikson's eight developmental stages or Havighurst's six periods of development is suggested to help one identify anticipated transitions and resulting conflicts or stressors that can occur at various times in life, especially during childhood or adolescence (Chapter 24).

Young children are considered quite vulnerable to stressors because of limited coping abilities and dependency on their environment. Vacationing with the family, starting school, and changing teachers are considered minimal-to-mild stressors, whereas the divorce of parents, hospitalization, the death of a peer, or a geographic move could be considered severe stressors. Examples of extreme stress in children include repeated physical or sexual abuse, or the death of a parent.

Adolescence has received attention as one of the most difficult adjustment periods. Breaking up with a steady significant other, being "cut" from a sport, experiencing the death of a peer, or leaving home for the first time are examples of stressors that may occur during adolescence, any of which may result in adjustment disorders. When the adolescent receives support during this developmental period, the likelihood of the onset of additional emotional disturbances is lessened.

CLINICAL SYMPTOMS AND DIAGNOSTIC CHARACTERISTICS /
CHILDHOOD AND ADOLESCENT DEPRESSION

CLINICAL SYMPTOMS OF CHILDHOOD DEPRESSION

- Pervasive sadness that is constantly present
- Withdrawal
- Irritable, negative behavior demonstrating the inability to have fun; destructive tendencies
- Low self-esteem
- Excessive guilt feelings, especially over minor incidents or situations that are not the child's fault
- Sleep disturbance such as insomnia, night terrors, or excessive napping
- Running-away behavior
- Changes in appetite such as decrease or lack of appetite or overeating
- Somatic or physical complaints such as headaches, stomachaches, or earaches
- Difficulty in school as evidenced by inattention, school anxiety, or a sudden change in performance, resulting in poor grades
- Preoccupation with death, such as undue concern about the health of a parent, persistent thoughts related to the death of a pet, or suicidal thoughts

CLINICAL SYMPTOMS OF ADOLESCENT DEPRESSION

- Sadness
- Fluctuation between apathy and talkativeness
- Anger and rage; verbal sarcasm and attack
- Overreaction to criticism

- Guilt
- Feelings of being unable to satisfy ideals
- Low self-esteem
- Loss of confidence
- Feelings of helplessness or hopelessness
- Intense ambivalence between dependence and independence
- Feelings of emptiness in life
- Restlessness and agitation
- Pessimism about the future
- Death wishes; suicidal thoughts, plans, or attempts
- Rebellious refusal to work in class or cooperate in general
- Sleep disturbances
- Increased or decreased appetite, severe weight loss or gain

DIAGNOSTIC CHARACTERISTICS

Same as those for adults; see Chapter 21.

THE NURSING PROCESS

ASSESSMENT

Winters and Tsai (2005) address pertinent issues that are important in the assessment of children and adolescents. For example, the rapid pace of children's development requires familiarity with the different competencies, vulnerabilities, and tasks of each developmental stage. Various methods of collecting data and interviewing the child apply at different ages. Assessment of an infant or toddler generally occurs in the presence of a parent or caregiver with special attention to their interactions, whereas adolescents usually provide more pertinent clinical information when assessed alone. Younger children may not have the understanding or ability to describe feeling states.

The assessment of a young person is often complicated by the interaction of psychopathology with the child's environment and with developmental processes. Presenting clinical symptoms determine the extent to which a medical history, physical, and neurologic examination are necessary, with laboratory testing as indicated. Schopick (2005) warns that children and adolescents who have a history of taking atypical antipsychotics to control mood or behavior disorders should be assessed for extrapyramidal symp-

BOX 29.2 SUMMARY OF A COMPREHENSIVE ASSESSMENT OF CHILDREN AND ADOLESCENTS

REASON FOR REFERRAL

Why and by whom

HISTORY OF CURRENT PROBLEM

Present problem and response to any past psychological and pharmacologic treatment

MEDICAL HISTORY AND PHYSICAL EXAMINATION

Include family history of any medical or psychiatric problems

Include history of physical, sexual, or substance abuse or violence experiences

NEUROLOGIC EVALUATION WHEN INDICATED

DEVELOPMENTAL HISTORY

Current developmental level

MENTAL STATUS AND EMOTIONAL ASSESSMENT

Current cognitive functioning, coping, and critical thinking skills

Recent stressors or losses, suicidal ideation and attempts

RELATIONSHIP WITH FAMILY

Roles, relationships, and communication styles

Cultural and religious observances

ENVIRONMENTAL SUPPORTS, CHANGES, AND EVENTS

Personal changes and community influences

NOTE: This summary is not intended to be all-inclusive. Additional information may be necessary to formulate a working diagnosis and to develop a plan of care.

---

toms because all of the atypicals have been implicated in neuromuscular or neurologic adverse effects. Gaffney (1996) discusses the essential components of a comprehensive assessment and notes that data are best obtained through semi-structured, open interviews (Box 29-2).

Assessment also focuses on the development of cognitive, communicative, physical, social, emotional, and adaptive self-help skills. Psychoeducational testing is conducted when the client's school functioning is impaired (Dulcan, Bregman, Weller, & Weller, 1998; Walsh, 2002). Examples of clinical assessment tools for children and adolescents are described in Box 29-3.

Assessment of a Child

Communication with children takes skill, thoughtfulness, and practice. Toddlers and preschoolers need time to complete their thoughts without interruption. This requires patience because the child's thoughts often don't seem logical. School-age children can grasp the seriousness of events around them and comprehend the impact of various stressors on themselves and others (Deering & Cody, 2002).

When assessing a child, interviewing at least one parent or adult caretaker is desirable to integrate information regarding the child's internalizing symptoms. Play therapy is often used because children have a limited ability to express themselves verbally. In this therapy, play materials are provided for the child to act out feelings and behaviors. The use of board games during the assessment of a school-age child may facilitate verbal interaction, especially regarding rules.

Attempt to explore all of the possibilities that could explain a child's behavior to determine if any additional problems such as learning disabilities, conduct disorders, or depression may be present. Exploration also helps to provide information about the family structure and classroom situation and to determine the child's thinking ability and academic skills.

Assessment, although challenging, can be completed. Additional challenges are presented when the child is suspected of having an autistic disorder, ADHD, or psychosis.

Assessment of a Child With Autistic Disorder.

Assessment for autism is based on evidence of specific behaviors indicated by direct observation and through

BOX 29.3 CLINICAL ASSESSMENT TOOLS FOR CHILDREN AND ADOLESCENTS

MENTAL STATUS

Mini-Mental Status Examination for a Child: Focuses on orientation, sexual identity, relationships with parents and peers, fantasy life, ability to identify feelings, risk behavior (suicide, homicide, chemical abuse), and history of physical or sexual abuse

ADAPTIVE BEHAVIOR

Vineland Adaptive Behavior Scales: Assesses children, adolescents to 18 years, and low-functioning adults. Focuses on four behavior domains: communication, daily living skills, socialization, and motor skills

AUTISM

Childhood Autism Rating Scale (CARS): Focuses on ability to relate to people, body use, adaptation to change, listening responses, and verbal communication. Estimates severity of disorder

Gilliam Autism Rating Scale (GARS): Assesses ages 3 through 22. Focuses on stereotyped behaviors, communication, social interaction, and developmental disturbances. Estimates severity of problem

ATTENTION SPAN

Tests of Variables of Attention (TOVA): Objective, standardized, continuous performance tests used to assess attention. There are two versions: TOVA is the visual version and TOVAA is the auditory version.

ADHD

Conners Parent Questionnaire: A 48-item scale completed by a parent.

Conners Teacher Questionnaire: A 28-item scale completed by a teacher.

ADHD Rating Scale: A scale related to *DSM-IV-TR* criteria completed by parents or teachers

Child Behavior Checklist (CBL): A 118-item questionnaire completed by a parent. Also includes questions about specific behaviors and psychiatric symptoms.

DISRUPTIVE BEHAVIORS

Disruptive Behavior Disorder Rating Scale (DBD): This 45-item scale is a checklist completed by parents and teachers to determine whether a child or adolescent meets the symptom criteria of *DSM-IV-TR* diagnoses of ADHD, oppositional defiant disorder, or conduct disorder.

DEPRESSION

Children's Depression Inventory (CDI): For ages 7–17 years, this seven-item scale rates feelings and behaviors over the last 2-week period.

Reynolds Child Depression Scale (RCDS): For ages 8–13 years, this 30-item scale rates frequency of depressive symptoms over the last 2-week period.

Reynolds Adolescent Depression Scale (RADS): For ages 12–18 years, this 30-item scale rates severity of current depressive symptoms.

SUICIDE

Reynolds Suicide Ideation Questionnaire Junior (SIQ-JR): For ages 13–19 years, this 15-item self-report questionnaire indicates the current level of suicidal ideation.

OTHER

Guidelines for Adolescent Preventive Services (GAPS): For ages 11–21 years, this is a primary-care screening tool highlighting topics or conditions common among adolescents.

Teacher Report Form (TRF): For school-age children, this tool assesses social competencies and childhood problems.

HEADSS

For children and adolescents. Assesses home environment; education/employment; activities; use of drugs by client, family members, or peers; sexuality, behavior, and orientation; history or presence of clinical symptoms of depressed mood and suicidal ideation or attempts.

parent consultation. Functional assessment and play-based assessment combined with parent interviews may help determine the diagnosis of an autistic disorder (Mercer, 2002).

Children suspected of having autistic disorder or a related developmental disorder may also be evaluated by a treatment team consisting of a developmental specialist, pediatrician or neurologist, psychologist, speech–language pathologist, and physician or occupational therapist. The most prevalent diagnostic tool is the Childhood Autism Rating Scale (CARS) described in Box 29-3. Although there are no specific medical tests or procedures to confirm a diagnosis of autism, medical tests that might be administered to rule out coexisting conditions include metabolic screening, and hearing, electroencephalographic (EEG), and genetic testing (Church, 1996; Mercer, 2002).

In a recent study published in the August 10, 2004, *Proceedings of the National Academy of Sciences,* researchers described the use of home videos as part of the assessment to differentiate Asperger's disorder from autism. According to the researchers, the persistent presence or total absence of motor reflexes serve as early detection markers for abnormal neurologic development in Asperger's disorder and autism (Literature Monitor, 2004).

Assessment of a Child With ADHD. The assessment of a child with ADHD primarily consists of a detailed history provided by parents and teachers if the child attends school; observation; the use of behavior-rating scales to quantify behavioral information; and a medical examination including ophthalmologic and hearing evaluations. In most cases no laboratory tests or other medical studies are warranted. An EEG is performed if the history of physical examination suggests the possibility of seizures. Psychoeducational testing by a psychologist is important to identify learning disabilities or general intellectual deficiency. A combination of assessment tools as described in Box 29-3 may be used to rule out the possibility of coexisting conditions such as learning disabilities, behavior problems, developmental disorders, food allergies, sleep disorder, mood disorder, anxiety disorder, conduct disorder, or ODD (Colyar, 2002; Glod, 2001; Myers et al.,2003).

For example, many symptoms of ADHD and bipolar disorder overlap, including distractibility, physical hyperactivity, and talkativeness. Comorbid ADHD is nearly universal in youths with bipolar disorder; and comorbid mania has been noted in 16% of children with ADHD. An accurate assessment is essential because planning interventions, especially choosing medication, for these complex clients is difficult. Psychostimulants may worsen mania, and mood stabilizers may not resolve ADHD symptoms (Patel & Sallee, 2005).

Assessment of a Child or Adolescent With Psychosis. The American Academy of Child and Adolescent Psychiatry guidelines recommend that all medical disorders be ruled out before establishing the diagnosis of a psychotic disorder, such as early onset schizophrenia, but the guidelines do not specify which medical conditions should be considered. The following questions, developed to supplement existing guidelines, are asked to rule out substance-induced, pharmacologic, and general medical conditions that may cause or exacerbate psychotic symptoms in children between the ages of 3 and 18 years (Fohrman & Stein, 2006). Does the child or adolescent:

1. Take substances that may cause or exacerbate psychotic symptoms (see Box 29-1)?
2. Take medications that may cause or exacerbate psychotic symptoms?
3. Have a medical condition that may cause psychotic symptoms (see Box 29-1)?
4. Exhibit unexplained somatic signs or symptoms that suggest delirium or a neurologic, rheumatologic, infectious, or toxic cause?
5. Function significantly below age-expected norms developmentally?
6. Have an atypical clinical presentation such as severe psychomotor retardation, or is the client treatment resistant?

If the client displays a positive response to any of the questions, a complete physical examination, consultation with colleagues, diagnostic tests, or a referral should be performed to rule out potential medical conditions. If the responses to all of the questions are negative, psychosis is considered to be the primary psychiatric disorder. The essential features for schizophrenia are the same for children, adolescents, and adults; however, in children, delusional content revolves around ideas of reference, somatic preoccupations, or delusions of persecution. Hallucinations may be less elaborate than those observed in adolescents and adults, and visual hallucinations may be more common. Disorganized speech is observed in a number of disorders with childhood onset as is disorganized behavior. These symptoms should not be attributed to schizophrenia without due consideration of the more common disorders of childhood (APA, 2000). Atypical psychotic symptoms may represent a number of phenomena, including post-traumatic stress disorder (PTSD), factitious or conversion disorders, or developmental delays that interfere with the accurate reporting of internal experiences, difficulty distinguishing fantasy from reality, and/or misunderstanding the questions being asked (Hlastala & McClellan, 2005). (See Chapter 22 for additional information regarding clinical symptoms of schizophrenia).

Assessment of an Adolescent

Privacy is the single most important criterion by which adolescents judge their interactions with health care providers. Adolescents perceive people and events in extreme terms. They often have difficulty trusting that adults will treat them with respect and consider their viewpoints (Deering & Cody, 2002). Failure to offer a promise of confidentiality can almost guarantee suspicion and evasiveness by the teen-aged client.

The significance of the nurse's approach during the assessment of an adolescent cannot be overstated. A nonjudgmental approach that makes no assumptions is important. Listening and waiting patiently for responses to open-ended questions also are key. Cohen and colleagues developed the HEADSS assessment tool for obtaining a psychosocial history from teens (see Box 29-3). The acronym stands for Home, Education/employment, Activities, Drugs, Sexuality, and Suicide/depression (Deering & Cody, 2002). This tool provides a natural pattern of progression during the assessment process, beginning with assessment of the adolescent's home situation and ending with discussion about clinical symptoms related to suicide and depression. The tool also allows the nurse to organize and remember important elements of the adolescent's psychosocial history.

Transcultural Considerations

Attention to ethnic and cultural background is important with intelligence testing to avoid a misdiagnosis such as mental retardation. Also consider cultural habits when assessing for disorders such as mental retardation or a pervasive developmental disorder. Immigrant children may be diagnosed with a communication disorder because of refusal to speak to strangers or inability to speak the language of the host country. The diagnosis of conduct disorder may be given to a teenager who, in fact, is exhibiting a specific behavior necessary for survival. The environment, including social and economic context, requires assessment before a diagnosis is made.

NURSING DIAGNOSES

Nursing diagnoses for children and adolescents are based on the client's problems, strengths, and coping abilities; adaptiveness of the symptoms; and inferences about the etiology of the specific disorder. Developing nursing diagnoses for a child with a psychiatric–mental health disorder often is difficult because:

- Children can be inconsistent and unpredictable in behavior
- The relationship and degree of comfort with the examiner affects the results of data collected
- Children are developing constantly
- Children are affected and shaped by their parents (Johnson, 1997)

See the accompanying box, Examples of North American Nursing Diagnosis Association (NANDA) Nursing Diagnoses: Disorders of Infancy, Childhood, and Adolescence.

OUTCOME IDENTIFICATION

Outcomes generally focus on a reduction of clinical symptoms; decreased stress; progression of normal developmental stages; and therapeutic changes. Outcomes are individualized to the child or adolescent, family, social environment, and school; measurable; and time-limited to goals. Given the long-term nature of childhood and adolescent disorders, outcomes may change several times (Johnson, 1997; Scahill, Hamrin, & Deering, 2002).

PLANNING INTERVENTIONS

Planning interventions is a collaborative effort with the client and parents, possibly requiring the involvement of other disciplines or community supports. To ensure continuity of care and prevent fragmentation of care, the psychiatric–mental health nurse assumes the role of case manager.

Treatment is based on the needs and problems of the client and family. Planning interventions includes prioritizing the target symptoms and determining which treatment methods are best suited to reduce them. Clinicians involved in the planning and implementation of care must collaborate with the family toward the same general outcomes.

As stated earlier, the relationship and degree of comfort the child or adolescent feels with the psychiatric nurse affect the type of data collected. The same can be said for the response of a child or adolescent during the planning and implementing of nursing interventions. Following are a list of guidelines to be considered when planning therapeutic interventions for children or adolescents:

EXAMPLES OF NANDA NURSING DIAGNOSES/ DISORDERS OF INFANCY, CHILDHOOD, AND ADOLESCENCE

ADHD

- Disturbed Sleep Pattern related to excessive hyperactivity secondary to ADHD
- Interrupted Family Processes related to disruption of family routines due to time-consuming care of child with ADHD
- Risk for Injury related to poor safety awareness as evidenced by hyperactivity, impulsivity, and distractibility

Conduct Disorder

- Risk for Other-Directed Violence related to history of aggressive acts secondary to temporal lobe epilepsy
- Impaired Social Interaction related to alienation from others secondary to impulsive behavior and overt hostility
- Hopelessness related to separation from parents as evidenced by "giving-up complex"

Autistic Disorder

- Disturbed Sensory Perception related to diminished awareness of environmental stimuli
- Self-Mutilation as evidenced by repetitive head-banging and scratching
- Impaired Social Interaction with peers and parents related to withdrawal
- Impaired Verbal Communication related to inadequate verbal skills as evidenced by repetitive, idiosyncratic speech
- Self-Care Deficit related to repetitive, ritualistic behavior

Separation Anxiety Disorder

- Disturbed Sleep Pattern related to anxiety as evidenced by verbalizing fear and nightmares
- Anxiety related to separation from mother as evidenced by crying and regressive behavior

Note: See specific chapters for Nursing Diagnoses related to Depression, Anxiety, and Psychosis.

- Accept the child or adolescent client as an equal when able, keeping in mind the person's age.
- Do not use baby talk or substandard English, or talk down while communicating with the child or adolescent. Listen to the emotions expressed and encourage verbalization of feelings.
- Do not force yourself on the client or push him or her to confide in you.
- Accept the client but discuss any undesirable behavior. Ignoring behavior such as tics also may be acceptable. Each behavior needs to be evaluated to decide the appropriate approach.
- Be a good role model.
- Be aware of body language and nonverbal communication. Children and adolescents are quite observant of what adults say and how they communicate feelings both verbally and nonverbally. They should know that adults have good and bad days that can affect their interpersonal relationships, especially in the area of communication.

Typically, adults are viewed as role models for children and adolescents. The following rules to live by for adult role models were written by boys in a reform school for delinquent behavior. Such suggestions can serve as guidelines for nurses as they plan interventions for children and adolescents in the psychiatric setting:

- Do not lose control in stressful situations because children are great imitators of parental behavior.
- Do not use alcohol or pills as a crutch. Your behavior tells children that it is okay to do the same.
- Be a strict and consistent disciplinarian. Call a bluff. Do not compromise. Such an attitude denotes love and provides security. Children do not always want what they ask for; they just test adults.
- Set a good spiritual example. Children need to know that a supreme being exists.
- Do not try to imitate children by dressing, talking, or acting younger. Children need good role models, not adults who try to be peers.
- Be honest and give a few compliments if they are deserved.

Other aspects when planning nursing interventions include (1) helping the child or adolescent master developmental tasks to overcome regressive, slow, or impaired developmental behavior; (2) establishing a method of communication with clients who have difficulty communicating, such as the withdrawn, disoriented, mute, hostile, preoccupied, or autistic child or adolescent; (3) identifying stimuli that might foster abusive, destructive, or otherwise negative behavior; and (4) allowing time for the client to respond to therapeutic interventions.

Nurses should be aware of their own reactions to clients' behaviors as they plan interventions. If unable to handle feelings or behaviors, seek assistance from peers or supervisory personnel. Also plan interventions that demonstrate respect for the child or adolescent's spatial territory and do not invade his or her privacy. Consider the use of therapeutic touch only after exploring the client's feelings about being touched (eg, a battered or abused child would probably withdraw and resist touch).

Activities are planned that are appropriate for the client's developmental level and age. This activity planning must consider the client's energy level and need to calm down after an activity.

IMPLEMENTATION

Specific nursing interventions are discussed for the following disorders of infancy, childhood, and adolescence: mental retardation, ADHD, conduct disorder, autistic disorder, childhood and adolescent depression, and anxiety.

Interventions for Mental Retardation

As stated previously, clients with mental retardation may be educable or trainable, or require custodial care. Such persons may have a dual diagnosis of mental retardation and mental illness, as well as a physical disability or limitation. Treatment is based on the needs of the client as well as attention to comorbid medical conditions.

Assistance in Meeting Basic Needs. The nurse working in an institutional setting is challenged to provide environmental stimulation as well as meet the emotional and physical needs of the child because clients with mental retardation do not always communicate physical symptoms or needs. Helping the child master activities of daily living may be a slow process involving behavioral therapy. Cognitive therapy has been used when clients are able to follow instructions. Psychodynamic therapy may be used to assist the client in dealing with conflicts that result in persistent anger, rage, resentment, or depression. Protective care may be necessary if the client experiences seizures, is prone to acting-out behavior, is disoriented, or engages in self-mutilating behaviors such as head-banging or biting oneself. The administration of anticonvulsant and psychotropic drugs may be necessary to stabilize behavior and clinical symptoms of any comorbid medical or psychiatric disorders (Sadock & Sadock, 2003).

Client and Family Education. Education of clients who are mentally retarded requires a comprehensive program that addresses communication skills, social skills, and vocational training to prepare clients for real-life situations and provide supportive feedback (Sadock & Sadock, 2003).

Education of the family is an important factor not to be overlooked, because some clients who are mentally retarded attend an institution during the week but go home for weekend or holiday visits. Others attend a day hospital, special school, or sheltered workshop, and return home at night as well as on weekends. The nurse is the client's advocate, both in the institutional setting and when relating to the family. Identifying the family's ability to cope and continue with the therapy at home is important to promote progress, thereby minimizing the stress and conflicts associated with family expectations that can occur when changing environments (Sadock & Sadock, 2003).

Interventions for Attention-Deficit Hyperactivity Disorder

ADHD is a complex disorder affecting every area of functioning and thereby requires a comprehensive treatment program. Unsuccessful treatment often occurs when comorbid diagnoses are not identified and addressed. Collaboration with a child's school is usually critical to ensure academic progress (Stubbe, 2005).

In 2001, the American Academy of Pediatrics published practice guidelines for treatment of school-age children with ADHD (American Pediatric Association, 2001). Traditionally, the most common therapy for ADHD has been stimulant medication. A multifactorial approach of behavioral therapy, group therapy, classroom interventions, client education about medication management, and family education is now recommended (Myers et al., 2003; Pelham, 2001).

Experiencing nature after school and during weekend activities may be considered a therapeutic intervention for children with ADHD. The result of a research study comparing the therapeutic effects of indoor and outdoor settings in the treatment of ADHD were recently reviewed. Parents were asked to compare the aftereffects of three different types of environment: indoor, green outdoor (eg, parks, farms), and built outdoor settings (eg, parking lots, school grounds). The findings suggested that green outdoor settings reduced ADHD symptoms significantly more than indoor or built outdoor settings (Foley, 2005).

Assistance in Meeting Basic Needs. The nurse's role is to provide a safe, structured environment that reduces anxiety and the possibility of injury resulting from impulsive, unpredictable behavior. Such an environment also provides the client with an opportunity to complete tasks that the client commonly fails to finish (eg, activities of daily living) because of poor self-regulation and easy distractibility. Sleep hygiene measures (eg, establishment of a consistent bedtime routine and avoidance of stimulating activities just before bedtime) may be necessary because sleep problems are common among children with ADHD (Efron & Pearl, 2003).

Working with the family or teachers also is important to plan a firm, consistent environment in which limits and standards are set. Behavior modification and behavior contracts are used to promote positive behavior. Social-skills training is used with children who exhibit aggressive, impulsive, and socially damaging behaviors. The goal is to change the relationships between children who are socially isolated and their peer groups by showing children how their behavior affects others.

Some children or adolescents with ADHD exhibit anxiety, depression, self-esteem problems, and other emotional difficulties. Therefore, psychotherapy may be provided by the psychiatric–mental health nurse practitioner. Family therapy also may be helpful to deal with sibling concerns or other family problems such as divorce or the loss of a loved one (Sadock & Sadock, 2003).

Client and Family Education. Medication therapy remains one of the most successful treatments for the client with ADHD. The child or adolescent, family, and school personnel (when necessary) are taught about the various types of medication used. Psychostimulants stimulate the areas of the brain that control attention, impulses, and self-regulation of behavior (See Chapter 16 for additional information). Other medications may be given to stabilize clinical symptoms of comorbid disorders such as depression, tic disorders, psychosis, anxiety, and obsessive–compulsive traits. Drug Summary Table 29-1 highlights selected drugs used for childhood and adolescent disorders. The parents and teachers are then asked to complete a form to evaluate the client's response to medication. These observations enable the nurse to determine which medication and dose are most efficacious.

Children do not typically outgrow ADHD; it often persists into adult life. When this occurs, intervention strategies focus on addressing psychosocial issues (eg, relationships and social functioning) and symptom management of hyperactivity, inattention, and impulsivity. As with children and adolescents, stimulant medication may be prescribed (Waite, 2004).

DRUG SUMMARY TABLE 29-1 Drugs Used for Childhood and Adolescent Disorders

GENERIC (TRADE) NAME	DAILY DOSAGE RANGE	IMPLEMENTATION
Drug Class: Stimulants		
amphetamine (Adderal)	5–60 mg (Dosage is age related; ages 3 and older)	Know that dosing depends upon age of client; give drug upon awakening and 4–6 hours apart, avoid late-evening dosing; administer Adderal XR once daily; tell client to swallow whole or sprinkle contents of capsule on food; monitor for anorexia, insomnia, GI upset, emotional liability, dizziness, tachycardia, and headache.
methylphenidate (Concerta)	18–72 mg (Dosage is age related)	Contraindicated in anxiety, motor tics, Tourette's syndrome, glaucoma, or during or within 14 days of MAOI use; monitor for paradoxical excitation, seizures, headache, anorexia, insomnia, dyskinesia, rash, and visual disturbances.

(Continued on following page)

DRUG SUMMARY TABLE 29-1 Drugs Used for Childhood and Adolescent Disorders *(Cont'd)*

GENERIC (TRADE) NAME	DAILY DOSAGE RANGE	IMPLEMENTATION
Drug Class: Nonstimulant SNRI		
atomoxetine (Strattera)	0.5–100 mg (Dosage is age related)	Monitor for GI disturbances, decreased appetite, dizziness, headache, fatigue, and mood swings; use is contraindicated during or within 14 days of MAOI therapy.
Drug Class: Antidepressants		
fluoxetine (Prozac)	10–80 mg (Dosage is age related; not recommended for younger than 8 years of age)	Contraindicated during or within 14 days of MAOI therapy; discontinue if unexplained allergic reaction occurs; monitor for GI disturbance, CNS stimulation, headache, weight loss, tremor, thirst, hyperkinesias, epistaxis, and urinary frequency.
bupropion (Wellbutrin)	150–300 mg	Know that dosage is 3–6 mg/kg given in divided doses b.i.d. or t.i.d.; monitor for CNS stimulant effects (eg, agitation, increased motor activity), dry mouth, headache, nausea and vomiting, and constipation.
venlafaxine (Effexor)	25–150 mg	Give in divided doses not to exceed total daily dose of 150 mg; should not be taken concurrently or within 14 days of MAOI therapy; monitor for hypertension, dreams, tremor, dizziness, somnolence, GI disturbance, and dry mouth.
Drug Class: Antipsychotics		
olanzapine (Zyprexa)	2.5–10 mg	Monitor for weight gain, EPS, TD, NMS, orthostatic hypotension, agranulocytosis, changes in blood sugar and serum lipid levels, constipation, dry mouth, seizures, and somnolence.
risperidone (Risperdal)	0.5–4 mg	Mix oral solution with water, juice, or low-fat milk; monitor for weight gain and adverse effects listed above for Zyprexa.
ziprasidone (Geodon)	20–160 mg	Monitor ECG for Q-T changes; monitor for adverse effects similar to those of Zyprexa.
Drug Class: Anticonvulsants		
carbamazepine (Tegretol) (Available as Tegretol-XR and Tegretol suspension, also)	20–1200 mg (Dosage is age related)	Target serum carbamazepine level is 7.0; monitor CBC, LFTs, BUN, thyroid, and sodium levels; contraindicated in sensitivity to TCAs and during or within 14 days of MAOI therapy; monitor for adverse effects such as rash, photosensitivity, dizziness, drowsiness; advise parents to report fever, infection, sore throat, or mouth ulcers.

Interventions for Oppositional Defiant Disorder and Conduct Disorder

Both ODD and conduct disorder require interventions that address overt and covert behaviors. Multimodality treatment programs using family and community resources are considered to be the most successful forms of intervention (Sadock & Sadock, 2003).

Providing nursing interventions for a client with ODD can be quite challenging because the client may have a chronologic age of 10 years, maturational age as that of a teenager, and frustration tolerance of a 2-year-old (Imperio, 2001). Inpatient treatment is used if the client is unmanageable at home or has been placed in a treatment center by a judge's order of detention (eg, juvenile detention center or residential treatment center).

The primary treatment is family intervention focusing on assessment of family interactions and direct training of parents in child management skills. All areas and settings in which the client exhibits behavior problems should be identified and addressed. Clients may benefit from behavioral therapy designed to discourage oppositional behavior and to encourage appropriate behavior. Individual psychotherapy provides the client with an opportunity to restore self-esteem and practice adaptive responses to adult or authority figures (eg, role-playing). Anger-management training is recommended but not widely available (Imperio, 2001; Sadock & Sadock, 2003; Perepletchikova & Kazdin, 2005).

Providing interventions for clients with the diagnosis of conduct disorder can also be quite challenging. The following nursing interventions incorporate the suggestions of boys with the diagnosis of conduct disorder and living in a reform school:

- Establish trust by being honest.
- Maintain control by setting limits for manipulative, acting-out behavior.
- Be consistent with limit-setting.
- Respect the client's age and maintain an adult–child or adult–adult relationship, whichever is appropriate.
- Establish realistic expectations. Discuss such expectations with the client and encourage verbalization of feelings.

Assistance in Meeting Basic Needs. Nursing interventions for ODD and conduct disorder focus on maintaining safety and helping the child or adolescent develop internal limits, problem-solving skills, and self-responsibility for acts of antisocial behavior, which may include physical violence, theft, fire-setting, assault, or callous or manipulative behavior. The client may have to be removed from home to benefit from a consistent therapeutic environment.

Young clients with conduct disorder often have underlying medical problems; therefore, nursing interventions may include treatment for a medical condition such as epilepsy or a closed head injury. Because conduct disorders do not resolve without intervention, appropriate planning and treatment are essential.

Additional nursing interventions aimed at helping young people realize and understand the effect their behavior has on others may include cognitive problem solving/skills training in either individual or group sessions. Medication may also be used to alleviate clinical symptoms of overt explosive or aggressive behavior; depression; or other comorbid disorders such as ADHD and PTSD. Examples of psychopharmacologic therapy are given in Drug Summary Table 29-1.

Client and Family Education. Both the client and family require education about the etiology of conduct disorder or ODD, and should be informed that adequate treatment of the client's clinical symptoms and any comorbid psychiatric disorders such as depression, PTSD, or seizure disorder often make such disruptive disorders go away. The rationale for the use of any psychoactive medication is explained and reinforced. Family interactions and parenting skills are explored because most children or adolescents with the diagnosis of conduct disorder or ODD come from households in which discipline was inconsistent and sometimes brutal. Rarely are such children held accountable for their actions; parents often surrender to the demands of the child or adolescent. Children said to have conduct disorder or ODD may just need help fitting into society through discipline, mentoring, job training, and coaching in independent living skills (Bates, 1999).

Interventions for Autistic Disorder

Autism is very difficult to treat because it is considered the most irreversible childhood disorder. The most clinically relevant interventions in the treatment of autistic disorder are speech–language therapy to promote communication development; behavioral therapy to stabilize behavioral difficulties; and educational placement to enhance and support social and academic skills. Although there is no specific pharmacologic treatment for autism, selective serotonin reuptake inhibitors (SSRIs) have proven effective to control repetitive, self-stimulating habits and tics. The use of psychotropic medications is aimed primarily at treating comorbid psychiatric disorders or to augment psychosocial interventions (Mercer, 2002; Stubbs & Cheng, 2005).

According to a Boston study led by Ellen Hanson, the use of complementary and alternative medicine (CAM) is very common among children with autistic spectrum disorders. The most common therapies include a modified diet, vitamins/minerals/food supplements, and prayer/shaman. The use of CAM is believed to help the family find some peace when they are working so hard to help their children (Wendling, 2005).

Assistance in Meeting Basic Needs. The nurse faces several challenges when implementing interventions, resulting from the child's inability to develop normal relationships with anyone; inability to verbalize needs; preoccupation with objects; and unpredictable behavioral changes. Remember that not all autistic individuals respond alike. Feedback from family members and/or previous care providers is invaluable to help individualize the client's care.

Determining the most effective mode of communication will greatly aid in client interaction. Speak calmly when giving instructions in direct, short phases, and repeat instructions if necessary. Allow adequate time for delayed responses to questions or directions.

A safe, consistent environment is provided to prevent self-destructive behavior and to minimize unpredictable behavior caused by hypersensitivity to certain environmental stimuli. Medication may be given to provide symptomatic relief of anxiety, hyperactivity, stereotypical, or self-destructive behavior. The environment gives the client an opportunity to develop tolerance for physical closeness and to establish a meaningful interpersonal relationship. The client is also encouraged to participate in self-care.

Behavior Management. Behavior management is implemented in a variety of ways. Grandin (2002) discusses therapeutic interventions for children with autism, recommending that hyperactive autistic clients who fidget all the time wear a "padded, weighted" vest. Pressure from the garment helps to calm the child. Desired behavior may be achieved by reading "social stories" to the child or adolescent. Such stories are used to describe step-by-step directions for completing an activity in a social setting. The psychiatric–mental health nurse helps the client's family develop strategies to minimize difficult behavior effectively by employing behavioral therapy at home.

Client and Family Education. The client and family members are educated about the newest and different forms of educational interventions available in the treatment of autistic disorder. Occupational therapy is used to develop or improve fine motor or sensory skills. Physical therapy is provided to improve gross motor skills. Virtual reality may be used to create a simplified world made up of only what the client is taught. For example, two autistic children ages 7 and 9

years were taught by a word recognition therapist to walk to a stop sign, look for cars, recognize cars, follow their motion, and cross the street only when the cars passed. The client may also be enrolled in special-education classes or extended day services that incorporate behavioral methods in their curriculums.

Family members are also taught the concepts and skills of behavior modification. They may also be instructed in the use of facilitated communication techniques in which a child is taught to pick out letters or pictures on a computer or letter/picture board to indicate their needs or express their feelings (Mercer, 2002; Sadock & Sadock, 2003). Family caregivers are also educated about the benefits of respite services.

Interventions for Mood Disorders

It is important that intervention includes psychoeducation about the disease process of a mood disorder, the nature of the treatment available, prognosis of the disorder, and the impact of a mood disorder on the life of the client and family. Unlike adults, children may not have the vocabulary to accurately describe how they feel. Up to a certain age, they simply do not understand such complex concepts as self-esteem, guilt, or concentration. If they do not understand the concepts, they cannot express these feelings to the psychiatric–mental health nurse. Complicating matters is that—again, unlike adult clients—children and adolescents may not even recognize that they need help. Further, there is a higher percentage of suicidal ideation in children and adolescents than that which is observed in adults (Chapter 31). Thus, treatment for this younger group of clients is absolutely essential.

Assistance in Meeting Basic Needs. If an organic cause of the mood disorder such as depression has been identified (eg, anemia, chronic fatigue syndrome, endocrine disorder, premenstrual syndrome), interventions are provided to meet the medical and emotional needs of the client. Meeting the basic needs of the client may be challenging as the client may also be experiencing clinical symptoms of bipolar disorder (eg, mania, dysphoric mood, grandiosity, psychosis, impaired cognition).

According to the American Academy of Child and Adolescent Psychiatry (AACAP), an estimated one third of the 3.4 million children who experience depression also manifest clinical symptoms of bipolar disorder. In addition, more than 50% of pediatric clients with bipolar symptoms experienced major depressive disorder before the onset of their mania. Unfortunately, no test can diagnose pediatric bipolar disorder (Birmaher, 2004; Ferguson-Noyes, 2005).

Nursing interventions for clients with a mood disorder such as depression are similar to those provided for adult clients. A safe and therapeutic environment, a therapeutic relationship with the child or adolescent, and verbalization of feelings such as suicidal ideation or anger by the depressed client are the primary focus of care. Play or art therapy is used with children who are unable to verbalize their needs or feelings. Individual, cognitive, and group therapy may be used to explore issues related to low-self esteem. Family therapy is important to address any issues related to dysfunctional behavior and to increase available psychosocial support. Antidepressant medication may be utilized as an additional option if there is no significant improvement in the client's clinical symptoms. Although the SSRI fluoxetine (Prozac) is the only drug approved by the U.S. Food and Drug Administration (FDA) to treat depression in children ages 8 to 17 years, other SSRIs are also being used.

Consensus guidelines for the treatment of children with bipolar disorder were published in the March 2004 issue of the *Journal of the American Academy of Child and Adolescent Psychiatry*. Monotherapy with the traditional mood stabilizers and the atypical antipsychotics are recommended as the first-line treatment. Long-term interventions include pharmacotherapy, psychotherapy, and lifestyle modifications that promote stress reduction, sleep hygiene, supportive accommodations at school, and avoidance of the use of caffeine, alcohol, and illegal drugs. The guidelines are not intended to serve as an absolute standard of care but rather to assist in the evaluation and treatment of pediatric clients (Barclay & Vega, 2005). If antidepressant medication is prescribed, the client and family receive education about the drug(s) being taken.

According to the statistics based on an analysis of data from the National Ambulatory Medical Care survey (1990–2001), the rate of SSRI-prescribing for depressed children ages 5 to 18 years has increased significantly. Between 1990 and 1993, fluoxetine (Prozac) was considered to be the drug of choice prescribed for about 3% of children in that age group. By 1998 through 2001, SSRIs were prescribed for approximately 12% of children. Fluoxetine continued to be the drug of choice, followed by paroxetine (Paxil), sertraline (Zoloft), and citalopram (Celexa) (Foley & Reis, 2005). As noted in Chapter 16, the FDA has issued "black box" warnings that antidepressant drugs are associated with a risk of suicide in children. Advisers to the FDA have suggested that antidepressants should be sold with a guide that tells parents of children taking the drugs to monitor them for suicidal tendencies. Drug Summary Table 29-1 earlier in this chapter and Chapter 16 provide information about the use of antidepressant medication. Chapter 21 provides additional information regarding the treatment of depression.

Interventions for Childhood or Adolescent Psychosis

Usual and customary care of clients with childhood or adolescent psychosis focuses on pharmacotherapy to decrease the more impairing symptoms such as hallucinations, delusions, and bizarre ideation, as well as to improve mood and school performance. Adjunctive psychosocial interventions include psychoeducation of families, individual cognitive-behavioral strategies to help clients optimize their functioning and enjoyment of life, reduction of negative home environments; and collaboration with schools (Hlastala & McClellan, 2005).

Assistance in Meeting Basic Needs. Interventions similar to those provided for adult clients with psychotic symptoms are provided. They include the provision of a safe, structured environment to maintain biologic integrity and to protect the client from self-harm (see Chapter 22).

The most recent American Academy of Child and Adolescent Psychiatry (AACAP) treatment guidelines regarding the use of psychotropic medication to manage clinical symptoms of childhood psychosis (eg, early-onset schizophrenia) are based on the acute, recuperative, and recovery/residual phases of the psychotic disorder. For example, during the acute phase, when the client exhibits positive symptoms of psychosis and requires assistance with basic needs, atypical antipsychotic therapy (eg, olanzapine [Zyprexa] or risperidone [Risperdal]) should be used for at least 4 to 6 weeks before a determination is made regarding the efficacy of the agent. The use of a short-term benzodiazepine (eg, lorazepam [Ativan] or alprazolam [Xanax]) may be necessary as an adjunct to stabilize positive symptoms and agitation.

As positive symptoms improve during the recuperative phase, a gradual reduction of the dosage of the atypical antipsychotic may be indicated. If the client exhibits dysphoria, the client may benefit from an antidepressant, as noted earlier in the section regarding the treatment of mood disorder. A medication-free trial may be considered in newly diagnosed youths during the recovery phase if the client has been symptom free for at least 6 to 12 months (APA, 1997; Hlastala & McClellan, 2005).

Client and Family Education. Client and family psychoeducation generally focuses on developing strategies to cope with the effects of the illness, treatment options, and relapse prevention. The importance of medication compliance is stressed. Adverse effects of medication are discussed. Discuss the potential for weight gain secondary to the use of antipsychotic agents. Explain the importance of a healthy, balanced diet and exercise to maintain a normal weight and avoid weight gain that can cause serious health problems.

Various psychosocial interventions are utilized in the treatment of childhood psychosis. Individual psychotherapy alone has not proven effective; however, the combination of psychoeducation, family therapy with a focus on behavior management, and cognitive-behavioral therapy has been shown to reduce relapse rates (Hlastala & McClellan, 2006).

Interventions for Anxiety

A multimodal treatment plan in the initial management of anxiety disorder in children and adolescents consists of cognitive-behavioral therapy, family psychosocial intervention, and family education. Collaboration with school staff or counselors to maintain consistent intervention strategies is also important (Sadock & Sadock, 2003).

Assistance in Meeting Basic Needs. Nursing interventions focus on providing support and understanding. A stress-free environment enables the client to develop coping skills and gradually experience safe exposure to feared situations. Since the terrorist attacks on September 11, 2001, children feel especially fearful when there are media reports about threats of terrorism and war. Minor anxieties can develop into more severe problems (eg, nightmares, insomnia, nocturnal enuresis, aggression, withdrawal, or separation anxiety) if children are not encouraged to talk about their worries or fears.

Pharmacologic intervention may be utilized in symptom management; however, it should never be used as the sole intervention. SSRIs are considered to be the agents of choice. Benzodiazepines may be given concurrently with an SSRI until therapeutic level of the SSRI is achieved. They may also be used alone in the short-term treatment of anxiety (eg, school phobia). Anticonvulsant or antipsychotic agents may be useful when all other medications have not been successful or in children with borderline reality testing. Drug Summary Table 29-1 earlier in this chapter and Chapter 16 provide information about the use of medications used in the treatment of anxiety. Children should also be given an opportunity to describe interventions that would make them feel better or safer (Pearson, 2003; Sadock & Sadock, 2003; Bryant & Cheng, 2005).

Client and Family Education. Give parents reassurance that anxiety disorders are readily and effectively treated. Family interventions are critical in the management of phobias or separation anxiety disorder, especially in children who refuse to socialize or attend school. Parents are educated about the nature of anxiety and its impact on the family. They are taught how to identify antecedents to separation symptoms and the types of effective interventions. They are also taught how to provide firm encouragement of school attendance while obtaining available, appropriate mental health support. (Pearson, 2003; Sadock & Sadock, 2003; Bryant & Cheng, 2005).

Special Needs of Adolescents

Adolescent behavior during inpatient or outpatient treatment can be frustrating as well as challenging to the psychiatric–mental health nurse. During adolescence, the teenager faces two major conflicts, identity versus role confusion and independence versus dependence, as he or she attempts to establish a stable self-concept, make a career or vocational choice, and adjust to a comfortable sexual role.

Psychological needs that must be met include peer interactions, privacy, autonomy, and the opportunity to verbalize concerns about body image, sexual identity, and self-worth. Such needs may result in reactions of anger, dependency, embarrassment, fear, guilt, hostility, regression, or resentment. The adolescent may also display noncompliance with nursing interventions because of fear of losing control if the illness interrupts school and social life (Muscari, 1998). Table 29-4 provides a list of nursing interventions for emotional responses and behaviors of adolescents undergoing psychiatric–mental health treatment.

TABLE 29.4 Nursing Interventions for Emotional Responses and Behaviors of Adolescents

ADOLESCENT EMOTIONAL RESPONSES/BEHAVIORS	NURSING INTERVENTIONS
Fear	Accept defenses or behavior used to retain control. Discuss with the client when able. Give detailed explanations regarding treatment, nursing care, and progress.
	Encourage participation in care.
	Encourage questions and discuss concerns.
	Interpret medical terminology to decrease fears.
	Maintain consistency in care to discourage manipulative behavior.
Resentment	Explore feelings of resentment to identify underlying cause.
	Encourage visits with peers.
	Allow young siblings to visit.
	Permit flexible visiting hours when appropriate.
	Make arrangements for school work to continue.
	Do not "side" with parents if the adolescent displays hostility.
Embarrassment	Explain and maintain confidentiality.
	Provide an opportunity to discuss concerns, without family present if necessary.
	Be alert to feelings regarding body image and need for privacy.
	Encourage as much self-care as possible.
	Provide for personal space and minimal body exposure during care.
	Explain treatments, procedures, or surgery and impact on the body.
Homesickness	Provide, if possible, for home conveniences such as TV, telephone, and snacks.
	Arrange for dietary preferences when appropriate.
	Allow family members to bring in favorite foods if they are part of the diet prescribed by the attending physician.
	See that the client is kept informed of news at home.
Guilt	Give appropriate detailed explanations regarding illness and causative factors.
	Be positive in approaches and comments to reinforce interest in the client.
	Explain that hospitals are to help people, not punish them.
Manipulative behavior	Be consistent in expectations regarding rules and regulations for all clients.
	State the limits and behaviors expected from the client.
	Explore the client's perceptions and feelings.
	Avoid arguing, debating, or bargaining with the client.
	Confront the client, if necessary, regarding any manipulative ploys.
	Avoid a personal relationship.
Hostile, aggressive behavior	Be firm and consistent in treatment approaches.
	Accept the client but make it clear that certain behaviors are unacceptable.
	Try to determine what precipitated these feelings.
	Assist the client to explore alternative ways in handling feelings.
	Inform the client that he or she is to take responsibility for his or her actions.
	Be supportive and provide positive feedback when the client controls hostile or aggressive behavior.

CONTINUUM OF CARE

Various treatment options are available to provide continuity of care for children and adolescents with psychiatric-mental health disorders. The different interactive therapies for children and adolescents referenced in the text are also described.

Inpatient Hospitalization

Inpatient hospitalization of children or adolescents serves various purposes such as removing the child from a dysfunctional environment; treating severely disturbed behavior (eg, psychosis) in a controlled setting; providing protective care for suicidal, destructive, aggressive, or hyperactive behavior; or treating severe anxiety disorders.

Day-Treatment Hospitals

Treatment in a day hospital setting (partial hospitalization program) provides a therapeutic milieu for children and adolescents. It serves as an extended outpatient clinic during the day, yet allows children to return home to their families on evenings, nights, and weekends. Classrooms or special education programs are structured so that the child is able to continue his or her education while receiving psychiatric care.

Alternative Families

Runaways, delinquents, and disturbed children and adolescents often benefit from placement in the homes of alternative families. Children's services, group homes, and foster homes may provide much-needed physical and emotional care.

Individual Psychotherapy

Individual psychotherapy should include the following principles, which may serve as guidelines for a therapeutic nurse-client relationship:

- Accept the client but not necessarily the behavior. Remember that all behavior has meaning. The client may be acting out to receive attention or love. Limit-setting may be necessary to protect the client or therapist.
- Do not criticize the client.
- Avoid discussing symptoms with the client unless the client refers to them.

- Attempt to understand the client's feelings and point of view.

Individual psychotherapy may focus on specific problems, such as poor self-concept, feelings of depression, extreme dependency, or the inability to communicate.

Family Therapy (Systems Therapy)

In family or systems therapy, the family is viewed as a biosocial subsystem that may be functional or dysfunctional (faultily integrated). Dysfunctional families may display poor interpersonal relationships, power struggles, extreme interdependency, or disintegration. Disturbed behavior often is seen in children and adolescents who become the focus of family problems. Family therapists attempt to provide help for disturbed children and families as a whole. This may include altering the family situation rather than treating the child individually.

Group Therapy

Children and adolescents may be treated in groups. Peer relationships play an important part in group therapy because peers often help each other by exchanging information, identifying with the group, expressing feelings openly, and suggesting solutions to problems. Group therapy is used in the treatment of disorders such as substance abuse, oppositional disorders, depression, and anorexia nervosa.

Play Therapy

Play therapy usually is used with children between the ages of 3 and 12 years. The child is given the opportunity to act out feelings such as anger, hostility, frustration, and fear. Various toys, puppets, or materials such as crayons and finger paints may be used. A dollhouse and dolls can be used to simulate family, sibling, or peer relationships. For example, a young girl may play with a doll and punish it or refer to it as a "bad girl," treating the doll the way she is treated by her parents. Watching a child at play gives the caregiver the opportunity to learn about a child's real and imaginary emotional life.

Behavioral Therapy

Behavioral therapy attempts to alter a client's behavior and modify or remove symptoms such as temper tantrums or bed-wetting. It often is used with children who are hyperactive to reduce their activity and to organize play, by employing learning theory to alter the circumstances before or after a particular behavior.

Operant conditioning, or behavior modification, is a second type of behavioral therapy used to modify behavior through manipulation. The client is given a reward or positive reinforcement for desired behavior and negative reinforcement for undesired behavior. This type of therapy is used in the treatment of anorexia nervosa, delinquent behavior, enuresis, mental retardation, and several other disorders or problems. Cognitive-behavior therapy (see Chapters 12 and 14) and dialectic behavior therapy (see Chapter 14) are also utilized in the treatment of child and adolescent disorders.

Art and Music Therapy

Therapies involving art or music allow the child or adolescent to express her- or himself in these disciplines and can be effective with those who have difficulty communicating with others. For example, a 7-year-old depressed child is able to draw a picture of his fear of death after separation from his father, who is hospitalized for treatment of Hodgkin's disease. He had overheard family conversations regarding the seriousness of his father's condition and feared that his father would never return home.

Community and School-Based Interventions

Community and school-based collaborative mental health programs have been developed to meet the needs of children and adolescents with behavioral and mental health problems. For example, mental health professionals employed by a psychiatric institute and clinic have teamed with clinicians and administrators of a pediatric center in Pennsylvania. Staffing involves a full-time advanced nurse practitioner who serves as the care manager, a full-time psychiatric social worker, and a pediatric psychiatrist who is available one day per week. Referrals are made to the collaborative care team when a primary care provider identifies a child

with acute or chronic emotional or behavioral problems (Mahoney, 2004).

School nurses can have a positive impact on the life of a child with mental illness. Puskar, Sereika, and Tusaid-Mumford (2003) describe a rural school-based intervention program, Teaching Kids to Cope, for adolescents with clinical symptoms of depression. The research study included weekly group sessions, led by master's-level nurses, and involved role-playing and discussion to cover topics of trust, self-image, life stressors, communication with parents and family, school issues, and peer relationships. Statistics revealed that depression scores of the participants improved and more than 90% of the 89 participants rated the intervention program as good or very good. Researchers concluded that school nurses are in a position to provide interventions for students at risk for, or suffering from, depression.

Claude M. Chemtob, of Mt. Sinai School of Medicine, and his colleagues worked with Hawaiian school officials to identify children experiencing post-hurricane–related trauma symptoms. Students who were identified to be highly symptomatic received four weekly sessions of group or individual therapy. Interventions by trained school counselors included play and art therapy to focus on issues such as safety and helplessness, loss, mobilizing competence, anger, and gaining closure. Significant reductions in trauma symptoms were noted for students immediately post-intervention and at 1 year follow-up, suggesting that school-based screening and treatment delivery to children is feasible (Mahoney, 2005).

EVALUATION

The evaluation of nursing interventions for children and adolescents who are seen in the clinical setting for the treatment of psychiatric–mental disorders is an ongoing process. Consideration is given to the developmental stage of the client and to whether any changes in mood or behavior have occurred since the initial assessment. The efficacy of prescribed medication is reviewed. Family dynamics are reassessed. Socialization and progress in school are discussed. See Nursing Plan of Care 29-1: The Depressed Adolescent Client.

THE DEPRESSED ADOLESCENT CLIENT

Nick, a 17-year-old male high school honor student, had qualified for the state swimming finals in the 100-meter free-style event and as a member of the 200-meter medley relay team. The weekend before the scheduled finals, Nick was a passenger in an automobile accident and sustained minor injuries. The driver of the automobile, his best friend, was critically injured. Nick became despondent, withdrawn, easily angered, and lost interest in his academics and sports activities. He informed the swimming coach that he intended to withdraw from the state finals. The coach overheard Nick tell a peer that if his friend died, life would not be worth living. The coach spoke to Nick privately and suggested a referral to the school nurse practitioner. Nick agreed and was seen that same day.

DSM-IV-TR DIAGNOSIS: Adjustment disorder with depressed mood

ASSESSMENT: Personal strengths: Supportive coach, active in sports, honor student, good physical health, socially active prior to accident, willing to seek help suggested by coach

Weaknesses: Difficulty coping with friend's injuries, low-self esteem

---

NURSING DIAGNOSIS: Ineffective Coping related to friend's injuries as evidenced by despondent, withdrawn behavior

OUTCOME: The client will verbalize feelings related to his emotional state.

Planning/Implementation	Rationale
Encourage the client to verbalize feelings.	Verbalizing feelings is difficult for an adolescent but it is necessary if effective coping skills are to be developed.

NURSING DIAGNOSIS: Situational Low Self-Esteem related to injury of friend as evidenced by anger, withdrawal, and verbalization of negative feeling about self

OUTCOME: The client will verbalize increased feelings of self-worth.

Planning/Implementation	Rationale
Do not allow client to dwell on past events.	The client may be blaming himself for the accident and his friend's critical injuries.
Provide realistic feedback about the accident.	The client may not have had realistic feedback about the cause of the accident. Realistic feedback reinforces the client's feelings of self-worth.

NURSING DIAGNOSIS: Anticipatory Grieving regarding the potential death of his peer as evidenced by statement that if his friend died, life would not be worth living

OUTCOME: The client will express his grief without verbalizing self-blame.

Planning/Implementation	Rationale
Assess for prior experiences with loss.	The client may be overwhelmed by his friend's injuries.
Explain grief reactions to loss.	Understanding the grief process can help the client work through his feelings.

NURSING DIAGNOSIS: Risk for Self-Directed Violence related to ineffective coping as evidenced by statement that life would not be worth living if his friend died

OUTCOME: The client will learn to identify and tolerate uncomfortable feelings properly.

Planning/Implementation	Rationale
Provide a safe environment	The client has verbalized that life would not be worth living if his friend died. The client's safety is a priority.
Initiate support systems such as the client's teacher, coach, and family, and 24-hour emergency hotline.	The client may feel more comfortable discussing his feelings with individuals who know him and his friend.

EVALUATION: Evaluation focuses on Nick's understanding of the grief process in relation to a potential or real loss, his development of positive coping skills, his use of support systems, and improvement in his self-esteem. Adjustment disorders are generally self-limited but can develop into major disorders. Nick's clinical symptoms should be monitored on an ongoing basis until his friend's injuries and medical condition are stabilized.

KEY CONCEPTS

◆ Although studies regarding the development of psychiatric–mental disorders in children and adolescents have been limited due to the overlap of one or more syndromes, theorists have identified some genetic and biologic factors contributing to the development of disorders such as mental retardation, pervasive developmental disorders (eg, Rett's disorder, autistic disorder, and Asperger's disorder), attention-deficit hyperactivity disorder (ADHD), conduct disorder, childhood psychosis, anxiety disorders, and mood disorders.

◆ According to Bowlby's Attachment theory, normal attachment in infancy is crucial to a person's healthy development. Attachment occurs when there is a warm, intimate and continuous relationship with the mother in which both the infant and mother find satisfaction and enjoyment.

◆ Seven specific groups of children considered to be at high risk for mental and emotional disorders due to psychosocial factors have been identified. They include children in families with conflict or divorce, children who experience poverty, children of minority ethnic status, children who are abused, children of substance-abusing and mentally ill parents, children of teenaged parents, and children with chronic illness or disability.

◆ Environmental factors that place children at risk for the development of psychiatric–mental health disorders include public schools and neighborhoods.

◆ Mental retardation is a developmental disorder in which the client exhibits subaverage general intellectual functioning associated with impairment in areas such as communication, activities of daily living, socialization, and functional academic or occupational skills.

◆ The incidence of autistic disorder, an incurable and life-long pervasive developmental disorder, has increased during the last 5 years.

◆ Asperger's disorder is considered a mild form of autism in which verbal intelligence quotient (IQ) is higher than performance IQ and developmental delay may not be recognized until the child exhibits social deficits in school.

◆ Although symptoms of ADHD are typically present before age 3 years and affect approximately 3% to 7% of prepubertal elementary school children, diagnosis is usually not made until academic and social functioning are impaired. Recent research supports the diagnostic continuity of ADHD throughout the life cycle.

◆ Children with disruptive behavior disorders (eg, oppositional defiant disorder and conduct disorders) are impaired by frequent, severe disruptive behavior.

◆ Tic disorders, manifested by involuntary movements or noise, are relatively common in childhood and last less than 1 year.

◆ Although the symptoms differ and may not be readily recognizable, children and adolescents experience anxiety disorders, mood disorders, psychotic disorders, and adjustment disorders similar to those experienced by adults.

◆ The assessment of a young client is often complicated by the interaction of psychopathology with the child's environment and developmental processes.

◆ Communication with children takes skill, thoughtfulness, and practice. Privacy is the single most important criterion by which adolescents judge their interactions with health care providers.

◆ Stating a nursing diagnosis for children or adolescents who exhibit a psychiatric–mental health disorder can be difficult because of changing or inconsistent behavior, discomfort in the presence of the examiner, developmental changes, and influence of parents.

◆ Planning interventions is a collaborative effort with the client and parents and may require the involvement of other disciplines or community supports. Interventions are individualized to meet the needs of each client.

◆ Psychopharmacology has been approved as adjunctive therapy in the treatment of certain disorders and remains one of the most successful treatments for ADHD.

◆ Continuum of care may include hospitalization, partial or day hospitalization, and placement with an alternative family if the client is unable to live with his or hers during a crisis. Various interactive therapies can be provided on an inpatient or outpatient basis.

◆ Community and school-based collaborative mental health programs have been developed to meet the needs of children and adolescents with behavioral and mental health problems.

◆ Evaluation is an ongoing process requiring consideration of the client's developmental stage and any changes that have occurred in mood or behavior since the initial assessment.

For additional study materials, please refer to the Student Resource CD-ROM located in the back of this textbook.

CHAPTER WORKSHEET

CRITICAL THINKING QUESTIONS

1. Watch a current movie involving gangs or troubled or delinquent adolescents. Can you identify characters in the movie with conduct or attention-deficit hyperactivity disorders? What causative factors would you identify if one of these characters were your client?

2. A friend comes to you for advice. Her 5-year-old son has been wetting the bed every night for the last several months. She is at her "wits' end" and says she "can't understand why he keeps doing this—after all, he's been toilet trained for 2 years." Identify some common causes for this type of behavior regression. What questions would you ask your friend? What interventions would be appropriate?

3. Read several articles or chapters about family systems therapy. What principles can you apply with any family you assess and work with?

REFLECTION

Reflect on the chapter opening quote. What does the author imply in the final statement "For behind the parent stood the school and behind the teacher, the home"?

NCLEX-STYLE QUESTIONS

1. The nurse interviews a 16-year-old female admitted to the psychiatric inpatient unit with a diagnosis of major depressive disorder. Which action would be the priority for the initial assessment?

   a. Determining educational experiences
   b. Determining social support system
   c. Questioning suicidal thoughts
   d. Questioning sexual experiences

2. Which intervention would the nurse include as the priority when planning the care for an adolescent with a diagnosis of conduct disorder?

   a. Discussion of feelings
   b. Maintenance of safety
   c. Medication evaluation
   d. Stabilization of mood

3. When assessing a 10-year-old child, which information would the nurse interpret as representing a significant risk factor for development of a psychiatric disorder in this child?

   a. Childhood obesity
   b. Early onset of puberty
   c. Poor school achievement
   d. Parental mental illness

4. Which treatment modality would the nurse expect to use when assisting a younger child to verbalize difficult feelings?

   a. Behavioral techniques
   b. Cognitive therapy
   c. Play therapy
   d. Recreational activities

5. When assessing a child with a history of Tourette's syndrome, which of the following would the nurse expect to find?

   a. Aggressive behaviors
   b. Aversion to touch
   c. Motor or vocal tics
   d. Poor educational achievement

6. The following events are associated with the development of child and adolescent psychiatry. Place the events in the order that they occurred from earliest to latest.

   a. Creation of the Juvenile Psychopathic Institute
   b. Founding of American Academy of Child Psychiatry
   c. Identification of a condition later termed Asperger's syndrome
   d. Publication of *Child Psychiatry* by Kanner
   e. Creation of American Academy of Child and Adolescent Psychiatry

Selected References

About.com. (2006). History of ADHD.Retrieved March 3, 2006, from http://add.about.com/cs/addthebasics/a/history.htm

AdultADD.com. (2006). What is adult ADD? Retrieved March 4, 2005, from http://www.adultadd.com

American Pediatric Association. (2001). Clinical practice guideline: Treatment of the school-aged child with attention-deficit/hyperactivity disorder. *Pediatrics, 108,* 1033.

American Psychiatric Association. (1997). Practice guideline for the treatment of patients with schizophrenia. *American Journal of Psychiatry, 154* (Supplement 4), 1–63

American Psychiatric Association. (2000). *Diagnostic and statistical manual of mental disorders* (4th ed., text revision). Washington, DC: Author.

Andrews, M. M., & Boyle, J. S. (2003). *Transcultural concepts in nursing care* (4th ed.). Philadelphia: Lippincott Williams & Wilkins.

Anxiety Disorders Association of America. (2003). Anxiety disorders in children and adolescents. Retrieved February 22, 2003, from http://www.adaa.org/anxietydisorderinfor/childrenado.cfm

Autism Society of America. (2002). What is autism? Retrieved May 22, 2003, from http://www.autism-society.org/whatisautism

Baker, B. (2000). Genetic test now available for diagnosis of Rett syndrome. *Clinical Psychiatry News, 28* (1), 5.

Barclay, L., & Vega, C. (2005). Consensus guidelines issued for diagnosis and treatment of bipolar disorder in children. Retrieved March 8, 2005, from http://www. medscape.com/viewarticle/500273_print

Baren, M. (2000). *Hyperactivity and attention disorders in children.* San Ramon, CA: Health Information Network.

Barker, P. (1995). *Basic child psychiatry* (6th ed.). Baltimore: University Park Press.

Bates, B. (1999). Conduct disorder seen as label of hopelessness. *Clinical Psychiatry News, 27*(12), 20.

Biederman, J. (1999, November 11-14). *Current concepts on neurobiology and psychopharmacology of ADHD.* Paper presented at the 12th Annual United States Psychiatric & Mental Health Congress, Atlanta, GA.

Birmaher, B. (2004). *New hope for children and teens with bipolar disorder.* New York: Three Rivers Press.

Bryant, B. J., & Cheng, K. (2005). Anxiety disorders. In K. Cheng & K. M. Myers (Eds.), *Child and adolescent psychiatry* (pp. 111-132). Philadelphia: Lippincott Williams & Wilkins.

Church, C. C. (1996). Unlocking the mystery: An overview of autism in children. *ADVANCE for Nurse Practitioners, 4*(2).

Colyar, M. R. (2002). ADHD testing. *ADVANCE for Nurse Practitioners, 10*(11), 26-27.

Deering, C. G., & Cody, D. J. (2002). Communicating with children and adolescents. *American Journal of Nursing, 102*(3), 34-41.

Dulcan, M. K., Bregman, J. D., Weller, E. B., & Weller, R. A. (1998). Treatment of childhood and adolescent disorders. In A. F. Schatzberg & C. B. Nemeroff (Eds.), *The American Psychiatric Press textbook of psychopharmacology* (2nd ed., pp. 669-706). Washington, DC: American Psychiatric Press.

Efron, L. A., & Pearl, P. L. (2003). Too much energy for rest: Sleep problems in children with ADHD. *ADVANCE for Nurse Practitioners, 11*(2), 57-59.

Elster, A. B., & Marcell, A. V. (2003). Health Care of Adolescent Males: Overview, Rationale, and Recommendations. *Adolescent Medicine: State of The Art Professional Reviews, 14*(3), 525-540.

Erikson, E. (1964). *Childhood and society* (Rev. ed.). New York: W. W. Norton.

Ferguson-Noyes, N. (2005). Bipolar disorder in children: Diagnostic and treatment issues. *ADVANCE for Nurse Practitioners, 13*(3), 35-36, 38-40, 42.

Flick, G. L. (2002). Controversies in ADHD. *ADVANCE for Nurse Practitioners, 10*(2), 34-43.

Fohrman, D. A., & Stein, M. T. (2006). Psychosis: 6 steps rule out medical causes in kids. *Current Psychiatry, 5*(2), 35-38, 41-44.

Foley, K. (2005). Experiencing nature may help to quell ADHD. *Clinical Psychiatry News, 33*(2), 34.

Foley, K., & Keller, J. (2006). Data watch: Top triggers for stress in children. *Clinical Psychiatry News, 34*(1), 40.

Foley, K., & Reis, A. (2005). Data watch: Rate of SSRI prescribing per 1,000 depressed 5- to 18-year-olds. *Clinical Psychiatry News, 33*(1), 44.

Gaffney, D. A. (1996). Individual therapy with children. In S. Lego (Ed.), *Psychiatric nursing: A comprehensive reference* (2nd ed., pp. 79-86). Philadelphia: Lippincott-Raven.

Glod, C. A. (2001). Attention deficit-hyperactivity disorder: An overview of assessment and treatment issues. *ADVANCE for Nurse Practitioners, 9*(2), 52-57.

Grandin, T. (2002). Teaching tips for children and adults with autism. Autism Society. Retrieved December 14, 2003, from http://www.autism.org/temple/tips.html

Hales, A., Karshmer, J., Monter-Sandoval, L., et al. (2003). Psychiatric-mental health clinical nurse specialist practice in a public school setting. *Clinical Nurse Specialist, 17*(2), 95-100.

Hendren, R. L. (1997, November 13-15). *An update on childhood psychosis.* Paper presented at the 10th Annual United States Psychiatric & Mental Health Congress, Orlando, FL.

Hendricks, C. S., Tavakoli, A., Hendricks, D. L., et al. (2001). Self-esteem matters: Racial and gender differences among rural southern adolescents. *Journal of National Black Nurses Association, 12,* 15-22. Retrieved August 20, 2002, from http://www.medscape.com/viewarticle/438822_4

Hlastala, S. A., & McClellan, J. (2005). Early onset schizophrenia and related psychotic disorders. In K. Cheng & K. M. Myers (Eds.), *Child and Adolescent Psychiatry: The Essentials* (pp. 211-226). Philadelphia: Lippincott Williams & Wilkins.

Imperio, W. A. (2001). Surgeon general confronts gaps in mental health care. *Clinical Psychiatry News, 29*(2), 1, 8, 11.

Jeffrey, D. A., Sava Bianca, D., & Winters, N. C. (2005). Depressive disorders. In K. Cheng & K. M. Myers (Eds.), *Child and adolescent psychiatry: The essentials* (pp. 169-190). Philadelphia: Lippincott Williams & Wilkins.

Jetmalani, A. (2005). Tourette disorder. In K. Cheng & K. M. Myers (Eds.), *Child and adolescent psychiatry: The essentials* (pp. 151-168). Philadelphia: Lippincott Williams & Wilkins.

Johnson, B. S. (1997). *Psychiatric-mental health nursing: Adaptation and growth* (4th ed.). Philadelphia: Lippincott-Raven.

Johnson, C., & Dorman, B. (1998). What is autism? Autism Society. Retrieved September 10, 2000, from http://www.autism-society.org/whatisautism

Kaplan, A. (2000). Meeting advances Surgeon General's recommendations on children's mental health. *Psychiatric Times, 17*(7), 22-23.

Li, J., & Bennett, N. (1994). *Young children in poverty: A statistical update.* New York: National Center for Children in Poverty, Columbia University School of Public Health.

Literature Monitor. (2004). Home videos help detect Asperger's syndrome. *Neuropsychiatry Reviews, 5*(6), 21-22.

Little, L. (2005). Consider genetic disorder in some milder autism cases. *Clinical Psychiatry News, 33*(8), 51.

McDonnell, M. A., & Dougherty, M. (2005). Righting a troubled course: Diagnosing and treating ADHD in adults. *ADVANCE for Nurse Practitioners, 3*(8), 53-56.

Mahoney, D. (2004). Team meets kids where they are. *Clinical Psychiatry News, 32*(12), 1, 32.

Mahoney, D. (2005). Psychiatric first aid: A necessity. *Clinical Psychiatry News, 33*(10), 55-56.

Melnyk, B. M., & Moldenbauer, Z. (1999). Current approaches to depression in children and adolescents. *ADVANCE for Nurse Practitioners, 7*(2), 24-29, 97.

Mercer, R. (2003). Dry at night: Treating nocturnal enuresis. *ADVANCE for Nurse Practitioners, 11*(2), 26-31.

Mercer, T. A. (2002). Brand new world: Recent research and attention is shedding light on autism. *ADVANCE for Nurses, 3*(12), 18-21, 33.

Moore, H. W. (2005). Adult ADHD: In the office and on the road. *Neuropsychiatry Reviews, 6*(8), 1, 16.

Muscari, M. E. (1998). When to worry about adolescent angst. *American Journal of Nursing, 98*(3), 22-23.

Myers, S. M., Eisenhauer, N. J., & Ryan, M. E. (2003). ADHD: It is real and it can be treated. *The Clinical Advisor, 6*(3), 15-18, 21-22, 25.

National Alliance for Autism Research. (2006). What is autism? History. Retrieved March 3, 2006, from http://www.naar.org/aboutaut/whatis_hist.htm

National Institute of Mental Health. (2003). Depression in children and adolescents. Retrieved February 27, 2004, from http://www.nimh.nih.gov

Neuropsychiatry Reviews. (2005). Multiple mutations may explain autism. *Neuropsychiatry Reviews, 6*(9), 15.

NPR online. (2003). Americans willing to pay for improving schools. Retrieved September 1, 2003, from http://www.npr.org/programs/specials/poll/education/education.front.html

Patel, N. C., & Sallee, F. R. (2005). What's the best treatment for comorbid ADHD/bipolar mania? *Current Psychiatry, 4*(4), 27-28, 33-34, 36-37.

Pearson, D. A. (2003). Kids, stress, & war. *ADVANCE for Nurses, 4*(9), 25-26.

Pelham, W. E. (2001). Treatment approaches: ADHD and behavioral modification. *Supplement to Consultations in Primary Care, 41*(14), 11-14.

Perepletchikova, F., & Kazdin, A. L. (2005). Oppositional defiant disorder and conduct disorder. In K. Cheng & K. M. Myers (Eds.), *Child and adolescent psychiatry: The essentials* (pp. 73-88). Philadelphia: Lippincott Williams & Wilkins.

Puskar, K., Serika, S., & Tusaid-Mumford, K. (2003). Effect of teaching kids to cope (TKC) program on outcomes of depression and coping among rural adolescents. *Journal of Child and Adolescent Psychiatric Nursing, 16*, 71-80.

Reed, B. (2001). Alike yet different somehow. *ADVANCE for Nurse Practitioners, 9*(2), 93-94, 112.

Romano, C. J. (2004). Imaging insights into the pathogenesis of adolescent psychiatric disorders. *Neuropsychiatry Reviews, 5*(8), 8.

Ryan, R., & Sunada, K. (1997). Medical evaluation of persons with mental retardation referred for psychiatric assessment. *General Hospital Psychiatry 19*(4), 274-280.

Sadock, B. J., & Sadock, V. A. (2003). *Kaplan & Sadock's synopsis of psychiatry: Behavioral sciences/clinical psychiatry* (9th ed.). Philadelphia: Lippincott Williams & Wilkins.

Scahill, L., Hamrin, V., & Deering, C. G. (2002). Care of children and adolescents with psychiatric disorders. In M. A. Boyd (Ed.), *Psychiatric nursing: Contemporary practice* (2nd ed., pp. 870-910). Philadelphia: Lippincott Williams & Wilkins.

Schopick, D. (2005). Watch for TD in children and teens. *Clinical Psychiatry News, 33*(7), 17.

Schowalter, J. E. (2006). A history of child and adolescent psychiatry in the United States. Retrieved March 3, 2006, from http://www.psychiatrictimes.com/p030943.html

Sherman, C. (2000). Core features identify Asperger's syndrome. *Clinical Psychiatry News, 28*(3), 31.

Sobsey, D. (1997). *Violence and abuse in the lives of people with disabilities: The end of silent acceptance?* Baltimore: P. H. Brookes.

Spittler, K. L. (2005). Unique immune response in children with autism. *Neuropsychiatry Reviews, 6*(6), 10-11.

Stubbe, D. E. (2005). Attention deficit hyperactivity disorder. In K. Cheng & K. M. Myers (Eds.), *Child and adolescent psychiatry: The essentials* (pp. 53-72). Philadelphia: Lippincott Williams & Wilkins.

Stubbs, E. G., & Cheng, K. (2005). Autism spectrum disorders. In K. Cheng & K. M. Myers (Eds.), *Child and adolescent psychiatry: The essentials* (pp. 227-246). Philadelphia: Lippincott Williams & Wilkins.

Sullivan, M. G. (2004). Attachment disorders can be spotted early. *Clinical Psychiatry News, 32*(3), 51.

United States Congress, Office of Technology Assessment. (1986). *Children's mental health: Problems and services— A background paper* (Report No. OTA-BP-H-33). Washington, DC: U.S. Government Printing Office.

United States Department of Health and Human Services. (1999). *Mental health: A report of the Surgeon General.* Rockville, MD: DHHS, Substance Abuse and Mental Health Services Administration, Center for Mental Health Services, NIH, NIMH.

Waite, R. L. (2004). Adult ADHD. *ADVANCE for Nurses, 5*(14), 21-22, 24.

Walsh, M. (2002). New screening program expected to improve early detection of autism. *Clinical Psychiatry News, 30*(1), 29.

Wendling, P. (2005). CAM use is common among families with autistic children. *Clinical Psychiatry News, 33*(12), 36.

Wikipedia.org. (2006). Attachment theory. Retrieved March 3, 2006, from http://en.wikipedia.org/wiki/Attachment_theory

Winters, N. C., & Tsai, J. (2005). Psychiatric assessment of children and adolescents. In K. Cheny & K. M. Myers (Eds.), *Child and adolescent psychiatry* (pp. 3-16). Philadelphia: Lippincott Williams & Wilkins.

Zoler, M. L. (2004). 10-year study: ADHD persists as boys become men. *Clinical Psychiatry News, 32*(8), 1, 4.

Zolot, J. S., & Sofer, D. (2001). Anxiety is increasing in children. *American Journal of Nursing, 101*(3), 18.

Suggested Readings

Barkley, R. A. (2000). *Taking charge of ADHD.* New York: Guilford.

Carpenito-Moyet, L. J. (2006). *Handbook of nursing diagnosis* (11th ed.). Philadelphia: Lippincott Williams & Wilkins.

Dubovsky, S. L. (2005). How to reduce mania risk when prescribing stimulants. *Current Psychiatry, 4*(10), 36-38, 47-50, 54.

Gaffney, D. A. (1996). Group therapy with children. In S. Lego (Ed.), *Psychiatric nursing: A comprehensive reference* (2nd ed., pp. 87-96). Philadelphia: Lippincott-Raven.

Homeyer, L. E. (2000). When is group play therapy appropriate? *Psychiatric Times, 17*(9), 49–51.

James, K. S. (2001). All in the family: Treating obesity in children and adolescents. *ADVANCE for Nurse Practitioners, 9*(1), 26–31.

Johnson, D. (2000). Parents' conflict resolution styles shape teens. *Clinical Psychiatry News, 28*(5), 42.

Kelly, P. (2003). Family support for children with ADHD. *ADVANCE for Nurse Practitioners, 11*(2), 53–56.

Klin, A., Volkmar, F. R., & Sparrow, S. S. (Eds.). (2000). *Asperger syndrome.* New York: Guilford.

Lawrence, P. R. (1999). Nocturnal enuresis in children: Treatment is a family matter. *ADVANCE for Nurse Practitioners, 7*(2), 41–43, 96.

Ludwikowski, K. L. (2004). All that moves or is inattentive is not ADHD. *ADVANCE for Nurse Practitioners, 12*(2), 57–58, 62–64.

Melnyk, B. M., Moldenbauer, Z., Tuttle, J., Veenema, T. G., Jones, D., & Novak, J. (2003). Improving child and adolescent mental health: An evidence-based approach. *ADVANCE for Nurse Practitioners, 11*(2), 47–52.

Moore, H. W. (2004). ADHD may continue into adulthood. *Neuropsychiatry Reviews, 5*(8), 1, 19.

Murphy, J. L. (Ed.). (2000). *Nurse practitioners' prescribing reference.* New York: Prescribing Reference.

Scheffer, R. E., & Apps, J. N. (2005). ADHD or bipolar disorder? Age-specific manic symptoms are key. *Current Psychiatry, 4*(5), 42–46, 51–52.

Schultz, J. M., & Videbeck, S. L. (2005). *Lippincott's manual of psychiatric nursing care plans* (7th ed.). Philadelphia: Lippincott Williams & Wilkins.

Sherman, C. (2000a). Assessment is good opportunity to change family dynamics. *Clinical Psychiatry News, 28*(3), 25.

Sherman, C. (2000b). Grasping the subjective dimension of ADHD. *Clinical Psychiatry News, 28*(3), 30.

Stabler, S. (2005). Adolescence and depression. *ADVANCE for Nurses, 6*(3), 32–33.

Waldrop, J. (2004). SSRI debate hurts kids. *ADVANCE for Nurse Practitioners, 12*(12), 65.

Zeanah, C. H. (Ed.). (2000). *Handbook of infant mental health.* New York: Guilford.

CHAPTER 30 / AGING CLIENTS WITH PSYCHOSOCIAL NEEDS

Elderly Americans are the fastest growing segment of the American population. By 2050, 1 in every 20 will be 85 years of age or older and 1 in every 5 will be retired. —U.S. CENSUS BUREAU, 1997
Psychiatric syndromes—rather than discrete disorders—are more realistic as diagnostic entities in geriatric psychiatry. The most common of these syndromes are memory loss, depression, anxiety, suspicions and agitation, sleep disorders, and hypochondriasis. —BLAZER, 1994

LEARNING OBJECTIVES

AFTER STUDYING THIS CHAPTER, YOU SHOULD BE ABLE TO:

1. Differentiate between the primary or intrinsic and secondary or extrinsic factors influencing the aging process.
2. Articulate Duvall's developmental tasks of aging.
3. Compare and contrast the more common psychiatric–mental health disorders among Native Americans, African Americans, Hispanic, and Asian American elderly.
4. Describe at least four patterns of behavior or emotional reactions that elderly clients exhibit as a result of experiencing despair.
5. Define *failure to thrive*.
6. Identify at least three causes of loneliness in the elderly.
7. Compare and contrast dementia and dementia syndrome of depression.
8. Explain the elements of a comprehensive assessment of geropsychiatric clients.
9. Identify provider-, client-, and illness-related barriers to the assessment of elderly clients.
10. State the rationale for prescribing low doses of psychoactive agents for elderly clients.
11. Explain the purpose of the life-review process and of reminiscence.
12. Develop a list of nursing diagnoses commonly used when planning care for elderly clients ineffectively coping with the psychosocial aspects of aging.
13. Plan nursing interventions for elderly clients who, according to Maslow's theory of motivation, demonstrate basic needs for survival, safety and security, love and belonging, self-esteem, and self-actualization.

KEY TERMS

Aging
Dementia syndrome of
   depression
Ego preoccupation
Ego transcendence
Failure to thrive
Polypharmacy
Primary aging
Reminiscence
Secondary aging
Self-actualization

The number of individuals over the age of 65 years (referred to as *late adulthood*) is rapidly expanding. In 2002, 35.6 million people in the United States were ages 65 years and older. It is estimated that by the year 2020, approximately 52 million persons will be 65 years of age or older, and by 2030 that number is expected to reach 71.5 million (Administration on Aging [AOA], 2003). Although data regarding the prevalence of mental disorders in elderly adults vary widely, in the year 2000, the number of mentally ill elderly persons was estimated to be about 9 million. This figure is expected to rise to 20 million by the middle of the 21st century. Diagnosing and treating older adults with first onset or chronic psychiatric disorders often presents more difficulties than treating younger individuals because older persons may have coexisting chronic medical conditions. For example, the most frequently occurring medical conditions in adults 65 years of age and over include hypertension, arthritis, heart disease, cancer, sinusitis, and diabetes. Psychiatric illnesses can be aggravated by concurrent medical problems and similarly, medical conditions and their associated disabilities can be aggravated by psychiatric illness (Sadock & Sadock, 2003).

The public has become increasingly sophisticated in its knowledge and expectations of older-adult health care. As a result, the health care profession has been required to pay greater attention to specialization, thereby responding to the increasing consumer demand. Public pressure is enhanced further when families themselves form organizations to better highlight these needs and focus attention on various areas. For example, the Alzheimer's Association in the United States, formed in 1980, now has over 200 local chapters across the country (Alzheimer's Association, 2003).

Nursing has also addressed the issue of health care for the elderly. The aging person, like any other younger human being, has certain psychosocial, physical, and environmental needs that he or she strives to satisfy throughout life. Therefore, an understanding of the aging person's life experiences and goal achievements is necessary for the development of a therapeutic milieu to meet the aging person's needs as he or she continues to achieve his or her goals.

The American Nurses Association (ANA) first acknowledged nursing of older adults as a specialty in 1966. In 1970, the ANA established the Standards of Geriatric Nursing Practice. In 1976, the title of the ANA's Geriatric Nursing Division was changed to the Gerontological Nursing Division. Today, gerontologic and psychiatric–mental health advanced nurse practitioners, as well as clinical nurse specialists, address the psychosocial needs of the elderly.

The compelling importance of psychiatric–mental health nursing of the elderly stems from the growing number and proportion of the elderly and from gains in longevity and active life expectancy. As a result, old age occupies a larger proportion of the average person's life. Consequently, the quality of life in old age and the impact of psychiatric–mental health problems on that quality of life are growing in relevance to the whole of a person's life. This chapter reviews the history of geriatric psychiatry, etiology of aging, and the developmental tasks for this group, focusing on the psychosocial aspects of aging. It provides information related to elderly clients who are ineffectively coping with the psychosocial aspects of aging, including application of the nursing process. The reader is referred to specific chapters in the text for additional information regarding specific psychiatric disorders experienced by the elderly.

History of Geriatric Psychiatry

A literature search regarding the history of geriatric psychiatry revealed interesting information. According to the Bible (Psalms 31:9–12), King David experienced clinical symptoms of depression. Historians believe this story indicates that the beginning of geriatric psychiatry is rooted in biblical times.

The presence of mental health, dementia, and mental illness in Egyptian, Roman, and French societies has been documented as early as the 7th century BC. The statue of an Egyptian elder is engraved with a message that states the elder spent his life in happiness, without worry or illness. A Roman, Cicero, at the age of 62, wrote an essay on senescence in which he stated the problems and goals of older adults. He acknowledged ageism in Roman society and described the severe regression that can occur with dementia. Father Jean Cassien published a book that described paranoid psychosis in a French monk who committed suicide during a delusional state (Sadavoy, Lazarus, & Jarvik, 1991).

During the Middle Ages (400–1500 AD), several individuals published articles about mental health and the aging process. For example, Berios, author of *Mont-*

pelier, differentiated depression and dementia. In the late 1890s, Freud, in an article about sexuality and neuroses, stated that the application of psychoanalytic techniques to older people was ineffective because too much time would be required to reach a cure in older persons who no longer were concerned about their "nervous health." About 20 years later, Abraham, in an article about psychoanalysis, described success in the employment of psychoanalytic techniques in the treatment of older adults. During the same time, Ferenczi described psychodynamic changes that he observed in older adults during therapy (Sadavoy, Lazarus, & Jarvik, 1991).

In 1906, Alzheimer published his classic description of dementia and Gaupp differentiated dementias from non-dementias or depression. In 1946, the Group for the Advancement of Psychiatry (GAP) was founded to collect and appraise significant data in the field of psychiatry. In 1950, this group published a paper regarding the problem of the aged patient in the public psychiatric hospital. During this same time period, the first geriatric psychiatric position emerged in England at the Bethlem Hospital (also known as Bethlehem Hospital), and between 1950 and 1951, an entire ward of the hospital was devoted to the psychiatric care of clients over the age of 60 years.

The 1960s to 1970s marked a significant worldwide interest in the field of geriatric psychiatry. The AOA was established in 1965; the National Institute of Mental Health (NIMH) sponsored research on mental health of the aging between 1960 and 1976; in 1977, U.S. President Jimmy Carter established a task force to address issues related to mental health and mental illness in late life; and by 1978, the need for an American organization with a focus on geriatric psychiatry was identified.

During the 1980s, assessment scales such as the Global Deterioration Scale, Geriatric Depression Scale, and a variety of brief mental status scales were developed. Research activity in the 1990s provided more knowledge about the relationship between mental health and aging than in all the history of psychogeriatrics before 1990 (Sadavoy, Lazarus, & Jarvik, 1991). In 1991, the American Board of Psychiatry and Neurology established geropsychiatry, which is now one of the fastest growing fields in psychiatry, as a subspecialty. Furthermore, the emergence of sophisticated diagnostic equipment (eg, magnetic resonance imaging, positron emission tomography scan) and the knowledge of pharmacodynamics and pharmacokinetics have played an important role in identifying and treating the psychosocial needs of the elderly (Sadock & Sadock, 2003).

Etiology of Aging

Aging has been defined as a process involving a gradual decline in the functioning of all the body's systems (eg, cardiovascular, endocrine, genitourinary, and so forth) (Sadock & Sadock, 2003). Busse (1996) states that aging usually refers to the adverse effects of the passage of time, but it can also refer to the positive processes of maturation or acquiring a desirable quality. The adverse effects or processes of decline associated with growing old are separated into primary and secondary aging. **Primary aging** is intrinsic and is determined by inherent or hereditary influences. **Secondary aging** refers to extrinsic changes (defects and disabilities) caused by hostile factors in the environment, including trauma and acquired disease.

Primary or Intrinsic Factors of Aging

Primary or intrinsic factors of aging include biologic and physiologic changes that are influenced by one's gender; ethnicity and race; intelligence and personality; familial longevity patterns; and genetic disease. These changes are the underlying basis for the biologic theories of aging. Table 30-1 summarizes the biologic theories of aging.

Gender

According to statistics provided by the AOA, women live longer than men by approximately 7 years and will continue to do so until the year 2050. By the year 2050, the composition of the U.S. population is estimated to differ markedly from that of today (AOA, 2001). Factors assumed to influence or contribute to women's longevity include endocrine metabolism before menopause that protects against circulatory or cardiovascular diseases, higher activity level, less occupational stress, better weight control, and less use of tobacco.

Culture, Ethnicity, and Race

Although the life expectancy for whites is approximately 5 years longer than for all other races, the death rate for the white population older than age 75 years is higher than for all other races. Mortality from cancer

TABLE 30.1 Biologic Theories of Aging

THEORY	BIOLOGIC CHANGES
Damage Theories	
Free radical theory	Unstable free radicals from environmental pollution and oxidation of certain elements produce deleterious effects on the biologic system.
Cross-link theory	Strong chemical bonding among different organic molecules in the body causes increased stiffness, chemical instability, and insolubility of connective tissue and DNA.
Immunologic theory	Erratic cellular mechanisms precipitate attacks on various tissues through auto-aggression or immunodeficiencies.
Somatic mutation	Failure of DNA to replicate, transcribe, or translate between cells
Error theory	Malfunction of RNA or related enzymes
Program Theory	Organisms are capable of a specific number of cell divisions that remain relatively constant.
Popular Theories	
Wear-and-tear theory	Body functions and structures wear out or are overused.
Stress-adaptation theory	The body is unable to resist stress due to residual damage.

SOURCES: Ebersole, P., & Hess, P. (1997). *Toward healthy aging: Human needs and nursing response* (5th ed.). St. Louis, MO: C.V. Mosby; and Sadock, B.J., & Sadock, V. A. (2003). *Kaplan & Sadock's synopsis of psychiatry: Behavioral sciences-clinical psychiatry* (9th ed.). Philadelphia: Lippincott Williams & Wilkins.

rises steeply with age and may contribute to the increase in death rate among white clients older than 75 years. The overall life expectancy of the Native American is shorter than that of all other U.S. races, at 65 years of age. Adherence to a set of cultural beliefs, values, and practices makes outside intervention for treatment of conditions such as malnutrition, alcohol abuse, and tuberculosis for Native Americans difficult at best (AOA, 2001; Sadock & Sadock, 2003, University of Missouri, 2003c).

Intelligence and Personality

Most older persons retain their cognitive abilities to a remarkable degree. However, persons with higher levels of intelligence appear to live longer than persons with lower levels of intelligence (AOA, 2001). This may be due, in part, to lifestyle choices of those with higher intelligence quotients (IQs). Such persons may remain physically active by participating in events that promote physical, mental, and social well-being, thereby contributing to longer life.

In addition, different personality types may affect longevity. Persons with type A personality may seldom relax or enjoy themselves because of a drive-to-succeed quality. They are prime candidates for heart attacks. In contrast, the person with type B personality is an easygoing individual who takes life in stride. Personality also influences the adoption of certain behaviors, such as overeating, tobacco dependence, and alcohol abuse, which impair physical health and shorten one's lifespan.

Familial Longevity

Familial longevity patterns are indicators of potential lifespan. A 45-year-old man from a family with a record of long-lived great-grandparents, grandparents, and parents probably will live longer than a man of the same age whose family history includes heart attacks by his father and grandfather in middle age. Many conditions that contribute to a shortened lifespan can be prevented, delayed, or minimized with effective interventions such as regular medical checkups; minimal use of substances such as coffee, cigarettes, or alcohol; work satisfaction; healthy eating habits; and adequate exercise (Sadock & Sadock, 2003).

Genetic Influences

Genetic disease may also affect lifespan. For example, persons with Down syndrome, cystic fibrosis, or Tay-Sachs disease typically experience shortened lifespans. Genetic factors have also been implicated in disorders commonly occurring in older adults (eg, coronary artery disease, hypertension, arteriosclerosis). Although people have minimal, if any, control over intrinsic factors influencing the aging process, a high quality of life can possibly promote one's sense of physical, mental, and social well-being (Sadock & Sadock, 2003).

Secondary or Extrinsic Factors

To some degree, people can control secondary or extrinsic factors of aging. Examples include:

- Employment
- Economic level
- Education
- Health practices and related diseases
- Societal attitude

Income, economic level, and educational level partially determine how one lives. For example, people may not seek health care because of high medical–surgical costs, lack of insurance, or ignorance about contributing factors to or symptoms of various diseases. People who have a poor diet, experience poor living conditions, have a substance-abuse problem, or ignore or minimize health problems also are at risk for a shortened lifespan. These practices have a negative effect on health and have been proven to contribute to deaths at earlier ages. Finally, societal attitudes affect persons psychologically, thus affecting the aging process. Most persons seek the approval of society, behaving in a manner based on societal expectations. Such thinking could lead to a lifestyle that is detrimental to one's health. For example, individuals in a busy law firm who believe it is necessary to drink alcoholic beverages when entertaining clients could develop a drinking problem (alcoholism) over a period of time. Older adults should seek intellectual, emotional, and physical stimulation to maintain an optimal level of health and longevity.

Developmental Tasks of Aging

Several theories have been proposed to explain aging on a psychological level. These theories are highlighted in Table 30-2. In addition, theorists have identified specific developmental tasks to be achieved by the older adult. Duvall (1977) lists developmental tasks of aging that influence the emotional needs of the elderly:

- Establishing satisfactory living arrangements
- Adjusting to retirement income
- Establishing comfortable routines

TABLE 30.2 Psychological Theories of Aging

THEORIST	SUMMARY OF THEORY
Piaget (1961)	Elderly adults experience a gradual progression of unique, cognitive development that should not be measured against the norms of young or middle-aged people.
Erikson (1963)	Elderly adults experience the last stage of life, from which they can look back with integrity or despair.
Peck (1968)	Elderly adults experience three discrete tasks of old age related to the establishment of integrity: Ego differentiation versus work role preoccupation Body transcendence versus body preoccupation Ego transcendence versus ego preoccupation
Neugarten (1968)	"Interiority" is characteristic of aged persons and indicates a growing interest in inner development during later life.
Jung (1971)	The last half of life has a purpose of its own; it is characterized by inner discovery, as opposed to the first half, which is oriented to biologic and social issues.
Kohlberg (1973)	Crises and turning points of adult life are moral dilemmas.

- Maintaining love, sex, and marital relationships
- Keeping active and involved
- Staying in touch with other family members
- Sustaining and maintaining physical and mental health
- Finding meaning in life

These tasks are summarized in the following sections. In addition, comparisons of the completion of these tasks by minority groups such as elderly Native Americans, African Americans, Hispanics, and Asian Americans (Asians and Pacific Islanders) are included.

Establishing Satisfactory Living Arrangements

Many factors influence this developmental task. The following questions are examples of some issues that the family and the aging client need to consider, related to satisfactory living arrangements:

- Is the elderly person single, widowed, divorced, or married?
- Does the elderly person have an incapacitating illness or handicap?
- Does the elderly person require assistance or supervision with activities of daily living (ADLs)?
- Are the grocery store, pharmacy, doctor's office, and church located close by or within walking distance?
- Is the elderly person able to stay in her or his own home, or does the person need to be relocated?

Loneliness, anxiety, depression, and other emotional reactions may occur if these needs are not met.

Native American Elderly

As a result of their limited adoption of mainstream society's values and ways of life, living arrangements of elderly Native Americans may differ greatly from those of elders of other cultures. All members of a tribe care for the elderly, who may have lived on reservations their entire lives and may have been isolated from mainstream society. Consequently, the above-mentioned considerations for satisfactory living arrangements may not apply for the elderly Native American (University of Missouri, 2003c).

African American Elderly

Approximately 33% of African American elderly live in poverty. More than twice as many elderly African American males as elderly white males are divorced or separated. African American elderly females with declining health are frequently the sole head of household. If elders live with their children, family networks provide the main source of needed assistance later in life. The possibility of being institutionalized for physical or mental disabilities decreases (University of Missouri, 2003a).

Hispanic Elderly

Compared with white and African American elderly, more Hispanic elderly are found living within neighborhood communities or "barrios" with their children or other members of their extended family, rather than in nursing homes or other institutional settings. Unfortunately, these neighborhoods are often densely populated, economically depressed metropolitan areas in which high crime rates occur, posing a threat to the Hispanic elderly's safety and security (University of Missouri, 2003b).

Asian American Elderly

The number of Asian American elders living below the poverty level (13%) is slightly higher than that of the white older population (10%). Approximately 80% of Asian American elderly live alone, as more adult married children work and become Westernized. This creates a pressing need for more affordable housing, congregate housing, and nursing facilities (American Association of Retired Persons [AARP], 2003; DuPuy, 2002).

Adjusting to Retirement Income

Retirement may be a time planned for relaxation and leisure activities, or it may pose a financial crisis. Not all people are fortunate enough to have a savings account and receive Social Security payments, retirement benefits, or some other form of supplemental income. Marriages may be strained by role changes related to retirement or to caring for a physically frail or cognitively impaired partner. Problems of adult children or grandchildren (eg, illnesses, unemployment) can burden retired elders, especially if families expect financial support, child-care help, or cohabitation. Many individuals who retire re-enter the work force when economic hardships occur. Adjusting one's standard of living to a reduced income can be quite stressful for the elderly when the cost of living continues to rise (Sadock & Sadock, 2003; Miller, 2005).

Native American Elderly

The average Native American barely lives long enough to reach the age of eligibility for most age-related benefit programs. Time takes on new meaning for the elderly Native American. Time is measured according to natural phenomena such as seasonal change, and the "right time" is viewed as when one is ready. Living in the present takes precedence over planning for the future. As noted earlier, the average life expectancy of the Native American person is 65 years (University of Missouri, 2003c).

African American Elderly

African American male elders generally have fewer personal post-retirement resources than white males and are more dependent on Social Security and Supplemental Security Income. Many African American elderly males regard themselves as "unretired-retired" because they generally continue to work after retirement age unless they are forced to retire because of a physical or mental disability (University of Missouri, 2003a). No information is available concerning retirement and African American elderly females.

Hispanic Elderly

Many Hispanic elderly have confronted educational and employment barriers throughout their younger years. A history of unemployment or a lifetime of hard work in unskilled labor positions, with deficient or nonexistent retirement programs, prevents the accumulation of sufficient wealth to sustain them in their later years (University of Missouri, 2003b). Hispanic elders are less likely to receive Social Security than their African American and white counterparts. If eligible, they are more likely to receive the minimum benefit because of a history of low-paying jobs (AARP, 2003).

Asian American Elderly

Asian Americans are more likely than white elderly to continue working after age 65 years. Social Security is the only source of retirement income for 34% of elderly Asian Americans (Social Security Administration, 2003). The vast majority of Asian American seniors do not speak English as a first language, and often struggle with the bureaucracy of social service and Medicaid programs (Ho, 2002).

Establishing Comfortable Routines

Retirement is a time for the pursuit of leisure and for freedom from the responsibility of previous working commitments. It allows one to establish a comfortable routine such as participating in a weekly bowling league during the day, doing volunteer work, or developing new hobbies. Conversely, retirement may be a time of stress, especially for the "workaholic" or type A personality, who needs to be busy all the time. "All my husband does is get in my way. He's always underfoot like a little puppy dog. I wish he were still working," "I thought we'd do things together such as golf, bowl, or play bridge. He's not interested in doing anything," and "I don't enjoy life any more. There's nothing to look forward to now that I am retired," are just a few comments by persons having difficulty adjusting to new routines during retirement. On the positive side, a senior citizen thoroughly enjoying retirement made the following comment: "I don't know how I managed to work before. I don't have enough time in the day to do everything."

Native American Elderly

The lifestyle of elderly Native Americans differs greatly in comparison with the lifestyle of mainstream society. Elderly Native Americans believe that each being has its own unique function and place in the universe. God is part of everything, including the routine of daily living. In traditional families, part of the elderly Native American's comfortable "aging routine" is spending time with members of the extended family and passing down one's wisdom and knowledge to the young (University of Missouri, 2003c).

African American Elderly

Retired African American elderly grandparents are often compelled to act as substitute parents for orphaned grandchildren or grandchildren of single parents. Instead of the retirement time they had looked forward to, they may be faced with the task of raising young children again (University of Missouri, 2003a).

Hispanic Elderly

Hispanic elderly tend to view themselves as old much earlier in life (eg, 60 years of age as compared with age 65 years for African Americans and white Americans) and expect fewer remaining years of life than any other group. Established negative attitudes and expectations about aging limit their ability to establish comfortable routines enjoyed by their elderly counterparts (University of Missouri, 2003b).

Asian American Elderly

Asian American men can expect to live to age 84 and women can expect to live to age 88. With longer life expectancies, they will live more years in retirement, allowing them the opportunity to establish a comfortable retirement routine. As a result of longer life expectancy, there is a demand for social and community outreach programs to provide bilingual, bicultural services (DuPuy, 2002).

Maintaining Love, Sex, and Marital Relationships

"Most older people want—and are able to lead—an active, satisfying sex life…When problems occur they should not be viewed as inevitable, but rather as the result of disease, disability, drug reactions, or emotional upset—and as requiring medical care" (National Institute on Aging, 1981).

Walker (1982, p. 171) states, "The notion that old age will be sexless has been proven false in study after study. Provided that they are healthy, elderly people are capable of an active sex life into their 80s and 90s. Sexual performance may be slowed somewhat with aging, but sexual pleasure and capacity remain intact."

Sexual problems can arise in later years due to physiologic changes, fear of impotence, fear of a heart attack because of physical exertion, or boredom. An older widowed man is able to establish a new marital relationship more readily than an older woman because of the availability of women in his age group or younger women. Stereotypically, older women are generally frowned upon if they marry a much younger man.

Kanapaux (2003) addresses the issues of fear and stigma as homosexual seniors progress through this developmental stage. Although gay and lesbian clients may encounter negative reactions from service providers at all ages, the experience can be especially difficult for seniors. Overt discrimination by the public and medical professionals has caused them to adopt a strategy of keeping their sexual orientation hidden. Most gay and lesbian seniors have support networks; however, same-sex partners lack the rights given to family members in terms of visitations, decision-making, and care-giving. Senior Action in a Gay Environment (SAGE) is the nation's oldest and largest social service agency for lesbian, gay, bisexual, and transgender seniors. SAGE has created a training guide for social service agencies to recognize the needs of gay and lesbian clients. Its mission is to eliminate the institutionalized homophobia that may exist within various organizations that provide services to elderly clients.

Native American Elderly

Self-disclosure about personal concerns (eg, love, sex, and marital relationships) to someone outside of the traditional family is not normally done by Native American elderly. The husband is the head of the household, although the wife has a voice in decision-making (University of Missouri, 2003c).

African American Elderly

African American elderly are the most unpartnered group in America. According to year 2000 census figures, 54% of African Americans have never married. Furthermore, approximately 36% of African Americans have divorced, compared with 34% of whites. The "sexual revolution" of the last two decades has wreaked havoc on African American relationships. Many African American men say they prefer companionship to long-term commitments (Peterson, 2000).

Hispanic Elderly

Nearly twice as many Hispanic men as women age 65 years and older are married and living with their spouse, a pattern mirrored in the white older population. It appears that elderly Hispanic men have a more favorable chance of completing this developmental task than do elderly Hispanic women (ie, there are 71 men for every 100 women). About the same proportion of Hispanic and white women are widowed (AARP, 2003).

Asian American Elderly

The developmental task of maintaining love, sex, and marital relationships may not be completed by many Asian American elders, especially elderly women. According to research, the majority of Asian American elderly women are widowed and living in isolation. A smaller proportion remain single in their later years (AARP, 2003; Ho, 2002).

Keeping Active and Involved

Butler and Lewis (1982) have identified special characteristics that demonstrate the ability of the elderly to keep active. These characteristics include the desire to leave a legacy; the desire to share knowledge and experience with younger generations; the ability to demonstrate an increased emotional investment in the environment; a sense of immediacy or "here-and-now" due to the decreased number of years left; the ability to experience an entire life cycle; increased creativity and curiosity; and a satisfaction with life. Physical illness may prevent a client from being active and becoming involved with others. The *theory of disengagement* assumes that society expects and older people desire to disengage or remove themselves from important activities such as employment, a figurehead role in the family, and civic responsibility. Supporting Evidence for Practice 30-1 highlights a study addressing the relationships among aging, social factors, lifestyle, and memory.

Active senior citizens may participate in volunteer employment programs such as Retired Senior Volunteer Program (RSVP), Service Corps of Retired Executives (SCORE), Volunteers in Service to America (VISTA), Peace Corps, Foster Grandparents Programs, and Senior Opportunities and Service (SOS) programs.

Native American Elderly

Keeping active and involved can be a challenge for elderly Native Americans because more than 80% of elderly Native Americans do not have telephones. The majority also do not receive newspapers or have television sets. According to tradition, knowledge and experience is shared with younger generations; however, there is minimal involvement with the outside world. Life-cycle events are marked by special rituals. Tribal and family ties are strong, contributing to a sense of belonging to a social group (Boyle, 2003; University of Missouri, 2003c).

African American Elderly

In general, elderly African Americans do not participate in social or recreational activities that are outside

---

SUPPORTING EVIDENCE FOR PRACTICE 30.1

Understanding the Effect of Aging and Socialization on Memory

PROBLEM UNDER INVESTIGATION / What is the relationship among aging, social factors, lifestyle, and memory?

SUMMARY OF RESEARCH / Subjects included 497 participants aged 25 to 80 years who had participated in the Maastricht Aging Study, a longitudinal representative study of cognitive aging in the Netherlands. Memory change, memory anxiety, and memory capacity were evaluated. Lifestyle was measured by the number of hours per week the subjects spent in sports activities, how active the subjects perceived themselves to be, participation in voluntary organizations, and contact with available family and friends. Subjects were also asked if they had children, a partner, or a full-time or part-time job. A nine-item version of the Health Locus of Control instrument was used to obtain data. Results of the study indicated that better subjective memory was associated with youth, health, education, and internal orientation. Higher memory capacity was associated with younger age, fewer health problems,

being female, frequent contact with family/friend, higher internal locus of control, and self-perception as active. Intact memory capacity was associated with being female and self-perception as active. Self-perception had greater impact than the hours per week the subject was engaged in activity. The researchers suggest that increasing an elder's social activity may support successful aging.

SUPPORT FOR PRACTICE / Psychiatric–mental health nurses working with older clients need to keep this study in mind and design nursing interventions to improve cognitive functioning and reduce anxiety about memory loss. Furthermore, the nurse should encourage elder clients to engage in physical and social activities.

SOURCE: Stevens, F. C. J., Kaplan, C. D., Ponds, R. W., Diederiks, J. P. M., & Jolles, J. (1999). How ageing and social factors affect memory. Age and Ageing, *28(4), 379–384.*

the realm of their individual cultural traditions, backgrounds, or experiences. Spirituality, faith in God, and increased participation in religious activities play an important role in elderly African Americans' ability to keep active and involved during the aging process (University of Missouri, 2003a).

Hispanic Elderly

Of all minority older persons age 65 years and older, Hispanic elderly are the least educated. Approximately 10% have had no education, and only 27% have graduated from high school. Language and transportation barriers, living in isolated areas, living on an inadequate income, and functional limitations can contribute to lack of motivation, thus preventing Hispanic elderly from becoming active and involved within the community (AARP, 2003).

Asian American Elderly

Although a large number of recent Asian American elderly immigrants are high-school graduates and are well educated professionally, cultural and language differences may provide barriers to their ability to remain active and involved in their communities (AARP, 2003).

Staying in Touch With Other Family Members

A 94-year-old woman placed in a nursing home by her family made this statement:"I cry inside every day. Each time they come to visit me, I beseech them to take me home... All I want...is to hold my daughter's hand and be surrounded by those people and things I love."

The following poem appeared in a local newspaper along with a drawing of a forlorn-looking elderly woman sitting alone in her home:

> *Next year.*
> *They said they'll come down for Christmas next*
> *   year.*
> *Excuses again.*
> *It's warm today.*
> *Too warm for Christmas anyway.*
> *I don't think I can wait another year.*
> — *Larry Moore, 1983*

This verse depicts the loneliness experienced by many elderly people without family or a substitute support system, especially on holidays, anniversary dates, and birthdays.

Loneliness can lead to depression and thoughts of suicide. The elderly are considered to account for approximately 25% of suicides reported yearly (American Psychiatric Association [APA], 2000; Blazer, 1996). Persons who meet the developmental tasks of maintaining love, sex, and marital relationships, and who keep active and involved, probably would be able to cope with separation from family members more readily than those who choose to disengage themselves from society.

Native American Elderly

Most elderly Native Americans have large extended families and are able to stay in touch with family members. Sharing of responsibilities by family members, respect for others, and allowing for individual freedom are integral parts of the Native American lifestyle. Generosity is valued, especially in helping family members and others who are less fortunate (University of Missouri, 2003c).

African American Elderly

As noted earlier, many elderly African Americans are divorced or live alone and do not have family members with whom they can visit. In addition to the lack of a family support group, prejudice and discrimination experienced by several minority groups within our society can also be factors that affect the quality of life of elderly African Americans, leading to loneliness or depression (University of Missouri, 2003a).

Hispanic Elderly

Hispanic family values are becoming increasingly vulnerable to acculturation, creating an increased need for housing in metropolitan areas because Hispanic elderly continue to prefer to remain in familiar neighborhoods, close to family. Living with family gives the Hispanic elderly social contact and an opportunity to attend functions important in the Hispanic family system. It also provides the Hispanic elderly with an opportunity to serve as a role model for younger members of the family (University of Missouri, 2003b).

Asian American Elderly

An increasing number of Asian American elderly are no longer living with their adult children. This break in tradition (ie, that of keeping in close touch with other family members) is leading to a critical need of various agency support services (eg, home care, education, transportation, translation, and public health) and companionship (DuPuy, 2002; Ho, 2002).

Sustaining and Maintaining Physical and Mental Health

Various emotional and behavioral reactions occur as people undergo the physiologic changes of the aging process such as impaired vision and hearing, limited mobility, incontinence, and a decline in cognitive abilities. These reactions include anxiety, frustration, fear, depression, intolerance, stubbornness, loneliness, decreased independence, decreased productivity, low self-esteem, and numerous somatic complaints (also referred to as *hypochondriasis*). Older clients often experience a slowing of their mental and physical reactions, and are unable to do anything about it. Reactions to aging are further compounded by the sight of younger people performing their job and assuming their role.

Loss is a predominant theme characterizing the emotional experiences of older people. The aged person fears loss of control over daily routines, loss of identity, confinement (eg, placement in a nursing home or hospital), social isolation because of failing health, and death (20% to 25% of the elderly occupy nursing homes when they die) (Brozovic & Wald, 2000).

Native American Elderly

Although elderly Native Americans are cared for by members of their tribe and receive extended family support, many elderly Native Americans enter their later years as survivors of significant stressors (eg, economic strife and discrimination) that take a toll on their physical and mental health. The geographic locations of reservations often provide a barrier to accessing health care. Death rates among elderly Native Americans are attributed to tuberculosis, diabetes, pneumonia, influenza, heart disease, malignant neoplasms, accidents, alcoholism, suicide, and homicide (Boyle, 2003; University of Missouri, 2003c).

African American Elderly

More than 50% of African American elderly are in poor health. They experience multiple chronic illnesses (eg, diabetes, hypertension, and obesity) that can progress into more severe complications. Also, they tend to be institutionalized for psychiatric–mental health

disorders (eg, multi-infarct and alcoholic dementia) more often than white elderly. Their admissions to psychiatric–mental health facilities are less likely to be voluntary (University of Missouri, 2003a).

Hispanic Elderly

Physical health is ranked as the most serious concern and fear that Hispanic elderly face. Their work, primarily unskilled labor, which often involved hard physical labor, has left them vulnerable to a variety of illnesses and disabilities. Hypertension, cancer, diabetes, arthritis, and high cholesterol are the leading medical problems found among the Hispanic elderly. In addition, Hispanic elderly who experienced functional limitations are at risk for mood disorders, such as depression (University of Missouri, 2003b).

Buki (2005), a psychiatrist of Latin American origin, states that the Hispanic immigrants in the United States have unique mental health needs. The most frequent complaints are insomnia and trouble concentrating. Although some men report a history of physical and verbal abuse as political prisoners and a few women report experiencing sexual abuse or rape as adolescents, few of these individuals have ever seen a psychiatrist because of the stigma and cost of treatment. Buki lists the most common psychiatric disorders experienced by Hispanic elderly immigrants as anxiety disorders, mood disorders, and age-related cognitive decline and dementias, whereas the least common disorders are alcohol and substance abuse.

Asian American Elderly

Although depression exists among Asian American elders, with 40% of them reporting symptoms of the condition, a deficiency in psychiatric–mental health services emphasizes the need for bicultural and bilingual psychiatric care. Certain types of cancers, hypertension, and tuberculosis are major health concerns of Asian American elderly. Relatively few data exist regarding the use of medical health care services by Asian American elderly. However, approximately 50% of Asian American elders have health insurance through Medicare, 41% receive Medicaid benefits, and 24% are covered by health maintenance organization (HMO) plans. Cultural and language differences, a reliance on folk medicine, and a distrust of Western medicine help explain why Asian American elderly are less likely to use formal health care services (AARP, 2003; Asian American Federation of New York, 2003; DuPuy, 2002).

Imagine what your own emotional or behavioral reactions would be to the following physical impairments: loss of hearing or sight, inability to speak because of a stroke, inability to perform activities of daily living (ADLs) because of left-side paralysis or disorientation, and incontinence of urine or stool due to loss of bladder or bowel control. How would you cope? What activities that you currently enjoy would be impeded by these impairments? What if you had no direct family members to care for you?

Finding Meaning in Life

"Listen to the aged. They will teach you. They are a distinguished faculty who teach not from books but from long experience in living" (Burnside, 1975, p. 1800).

The elderly reminisce frequently as they adapt to the aging process. They are eager to talk about days gone by. Schrock (1980) refers to Roger C. Peck's concept of ego transcendence versus ego preoccupation in her discussion of the elderly person's outlook on life. **Ego transcendence** describes a positive approach to finding meaning in life as aging persons talk about past life experiences and realize that they have the wisdom and knowledge to serve as resource persons. They are willing to share themselves with others, remain active, and look to the future. Persons exhibiting **ego preoccupation** resign themselves to the aging process, become inactive, feel they have no future, and wait to die. They do not feel their lives have any significant meaning to themselves or others as they disengage themselves from society.

Neugarten (in Schrock, 1980) discusses five components of measuring the elderly person's satisfaction with life:

1. Zest versus apathy
2. Resolution and fortitude versus passivity
3. Congruence between desired and achieved goals
4. Self-concept
5. Mood tone

Table 30-3 compares ego transcendence and ego preoccupation using Neugarten's five components of life satisfaction, which is a helpful tool for assessing older clients.

Native American Elderly

The meaning of life for elderly Native Americans does not rely upon individual success. Ego transcendence occurs as the elderly present themselves with respect to the world, provide security to the extended family, consider the extended family's welfare when making decisions, and pass down their wisdom and learning to the young. When ego transcendence is accomplished, the elderly Native American views him- or herself as brave, patient, honest, and respectful of others, and believes the self to be in balance with nature (University of Missouri, 2003c).

African American Elderly

African American elderly who experience external stressors (eg, lack of a family support system, chronic medical problems, socioeconomic disadvantages, prejudicial treatment, or unresolved personal conflicts) are at risk for the development of ego preoccupation rather than ego transcendence. Ego transcendence may be accomplished when the elderly learn to cope with external stressors, manage chronic medical problems, and utilize community resources that focus on meeting their needs.

Hispanic Elderly

Similar to their African American counterparts, the Hispanic elderly often resign themselves to the aging process, feeling useless and unmotivated. Hispanic family structure is traditionally hierarchical in nature, placing respected elder members at the top. However, emotional overinvolvement, divided loyalties among family members, and the need to keep the family together can create added stress for the elderly and place them at risk for the development of ego preoccupation (University of Missouri, 2003b).

Asian American Elderly

Many Asian American elderly have experienced rejection by their Americanized children. Consequently, they live alone and depend more on friends and neighbors than their adult children for support. They feel ashamed to seek help and are reluctant to reveal their physical or psychological needs. If these circumstances prevail, the Asian American elderly have difficulty finding meaning in life and are at risk for

TABLE 30.3 Neugarten's Five Components of Life

EGO TRANSCENDENCE	EGO PREOCCUPATION
Zest Enthusiastic and personally involved in activities around him or her	*Apathy* Bored, lacks energy and interest in others and activities around him or her
Resolution and fortitude Assumes an active responsibility for one's life and actions. Maslow describes this self-actualized person as realistic; accepting of others; spontaneous in actions; displaying a need for privacy, autonomy, and independence; democratic; and humorous (Schrock, 1980).	*Passivity* Does not assume an active responsibility for one's life and action; remains inactive and passive, allowing things to happen
Goal congruence (has achieved goals) Satisfied with the way goals have been met Feels successful as a person	*Goal incongruence (has not achieved goals)* Regrets action taken to achieve goals; dissatisfied with the way life is treating her or him
Positive self-concept Likes one's physical appearance and cares about how one presents self to others Feels competent; is able to socialize with others without feeling like a "third party"	*Negative self-concept* Does not place much emphasis or concern on physical appearance; feels incompetent; is unable to relate to others socially without feeling as if he or she is imposing
Positive mood tone Has the ability to appreciate life, displays a sense of humor, is optimistic and happy	*Negative mood tone* Is unable to appreciate life; displays a pessimistic attitude; may be irritable, bitter, or gloomy in emotional reactions

exhibiting ego preoccupation rather than ego transcendence (Ohio State University Extension, 2003).

Psychodynamics of Aging

According to Erikson (1963), the elderly experience the last stage of psychological development, identified as ego integrity versus despair. Individuals who experience ego integrity develop a sense of satisfaction with life and its meaning and believe that life is fulfilling and successful. They adapt to the changing environment and strive toward personhood as they adjust to and overcome what has been referred to as a "season of losses." Such losses include physical attractiveness, friends and affiliations, occupation, material prosperity, physical abilities, power, prestige, sexual opportunities, intimacy, and strength. Those elderly individuals who experience despair may exhibit patterns of behavior or emotional reactions such as those listed in Box 30-1.

A nonspecific condition often seen in elderly clients is referred to as **failure to thrive.** This syndrome, diagnosed in newborns and resulting from conditions that interfere with normal metabolism, appetite, and activity, also occurs in the elderly as a result of systemic disease, acute or chronic illness, or psychological stress. Clinical symptoms include unexplained weight loss, deterioration in mental status and functional ability, and

---

BOX 30.1 ELDERLY RESPONSES TO DESPAIR*

- Hypersomnia: Sleepy all day
- Insomnia: Inability to stay asleep
- Insomnia: Difficulty falling asleep
- Suspiciousness
- Persecutory thoughts
- Depressed mood
- Hypochondriasis
- Anxiety

*Reactions are listed in order of descending prevalence.

social isolation. The more common psychodynamics of aging (eg, emotional reactions, cognitive changes, and behavioral disturbances) that occur in the elderly are discussed in this chapter. They include anxiety, loneliness, guilt, depression, somatic complaints, paranoid reactions, dementia, and delirium.

Anxiety

Anxiety disorders were believed to decline with age. Experts are now beginning to recognize that anxiety and aging are not mutually exclusive. Although anxiety is as common in the elderly as in the young, how and when it appears can be distinctly different in older adults. Most older adults with an anxiety disorder had one when they were younger. The loss of mental acuity, admission to a nursing home, loss of a spouse, emergency surgery, confinement to bed because of a physical illness, and the diagnosis of a terminal illness are examples of the stressors and vulnerabilities unique to the aging process that may precipitate anxiety or exacerbate an existing anxiety disorder (Anxiety Disorders Association of America, 2003).

Because older adults may be unaccustomed to expressing their feelings openly, pent-up feelings and concerns or reactions to loss may manifest themselves as physical or somatic complaints, insomnia, restlessness, fatigue, hostility, dependency, and isolation. (See Chapters 19 and 20 for additional information on anxiety.)

Loneliness

Loneliness is considered the "reactive response to separation from persons and things in which one has invested oneself and one's energy" (Burnside, 1981, p. 66). Burnside lists five causes of loneliness in the elderly (from most common and severe to least common and severe):

1. Death of a spouse, relative, or friend.
2. Loss of a pet: Some elderly persons relate to pets as though they are family members, and the death of a longtime pet can be very traumatic.
3. The inability to communicate in the English language: People feel isolated and lonely if they are in a foreign environment or are unable to understand what is being said.
4. Pain: People often complain of loneliness when pain occurs during the late-evening or early-morning hours because no one is around to provide comfort.

5. Certain times of the day or night: Changes in living habits due to institutionalization in a nursing home may cause loneliness because the elderly are no longer able to perform daily or nightly rituals. Daily activities generally provide some stimulation for the elderly, whereas quiet evenings can seem quite long, especially if no relatives or friends visit.

Elderly clients who experience loneliness often feel that they no longer have a purpose in life, and are at risk for the development of late-life depression and suicide.

Guilt

As elderly clients experience the life-review process, reminiscing about the past, guilt feelings may emerge from past conflicts or regrets. For example, an elderly man revealed guilt about not lending his daughter and son-in-law money several years ago when they were in a financial bind. At the time of the request, the man felt that the couple should be able to support themselves. "Young people don't appreciate things given to them on a silver platter. They need to work for what they get. Then they'll take care of it," were his words of advice when they asked for help. He went on to state that they had plenty of money now, but "money doesn't keep one company." Feelings of guilt may also occur when a client considers past grudges, actions taken against others, outliving others, or unemployment or retirement.

Late-life Depression

Late-life depression is a major public health problem. As the elderly population grows, the number afflicted increases. The problem is further compounded because rates of depression are especially high in elderly individuals who are medically ill (Nelson & Battista, 2001). More than 2 million of approximately 34 million adults age 65 years or older in the United States suffer from depression (AOA, 2001). Bipolar disorder may also surface as a late-onset disorder and significantly interfere with personal relationships and social functioning. Experts predict that the incidence will increase significantly as the baby boomer generation grows older. Although bipolar disorder is either misdiagnosed or under-diagnosed in the elderly population, awareness about bipolar disorder in older individuals is increasing because of the documentation of statistics worldwide (Luggen, 2005).

Although medical illness is a common cause, loss, unresolved grief or guilt, changes in living situation, limited coping skills, or altered perceptions of one's physical capabilities may leave elderly persons with low self-esteem and feelings of helplessness, precipitating a reactive depression. Medications taken by the elderly (eg, pain medication, steroids used to treat medical conditions) or the use of alcohol also may precipitate or enhance a depressive reaction (Monarch Pharmaceuticals, 2000; Resnick, 2001). Elderly persons most at risk are white men older than 85 years, isolated elderly persons, older persons experiencing increased dependency and changes in body function, and older persons diagnosed with a terminal illness. Indeed, approximately 25% of all suicides committed yearly are by persons 65 years of age or older (APA, 2000; Blazer, 1996). Diagnoses frequently used to describe depression in older adults include dysthymic disorder, major depressive disorder, bereavement, and adjustment disorder with depressed mood (APA, 2000). (See Chapter 21 for additional information about depression.)

Somatic Complaints

Hypochondriasis—or preoccupation with one's physical and emotional health, resulting in bodily or somatic complaints—is common in the elderly client. The aging person re-channels stress and anxiety into bodily concerns as he or she assumes the "sick" role. Support, concern, and interest conveyed to the client serve as secondary gains, reinforcing a sense of control. The caregiver should assess all complaints thoroughly, in a matter-of-fact manner, and avoid stereotyping the person as a "chronic complainer." Common somatic complaints include pain, insomnia, and involuntary weight loss. (See Chapter 20 for additional information about anxiety-related disorders such as hypochondriasis and pain disorder.)

Paranoid Reactions

Loss of sight or hearing, sensory deprivation, and physical impairment often contribute to suspiciousness in elderly persons. Aging persons may feel that others are talking about them or conspiring against them. Various medications that have anticholinergic effects such as atropine sulfate (Atropine) or amitriptyline (Elavil), or antihistaminic effects such as cyproheptadine (Periactin) or diphenhydramine hydrochloride (Benadryl), have been known to cause adverse reactions such as blurred vision and confusion, leading to paranoid reactions in the elderly. A strange environment also may contribute to confusion and suspicious behavior among the elderly. (See Chapter 16 regarding medications and Chapter 28 for additional information about delusional disorders.)

Dementia

As noted in Chapter 27, dementia is an acquired organic syndrome defined by the presence of cognitive deficits such as impairment of memory, abstract thinking, and judgment. The elderly are at risk for dementia resulting from irreversible deterioration of the brain, mini-strokes caused by hypertension, chronic substance abuse, neurologic diseases, brain tumors, and metabolic diseases.

However, elderly clients have also been mistakenly diagnosed with dementia because of a failure in recognizing a psychiatric disorder. Depression by far remains the most frequent psychiatric disorder mimicking or associated with dementia in the elderly. Clinical symptoms of mania, psychosis, anxiety, personality disorders, and conversion disorders also have been misdiagnosed as dementia (Read, 1991). Table 30-4 distinguishes the characteristics of dementia from the **dementia syn-**

TABLE 30.4 Comparison of Dementia and Dementia Syndrome of Depression

DEMENTIA	DEMENTIA SYNDROME OF DEPRESSION
Insidious, indeterminate onset	Rapid onset
Symptoms of long duration	Symptoms of short duration
Mood and behavior fluctuate	Depressed mood
Client gives "near-miss" answers	Client replies "I don't know"
Client conceals disabilities	Client focuses on disabilities
Level of cognitive impairment relatively stable	Fluctuation in level of cognitive impairment

drome of depression (the rapid onset and short duration of clinical symptoms that are often misdiagnosed as dementia in clients who are severely depressed).

Delirium

Delirium is characterized by a disturbance of consciousness and impairment of attention that fluctuates during the course of the day. It is usually caused by disturbance of brain physiology by a medical disorder or ingested substance. It is one of the most common psychiatric–mental health diagnoses in the elderly population.

Delirium is particularly important to identify because it is assumed to be a reversible disorder, although it may persist for months in hospitalized medical or surgical clients. Common causes of delirium in the elderly as identified by Peskind and Raskind (1996) and Jung and Grossberg (1993) are classified as systemic illness, metabolic disorders, neurologic disorders, pharmacologic adverse effects, and miscellaneous causes.

Common clinical symptoms frequently seen include hallucinations, illusions, delusions, agitation, disorientation, memory impairment, anxiety, and abnormal vital signs. (See Chapter 27 for additional information on delirium.)

THE NURSING PROCESS

ASSESSMENT

The assessment of the psychosocial needs of elderly clients is multifaceted, focusing on the collection of demographic data, the interview process, and the review of medical records. Many long-standing psychosocial issues not addressed in earlier years, as well as the psychodynamics of aging discussed previously, may be present. These issues may cause serious problems for family members or caregivers to cope with. In addition, what looks like dementia or a similar mental syndrome may, in fact, be clinical symptoms of heart failure, pneumonia, or another medical disorder.

The following discussion focuses on the assessment setting, assessment interview, use of assessment tools, special assessment concerns (eg, pain, polypharmacy, sleep–rest activity, involuntary weight loss), barriers to assessment, and transcultural considerations. The assessment and nursing interventions for elderly clients who exhibit clinical symptoms of disorders such as anxiety, depression, substance abuse, and impaired cognition are discussed in separate chapters in this text.

The Assessment Setting

Assessment of the elderly client may take place in various settings depending on the physical and mental status of the client and access to health care. Common settings include the client's home, an assisted-living facility, senior wellness center, nursing home, medical–psychiatric unit, and acute care hospital. When assessing elderly clients, outcomes focus on providing the best treatment and services available to the client, achieving the best outcome, minimizing cost and time, advocating for identified necessary services to promote wellness, and reducing stress and frustration of both the client and caregivers (Edelson, 1999).

The Interview

When interviewing the older client, the physical setting may be a decisive factor in determining effectiveness of the interview or assessment. Adequate lighting is necessary because of possible reduction in the client's visual acuity. Additionally, the nurse should speak clearly and distinctly, facing the client, making sure to introduce oneself initially and establish how the client prefers to be addressed (surname or first name). If the client wears dentures, ensure that he or she is wearing them to avoid embarrassment or impaired communication.

Open-ended questions allow the client to respond without difficulty or fear of giving incorrect responses that could result in institutionalization or hospitalization. Initially, older adults may be resistant to or resent questions regarding personal problems (eg, sexual, marital). Explain the reason that specific questions are asked and reassure the client that the information obtained will be kept confidential. Clients with memory impairment may reminisce because they cannot converse in the here-and-now. Therefore, consider whether a family member or health care surrogate should be interviewed to validate data or obtain additional information as needed.

Assessment Tools

Format for a comprehensive nursing assessment tool takes into consideration the complexity of the multifaceted problems of older clients and provides a guide for holistic assessment by the psychiatric–mental health nurse (Neff, 1996). The tool assesses mental status, func-

BOX 30.2 COMPREHENSIVE GEROPSYCHIATRIC ASSESSMENT

Name:

Date of Birth:

Sex:

Marital Status:

Religion:

Educational Level:

Medical Diagnosis:

Medications (include start dates, dosage adjustments and medications previously taken, including all over-the-counter medications):

Allergies:

Laboratory Findings (include dates obtained):

Neurologic Findings (include tests performed):

Presenting Symptoms:

    Mental Status:

    Functional Status:

    Behavioral Assessment:

History of Previous Psychiatric Treatment:

Support Systems (include social functioning, religious preference/belief/support, cultural beliefs, financial resources, and family dynamics):

Family Input:

Review of Medical Records:

tional status, behavior, family dynamics, and social history. Demographic and health–illness data collection complete the comprehensive assessment of the elderly client. Box 30-2 lists the components of a comprehensive geropsychiatric assessment for clients who present with emotional or behavioral disturbances.

As noted earlier in this chapter, older adults may have difficulty with the developmental task of maintaining love, sex, and marital relationships. Wallace (2003) discusses the use of the PLISSIT model to assess and manage sexuality issues of older adults. As sexuality is discussed, the model and questions help the nurse to initiate and maintain discussions of sexuality. For example, the nurse might ask the client to state what concerns or questions the client has about fulfilling continuing sexual needs. The goal of such an assessment is to gather information that allows the client to express his or her sexuality safely and to feel uninhibited by normal or pathologic problems.

The acronym PLISSIT stands for the following actions by the nurse:

- **P: P**ermission is obtained to initiate sexual discussion during the assessment.
- **LI: L**imited **I**nformation is provided to assess normal aging changes and any medical conditions or medications that may interfere with the client's ability to function sexually.
- **SS: S**pecific **S**uggestions regarding sexual relations are discussed. This action allows the nurse to assess the client's comfort level and knowledge about sexual relationships among older adults
- **IT: I**ntensive **T**herapy is available as needed to address the issues of sexuality.

Various assessment tools used to determine *Diagnostic and Statistical Manual of Mental Disorders, 4th Edition, Text Revision (DSM-IV-TR)* clinical diagnoses have been discussed or referred to throughout the text. Examples of tools used to assess the elderly client include the Geriatric Depression Scale, Beck Depression Scale, Beck Anxiety Scale, Annotated Mini-Mental State Examination, Short Portable Mental Status Questionnaire, Global Deterioration Rating Scale, and Suicide Intention Rating Scale.

Special Assessment Concerns

The management of pain, **polypharmacy** (use of multiple over-the-counter drugs, prescription drugs, or a combination of both), getting a good night's sleep, and loss of appetite or involuntary weight loss are four recurring special concerns that may be identified during the assessment of psychosocial needs of the elderly.

Pain. The elderly, who have medical problems or chronic diseases, are twice as likely to experience pain when compared with younger adults. Moreover, elderly clients who experience unrelieved pain are prone to the development of behavioral disturbances, depression, or anxiety. Behavioral disturbances are often seen in elderly clients who are unable to verbally express that they are in pain (eg, clients with aphasia, clients who are delirious, or clients with impaired cognition) or who are unable to express anger regarding their medical condition. Clients experiencing pain may also develop depression or anxiety resulting from separation from family or fear of the unknown prognosis of their medical condition. Assessment of pain is the key to proper diagnosis and treatment. Because there are no biologic markers for the presence of pain, an accurate conclusion about a client's pain can be determined only by assessment and a thorough interview (Battista, 2002). Failure to recognize pain as the underlying cause of changes in the elderly person's behavior, mood, or affect may result in the inappropriate treatment of clinical symptoms with psychoactive drugs instead of pain medication.

Pain assessment includes an evaluation of the onset, location, intensity, pattern, duration, quality of pain, precipitating and relieving factors, and the effect pain has on function, mood, and sleep (American Geriatric Society, 1998). In addition to pain assessment, the psychiatric–mental health nurse collects data about the type and quantity of medication that the elderly client takes to provide information about possible adverse effects or interactions that may complicate the client's situation. (See Chapter 9 for additional information regarding pain assessment.)

Polypharmacy and Substance Abuse. A history of polypharmacy to treat pain or other conditions such as heart failure, hypertension, or arthritis can place clients at risk for adverse effects of drug interactions (eg, dizziness, confusion, or unstable gait) or physiologic changes (eg, electrolyte or metabolic imbalance, liver damage, or renal failure). Absorption of drugs is generally complete, but slower; toxic levels may occur more quickly; and clearance and excretion of drugs take longer. Furthermore, polypharmacy is a significant factor in the morbidity and mortality of elderly clients. Adverse events are detrimental to physical outcomes, causing approximately one death per 1,000 hospitalized clients. Therefore, be sure to obtain accurate information regarding the client's use of medication.

Polypharmacy places clients at risk for the development of depression and possible polysubstance abuse. According to a retrospective analysis of more than 875,000 clients in long-term care, polypharmacy is a strong predictor of depression in elderly clients. The relationship between depression and polypharmacy, appears to be bi-directional. For example, people who are depressed generally have more somatic complaints. When their doctors prescribe more medication in an effort to treat those symptoms, clinical symptoms of depression are exacerbated (MacReady, 2005). As this cycle continues, the client may develop clinical symptoms of polysubstance abuse.

In addition, attempt to determine whether the client drinks alcoholic beverages socially or as a means to cope with stress. Alcohol abuse that begins before the age of 60 years is referred to as early-onset and is generally associated with personality disorders, schizophrenia, mood disorders, or poverty. Conversely, late-onset alcohol abuse usually begins after age 60, years and is frequently associated with medical and psychosocial issues faced by senior citizens. Alcohol interferes with the actions of numerous medications, and elderly clients who use alcohol may be unaware of the risk factors associated with mixing medication with alcohol (Lemieux, 2005). (See Chapter 25 for additional information related to assessment of clients with substance-related disorders.)

Be knowledgeable about physical conditions that impair absorption of drugs; which drugs require sufficient serum protein levels for binding; and which drugs have prolonged half-lives that cause physiologic changes or an alteration in mental status. Psychiatric symptoms indicative of delirium, dementia, or psychosis may result from impaired drug clearance, increased serum drug levels caused by failure to follow the directions of the prescribing clinician, or drug–drug interactions. Chapter 16 discusses other issues related to psychopharmacology.

Sleep–Rest Activity (Insomnia). The elderly client may experience episodic, acute insomnia that lasts from one night to a few weeks, or chronic insomnia that lasts for 1 month or longer. The consequences of lost sleep include fatigue, lack of energy, difficulty concentrating, and irritability. Lack of sleep, which has an adverse effect on occupational and social functioning, also leads to accidents and traffic fatalities (Nadolski, 2003). Common causes of insomnia in the elderly client may include environmental changes; disruption in the client's sleeping environment (eg, phone calls or noise), emotional stress, medical conditions (eg, pain disorder, chronic obstructive pulmonary disease [COPD], or heart failure), medication (eg, central nervous system stimulants, diuretics, or decongestants), poor sleep hygiene, or the presence of a specific sleep disorder. (Chapter 9 discusses primary and secondary insomnia.)

When assessing the client's sleep problems, ask the client to describe:

- When the problem began
- His or her sleep hygiene habits
- Usual retirement and wake-up time

- His or her sleep environment
- The effect of the lack of sleep on his or her daily activities
- Any medication that the client takes at bedtime

The nurse clarifies the responses with the client and explains that the information will be used to plan interventions to promote sleep.

Involuntary Weight Loss. Involuntary weight loss (IWL), frequently observed in the older population, is an indicator of significant decline in health and function. It has been estimated that approximately 13% of ambulatory elderly clients and 50% to 65% of long-term care residents exhibit IWL (Bouras, Lange, & Scolapio, 2001).

Assessing IWL is challenging and generally includes a multidisciplinary team approach. Assessment should cover the potential pathophysiologic etiologies (eg, pain, difficulty swallowing, loss of taste or smell), psychosocial status (eg, depression, memory impairment, delusions, alcoholism), and functional status (eg, ability to perform ADLs, dexterity, mobility), along with normal aging considerations. The client's medication regimen also must be assessed because several medications are associated with weight loss, including selective serotonin reuptake inhibitor (SSRI) antidepressants, cardiac agents (eg, digoxin or ace inhibitors), theophylline, antibiotics, stimulants, anticonvulsants, cholinesterase inhibitors, appetite suppressants, neuroleptics, and some benzodiazepines (Saffel-Shrier, Gay, Oderda, & Thiese, 2003; McNamara, 2004). (Chapter 23 discusses additional information regarding disturbances of appetite.)

Barriers to Assessment

Barriers to the assessment of elderly clients have been identified. Typically they are classified as related to the provider, client, or illness.

Provider-Related Barriers. Provider-related barriers involve the health care professional. The health care professional may have limited experience working with elderly clients or may feel uncomfortable working with older adults. Provider-related barriers may include the nurse's concern about stigmatizing the client, especially if the client has never been treated by a mental health professional, or the nurse's uncertainty about when to initiate an assessment for mental health problems. In addition, time constraints imposed on the nurse may lead to feelings of being rushed and obtaining incomplete data when discussing mental health issues with elderly clients. Other barriers include lack of provider or referral access due to limitations of health care coverage; and reimbursement considerations such as precertification requirements for a mental health consultation.

Client-Related Barriers. Client-related barriers, as the name implies, involve the client. These barriers may include the presence of a wide variety of symptoms that are difficult to prioritize and diagnose. Because of cultural differences between the psychiatric–mental health nurse and client, the client may not present an accurate picture of his or her clinical symptoms. For example, Native Americans are generally very stoic and do not maintain eye contact during an assessment, and many Hispanics, mainly Cubans and Nicaraguans, know neither what depression and anxiety are nor how these illnesses can be managed (Buki, 2005). Language barriers may also make it difficult for the client to accurately describe emotions or thoughts. The client may be unfamiliar with or reluctant to discuss words such as "sadness" or "depression." Somatic symptoms may be amplified by the client for secondary gain. The elderly client, or the family member accompanying the client, may refuse to answer questions because of the stigma attached to mental illness. It is common for a caregiver to describe a client as mentally healthy when, in fact, the client reveals feelings of depression or suicidal ideation during the assessment process. The same can be said for significant others who deny the presence of dementia in a loved one although clinical symptoms are evident.

Illness-Related Barriers. Illness-related barriers typically involve medical or psychological problems. It is not uncommon for the psychiatric–mental health nurse to receive a request to assess an elderly client with a medical condition or psychological problems. The nurse may encounter illness-related barriers due to acute change in the client's health, neurologic (eg, Parkinson's disease) or metabolic (eg, diabetes mellitus) disorders, drug–drug interactions (eg, metoclopramide [Reglan] and phenelzine [Nardil]), or undisclosed drug or alcohol use. For example, a client may be admitted to the hospital for treatment of diabetes and comorbid depression. Because the client presents with clinical symptoms of agitation, confusion, and impaired cognition due to metabolic acidosis, the nurse is unable to assess the client. Unmet psychosocial needs can also cause illness-related barriers. For example, an elderly client who lives alone, is depressed, and has a dysfunctional family relationship may desire—but not have access to—mental health care.

Transcultural Considerations. Nurses assessing elderly persons in culturally diverse settings should speak the language of the population being served. If necessary, a translator should be used to obtain adequate, accurate information. It may be beneficial to include a family member or caretaker to validate information obtained during the assessment. (See Chapter 4 for additional information regarding the assessment of culturally diverse clients.)

Elderly persons who achieve integrity (ie, developmental task of integrity vs. despair) view aging as a positive experience. They find meaning in their lives by sharing their traditions and values with others. When assessing elderly clients, be sure to consider the culturally diverse elderly client's perspective on aging in at least three general areas:

1. How the person perceives health and illness
2. What expectations of care the person has
3. How nursing can support culturally determined patterns of dealing with health and coping with illness

NURSING DIAGNOSES AND OUTCOME IDENTIFICATION

The formulation of nursing diagnoses and statements of outcome for elderly clients with psychiatric–mental health issues can be challenging because of the coexistence of at least one medical condition. Moreover, elderly clients commonly have at least three or four medical diagnoses, requiring the client to take six or seven different medications, which could lead to an increase in adverse effects or possible interactions. The complexity of an elderly client's medical history, including the investigation of underlying factors, can make the determination of an appropriate nursing diagnosis and subsequent outcome identification difficult.

Psychiatric–mental health nursing diagnoses and outcomes generally focus on issues of loss or grief, social isolation, alteration in affect or mood, low self-concept, changes in behavior or cognition, and special concerns related to pain, disturbance in sleep–rest activity, and IWL. Other issues that are not as commonly disclosed during assessment include chemical dependence and chronic mental illness. See the accompanying

box, Examples of North American Nursing Diagnosis Association (NANDA) Nursing Diagnoses: Elderly Clients With Psychosocial Needs.

PLANNING INTERVENTIONS AND IMPLEMENTATION

Emphasis is placed on maximizing the older person's independence by assisting with the basic human needs identified by Maslow (1968); meeting emotional needs; and maintaining life with dignity and comfort until death.

Assisting With Meeting Basic Human Needs

Geropsychiatric–mental health nursing interventions focus on Maslow's (1968) theory of motivation, in which he identified these basic human needs: the need for survival, safety, and security; love and belonging; positive self-esteem; and self-actualization. Using

---

EXAMPLES OF NANDA NURSING DIAGNOSES/ ELDERLY CLIENT WITH PSYCHOSOCIAL NEEDS

- Acute Confusion related to disturbance in cerebral metabolism secondary to adverse effects of pain medication
- Adult Failure to Thrive related to limited ability to adapt to effects of aging
- Anxiety related to perceived change in socioeconomic status secondary to retirement
- Ineffective Coping related to changes in physical environment secondary to relocation
- Disturbed Sleep Pattern related to pain secondary to arthritis
- Ineffective Health Maintenance related to lack of motivation secondary to divorce
- Risk For Loneliness related to loss of usual social contacts secondary to loss of driving ability
- Powerlessness related to unmet dependency needs secondary to death of spouse
- Risk for Relocation Stress related to high degree of environmental change secondary to change in available caregiver

Maslow's concept enables the caregiver to meet more than just survival needs, a condition that occurs too frequently in nursing care. The following points about the aging process may be helpful as one plans and implements nursing care to meet the basic human needs of elderly clients, whether they are seen as outpatients or inpatients.

Need for Survival. Physical illness can be traumatic, especially if the onset of illness is sudden and affects the elderly client's mobility and ability to perform personal ADLs. The elderly client, in his or her need for survival, may become angry or frustrated if recovery is slow or physiologic needs are not met. Pain, insomnia, and IWL, noted during the psychosocial assessment, may have a negative impact on the elderly client's need for survival. A brief discussion of interventions used to manage pain, insomnia, and IWL is presented.

Pain Management. Pain in the absence of disease is not a normal part of aging, yet it is experienced daily by a majority of older adults. Untreated or poorly managed pain can affect the physical, psychological, social, emotional, and spiritual well-being of older adults who are at high risk for undertreatment of pain resulting from a variety of barriers such as lack of adequate pain management education of health care professionals, the expense of pain management, or the reluctance of the older adult to report pain or take analgesics. Common causes of pain in the elderly include fibromyalgia, gout, neuropathies, osteoarthritis, osteoporosis and fractures, and polymyalgia rheumatica (Hanks-Bell, Halvey, & Paice, 2004).

Pain management with the elderly can be challenging. With increasing age, individuals experience decreased liver functioning and develop lower levels of body water as a reflection of the increasing percentage of their body weight attributed to fat. These changes affect the body's ability to metabolize medication placing the elderly at risk for adverse effects of drug interactions. Also, the brain becomes more sensitive to the sedating effects of most medications.

Because the rate of cognitive processing diminishes with increasing age, appropriate time must be taken to explain each of the issues related to the client's diagnosis and use of pain medication.

Impaired vision (including color vision), hearing, smell, and taste might contribute to the client's inadvertently taking the wrong medication. Printed or written instructions, in large print, may be necessary. Review of the instructions with a family member or significant other lessens the possibility of medication confusion or noncompliance (Schuckit, 1997).

In 1998, the American Geriatric Society published guidelines for the chronic pain management. The following year, the American Medical Directors Association (AMDA) published similar guidelines stating that, whenever possible, use the least invasive route to administer pain medication, identify the underlying cause of pain, and use a cautious approach to prevent oversedation. For example, short-acting analgesics such as acetaminophen (Tylenol) are best for acute flare-ups of minor or mild pain related to chronic conditions. Regularly scheduled dosing (eg, every 6–8 hours) is more effective than as-needed dosing. Table 30-5 lists examples of agents used to treat pain in the elderly (Feldt, 2005). (See Chapter 12 for additional information regarding pain management.)

Stabilization of Sleep–Rest Activity. The goals of treatment for elderly clients with sleep, rest, and activity problems and insomnia are to resolve the underlying problem(s), prevent progression to a chronic state, restore and improve the client's quality and duration of sleep, and improve the client's quality of life (Nadolski, 2003).

According to the National Sleep Foundation (2006), older adults are likely to suffer both medical and psychiatric disorders that may disrupt sleep. It is not unusual for elderly clients to experience a specific sleep disorder (eg, restless leg syndrome or sleep apnea). Medical problems (eg, asthma, heartburn, incontinence, COPD) can interrupt, delay, and/or shorten sleep. Examples of psychiatric disorders that may cause insomnia include depression, anxiety, and substance abuse.

Nursing interventions depend upon the severity of the client's symptoms. If the client does not respond to nonpharmacologic interventions for insomnia (eg, sleep hygiene, relaxation therapy, psychotherapy for underlying anxiety), pharmacologic measures (eg, the use of sedating antidepressants or the natural hormone melatonin) may be necessary. Drugs of choice in the treatment for restless leg syndrome include dopamine agonists such as ropinirole (Requip) and pramipexole (Mirapex). Other considerations include dopamine precursors such as levodopa (Sinemet); anticonvulsants such as gabapentin (Neurontin); or short-acting benzodiazepines. (See Chapters 12 and 16 for additional information regarding the treatment of sleep disorders.)

TABLE 30.5 Examples of Agents Used to Treat Pain in the Elderly

CLASSIFICATION	GENERIC (TRADE)	TOTAL DAILY DOSAGE
Antipyretic/analgesic	acetaminophen (Tylenol)	4000 mg
Nonsteroidal anti-inflammatory	celecoxib (Celebrex)	400 mg
	etodolac (Lodine)	1000 mg
	ketoprofen (Oruvail)	2000 mg
	naproxen (Naprosyn)	1000 mg
	rofecoxib (Vioxx)	50 mg
Opioid analgesic	dextropropoxyphene (Darvon)	390 mg
	dihydrocodeine (Panlor SS)	5 tabs
Anticonvulsant	carbamazepine (Tegretol)	1200 mg
	gabapentin (Neurontin)	1800 mg

NOTE: Low-dose tricyclic antidepressants such as nortriptyline (Pamelor) and amitriptyline (Elavil) have been used; however, the risks outweigh the benefits in the presence of comorbid medical disorders.

SOURCE: National Council on the Aging. (2003). *Facts about older Americans and pain*. Retrieved August 17, 2003, from http://www.ortho-mcneil.com/resources/misc/seniors_facts_bottom.htm

Interventions for Involuntary Weight Loss. After the diagnosis of IWL has been confirmed and no medical problems have been identified, the psychiatric–mental health nurse discusses the treatment approaches with the client. If the client lives alone, nonpharmacologic interventions such as the use of local community agencies (eg, Meals on Wheels or home health care) may be used to provide meals and an opportunity for the client to socialize during meal time. If the IWL is caused by psychosocial issues, the client may agree to individual therapy with the nurse–therapist. Pharmacologic interventions may include the use of an appetite stimulant such as megestrol acetate (Megace) or dronabinol (Marinol). If the psychiatric–mental health nurse has determined that the IWL is secondary to depression, the use of mirtazapine (Remeron) or a similar antidepressant that also stimulates the appetite may be used. (See Chapters 16 and 23 for additional information regarding interventions to stabilize weight loss and promote weight gain.)

Need for Safety and Security. People who have difficulty adjusting during the aging process may have been somewhat emotionally frail all their lives and dependent on others due to unmet needs of survival, and safety and security. For example, the elderly client may have difficulty establishing satisfactory living arrangements, adjusting to retirement income, or keeping in touch

with family members after the unexpected death of a spouse. Nursing care is planned to meet the client's needs by:

- Minimizing the amount of change to which the client is exposed
- Introducing change gradually
- Determining the client's previous lifestyle and making adjustments as needed to ensure that the need for safety and security is met
- Encouraging the client or family members to bring familiar items from home if the client relocates, is hospitalized, or is institutionalized
- Explaining new routines, medications, or treatments when providing care
- Including the client in decision-making regarding such issues as medical treatment, relocation, or finances

Need for Love and Belonging. Older persons have a need for love and belonging as well as a need to maintain their status in society. As they become older, it may be increasingly difficult for them to remain active and involved or to make contributions to society. The widowed or divorced client may not be able to achieve the developmental task of maintaining love, sex, and marital relationships. If the client feels unwanted, he or she may resort to telling stories about earlier achievements. Nursing interventions to meet the need for love and belonging include:

- Encouraging expression of affection, touch, and human sexuality
- Permitting the client to select a roommate when appropriate
- Providing opportunities to form new friendships and relationships with persons of varying ages
- Permitting flexible visiting hours with family or friends
- Providing privacy when desired
- Encouraging expression of feelings such as loneliness and the need to be loved

Need for Positive Self-Esteem. Irritating behavior usually is related to the elderly person's frustration, fear, or awareness of limitations rather than a physiologic deficit or the actual issue at hand. The older person needs to feel a sense of self-worth, to take pride in her or his abilities and accomplishments (ie, find meaning in life), and to be respected by others. Nursing interventions are planned to restore, preserve, and protect the elderly person's self-esteem. Include the client in the development of the plan of care, especially ADLs. Provide positive feedback when the client accomplishes identified goals. Encourage the client to take pride in personal appearance. Identify personal strengths to promote self-confidence and independence. Communicate with the client on an adult level when seeking the client's advice or listening to the client reminisce about life experiences.

Need for Self-Actualization. Self-actualization or self-fulfillment occurs only after the more basic needs of survival, safety and security, love and belonging, and a positive sense of self-esteem have been met. Peck's concept of ego transcendence, discussed earlier in this chapter, describes the self-actualized person. Nursing interventions to promote self-actualization in the elderly include encouraging the client to participate in activities or develop hobbies to promote socialization, productivity, and creativity. Doing so also helps to foster a sense of accomplishment in the client. Also encourage the client to be a resource person as well as a teacher of skills or crafts to younger generations. Such activities serve a useful purpose and earn the elderly person recognition. In addition, the nurse works with the elderly client to meet the developmental task of dying.

Life-Review Process. As aging persons prepare to complete the task of self-actualization or self-fulfillment,

they experience a mental life-review process in which they may address unresolved conflicts or reflect on their purpose in life. They may be motivated to read philosophy, study religion, take college courses, or use computers to expand their knowledge base.

Computers have found their way into the hands of elderly persons who are willing to use them. According to a 1999 survey, at least 25% of individuals between the ages of 60 and 69 years own a computer. This number drops to 16% for those between the ages of 70 and 79 years. Research has shown that elderly clients who use the Internet demonstrate some improvement in mood and a sense of well-being as a result of increased socialization, communication, and intellectual stimulation (Schuman, 2000).

The nurse can enhance the life-review process of the client in a private or group setting by encouraging him or her to discuss accomplishments, record an autobiography, review and discuss photographs, discuss work accomplishments, or discuss concerns about the final stage of life (Neff, 1996).

Reminiscence. Self-actualization may also be achieved through reminiscence. In contrast to the life-review process, **reminiscence** is a therapeutic process of consciously seeking and sharing memories of past significant experiences and events. This process may occur with an individual client or in groups. Nursing interventions are similar to those used in the life-review process (Neff, 1996).

Grief Work. The loss of a spouse has been rated as the most stressful life event across all ages and all cultural backgrounds. Loss of an adult child is equally as stressful to many elderly individuals who rely on their children to provide emotional or financial support. Some elderly clients are unable to complete the task of self-actualization until they work through the grief process.

Each individual reacts differently to the loss of a loved one. The role of the nurse as the facilitator in grief work is to help the client accept the loss, express feelings about the loss, and learn and grow from the experience. If grief work is unresolved, the client may exhibit clinical symptoms of bereavement, which has long-term effects on the survivor's social, interpersonal, and economic performance in the months and years following the loss (Khin & Sunderland, 2000). (See Chapter 7 for additional information related to Loss and Grief.)

Psychotherapy. Integrated psychotherapy may be the best method for addressing complex issues that are often unique to geriatric clients. Older adults are less likely than younger individuals to have support since they are no longer married, are retired from the work that defined their identity and purpose in life, and have lower physical health and strength. *Integrated psychotherapy* is the concurrent application of more than one psychotherapeutic technique to address symptoms that arise from various sources such as lack of understanding and knowledge about illness and aging, maladaptive thoughts and actions that interfere with problem-solving ability, and reactions and emotions that originate from lifelong, unconscious conflicts and perceptions (Evans, 2006).

Psychotherapy is provided in individual or group settings to help elderly clients examine their purpose and goals in life as they achieve self-actualization through creativity and satisfying life experiences.

The nurse's role is to encourage clients to talk about their lives, describe any abandonment issues, and interpret any fantasies and dreams they may have; as well as help clients verbalize feelings such as anger, envy, or jealousy. It is hoped that clients will exhibit an increase in self-worth, improvement in morale, and a sense of having made a contribution to others (Neff, 1996). (See Chapter 14 for additional information regarding psychotherapy.)

Medication Management

If the elderly client requires psychotropic medication, certain guidelines should be followed when medication is prescribed and administered. As noted earlier, the pharmacokinetics and pharmacodynamics that are inherent in the aging process place elderly clients at risk for adverse effects. Antipsychotic drugs are used cautiously because elderly clients are more sensitive to the adverse effects than young clients are. In addition, anti-manic drugs are generally considered to be contraindicated because of physiologic changes that occur in the heart, thyroid, and kidneys of elderly clients. A pretreatment history and physical examination, as well as baseline laboratory testing and electrocardiogram (ECG), are imperative. Nonspecific complaints of confusion, lethargy, dizziness, incontinence, depression, and falls strongly suggest an older client is experiencing some type of drug–drug interaction. If a client is already taking a psychotropic drug, it is desirable that the drug be discontinued to allow its removal from the client's system so that baseline clinical symptoms can be observed before a different psychotropic agent is prescribed. Most agents are usually given in divided dosages over a 24-hour period. Drug Summary Table 30-1 highlights commonly used drugs for elderly clients.

GENERIC (TRADE) NAME	DAILY DOSAGE RANGE	IMPLEMENTATION
DRUG SUMMARY TABLE 30-1 ▪ Selected Drugs Used for Elderly Clients		
Drug Class: TCAs (for depression)		
desipramine (Norpramin)	1.5–2 mg/kg	Know that more than 150 mg per day in divided doses is not recommended; monitor for anticholinergic effects, confusion, and orthostatic hypotension; be aware of potential for several adverse effects of drug–drug interactions; give major portion of drug at h.s. if drowsiness occurs; instruct client to avoid alcohol and sleep-inducing and OTC drugs.
nortriptylene (Pamelor)	1–1.2 mg/kg	Do not exceed 50 mg per day in divided doses; be aware of potential for several adverse effects of drug–drug interactions; monitor for anticholinergic effects, sedation, confusion, orthostatic hypotension, and GI disturbances, including paralytic ileus.

DRUG SUMMARY TABLE 30-1 Selected Drugs Used for Elderly Clients (Continued)

GENERIC (TRADE) NAME	DAILY DOSAGE RANGE	IMPLEMENTATION
Drug Class: SSRIs (for depression and anxiety)		
citalopram (Celexa)	10–30 mg	Give once a day in the morning; inform client of severe drug–drug reaction if taken with St. John's wort therapy; monitor for somnolence, dizziness, insomnia, tremor, sweating, and GI disturbances.
sertraline (Zoloft)	25–75 mg	Give drug in the morning; monitor for insomnia, akathisia, nausea, anorexia, pseudoparkinsonism, and hyponatremia; increased risk of severe adverse effects if combined with St. John's wort therapy.
Drug Class: Stimulants (for depression)		
methylphenilate (Ritalin)	2.5–20 mg	Use with caution in presence of seizure disorders; obtain ECG; give in the morning or before 6 PM to prevent insomnia; monitor CBC and platelet count if utilized as long-term therapy; instruct client to report nervousness, palpitations, or fever.
Drug Class: SNRIs (for depression)		
atomoxetine (Strattera)	10–100 mg	Contraindicated during or within 14 days of MAOI therapy and in the presence of narrow-angle glaucoma; monitor vital signs and for adverse effects such as GI upset, weight loss, headache, mood swings, and insomnia. Discontinue if jaundice or elevated liver enzymes occur.

NOTE: Additional drugs used to treat elderly clients with anxiety, depression, psychosis, and cognitive impairment are discussed in Chapter 16: Psychopharmacology and in specific disorder chapters.

Continuum of Care

Most communities provide continuum of care in various settings to the elderly client who has experienced difficulty with the developmental tasks of later maturity. Assisted-living facilities, adult daycare centers, community mental health centers, and senior centers offer several interventions, such as those listed in Box 30-3. After the client's physical and mental conditions have stabilized, emphasis is placed on the development of new interests, hobbies, and friendships that will help the client fill the day's extra hours due to retirement, widowhood, or an illness, when appropriate.

EVALUATION

During the evaluation process, the nurse determines whether any barriers have interfered with the plan of care. The nurse and client evaluate whether the client's psychosocial needs have been met, and if they have not, what changes are necessary. Input may be solicited from family or a significant other.

BOX 30.3 | **COMMUNITY CONTINUUM OF CARE INTERVENTIONS**

Counseling: Individual, group, family, marital, or remotivation therapy as well as legal, financial, or spiritual counseling

Cultural activities and recreation: Promotion of socialization, intellectual stimulation, and self-actualization

Education: Programs to encourage learning new information or skills

Exercise: Scheduled walks, aerobics, sports, dance, and so forth to improve health status

Health screening: Tests to identify and prevent physical or mental disorders and promote health

Meals: Provision of meals, supplements, or both to meet nutritional needs

Medical and social evaluation: Assessment to determine special needs and monitor progress

Medication assessment: Evaluation of all medications, their purposes, interactions, and efficacy

Occupational, physical, and speech therapy: Assessment to determine needs and provide therapy

Transportation: Rides to and from various appointments, grocery shopping, banking, and so forth

KEY CONCEPTS

◆ The importance of psychiatric–mental health nursing of the elderly stems both from the growing number and proportion of the elderly and from gains in longevity and active life expectancy.

◆ *Primary aging* is intrinsic and is determined by inherent or hereditary influences such as gender; culture, ethnicity, and race; intelligence and personality; familial longevity patterns; and genetic disease.

◆ *Secondary aging* refers to extrinsic factors such as employment, economic level, education, health practices and related diseases, and societal attitude.

◆ Several developmental tasks of the elderly influence their emotional needs: establishing satisfactory living arrangements; adjusting to retirement income; establishing comfortable routines; maintaining love, sex, and marital relationships; keeping active and

involved; staying in touch with other family members; sustaining and maintaining physical and mental health; and finding meaning in life. Not all elderly clients of diverse cultures, such as Native Americans, African Americans, Hispanics, and Asian Americans, successfully complete these developmental tasks.

◆ Erikson (1963) describes the elderly as experiencing a developmental stage of ego integrity versus despair. Individuals experiencing despair may exhibit patterns of behavior or emotional reactions such as hypersomnia, suspiciousness, hypochondriasis, depressed mood, or anxiety.

◆ Common emotional reactions, cognitive changes, or behavioral disturbances that occur in the elderly include anxiety, loneliness, guilt, depression, somatic complaints, paranoid reactions, dementia, and delirium.

◆ Assessment of the psychosocial needs of elderly clients is multifaceted and may take place in various settings. Long-standing psychosocial issues may not have been addressed in earlier years. The client's attempt to adapt to the developmental task of ego integrity versus despair may present with serious adverse effects that family members or caregivers find troublesome to live and work with. Special concerns such as pain, polypharmacy, insomnia, or involuntary weight loss may also require assessment.

◆ Barriers to the assessment of the elderly are classified as provider related, client related, or illness related.

◆ The formulation of nursing diagnoses and statements of outcome for elderly clients with psychiatric issues can be challenging because of the coexistence of at least one medical condition.

◆ Psychiatric–mental health nursing interventions for older adults focus on Maslow's theory of motivation and assist the client in meeting the basic human needs of survival (eg, pain management, adequate rest, adequate nutrition), safety and security, love and belonging, self-worth, and self-actualization or self-fulfillment; meeting the client's emotional needs (eg, loss or unresolved grief); and assisting the client in maintaining life with dignity and comfort until death.

◆ The goal of continuum of care is to assist the client in accessing support systems for physical or mental problems and in the development of new interests, hobbies, and friendships to decrease social isolation and increase self-esteem.

For additional study materials, please refer to the Student Resource CD-ROM located in the back of this textbook.

CHAPTER WORKSHEET

CRITICAL THINKING QUESTIONS

1. Visit a local retirement community. Interview several people about what it is like to get older and how they cope. What conclusions can you draw about coping skills and healthy aging?
2. Using Peck's concept of ego transcendence, how might an elderly person help you and your classmates understand aging?

REFLECTION

According to the chapter opening quote by the U.S. Census Bureau, by the year 2050, one in every 20 Americans will be 85 years of age or older, and one in every five will be retired. What do you plan to be doing in the year 2050? What preparations have you made or are you making? What developmental task(s) of aging, if any, do you think will be problematic for you? Explain your answer.

NCLEX-STYLE QUESTIONS

1. The community health nurse plans a teaching program on healthy living for members of a senior citizens' center. Which topic would be essential to include?
   a. Controlling intrinsic factors of aging process
   b. Monitoring blood pressure every month
   c. Obtaining adequate health insurance
   d. Refraining from use of abusive substances

2. The charge nurse in a nursing home teaches the certified nursing assistants to identify residents at high risk for depression to help in establishing a plan of care. Which factor would be of highest priority in determining this risk?
   a. Decreased productivity
   b. Lack of a support system
   c. Sensory impairment
   d. Rigid lifestyle

3. The nurse understands that an elderly client who has a positive approach and finds meaning in life possesses which of the following characteristics?
   a. Ego preoccupation
   b. Ego transcendence
   c. Passive acceptance
   d. Reminiscence ability

4. When assessing an aging client, the nurse focuses questions to elicit information about primary factors related to aging. Which factors would the nurse address? Select all that apply.
   a. Gender
   b. Employment
   c. Educational level
   d. Culture
   e. Intelligence
   f. Health practices

5. The nurse assesses an elderly client who presents with symptoms of decreased concentration, sadness, and somatic complaints for the ability to complete the Annotated Mini-Mental State Examination. This assessment is for the purpose of differentiating depression from which of the following?
   a. Anxiety
   b. Dementia
   c. Paranoia
   d. Somatization

6. Which of the following nursing interventions would be most appropriate in assisting an elderly client to meet the need for love and belonging?
   a. Communicating clearly on an adult level
   b. Encouraging participation in decision-making
   c. Mobilizing strengths and ability for independence
   d. Using therapeutic affection and touch

Selected References

Administration on Aging. (2001). The 65 years and over population 2000. Retrieved March 4, 2004, from http://www.census.gov/prod/2001pubs/c2kb101-10.pdf

Alzheimer's Association (Alzheimer's Disease and Education Center). (2003). General information about AD. Retrieved March 4, 2004, from http://www.alzheimers.org/

American Association of Retired Persons. (2003). AARP research: A portrait of older minorities. Retrieved December 16, 2003, from http://research.aarp.org/general/portmino.html

American Geriatric Society Panel on Chronic Pain in Older Persons. (1998). The management of chronic pain: A study of related variables and age differences. *Journal of American Geriatric Society, 46,* 635-651.

American Psychiatric Association. (2000). *Diagnostic and statistical manual of mental disorders* (4th ed., test revision). Washington, DC: Author.

Anxiety Disorders Association of America. (2003). Anxiety in the elderly. Retrieved December 16, 2003, from http://www.adaa.org/AnxietyDisorderInfor/AnxietyElderly.cfm

Asian American Federation of New York. (2003). Elderly Asian American New Yorkers face higher levels of poverty and depression, Asian American Federation reports. Retrieved December 16, 2003, from http://www.aafny.org/proom/pr/pr20030219.asp

Battista, E. M. (2002). The assessment and management of chronic pain in the elderly: A guide for practice. *ADVANCE for Nurse Practitioners, 10*(11), 29-32.

Blazer, D. G. (1994). Geriatric psychiatry. In R. E. Hales, S. C. Yudofsky, & J. A. Talbott (Eds.), *The American Psychiatric Press textbook of psychiatry* (2nd ed.). Washington, DC: American Psychiatric Press.

Blazer, D. G. (1996). Epidemiology of psychiatric disorders in late life. In E. W. Busse & D. G. Blazer (Eds.), *Textbook of geriatric psychiatry* (2nd ed., pp. 155-171). Washington, DC: American Psychiatric Press.

Bouras, E. P., Lange, S. M., & Scolapio, J. S. (2001). Rational approach to patients with unintentional weight loss. *Mayo Clinic Proceedings, 76*(9), 923-929.

Boyle, J. S. (2003). Culture, family, and community. In M. M. Andrews & J. S. Boyle (Eds.), *Transcultural concepts in nursing care* (4th ed., pp. 315-360). Philadelphia: Lippincott Williams & Wilkins.

Brozovic, B., & Wald, K. (2000, November/December). Managing depression in nursing home elderly. *Clinical Advisor, 3,* 42, 45-46, 49-51.

Buki, V. M. V. (2005). Treating the Hispanic elderly. *Clinical Psychiatry News, 33*(4), 8.

Burnside, I. (1975). Listen to the aged. *American Journal of Nursing, 75*(11), 1800.

Burnside, I. (1981). *Nursing and the aged* (2nd ed.). New York: McGraw-Hill.

Busse, E. W. (1996). The myth, history, and science of aging. In E. W. Busse & D. G. Blazer (Eds.), *Textbook of geriatric psychiatry* (2nd ed., pp. 3-24). Washington, DC: American Psychiatric Press.

Butler, R., & Lewis, M. (1982). *Aging and mental health: Positive psychosocial and biomedical approaches* (3rd ed.). St Louis, MO: C. V. Mosby.

DuPuy, L. (2002). UMass Boston study identifies critical lapses in services for elderly Asian American women. Retrieved December 16, 2003, from http:// www.umb.edu/news/2002news/reporter/december/asian.html

Duvall, E. M. (1977). *Marriage and family development* (5th ed.). Philadelphia: J. B. Lippincott.

Ebersole, P., & Hess, P. (1997). *Toward healthy aging: Human needs and nursing response* (5th ed.). St. Louis, MO: C. V. Mosby.

Edelson, F. (1999, November 11-14). *Integrating geriatric primary care givers into the treatment team.* Paper presented at the 12th Annual United States Psychiatric & Mental Health Congress, Atlanta, GA.

Erikson, E. H. (1963). *Childhood and society* (2nd ed.). New York: W. W. Norton.

Evans, J. (2006). Try integrated psychotherapy for complex issues. *Clinical Psychiatry News, 34*(2), 44.

Feldt, K. S. (2005). Pain in the elderly. *ADVANCE for Nurse Practitioners, 13*(6), 51-52, 54.

Hanks-Bell, M., Halvey, K., & Paice, J. A. (2004). Pain assessment and management in aging. *Online Journal Issues in Nursing, 9*(3). Retrieved December 17, 2004, from http://www.medscape.com/viewarticle/490773_print

Ho, V. (2002, April 3). Culture shift strains social services as elderly Asians' numbers rise. *Seattle Post-Intelligence.* Retrieved September 14, 2006, from http://seattlepi.nwsource.com/local/65060_census03.shtml

Jung, R. J., & Grossberg, G. T. (1993, July/August). Diagnosis and treatment of psychiatric disorders in the nursing home. *Nursing Home Medicine: The Annals of Long-Term Care, 1*(3), 24-35.

Kanapaux, W. (2003). Homosexual seniors face stigma. *Geriatric Times, 4*(6), 3-4

Khin, N. A., & Sunderland, T., III. (2000). Geriatric treatment. *Psychiatric Times, 27*(1), 47-48.

Lemieux, P. (2005). Substance abuse in the elderly. *ADVANCE for Nurses, 6*(12), 19-20.

Luggen, A. S. (2005). Bipolar disorder in older adults: An overview of recognition and management. *ADVANCE for Nurse Practitioners, 13*(3), 43-44, 46, 48.

MacReady, N. (2005). Polypharmacy may be linked to depression in the elderly. *Clinical Psychiatry News, 33*(1), 13.

Maslow, A. H. (1968). *Toward a psychology of being.* New York: D. Van Nostrand.

McNamara, D. (2004). Intervene to counter weight loss in elderly. *Clinical Psychiatry News, 12*(6), 1-2.

Miller, M. D. (2005). Late-life depression: Focused IPT eases loss and role changes. *Current Psychiatry, 4*(11), 40-42, 47-50.

Monarch Pharmaceuticals. (2000). Trend watch: Depression and the elderly. *Clinical Geriatrics, 8*(6), 72-75.

Nadolski, N. (2003). Getting a good night's sleep: Diagnosing and treating insomnia. *American Journal for Nurse Practitioners Spring Supplement,* s2-s14.

National Council on Aging. (2003). Facts about older Americans and pain. Retrieved August 17, 2003, from http://www.orthomcneil.com/resources/misc/seniors_facts_bottom.htm

National Institute on Aging. (1981, Oct). *Age page: Sexuality in later life.* Washington, DC: U.S. Department of Health and Human Services.

National Sleep Foundation. (2006). Medical problems affecting sleep.Retrieved March 14, 2006, from http://www.sleep foundation.org/hottopics/index.php?secid=12&id=187

Neff, D. F. (1996). Gerontological counseling. In S. Lego (Ed.), *Psychiatric nursing: A comprehensive reference* (2nd ed., pp. 165–174). Philadelphia: Lippincott-Raven.

Nelson, J. C., & Battista, D. M. (2001). Diagnosis and treatment of late-life depression. *CNS News, 3*(7), 18–20.

Neugarten, B. (1968). Adult personality: Toward a psychology of life cycle. In B. Neugarten (Ed.), *Middle age and aging.* Chicago: University of Chicago Press.

Ohio State University Extension. (2003). Senior series: Asian American older adults.Retrieved December 16, 2003, from http://ohioline.osu.edu/ss-fact/0194.html

Peskind, E. R., & Raskind, M. A. (1996). Cognitive disorders. In E. W. Busse & D. G. Blazer (Eds.), *Textbook of geriatric psychiatry* (2nd ed., pp. 213–234). Washington, DC: American Psychiatric Press.

Peterson, K. S. (2000, March 7). Black couples stay the course. *USA Today*.

Read, S. (1991). The dementias. In J. Sadavoy, L. W. Lazarus, & L. F. Jarvik (Eds.), *Comprehensive review of geriatric psychiatry* (pp. 287–310). Washington, DC: American Psychiatric Press.

Resnick, B. (2001). Depression in older adults. *ADVANCE for Nurses, 2*(14), 23–26.

Sadavoy, J., Lazarus, L. W., & Jarvick, L. F. (1991). The aging process: Introduction. In J. Sadavoy, L. W. Lazarus, & L. F. Lissy (Eds.), *Comprehensive review of psychiatry* (pp. 3–24). Washington, DC: American Psychiatry Press.

Sadock, B. J., & Sadock, V. A. (2003). *Kaplan & Sadock's synopsis of psychiatry: Behavioral science/clinical psychiatry* (9th ed.). Philadelphia: Lippincott Williams & Wilkins.

Saffel-Shrier, S., Gay, C., Oderda, L., & Thiese, M. S. (2003). Involuntary weight loss and malnutrition: Screening, evaluation and treatment. *Geriatric Times, 4*(3), 29–33.

Schrock, M. M. (1980). *Holistic assessment of the healthy aged.* New York: John Wiley & Sons.

Schuckit, M. (1997, November 13–15). *A review of geriatric psychopharmacology.* Paper presented at the 10th Annual United States Psychiatric & Mental Health Congress, Orlando, FL.

Schuman, J. (2000). The computer as a resident's communicative bridge: Its use in long-term care facilities. *Long-Term Care Interface, 1*(4), 30–34.

Social Security Administration. (2003). *Social Security is important to Asian Americans.* Retrieved December 16, 2003, from http://www.ssa.gov/organizations/asianfact sheet.htm

Stevens, F. C. J., Kaplan, C. D., Ponds, R. W., Diederiks, J. P. M., & Jolles, J. (1999). How ageing and social factors affect memory. *Age and Ageing, 28*(4), 379–384.

United States Census Bureau. (1997). Demographic state of the nation, 1997.Retrieved March 4, 2004, from http://www.census.gov/prod/2/pop/23/p23-193.pdf

University of Missouri. (2003a). Black elderly. Retrieved December 16, 2003, from http://iml.umkc.edu/casww/blackeld.htm

University of Missouri. (2003b). Hispanic elderly. Retrieved December 16, 2003, from http://iml.umkc.edu/casww/hispanic.htm

University of Missouri. (2003c). Native American elderly. Retrieved December 16, 2003, from http://iml.umkc.edu/casww/natamers.htm

Walker, J. I. (1982). *Everybody's guide to emotional well-being.* San Francisco: Harbor.

Wallace, M. (2003). Best practices in nursing care to older adults: Sexuality. *Dermatological Nursing, 15*(6), 570–571.

Suggested Readings

Antai-Otong, D. (2005). Psychotropic use in older adults. *ADVANCE for Nurses, 6*(1), 13–17.

Butcher, H. K., & McGonigal-Kenney, M. (2005). Depression & dispiritedness in later life. *American Journal of Nursing, 105*(12), 52–62.

Carpenito-Moyet, L. M. (2006). *Handbook of nursing diagnosis* (11th ed.). Philadelphia: Lippincott Williams & Wilkins.

Collins, N., & Schafer, P. (2002, Jan/Feb). Appetite stimulants: An overview. *Extended Care Product News, 1,* 16–17.

Cook-Flannery, J. (2003). The aging society. *ADVANCE for Nurses, 4*(14), 19–20, 25.

Crutchfield, D. B. (2002). Pain in the elderly: Recognition and treatment guidelines. *Geriatric Times, 3*(6), 28.

Keefe, S. (2002). Medication 01: Nurses play pivotal role in educating seniors about their medication. *ADVANCE for Nurses, 3*(25), 23–24.

Logue, R. (2002a). The impact of advanced practice nursing on improving medication adherence in the elderly: An educational intervention. *American Journal for Nurse Practitioners, 6*(5), 9–15.

Logue, R. (2002b). Self-medication and the elderly: How technology can help. *American Journal of Nursing, 102*(7), 51, 54–55.

McKenna, M. A. (2003). Transcultural nursing care in older adults. In M. M. Andrews & J. S. Boyle (Eds.), *Transcultural concepts in nursing care* (4th ed., pp. 209–246). Philadelphia: Lippincott Williams & Wilkins.

McNamara, D. (2005). Intervention's benefits persist in depressed elderly. *Clinical Psychiatry News, 33*(1), 1, 13.

Scanland, S., & Stucke, S. (2005). Common geriatric syndromes. *ADVANCE for Nurse Practitioners, 13*(1), 47–51.

Schultz, J. M., & Videbeck, S. L. (2005). *Lippincott's manual of psychiatric nursing care plans* (7th ed.). Philadelphia: Lippincott Williams & Wilkins.

Scott, A. (2002). No time for the pain: Improvement needed in pain management for the elderly. *ADVANCE for Nurses, 3*(4), 25-27.

Selman, J. E. (2005). Restless legs syndrome is too often ignored. *Clinical Advisor, 8*(10), 68, 72-74, 77-78.

Sherer, R. A. (2001). Assisted living offers independence, but health care needs may be unmet. *Geriatric Times, 2*(2), 4-6.

Stotts, N. A., & Deitrich, C. E. (2004). The challenge to come: The care of older adults. *American Journal of Nursing, 104*(8), 40-48.

Sussman, N., Hardy, M., & Magid, S. (2002). Psychiatric manifestations of NSAIDs in older adults. *Geriatric Times, 3*(1), 29-32.

Thomas, M. (2003). Epidemiology and psychosocial aspects of chronic pain in older adults. *Geriatric Times, 4*(4), 29-31.

CHAPTER 31 / SUICIDAL CLIENTS

*Suicide is associated with thwarted or unfulfilled needs, feelings of hopelessness
and helplessness, ambivalent conflicts between survival and unbearable stress,
a narrowing of perceived options, and a need to escape.* —Shneidman, 1996

*Suicide may be the culmination of self-destructive urges that have resulted from the client's
internalizing his or her anger or a desperate act by which to escape a perceived intolerable
psychological state or life situation. The client may be asking for help by attempting suicide, seeking
attention, or attempting to manipulate someone with suicidal behavior.* —Schultz & Videbeck, 2005

LEARNING OBJECTIVES

AFTER STUDYING THIS CHAPTER, YOU SHOULD BE ABLE TO:

1. Describe the genetic, biologic, sociologic, and psychological factors believed to precipitate suicidal behavior.
2. Compare and contrast the theory of self with the theory of parasuicidal behavior.
3. Identify those clients or groups of individuals considered to be at risk for suicide.
4. State at least two examples of verbal, behavioral, and situational suicidal clues.
5. Distinguish among suicidal ideation, intent, threat, gesture, and attempt.
6. Differentiate among three cultural beliefs about suicide.
7. Explain primary, secondary, and tertiary suicide prevention.
8. Describe the purpose of suicide precautions, no-suicide contracts, and seclusion and restraints in the clinical setting.
9. Explain the rationale for the use of medication, interactive therapies, and family and client education when providing care for clients who are exhibiting suicidal behavior.
10. Articulate the importance of self-assessment when providing care for suicidal clients.
11. State the purpose of a psychological autopsy.
12. Define the term *postvention*.
13. Reflect on the impact of physician-assisted suicide on the nursing profession.

KEY TERMS

Alexithymia
Altruistic suicide
Anomic suicide
Egoistic suicide
Euthanasia
Parasuicide
Physician-assisted suicide (PAS)
Postvention
Primary prevention
Psychological autopsy
Secondary prevention
Tertiary prevention
Theory of Self
Trichotillomania

Suicide is a tragic and potentially preventable public health problem. Since the year 2000, suicide has remained the 11th cause of death; homicide ranks 15th. According to the 2003 statistics prepared for the American Association of Suicidology by J. L. McIntosh, firearms were responsible for 53.7% of the 31,484 suicides followed by suffocation/hanging (21.1%), poisoning (17.3%), cutting or piercing (1.8%), and drowning (1.2%). Although there were three female attempts for each male attempt, the ratio of completed suicides was 2.1% males to 0.5% females.

Suicide continues to be the third leading cause of death among children and youth after accidents and homicide. Statistics indicate that 11.9% of the suicides in 2003 were by the young (ages 15–24 years) who comprised 14.2% of the population. The suicide rate for youth ages 5 to 14 years was 0.6%.

Older adults are disproportionately likely to die by suicide. Comprising 12.4% of the 2003 population, individuals age 65 years and over represented 16.7% of the suicides (American Association of Suicidology, 2006). This chapter addresses the etiology of suicide and identifies those individuals or groups at risk for attempting suicide. It focuses on the role of the nurse in the treatment and prevention of suicide.

Etiology

The need to be loved and accepted, along with a desperate wish to communicate feelings of loneliness, alienation, worthlessness, helplessness, and hopelessness, often results in intense feelings of anxiety, depression, and anger or hostility directed toward the self. If no one is available to talk to or listen to such feelings of insecurity or inadequacy, a suicide attempt may occur in an effort to seek help or end an emotional conflict. Various theories have been proposed to explain the possible factors that influence suicidal behavior. A summary of the major ideas of these theories follows.

Genetic and Biologic Theories

In medicine, the strongest evidence for involvement of genetic and biologic factors in suicidal behavior is suggested by analyses of several different areas. These areas include genetic markers, studies on the relationship of neurochemical binding sites, and suicidal behavior among twins and adopted individuals.

Genetic Markers

Researchers have discovered a genetic marker for suicidal ideation. DNA analysis showed that the 102T/C polymorphism in 5-HT2a receptor gene is significantly associated with major depression. In this study, individuals were evaluated using the Hamilton Rating Scale for Depression. Results revealed that persons with a 102C/C genotype scored significantly higher (a high score on item three of the scale indicates suicidal ideation) than did individuals with T/C or T/T genotypes. In addition, serotonin receptor levels did not normalize after the depression was treated successfully (Muller, 2000a). Such findings suggest that individuals may be biologically predisposed to suicidal thoughts, versus the view of suicide as a character flaw. Perhaps if clients knew that their suicidal urges had a genetic component, they might seek help more readily.

Endocrine Basis

Researchers, striving to identify an endocrine basis for suicide, have demonstrated that a dexamethasone suppression test can identify suicide risk. In a clinical study that spanned 15 years, 114 participants initially received 1 milligram of dexamethasone at 11 p.m. on day one, followed by three measurements of serum cortisol on day 2. The researchers looked at death records an average of more than 15 years later to determine the number of suicides in each group. Of the 56 individuals in the cortisol-suppressor group, 45 participants were still alive and 11 were dead, including one suicide. In the cortisol-nonsuppressor group, 40 of the 58 participants were still alive and 18 were dead, including six suicides. Researchers concluded that the participants in the cortisol-nonsuppressor group experienced a hyperarousal of the hypothalamic–pituitary–adrenal (HPA) axis that affected the brain's ability to modulate stress states. Disturbances in the regulation of anxiety and aggression due to increased levels of cortisol placed the participants at an increased risk for suicide (McNamara, 2004a).

Relationship of Neurochemical Binding Sites

The relationship among serotonin and postsynaptic frontal cortices' binding sites, 5-HIAA (a metabolite of serotonin normally found in spinal fluid), and serum cholesterol has been the focus of research studies. Results concluded that the presence of increased binding sites decreases the availability of serotonin for regulation of aggressive behavior. Low fluid levels of 5-HIAA predict short-range suicide risk, thereby supporting the serotonin hypothesis of suicide risk. Low levels of cholesterol suggest low serotonin availability and reduced inhibition of aggressive behavior (Mericle, 1997; Sadock & Sadock, 2003).

Protein Kinase C Abnormality

Teenage suicide may be associated with abnormalities of protein kinase C. Postmortem brains of teenage suicide victims revealed a significant decrease in protein kinase C activity in the prefrontal cortex and hippocampus compared with postmortem brains of teenagers who were free of psychiatric illness and did not commit suicide. Researchers believe that protein kinase C may be a target for therapeutic intervention in clients with suicidal behavior (Stong, 2004).

Familial Suicidal Behavior

Studies show that suicidal behavior is familial, but the risk factors for transmission from parent to child are unclear. Researchers are attempting to clarify the difference between the development of a mood disorder, which tends to run in families, and the development of suicidal behavior. They are investigating genetic data and neurobiologic factors (eg, endophenotypes) believed to precipitate behaviors (eg, impulsive aggression or cortical responses to stress) that result in suicidal behavior (Kennedy, 2004).

Twin and Adoption Studies

Studies also have focused on suicidal behavior among twins and adoptees (Sadock & Sadock, 2003). According to the studies of twins, suicide among identical twins was significantly higher (11.3%) than suicide among fraternal twins (1.8%). A Danish–American adoption study revealed that adoptee suicide victims experiencing a situational crisis or impulsive suicide attempt or both had more biologic relatives who had committed suicide than did members of the control group.

Sociologic Theories

Emile Durkheim, a French sociologist, identified society as an influencing factor on suicide rates. He divided suicides into three categories based on the degree of an individual's socialization: egoistic, altruistic, and anomic. **Egoistic suicide** refers to suicide by individuals who are not strongly integrated into any social group (eg, a divorced male, who has no children and who lives alone, commits suicide). **Altruistic suicide** describes suicide by persons who believe sacrificing their lives will benefit society. For example, a fireman who knows his life is in danger and that he could die, sacrifices his life while attempting to save the lives of others during the attack on the World Trade Center; a suicide bomber in Palestine dies while fighting for independence from Israel. **Anomic suicide** refers to suicide that occurs when an individual has difficulty relating to others, adapting to a world of overwhelming stressors, or adjusting to expected normal social behavior (eg, a college student who was popular in high school has difficulty adjusting to college life, feels socially unaccepted on campus, and commits suicide).

Psychological Theories

Both Sigmund Freud and Karl Menninger believed suicide was a result of anger turned inward. According to Freud, suicide represented aggression against an introjected love object. He also doubted that suicide would occur without an earlier repressed desire to kill someone else. Menninger, building on Freud's theory, believed that suicide was an inverted homicide act because of anger toward another person. He also believed that an individual has a self-directed death instinct composed of the wish to kill, the wish to be killed, and the wish to die (Sadock & Sadock, 2003).

Theory of Self

Of all the perceptions we experience, none has more profound significance than the perceptions we hold regarding our view of who we are and how we fit into the world. This internal view of personal existence is called "the self." According to the **Theory of Self**, "the self" tries to maximize its own self-esteem, seeks pleasure, and avoids pain. The maintenance, protection, and enhancement of "the self" may be the basic motive for behavior. "The self" takes precedence over the physical body as individuals often sacrifice physical comfort and safety for psychological satisfaction.

In healthy individuals there is a constant assimilation of new ideas and expulsion of old ideas through life. "The self" continuously guards against perceived threats. If "the self" remains in a defense mode, feelings of disappointment, guilt, shame, depression, or anxiety may occur. Chronic negative feelings result in low self esteem, cognitive distortions, and irrational beliefs. Social psychologists believe suicide occurs when "the self" is unsuccessful at achieving self-actualization or psychological satisfaction (McNamara, 2004b).

Theory of Parasuicidal Behavior

The term **parasuicide** describes individuals who engage in self-inflicted injury or mutilation but usually do not wish to die. Self-inflicted injury is often associated with childhood trauma. It is a coping method used to deal with situations that produce feelings of rejection, anger, helplessness, and guilt. Self-inflicted injury represents an attempt to relieve tension or bear intolerable emotional pain when everything else fails. This behavior may be an attempt to communicate hurt to others, exert control in an out-of-control life, or to experience a pleasurable analgesic effect as opiates are released into the body after trauma (Starr, 2004; Tumolo, 2005).

Clients who self-inflict generally claim to experience no pain and state they are angry at themselves or others. The incidence of self-injury in the psychiatric setting has been estimated to be more than 50 times that of self-injury in the general population. Self-injury occurs in approximately 30% of clients who abuse substances orally and 10% of clients who abuse intravenous substances before admission to a substance-abuse unit (Johnston, 2002; Sadock & Sadock, 2003).

Although controversy exists over its classification (ie, impulse control disorder, mood disorder, obsessive-compulsive disorder, or tic disorder), **trichotillomania** (TTM), or compulsive hair pulling, is a form of self-injury that may affect as many as 3% of the U.S. population. Compulsive hair pulling affects young children, adolescents, and adults alike. Persons with TTM most often pull hair from the scalp, but may also pull hair from the eyebrows, eyelashes, pubis, and body (Whitaker, Wolf, & Keuthen, 2003). Individuals who exhibit this behavior claim that they experience an increasing sense of tension immediately before pulling out the hair, followed by pleasure, gratification, or relief. Pulling of hair may continue until external events, self-loathing, or soreness intervenes or an elusive "just-right" feeling is achieved. Physical disfigurement and the inability to control one's behavior can lead to shame and isolation, as well as avoidance of needed health care services. The social consequences to self-esteem resulting from the hair loss may precipitate

depression, contribute to the use of alcohol or drugs to cope with feelings, or place the client at risk for suicidal behavior (Buchanan, 2002; King & Scahill, 1998).

Other Psychological Factors

Additional psychosocial factors or motives believed to precipitate suicidal behavior have been identified and explained. Briefly summarized, these factors may include:

- *A reunion wish or fantasy:* A newspaper article described the death of an elderly man whose wife had just died. He left a note to his children stating that he did not want to live without his wife, and because of his belief in life after death, he planned to join his wife.
- *A way to end one's feelings of hopelessness and helplessness:* Hope infers a sense of the possible, giving promise for the future and an expectation of fulfillment. Persons who experience hopelessness feel insecure, believing that there are no solutions to problems. They experience a sense of the impossible. Helplessness is a feeling that everything that can be done has been done; there is nothing left to sustain hope.
- *A cry for help:* Some people attempt suicide hoping to draw attention to themselves to receive help. For example, a 49-year-old woman in financial distress attempts suicide by taking a moderate overdose of sleeping pills, hoping that her boyfriend, who never displayed an interest in her business, will come to her rescue financially as well as emotionally.
- *An attempt to "save face" or seek a release to a better life:* Persons who were involved in the stock market crash of 1929 precipitating the Great Depression jumped from windows in suicide attempts caused by feelings of failure. These people had viewed themselves as competent, successful, and respected before the crash. The suicides were an effort to save face, relieving them of the responsibility of dealing with business failures.

Individuals at Risk for Self-Destructive Behavior

One of every ten persons entertains recurrent or persistent thoughts of suicide. Overall, there may be between 8 and 25 attempted suicides for every suicide death. Suicide attempts generally are reported as accidents to spare families the stigmatizing impact of suicide and to facilitate insurance coverage that otherwise would not occur in the event of suicide (National Institute of Mental Health [NIMH], 2003).

Approximately 80% of persons attempting suicide give clues, which are categorized as verbal, behavioral, or situational. *Verbal suicidal clues* include talking about death, making comments that significant others would be "better off without" the person, and asking questions about lethal dosages of drugs. *Behavioral suicidal clues* include writing forlorn love notes, directing angry messages at a significant other who has rejected the person, giving away personal items, or taking out a large life-insurance policy. *Situational suicidal clues* describe events or situations that present themselves either around or within the person, such as the unexpected death of a loved one, divorce, job failure, or diagnosis of a malignant tumor. Such situational clues may place the person at high risk for suicide. Supporting Evidence for Practice 31-1 highlights a study addressing the risk of suicidal ideation in parents who have suffered the loss of a child.

Suicidal behavior is complex. Various individuals or groups of individuals are at risk for self-destructive behavior. Although risk factors vary with age, gender, and ethnic group and may even change over time, the risk factors frequently occur in combination. Specific client groups with an increased risk for suicide are described in the following sections.

Clients With a Psychiatric Disorder

At some point in their career, clinicians face a 50% risk that a client will commit suicide. Psychiatric disorders, such as major depression, bipolar disorder, schizophrenia, schizoaffective disorder, personality disorders, eating disorders, and alcoholism or drug abuse are considered among the most serious of risk factors. (Ayd & Palma, 1999; Lott, 2000). For example, male clients who are depressed successfully commit suicide approximately five times more frequently than females who are depressed. Approximately 4,000 clients with the diagnosis of schizophrenia commit suicide per year; approximately 5% of clients diagnosed with antisocial personality disorder commit suicide per year; and approximately 10% to 15% of individuals who abuse alcohol commit suicide per year. Although 20% of clients with the diagnosis of anxiety attempt suicide, they are usually unsuccessful (Sadock & Sadock, 2003).

Research has shown that more than 90% of people who kill themselves have a diagnosable depression or another diagnosable mental or substance abuse disorder (NIMH, 2003). For example, command hallucinations, delusions of grandeur, lack of impulse control,

---

SUPPORTING EVIDENCE FOR PRACTICE 31.1

The Sudden, Violent Death of a Child and Parental Suicidal Ideation

PROBLEM UNDER INVESTIGATION / What factors precipitate suicidal ideation among parents after the sudden, violent death of a child?

SUMMARY OF THE RESEARCH / This 5-year study by nurse researchers followed up with 261 parents whose children (average age was 20 years) experienced a sudden, violent death. The sample consisted of parents whose age ranged from 32 to 61 years; 86% were white; and most were considered to be well educated and employed. There were 171 mothers and 90 fathers, with 69 couples; 90% were biological parents, 5% were adoptive parents, and 5% were step-parents. Sixty-five percent of the deceased children were male and the causes of death included accidents (58%), suicides (24%), and homicides (10%). The subjects who reported suicidal ideation reported three patterns:

within the first year of the child's death (75%); delayed reaction after the first year (9%); and continuous ideation throughout the study period (16%). Results indicated that parents with suicidal ideation were less able to accept the death and scored higher for distress, depression, and trauma and lower in self-esteem, self-efficacy, and coping compared with parents who reported no suicidal ideation.

SUPPORT FOR PRACTICE / Psychiatric–mental health nurses must assess for depression, distress, and suicidal ideation in clients who have experienced the sudden, violent death of a child. Furthermore, assessment may need to be repeated over time.

SOURCE: Murphy, S. A., Tapper, V. J., Johnson, L. C., & Loban, J. (2003). *Suicide ideation among parents bereaved by the violent deaths of their children.* Issues in Mental Health Nursing, 24, 5–25.

and manipulative behavior may precipitate suicide attempts in clients with psychotic disorders. Overwhelming grief, severe anxiety, panic attacks, agitation, or a chemical imbalance are linked to suicide risk in clients with depression. Individuals with severe depression have been known to commit suicide after treatment and during the recovery process, a time during which the client experiences the energy level to follow through with self-destructive thoughts (Jancin, 1999). Individuals with anorexia nervosa or bulimia nervosa exhibit a passive form of suicide that could become active due to feelings of frustration, guilt, anger, or manipulation and loss of control.

Alcohol and certain drugs are known to cause central nervous system depression. The mixing of drugs and alcohol may cause a drug–alcohol interaction that could result in death. Many drugs cause psychological or physiologic dependency, thus creating emotional conflict and depression as well as physiologic deterioration. Drug–drug interactions also increase the likelihood of death as a result of self-destructive impulses.

Clients With Alexithymia

Alexithymia is not a psychiatric diagnosis, but a construct introduced in 1972 by Peter Sifneos. Derived from the Greek language, it literally means "having no word for emotions." This construct is useful for characterizing clients who seem not to understand the feelings they experience and who seem to lack the words to describe their feelings to others. It is a real phenomenon and identifies a deficit of self. Individuals who experience this phenomenon have been found to be at risk for self-mutilation and suicidal behavior (Muller, 2000b).

Clients With Medical Illnesses

The suicide rate among non-psychiatric general hospital clients after discharge has been reported to be three times higher than it is among the general population. Individuals with a chronic or terminal medical illness have verbalized several reasons for suicidal ideation. They include pain, suffering (eg, fear of a "horrible death" caused by dyspnea, dysphagia, or another cause), fatigue, loss of independence, and decreased quality of life. Furthermore, some non-psychiatric health problems are linked to risk of suicide in the elderly. These include congestive heart failure, chronic obstructive lung disease, seizure disorder, urinary incontinence, and moderate or severe pain. Clients

have solicited help from caregivers, including medical and nursing professionals, to perform euthanasia or physician-assisted suicide (Knowlton, 1998).

The presence of a neurologic disorder raises the overall suicide risk. Suicide is more frequent at particular moments of a disease's natural course, such as the period after diagnosis and the period after hospitalization. For example, suicides have been reported to account for up to 13 times the expected death rate in clients with Huntington's disease. Epilepsy raises the expected death rate due to suicide fivefold in men and twofold in women. Suicide after traumatic brain injury is two to three times higher than in the general population. In clients with spinal cord injury, the period immediately after the injury is one of particular vulnerability. Approximately 83% of the suicides occur within 6 months of the injury and 90% occur within 5 years (Sherman, 2000).

Euthanasia and Physician-Assisted Suicide

Euthanasia, defined as a health care provider's deliberate act to cause a client's death, and **physician-assisted suicide (PAS),** defined as the imparting of information or means to enable suicide to occur, have become controversial issues in the health care industry (Sadock & Sadock, 2003). The increase in human longevity, development of modern medical technology, and use of life-support systems have created an ethical dilemma for health care providers who are often confronted with their responsibility to relieve pain and suffering as well as their obligation to preserve life. Nurses who provide palliative care for dying clients have difficulty distinguishing among allowing, hastening, or causing death when their only goal is to help clients die with peace and dignity (Schwartz, 2002).

In 1997, voters in the state of Oregon approved a Death With Dignity Act. This act applies to adults diagnosed with a terminal illness that is expected to cause death within 6 months. It requires a client to make two oral requests and one written request to a physician and to wait at least 15 days after the initial oral request before receiving a prescription for lethal drugs. A second physician's opinion is required to verify the initial diagnosis; that the client is capable of and did make an informed decision; and that the decision was made voluntarily. Factors affecting client requests in Oregon for assistance with suicide included pain, fatigue, dyspnea, loss of independence, and poor quality of life (Kirk, 1998; Libow, 2000).

Individuals intent on self-destructive behavior are able to obtain information through books such as *Final Exit,* a 1991 publication by the Hemlock Society. In 1993, the Hemlock Society held a suicide workshop in San Francisco attended by homosexual males infected with the human immunodeficiency virus (HIV). Internet resources also provide information to educate people on how to commit suicide.

Regardless of the situation, nurses are ethically bound to protect clients who are at risk for self-harm, with the assumption that nurses will do nothing to harm or shorten the lives of clients in their care. The question, though, is raised: "Is it ethical to participate in physician-assisted suicide?" Caring for clients who make such a request may conflict with a nurse's personal moral beliefs. Although a nurse has the right to choose whether to participate, the nurse may not be aware of a client's request and therefore become an unknowing participant in PAS.

Knowlton (1998) also discusses the controversy of PAS after a survey of surgical and medical residents who were asked questions such as "Should physicians act on patient requests to die, or should they address patient needs through other measures?" and "What factors other than patient suffering influence requests for assisted death?" The conclusion was reached that further investigation is imperative so that care of severely ill clients is derived from explicit clinically and ethically sound principles of medicine and not based on uncertain motive, incorrect information, or prejudicial attitudes.

Libow (2000) discusses an alternative to PAS, the establishment of a palliative care and ethics team. Such a team would be available to help ease the last days of clients and provide support for family members.

Adolescent Clients

Adolescent suicide is not usually a spur-of-the-moment act. According to the latest statistics, for every teen who is successful at committing suicide, more than 2,000 consider it, and nearly 66% of those who kill themselves show psychiatric symptoms more than a year before their death. During the year 2003, one young person between the ages of 15 and 24 years committed suicide every 2 hours and 11.8 minutes. Additionally, more than 12,000 children and adolescents are hospitalized in the U.S. each year as a result of suicidal threats or behavior (American Association of Suicidology, 2006; National Center for Health Statistics, 2003; Perlstein, 2004; Sadock & Sadock, 2003).

Suicidal ideation, gestures, and attempts are associated with adolescent depression and have become a growing mental health problem. Risk factors for adolescent suicide include male gender; age 16 years or older; living alone; history of impulsivity, aggression, or previous attempt; history of physical or emotional abuse, mood disorder, substance abuse disorder, or preoccupation with death or dying; recent change in mental status or personality; and psychosocial crisis. Suicidal behaviors are often linked to school performance, making potential high-school dropouts a high-risk group.

High-Risk Population Groups

High-risk populations include ethnic minorities, homosexuals, the incarcerated, and the elderly. Between 1980 and 1996, suicide rates doubled among African American males between the ages of 15 and 19 years. People of Native American and Alaskan native heritage continue to have high suicide rates. Unusually high rates of attempted suicide have been found among homosexual individuals (20%–42%), particularly men. Suicide is the third leading cause of death in prison, after natural causes and AIDS-related deaths. The suicide rate is three times more common among incarcerated individuals than among the general population. Approximately 39% of all suicide victims are persons 65 years of age and older. Men accounted for 84% of suicide victims among persons aged 65 years and older in the year 2000 (Frieden, 2005b; Lindsay, 1999, 2000; National Center for Injury Prevention and Control, 2003).

Additionally, persons who are divorced, separated, widowed, unemployed, or socially isolated are also at high risk because of feelings of dependency, loneliness, and worthlessness as they attempt to care for themselves in a society that places much emphasis on youth, success, and independence.

Individuals whose occupations require selfless public service and dedication and who work under pressure are also at risk for suicide. For example, police officers and air-traffic controllers who work long hours and often experience disruptions of family and social life may develop a major depressive disorder or substance-related disorder due to ineffective coping. Thus, suicide may be a means for them to escape feelings of hopelessness or helplessness. Several studies have indicated that occupations with the highest risk of suicide include anesthesiologists, psychiatrists, and dentists (Crisis Intervention Network, 2002).

Persons who engage in masochistic sexual acts by using devices to enhance autoerotic feelings, and "daredevils" such as Evel Knievel who attempt death-defying acts, are thought to be risking their lives by engaging in passive suicidal behavior. Finally, individuals who have a history of previous suicide attempts, and who have not developed adequate coping skills or who lack sufficient support systems, are at risk each time they experience increased stress.

THE NURSING PROCESS

ASSESSMENT

Suicide is considered more preventable than any other cause of death (Badger, 1995). This statement is based on the assumption that all suicidal persons are ambivalent about life and therefore are never 100% suicidal. The decision to provide care for a suicidal client requires the use of excellent assessment skills and crisis intervention techniques (see Chapter 13 for information about crisis intervention).

Assessment of the client who is self-destructive involves close observation and acute listening. It is acceptable to ask the following questions during the assessment process to detect any suicide clues, assess the motive for suicide (eg, escape from pain, manipulation of others, both), and gain information regarding the specificity of the plan, and its degree of lethality:

- Have you had thoughts that life is not worth living?
- What worries do you have?
- Do you want to die?
- Do you have a specific plan? If so, what is your plan?
- What keeps you from acting out your plan?
- Have you attempted suicide before? If so, how?

The following terminology, often referred to as "the suicide lexicon," is commonly used to describe the range of suicidal thoughts and behavior identified during assessment:

- *Suicidal ideation,* or vague, fleeting thoughts about wanting to die
- *Suicidal intent,* or thoughts about a concrete plan to commit suicide
- *Suicidal threat,* or the expression of a person's desire to end his or her life
- *Suicidal gesture,* or intentional self-destructive behavior that is clearly not life-threatening but does resemble an attempted suicide
- *Suicidal attempt,* or self-destructive behavior by which an individual responds to ambivalent feelings about living (Badger, 1995)

Assessment of Suicide Risk

A client's degree of suicidality is not a static quality, possibly fluctuating quickly and unpredictably. Therefore, assessment of suicide risk is an ongoing process, not a single event. Assessing individual suicide risk factors generally requires in-depth knowledge of a client. Also, obtaining information from other sources (eg, family, significant other, family physician, teacher, or therapist if the client is being seen as an outpatient client) may be necessary before the degree of suicidal risk can be determined (Lott, 2000). Table 31-1 presents some key behaviors or symptoms and the degree of suicide risk associated with each.

When assessing a client's suicide risk, keep in mind that approximately 80% of all potential suicide victims give some clue before exhibiting self-destructive behavior. Regard all behaviors and comments about suicide seriously. Clues may provide an indication of a client's suicidal intent. Be alert when the client:

- Talks about death, suicide, and wanting to be dead, and appears to be in deep thought
- Asks suspicious questions such as, "How often do the night personnel make rounds?" "How many of these pills would it take to kill a person?" "How high is this window from the ground?" "How long does it take to bleed to death?" and so forth
- Fears being unable to sleep and fears the night
- Is depressed and cries frequently
- Keeps away from others due to self-imposed isolation, especially in secluded areas or behind locked doors
- Is tense and worried and has a hopeless, helpless attitude
- Imagines he or she has some serious physical illness

TABLE 31.1 Assessing the Degree of Suicide Risk

BEHAVIOR OR SYMPTOM	INTENSITY OF RISK		
	Low	Moderate	High
Anxiety	Mild	Moderate	High, or panic state
Depression	Mild	Moderate	Severe
Isolation, withdrawal	Some feelings of isolation, no withdrawal	Some feelings of helplessness, hoplessness, and withdrawal	Hopeless, helpless, withdrawn, and self-deprecating
Daily functioning	Fairly good in most activities	Moderately good in some activities	Not good in any activities
Resources	Several	Some	Few or none
Coping strategies, devices being used	Generally constructive	Some that are constructive	Predominantly destructive
Significant others	Several who are available	Few or only one available	Only one or none available
Psychiatric help in past	None, or positive attitude toward	Yes, and moderately satisfied	Negative view of help received
Lifestyle	Stable	Moderately stable	Unstable
Alcohol or drug use	Infrequently to excess	Frequently to excess	Continual abuse
Previous suicide attempts	None, or of low lethality	One or more, of moderate lethality	Multiple attempts of high lethality
Disorientation, disorganization	None	Some	Marked
Hostility	Little or none	Some	Marked
Suicide plan	Vague, fleeting thoughts but no plan	Frequent thoughts, occasional ideas about a plan	Frequent or constant thought with a specific plan

such as cancer or tuberculosis. (The person may want to end the suffering or decrease the imagined burden to the family.)
- Feels very guilty about something real or imaginary or feels worthless. (The person may feel she or he is not worthy to live.)
- Talks or thinks about punishment, torture, and being persecuted
- Is listening to voices. (The voices may tell the person to try to take his or her life.)
- Suddenly seems very happy, without any apparent reason, after being very depressed for some time. (The person may be happy now that she or he has figured out a method of committing suicide.)
- Collects and hoards strings, pieces of glass, a knife, or anything else sharp that might be used for self-harm
- Is very aggressive or very impulsive, acting suddenly and unexpectedly

- Shows an unusual amount of interest in getting his or her affairs in order
- Gives away personal belongings
- Has a history of suicide attempts

Establishing a therapeutic relationship during the assessment process is crucial. Demonstrate an attitude of acceptance, empathy, and support, especially important to clients who experience feelings of worthlessness, helplessness, and hopelessness. Encourage the client to verbalize negative feelings. Collection of data also involves review of any available medical records regarding the client's physical condition and previous hospital admissions.

Assessment After a Suicide Attempt

If assessment reveals a suicide attempt or the client has experienced injury resulting from the attempt, then additional assessments are completed to determine the most appropriate setting for the client's care. For example, a client who attempted suicide by shooting himself in the head may need to be monitored closely in the critical care unit. A female client who attempted suicide by overdosing on sleeping pills refuses inpatient hospitalization after being treated in the emergency department. Her husband, who is present during the assessment, informs the nurse that his mother-in-law lives with them and that she is willing to stay with his wife during the day until he returns home from work. The nurse assesses the client's home environment, relationship with her husband and mother-in-law, and motivation to receive treatment on an outpatient basis. The nurse also discusses a proposed plan of care with the husband and client, with the understanding that a reassessment may be conducted at the discretion of the nurse.

Assessment Tools

An essential aspect of assessment is direct questioning about suicidal intent. An assessment tool referred to as the SAD PERSONS Assessment Scale is often used to determine suicidal intent (Box 31-1).

Another tool that may be used in clinical practice to assess a client's levels of optimism and pessimism is a self-rating hopelessness form, the Beck Hopelessness Scale (Beck, Steer, Beck, & Newman, 1993). This tool is helpful because hopelessness is considered the best-proven clinical predictor of eventual suicide other than a previous attempt. Also inquire about the symptoms of subjective (emotional) intent and objective (purpose of) suicidal planning to aid in assessing actual suicidal intent. Ask the client whether fatality is perceived, and how rescuable the client thinks he or she would be if medical attention were immediately available. Although suicide attempts ultimately may be carried out impulsively, most are well planned.

Assessment Tools for Adolescents. The Suicidal Ideation Questionnaire (SIQ) is a tool used to screen for suicidal ideation in adolescents age 13 to 18 years. The SIQ is designed for grades 10 through 12, and the SIQ-JR version is for grades 7 through 9. Both assess the frequency of suicidal thoughts in adolescents and may be used to evaluate or monitor troubled youths. They can be administered individually or in a group, and each takes 10 minutes or less to complete.

The Multi-Attitude Suicide Tendency Scale for Adolescents (MAST), developed in 1991, is a 30-item measure assessing risk for suicidal behavior that evolves as a

---

BOX 31.1 SAD PERSONS ASSESSMENT SCALE

Sex: Men commit suicide more frequently than women do; however, women make more suicide attempts.

Age: Those at greater risk of suicide are younger than 19 and older than 45 years.

Depression: The risk of suicide increases with depresssion.

Previous attempts: The rate of suicide increases among people with a history of suicide attempts.

Ethanol or alcohol abuse: The rate of suicide is higher among alcoholics than among the *general population.*

Rational thinking: Individuals who experience impaired judgement (eg, psychosis, substance abuse, neurologic disorder) are at greater risk.

Social support: Individuals who lack support systems are at greater risk.

Organized plan: The more organized the plan for committing suicide, the greater the risk.

No spouse: Single, divorced, widowed, or separated individuals are at greater risk for suicide than those who are married.

Sickness: Individuals who experience a chronic or debilitating illness are at greater risk.

---

result of a basic conflict among attitudes toward life and death. Four sets of attitudes are measured: attraction toward life (arising from one's sense of security and the fulfillment of needs); repulsion by life (arising from pain, suffering, and unresolvable problems); attraction to death (arising from the notion that aspects of death might be preferable to life); and repulsion by death (arising from fear of death and permanent cessation). An earlier version of this test (the Fairy Tales Test) was developed for younger children in 1983 (EndingSuicide.com, 2006).

Transcultural Considerations

Although minimal information is available pertaining to cultural beliefs about suicide, nurses need to be aware of possible cultural influences. For example, suicide is forbidden under Islamic law and is considered shameful in the Filipino culture. However, the suicide of elderly Eskimos who could no longer participate as productive members of a tribe was expected (Andrews & Hanson, 2003).

Culturally sanctioned suicide has been practiced by the Japanese ("hara-kiri") and Hindu widows ("suttee"). Members of militant groups in the Middle East (eg, Palestine and Iraq) still practice culturally sanctioned suicide, such as by attaching explosives to themselves and detonating them when approaching specific targets. Suicide patterns among Native American youths vary widely among tribes, depending on physical environment, the process of imitation, social environment (ie, group integration, cohesion, and regulation), poverty, and economic change. Suicide is the second leading cause of death among Native American adolescents. Nearly half of emotionally distressed Native American adolescents have attempted suicide, compared with 16.9% of youths in general (Boyle, 2003).

Two of every three suicide victims are white males; however, the suicide rate among African Americans is rising. Suicide rates among immigrants are higher than those among the native-born population (Sadock & Sadock, 2003).

NURSING DIAGNOSES

Several nursing diagnoses are appropriate when dealing with a suicidal client. The diagnosis is based on the client's potential for self-harm, level of coping skills, degree of hopelessness, and use of support systems (Mericle, 1997). Examples of North American Nursing Diagnosis Association (NANDA) Nursing Diagnoses: Suicide are presented in the accompanying box.

OUTCOME IDENTIFICATION

Outcomes focus on the client's safety, development of positive coping skills and self-esteem, ability to interact with staff and disclose feelings regarding suicidal intent or plan, and the client's willingness to take steps to resolve any relationship or lifestyle issues that increase the risk of suicide. Long-term outcomes focus on the client's ability to be free of suicidal ideation, his or her use of task-oriented reactions to stress, and the resolution of issues that increase the risk of suicide (Mericle, 1997).

EXAMPLES OF NANDA NURSING DIAGNOSES/ SUICIDE

- Risk for Injury related to a recent suicide attempt and the verbalization, "Next time, I won't fail."
- Risk for Suicide related to stated desire to "end it all" and recent purchase of a handgun
- Risk for Violence: Self-directed related to multiple losses secondary to retirement
- Hopelessness related to diagnosis of terminal cancer as evidenced by the statement, "I'd rather be dead."
- Impaired Social Interaction related to alienation from others secondary to depressive behavior
- Ineffective Coping related to inadequate psychological resources as evidenced by impulsive, suicidal behavior
- Chronic Low Self-Esteem related to feelings of failure secondary to marital discord

---

PLANNING INTERVENTIONS

The psychiatric–mental health nurse may encounter a suicidal client in a variety of settings such as the home, hospital emergency room, private practice, mental health clinic, long-term care facility, or inpatient psychiatric setting. In any of these environments, the role of the psychiatric–mental health nurse is to plan interventions to establish a safe environment, assist the client in meeting basic needs, administer and monitor the use of prescribed medication, assist with interactive therapies, provide client and family education, and provide continuum of care as needed. Nurses who provide care for at-risk clients may have difficulty being objective as they plan interventions, because of their own religious or cultural values and beliefs about the sanctity of life. Unintentional disclosure of such a conflict to the client could have a negative effect on the client's response to treatment. Self-assessment is imperative if the nurse expects to work effectively with clients who exhibit self-destructive behavior.

IMPLEMENTATION

Interventions are individualized according to the client's medical status after a suicide attempt. Consideration is also given to the client's mental status, assessed degree of suicide risk, and motivation for treatment.

Establishment of a Safe Environment

The risk of a completed suicide increases in vulnerable clients when:

- There is a history of suicide attempts.
- There is a family history of suicide.
- A suicide plan has been formulated.
- The client has the means to carry out the plan.
- The client's mood or activity level suddenly changes.
- The client is alone.

Several approaches, such as suicide prevention measures, suicide precautions, a no-suicide contract, or seclusion and restraint may be used to provide a safe environment. The involuntary admission of a client to a psychiatric facility to provide a safe environment is discussed in Chapter 5, Ethical and Legal Issues.

Suicide Prevention. Nursing interventions focus on the prevention of self-destruction and are classified as primary, secondary, and tertiary prevention depending on risk factors identified during assessment. The purpose of **primary prevention** is to identify and eliminate factors that cause or contribute to the development of an illness or disorder that could lead to suicide. For example, a 17-year-old male student is injured in a diving accident and faces the possibility of being confined to a wheelchair. Recognizing that teenagers with disabilities are at risk for depression and suicide, primary prevention focuses on providing a support system, promoting the development of positive coping skills, and educating the student about his rehabilitation.

Secondary prevention involves attempts to identify and treat physical or emotional disorders in the early stages before they become disturbing to an individual. For example, a 24-year-old schoolteacher experiences feelings of increased anxiety and mild depression when told by her fiancé that he is breaking their engagement. Secondary prevention such as individual therapy or couple therapy, if the fiancé agrees to attend, should alleviate such symptoms and prevent the onset of self-destructive behavior.

Tertiary prevention is used to reduce residual disability after an illness. For example, a residential treatment center, halfway house, or rehabilitation center may be used to treat a recovering alcoholic client who previously attempted suicide and is recovering from severe depression, but needs the supervision and support of others to avoid a relapse.

Suicide Precautions. Clients at risk for suicide need either constant (one-to-one visual supervision) or close (visual check every 15 minutes) observation in a safe, secure environment. Suicide precautions and level of observation vary according to the client's intention of suicide and established protocol of the facility or agency providing care. Constant or close monitoring of the client's behavior is important because a suicidal client's mental state often fluctuates.

Bailey and Dreyer (1977) discuss a suicidal intention rating scale (SIRS) that provides a guide for managing clients considered to be self-destructive. Table 31-2 summarizes this rating scale, clinical symptoms, and nursing interventions for each level.

No-Suicide Contract. Since 1973, nurses, social workers, psychologists, and psychiatrists have endorsed the use of no-harm or no-suicide contracts, believing them beneficial in treating suicidal clients. In such a contract, the client is asked to agree to control suicidal impulses or to contact a nurse or therapist before attempting suicide. Some advocates of such contracts contend they reduce the risk and incidence of suicide (Figure 31-1).

No-suicide contracts must be used with caution because they may give a false sense of security to therapists and staff personnel, who may overlook the impact of depression on a client's mental functions, cognitive and perceptual processes, and capacity to exercise self-control, judgment, and discretion. Contracts are often made with clients whose suicidal risks are underestimated (Ayd & Palma, 1999).

Seclusion and Restraint. The hospitalized client may require confinement to a secure room to allow staff to observe the client's behavior more readily. Objects that could prove to be dangerous to the client are removed by searching the client's clothing, carry-in items, and body in a dignified and professional manner. The body search includes checking any part of the body in which harmful objects might be stored, such as body orifices and the hair.

Street clothes are removed, and the client is placed in a seclusion gown. Clothing and bed linens are removed from the room because these items have been used to attempt suicide by hanging oneself. The door to the seclusion room is locked whenever the client is left alone, and frequent, periodic checks are made according to established protocol.

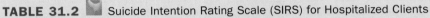

TABLE 31.2 Suicide Intention Rating Scale (SIRS) for Hospitalized Clients

RATING	SYMPTOMS	INTERVENTIONS
Zero	No evidence of past or present suicidal ideation	Implement interventions per nursing plan of care
One plus	Suicidal ideation but no attempt or threat	Observe and evaluate for evidence of development of a plan Provide routine care
Two plus	Actively thinking about suicide or history	Protect from self-destructive impulses of previous attempt Remove potentially dangerous personal items from room
Three plus	Suicidal threat verbalized	Search client and room; remove potentially dangerous items such as razor, mirror, or nail file. Provide protective care per protocol Periodically check, per protocol (eg, every 15–30 minutes) Allow limited visits by family members Confine to unit unless accompanied by a member of staff
Four plus	Actively attempted suicide or hospitalized to prevent self-destructive impulses	Implement protective care per protocol for a high-risk suicidal client

NOTE: An explanation should be given to the client so that he or she understands that the nurse is legally bound to follow policies and procedures to provide protective care.

Although the law requires the use of least-restrictive interventions to manage psychotic or suicidal clients, the use of restraints, full or belt, may be necessary to immobilize agitated, self-destructive clients. When restraints are necessary, periodic checks (eg, every 15 minutes) are made to assess and document the client's location, behavior, interventions to meet the client's needs, and the reason for the continued use of restraints.

FIGURE 31.1 The nurse reviewing a no-suicide contract with a client diagnosed with major depression.

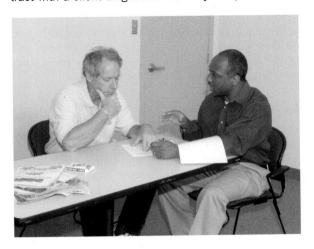

Assistance in Meeting Basic Human Needs

Clients at risk for suicide often neglect personal care. Therefore, provide assistance with activities of daily living until the client is able to assume responsibility for self-care. In addition, assist with meeting the client's nutritional needs and establishing an adequate sleep–rest–activity schedule. Medical care is provided as needed.

Visitation by family or significant others often is restricted. However, the attending physician may grant special permission for visits. After visitors have departed, be sure to check the client for items that may have been accidentally left behind or innocently given to the client.

Medication Management

The use of psychotropic medication to manage behavior is, unfortunately, sometimes referred to as *chemical restraint*. Individuals at risk for suicide, self-abusive behavior, or extreme agitation may require medications parenterally to facilitate rapid absorption of medication, stabilize mood and behavior, and prevent noncompliance (such as refusal to take oral medication or the hoarding of it).

Research studies have identified various psychotropic "drugs of choice" in the treatment of suicidal or self-injurious behavior. For example, clozapine (Clozaril) is considered to be a highly effective medication for suicidal clients with the diagnosis of schizophrenia; lithium has proven to lower suicide rates in clients with the diagnosis of bipolar disorder; and naltrexone (ReVia) has been effective in the reduction of self-injurious behavior in clients with developmental disorders. Selective serotonin reuptake inhibitors remain the treatment of choice for depressive disorders, particularly because there is a low risk of overdose. Slow titration may be necessary to minimize adverse effects (Leard-Hansson & Guttmacher, 2004; Sherman, 2004; Sullivan, 2004; Zoler, 2006). Monitor the client's response to medication, including the presence of any adverse effects (see Chapter 16, Psychopharmacology).

Interactive Therapies

After the initial threat of suicide is believed to be contained, different treatment modalities may be used. Interactive therapies, such as cognitive behavioral therapy, are provided to help the client explore the reasons behind suicidal ideation and to provide the client with adequate situational support (see Chapters 12 and 13) by parents, friends, or clergy. Feelings of anger, helplessness, and hopelessness; sources of pain; the status of relationships; and problem-solving techniques are addressed in individual, group, or family therapy.

Encourage the client to engage in an activity that is an outlet for tension and anger. For example, a sport such as volleyball or running, or an activity such as working with sandpaper or pounding wood, allows the client to express feelings while also providing him or her with an opportunity to interact with staff and peers.

Client and Family Education

Commonly, health care providers tend to believe that suicidal clients or their family members know all about the factors that place an individual at risk for suicidal

---

BOX 31.2 EXAMPLES OF FAMILY INTERVENTION AND PREVENTION STRATEGIES

1. Provide a safe home environment by removing objects or items that could be used to inflict self-injury (eg, knives, guns, medication, alcohol, or razors).
2. Have client sign a written no-suicide contract.
3. Obtain permission from client to contact the client's health care provider in the event of a crisis or an emergency.
4. Recognize changes in mood or behavior that could indicate a plan for self-injury (eg, irritability, anger, agitation, withdrawal, or self-deprecating comments) and notify the client's health care provider.
5. Anticipate future stressors and assist client to use appropriate coping skills.
6. Set limits on repeated discussions about suicide or previous attempts.
7. Keep a 24-hour emergency hotline phone number readily available.
8. Encourage the client to continue with outpatient treatment.
9. Attend a family caregiver support group meeting.
10. Do not hesitate to notify the police if the client exhibits unmanageable self-destructive behavior.

---

behavior, especially if the client has a history of previous psychiatric treatment. However, the client or family member may be too polite, withdrawn, or embarrassed to initiate a conversation with the psychiatric–mental health nurse or other health care providers. Although no immediate "cure" exists, educating the client and family members about intervention and prevention strategies can provide great relief (Box 31-2).

Continuum of Care

After the acute situation has stabilized, continuum of care is addressed. Assist the client and family with scheduling appointments for continuation of interactive therapies and medication management as needed. Social service referrals regarding financial assistance, housing, and transportation may be necessary. Discuss the importance of support services such as a 24-hour suicide hotline and the community mental health agency. Review signs and symptoms of depression, warning signs of suicidal thoughts, and effects of medication, including any special precautions, with the client and family prior to the client's discharge.

Special Considerations: Adolescent Clients

The emergency department is a pivotal point in working with suicidal adolescents, because 50% leave treatment immediately afterward and are lost to follow-up interventions. Appropriate interventions for suicidal teens who do agree to enter treatment as outpatients and cooperate with the psychiatric–mental health nurse's plan of care (Jancin, 1999) include the following:

- Repeating risk assessment throughout treatment
- Calling the child or adolescent after a missed session and rescheduling an appointment for the same day or evening
- Insisting on family therapy
- Encouraging family therapy and cognitive–behavioral therapy coupled with a good working knowledge of medication
- Working with the teen's school counselors on a weekly basis initially and then at regularly scheduled, less frequent intervals
- Being aware that finances may be an issue; however, risk is the key consideration for continuing with treatment

Signs of Suicide (SOS) Prevention Program

As noted earlier, suicide is the third leading cause of death in youth ages 15 to 24 years. Unfortunately, many youths who entertain suicidal thoughts do not seek professional help or, when they do, they do not follow through with treatment recommendations.

Signs of Suicide (SOS) is a pilot school-based prevention program in Hartford, Connecticut, and Columbus, Georgia, that has significantly reduced self-reported suicide attempts among high-school students in high-risk settings. SOS promotes the idea that suicide is directly related to mental illness such as depression and is not a normal reaction to stress or emotional upset. Peer intervention is one of the advantages of the program. Students are taught to recognize the signs of

suicide and depression in themselves and others and to respond to those signs with the following specific action steps referred to as ACT:

- **A**cknowledge the signs of suicide that others display and take them seriously.
- Let others know that they **C**are and want to help.
- **T**ell a responsible adult.

The objective of this program make the action steps of ACT as instinctual a response as the Heimlich maneuver and as familiar as CPR (Norton, 2004).

Interventions After a Successful Suicide Attempt

It would be wrong to suggest that clients do not succeed in suicide attempts. Clinical Example 31-1 describes a client who did succeed in a suicide attempt after suicide precautions were lifted.

CLINICAL EXAMPLE 31.1

THE CLIENT WHO COMMITS SUICIDE

SM, a 35-year-old teacher and father of three children, had been admitted to the neuropsychiatric unit with the diagnosis of depression. During the intake interview, SM exhibited symptoms of suicidal ideation because he made statements such as "I'd be better off dead," "My family would be better off without me," and "Yes, I have thought about killing myself." SM was placed on strict suicide precautions and antidepressant medication and began attending therapy sessions on the unit. Within 3 weeks, the suicidal precautions were lifted, and SM was granted lawn privileges but was to be supervised by one of the unit's employees. SM appeared to be improving and was granted a day pass to visit his family 4 weeks after his admission. At approximately 3:00 PM the day after SM visited his family, he asked for lawn privileges to play tennis. Although SM was supervised by a hospital employee, he was able to run away and leave the facility's grounds. Later that evening, SM's family notified the facility that he had secured a handgun and committed suicide.

Psychological Autopsy. The client described in Clinical Example 31-1 was being cared for by a female student nurse who had begun to develop a therapeutic relationship with SM. The student was shocked by the news of his suicide and immediately experienced guilt, wondering whether she had said something to upset him. She also questioned whether there had been verbal clues that she should have noticed. The staff was helpful in explaining to the student that clients may commit suicide despite all the precautions taken during hospitalization. They further explained that in the capacity of being a student, she was not with the client 24 hours a day to observe him continuously as the three shifts did. She should therefore not blame herself for his actions.

This interaction among the staff, in which the staff reviews the client's behaviors and suicidal act, is referred to as a **psychological autopsy.** It is a process used to examine what clues, if any, were missed so that staff members can learn from the evaluation of a particular situation. This process also provides staff with an opportunity to self-assess their behavior and responses and discuss their concerns with peers.

Postvention for Bereaved Survivors. Survivors of a successful suicide attempt are also victims, commonly experiencing feelings of confusion, shock, and disbelief initially. When they recover from the psychological impact of a loved one's death, feelings of anger, ambivalence, guilt, grief, and possible rejection emerge.

Postvention is a therapeutic program for bereaved survivors of a suicide. It allows family members or other survivors to vent their feelings. Emphasis needs to be placed on one unusual dynamic associated with suicide; that is, often the non–family members, such as coworkers or significant others, may be more closely involved in the death than the spouse, children, siblings, or parents of the victim. For this reason, it is extremely important for these individuals to be recognized as survivors with legitimate needs of their own. In most cases, the non–family survivors should be included in the network of the family (Staudacher, 1987).

Postvention involves three phases. In the first phase, survivors are contacted immediately (within 24 hours) to assist them in coping with their feelings of shock and grief. During the second phase, survivors are given the opportunity to develop new coping methods to help prevent the development of maladaptive or destructive behaviors. The survivor learns to cope with feelings of lowered self-esteem, depression, and the fear of devel-

oping a close interpersonal relationship. The third phase focuses on helping the survivor view the grief experience as a growth-promoting experience. This last phase ends on the first anniversary of the suicide.

Children who are survivors require special attention because they are quite vulnerable to the death of a parent, relative, peer, or close family friend. They may feel that they caused the death by "wishing Daddy dead" or "telling the person that I hate her." As a result of such feelings, children may be unable to work through the grieving process, become preoccupied with the subject of suicide, develop self-destructive behavior, exhibit signs of depression, or have difficulty working through the developmental tasks of childhood. The following are helpful as preventive and postventive measures with children who are survivors:

- Allow the child to express feelings.
- Assist the child in developing a meaningful relationship with others.
- Encourage the development of positive coping skills.
- Teach the child assertiveness.
- Allow the child to develop ideas and values.
- Expose the child to principles on human behavior during the preventive or postventive process.

Empowering Survivors of Suicide. According to the American Association of Suicidology, transforming grief into action after the suicide of a loved one can empower survivors. Participation in support groups such as the Suicide Prevention Action Network USA, Inc., provides an outlet for talking with individuals who have had similar experiences and promotes letting go of self-imposed guilt (McNamara, 2005).

A brief forensic psychiatric intervention may also help survivors understand why a loved one committed suicide. The main object of the consultation is to foster a supportive process of communication among family members and friends in their struggle to understand the suicide. Community resources, individual therapy, local survivor groups, or Internet sites such as EndingSuicide.com may be recommended at the end of the intervention (Frieden, 2005a).

EVALUATION

Evaluation of the client's progress in attaining expected outcomes is an ongoing process because the client's mood, affect, and behavior may fluctuate quickly and unpredictably. If the client is hospitalized, information obtained daily forms the basis for determining whether the client continues to be at risk. Reassessment includes reevaluation of the goals of therapy, the effectiveness of interventions, and the progress the client is making (Mericle, 1997; Robie, Edgemon-Hill, Phelps, Schmitz, & Laughlin, 1999).

If the client is not hospitalized, information is obtained from the client and family or significant others who have agreed to provide supportive care. The efficacy of an outpatient plan of care and continuum of care is evaluated. See Nursing Plan of Care 31-1: The Client With a History of Suicide Attempts.

NURSING PLAN OF CARE 31.1

THE CLIENT WITH A HISTORY OF SUICIDE ATTEMPTS

Carol, a 29-year-old engineer, was recently hospitalized for treatment of major depressive disorder following an overdose of over-the-counter pain medication. During the assessment, she admitted to attempting suicide at the age of 24 when her younger brother was accidentally killed in an automobile accident. Her brother was a passenger in the car she was driving and she blamed herself for his death, although the driver of the other car was cited for failure to yield the right of way. Carol stated that she felt alienated from her parents because her brother was their favorite child and they still question her about the details of the accident. She commented that she believed her parents wished she had died rather than her brother. Carol informed the nurse during the assessment that she was tired of being depressed and was willing to seek help. Her employer had promised her that her job will be available when she is ready to return to work.

DSM-IV-TR DIAGNOSIS: Major depressive disorder, severe, without psychotic features

ASSESSMENT: Personal strengths: Recognizes the need for help, motivated for treatment, supportive employer

Weaknesses: Low self-esteem, feels alienated from parents and guilt regarding her brother's death

---

NURSING DIAGNOSIS: Risk for Violence: Self-Directed as evidenced by a history of two suicide attempts

OUTCOME: The client will remain free of self-inflicted harm.

Planning/Implementation	Rationale
Determine and implement the appropriate level of suicide precautions for the client.	A safe environment promotes physical safety.
Involve the client in planning her own treatment.	This intervention encourages the client to assume responsibility for and control of her behavior.

NURSING DIAGNOSIS: Chronic Low Self-Esteem as evidenced by self-blame for her brother's death and belief that her parents wished she had died instead of her brother

OUTCOME: The client will identify source of threat to self-esteem and work through the issue.

(Continued on following page)

Planning/Implementation	Rationale
Convey to the client that she is a worthwhile human being.	The client should understand that she is acceptable as a person.
Encourage verbalization of feelings.	Verbalization of feelings enables the client to explore the cause of self-blame and low self-esteem.
Encourage continued therapy for chronic low self-esteem issues.	Low self-esteem issues may be deeply rooted and require long-term therapy.

NURSING DIAGNOSIS: Dysfunctional Grieving related to unexpected death of brother and perceived lack of support by parents

OUTCOME: The client will demonstrate an understanding of the grief process.

Planning/Implementation	Rationale
Educate the client about the normal phases of the grief process.	The client may have little knowledge about the grief process.
Encourage expressions of anger or guilt about the accident.	Encouraging the client to express her feelings facilitates a functional grief process.
Refer client to a spiritual resource person to discuss her brother's death.	The client may feel more comfortable discussing her brother's death with an advisor who shares her beliefs.

EVALUATION: Evaluation focuses on Carol's progress during hospitalization. Assessment is an ongoing process in which stated outcomes are reviewed to determine if they have been met. The effectiveness of interventions, the progress Carol has made, and the availability of 24-hour support are reassessed prior to discharge.

KEY CONCEPTS

◆ Several factors have been identified as contributing to suicidal behavior. Researchers have identified a genetic marker for suicidal ideation. Biologic theories regarding suicidal behavior focus on the relationship between high cortisol levels and the hypothalamic–pituitary–adrenal axis; the relationship among serotonin and postsynaptic frontal cortices' binding sites and serum cholesterol; the result of decreased protein kinase C activity; and the relationship between genetic data and endophenotypes. Sociologic and psychological factors such as isolation, internalized anger, or chronic negative feelings believed to precipitate suicidal behavior have also been identified.

◆ The term *parasuicide* is used to describe individuals who self-inflict wounds (eg, hair pulling or cutting of the skin with a sharp object) to cope with disturbing thoughts or emotions, or to relieve tension.

◆ The incidence of suicide increases in the presence of certain psychiatric and neurologic disorders, alexithymia, and the presence of chronic or terminal medical illness.

◆ High-risk populations include adolescents, ethnic minorities, homosexuals, the incarcerated, and the elderly.

◆ The act of physician-assisted suicide may conflict with a nurse's personal moral beliefs or may cause a nurse to be an unknowing participant if the nurse is not aware of the client's request.

◆ Commonly used assessment terminology to describe the range of suicidal thoughts and behaviors include ideation, intent, threat, gesture, and attempt.

◆ Various assessment tools are used during the collection of data, such as SAD PERSONS and the Beck Hopelessness Scale. Assessment tools designed to screen adolescents include the Suicidal Ideation Questionnaire and the Multi-Attitude Suicide Tendency Scale for Adolescents.

◆ Nursing interventions focus on the establishment of a safe environment, including primary, secondary, or tertiary suicide prevention; implementation of suicide precautions; development of a no-suicide contract; use of seclusion and restraints; assistance in meeting basic human needs; medication management; employment of interactive therapies; and the provision of client and family education.

◆ Continuum of care is designed to provide support services on a 24-hour basis. Suicidal adolescents require special considerations because approximately 50% leave treatment immediately after they receive emergency treatment and are lost to follow-up interventions.

◆ Psychological autopsy is a process used to review a client's behaviors and completed suicidal act despite all the precautions taken in a controlled environment.

◆ Postvention is a therapeutic program for bereaved survivors of a suicide victim. It begins within 24 hours of the suicide and ends on the first anniversary of the suicide. The American Association of Suicidology believes transforming grief into action after the suicide of a loved one can empower survivors. Empowerment may be achieved through participation in forensic psychiatric intervention, community resources, individual therapy, local survivor groups, or Internet sites such as EndingSuicide.com.

◆ Evaluation is an ongoing process that considers the client's progress in attaining expected outcomes as stated in the inpatient or outpatient plan of care and continuum of care.

For additional study materials, please refer to the Student Resource CD-ROM located in the back of this textbook.

CHAPTER WORKSHEET

CRITICAL THINKING QUESTIONS

1. Write a journal of your feelings, thoughts, stressors, and coping methods for several weeks. Review it for patterns; that is, identify events, situations, or individuals who are stressors (eg, what makes you mad or sad). What do you do to cope? Are your coping methods healthy? Do they work?

2. Team up with a classmate and interview each other about your values and beliefs concerning life, death, and suicide. What differences and similarities do you have?

3. You notice that your 13-year-old neighbor always wears black, refuses to make eye contact, is often alone, and has a defeated posture. Your mother and the boy's mother are good friends. You are concerned about the teen's increasing isolation. Describe several interventions that might be appropriate in this situation and explain your rationale for selecting them.

REFLECTION

Think back to the quotes presented at the beginning of the chapter. Incorporate these quotes in the following scenario: The parent of an adolescent client who attempted suicide approaches you privately and asks you to explain how suicide can be considered manipulative behavior. What explanation could you give to the client's parent? What additional educational material could you provide to support your response?

NCLEX-STYLE QUESTIONS

1. The nurse on an alcohol and drug rehabilitation unit teaches a client group about depression and suicide. Which behavioral clue would the nurse identify as suggestive of suicide?

   a. Joking about stressful situations
   b. Verbalizing feelings of hopelessness and helplessness about problems
   c. Engaging in weekend drinking episodes
   d. Seeking help for symptoms of depression

2. The nursing plan of care for a client with depression who has verbalized the wish to die identifies the period of greatest suicide risk as which of the following?

   a. During the period of recovery from depression
   b. During the period of deepest depression
   c. Prior to effective onset of action of antidepressants
   d. When the client continues to ruminate about problems

3. The nursing assessment of a client who expresses suicidal intent is made based on which of the following principles about suicide prevention?

   a. Clients expressing intentions of suicide rarely follow through with the action.
   b. Degree of suicidal intent is not a static quality and may change from day to day.
   c. After a suicidal gesture, the client will be grateful to be alive.
   d. Questions related to the specific details of a suicide plan are not therapeutic.

4. Which nursing intervention would be the priority for a client with suicidal intent?

   a. Encouraging verbalization of negative feelings
   b. Pointing out the positive aspects of living
   c. Providing activities to keep the client busy
   d. Reassuring the client that thoughts of suicide will decrease

5. A client has committed suicide while hospitalized on an inpatient psychiatric unit. The nursing staff and treatment team participate in a process of reviewing the client's behaviors and the completed suicide despite all precautions implemented on the unit. The staff is engaging in which of the following?

   a. Psychological autopsy
   b. Postvention process
   c. Treatment analysis
   d. Team discussion

6. Which assessment findings would lead the nurse to suspect that a client is at a high risk for suicide? Select all that apply.

   a. Hopelessness accompanied by withdrawal
   b. Several available support persons
   c. Marked degree of hostility

   d. Mostly constructive coping mechanisms
   e. Continual abuse of alcohol
   f. History of multiple previous lethal attempts

Selected References

American Association of Suicidology. (2006). U.S.A. suicide: 2003 official final data prepared by John L. McIntosh, Ph.D. Retrieved March 21, 2006, from http://www.suicidology.org

Andrews, M. M., & Hanson, P. A. (2003). Religion, culture, and nursing. In M. M. Andrews & J. S. Boyle (Eds.), *Transcultural concepts in nursing care* (4th ed., pp. 432–502). Philadelphia: Lippincott Williams & Wilkins.

Ayd, F. J., Jr., & Palma, J. M. (1999). Suicide: Risk recognition and prevention. *Psychiatric Times, 16*(5), 36–41.

Badger, J. M. (1995). Reaching out to the suicidal patient. *American Journal of Nursing, 95*(3).

Bailey, D., & Dreyer, S. (1977). *Care of the mentally ill.* Philadelphia: F.A. Davis.

Beck, A.T., Steer, R.A., Beck, J.S., & Newman, C.F. (1993). Hopelessness, depression, suicidal ideation, and clinical diagnosis of depression. *Suicide and Life-Threatening Behavior,* (2).

Boyle, J. S. (2003). Culture, family, and community. In M. M. Andrews & J. S. Boyle (Eds.), *Transcultural concepts in nursing care* (4th ed., pp. 315–360). Philadelphia: Lippincott Williams & Wilkins.

Buchanan, M. J. (2002). Leaving the root intact. *ADVANCE for Nurses, 3*(4), 21–22.

Crisis Intervention Network. (2002). Suicide fact sheet. Retrieved October 18, 2002, from http://www.crisisintervention network.com/resources_sfs.html

EndingSuicide.com. (2006). Online education on suicide prevention for professionals. Retrieved March 21, 2006, from http://www1.endingsuicide.com/PageReq?idj=1940:9829

Frieden, J. (2005a). Brief consults help suicide survivors. *Clinical Psychiatry News, 33*(12), 1, 50.

Frieden, J. (2005b). Suicide risk assessment difficult in jails, prisons. *Clinical Psychiatry News, 33*(1), 63.

Jancin, B. (1999). Ten tips for working with suicidal teens. *Clinical Psychiatry News, 27*(6), 25.

Johnston, M. (2002). Patients who self-injure. *American Journal of Nursing, 102*(12), 11.

Kennedy, R. (2004). Familial suicidal behavior: A newsmaker interview with Maria Oquendo, MD. *Medscape Medical News.* Retrieved February 18, 2004, from http://www.medscape.com/viewarticle/469167

King, A. A., & Scahill, L. (1998). Understanding and treating trichotillomania. *Masters in Psychiatry,* 2–3.

Kirk, K. (1998). How Oregon's death with dignity act affects practice. *American Journal of Nursing, 98*(8), 54–55.

Knowlton, L. (1998). Is it ethical? Residents uncertain about assisted suicide. *Psychiatric Times, 14*(6), 53–54.

Leard-Hansson, J., & Guttmacher, L. (2004). Naltrexone and self-injurious behavior. *Clinical Psychiatry News, 32*(6), 20.

Libow, L. S. (2000, May/June). Physician-assisted suicide for older patients in the LTC setting. *Long-Term Care Interface, 1,* 10-11.

Lindsay, H. (1999). Surgeon general proposes national strategy for suicide prevention. *Clinical Psychiatry News, 27*(10), 2.

Lindsay, H. (2000). Homosexuals at risk of suicide, mental illness. *Clinical Psychiatry News, 28*(1), 34.

Lott, D. A. (2000). Risk management with the suicidal patient. *Psychiatric Times, 17*(8), 9-12.

McNamara, D. (2004a). Dexamethasone suppression test can indicate suicide risk. *Clinical Psychiatry News, 32*(9), 60.

McNamara, D. (2004b). Suicide for some is an escape from 'the self.' *Clinical Psychiatry News, 32*(7), 48.

McNamara, D. (2005). Action, advocacy empower survivors of suicide. *Clinical Psychiatry News, 33*(2), 47.

Mericle, B. P. (1997). Suicide. In B. S. Johnson (Ed.), *Psychiatric-mental health nursing: Adaptation and growth* (4th ed., pp. 857-875). Philadelphia: Lippincott-Raven.

Muller, R. J. (2000a). Researchers identify gene for suicidality. *Psychiatric Times, 17*(3), 78.

Muller, R. J. (2000b). When a patient has no story to tell: Alexithymia. *Psychiatric Times, 17*(7), 71-72.

Murphy, S. A., Tapper, V. J., Johnson, L. C., & Lohan, J. (2003). Suicide ideation among parents bereaved by the violent deaths of their children. *Issues in Mental Health Nursing, 24,* 5-25.

National Center for Health Statistics. (2003). Fast stats: Suicide. Retrieved July 1, 2003, from http://www.cdc.gov/nchs/fastats/suicide.htm

National Center for Injury Prevention and Control. (2003). Suicide in the United States. Retrieved July 1, 2003, from http://www.cdc.gov/ncipc/factsheets/suifacts.htm

National Institute of Mental Health. (2003). In harm's way: Suicide in America. Retrieved October 20, 2004, from http://www.nimh.nih.gov/publicat/harmsway.cfm?output=print

Norton, P. G. W. (2004). Prevention plan reduces teen suicide attempts. *Clinical Psychiatry News, 32*(5), 34.

Perlstein, S. (2004). Teen screen flags adolescents at risk of suicide. *Clinical Psychiatry News, 32*(4), 43.

Robie, D., Edgemon-Hill, E. J., Phelps, B., Schmitz, C., & Laughlin, J. A. (1999). Suicide prevention protocol. *American Journal of Nursing, 99*(12), 53-57.

Sadock, B. J., & Sadock, V. A. (2003). *Kaplan and Sadock's synopsis of psychiatry: Behavioral sciences/clinical psychiatry* (9th ed.). Philadelphia: Lippincott Williams & Wilkins.

Schultz, J. M., & Videbeck, S. D. (2005). *Lippincott's manual of psychiatric nursing care plans* (7th ed.). Philadelphia: Lippincott Williams & Wilkins.

Schwartz, J. K. (2002). The war on assisted suicide. *American Journal of Nursing, 102*(3), 11.

Sherman, C. (2000). Neurologic disorders raise overall suicide risk. *Clinical Psychiatry News, 28*(5), 44.

Sherman, C. (2004). Depression and suicide. *Clinical Psychiatry News, 32*(7), 16.

Shneidman, E. S. (1996). *The suicidal mind.* New York: Oxford University Press.

Starr, D. L. (2004). Understanding those who self-mutilate. *Journal of Psychosocial Nursing and Mental Health Services, 42*(6). Retrieved January 24, 2005, from http://www.jpnonline.com/keypoints/kp0406_starr.asp

Staudacher, C. (1987). *Beyond grief: A guide for recovering from the death of a loved one.* Oakland, CA: New Harbinger Publications.

Stong, C. (2004). News roundup: Pathogenesis of teenage suicide. *Neuropsychiatry Reviews, 5*(6), 4.

Sullivan, M. G. (2004). Clozapine is a proven choice for suicidal patients. *Clinical Psychiatry News, 32*(12), 53.

Tumolo, J. (2005). Slice at life. *ADVANCE for Nurse Practitioners, 13*(12), 54-56.

Whitaker, H., Wolf, K. A., & Keuthen, N. (2003). Chronic hair pulling: Recognizing trichotillomania. *Clinician Reviews, 13*(3), 37-38, 40, 43-44.

Zoler, M. L. (2006). Lithium lowers suicide rates in bipolar disorder. *Clinical Psychiatry News, 34*(2), 28.

Suggested Readings

Carpenito-Moyet, L. J. (2006). *Handbook of nursing diagnosis* (11th ed.). Philadelphia: Lippincott Williams & Wilkins.

Chlebus, P. M. (2004). Risk factors for adolescent suicide. *ADVANCE for Nurse Practitioners, 12*(2), 49-52, 54, 56.

Crow, S., & Parks, L. (2006). Suicide assessment in the ED. *ADVANCE for Nurses, 7*(5), 15-18.

Fawcett, J. A. (2005). Suicide and bipolar disorder. *Medscape Psychiatry & Mental Health, 8*(2). Retrieved September 23, 2005, from http://www.medscape.com/viewarticle/510318

Franklin, D. (2004). Education key to suicide prevention on campus. *Clinical Psychiatry News, 32*(10), 35.

Freeman, A., & Alaimo, C. (2001). Prevention of suicide in a large urban jail. *Psychiatric Annals, 31*(7), 447-452.

Grant, J. E. (2005). Malpractice verdicts: Restraint and monitoring of psychotic or suicidal patients. *Current Psychiatry, 4*(11), 84-86.

Lantz, M. S. (2001). Suicide in late life: Identifying and managing at-risk older patients. *Geriatrics, 56*(7), 47-48.

Mahoney, D. (2005). Psychosis duration affects suicidality. *Clinical Psychiatry News, 33*(7), 1, 8.

Reed, M. (2002). Preventing teen suicide. *ADVANCE for Nurses, 3*(21), 27-29.

Schwartz, J. K. (2002). The war on assisted suicide. *American Journal of Nursing, 102*(3), 11.

Sherman, C. (2000). Adolescent suicide pacts are rare, but lethal. *Clinical Psychiatry News, 28*(2), 26.

Specht, J., Singer, A. J., & Henry, M. C. (2005). Self-inflicted injuries in adolescents presenting to a suburban emergency department. *Journal of Forensic Nursing, 1*(1), 20-22.

U.S. Preventive Services Task Force. (2005). Screening for suicide risk: Recommendation and rationale. *American Journal for Nurse Practitioners, 9*(3), 46, 51-54.

CHAPTER 32 / CLIENTS WITH A DUAL DIAGNOSIS

According to the National Mental Health Association, 29% of all people diagnosed as mentally ill abuse either alcohol or drugs. —NATIONAL MENTAL HEALTH ASSOCIATION, 2003
Chemical dependency is a serious public health problem. For people with mental illness, comorbid chemical dependency can be a catastrophic life problem. —VACCARO, 1999

AFTER STUDYING THIS CHAPTER, YOU SHOULD BE ABLE TO:

1. Define the term *dual diagnosis*.
2. Explain the acronyms MICAA, MICA, and CAMI.
3. Differentiate the two main theories related to the development of a dual diagnosis.
4. Describe the defining characteristics of clients with a dual diagnosis.
5. Articulate the barriers to effective treatment of a client with a dual diagnosis.
6. Interpret the four categories that have been developed to describe the dually diagnosed client.
7. State why it is difficult to assess a client with a dual diagnosis.
8. Summarize the following phases of treatment for clients with a dual diagnosis: acute stabilization, engagement, prolonged stabilization, rehabilitation and recovery including continuum of care.
9. Explain why evaluation of a dually diagnosed client's progress is an ongoing process.

CAMI
Dual diagnosis
MICA
MICAA
Persuasion
Self-medication hypothesis
Vulnerability model

The term **dual diagnosis** is used to refer to coexisting or comorbid conditions. In the field of psychiatry, dual diagnosis refers to the existence of a serious mental illness and the problematic use of alcohol or other drugs, or both. (Please note that this term has also been used to describe the presence of a psychiatric illness in developmentally disabled clients. These clients are not included in this discussion.) It has been estimated that approximately 50% to 75% of severely mentally ill clients have a dual diagnosis. For example, approximately 1 in 12 clients (7.8%) with a psychiatric diagnosis such as schizophrenia abuses substances and is human immunodeficiency virus (HIV)-positive. Furthermore, approximately 37% of clients who abuse alcohol and 53% of clients who abuse drugs have at least one serious mental illness such as bipolar disorder or an eating disorder. Children with conduct disorder are at risk for abuse of drugs or alcohol, and individuals with depression or anxiety often use alcohol or substances to alleviate symptoms. In addition, approximately 20% of incarcerated substance abusers have a history of mental illness (Baker, 2002; Blinder, Blinder, & Sanathara, 1998; Finkelstein, 1999a, 1999b; Kirn, 1999; National Alliance for the Mentally Ill, 2006; Vaccaro, 1999). Table 32-1 ranks the prevalence of substance-related disorders in clients with a *Diagnostic and Statistical Manual of Mental Disorders, 4th Edition, Text Revision (DSM-IV-TR)* diagnosis.

Various acronyms have been used to describe dual diagnosis. The first acronym is **MICAA** (Mentally Ill, Chemically Abusing, and Addicted), which implies that the primary diagnosis is severe mental illness and the secondary diagnosis is chemical abuse or addiction. The drug most commonly used is alcohol, followed by marijuana and cocaine. Prescription drugs such as tranquilizers and sleeping medicines may also be abused. For example, the term MICAA would be used to refer to a client with schizophrenia who abuses alcohol. This acronym has been shortened to **MICA** (Mentally Ill, Chemically Abusing) by some professionals. The acronym **CAMI** (Chemically Abusing, Mentally Ill) implies that the primary diagnosis is chemical abuse and the secondary diagnosis is mental illness. Nearly all the psychiatric disorders, such as delirium, dementia, or depression, can be precipitated by the use of addictive substances. An example of CAMI is the client who abuses alcohol and develops alcohol-related dementia or Korsakoff's psychosis.

Planning care for clients with a dual diagnosis is a difficult challenge because such clients often have medical problems that require immediate attention. Detoxification may be necessary before clinical symptoms of disorders such as depression, anxiety, or schizophrenia are treated. Furthermore, clients with a dual diagnosis have a statistically greater propensity for violence, medication noncompliance, and failure to respond to treatment than do clients with a solitary diagnosis of mental illness or substance abuse. Clients are frequently hospitalized because they lack motivation to participate in treatment. Unfortunately, failure to respond to treatment also affects family members, friends, and co-workers (National Alliance for the Mentally Ill, 2006). Chapter 35 addresses issues of seriously and persistently mentally ill, homeless, or incarcerated clients.

This chapter reviews the two main etiologic theories associated with dual diagnosis and describes the

TABLE 32.1 Prevalence of Substance-Related Disorders in Clients With a *DSM-IV-TR* Diagnosis

DSM-IV-TR DIAGNOSIS	PREVALENCE OF SUBSTANCE-RELATED DISORDER*
Antisocial personality disorder	80%
Schizophrenia	60%
Bipolar disorder	40%
Major depressive disorder	30%
Anxiety disorders	30%
Eating disorders	25.7%
Phobic disorders	25%

*The percentages were averaged based on data obtained from several sources during the period 1990–2000. (Blinder, Blinder, & Sanathara, 1998; Finkelstein, 1999a, 1999b; Miller, 1994; Vaccaro, 1999; Zahourek, 1996; Zwillich, 1999.)

clinical symptoms and diagnostic characteristics. The chapter then focuses on the application of the nursing process to clients with a dual diagnosis.

Etiology of Dual Diagnosis

The etiologies of substance-related disorders and different psychiatric disorders have been presented in other chapters. Two main theories have been proposed about the development of a dual diagnosis (Faltz & Callahan, 2002; Zahourek, 1996).

Vulnerability Model

The **vulnerability model** of dual diagnosis is based on the assumption that drug use causes a mental disorder. For example, daily marijuana use doubles the risk for psychosis; daily cocaine users have a seven times greater risk of a psychotic episode than nonusers; and dependence on alcohol doubles the risk of psychosis (Kosta, 2002; Miller, 1994; Miller, Eriksen, & Owley, 1994).

Attempts to identify what determines vulnerability are numerous. For example, alcoholic personality subtypes have been identified, and several personality traits have been described. They include emotional insecurity, anxiety, unsatisfied dependence needs, narcissism, externalization of blame, and the use of defense mechanisms such as denial.

Self-Medication Hypothesis

The **self-medication hypothesis** of dual diagnosis is based on the assumption that individuals with a psychiatric disorder use drugs to help them feel calmer or to alleviate clinical symptoms to achieve emotional homeostasis. Self-medication often leads to physical or psychological dependency on drugs or alcohol, creating a complex dual diagnosis problem (Kosta, 2002). For example, clients with schizophrenia self-medicate with alcohol or drugs to decrease anxiety (positive symptom) and the intensity of hallucinations (negative symptoms). Using substances does not result in the uncomfortable adverse effects of neuroleptic drugs, and to some degree is a socially accepted behavior. Table 32-2 lists seven major psychiatric disorders and shows how much each one increases an individual's risk for substance-related disorders (National Mental Health Association, 2003).

TABLE 32.2 Psychiatric Disorders and Increased Risk for Substance-Related Disorders

PSYCHIATRIC DISORDERS	INCREASED RISK FOR SUBSTANCE-RELATED DISORDERS
Antisocial personality disorder	15.5%
Manic episode	14.5%
Schizophrenia	10.1%
Panic disorder	4.3%
Major depressive episode	4.1%
Obsessive–compulsive disorder	3.4%
Phobias	2.4%

SOURCE: National Mental Health Association. (2003). *Substance abuse: Dual diagnosis.* Retrieved July 4, 2003, from http://www.nmha.org/infoctr/factsheets/03.cfm

Clinical Symptoms and Diagnostic Characteristics

Clients with a dual diagnosis often are dissatisfied with life circumstances, have inadequate or ineffective support systems, live in a nontherapeutic home environment, and have a history of self-medication (National Alliance for the Mentally Ill, 2006; Zahourek, 1996).

The frequent use of drugs and alcohol interferes with the action of any psychiatric medications the client may be taking. Substance-related disorders often exacerbate clinical symptoms of an existing disorder or precipitate additional symptoms. Symptoms commonly seen include irritability, depression, sedation, hostility, aggression, delusions, hallucinations, poor impulse control, and suicidal or violent behavior. Lack of self-esteem and social skills contributes to disinterest in activities of daily living. Clients also have little interest in the future.

As noted earlier, many individuals are at risk for health problems, may have medical problems including acquired immunodeficiency syndrome (AIDS) or tuberculosis, are homeless, and are not motivated to receive treatment. If they do enter treatment, they often fail to keep scheduled appointments or follow through on referrals. Relapses and repeated institutionalizations are not uncommon. Several barriers to effective treatment have been identified. These are listed in Box 32-1.

BOX 32.1 BARRIERS TO EFFECTIVE TREATMENT OF DUAL DIAGNOSIS

Nature of substance-related disorder: The dually diagnosed (CAMI) client faces two options:

1. Continue with illicit drug of choice for brief moments of calmness, joy, and escape from problems, which can result in a decline in overall function and potentially increase the severity of psychiatric symptoms, or
2. Accept prescribed treatments to cease illicit drug use, which might include the use of medication to promote improved functioning and treatment outcome.

Countertransference: The nurse's emotional reactions to the client are based on the nurse's unconscious needs, conflicts, and misunderstanding of or prejudice about behaviors or the legal status of clients with a dual diagnosis. Countertransference can precipitate relapse secondary to inappropriate treatment.

Refusal by substance-related disorder treatment professionals to accept dually diagnosed clients into programs.

Health issues: Clients are often underserved and only partially treated because of the complexity of health issues they present, noncompliance with plan of care, and potential for drug–drug interactions secondary to the use of substances in addition to medication prescribed to stabilize clinical symptoms of a mental illness.

SOURCE: Faltz, B. G., & Callahan, P. (2002). Special care concerns for patients with dual disorders. In M.A. Boyd (Ed), *Psychiatric nursing: Contemporary practice* (2nd ed., pp. 874–893). Philadelphia: Lippincott Williams & Wilkins.

The *DSM-IV-TR* does not have a specific classification or category for dual diagnosis. The multiaxial system (discussed in Chapter 10) is used to list the clinical diagnosis or diagnoses and the presence of any comorbid personality disorder.

Four categories have been developed to describe the client with a dual diagnosis (Krausz, 1996; Sciacca, 2003):

- Category 1: The primary diagnosis is a major mental illness such as schizophrenia with a subsequent secondary diagnosis of a substance-related disorder such as alcohol dependence.
- Category 2: The primary diagnosis is a substance-related disorder such as cocaine abuse that results in a secondary mental illness such as organic mood disorder, organic anxiety disorder, organic delusional disorder, or antisocial behaviors that decrease or disappear when substance abuse is discontinued.
- Category 3: Mental illness and substance-related disorder occur simultaneously with no apparent etiologic relationship.
- Category 4: Substance-related disorder and mood disorder occur due to an underlying traumatic experience.

Identification of the primary diagnosis may be problematic because the signs and symptoms of the mental illness may mimic the signs of intoxication and withdrawal of the substance-related disorder. Misdiagnosis may occur.

THE NURSING PROCESS

ASSESSMENT

Clients with a dual diagnosis are difficult to assess because they are not a homogenous group. In addition, clients often are poor historians and are non-compliant during the assessment process. They may present for assessment on a voluntary basis because they desire help (eg, the client who utilizes alcohol to cope with clinical symptoms of depression recognizes the fact that he or she is dependent on alcohol); they may be adjudicated by the court system to be evaluated prior to sentencing for a crime (eg, the client has a personality disorder, is addicted to cocaine, and has committed a felony); or they may be referred by another health care professional to rule out the presence of a comorbid psychiatric disorder (eg, a family practitioner refers a client to rule out addiction to benzodiazepines initially prescribed to treat clinical symptoms of anxiety) (Kosta, 2002).

The severity of each client's psychological problems and his or her level of functioning vary depending on the specific combination of psychiatric disorder and substance-related disorder. The most common mental disorders that coexist in clients who abuse substances include anxiety disorders, depressive disorders, personality disorders, and schizophrenia. Nurses need to identify the relative contribution of each diagnosis to the severity of the current symptoms presented and prioritize data accordingly (Faltz & Callahan, 2002). For example, the nurse may have difficulty distinguishing the manifestations of schizophrenia from those of intoxication and withdrawal in a client with dual diagnosis.

Substance-related disorder assessment tools (discussed in Chapter 25), a mental status exam (discussed in Chapter 9), and laboratory testing are useful when collecting data. Additional methods included in a comprehensive assessment of dually diagnosed clients include:

- Review of court records, medical records, and previous treatment records
- Interview of social worker familiar with client's history
- Revision of initial assessment by observation of the client in the clinical setting, because full assessment of underlying psychiatric problems may not be possible until abstinence has occurred
- Assessment of client's motivation to seek treatment, desire to change behavior, and understanding of diagnosis (Faltz & Callahan, 2002)

NURSING DIAGNOSES

Differences in the philosophies and approaches of treatment models for mental illness and substance-related disorders can affect the formulation of nursing diagnosis, outcome statements, planning and implementation, and evaluation. The issue of diagnosing mood, cognitive, or psychotic disorders among substance abusers has been controversial as some health care professionals attempt to ascertain which disorder came first or which disorder is the primary disorder. For example, clients with cognitive impairment, limited insight, or decreased ability to process abstract concepts have little success in substance-abuse treatment programs. Conversely, treatment designed to manage psychotic symptoms is less successful when the client drinks alcohol or uses substances that can exacerbate psychotic symptoms. In such a situation, the presence of one illness may adversely affect the nursing diagnosis and course of treatment of the other disorder. Furthermore, many clients with a dual diagnosis have concomitant Axis III disorders (eg, a general medical disorder such as cirrhosis of the liver, peptic ulcer disease, or cardiovascular disease) either directly related to substance use or to self-care deficits stemming from a psychiatric disorder and substance abuse (Albanese, 2001). Examples of the more common nursing diagnoses associated with clients who have a dual diagnosis are highlighted in the accompanying box.

OUTCOME IDENTIFICATION

Outcomes focus on the client's willingness to participate in treatment, including compliance with the plan of care. The development of positive coping skills, verbalization of feelings of increased self-worth, development of appropriate social skills, desire to establish and maintain contact or relationship with a professional in the community, and desire to socialize in drug- and alcohol-free environments are examples of appropriate outcomes.

PLANNING INTERVENTIONS

Because clients with a dual diagnosis have to proceed at their own pace in treatment, interventions are based on the individual client's needs. Consideration is given to the type of substance-related disorder involved, the presence or absence of cognitive impairment, ability to process abstract concepts, motivation for treatment, and availability of social support (Schultz & Videbeck, 2005). Detoxification may be necessary before clinical symptoms of the comorbid diagnosis, such as schizophrenia or depression, can be treated.

EXAMPLES OF NANDA NURSING DIAGNOSES/ DUAL DIAGNOSIS

- Ineffective Health Maintenance related to lack of motivation to participate in a dual diagnosis treatment program (schizophrenia and cocaine abuse)
- Ineffective Health Maintenance related to lack of access to adequate health care services for medical treatment of a dual diagnosis (abuse of pain medication and AIDS)
- Disturbed Thought Processes related to physiologic changes secondary to self-medicating with substances to reduce anxiety
- Impaired Social Interaction related to alienation from others secondary to drug-seeking behavior and high level of anxiety
- Ineffective Coping related to altered appearance (significant weight loss) due to substance abuse and self-induced vomiting
- Noncompliance related to barriers to accessing treatment for a dual diagnosis secondary to underlying health issues and lack of finances
- Situational Low Self-Esteem related to feelings of failure secondary to relapse following treatment for a dual diagnosis of substance abuse and depression

Therefore, the client's clinical symptoms may dictate the setting in which treatment occurs.

Treatment is available in a variety of settings, including outpatient medical units, inpatient psychiatric units, inpatient substance-abuse units, community mental health centers, general hospitals, and day- and evening-treatment programs. The location of treatment is often determined by the severity of the client's symptoms and his or her ability to pay for services due to the limited insurance coverage for inpatient treatment that has occurred over the past several years.

Research has addressed additional problems and concerns that can arise during the planning and implementation of care for youth and adults with a dual diagnosis. Summarized, they include disrupted motivation and increased risk of relapse, unstable living arrangements resulting from loss of family or support networks, failure to develop appropriate social skills, and disruptive behavior or violence that necessitates contact with the criminal justice system (Youth Action and Policy Association, 2003, 2006).

IMPLEMENTATION

Clients enter treatment at various stages of their disorders. Although the concept of integrated treatment is increasingly recognized as preferential over sequential and parallel models for individuals with dual diagnosis, research, and attendant documentation, on integrated approaches is still in an infancy stage. Case management and provision of care must be balanced with empathetic detachment and confrontation in accordance with the client's level of functioning, disability, and capacity for treatment adherence. Therefore, flexible treatment programs that can meet the individual needs of each client are considered the most effective (Raby, Doub, & Cartwright, 2003). Box 32-2 summarizes treatment approaches for dually diagnosed clients.

Different phases of treatment are provided for clients with a dual diagnosis. These phases (referred to as a "disease and recovery model") include acute stabilization, engagement, prolonged stabilization, and rehabilitation and recovery (Minkoff, 2000; Osher and Olfed, 1989).

Acute Stabilization

During the acute stabilization phase, a safe environment is provided for clients who are at risk for suicidal or homicidal ideation, exhibit psychotic disorganization, or exhibit clinical symptoms of other serious psychiatric disorders, such as post-traumatic stress disorder or bipolar disorder. In addition, the medical needs of clients requiring detoxification, such as the pregnant client who continues to abuse substances, or clients who have an exacerbated medical disorder or illness that interferes with outpatient treatment, such as the client with HIV infection who is addicted to pain medication, are met. Psychopharmacologic agents may be used depending on the client's underlying psychiatric–mental health disorder. There is some indication that medications such as clozapine (Clozaril), risperidone (Risperdal), and olanzapine (Zyprexa) can ameliorate substance abuse problems. Keep in mind that the impact of alcohol and drugs of abuse may alter pharmacokinetics and exacerbate adverse effects when psychotropic medication is administered. For example, liver dysfunction and anemia secondary to alcohol abuse can disrupt drug metabolism and generate what seem like negative symptoms (Sherman, 2004). (See Chapter 16, Psychopharmacology; Chapter 22, Schizophrenia and Schizophrenic-like Disorders; and Chapter 25, Substance-Related Disorders for information about medication management.)

BOX 32.2 | **TREATMENT APPROACHES FOR DUALLY DIAGNOSED CLIENTS**

Serial or sequential model: Treatment for one disorder (eg, substance abuse) follows treatment for another (eg, depression or anxiety) in different sites with different staff. Treatment is often fragmented, dropout rates are high, and relapse occurs.

Parallel model: Concurrent treatment for both problems occurs in separate facilities or separate programs with separate staff. Treatment can be stressful if the programs are not easily accessible, if staff in each program do not communicate with each other, or if the client receives conflicting messages.

Integrated or unified model: Both diagnoses are considered primary and staff members are trained and experienced in providing care for clients with a dual diagnosis. Caution is exercised to avoid the overdiagnosis of a psychiatric disorder in clients who have a primary addictive disorder but who sought help for depressive or anxious symptoms related to substance abuse.

Treatment modalities: Frequently used modalities in the above-mentioned models include cognitive-behavioral or brief interactive therapy, family therapy, psychoeducation including medication management, case management, skills training, vocational counseling, referrals to community resources, and referrals to self-help groups such as Anger Management, AA, NA, Rational Recovery, and Women for Sobriety.

SOURCES: Miller, N. (1994). Prevalence and treatment models for addiction in psychiatric populations. *Psychiatric Annals, 24,* 394–06; Minkoff, K. (1994). Models of addition treatment in psychiatric population. *Psychiatric Annals, 24,* 413–418; Zahourek, R. P. (1996). The client with dual diagnosis. In S. Lego (Ed.), *Psychiatric nursing: A comprehensive reference* (2nd ed., pp. 275–284). Philadelphia: Lippincott-Raven; Youth Action and Policy Association NSW (YAPA). (2003). *Fact sheet: Take action now on dual diagnosis.* Retrieved September 4, 2003, from http://www.yapa.org.au/facts/DualDiagnosis.pdf; and Dual diagnosis info sheet: Concepts and treatment issues. (2003). Retrieved September 4, 2003, from http://www.dlcas.com/course5.html

---

Engagement

Engagement involves four steps: establishing a treatment relationship with the client; educating the client (referred to as **persuasion**) about the illnesses; active treatment, when the nurse provides various interventions to enable the client to maintain stabilization by complying with treatment; and relapse prevention, in which the nurse helps the client overcome denial and other resistances to treatment.

Establishing a treatment relationship with a client may require many contacts by the psychiatric–mental health nurse. Clients often struggle with issues of authority and control and feel threatened. Nonconfrontational, nonthreatening approaches such as the expression of empathy and acceptance of the client are effective interventions during this step. The nurse utilizes reflective listening without judging, criticizing, or blaming and accepts any ambivalence as a normal part of the client's human experience not as psychopathology (Sciacca, 1997).

Education (persuasion) focuses on helping clients recognize problematic behaviors and symptoms and identifying methods to activate change. Awareness of consequences is important. A discrepancy between present behavior and important goals will motivate change. The client is encouraged to present arguments for change. Medication management is stressed to help clients maintain stability. Medication noncompliance is associated with increased behavior problems after discharge and accounts for frequent relapse and rehospitalization. Peer-group discussions, family education, social-network interventions, and self-help groups are just a few of the educational interventions provided.

During active treatment, specific abstinence-related strategies, such as the identification of specific stressors and development of positive coping skills, are targeted. Individual, cognitive–behavioral, or group therapy may be used to promote positive coping patterns and cognitive and behavioral skills. The client is encouraged to improve social-network strengths. Family support and involvement also is encouraged.

Nursing interventions during relapse prevention include teaching the client signs and symptoms of relapse, helping the client identify problems caused by the use of drugs and alcohol, identifying risk factors such as dangerous people or places to avoid, reinforcing behavioral change, and encouraging the adoption of wellness activities such as healthy diet and exercise. During this step, the client is encouraged to participate in support groups such as Alcoholics Anonymous (AA), Narcotics Anonymous (NA), or Dual Recovery Anonymous (DRA). If the client is unable to attend such groups, special peer groups based on AA principles might be beneficial.

Prolonged Stabilization

The interventions used during engagement continue during this phase. The focus is on discussing potential crises and exploring crisis management skills for the client and family to develop.

Rehabilitation and Recovery

Rehabilitation and recovery are viewed as a long-term, community based process, one that can take months or, more likely, years to undergo. The client is encouraged to return to work if he or she was previously employed. Alternatively, the client may be referred to a community vocational rehabilitation program. Participation in self-help groups and reaching out to others in a giving way are also encouraged. Establishing a positive social network prevents isolation and alienation, a problem that most chronic dually diagnosed clients share.

During the rehabilitation and recovery phase, continuum of care begins. A case manager may be assigned to the client before discharge from a mental health facility. The case manager serves as a link with several services, monitors the client's progress, provides client education when necessary, reiterates treatment recommendations, and coordinates treatment planning with other providers. Community organizations are considered a valuable source of support for clients with a dual diagnosis (Faltz & Callahan, 2002).

EVALUATION

Evaluation of the client's progress is an ongoing process that can be challenging because of the potential for relapse or recidivism. Obtain information from the client, family, or significant others as well as providers of outpatient services. Evaluation focuses on compliance by the client, the stated outcomes, the effectiveness of interventions, and the progress the client is making. See Clinical Example 32-1: The Dually Diagnosed Client.

CLINICAL EXAMPLE 32.1

THE DUALLY DIAGNOSED CLIENT

PJ, a 53-year-old African American male resident of a local nursing home, was referred for a psychiatric evaluation because of behavioral changes that included spitting, scratching, and unpredictable combativeness. His past medical history included a stroke, hypertension, non–insulin-dependent diabetes, and chronic renal failure. Psychiatric history included the diagnoses of vascular dementia, schizophrenia (type unspecified), and polysubstance dependence, including cocaine.

PJ was recently transferred from a general hospital's medical–psychiatric unit following treatment for a dual diagnosis. The hospital history and physical examination indicated the presence of cocaine in his urine. His ECG was abnormal and the CT scan of the brain revealed small vessel disease and subcortical atrophy. His Annotated Mini-Mental Status Exam score was 10/30, indicative of severe dementia, the presence of delirium superimposed on vascular dementia during hospitalization, or the result of his refusal to cooperate during the assessment. He required haloperidol (Haldol) for hallucinations and lorazepam (Ativan) for agitation in the hospital. His past psychiatric treatment included inpatient treatment at a local community mental health center at least twice prior to his recent admission to the medical psychiatric unit.

Prior to the most recent hospitalization, PJ was unemployed and lived alone. Nursing staff and a social worker were unable to obtain any significant demographic or personal data due to PJ's refusal to speak to staff. He appeared to be selectively mute, as he would verbalize his needs but would not respond to personal questions.

PJ's present medications included an antihypertensive drug, aspirin for prevention of a stroke, and alprazolam (Xanax), if needed, for agitation. He was not receiving any antipsychotic medication.

During the attempt to interview PJ, he presented with a flat affect, avoidant eye contact but hypervigilance regarding his environment, and

(Continued on following page)

CLINICAL EXAMPLE 32.1 (continued)

appeared to be selectively mute. He became some-what restless and was easily distracted during the interview, but denied being afraid, suspicious, or unhappy. PJ was able to follow directions, but could not be engaged in any detailed conversation.

Following is a summary of the clinical impressions and recommendations that were listed in the client's medical record:

DSM-IV-TR Diagnoses	Vascular dementia secondary to small vessel disease and history of CVA
	Dementia secondary to history of polysubstance abuse noted in medical record
	Schizophrenia, type unknown, noted in medical record
	Rule out delirium secondary to recent hospitalization and use of cocaine.
Recommendations	Discontinue alprazolam (Xanax), which is a benzodiazepine, because client has a history of polysubstance abuse.
	Give risperidone (Risperdal) 0.5 mg every 12 hours for 10 days. May require dosage adjustment if clinical symptoms do not subside.
	Document behavior on all three shifts for 1 week to determine baseline symptoms and efficacy of risperidone.
	Reevaluate clinical symptoms in 1 week.
	Obtain records from local community mental health center.

KEY CONCEPTS

◆ The term dual diagnosis is used to designate mentally ill clients who show a comorbid substance-related disorder.

◆ Two main theories, referred to as models, discuss the etiology of dual diagnosis: vulnerability model and self-medication hypothesis.

◆ Clients with a dual diagnosis exhibit characteristics indicating that they are dissatisfied with life circumstances, have inadequate or ineffective support systems, live in a nontherapeutic home environment, and have a history of self-medication.

◆ Several barriers to treatment, such as counter-transference, misunderstandings and prejudice about mental illness behaviors and underlying health issues, have been identified.

◆ There are no *DSM-IV-TR* diagnostic criteria for dual diagnosis. However, four categories have been developed to describe the dually diagnosed client.

◆ Clients with a dual diagnosis are difficult to assess because they are not a homogenous group, often are poor historians, and often are noncompliant during the assessment process. Assessment involves identifying the relative contribution of each diagnosis to the severity of the current symptoms and prioritizing data accordingly.

◆ Differences in philosophies and approaches of treatment models for mental illness and substance-related disorders can affect how the nursing process is applied.

◆ Treatment is available in a variety of settings and is often determined by the severity of the client's symptoms and the ability to pay for services. Insurance coverage for inpatient treatment has become limited over the past several years.

◆ Flexible treatment programs meet the individual needs of each client. Phases of treatment for dually diagnosed clients include acute stabilization, engagement, prolonged stabilization, and rehabilitation and recovery, including continuum of care.

For additional study materials, please refer to the Student Resource CD-ROM located in the back of this textbook.

CHAPTER WORKSHEET

CRITICAL THINKING QUESTIONS

1. Review the barriers to treatment listed in Box 32-1. Describe several interventions that might be appropriate to lower the barriers and enable clients to enter treatment.

2. With the assistance of another classmate, develop a list of at least five topics to be discussed during an education group for dually diagnosed clients. Develop a teaching plan for two of the topics, and share the information with your classmates.

REFLECTION

Reflect on the opening chapter quote by Vaccaro. Explain your interpretation of the phrase "catastrophic life problem." What nursing challenges do you think you would encounter if you were to develop a nursing plan of care for such a client? Do you feel adequately prepared to provide care for such a client? Explain your answer.

NCLEX-STYLE QUESTIONS

1. A client with a history of marijuana abuse has recently been diagnosed with bipolar disorder. When reviewing client data to formulate the nursing plan of care, the nurse understands that the client with a substance-abuse history can subsequently develop a major mental illness. The nurse is incorporating which etiologic theory?
   a. Comorbidity model
   b. Behavioral model
   c. Self-medication model
   d. Vulnerability model

2. Which piece of nursing assessment data would the nurse be least likely to identify in a client with a dual diagnosis?
   a. Dissatisfaction with life circumstances
   b. Good life adjustment prior to diagnosis
   c. Inadequate support systems
   d. History of self-medication

3. Clients hospitalized on an inpatient unit have a dual diagnosis of alcohol dependence and another major mental illness. The staff nurse facilitates a client group discussion as part of the initial treatment plan. Nursing interventions in this group would focus on which of the following?
   a. Identifying signs and symptoms of relapse
   b. Teaching importance of diet and exercise
   c. Facilitating client recognition of problematic behaviors
   d. Planning work-related strategies to decrease stress

4. The nurse anticipates that the process of engaging the client with a dual diagnosis in a therapeutic nurse–client relationship may be difficult and requires which of the following?
   a. Ability of the nurse to provide sympathy for the client
   b. Assessment of the client's problems and symptoms
   c. Educational materials for teaching about substance abuse
   d. Strategies to handle client's problems with authority and control

5. The nurse plans interventions to prevent relapse for the client who has a dual diagnosis of a substance-abuse problem and major depressive disorder. Which of the following has priority?
   a. Identifying risk factors such as dangerous people or places to avoid
   b. Facilitating relationships with family who may be disengaged from the client
   c. Encouraging client to identify symptoms of the mental illness
   d. Teaching the purpose of antidepressant therapy as well as major adverse effects

6. A client with a dual diagnosis is entering the engagement phase of treatment. Which interventions would the nurse include in the plan of care? Select all that apply.
   a. Establishing a treatment relationship
   b. Educating the client about the illness
   c. Implementing measures to stabilize the client
   d. Using measures to help client overcome denial
   e. Providing detoxification for substance abuse
   f. Ensuring a safe environment

Selected References

Albanese, M. J. (2001). Assessing and treating comorbid mood and substance use disorders. *Psychiatric Times, 18*(4), 55–58.

American Psychiatric Association. (2000). *Diagnostic and statistical manual of mental disorders* (4th ed., Text Revision). Washington, DC: Author.

Baker, W. C. (2002). A triple threat: HIV, mental illness and chemical addiction. *ADVANCE for Nurse Practition-ers, 10*(9), 28–34.

Blinder, B. J., Blinder, M. C., & Sanathara, V. A. (1998). Eating disorders and addiction. Psychiatric Times, *15*(12), 30–33.

Dual diagnosis info sheet: Concepts and treatment issues. (2003). Retrieved September 4, 2003, from http://www.dlcas.com/course5.html

Faltz, B. G., & Callahan, P. (2002). Special care concerns for patients with dual disorders. In M. A. Boyd (Ed.), *Psychiatric nursing: Contemporary practice* (2nd ed., pp. 874–893). Philadelphia: Lippincott Williams & Wilkins.

Finkelstein, J. B. (1999a). Alcohol use in bipolar patients turns destructive. *Clinical Psychiatry News, 27*(8), 24.

Finkelstein, J. B. (1999b). Substance abusing ex-convicts: Continuity of care. *Clinical Psychiatry News, 27*(4), 11.

Kirn, T. F. (1999). Conduct disorder links ADHD, drug abuse. *Clinical Psychiatry News, 27*(5), 24.

Kosta, K. (2002). Dual diagnosis. *ADVANCE for Nurses, 3*(24), 13–12.

Krausz, M. (1996). Categories of dual diagnosis. In *Models of care for the treatment of drug misusers*. Retrieved September 3, 2003, from http://www.nta.nhs.uk/publications/mocpart2/chapter4_3.htm

Miller, N. (1994). Prevalence and treatment models for addiction in psychiatric populations. *Psychiatric Annals, 24,* 394–406.

Miller, N., Eriksen, A., & Owley, T. T. (1994). Psychosis and schizophrenia in alcohol and drug dependence. *Psychiatric Annals, 24,* 418–424.

Minkoff, K. (1994). Models of addiction treatment in psychiatric populations. *Psychiatric Annals, 24,* 413–418.

Minkoff, K. (2000, November). An integrated model for the management of co-occurring psychiatric and substance disorders in managed care systems. *Disease Management & Health Outcomes, 8*(5), 251–257.

National Alliance for the Mentally Ill. (2006). Dual diagnosis and integrated treatment of mental illness and substance abuse disorder. Retrieved March 26, 2006, from http://www.nami.org

National Mental Health Association. (2003). Substance abuse: Dual diagnosis. Retrieved July 4, 2003, from http://www.nmha.org/infoctr/factsheets/03.cfm

Osher, F. C., & Olfed, K. L. (1989). Treatment of patients with psychiatric and psychoactive substance abuse. *Hospital and Community Psychiatry, 40,* 1025–1030.

Raby, P., Doub, T. W., & Cartwright, M. (2003). *Techniques in an integrated residential service model.* Retrieved September 3, 2003, from http://www.dualdiagnosis.org

Schultz, J. M., & Videbeck, S. D. (2005). *Lippincott's manual of psychiatric nursing care plans* (7th ed.). Philadelphia: Lippincott Williams & Wilkins.

Sciacca, K. (1997). Removing barriers: Dual diagnosis and motivational interviewing. *Professional Counselor, 12*(1), 41–46.

Sciacca, K. (2003). Dual diagnosis: Glossary of terms. Retrieved July 4, 2003, from http://users.erols.com/ksciacca/ glossary.htm

Sherman, C. (2004). Substance abuse, schizophrenia often coexist. *Clinical Psychiatry News, 32*(6), 56.

Vaccaro, J. V. (1999). Integrated treatment of comorbid chemical dependency, psychiatric disorders. *Psychiatric Times, 16*(12), 48–50.

Youth Action and Policy Association NSW. (2003). Fact sheet: Take action now on dual diagnosis. Retrieved September 4, 2003, from http://www.yapa.org.au/facts/DualDiagnosis.pdf

Youth Action and Policy Association NSW. (2006). Take action on dual diagnosis. Retrieved March 13, 2006, from http://www.yapa.org.au

Zahourek, R. P. (1996). The client with dual diagnosis. In S. Lego (Ed.), *Psychiatric nursing: A comprehensive reference* (2nd ed., pp. 275–284). Philadelphia: Lippincott-Raven.

Zwillich, T. (1999). Clozapine may cut substance use in schizophrenics. *Clinical Psychiatry News, 27*(6), 1–2.

Suggested Readings

Becker, M. (2003). The mentally ill chemical abuser. *ADVANCE for Nurses, 4*(14), 13–15.

Carpenito-Moyet, L. J. (2006). *Handbook of nursing diagnosis* (11th ed). Philadelphia: Lippincott Williams & Wilkins.

Drake, R. E., Wallach, M. A., Alverson, H. S., & Mueser, K. T. (2002). Psychosocial aspects of substance abuse by clients with severe mental illness. *Journal of Nervous & Mental Disease, 190*(2), 100–106.

Goswami S., Mattoo S., Basu, D., & Singh, G. (2004). Substance-abusing schizophrenics: Do they self-medicate? *American Journal on Addictions, 13*(2), 139–50.

Laudet, A. B., Magura, S., Vogel, H. S., & Knight, E. L. (2000). Recovery challenges among dually diagnosed individuals. *Journal of Substance Abuse Treatment, 18*(4), 321–29

Laudet, A. B., Magura, S., Vogel, H. S., & Knight, E. L. (2003). Participation in 12-step-based fellowships among dually-diagnosed persons. *Alcoholism Treatment Quarterly, 21*(2), 19–40.

Rassool, G. H. (2002). Substance misuse and mental health: An overview. *Nursing Standard, 16*(50), 47–55.

Riggs, P. D. (2003). Treating adolescents for substance abuse and comorbid psychiatric disorders. *Science & Practice Perspectives, 2*(1), 18–28.

Todd, F. C., Sellman, J. D., & Robertson, P. J. (2002). Barriers to optimal care for patients with coexisting substance use and mental health disorders. *Australian and New Zealand Journal of Psychiatry, 36*(6), 792–799.

Please, Mom and Dad
My hands are small—I don't mean to spill my milk.
My legs are short—please slow down so I can keep up with you.
Don't slap my hands when I touch something bright and pretty—I don't understand.
Please look at me when I talk to you—it lets me know you are really listening.
My feelings are tender—don't nag me all day—let me make mistakes without feeling stupid.
Don't expect the bed I make or the picture I draw to be perfect—just love me for trying.
Remember I am a child not a small adult—sometimes I don't understand what you are saying.
I love you so much. Please love me just for being me—not just for the things I can do.
—J. RICHARDSON & J. RICHARDSON,
POSTER FUNDED BY HEALTH AND REHABILITATIVE SERVICES,
STATE OF FLORIDA

LEARNING OBJECTIVES

AFTER STUDYING THIS CHAPTER, YOU SHOULD BE ABLE TO:

1. Identify risk factors that create an environment in which the abuse of a child may occur.
2. Differentiate between child abuse and child neglect, and cite an example of each.
3. Recognize at least five common physical findings indicating physical abuse of a child.
4. Explain at least four causative factors related to domestic violence.
5. Discuss the dynamics of intimate partner or spousal abuse.
6. Differentiate among sexual harassment, sexual assault, rape, and statutory rape.
7. Articulate the dynamics of rape-trauma syndrome.
8. Explain ways in which elderly persons are abused.
9. Construct a profile of an individual who may become violent in the work setting.
10. Describe the emotional and behavioral reactions of the following victims of physical abuse or domestic violence: children, women, men, and the elderly.
11. Develop an assessment tool for the following clients: a victim of child abuse, an elderly victim of domestic violence, and a teen-aged victim of rape.

KEY TERMS

Abduction
Abuse
Attempted rape
Child abuse
Discipline
Domestic violence
Emotional abuse
Emotional neglect
Family violence
Hate crime
Incest
Intimate partner violence
Munchausen's syndrome by proxy
Neglect
Rape
Rape-trauma syndrome
Sexual abuse
Sexual coercion

Sexual harassment	Silent rape syndrome	Statutory rape
Sexual misuse of a child	Sodomy	Violence
Shaken baby syndrome	Stalking	Workplace violence

Much has been written and a great deal of public concern has been expressed about the physical or sexual abuse of children, women, and the elderly. In addition, youth and workplace violence, as well as hate crimes, have been recognized as serious and widespread public health problems affecting individuals of all ethnic and socioeconomic backgrounds. Consider the following stories recently covered by the news media:

- High school teacher accused of child abuse and pornography
- Young minister killed by wife
- KKK demonstration spurs riot
- Estranged husband suspected of murder of wife, three children, and mother-in-law
- Lacrosse players accused of gang rape of exotic dancer
- Friends of 81-year-old female illegally withdrew $30,000 from her bank account
- Angry postal worker kills fellow employees in mailroom
- Abduction of 14-year-old female recorded on surveillance camera
- Youth kills six and commits suicide at Minnesota house party

Although epidemiologic studies have shown that aggressive or abusive behavior may occur in adults with the diagnosis of schizophrenia, affective disorder, posttraumatic stress disorder, and personality disorders, recent research has shown that the vast majority of people who are abusive or who commit violent acts do not suffer from mental illness. A certain small subgroup of people, such as clients with neurologic impairment due to head injury; a disease such as Huntington's chorea; or a psychotic disorder are at risk of becoming abusive or violent (eg, threatening, hitting, fighting, or otherwise hurting another person). However, the conditions likely to increase the risk of violence are the same whether a person has a mental illness or not (American Psychiatric Association [APA], 2003).

This chapter discusses the etiology of abuse and violence. General topics include child abuse, domestic violence or intimate partner violence, adult sexual abuse, elder abuse, youth violence, workplace violence, and hate crimes. Although the focus of domestic violence and sexual abuse is primarily on women, information about male victims is incorporated when appropriate. The chapter concludes with an application of the nursing process to victims of abuse and violence.

Abuse

The term **abuse** is used in psychiatric–mental health nursing to describe behaviors in which an individual misuses, attacks, or injures another individual. Abuse may be sexual, physical, or emotional. Neglect is also a form of abuse. The term **violence** is used to describe behaviors in which an individual displays an intensive destructive or uncontrolled force to injure a person (Sadock & Sadock, 2003; Shahrokh & Hales, 2003). Examples of abuse and violence were cited in the introduction to this chapter.

Elements of Abuse

Three elements generally create the environment for an incident of abuse to occur: the abuser or perpetrator, the abused, and a crisis.

The Abuser

A profile of abusive individuals has been described by several agencies such as the National Coalition Against Domestic Violence (NCADV) and the National Center for Injury Prevention and Control (NCIPC). The abuser, or perpetrator, is usually an individual who grew up in an abusive family. Research findings indicate that children who observed or were victims of beatings and violence when young believe that abuse is normal behavior and will reenact these behaviors later as adults.

Statistically, abusive individuals usually are young and live in lower socioeconomic environments; however, those individuals who live in higher classes are not immune. Perpetrators of intimate partner abuse or domestic violence are generally male, whereas perpetrators of child abuse are generally female. Both male and female perpetrators abuse the elderly. Common characteristics of abusive individuals include low self-concept, immaturity, fear of authority, lack of skills to meet their own emotional needs, belief in harsh physical discipline, and poor impulse control. Abusers lack parenting or relationship skills and often use alcohol or other substances to cope with stress. In the event of child or elder abuse, the partner, who usually knows about the abuse, either ignores it or may even participate in it (NCADV, 2003; NCIPC, 2006a.)

The Abused

Abused individuals often demonstrate a pattern of learned helplessness, manifest characteristics of low-self esteem and shame, and often experience feelings of increased dependence, isolation, guilt, and entrapment (NCADV, 2003; Quillian, 1995).

A Crisis

A crisis (eg, loss of job, divorce, illness, death in the family) is usually the precipitating event that sets the abusive person into action. The individual overreacts because he or she is unable to cope with numerous or complex stressors. The person becomes frustrated and anxious and suddenly loses control. (Chapter 13 discusses crisis intervention.)

Child Abuse

The Child Abuse Prevention and Treatment Act (CAPTA), enacted in 1974, and reauthorized in 1996, provides federal funding to states to prevent, identify, and treat the abuse and neglect of children and adolescents. **Child abuse**, also referred to as *maltreatment*, is described as any recent act or failure to act, resulting in imminent risk of serious physical harm or death, emotional harm, sexual abuse, neglect, or exploitation of a child under the age of 18 years by a parent, caretaker, or other person (CAPTA, 2003). Bullying is the most common form of abuse children and adolescents experi-

ence. It is estimated that 160,000 students in American schools are absent every day because of fear of being bullied either physically or verbally (Voors, 2004). Child abuse is not to be confused with **discipline.** Discipline is a purposeful action to restrain or correct a child's behavior. It is done to teach, not to punish, and it is not designed to hurt the child or result in injury. **Neglect** is an act of omission and refers to a parent's or other person's failure to meet a dependent's basic needs such as proper food, clothing, shelter, medical care, schooling, or attention; provide safe living conditions; provide physical or emotional care; or provide supervision, thus leaving the child unattended or abandoning him or her.

Children are also victims of intimate partner or family violence (eg, one parent kills the other), school violence (eg, a child brings a gun to school and kills a teacher), or public violence (eg, the terrorist attack on the World Trade Center and Pentagon on September 11, 2001).

The World Health Organization, Regional Office for Africa (WHO/AFRO) estimates that 40 million children younger than 15 years fall victim to various forms of child abuse and violence each year. The WHO subcategorizes child abuse into physical abuse, physical neglect or abandonment, emotional abuse, and sexual abuse including commercial or other forms of exploitation that cause actual or potential harm to the child's health, survival, development, or dignity (WHO/AFRO, 2002).

According to the NCIPC, an estimated 906,000 children in the United States experienced or were at risk for child abuse or violence in the year 2002, compared with 879,000 children in the year 2000. Of the 906,000 children:

- 61% experienced neglect
- 19% were physically abused
- 10% were sexually abused
- 5% were emotionally or psychologically abused.

Statistics provided by the NCIPC confirm that 1,500 children died from maltreatment: 36% from neglect, 28% from physical abuse, and 29% from multiple maltreatment types. In 2003, children younger than 4 years accounted for 79% of child maltreatment fatalities.

Etiology of Child Abuse

The etiology associated with child abuse is complex. Child abuse can occur mainly within the family, where the abusers are parents or parent substitutes; in the institutional setting, such as daycare centers, child-care agencies, schools, welfare departments, correctional settings, and residential centers; in society, which allows children to live in poverty or to be denied the basic necessities of life; or as a result of war. In times of war, children are exposed to various forms of abuse and violence. They may experience traumas that can interrupt their development, trigger serious psychiatric disorders, or predispose them to delinquency and life-long crime (WHO/AFRO, 2002).

Anyone can abuse or neglect a child under certain circumstances, such as stress due to illness, marital problems, financial difficulties, or parent–child conflict. Parents or other persons may lose control of their feelings of anger or frustration and direct such feelings toward a child.

Characteristics of Potentially Abusive Parents

No physical characteristics automatically identify the potential child abuser. The person may be rich or poor, of any racial origin, male (40.7%) or female (59.3%), and living in a rural area, a suburb, or a city.

Parents who are potentially abusive often display characteristic warning signs. However, evidence of these signs does not automatically imply that abuse will inevitably occur. Box 33-1 highlights some of the typical warning signs. Such characteristics displayed

---

BOX 33.1 PROFILE OF POTENTIALLY ABUSIVE PARENTS

- Denial of pregnancy by a mother who has made no plans for the birth of the child and refuses to talk about the pregnancy
- Depression during pregnancy
- Fear of delivery
- Lack of support from husband or family
- Undue concern about the unborn child's gender and how well it will perform
- Fear that the child will be one of too many children
- Birth of an unwanted child
- Indifference or a negative attitude toward the child by the parent after delivery
- Resentment toward the child by a jealous parent
- Inability to tolerate the child's crying; viewing child as being too demanding

---

for a short time may indicate anxiety in a new mother or father. However, if the characteristics persist, the parent should seek help.

Characteristics of an Abused Child

The abused or neglected child is usually younger than 6 years, is more vulnerable to abuse than others, and may have a physical or mental handicap. Emotionally disturbed, temperamental, hyperactive, or adopted children also demonstrate a higher incidence of abuse. Children with congenital anomalies or chronic medical conditions are also at risk for abuse because of the demands of care placed on the parents or caretakers. The child, in an attempt to get attention, unintentionally may irritate the parent, leading to a loss of control in the parent and possible reactions with abuse.

Classifications of Child Abuse

Abuse of children usually is classified as physical abuse; child neglect; emotional abuse or neglect; and sexual abuse.

Physical Abuse of a Child

Physical abuse of a child involves the infliction of bodily injury that results from punching, beating, kicking, biting, burning, shaking, or otherwise harming a child. Indicators of actual or potential physical abuse have been categorized as physical, behavioral, and environmental, briefly discussed in the following sections (Figure 33-1).

Physical Indicators. The most common indicators of physical abuse of a child are bruises involving no breaks in skin integrity. The bruises are usually seen on the posterior side of the body or on the face, in unusual patterns or clusters, and in various stages of healing, making it difficult to determine the exact age of a bruise. Burns also are seen frequently, and usually are due to immersion in hot water, contact with cigarettes, tying with a rope, or the application of a hot iron. Common burned areas include the buttocks, palms of hands, soles of feet, wrists, ankles, or genitals. Lacerations, abrasions, welts, and scars may be noted on the lips, eyes, face, and external genitalia.

Other indicators of physical abuse include missing or loosened teeth; skeletal injuries such as fractured bones, epiphyseal separation, or stiff, swollen, enlarged

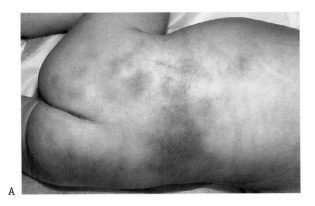

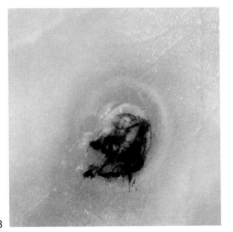

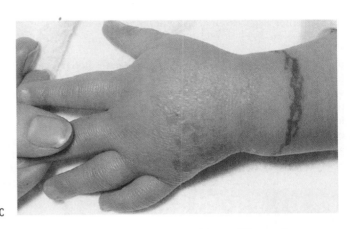

FIGURE 33.1 Examples of child abuse: (**A**) bruising on a child's body, (**B**) cigarette burns, (**C**) rope burn. (Source: Pillitteri, A. [2003]. *Maternal and child health nursing* [4th ed.]. Philadelphia: Lippincott Williams & Wilkins.)

joints; head injuries; and internal injuries. Such bodily injuries must be evaluated with respect to the child's medical history, developmental ability to injure self, and behavioral indicators (which are discussed later in this chapter).

Munchausen's Syndrome by Proxy. **Munchausen's syndrome by proxy** is now a well-known phenomenon in which the biologic mother (90%), the biologic father (5%), or a female caregiver (5%) systematically fabricates—or deliberately causes—illness or injury in the child in order to gain sympathy or attention for themselves (Thomas, 2003). The perpetrators have well-developed plans and act with malevolent intent to satisfy

craving for medical attention and psychological gain. Forms of fabricated or caused illnesses include poisonings, seizures, apparent bleeding from a variety of orifices, skin rashes, and pyrexia (Quisenberry, 2006; Skuse & Bentovim, 1994). Usually, the child is brought in for frequent and persistent medical examinations. However, when the child is separated from the parent, acute symptoms and the signs of illness cease. The perpetrator denies having any knowledge of the cause of the disorder. Comorbidity is a major problem because it is highly likely that the child will have more than one fabricated illness. Failure to thrive and nonaccidental injuries are also commonly noted. Approximately 21.8 months lapse from symptom presentation to definitive diagnosis. This allows ample time for substantial morbidity to occur while unnecessary tests and surgical procedures take place. The average age of death is at 18.8 months (Quisenberry, 2006; Sheridan, 2003).

Shaken Baby Syndrome. **Shaken baby syndrome** is a form of child abuse affecting between 1,200 and 1,600 children every year and is the leading cause of brain injury to infants (NCIPC, 2006a). It occurs when an adult loses control and violently shakes a child who has been crying incessantly. This syndrome has been documented in children up to 5 years of age. An estimated 20% to 25% of infant victims die from their injuries. The physical findings usually include bruising from being grabbed firmly, and major head injury such as subdural hematoma or cerebral edema. Nonfatal consequences include blindness due to retinal hemorrhage, cerebral palsy, and cognitive impairment (Brasseur, 1995; NCIPC, 2001).

Behavioral and Environmental Indicators. Behavioral indicators of physical abuse depend on the age at which the child is abused, as well as the frequency and the severity of abuse. The behavioral profile of a physically abused child is presented in Box 33-2. If a child exhibits such behaviors, observation for bodily injuries is crucial.

BOX 33.2 **BEHAVIORAL PROFILE OF A PHYSICALLY ABUSED CHILD**

- Fear of parents and fear of physical contact with adults
- Extremes in behavior such as passivity or aggressiveness, or crying very often or very seldom
- Sudden onset of regressive behavior such as thumb sucking, enuresis, or encopresis
- Learning problems that cannot be diagnosed
- Truancy from school or tardiness
- Fatigue causing the child to sleep in class
- Inappropriate dress to hide burns, bruises, or other marks of abuse
- Inappropriate dress, resulting in frostbite or illness due to exposure to inclement weather
- Excessive compliance to avoid confrontation
- Sporadic temper tantrums
- Violence toward other children or animals
- Demanding behavior

CLINICAL EXAMPLE 33.1

THE PHYSICALLY ABUSED CHILD

KW, the 22-year-old boyfriend of JN, was accused of beating JN's 5-year-old daughter severely enough to cause permanent brain damage. The child was beaten with a stick and forced to drink dishwashing liquid because she was "too sassy." After the beating, the child was kept on the floor of the apartment because she appeared to be unconscious at times. JN force-fed her daughter oatmeal and bananas in an effort to revive her. Two days later, the child was taken to the hospital and was found to have burn marks on her buttocks, a head injury, and bruises on her body. JN was charged with child abuse, and KW was sentenced to 15 years in prison for aggravated child abuse.

Environmental indicators of potential physical abuse in children include severe parental or caretaker problems such as drug addiction, alcoholism, and mental illness; crisis; and geographic or social isolation of the family. See Clinical Example 33-1: The Physically Abused Child.

Child Neglect

Child neglect is the failure to provide for a child's basic physical, medical, or educational needs. Examples of child neglect include withholding shelter, adequate nutrition, adequate clothing, access to education, and proper medical or dental care. Abandonment of a child or lack of adequate supervision also constitutes neglect. However, financial status, cultural values, and parental capacity must be considered before a parent or adult is accused of neglecting a child.

Physical Indicators. Potential physical indicators of child neglect may include weight loss resulting from inadequate nutrition, dental caries caused by lack of appropriate nutrition or dental care, or symptoms of an undiagnosed medical condition such as anemia or pneumonia. The child may also look unkempt and lack adequate clothing (eg, no shoes or adequate clothing for seasonal weather changes).

Behavioral and Environmental Indicators. Behavioral indicators of child neglect commonly seen include failure to thrive; learning difficulties caused by poor attention span, inability to concentrate, or autistic behavior; use of drugs or alcohol; delinquency; and sexual misconduct. Environmental indicators of child neglect by parents or caretakers include living in poverty; the presence of a large family with marital conflict; lack of material resources; or the lack of positive parental attitudes. Parents or caretakers may lack an adequate understanding of the developmental stages of childhood; fail to recognize physical or emotional needs of children; display a lack of interest in childhood activities; display poor parenting skills; or exhibit a lack of interest in personal hygiene. See Clinical Example 33-2: The Neglected Child.

Emotional Abuse or Neglect

Emotional abuse consists of verbal assaults or threats that provoke fear; poor communication that may send double messages; and blaming, confusing, or demeaning messages. Parents or caretakers who emotionally abuse children may tell the child that she or he is unwanted, unloved, or unworthy of care. The child may become the scapegoat of the family (ie, accused of causing family problems).

Conversely, **emotional neglect,** considered to be a form of child neglect discussed earlier, occurs when parents or other adults responsible for the child fail to provide an emotional climate that fosters feelings of love, belonging, recognition, and enhanced self-esteem. Examples of emotional neglect include ignoring the child, providing minimal human contact, and failing to provide opportunities to foster growth and development. Children who are emotionally abused or neglected may develop serious behavioral, cognitive, emotional, or mental disorders.

Behavioral and Environmental Indicators. The emotionally abused or neglected child often develops a low self-concept as he or she hears negative comments such as "If it weren't for your bad habits, Daddy wouldn't leave us!," "It's all your fault we don't have enough money. You're sick all the time," and "The family got along fine until you started to act so selfish." Behavioral indicators of an emotionally abused or neglected child are listed in Box 33-3.

Examples of environmental indicators of emotional abuse or neglect of a child include inadequate parenting skills; rejection or immature behavior by parents or caretakers; continuous friction or conflict in the home; discriminatory treatment of the children in the family; and abuse of drugs or alcohol by the parents or caretaker.

Child Sexual Abuse

Sexual abuse of a child includes fondling of a child's genitals, intercourse, incest, rape, sodomy, exhibitionism, and commercial exploitation through prostitution or the production of pornographic materials. Child

---

CLINICAL EXAMPLE 33.2

THE NEGLECTED CHILD

FR, a young, single working mother, entrusted the care of her 1- and 2-year-old children to her 8-year old daughter while she worked as a waitress from approximately 7:00 PM to midnight. Before she left for work each evening, FR locked the younger children in their bedrooms and instructed the older daughter to stay indoors and "keep an eye on the children." One evening, a fire began on the second floor of the apartment, killing the two younger children by smoke inhalation. The 8-year-old was able to escape the fire. FR told the authorities she made minimum wage and was unable to afford to pay a babysitter, so she worked at night while her older daughter was home.

BOX 33.3 **BEHAVIORAL INDICATORS OF AN EMOTIONALLY ABUSED OR NEGLECTED CHILD**

- Stuttering
- Enuresis or encopresis
- Delinquency, truancy, or other disciplinary problems
- Hypochondriasis
- Autism or failure to thrive
- Overeating
- Childhood depression
- Suicide attempts

sexual abuse is four times higher among female than male victims (NCIPC, 2002).

According to a 2001 study funded in part by the U.S. Department of Justice, titled "The Commercial Exploitation of Children in the U.S., Canada, and Mexico," approximately 300,000 to 400,000 U.S. children are victims of some type of sexual exploitation, particularly commercial sexual exploitation, every year (CNN.com, 2001). Sexual abuse has serious direct consequences such as emotional distress, behavioral problems, sexually transmitted diseases (STDs), unwanted pregnancies, and indirect consequences such as the development of a substance-use disorder, mood disorder, sexual deviance, or difficulty in establishing a satisfying intimate relationship later in life. Sexual abuse of a child is not easy to identify because the physical signs of abuse usually are not seen outside a clinical or medical setting. The child victim is usually reluctant to share information about the abuse because the child fears she or he may alienate or anger the person who provides food, shelter, and a family bond.

Children at high risk for sexual abuse include those who:

- Are 3 years of age or younger
- Suffer from a developmental delay
- Live in a home where substance abuse occurs
- Have adolescent parents or a single parent
- Are in foster care
- Have primary caretakers who were sexually abused themselves
- Have primary caretakers who are mentally ill or who have a developmental delay

Classifications of Child Sexual Abuse. Episodes of childhood sexual abuse are classified as acute, subacute, or nonacute. *Acute* episodes include cases of sexual abuse that have occurred within the previous 72 hours of examination by a clinician. Evidence of moderate-to-severe injury, such as vaginal bleeding or genital lacerations, may be present. *Subacute* episodes involve sexual abuse cases that have occurred more than 72 hours before an examination by a clinician. Symptoms such as minor abrasions or dysuria may be present. *Nonacute* episodes also involve sexual abuse cases that occur more than 72 hours before a clinician's examination; however, there are no significant injuries or symptoms.

Box 33-4 lists physical and behavioral indicators of a sexually abused child. Clinical Example 33-3 describes a case of sexual abuse by a father.

BOX 33.4 INDICATORS OF A SEXUALLY ABUSED CHILD

PHYSICAL INDICATORS

- Itching, pain, bruises, or bleeding in the external genitalia, vagina, or anal area
- Edema of the cervix, vulva, or perineum
- Torn, stained, or bloody undergarments
- Stretched hymen at a very young age
- Presence of semen or a sexually transmitted disease
- Pregnancy in an older child
- Bladder infections

BEHAVIORAL INDICATORS

- Fear of being touched
- Difficulty walking or sitting
- Reluctance to participate in recreational or physical activities
- Poor peer relationships
- Delinquency, truancy, acting-out, or running away
- Preoccupation with sexual organs of self or others (in younger children)
- Sexual promiscuity or prostitution (in older children)
- Change in sleeping patterns; nightmares; or sudden fear of falling asleep
- Bed-wetting or thumb-sucking (inappropriate to age)
- Use of drugs and alcohol

Terminology of Child Sexual Abuse. Three terms are frequently used to describe the sexual abuse of children: sexual misuse, rape, and incest. **Sexual misuse of a child** is defined as sexual activity that is inappropriate because of the child's age, development, and role within the family unit. Examples include fondling, genital manipulation, voyeurism, or exhibitionism.

Rape refers to actual penetration of an orifice of a child's body during sexual activity. Oral penetration is the most frequent type of penetration experienced by very young children.

Incest, defined as sexual intercourse or sexual behaviors that occur between family members who are so closely related as to be legally prohibited from marrying one another because of consanguinity (ie, they share the same ancestry and are referred to as "blood relatives"), is usually a well-guarded secret.

THE SEXUALLY ABUSED CHILD

CB, a 6-year-old girl, daughter of a well-liked and respected member of the community, was forced by her father to have oral sex with him when her mother was away at club meetings. The sexual encounters lasted a few months and had a profound effect on CB, whose parents divorced when she was 14. She loved her father but also hated him and swore that she would never tell anyone about the incest. A few years after CB married, her deteriorating sexual relationship with her husband prompted her to admit the incest and to seek therapy.

Approximately 100,000 cases of incest occur each year, but fewer than 25% are reported, according to statistics provided in the year 2000 by the American Academy of Child and Adolescent Psychiatry and the National Center on Child Abuse and Neglect. Victims of incest are usually very young. The average age of an incest victim is 11 years, although most child victims experience their first incestuous encounter between the ages of 5 and 8 years.

Child Abduction

Abduction or kidnapping occurs whenever a person is taken or detained against his or her will. Statistics reported by the Department of Justice in 2002 indicate that every 40 seconds in the United States, a child is reported missing or abducted. That statistic translates to more than 2,000 missing children per day or 800,000 per year. Approximately 69,000 of the missing children are abducted (KidsFightingChance.com, 2006).

Approximately 82% of abductions are committed by family (primarily parents), occur more frequently to children under the age of 6 years, equally victimize children and adolescents of both sexes, and most often originate in the home. Non-family or acquaintance abduction accounts for 18% of reported cases, has the largest percentage of female and teen-aged victims, is more often associated with crimes such as sexual and physical assault, occurs at homes and residences, and has the highest percentage of injured victims. Stranger kidnapping accounts for 37% of non-family abductions, occurs primarily in outdoor locations, victimizes more female than male children and adolescents, is often associated with sexual assaults and robberies, and generally involves the use of a firearm (KidsFightingChance.com, 2006; Klass Kids Foundation, 2006).

Domestic or Intimate Partner Violence

Domestic violence, also referred to at times as **intimate partner violence** or **family violence,** is a public health problem of epidemic proportions that crosses racial/ethnic boundaries and socioeconomic strata. It is designed to manipulate, control, and dominate the partner to achieve compliance and dependence. Domestic violence may include repeated battering and injury, psychological abuse, sexual assault, progressive social isolation, stalking, deprivation, and intimidation. Someone (ie, spouse, ex-spouse, or significant other) who is or was involved in an intimate relationship with the victim perpetrates these behaviors.

Groups at Risk

Although 95% of domestic violence is directed at women who are emotionally involved with the batterer, children, the elderly, men, and same-sex couples are also at risk. As noted earlier, children who are raised in homes where domestic violence occurs are often victims. They are referred to as "silent victims" who are at risk for abuse and the development of emotional or behavioral problems later in life. Domestic violence between elder partners may manifest as a long-standing pattern of marital violence or originate as the result of stress that accompanies disability and changing family relationships. Studies demonstrate that when men are victims of domestic violence, women usually act out of self-defense, or the defense of their children. Statistics also indicate that domestic violence exists in same sex couples. Women living with female intimate partners experience less domestic violence than women living with men; however, men living with male intimate partners experience more domestic violence than do men who live with female intimate partners (Makar, 2000; Allen, 2006). Figure 33-2 depicts the annual national morbidity rate associated with domestic violence.

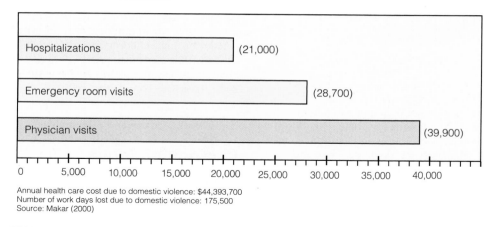

Annual health care cost due to domestic violence: $44,393,700
Number of work days lost due to domestic violence: 175,500
Source: Makar (2000)

FIGURE 33.2 Annual national domestic violence morbidity rates reported by The National Crime Survey.

Epidemiology

Domestic violence is the single greatest cause of injury to women. Although exact numbers of domestic violence incidents differ because this is such an underreported crime and a relatively new area of study, experts do agree on some statistics. The following statistics on domestic violence were compiled from the Journal of the American Medical Association, U.S. Department of Health and Human Services, Federal Bureau of Investigation (FBI), Medical College of Pennsylvania, and NCICP (NCIPC, 2006b; Women Against Abuse, 2003).

- Nearly 5.3 million women and 3.2 million men are victims of domestic violence each year.
- Approximately 1.5 million women and more than 800,000 men are raped or physically assaulted by an intimate partner.
- 20% of all emergency room visits by women are the result of domestic violence.
- 75% of women victims of domestic violence suffer additional injuries within a year.
- Every 15 seconds, a woman in this country is beaten by her current or former husband or intimate partner.
- In 2002, 76% of intimate partner homicide victims were female and 24% were male.
- Approximately 33% of all women with children in homeless shelters cite domestic violence as the primary cause of their homelessness.

- One of three teenagers reports having experienced violence in a dating relationship.
- The rate of domestic violence in gay and lesbian communities is approximately 25%.

Supporting Evidence for Practice 33-1 highlights a study addressing the need for identifying potential victims of domestic violence.

Factors Contributing to Domestic Violence

Physical abuse during domestic violence involves a willful, nonaccidental attempt to injure a person by way of a direct, overtly aggressive attack. Examples of abuse during domestic violence include throwing objects at one's husband, threatening to injure one's wife, or physically beating a significant other. Men usually push, shove, grab, slap, hit repeatedly, torture, or threaten with a lethal object. Women hit or throw objects, use fists, kick, bite, or scratch.

Various disciplines describe factors that contribute to domestic violence toward partners, children, and elderly parents. Box 33-5 lists these identified factors.

Profiles of the Abuser and the Abused

Although perpetrators of domestic violence can be male or female, most studies focus on the male as the

SUPPORTING EVIDENCE FOR PRACTICE 33.1
Identification of Potential Victims of Domestic Violence in the Primary Care Setting

PROBLEM UNDER INVESTIGATION / What attitudes, beliefs, and practices regarding domestic violence do primary health care providers exhibit?

SUMMARY OF THE RESEARCH / The sample consisted of 206 subjects including 33 medical students, 25 licensed practical nurses, 58 registered nurses, 6 nurse practitioners, 13 physician assistants, and 71 physicians recruited from five different primary care practices. Most of the participants were women (70%) and had been in health care for more than 10 years (72%). A self-administered questionnaire was administered and responses were grouped according to the type of clinician (eg, RN, NP, LPN). Results indicated that 10% of the sample had never identified a victim and 55% had never identified a batterer; 50% of the clinicians and 70% of the assistants believed domestic violence was rare or very rare in their practice; and 45.2% seldom or never asked about anxiety, depression, or chronic pelvic pain when evaluating an injured client. One fourth of the clinicians and approximately 50% of the

assistants reported that they did not feel confident in asking about domestic violence. Few (23%) felt that they had strategies to aid victims or felt comfortable referring victims (16.2% assistants, 37.1% clinicians) or batterers (14.6% assistants, 22.4% clinicians).

SUPPORT FOR PRACTICE / The identification, treatment, and referral of persons experiencing domestic violence is a priority for psychiatric–mental health nurses in any clinical setting. Furthermore, the nurse needs to develop techniques for effective management of the identified battered and batterer. Therefore, educational programs may be necessary to help nurses feel better equipped to identify potential victims and be more comfortable in asking about domestic violence. This study can serve as a guide as to the specific content that should be included in educational programs.

SOURCE: Sugg, N. K., Thompson, R. S., Thompson, D. C., Maiuro, R., & Rivars, R. P. (1999, Jul/Aug). Domestic violence and primary care: Attitudes, practices, and beliefs. Archives of Family Medicine, 8, 301-306.

abuser and the female as the abused. Professional staff who have worked with and studied men who physically abuse others have developed a profile of male abusers. Male abusers usually have low self-esteem, believing that a man should be the head of the household and have the final say in family decisions. Because of their insecurities and fears, batterers experience extreme jealousy. Because they grew up in violent homes, they have not developed positive ways to communicate feelings and needs, or the ability to compromise. They use force or violence to solve problems, typically blaming everyone and everything but themselves for their actions. Because batterers do not want to face the seriousness of their behavior and its consequences, denial is a common defense mechanism.

The profile of an abused client (either male or female) includes a history of being raised in insecure living conditions, experience of abuse as a child, and getting married as a teenager. Abused women often exhibit a pattern of learned helplessness as well as characteristics of low self-esteem and shame. They may

hold religious or cultural beliefs about the traditional gender roles of men and women.

Forms of Domestic Violence

Domestic violence takes many forms. In the Duluth, Minnesota, Minnesota Domestic Abuse Intervention Project, a power and control wheel was developed to serve as a teaching model for counseling groups of men who physically and emotionally abused their spouses or partners. Eight forms of abusive behavior were identified and described by women who lived with men who batter. These forms of behavior illustrate that domestic violence is part of a pattern of behavior, rather than isolated incidents of abuse or cyclical pent-up anger, frustration, or painful feelings experienced by the batterer (Medical Education Group Learning Systems, 1995). The behaviors of domestic violence include:

- Intimidation (eg, using looks, action, or gestures to instill fear in the victim)

BOX 33.5 FACTORS CONTRIBUTING TO DOMESTIC VIOLENCE

- Individuals with neurologic impairments, agitated depression, antisocial or borderline behavior, or who abuse drugs and alcohol are often unable to control impulsive behavior due to increased frustration or anxiety. They are prone to committing acts of domestic violence when they are under the influence of substances.
- Lack of nurturing and mothering during childhood results in the inability to nurture others as an adult.
- Poor socioeconomic conditions resulting in increased stress, anxiety, or frustration may precipitate domestic violence within the family.
- Poor communication skills may result in the use of verbal or physical abuse.
- Specific behaviors learned during various developmental stages become part of a person's interactions with spouse and family. For example, a child who lives in an environment in which spousal or parental abuse occurs probably will believe that domestic violence is normal unless intervention occurs to prohibit such behavior.
- Domestic violence may increase after the death of a significant family member, the loss of a job, a geographic move, the onset of physical or mental illness, a developmental change, or a family change such as pregnancy or the birth of a child.

- Threats (eg, threatening to do something harmful to the children, a pet, or self)
- Sexual abuse (eg, forcing unwanted sexual activity on the victim)
- Isolation (eg, controlling the victim's contacts and activities)
- Emotional abuse (eg, using put-downs or attacking the abused victim's self-confidence)
- Use of children (eg, using custody/visitation rights as a way to control or harass the victim)
- Male privilege (eg, expecting to be waited on by the victim)
- Economic abuse (eg, refusing to share money with or provide financial support for the victim)

Dynamics of Domestic Violence

Three phases of domestic violence are described: the tension-building phase, the acute battering phase, and the loving phase. Domestic violence usually occurs as a result of the inability to cope with an increase in daily stressors.

Tension-Building Phase

During the tension-building phase, disagreements may occur within a couple as the battered person withdraws rather than making any attempts to display anger verbally or nonverbally. The batterer becomes possessive, jealous, and fearful, sensing the battered partner's anger. As a result, emotional distancing occurs. The batterer rationalizes the battered partner's nonassertiveness as acceptance and permission to vent tensions. Minor physically abusive incidents may cause the battered person to cope with abuse by somatizing, whereas the batterer attempts to reduce tension by taking drugs or drinking alcohol, further decreasing inhibitions and precipitating abusive episodes.

Acute Battering Phase

During the acute battering phase, the batterer loses control of behavior because of blind rage. The battered person also loses control and is unable to stop the physical abusiveness experienced. Both persons are in a state of shock immediately after the incident. The batterer is unable to recall his or her behavior; the battered person depersonalizes during the abusive incident and is unable to recall in detail what occurred.

Loving Phase

As both calm down, the batterer may exhibit feelings of remorse, beg forgiveness, promise not to abuse in the future, and state that he or she cannot live without the battered partner. During this loving phase, the abused person believes the batterer's promises and forgives the batterer because the battered partner then feels less helpless. The batterer interprets such behavior as an act of love and acceptance by the battered partner.

Barriers to Leaving a Violent Relationship

According to the NCADV (2003), the reasons why women stay in a violent relationship fall into three major categories. They include lack of resources, lack of institutional responses, and traditional ideology.

Lack of Resources

Most victims of domestic violence have at least one dependent child and do not have the financial resources (eg, unemployed, lack access to cash or bank accounts) to maintain adequate living standards for themselves and their dependent children. If they leave home, women fear being charged with desertion, losing custody of their children, and losing any joint assets they may have with their spouse.

Lack of Institutional Responses

Many victims of domestic violence report negative experiences with the police and their clergy. Police often treat domestic violence as a domestic dispute instead of a crime and try to dissuade women from filing charges. Restraining orders rarely prevent a released abuser from returning and repeating an assault. Prosecutors are often reluctant to prosecute cases. Clergy and secular counselors usually focus on saving the marriage rather than the goal of stopping the violence.

Traditional Ideology

The victim may not believe that divorce is a viable option because her children need their father and a single-parent family is unacceptable. She may blame her husband's behavior on stress, problems at work, or other factors. She may not take assertive action to stop the abuse because she believes her husband will change; is afraid of more violence; lacks self-confidence; feels guilty, ashamed, embarrassed, helpless, or powerless; or rationalizes that life is "not so bad." See Clinical Example 33-4: Family Violence.

Adult Sexual Abuse

According to the American Medical Association (AMA, 2003), **sexual abuse** (also referred to as *sexual assault*) of both men and women continues to escalate at a dramatic rate, claiming a victim every 45 seconds. Because many of the sexual assaults go unreported and unrecognized, sexual abuse can be considered a "silent-violent epidemic" in the United States today. Terminology used to discuss sexual abuse of the adult includes sexual harassment, stalking, sexual coercion, and rape.

Sexual Harassment, Stalking, and Sexual Coercion

Sexual harassment is defined as any unwelcome sexual advance or conduct on the job that creates an intimidating or offensive working environment. **Stalking** is defined as a pattern of unwanted communication, such

---

CLINICAL EXAMPLE 33.4

FAMILY VIOLENCE

JW, a 43-year-old investment banker, was beaten, bruised, and afraid. She stood in her bedroom pointing a pistol at her angry, abusive husband. Both her eyes were swollen, choke marks were on her neck, and bruises were evident on several areas of her body. She killed her husband with the pistol. When questioned by police, she stated that he was totally out of control after drinking beer. His blood alcohol level was 0.236. (A person is considered legally intoxicated if the level is above 0.10.) JW described her husband as a hard worker and good father who was a loving person when he was sober but a totally different person when intoxicated. He had beaten her on several occasions in the past 6 months but never to the point of choking and punching her. In the past, JW's husband would wake up in the morning after physically abusing her and ask, "Did I do that?" He would promise such behavior "wouldn't happen again" and she would believe him.

---

as harassing or menacing behavior, coupled with a threat to do harm. Almost 60% of female victims and 30% of male victims are stalked by current or former intimate partners, with most of these cases occurring during the relationship. The average duration of stalking is 1.8 years. If stalking involves an intimate partner, the average duration increases to 2.2 years. Stalkers may use such means of communication as telephone calls, letters, e-mail, graffiti, or placing notices in the media. The stalker may approach or follow the victim, or keep the victim's residence under surveillance. **Sexual coercion** is a term used for incidents in which one person dominates another by force or compels the other person to perform a sexual act (Sadock & Sadock, 2003; National Center for Victims of Crime, 2004). Sexual harassment of women or men may range from sexual innuendo to coerced sexual relations (Davidhizar & Giger, 1995; Petrocelli & Repa, 1998). One much-publicized case in 1991 involved a female attorney who accused a Supreme Court nominee of sexually harassing her while they were working together. A second high-profile case in 1992 involved a Republican senator who allegedly harassed dozens of female employees and associates. In 1993, the Defense Department released its final report involving sexual harassment of 83 women and 7 men at the convention of the Navy's Tailhook Association, implicating 117 officers (Philbin, 2004).

Studies suggest anywhere between 40% and 70% of women and 10% and 20% of men have experienced sexual harassment in the workplace. Approximately 15,000 sexual harassment cases are brought to the office of the Equal Employment Opportunity Commission each year. The number of complaints filed by men has more than tripled in recent years. Currently, approximately 11% of claims involve men filing against female supervisors (D. B. Pargman Diversity Training, 2003).

Rape

Legally, the term *rape* has traditionally referred to forced vaginal penetration of a woman by a male assailant. Many states have now abandoned this concept in favor of the gender-neutral concept of sexual assault. Although the legal term for male rape is **sodomy,** many research articles use the terminology "sexual assault by an intimate partner" or simply state "male rape" (National Center for Victims of Crime [NCVC], 2003b).

The NCVC reports that over 700,000 women are raped or sexually assaulted annually. Of these victims, 61% are under the age of 18. Cases of male rape are so underreported that most people assume incorrectly that they do not exist (AMA, 2003; NCVC, 2003a). Male gender norms and related myths about men and sexual victimization may prevent a male from reporting sexual abuse. For example, a male may believe that males can't be sexually abused, that only "sissies and weaklings allow abuse," or that sexual abuse is always overt. The male might also believe that his masculinity is at stake if he is identified as a victim (Worcester, 2005). According to statistics cited in the National Violence Against Women Survey, 10% to 11% of rape victims are men. Approximately one of six boys is sexually assaulted by age 16 (Silent Tears, 2003).

Essential Elements of Rape

Three essential elements are necessary to legally define rape of a man or woman (NCVC, 2003b):

1. Use of force, threat, intimidation, or duress
2. Vaginal, oral, or anal penetration
3. Nonconsent by the victim

Rape statutes vary from state to state, and in some states, a wife may charge her husband with rape.

Attempted rape is defined as an assault in which oral, vaginal, or anal penetration is intended but does not occur. **Statutory rape** is the act of sexual intercourse or sexual assault on an individual younger than the age of consent (usually 16 years) (NCVC, 2003a; Roye & Coonan, 1997).

Adolescents who have been raped experience anxiety, traumatization, and physical pain, as well as fear of pregnancy, STDs, and possible retaliation from the assailant. They may have difficulty disclosing the rape, and feel embarrassed or responsible for what occurred. Some do not ask for health care until a few days after the crime (Roye & Coonan, 1997). Others may exhibit a series of behavioral manifestations such as brooding, verbal or physical aggression, outbursts of violence, or impulsive self-harm that continue for months to years until some form of intervention occurs (Matthews & Mossefin, 2006).

Rape-Victim Profile

There is no typical rape-victim profile. Every woman is a potential victim regardless of age, race, or socioeconomic status. Men who commit rape are from all walks of life and ethnic backgrounds, often from single-parent homes, usually younger than 25 years, and often married, leading otherwise normal sex lives. Persons at high risk to be a rape victim include single females between the ages of 11 and 25 years who are African American and come from a low socioeconomic background.

Although most victims are women, a far smaller proportion of men also experience rape. According to the National Institute of Justice and the Centers for Disease Control, 86% of heterosexual men raped and/or physically assaulted were raped/assaulted by other men who were strangers or acquaintances (NCVC, 2003b).

Both lesbians and homosexual males are also at risk for rape by their intimate partners; however, few data are available regarding the prevalence in lesbian or male homosexual relationships (Kimberg, 2001).

Elvik (1995) addresses rape of the developmentally disabled. Individuals with mild developmental delays usually want to be accepted and to fit in with "normal" society. Such a person may also exhibit some degree of impulsivity or gregariousness that could put him or her at risk for rape.

Motives for Rape

Theorists have described several patterns of rape or sexual assault according to the motive involved: anger rape, power rape, sadistic rape, and impulsive or opportunistic rape. In *anger rape,* sex is used as a means of expressing rage, hatred, and contempt toward the victim. The rapist exhibits physical brutality by beating, kicking, or choking, while he views the victim as a symbol of those women who wronged him at some point in life. Motives for *power rape* vary. Power rape is generally committed by persons with low self-esteem and a history of poor relationships with women, and is done in an attempt to prove manhood and strength. Intimidation may occur by means of a weapon, physical force, or threat of bodily harm. The victim may be tied up, held down by physical force, or otherwise rendered helpless. The offender forces the victim to become weak, helpless, and submissive—the exact qualities he despises in himself. Power rape is committed by a perpetrator who is impulsive, has no doubts about masculinity, and gives little or no thought to the crime beyond immediate gratification and a sense of entitlement. *Sadistic rape* occurs because the person feels a need to inflict pain and torment on his victim to achieve sexual satisfaction. The rapist misinterprets the victim's emotional anguish as sexual excitation rather than a refusal of his or her advances. Bizarre ritualistic behavior may occur during a sadistic rape. *Impulsive* or *opportunistic rape* may occur in conjunction with another antisocial act, such as a robbery. An antisocial person takes what he wants whenever he desires it; rape therefore becomes a form of stealing (North Carolina Rape Crisis, 2003; Brown, 2004).

Subclassifications of Rape

Rape is divided into five subclassifications:

1. Blitz rape, in which an unexpected surprise attack occurs in the absence of prior interaction with the victim
2. Confidence rape, in which the offender and victim have had a prior interaction
3. Marked victim rape, in which the offender assaults a woman he has been acquainted with in some way
4. Accessory-to-sex rape, which refers to a vulnerable victim's inability to give consent (as in the case of a person who is mentally retarded)
5. Date rape, which refers to the exploitation of an individual's friendliness or behavior during a date

Although not generally considered one of the official subclassifications of rape, gang rape is a distinctive category that should be discussed. *Gang rape* occurs when a group of offenders take turns assaulting the victim. Each member of the group is attempting to assert his manhood and power, and to gain acceptance by a group of his peers. Various levels of force occur during gang rape.

Emotional Reactions to Rape

The *Diagnostic and Statistical Manual of Mental Disorders, 4th Edition, Text Revision (DSM-IV-TR)* recognizes the reaction to rape as a post-traumatic stress disorder (PTSD) (APA, 2000). **Rape-trauma syndrome** is a North American Nursing Diagnosis Association (NANDA) nursing diagnosis used to describe a victim's response to rape, including an acute phase of disorganization and a longer phase of reorganization in the victim's life. Sadock and Sadock (2003) describe, in detail, the phases of rape trauma.

With the acute phase of rape trauma, the victim is disrupted by the crisis and displays emotional reactions of anger, guilt, embarrassment, humiliation, denial, shock, disbelief, or fear of death; multiple physical or somatic complaints; or a wish for revenge. After several weeks, the acute-phase reactions give way to deeper, more long-term feelings or reorganization that cause the victim to change daily life patterns, experience recurring dreams and nightmares, seek support from friends and family, initiate or refuse counseling, or develop irrational fears (phobias). One or more six major phobic reactions may occur: (1) fear of being indoors if the rape occurred in the home; (2) fear of the outdoors if the victim was sexually assaulted outside the home; (3) fear of crowds; (4) fear of being alone; (5) fear of people around the victim while the person engages in daily activities; and (6) fear of sexual activity if the person had no prior sexual experience (Sadock & Sadock, 2003).

Long-Term Reactions to Rape. Long-term reactions to rape and sexual assault may take several years to resolve, especially if the person goes through legal court action. During this time, the victim may move into a new residence, change his or her telephone number, change jobs, or move to a new state. If the victim is married, severe marital conflict may occur (Sadock & Sadock, 2003).

A maladaptive stress reaction referred to as **silent rape syndrome** may occur. The victim fails to disclose information about the rape to anyone, is unable to resolve feelings about the sexual assault, experiences increased anxiety, and may develop a sudden phobic reaction. Behavioral changes may include depression, suicidal behavior, somatization, and acting-out (eg, alcohol or drug abuse or sexual promiscuity) (Sadock & Sadock, 2003).

Adult Survivors of Childhood Sexual Abuse

Much attention has been paid in recent years to identifying and treating adult survivors of childhood sexual abuse or incest. Although most attention has been given to women, men suffer from childhood sexual abuse as well. Both male and female victims of abuse often go through life asking themselves what they did to deserve feelings of guilt, distrust, and alienation.

They may lack self-confidence or self-respect, or lose the ability to trust people. They may cope with the past abuse by using alcohol or other substances; engage in self-harming activities such as cutting, scratching, or burning oneself; or exhibit obsessive behavior and strict routines. Conversely, some survivors cope by breaking ties with or confronting the abuser; speaking about the abuse and seeking support; working to protect children from abuse; or writing about abuse (HealthyPlace.com, 2003). Adult survivors feel a need to control sexual situations. Some resort to promiscuity or prostitution as a means of seeking power over their partners. Others may turn to homosexuality because their trust in the opposite sex was permanently damaged from the abusive or incestuous act. Victims who do marry often find that fear and anxiety interfere with sustaining a successful marriage. Males often suppress their abusive experiences and carry abusive behaviors into their own families. Unfortunately, adult survivors who do not seek help at the time of victimization may experience clinical symptoms of rape-trauma syndrome (HealthyPlace.com, 2003).

Elder Abuse

Abuse of the elderly was ignored, overlooked, or perhaps thought not to exist until health care professionals began to appreciate the extent of the problem, long buried in family guilt, denial, and cover-up. Interest in elderly abuse increased in the 1980s, and a profile of elderly abuse that demanded attention and research interest emerged (Lachs & Pillemer, 1995). The National Elder Abuse Incidence Study, conducted in 1996, states that at least 500,000 persons age 60 years and older living in domestic settings were abused, neglected, or experienced self-neglect (National Center on Elder Abuse, 1998).

Major Types of Elder Abuse

Six types of elder abuse have been defined by the National Center on Elder Abuse (1998). They include physical abuse, sexual abuse, emotional or psychological abuse, abandonment (also referred to as *neglect*), financial or material exploitation, and self-neglect. Many states have adopted laws similar to child-abuse laws to prevent elder abuse. For example, in the state of Florida, Chapter 400 of the Florida Statutes mandates the standard of nursing care for residents of long-term care facilities, and violations of this chapter are reported to the Department of Children and Family Services or the long-term care ombudsman (advocate for the elderly). Unfortunately, the abuse of elderly individuals who reside alone or with family members often goes undetected (Douris & Pritchard, 1999).

The typical victim is female, with an average age of 76 years or older, is dependent on the abuser for basic needs, and is mentally or physically impaired. Abuse of the elderly may occur in a variety of settings, such as nursing homes, general hospitals, retirement centers, their own homes, or in the homes of adults who provide care for them. Types and examples of elder abuse are listed in Table 33-1.

Etiology of Elder Abuse

Most frequently, abusers of the elderly are adult children and caretakers. Causative factors eliciting abuse of the elderly include the presence of:

- Dependency on adult children or caretaker because of severe physical or mental disabilities
- Financial dependency on adult children or caretaker
- Personality conflicts with adult children or caretaker
- Societal attitudes toward aging (eg, considering the elderly person a burden)
- Frustration on the part of the adult children or caretaker

Emotional Response to Elder Abuse

Many times, elderly persons are expected to meet the needs of their grown children. These family members may become abusive if the elderly parent is unable to communicate clearly with them or is unable to meet their emotional needs.

TABLE 33.1 Types and Examples of Elder Abuse

FORMS	EXAMPLES
Physical	Direct beating, slapping, kicking, or shaking
	Overmedication
	Withholding life-sustaining medication
Emotional	Verbal assault or threats
	Intentional isolation by refusing to transport the elderly person who is unable to leave home unattended
Abandonment	Leaving disabled elderly person unsupervised
	Allowing the elder to live in unsanitary conditions
	Failure to provide food or personal care
	Withholding aids such as hearing aids, dentures, or eyeglasses
Financial exploitation or material abuse	Misuse of money or property by children or legal guardian
	Stealing of social security checks, credit cards, or property
Sexual abuse	Sexual assault of cognitively or physically impaired elder by caretaker or intruder
Self-neglect	Elder threatens own health through failure to take medication or to eat adequate amounts of food

SOURCE: National Center on Elder Abuse, Washington, DC.

Current statistics estimate that between 700,000 and 1.2 million older adults are victims of elder abuse and neglect. Furthermore, only one in ten cases of elder abuse and neglect are reported, and there is a serious underreporting by clinical professionals, likely due to the lack of appropriate screening instruments. Barriers to self-reporting abuse by elderly victims include cognitive impairment, the inability to communicate clearly or accurately what occurred, fear of rejection, low self-esteem (whereby they feel they deserve such treatment), loyalty to caretakers, lack of contact with helping persons, or reluctance to report the abuse due to fear of retaliation by the abuser (Burgess, Brown, Bell, Ledray, & Poarch, 2005; Fulmer, 2004).

Violence

The World Health Organization defines violence as the intentional use of physical force or power, threatened or actual, against oneself, another person or against a group or community, which either results in or has a high likelihood of resulting in injury, death, psychological harm, mal-development or deprivation. Statistics indicate that each year, more than 1.6 million people worldwide lose their lives to violence. It is among the leading causes of death for people ages 15 to 44 years worldwide, accounting for 14% of deaths among males and 7% of deaths among females. For every person who dies as a result of violence, many more are injured and suffer from a range of physical, sexual, reproductive and mental health problems (World Health Organization, 2006).

Both youth and workplace violence have emerged as important safety and health issues in today's society. Although high-profile school shootings have increased public concern for student safety, school-associated violent deaths account for less than 1% of homicides among school-aged children and youth. In addition to causing injury and death, youth violence affects communities by increasing the cost of health care, reducing productivity, decreasing property values, and disrupting social services (NCIPC, 2006c).

Homicide is the third-leading cause of fatal occupational injury in the United States (Occupational Safety & Health Administration [OSHA], 2003). Although the workplace was typically thought of as a safe environment, media coverage of workplace violence has heightened the underlying sense of insecurity about when, where, and how the next traumatic event will occur (Clements, DeRanieri, Clark, Manno, & Kuhn,

2005). Following is a discussion of youth and workplace violence.

Youth Violence

Youth violence may involve a youth victim, a youth perpetrator, or both. The rate of youth violence in America is unlike that in any other developed country. According to the Centers for Disease Control, 5,570 young people ages 10 to 24 years were murdered in 2003, an average of 15 each day. Of these victims, 82% were killed with firearms. In 2004, more than 750,000 young people ages 10 to 24 years were treated in emergency departments for injuries sustained as a result of violence. In a nationwide survey of high school students, 33% reported being in a physical fight one or more times in the 12 months preceding the survey, and 17% reported carrying a weapon (eg, gun, knife, or club) on one or more of the 30 days preceding the survey (NCIPC, 2006c).

Etiology of Youth Violence

Youth violence is not a race- or location-specific phenomenon. Violence between male youths usually involves one-on-one (or gang-against-gang) physical conflict. Violence between female youths generally occurs in groups or packs against one individual, is more relationship oriented, and usually consists of threatening or bullying behavior. Girls are not generally as violent as boys (Tumolo, 2003).

Lethal violence among youths has escalated during recent years because of the increased access to and use of firearms. Also, gang-related violence has increased rapidly since the 1960s. Status within and among gangs is a major issue, and threats to gang status may lead to violence between individuals or groups. Family problems such as poor monitoring or supervision of children, parental drug or alcohol abuse, and poor emotional attachment to parents or caretakers contribute significantly to delinquency. Exposure to violence at home is the most accurate predictor of membership in a delinquent group. Children who are themselves not victims of, but are witnesses to such violence, can subsequently become violent themselves (Reichlin, 2005; Thornton, Craft, Dahlberg, Lyncy, & Baer, 2000).

Those who study the etiology of criminal and violent adolescent behavior are looking beyond broad demographic characteristics such as race, age, and income level. Research findings support the conclusion that no single cause accounts for all episodes of violence. Almost always, youths who perpetrate acts of violence against others or themselves have a long history of mental illness. Comorbidity (eg, attention-deficit hyperactivity disorder, conduct disorder, mood disorder, psychosis, PTSD, substance abuse) is the rule, and often it is further compounded by destructive family relationship patterns (Danielsen, 1998; Koplewicz, 1999; Reichlin, 2005).

Research has also demonstrated a link between animal cruelty and human violence. A survey by the Humane Society in 2003 determined that teens were accountable for 22% of 1,682 cases of animal cruelty, and the vast majority of all abusers of animals were male. Law enforcement professionals, sociologists, and psychologists also recognize animal cruelty as a warning sign of potential human violence (Humane Society of the United States, 2003; Muscari, 2005a).

According to the APA, the one overriding finding in research on the mass media is that exposure to media portrayals of violence increases aggressive behavior in children. The National Institute of Mental Health (NIMH) has reported that exposure to television violence also causes desensitization, creates a climate of fear, and has been shown to be a risk factor to the health and well-being of the developing child, adolescent, and to the stability of their families (HealthyMinds.org, 2006; Reichlin, 2005).

Emotional Response of Victims of Youth Violence

Each year, many children and adolescents sustain injuries from violence, lose friends or family members to violence, or are adversely affected by witnessing a violent or catastrophic event. They are vulnerable to serious long-term problems. Their emotional responses, including fear, depression, withdrawal, or anger, can occur immediately or some time after the tragic event—resulting in PTSD. Research has shown that girls who have been bullied by female peers have a higher incidence of eating disorders, a higher incidence of depression, poorer school performance, and lower self-esteem. Furthermore, there have been suicides as a result of girl bullying (Tumolo, 2003).

Victims often need support from parents and teachers to avoid long-term emotional harm. The NIMH has supported studies regarding the impact of violence and disaster on children and adolescents. Research findings indicate that inner-city children experience the greatest exposure to violence, and youngsters who are exposed to community violence are more likely to exhibit aggressive behavior or depression within the following year (NIMH, 2000a, b).

Generally, the stigma surrounding mental illness is more pronounced among teenagers. Often, they are reluctant to seek or accept help. Moreover, parents, teachers, and administrators are far too willing to ignore or rationalize symptoms of a mental illness in students. As a result of this stigma, teenage perpetrators of youth violence, who have behavioral problems or conduct disorders, are also considered to be victims of violence (Koplewicz, 1999).

Workplace Violence

Workplace violence is defined as any physical assault, threatening behaviors, verbal abuse (eg, obscene phone calls, intimidation, harassment), stalking, and psychological trauma in the workplace (OSHA, 2003).

In 2001, the CDC reported that 13% of all homicides occurred in an office or factory. Most of the deaths occurred as a result of robbery (NCIPC, 2001). According to the Bureau of Labor Statistic's Census of Fatal Occupational Injuries, there were 551 workplace homicides in the year 2004 (OSHA, 2006). Recent statistics indicate that, in an average week in U. S. workplaces, one employee is killed and at least 25 are seriously injured in violent assaults by current or former co-workers (Armour, 2006).

Statistics regarding stalking (discussed earlier in this chapter in the content of sexual abuse) are also reported under the category of workplace violence. According to the National Center for Victims of Crime's Stalking Resource Center (2004), 28% of female victims and 10% of male victims obtained a protective order; however 69% of female victims and 81% of male victims had the order violated. Furthermore, 26% of stalking victims lost time from work, and 7% never returned to work. Statistics also revealed that 76% of female murder victims had been stalked by the individual who killed them.

The severity and frequency of assaults against employees in the health care setting have dramatically increased in the last decade. According to OSHA, health care and social-service workers are at high risk for workplace violence, with nursing staff in all work settings as the most frequent victims of assault. The National Institute for Occupational Safety and Health reports that 9,000 health care providers are attacked on the job daily. Other occupations that regularly face violence in the workplace include police officers, security guards, taxi drivers, prison guards, bartenders, and high-school teachers (OSHA, 2003).

Predictors of Workplace Violence

A consensus is emerging on the types of individuals who may become violent in work settings. The following characteristics are predictive of violence (Flannery, 1995, 1997; Resnick & Kausch, 1995):

- Angry customers dissatisfied with their treatment
- Clients with certain mental illnesses such as substance abuse, schizophrenia, delusional disorder, or depression
- Domestic batterers who may follow the spouse to work
- Women who experience severe cases of premenstrual tension
- Disgruntled older male employees who fear a potential loss of their job
- Juvenile delinquents
- Career criminals

Classification of Workplace Violence Incidents

In 1995, the California Occupational Safety and Health Administration developed Guidelines for Workplace Security. These guidelines classified violent workplace incidents into three types:

- Type I: Incidents of violent acts performed by someone who has no legitimate relationship to the workplace and who commits robbery or another criminally motivated act.
- Type II: Incidents of violent acts or threats by someone who receives services from the workplace or from the victim.
- Type III: Incidents of violent acts or threats by a current or former employee, supervisor, manager, spouse, lover, relative, or someone who has a dispute with the employee

Stalkers fall into the last category (Wiseman, 1999).

Emotional Responses of Victims of Workplace Violence

Victims of workplace violence may develop psychological trauma and PTSD with hypervigilance, sleep disturbance, exaggerated startle response, intrusive memories, and avoidance of others (Grinfield, 2000). Victims who are stalked experience a significant dis-

SELF-AWARENESS PROMPT

Do you know anyone who has been victimized by abuse or violence? How has it affected them? Do you consider yourself to be adequately prepared to provide nursing care to a client who has been sexually or physically abused? If not, what additional preparation do you feel is necessary?

ruption in their everyday living, including work, as they alter normal routines to avoid detection by the offender. Loss of job may occur as a result of poor job performance secondary to stress, excessive absenteeism, or the need to seek temporary or permanent relocation (Muscari, 2005b).

Hate Crimes

Hate crimes are crimes (eg, violent crime, hate speech, vandalism) that are motivated by feelings of hostility against any identifiable group of people within a society. If systematic, rather than spontaneous, instigators of such crimes are sometimes organized into hate groups.

In 1992, the U.S. Congress defined a hate crime as "a crime in which a defendant's conduct was motivated by hatred, bias or prejudice, based on the actual or perceived race, color, religion, national origin, ethnicity, gender, sexual orientation, or gender identity of another individual or group of individuals." In 1994, the Violent Crime Control and Law Enforcement Act added disabilities to the list. The actions considered criminal are using force or threat of force to willfully injure, intimidate, interfere with, oppress, or threaten another person in the free exercise of enjoyment of any right or privilege secured to him or her by the Constitution or laws of the state or the country (Wikipedia, 2006).

According to the 2003 FBI uniform crime statistics, there were 4,754 victims of race-related hate crimes; 1,489 victims of religion-related hate crimes; 1,479 victims of sexual orientation–related hate crimes; and 1,326 victims of ethnicity/national origin–related hate crimes. In addition, there were 43 victims of disability-related hate crimes (physical or mental) and nine victims of multiple-bias hate crimes as a result of two or more bias motivations (Infoplease.com, 2006).

THE NURSING PROCESS

ASSESSMENT

The assessment of victims of abuse or violence requires the nurse to display sensitivity, empathy, and confidentiality. Privacy is essential when collecting data.

Assessment of Abuse and Violence in Children and Adolescents

Parents, caretakers, or relatives of physically abused children brought to emergency room settings usually give a predictable history of the child's injuries: namely, falling out of bed, against a piece of furniture or household appliance, or down a flight of stairs. They are usually inconsistent in giving details that are nearly always incompatible with the child's injuries. The child may appear guarded or afraid of any physical contact with the examiner or parents while receiving treatment. Victims of sexual abuse usually try to protect the offender.

Assessment of adolescent victims of abuse or violence can be quite challenging. The nurse bases assessment strategies on several factors: chronological age, maturational age, physical development, medical condition, and emotional and behavioral manifestations of the victim. The adolescent victim may be accompanied by an adult (eg, parent or family member) or may have no support system. In either situation, the nurse assures the adolescent that all data will be considered confidential and provides for privacy during the assessment. (See Chapter 13 regarding assessment of children and adolescents during a crisis.)

Biopsychosocial Data. The assessment process for both children and adolescents includes a thorough physical and x-ray examination, including inspection of the genitals and anus. If sexual abuse is suspected, cultures of the oral, rectal, or vaginal area may be performed to determine the presence or absence of STDs. Testing for the human immunodeficiency virus (HIV) may be necessary if there is an indication that the perpetrator is at risk for HIV/acquired immunodeficiency virus (AIDS).

Play therapy and art therapy can serve as assessment tools when child abuse is suspected. A mature, patient, empathetic approach is used, focusing on physical, behavioral, and environmental indicators of abuse as well as family dynamics. Evidence of malnutrition, dehydration, old fractures, bruises, internal injuries, or intracranial hemorrhage may be present. Behaviorally, the child or adolescent may exhibit withdrawal, low self-esteem, oppositional behavior, compulsive behavior, hypervigilance or an increased awareness of the environment, and a fearful attitude toward parents. (See discussion of physical, behavioral, and environmental indicators earlier in the chapter.)

Documentation of the Assessment. Assessment findings must be well documented, with emphasis on the child's or adolescent's physical status, emotional status, developmental level or stage, interpersonal skills, and behavioral response to the family. Photographs taken before medical treatment help to document the initial appearance of the injuries.

Assessment of Adult Victims of Physical Abuse or Violence

Clinical assessment of victims of physical abuse or violence by the nurse and attending physician is performed to determine if the abused or assaulted victim is in any physical or life-threatening danger because of injuries requiring emergency medical care. The victim may present with multiple bruises or injuries, somatic complaints or symptoms associated with trauma that may not be observable, or characteristic behavioral reactions such as acute anxiety reaction, depression, or suicidal ideation. (See Chapter 13 for information on crisis intervention.)

Biopsychosocial Data. Determining the emotional status of the victim is imperative. Obtaining a medical history is also important to acquire additional clues to abuse and to make a tentative medical, psychological, and nursing diagnosis.

The abused person may describe a history of multiple injuries, psychiatric problems, medical problems, or self-destructive behavior (eg, alcohol abuse, drug abuse, or suicidal gestures).

Interview questions directed at victims of possible abuse must be carried out in a supportive and sensitive manner. Inquiries focus on any suspicious-looking injuries; how the injuries occurred; whether the victim is living with the abuser; the victim's emotional response to the abuser; a safe place for the victim and any children to go, such as a shelter; and whether the victim wants to press charges.

Assessment Tools. Although the U.S. Preventive Services Task Force (USPSTF, 2004) has found insufficient evidence to recommend for or against routine screening of women for abuse or intimate partner violence, the American College of Gynecologists and the AMA recommend that physicians routinely ask women direct, specific questions about abuse and domestic violence. Two instruments that are used to ask specific questions include the Danger Assessment Instrument and the Migrant Clinicians Network Domestic Violence Assessment Form.

Campbell (1986) developed the Danger Assessment Instrument for assessing the potential for homicide. The questions denote risk factors that have been statistically associated with homicides of abused women. They focus on the frequency of abuse, type of abuse, presence of lethal weapons in the home, forced sex, use of drugs or alcohol, jealous behavior or violence toward family members by the abuser, and suicidal ideation verbalized by the abused. Grant (1996a) refers to the Migrant Clinicians Network Domestic Violence Assessment Form developed by McFarlane for use in a migrant health center setting. Four questions are posed:

1. Within the last year, have you been hit, slapped, kicked, or otherwise physically hurt by someone? (The perpetrator is then identified, the frequency of abuse noted, and the area of injury noted on a body map.)
2. If pregnant, since the pregnancy began, have you been hit, slapped, kicked, or otherwise physically hurt by someone? (The frequency of abuse is noted, and the area of injury is noted on a body map.)
3. Within the last year, has anyone forced you to have sexual activities? (The perpetrator is then identified and the frequency of abuse is noted.)
4. Are you afraid of your partner or anyone you identified?

Figure 33-3, the Abuse Assessment Screen, is a similar form developed by the Nursing Research Consortium on Violence and Abuse.

Documentation of Data. During the assessment process, colored photographs are taken to complement the data noted on the body map. Laboratory and diagnostic tests as well as x-ray examinations may be ordered, and the results are placed on the client's medical record. Finally, if the police have been notified, the

1. Have you *ever* been emotionally or physically abused by your partner or someone important to you? ☐ YES ☐ NO

2. **WITHIN THE LAST YEAR,**
   Have you been hit, slapped, kicked, or otherwise physically hurt by someone? ☐ YES ☐ NO

   If YES, by whom? _____
   Total number of times _____

3. When pregnant, were you hit, slapped, kicked, or otherwise physically hurt by someone? ☐ YES ☐ NO

   If YES, by whom? _____
   Total number of times _____

MARK THE AREA OF INJURY ON THE BODY MAP. SCORE EACH INCIDENT ACCORDING TO THE FOLLOWING SCALE:

Score

1= Threats of abuse including use of a weapon _____

2= Slapping, pushing; no injuries and/or lasting pain _____

3= Punching, kicking, bruises, cuts and/or continuing pain _____

4= Beating up, severe contusions, burns, broken bones _____

5= Head injury, internal injury, permanent injury _____

6= Use of weapon; wound from weapon _____

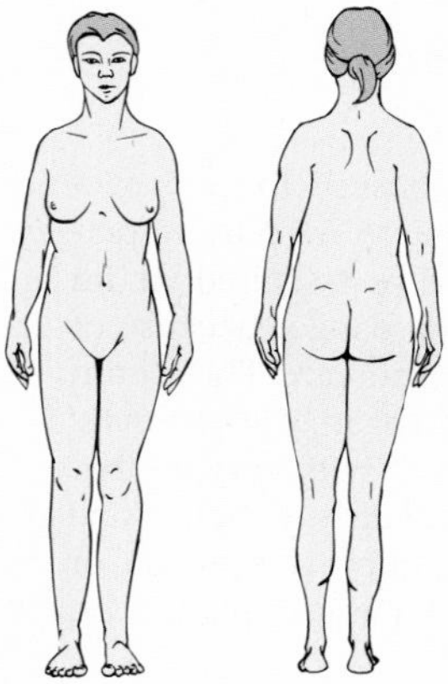

If any of the descriptions for the higher numbers apply, use the higher number.

4. **WITHIN THE LAST YEAR,**
   Has anyone forced you to have sexual activities? ☐ YES ☐ NO

   If YES, who? _____
   Total number of times _____

5. Are you afraid of your partner or anyone you listed above? ☐ YES ☐ NO

Source: Developed by the Nursing Research Consortium on Violence and Abuse. Readers are encouraged to reproduce and use this assessment tool.

FIGURE 33.3 Assessment screening tool for abuse.

name of the investigating officer and any action taken are documented.

Assessment of Victims of Sexual Abuse or Rape

During the initial assessment of victims of sexual abuse such as rape, the nurse may experience strong reactions, including conflict over who is to blame; anxiety about the possibility of becoming a sexual assault victim him- or herself; anger and hostility toward the victim, the rapist, and society for allowing such an act to occur; or a desire to learn more about rape to resolve personal feelings.

The victim may be reluctant to disclose information, feel guilty that he or she allowed the abuse or rape to happen, or feel that he or she didn't offer enough resistance. The victim may also be exhibiting symptoms of rape-trauma syndrome.

Guidelines for Collection of Data. Guidelines for interviewing rape victims in crisis have been identified by Grant (1996b). Assessment data to be collected if the client is able and willing to answer questions include the victim's recounting of the events of the rape or attempted rape; legal information, including the names of persons who have been notified, such as the police; what evidence has been preserved; and support persons or systems available to the abused person. Specific information focuses on demographic data, crisis status, type of assault, services needed or requested, and leading questions to consider. Available services usually include medical, police and legal, shelter, transportation, and counseling. Questions to consider during the interview include "Does she feel the rape was her fault?" "Does she believe any of the myths about rape?" and "Which ones and what are their impact on her?" The more common myths and facts about rape are presented in Table 33-2.

Medical Data. Assessment by the nurse, attending physician, or other health care professional is performed to determine if any physical or life-threatening danger exists. Emergency medical care may be given concurrently with assessment if multiple bruises or injuries are present. Keep in mind that the victim may have somatic complaints or symptoms associated with trauma that are not readily observable.

TABLE 33.2 Rape: Myths and Facts

MYTH	FACT
Attractive women provoke men into raping them.	70% to 80% of all rapes are violent, planned aggressive acts not based on physical attractiveness or age. Statistics show rape victims range in age from approximately 3 months to over 90 years.
If a woman struggles, rape can be avoided; no woman can be raped against her will.	Rapists frequently overpower smaller and physically weaker women and carry weapons to harm, mutilate, or kill their victims. Counterattack by the victim may cause more injury to occur.
Only women with bad reputations or who are friendly to strangers outside their homes are raped.	All women are potential sexual assault victims. The rapist's desire is control, not sex. Approximately one third to one half of all rapes occur in a victim's home. Rapists include husbands, ex-husbands, neighbors, and boyfriends.
Women "cry rape" to get revenge.	Rape is an underreported crime due to feelings of guilt. Only approximately 2% of all reported rape cases are false.
Most sexual assaults involve African American men raping white women.	The rapist and victim tend to be of the same race (intraracial) in most cases of sexual assault.

Behavioral and Emotional Responses. Behavioral and emotional responses to rape or sexual assault may vary according to the client's age and developmental stage. Therefore, the psychiatric–mental health nurse must have a thorough understanding of the developmental stages of the life cycle. Common behavioral responses of victims of all ages include nightmares, refusal to be left alone with certain individuals, poor social interactions, and problems in school or at work. Following are additional examples of responses to rape or sexual assault, according to developmental levels from childhood to older adulthood:

- Preoccupation with wrong or bad acts during childhood (4–7 years)
- Misperception of rape as a sexual act during latency (7 years to puberty)
- Confusion over normal sexual behavior and concern about pregnancy or STDs as an adolescent (puberty to 18 years)
- Concern over credibility, lifestyle, morality, and character as a young adult (18–24 years)
- Concern over how rape will affect family and lifestyle during adulthood (25–45 years)
- Concern over physical safety, fear of death, reputation, and respectability as an older adult (45 years and older)

Identification of the victim's response to the assault as acute stress reaction, maladaptive stress reaction, or reorganization stress reaction is important because not all rapes are reported immediately after the assault occurs.

Collection and Documentation of Physical Evidence. If the victim gives consent and is able to tolerate the procedure, a gynecologic examination usually is performed after a rape situation, along with a pregnancy test if indicated, and laboratory tests. The date of the victim's last menstrual period is obtained.

Documentation of physical evidence includes the presence of semen, stains, fiber, or hair on clothing or the body; fingernail scrapings; and pieces of torn clothing. The evidence or specimens are saved for analysis, according to hospital protocol. These findings are also important as evidence in any criminal investigation if charges are filed by the victim. (Refer to Chapter 6 for additional information regarding Forensic Nursing Practice.)

Transcultural Considerations

During assessment, keep in mind that abuse and violence affect individuals of all ethnic and socioeconomic backgrounds and cannot be predicted by demographic features. Certain cultural practices, however, do place women at risk for abuse. For example, in some cultures, the genitalia of females are mutilated when they reach puberty. Women are also abused and disfigured when they reject a marriage proposal, and physically abused or ostracized by family members if they are victims of rape. Women who refuse a marriage proposal or are victimized by rape are thought to bring shame to a family.

According to a national survey conducted in 1994, family income, ethnicity, region of residence, and type of metropolitan area all are associated with risk of victimization of children (Finkelhor & Leatherman, 1994). For example, Hispanic and African American children, those living in Mountain and Pacific states, and those from large cities were at greater risk for victimization. African American youths demonstrated elevated rates for sexual assault and kidnapping; low-income children demonstrated high rates of family assault and general violence. Approximately 6.2 million youths participated in this national survey. Additionally, cross-cultural variability in childrearing beliefs and behavior is so great that it would be difficult, although probably not impossible, to define a framework of acceptable childrearing practices that would be universally applicable (Skuse & Bentovim, 1994).

Be aware that treatment of the elderly by family members and caregivers is partially determined by cultural influence and values placed on aging. Culture defines who is old, establishes rituals for identifying the elderly, sets socially acceptable roles and expectations for behavior of the elderly, and influences attitudes toward the aged. However, the underreporting of elder abuse has resulted in a lack of cultural data related to victimization.

NURSING DIAGNOSES

Several nursing diagnoses are applicable to victims of abuse or violence, regardless of the victim's age or sex. They address issues of anxiety, powerlessness, fear, pain, impaired communication, ineffective coping, disturbance in self-esteem or self-concept, risk for injury or violence, or clinical symptoms of post-trauma response or rape-trauma syndrome. See the accompanying Examples of North American Nursing Diagnosis

EXAMPLES OF NANDA NURSING DIAGNOSES/ ABUSE AND VIOLENCE

- Anxiety related to actual threat to biologic integrity secondary to physical assault
- Impaired Verbal Communication related to psychological barrier (fear) secondary to sexual assault
- Ineffective Denial related to need to escape personal problems secondary to intimate partner abuse
- Disabled Family Coping related to impaired ability to manage stressors constructively secondary to history of abusive relationships with own parents
- Interrupted Family Processes related to social deviance by father threatening harm to family members
- Fear related to vulnerability to crime secondary to living in ghetto
- Rape-Trauma Syndrome related to traumatic event of forced rape by stranger
- Risk for Violence related to increase in stressors secondary to loss of job and restraining order issued at the request of wife

Association (NANDA) Nursing Diagnoses for abuse and violence.

OUTCOME IDENTIFICATION

Stated outcomes focus on reducing anxiety, fear, pain, and the potential for injury or violence; improving communication, coping, self-esteem, or self-concept; identifying members of support system(s) and the appropriate use of them; and assisting the victim in returning to a precrisis level of functioning.

PLANNING INTERVENTIONS AND IMPLEMENTATION

Nursing interventions may occur in a variety of settings such as in the school, by the school nurse; in the home, by the public health or home health care nurse; in the hospital, by the emergency room or staff nurse; or in the clinician's office, by the nurse. The hardest task for the nurse is to develop a trusting relationship with the victim and family, if a family member is present. Immediate

care should focus on meeting the client's physical and emotional needs, promoting homeostasis and comfort, and reducing fear. Clients who are victims of abuse and violence may experience anxiety and depression (See Chapter 16, Psychopharmacology; Chapter 19, Anxiety Disorders; Chapter 20, Somatoform and Dissociative Disorders; and Chapter 21, Mood Disorders).

Interventions for Victims of Child Abuse

Nursing personnel generally respond to child abuse with feelings of shock, anger, rage, or revulsion. People who have abused children anticipate such responses from helping persons and authority figures. Thus, they often resist efforts to become involved in therapy. Negative responses, such as frustration, hopelessness, sadness, or sympathy, interfere with objectivity and planning competent nursing interventions. Always keep in mind that abusive parents, as well as abused children, have severe unmet dependency needs, and accept abusive parents as vulnerable human beings.

Multidisciplinary Approach. Treatment of victims of child abuse or neglect requires a multidisciplinary approach, frequently beginning with crisis intervention. Members of the treatment team may include doctors, nurses, psychologists, psychiatrists, social workers, teachers, and law-enforcement officers. If child abuse is established, the most important intervention is to separate the child from the danger. The child welfare agency is generally responsible for the child's immediate welfare and decides whether to remove the child from his or her natural environment by placing the child in a hospital or foster home. A social worker from the child welfare agency usually investigates the family and recommends whether psychiatric treatment is needed for the child, family, or both. Interventions focus on symptoms that cause suffering, interfere with daily functioning, and negatively affect developmental progress. Psychotropic medication that may be used includes clonidine (Catapres), propranolol (Inderol), carbamazepine (Tegretol), selective serotonin reuptake inhibitors, and other antidepressants depending upon the age of the victim (Childers, 2005).

Behavioral Interventions. Behavioral strategies have been developed to help young children cope with traumatic events such as abuse, incest, and violence. Interventions are individualized, based on diagnoses generated from a complete developmental multidisci-plinary assessment, and focus on maximizing the child's abilities and strengths while addressing prob-lems and conflicts that affect the child's current func-tioning (Childers, 2005). Therapeutic approaches include deep-breathing exercises, progressive mus-cle relaxation, exposure techniques (exposure to reminders of a traumatic event), thought-replacement and thought-stopping, positive imagery, psychoeduca-tion and cognitive reframing, and addressing grief reac-tions including "survivor's guilt" (Bates, 1999).

Continuum of Care. Ideally, continuum of care focuses on treating the family as a unit to facilitate a healthy, safe environment for the child after treatment. Participation in family therapy and using community support systems help prevent the repetition of abuse. Support services available for victims of child abuse and their families include:

- Visiting or public health nurses
- Protective services for children
- Emergency shelters for children
- Daycare centers or nurseries
- Self-help groups such as Parents Anonymous
- Telephone hotlines
- Homemaker services
- Financial assistance such as the local welfare depart-ment
- Employment counseling
- Parent-education classes
- Foster-home care
- Transportation services
- Assertiveness-training classes and groups
- Mental health and other services through the provi-sions of the Individuals with Disabilities Education Act

Prevention of Child Abuse and Neglect. The nurse may help prevent child abuse by recognizing early signs of abuse, supporting and working for legislation to interrupt the child-abuse syndrome, promoting edu-cational courses on family interpersonal relationships and childrearing practices, promoting community awareness programs, participating in continuing-education courses, and participating in nursing research of child abuse and effective treatment meas-ures.

In most states, certain professionals are required by law to report suspected child abuse, neglect, or sexual abuse. Even if the law does not require nurses to report

such a case, they have an ethical obligation to protect a child from harm. It is not the intent of the law to remove a child from his or her home unless the child is in dan-ger. Parents are not punished unless undue harm has occurred. In most situations, the family is helped so that the parents and child can stay together.

When reporting child abuse, the report may be made by telephone, in person, or in writing to the children's services board of a local welfare department or to the local police department. The following infor-mation is stated:

- Name and address of the suspected victim
- Child's age
- Name and address of the child's parent or caretaker
- Name of the person suspected of abusing or neglecting the child
- Why abuse or neglect is suspected
- Any other helpful information
- Nurse's name, if she or he wishes (some states require a signature)

The case will be investigated whether the reporter remains anonymous or gives a name.

Interventions for Victims of Physical Abuse and Violence

Important interventions focus on providing a safe environment, including emergency medical care when necessary; empowering the victim through supportive therapies; and exploring continuum of care to assist the victim to regain control of his or her own life. Each victim's situation is unique, and the decision to take action varies among individuals.

Safe Environment. After the client's medical condi-tion is stabilized, often a referral to a local domestic-violence shelter may be made to ensure a safe environment and to assist the victim and the victim's family. If the situation is acute, law enforcement offi-cials should be notified immediately. However, some victims may refuse help or refuse to press charges due to fear of retaliation by the perpetrator. If an in-depth formal interview is planned, arrange for someone to stay with the victim. Inform the victim of his or her rights. Make arrangements so that the victim needs to tell the story in detail only once. This way the victim does not have to re-live the incident psychologically over and over again by repeating the story.

Supportive Therapies. Crisis counseling is provided to reduce anxiety and provide supportive care. Medication may be prescribed for symptoms of depression, anxiety, insomnia, agitation, or the presence of nightmares. Displaying a nonjudgmental attitude is essential while encouraging the client to verbalize feelings, allowing for the expression of both anger and possible affection toward the perpetrator or batterer. Past coping responses and adaptations to battering are discussed. Emphasis is placed on helping the victim develop a realistic and rational perception of the battering situation and to provide the victim with the information necessary to make an informed decision.

Interactive therapies that are available include individual, couples, and family therapy. Additionally, referrals may be made to self-help groups and a community mental health social worker who is familiar with additional services that are available.

Continuum of Care. If the victim prefers to return home, an action plan is developed in the event that the violence recurs (Box 33-6). The victim also is given emergency telephone numbers and informed of available options (Grant, 1996a). They include:

- Legal assistance to obtain a restraining or protective order
- Temporary custody of minor children
- Emergency financial assistance
- Temporary emergency housing
- Assistance from local women's organizations
- Advocacy services

BOX 33.6 ACTION PLAN TO AVERT DOMESTIC VIOLENCE

- Create an emergency kit containing money, car keys, medical records, medical cards, important phone numbers, clothing, and copies of pertinent papers to validate identity and eligibility for assistance.
- Secure access to emergency transportation.
- Identify a safe place to go.
- Pack clothing for children.
- List information about partner's place of employment, including name, address of company, and employer's name.

- Community counseling services
- Vocational counseling
- Legal-aid services

If the victim is an older adult, additional services such as alternate housing, nursing care by the visiting nurse, food from Meals on Wheels, assistance from a visiting homemaker program, visits by persons involved in a foster grandparent program, and transportation for the elderly provided by community organizations may be helpful.

Interventions for Victims of Sexual Abuse

Survivors of sexual assaults were treated much differently in the past than they are today. Many communities now employ what is known as a mobile sexual assault response team (SART), which consists of a law enforcement officer, nurse examiner, and victim advocate practicing in a freestanding facility no longer associated with a specific hospital. Initial contact with the team begins at the time the victim or a support person reports the assault. The report may be made to any member of the team, who then responds to the location of the victim, including the crime scene if necessary. The team approach is designed to provide a safe environment, empower the survivor, and begin the process of rehabilitation while simultaneously providing examination for evidence to assist in prosecution of the perpetrator (LoCascio, 2000).

In some emergency departments, sexual assault nurse examiners (SANEs) perform the entire examination and provide treatment to the victim. SANEs are registered nurses or nurse practitioners trained to collect forensic evidence from sexual assault survivors (Liddell, 2002). (Refer to Chapter 6, Forensic Nursing Practice, for more information.)

Crisis Intervention. The psychiatric–mental health nurse's role is to plan appropriate interventions to help the victim recover from the physical, emotional, social, or sexual disruption. During the acute stress reaction phase of rape, crisis intervention skills are used (see Chapter 13) to reduce anxiety and provide supportive care. It is imperative that a nurse stay with the victim, be supportive, listen carefully to what the victim has to say, encourage the victim to speak distinctly and clearly when describing the rape incident, and reassure the victim that the information given will be kept confidential and handled discreetly. The victim must be treated with respect and dignity during crisis intervention. Psychotropic agents may be prescribed to stabilize clinical symptoms of anxiety or depression.

Continuum of Care. After the victim's clinical symptoms have been stabilized, the psychiatric–mental health nurse focuses on continuum of care. The psychiatric–mental health nurse should ask the victim for permission to provide a crisis center with her telephone number, with the understanding that a follow-up person will take the initiative in contacting the victim.

The establishment of ongoing support systems, including medication management, is important if the victim is to resolve an abuse or rape experience. Such support systems include:

- Crisis hotlines that provide 24-hour crisis intervention and support
- Emergency shelters that provide safe refuge to victims of sexual assault
- Community outreach and prevention programs that provide education and awareness of sexual abuse
- Legal-advocacy services that provide support and information regarding criminal and civil court proceedings
- Advocacy services that provide individual counseling, medical treatment, assistance with basic needs, and coordination with other service providers

Sullivan (2005) discusses the use of spiritualized therapy and cognitive therapy to lessen symptoms in sex abuse survivors. A pilot nondenominational program, Solace for the Soul: Journey Towards Wholeness, introduced by Dr. Murray-Swank, focuses on a specific aspect of spirituality and its relationship to childhood sexual abuse: feelings of abandonment by God and associated anger; connecting with the spiritual; letting go of shame; seeing the body as a beautiful creation; and seeing sexuality as a sacred, life-affirming way of connecting to others. A significant decrease in symptom scores in all clients was reported during the program.

Care of Elderly Survivors of Sexual Abuse. Research is lacking regarding the impact of sexual abuse survival on older adults. This may be due in part to the relative unavailability of the elderly, disinterest in older adults, or the stigma associated with this type of victimization.

Older adult assessment forms may ask for information regarding elder abuse but do not assess for a past history of incest or sexual abuse. Many survivors exhibit symptoms of depression or anxiety.

The topic of elderly survivors of sexual abuse and their need for nursing interventions as they review the life process is addressed by Walker (1992). After an elderly person is identified as a survivor of sexual abuse, nursing care should focus on improving coping skills and increasing self-esteem. Encourage the individual to vent emotions, and provide supportive measures such as individual therapy as necessary.

Interventions for Victims of Youth or Workplace Violence and Hate Crimes

Developing an awareness of the problem and establishing a workplace-, school-, or community-violence program can help reduce the incidence and consequences of violent incidents. Trauma/crisis counseling or critical-incident stress debriefing may need to occur not only for the victims but for students, peers, parents, teachers, co-workers, or the public in general, depending on the location of the violence. Providing assistance to troubled individuals and counseling services for victims can help reduce the long-term effects of violence. The consequences of violence may not be fully realized until months, or even years, after the incident (Wiseman, 1999). Nursing interventions discussed earlier in the chapter regarding victims of physical abuse and domestic violence are also used when appropriate.

EVALUATION

Evaluation of the client's emotional and physical well-being after crisis intervention is an ongoing process because the consequences of abuse and violence may not be resolved for months or years. If the client agrees to enter into treatment, the nurse evaluates the effectiveness of interventions and the progress the client is making. Information is obtained from the client, family, significant others, or health care providers who continue to provide supportive care. If the client is taking medication to alleviate clinical symptoms of anxiety, depression, or other disorders, the efficacy of the medication is evaluated. See Nursing Plan of Care 33-1: The Victim of Domestic Violence.

NURSING PLAN OF CARE 33.1

THE VICTIM OF DOMESTIC VIOLENCE

Andrea, a 31-year-old mother of 3-year-old twins, brought her children to the clinic for their well-baby visits. The nurse practitioner noted Andrea was wearing sunglasses and long sleeves although it was the middle of July and the outside temperature was 85°F. She also appeared hypervigilant and easily distracted.

After the well-baby visits, Andrea asked the nurse if she could speak to her about a problem that she was having. Andrea related that her husband of 7 years had been under a considerable amount of stress at work for the past 6 months and had lost his temper on several occasions. He began drinking alcohol nightly and has become quite critical of her at times. She questions whether she and the children are to blame for his anger because they have purchased a larger home and incurred more bills since the birth of the twins.

Andrea revealed bruise marks on both upper extremities and a bruise directly under her right lower eyelid. She stated that her husband became angry when she confronted him about his behavior and she feared that he might injure the children.

DSM–IV–TR DIAGNOSIS: Physical abuse of adult

ASSESSMENT: Personal strengths: Recognizes the presence of domestic violence, provides good care for her children, desires help with her situation

Weaknesses: Self-blame or guilt regarding her husband's behavior, expressed fear that her husband could harm the children, ineffective communication with husband

---

NURSING DIAGNOSIS: Situational Low Self-Esteem as evidenced by self-blame and guilt related to her husband's drinking and battering behavior

OUTCOME: The client will identify the source of her situational low self-esteem and work through that issue.

Planning/Implementation	Rationale
Encourage verbalization of feelings, especially about the way the client views self and her role as a wife and mother.	Verbalization of feelings allows the client to identify, accept, and work through feelings.
Recognize the client's efforts to improve her self-esteem.	Positive feedback may reinforce the client's efforts and promote personal growth and self-esteem.

NURSING DIAGNOSIS: Fear related to change in behavior of spouse and possible escalation of abuse

OUTCOME: The client will verbalize feelings about husband without fear of reprisal.

(Continued on following page)

Planning/Implementation	Rationale
Educate the client about abusive behavior, including why domestic violence can occur.	Learning about abuse can help the client focus on feelings and face the reality of the abusive situation.
Identify and contact at least one support system available on a 24-hour basis.	Support systems can help the client feel less isolated, increase her self-respect, and address issues related to her husband's behavior.

NURSING DIAGNOSIS: Disabled Family Coping because of family conflict related to violence

OUTCOME: The client's family will be free of violence by using family discussions to resolve conflict.

Planning/Implementation	Rationale
Explore communication skills within the family unit.	Clients in abusive relationships often lack confidence and exhibit poor communication skills.
Refer the victim, her husband, and children to a family therapist to improve family coping skills.	Development of positive communication and coping skills within the family unit will enable the family to resolve conflict.

EVALUATION: Evaluation focuses on the ability of Andrea to regain control of her life and to live in an environment free of violence. The effectiveness of the interventions to improve Andrea's self-concept, reduce feelings of guilt and fear, and establish effective family coping skills and communication is included in the evaluation process.

KEY CONCEPTS

◆ Abuse of children, women, and the elderly; youth and workplace violence; and hate crimes have become widespread public health problems affecting individuals of all ethnic and socioeconomic backgrounds.

◆ Classification of child abuse includes physical abuse, child neglect, emotional abuse, and sexual abuse. Child abuse may occur in a variety of settings such as the home, institutional settings, or in society.

◆ Factors that may contribute to child abuse include parental stress, marital problems, financial difficulties, or parent–child conflict.

◆ Terms used to describe sexual abuse of a child include *sexual misuse*, *rape*, and *incest*.

◆ Classifications of child abduction, or kidnapping, include family, non-family or acquaintance, and stranger abduction. Approximately 69,000 children are abducted yearly.

◆ Domestic violence is defined as a pattern of coercive behaviors that may include repeated battering and injury, psychological abuse, sexual assault, progressive social isolation, deprivation, and intimidation.

◆ Identified factors that can contribute to domestic violence include neurologic impairments; various psychiatric disorders in which individuals are unable to control impulsive behaviors; the inability to nurture others; poor socioeconomic conditions; poor communication skills; learned abusive behaviors; and abusive behavior after a loss.

◆ Victims of domestic violence (intimate partner or spousal abuse) generally experience three phases: the tension-building phase, the acute battering phase, and the loving or honeymoon phase.

◆ Barriers to leaving a violent relationship include lack of resources, lack of institutional responses, and traditional ideology.

◆ Sexual harassment of women or men constitutes any unwelcome sexual advance or conduct on the job that creates an intimidating or offensive working environment.

◆ Three elements are necessary to define rape legally: the use of force, threat, intimidation, or duress; vaginal, oral, or anal penetration; and nonconsent by the victim.

◆ There is no typical rape-victim profile; every woman is a potential victim regardless of age, race, or socioeconomic status. Although most victims are women, men also experience sexual assault.

◆ Patterns of rape are classified as anger, power, sadistic, and impulsive or opportunistic rape according to motive involved.

◆ Dependency on adult children or the caretaker because of physical or mental disabilities, financial dependency, personality conflicts, or frustration on the part of adult children or the caretaker may predispose the elderly person to elder abuse.

◆ Youth and gang-related violence have escalated during recent years because of increased access to and use of firearms. Exposure to violence at home is the most accurate predictor of membership in a delinquent group.

◆ Predictors of workplace violence include angry or dissatisfied customers, clients with certain psychiatric disorders, domestic batterers, women with severe cases of premenstrual tension, disgruntled older male employees fearing a potential loss of their job, juvenile delinquents, and career criminals.

◆ Hate crimes are motivated by feelings of hostility against any identifiable group of people within a society (eg, race, religion, sexual orientation, ethnicity/national origin, disability).

◆ Assessment of victims of abuse or violence requires that the nurse display sensitivity, empathy, and confidentiality. Providing for privacy is essential during the collection of data.

◆ Nursing interventions address issues of anxiety, powerlessness, fear, pain, impaired communication, ineffective coping, disturbance in self-esteem or self-concept, risk for injury or violence, or clinical symptoms of post-trauma response or rape-trauma syndrome.

◆ Evaluation of the client's emotional and physical well-being after crisis intervention is an ongoing process because the consequences of abuse and violence may not be resolved for months or years.

For additional study materials, please refer to the Student Resource CD-ROM located in the back of this textbook.

CHAPTER WORKSHEET

CRITICAL THINKING QUESTIONS

1. Child abuse and neglect are epidemic in the United States. What might be the role and responsibility of nursing in responding to this crisis?
2. Explore your feelings about child abuse. How might you cope with meeting the parents of a child for whom you are caring and who you suspect is being abused?
3. As you perform a physical assessment on 78-year-old Mr. Brass, you notice bruises and tender areas on his upper arms and back. When you question him, he becomes agitated and tells you not to bother about them. You suspect elder abuse. What do you do?
4. Interview a layperson who has been trained as a rape counselor. How does her focus differ from a nursing focus? What can you teach each other about the care of a rape survivor?

REFLECTION

Reflect on the chapter opening quote by Richardson and Richardson. In your own words, interpret the message that the authors are relating. In what situations would it be appropriate to use this poster? Explain the rationale for your answer.

NCLEX-STYLE QUESTIONS

1. An 8-year-old boy is hospitalized on a psychiatric unit following aggressive, acting-out behavior in school and threatening to kill himself by running in front of a car. Nursing assessment identifies that the child has been the victim of physical abuse by his father. Which intervention would be the initial priority?

a. Helping the child describe the abuse in detail
b. Confronting the father with the child's allegations
c. Documenting complete assessment data in chart
d. Reporting the abuse to the appropriate community agency

2. Which of the following would the nurse interpret as most indicative of child abuse?
   a. Bruises on face or posterior side of body in various stages of healing
   b. Complaints of abdominal pain not accompanied by increased temperature
   c. Symptoms of dehydration after an episode of vomiting and diarrhea
   d. Temperature elevations unexplained by physical symptoms present

3. The community psychiatric nurse plans an educational program for a group of parents who have been abusive to their children. Which of the following topics would be most helpful in preventing future abusive incidents?
   a. Handling a child who is a "picky" eater
   b. Interacting with your child's teacher
   c. Importance of regular pediatric check-ups
   d. Managing stressful life events

4. A 35-year-old woman visits a family-planning clinic, and during interaction with the nurse reveals that her husband has frequently hit her when she visits friends or family members he does not like. Which intervention would be the priority?
   a. Encouraging the client to leave her husband before the situation becomes worse
   b. Instructing the client to talk about her feelings to her husband
   c. Providing the client with information about domestic violence and community resources
   d. Telling the client about the importance of obtaining marital counseling as soon as possible

5. Which nursing diagnosis would be most appropriate for an adult child who has admitted to abusing an elderly, dependent parent?

a. Anxiety
b. Caregiver Role Strain
c. Ineffective Coping
d. Ineffective Role Performance

6. The nurse is presenting a talk to a local community group about abuse and violence. Which statements would the nurse include? Select all that apply.
   a. Most perpetrators of child abuse are female
   b. More men than women abuse the elderly
   c. Men are typically the perpetrators of intimate partner abuse
   d. Individuals who abuse typically have no fear of authority
   e. Poor impulse control is a common trait with perpetrators of abuse

Selected References

Allen, M. C. (2006). Domestic violence: The Florida requirement. *CME resource: Continuing education for Florida nurses, 131*(2), 13–24.

American Medical Association. (2003). Sexual assault: The silent, violent epidemic. Retrieved July 12, 2003, from http://www.infoplease.com/ipa/A0001537.html

American Psychiatric Association. (2003). Violence and mentally ill clients. Retrieved July 12, 2003, from http://www.psych.org/public_info/violen~1.cfm

American Psychiatric Association. (2000). *Diagnostic and statistical manual of mental disorders* (4th ed., text revision). Washington, DC: Author.

Armour, S. (2006). Managers not prepared for workplace violence. Retrieved April 2, 2006, from http://usatoday.com

Bates, B. (1999). Behavioral strategies soothe traumatized children. *Clinical Psychiatry News, 27*(1), 32.

Brasseur, J. W. (1995, July/August). Child abuse: Identification and intervention. *Clinician Reviews, 5.*

Brown, K. (2004). Rape and sexual assault: Understanding the offense and the offender. *ADVANCE for Nurse Practitioners, 12*(8), 69–70.

Burgess, A. W., Brown, K., Bell, K., Ledray, L. E., & Poarch, J. C. (2005). Sexual abuse of older adults. *American Journal of Nursing, 105*(10), 66–71.

Campbell, J. (1986). Nursing assessment for risk of homicide in battered women. *Advances in Nursing Science,* (8).

Child Abuse Prevention and Treatment Act, Public Law 104-235, §111;42. U.S.C. 5106g (2003).

Childers, A. M. (2005). Child maltreatment. In K. Cheng & K. M. Myers (Eds.), *Child and adolescent psychiatry: The essen-*

tials (pp. 363–380). Philadelphia: Lippincott Williams & Wilkins.

Clements, P. T., DeRanieri, J. T., Clark, K., Manno, M. S., & Kuhn, D. E. (2005). Workplace violence and corporate policy for health care settings. *Nursing Economics, 23*(3), 119–124.

CNN.com. (2001). Study: Child sex abuse "epidemic" in U.S. Retrieved July 9, 2003, from http://www.cnn.com/2001/LAW/09/10/child.exploitation/index.html

Danielsen, R. D. (1998). Adolescent violence in America. *Clinician Reviews, 8*(5), 167–184.

Davidhizar, R., & Giger, J. N. (1995). Sexual harassment today: Workplace policy is the best form of prevention. *ADVANCE for Nurse Practitioners, 3*(12).

D. B. Pargman Diversity Training. (2003). Sexual harassment statistics. Retrieved July 12, 2003, from http://www.dbpargman.com/statssexual.htm

Douris, K., & Pritchard, M. (1999). When you suspect elder abuse. *ADVANCE for Nurse Practitioners, 7*(4), 22.

Elvik, S. L. (1995). Sexual abuse of the developmentally disabled. *ADVANCE for Nurse Practitioners, 3*(9).

Finkelhor, D., & Leatherman, J. D. (1994). Children as victims of violence: A national survey. *Pediatrics,* (10).

Flannery, R. B., Jr. (1995). *Violence in the workplace.* New York: Crossroad Press.

Flannery, R. B., Jr. (1997). *Violence in America: Coping with drugs, distressed families, inadequate schooling and acts of hate.* New York: Continuum.

Fulmer, T. (2004). Elder abuse and neglect assessment. *Dermatological Nursing, 16*(5), 473.

Grant, C. A. (1996a). The client who has been battered. In S. Lego (Ed.), *Psychiatric nursing: A comprehensive reference* (2nd ed., pp. 296–304). Philadelphia: Lippincott-Raven.

Grant, C. A. (1996b). The client who has been raped. In S. Lego (Ed.), *Psychiatric nursing: A comprehensive reference* (2nd ed., pp. 305–315). Philadelphia: Lippincott-Raven.

Grinfield, M. J. (2000). The big picture: Averting the course of violence. *Psychiatric Times, 17*(1), 1, 3–4.

HealthyMinds.org. (2006). Healthy minds, healthy lives. Psychiatric effects of media violence. Retrieved April 2, 2006, from http://healthyminds.org/mediaviolence.cfm

HealthyPlace.com. (2003). Safeline: Information for adult survivors of childhood sexual abuse. Retrieved September 14, 2003, from http://www.healthyplace.com/communities/abuse/safeline/survivors.htm

Humane Society of the United States. (2003). 2003 report of animal cruelty cases. Retrieved April 2, 2006, from http://www.hsus.org/ace/20929

Infoplease.com. (2006). Summary of hate crime statistics, 2003. Retrieved April 2, 2006, from http://www.infoplease.com/ipa/A0004885.html

KidsFightingChance.com. (2006). Statistics. Retrieved March 30, 2006, from http://www.kidsfightingchance.com/statistics.htm

Kimberg, L. (2001). Addressing intimate partner violence in primary care practice. *Medscape Women's Health, 6*(1).

Retrieved September 18, 2006, from http://www.medscape.com/viewarticle/408937

Klass Kids Foundation. (2006). Missing child statistics. Retrieved March 30, 2006, from http://www.klasskids.org/pg-mc-mcstatistics.htm

Koplewicz, H. S. (1999). Preempting teen violence. *Clinical Psychiatry News, 27*(11), 12.

Lachs, M. S., & Pillemer, K. (1995). Abuse and neglect of elderly persons. *New England Journal of Medicine,* (2).

Liddell, W. B. (2002). Does provider gender matter in sexual assault treatment? *ADVANCE for Nurse Practitioners, 10*(7), 51–52, 55–58, 75.

LoCascio, E. (2000). Sexual assault response teams: Current trends in care. *Vital Signs, 10*(12), 38–39.

Makar, M. C. (2000). *Domestic violence. Continuing education for Florida nurses, 2001.* Sacramento, CA: Continuing Medical Education Resource.

Matthews, A. M., & Mossefin, C. (2006). The "date" that changed her life. *Current Psychiatry, 9*(2), 75–76, 83–86.

Medical Education Group Learning Systems. (1995). *Nurse update: Domestic violence.* Jacksonville, FL: Author.

Muscari, M. E. (2005a). Animal cruelty as a predictor of human violence. *ADVANCE for Nurse Practitioners, 13*(4), 55–57, 63.

Muscari, M. E. (2005b). What should I do when a client is being stalked? Retrieved February 3, 2005, from http://www.medscape.com/viewarticle/497454

National Center for Injury Prevention and Control. (2001). Child maltreatment: Overview. Retrieved July 11, 2003, from http://www.cdc.gov/ncipc/factsheets/cmfacts.htm

National Center for Injury Prevention and Control. (2002). Youth risk behavior surveillance—U.S. Retrieved July 11, 2003, from http://www.cdc.gov/ncipc/factsheets/yvfacts.htm

National Center for Injury Prevention and Control. (2006a). Child maltreatment: Fact Sheet. Retrieved March 30, 2005, from http://www.cdc.gov/ncipc/factsheets/cmfacts.htm

National Center for Injury Prevention and Control. (2006b). Intimate partner violence: Fact sheet. Retrieved March 30, 2006, from http://www.cdc.gov/ncipc/factsheets/ipvfacts.htm

National Center for Injury Prevention and Control. (2006c). Youth violence: Fact sheet. Retrieved March 30, 2006, from http://www.cdc.gov/ncipc/factsheets/yvfacts.htm

National Center for Victims of Crime. (2003a). Get help on child victims and the law. Retrieved March 3, 2004, from http://www.ncvc.org/gethelp/childvictimsandthelaw

National Center for Victims of Crime. (2003b). Male rape. Retrieved September 14, 2003, from http://www.ncvc.org/gethelp/malerape/

National Center for Victims of Crime. (2004). Stalking. Retrieved May 17, 2004, from http://www.ncvc.org/stalkingandresourcecenter/

National Center on Elder Abuse. (1998). The national elder abuse incidence study. Retrieved December 13, 2003, from http://

www.aoa.gov/eldfam/Elder_Rights/Elder_Abuse/ABuseReport_Full.pdf

National Coalition Against Domestic Violence. (2003).The problem: Barriers to leaving a violent relationship.Retrieved July 7, 2003, from http://www.ncadv.org/problem/barriers.htm

National Institute of Mental Health. (2000a). Fact sheet: Child and adolescent violence research. Retrieved January 18, 2001, from http://www.nimh.nih.gov/publicat/violenceresfact.com

National Institute of Mental Health. (2000b). Fact sheet: Helping children and adolescents cope with violence and disasters. Retrieved January 18, 2001, from http://www.nimh.nih.gov/publication/violence.cfm

North Carolina Rape Crisis. (2003). What is rape? Retrieved March 3, 2004, from http://www.rapecrisisonline.com/articles.htm

Occupational Safety & Health Administration. (2003).Workplace violence. Retrieved July 13, 2003, from http://www.osha.gov/SLTC/workplaceviolence/

Occupational Safety & Health Administration. (2006). National census of fatal occupational injuries. Retrieved February 16, 2006, from http://www.osha.gov/SLTC/occupationalinjuries/

Petrocelli, W., & Repa, B. (1998). *Sexual harassment on the job. What it is and how to stop it.* Berkeley, CA: Nolo Press.

Philbin, G. S. (2004, March 24). Not too long on history. *Orlando Sentinel*, p. G10.

Pillitteri, A. (2003). *Maternal and child health nursing* (4th ed.). Philadelphia: Lippincott Williams & Wilkins.

Quillian, J. P. (1995). Domestic violence: Continuing education forum.*Journal of the American Academy of Nurse Practitioners*, 7(7), 351–359.

Quisenberry, S. (2006). Munchausen syndrome by proxy. *ADVANCE for Nurses*, 7(6), 13–16.

Reichlin, K. M. (2005).Violence by children and adolescents. In K. Cheng & K. M. Myers (Eds.), *Child and adolescent psychiatry: The essentials* (pp. 321–340). Philadelphia: Lippincott Williams & Wilkins.

Resnick, P. J., & Kausch, O. (1995). Violence in the workplace: Role of the consultant. *Consulting Psychology Journal: Practice and Research, 47*, 213–222.

Roye, C. F., & Coonan, P. R. (1997). Adolescent rape. *American Journal of Nursing*, 97(4), 45.

Sadock, B. J., & Sadock, V. A. (2003). *Kaplan & Sadock's synopsis of psychiatry: Behavioral sciences/clinical psychiatry.* Philadelphia: Lippincott Williams & Wilkins.

Shahrokh, N., & Hales, R. E. (Eds.). (2003). *American psychiatric glossary* (8th ed.). Washington, DC: American Psychiatric Press.

Sheridan, M. S. (2003). The deceit continues: An updated literature review of Munchausen syndrome by proxy. *Child Abuse & Neglect, 27*(4), 431–451.

Silent Tears. (2003). *Men are victims too!* Retrieved December 15, 2003, from http://silenttears.itgo.com/custom.html

Skuse, D., & Bentovim, A. (1994). Physical and emotional maltreatment. In M. Rutter, E. Taylor, & L. Hersov (Eds.), *Child and adolescent psychiatry* (3rd ed.). London: Blackwell Scientific.

Sugg, N. K., Thompson, R. S., Thompson, D. C., Maiuro, R., & Rivars, R. P. (1999, July/August). Domestic violence and primary care: Attitudes, practices, and beliefs. *Archives of Family Medicine, 8*, 301–306.

Sullivan, M. G. (2005). Spiritualized therapy may lessen symptoms in sex abuse survivors. *Clinical Psychiatry News, 33*(3), 18.

Thomas, K. (2003). Munchausen syndrome by proxy: Identification and diagnosis. *Journal of Pediatric Nursing, 18*(3), 174–180.

Thornton, T. N., Craft, C. A., Dahlberg, L. L., Lyncy, B. S., & Baer, K. (2000). *Best practices of youth violence prevention: A sourcebook for community action.* Atlanta, GA: National Center for Injury Prevention and Control.

Tumolo, J. (2003). Sticks and stones and slams: How girls use violence to tear each other down. *ADVANCE for Nurse Practitioners, 11*(11), 91–93.

U.S. Preventive Services Task Force. (2004). Screening for family and intimate partner violence: Recommendation statement. *American Journal for Nurse Practitioners, 8*(7), 31–38.

Voors, W. (2004). Dealing with bullying. *Clinician News, 8*(3), 15–16.

Walker, K. (1992). That was then: Elderly survivors of incest. *Journal of Psychosocial Nursing and Mental Health Services*, (1).

Wikipedia.org. (2006). Hate crimes.Retrieved April 2, 2006, from http://en.wikipedia.org/wiki/Hate_crimes

Wiseman, R. (1999). Violence in the workplace: Continuing education course #11. *Vital Signs, IX*(5).

Women Against Abuse. (2003). Statistics on domestic violence. Retrieved July 10, 2003, from http://www.libertynet.org/~waasafe/stats.html

Worcester, S. (2005). Gender myths that affect treatment. *Clinical Psychiatry News, 33*(1) 36.

World Health Organization. (2006). *Injuries and violence prevention.* Retrieved April 2, 2006, from http://www.who.int/violence_injury_prevention/violence/en/

World Health Organization, Regional Office for Africa. (2002). Press release: Trauma among children who are victims of violence. Retrieved July 7, 2003, from http://www.afro.who.int/press/2002/pr2002091602.html

Suggested Readings

Carpenito-Moyet, L. J. (2006). *Handbook of nursing diagnosis* (11th ed.). Philadelphia: Lippincott Williams & Wilkins.

Howard-Siewers, M. (2004). Crisis intervention in the workplace. *ADVANCE for Nurses, 5*(23), 27–29.

Kennedy, J. C., & Pollack, W. S. (2005). Adolescent violence: What school shooters feel and how psychiatrists can help. *Current Psychiatry, 4*(6), 12–16, 22.

Laubscher, A. L., & Corwin, El J. (2005). Inquiring about a history of childhood sexual abuse: Why NPS need to ask. *American Journal for Nurse Practitioners, 5*(9), 44–48, 53–54.

Muscari, M. E. (2003). Coach and activist: The NP's role in preventing youth violence. *ADVANCE for Nurse Practitioners, 11*(2), 37–41.

Muscari, M. E. (2004). Identifying victims and perpetrators of violence. *ADVANCE for Nurse Practitioners, 12*(4), 83–87.

National Center for Victims of Crime. (2003). Statistics: Workplace violence. Retrieved July 13, 2003, from http://www.ncvc.org/resources/statistics/workplaceviolence/

Paulk, D. (2001). Munchausen syndrome by proxy: Tall tales and real hurts. *Clinician Reviews, 11*(8), 51–57.

Paulk, D. (2004). How to recognize child abuse and neglect. *Clinical Advisor, 7*(10), 43–44, 47–49.

Schultz, J. M., & Videbeck, S. L. (2005). *Lippincott's manual of psychiatric nursing care plans* (7th ed.). Philadelphia: Lippincott Williams & Wilkins.

Thompson, R. (2005). Intimate partner violence: A culturally sensitive approach. *ADVANCE for Nurse Practitioners, 13*(5), 57–59.

Tumolo, J. (2001). Making children sick: Munchausen's syndrome by proxy. *ADVANCE for Nurse Practitioners, 9*(6), 103–106.

Walton-Moss, B. M., & Campbell, J. C. (2002). Intimate partner violence: Implications for nursing. *Online Journal of Issues in Nursing, 7*(1), Manuscript 5. Retrieved January 10, 2005, from http://www.nursingworld.org/ojin/topic17/tpc17_5.htm

Willis, D. G. (2004). Hate crimes against gay males: An overview. *Issues in Mental Health Nursing, 25*(2), 115–132.

CHAPTER 34 / CLIENTS COPING WITH ACQUIRED IMMUNODEFICIENCY SYNDROME (AIDS)

Although the central feature of HIV infection involves collapse of the body's ability to mount an appropriate cell-mediated immune response with attendant medical complications, neuropsychiatric phenomena can also be prominent. —SADOCK & SADOCK, 2003

AFTER STUDYING THIS CHAPTER, YOU SHOULD BE ABLE TO:

1. Explain the etiology of acquired immunodeficiency syndrome (AIDS).
2. Identify those groups of individuals at risk for AIDS.
3. Compare and contrast the following disease processes associated with AIDS: AIDS-related complex, secondary infectious diseases, and neuropsychiatric syndromes.
4. Describe the psychosocial impact of AIDS.
5. Discuss the effects of AIDS on family dynamics.
6. Recognize the clinical phenomena of each of the three phases of AIDS.
7. Formulate a plan of care for a client exhibiting clinical symptoms of the middle stage of AIDS.
8. Articulate the purpose of including interactive therapies in the plan of care for a client with AIDS.
9. Outline the types of community services available to provide continuum of care for clients with AIDS.

LEARNING OBJECTIVES

KEY TERMS

Acquired immunodeficiency syndrome (AIDS)

AIDS-related complex (ARC)

Homophobia

Human immunodeficiency virus (HIV)

Neuropsychiatric syndromes

Opportunistic infectious diseases

Secondary infectious diseases

Stigmatization

To be effective and provide compassionate care without undue fear or anxiety, health care professionals must be knowledgeable about the transmission, prevention, diagnosis, and treatment of individuals who have acquired immunodeficiency syndrome (AIDS) or who are infected with human immunodeficiency virus (HIV; Norman, 2006). AIDS is associated with numerous biopsychosocial complications, secondary infectious diseases, and AIDS-related disorders. The medical conditions (eg, persistent generalized lymphadenopathy, lymphoma, and pneumonia) and neuropsychiatric phenomena (eg, delirium, dementia, depression, and anxiety) associated with HIV-positive status and AIDS are pandemic (Sadock & Sadock, 2003).

Although neither a cure for the disease nor a preventive vaccine has been developed, therapeutic alternatives are providing benefit to many who are HIV-infected. Much has been learned about the complexities of HIV/AIDS, how to keep clients disease free longer, and how to manage their symptoms more effectively. As a result of these advances, individuals with HIV infection are living longer than before and the progression to AIDS has declined sharply (Norman, 2006; Tucker, 2006). Nurses play a key role in recognizing these conditions. Each of the conditions is usually treated by medication that puts the client at risk for the development of adverse effects on the central nervous system, as well as increases the risk for development of neuropsychiatric disorders.

This chapter focuses on the history, etiology, and epidemiology of AIDS; the clinical symptoms of AIDS, secondary infectious diseases, and AIDS-related disorders; the psychosocial impact of these disorders; and the effects of these disorders on family dynamics. The role of the psychiatric–mental health nurse and application of the nursing process are also discussed.

History and Etiology of HIV/AIDS

Beginning as a benign simian immunodeficiency virus (SIV) found in the African chimpanzee population, SIV evolved into a human-killer in the early 1930s, long before it was recognized as a disease. Analysis of a blood sample of a Bantu man who died of an unidentified illness in the Belgian Congo in 1959 made him the first human confirmed case of the SIV infection, later to be identified as HIV infection. The virus stayed in remote Africa until jet travel, big cities, and the sexual revolution spread it worldwide, according to Tanmoy Bhattachary, a researcher at the Los Alamos National Laboratory in Los Alamos, New Mexico (Associated Press, 2000).

In 1978, gay men in the United States and Sweden and heterosexuals in Tanzania and Haiti began to exhibit signs of the SIV infection. Between 1980 and 1983, there were 3,422 deaths in the United States attributed to the virus. During that time, doctors in New York and Los Angeles reported an unusual and deadly form of lung infection (*Pneumocystis carinii* pneumonia) and a rare skin cancer (Kaposi's sarcoma) among young homosexual men. In 1983, researchers at the Pasteur Institute, a private foundation dedicated to the prevention and treatment of diseases through biologic research, identified the cause of these conditions as the lymphadenopathy-associated virus. Referred to as HTLV-III (human T-cell lymphotropic virus), the virus was later renamed the **human immunodeficiency virus (HIV).** In 1986, HIV was identified as the virus that causes several conditions we now call **acquired immunodeficiency syndrome (AIDS).** In 1988, as an attempt to educate the public about this disease, the U.S. Surgeon General published and mailed a pamphlet, "Understanding AIDS," to more than a million citizens (Aegis.com, 2006; Avert.org, 2006; Fohn.net, 2006). Extensive research has led to the discovery that human immunodeficiency virus is carried in the blood, blood products, and body fluids such as semen. It is transmitted primarily through intimate sexual contact or through the sharing of needles by intravenous drug users.

Epidemiology

Global statistics, representative of cases in Africa, Asia, Europe, and North America, have remained fairly constant during the years 2001 through 2005. Figure 34-1 depicts the global distribution of HIV/AIDS as of 2001. In the year 2005, there were an estimated 39.4 million people living with HIV/AIDS worldwide compared with 40 million in 2001 (United Nations, 2006). Additionally, 2005 global statistics (MacNeil, 2006; United Nations, 2006) show that:

- 5 million individuals were infected. Of these 5 million, 2 million were children.
- Teenagers accounted for 50% of newly infected cases

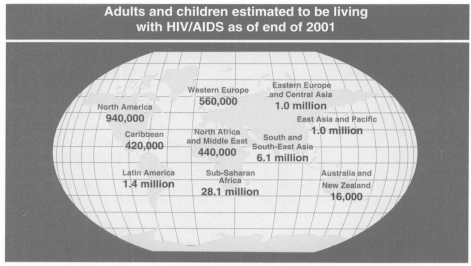

Total: 40 million

FIGURE 34.1   Global distribution of HIV/AIDS.

- 46% (or 18 million) to 50% (or 20 million) of infected cases were women and girls
- 25% to 33% of infected individuals were unaware of their status
- 3 million HIV/AIDS-related deaths occurred

In the United States, at the beginning of 2004, approximately 1,039,000 to 1,185,000 individuals were infected with HIV, and an estimated 405,925 individuals were living with AIDS. Approximately 25% of those individuals affected were women, compared with 20% in 2001. An estimated 21.8 million deaths have occurred since the first cases of AIDS were identified in 1981 (Seattle Biomedical Research Institute, 2003; United Nations, 2006).

Groups at Risk for AIDS

Approximately 2% to 4% of the U.S. population, or 4 to 5 million people, are at high risk for AIDS because of unsafe sexual practices or injection drug use. Groups at risk for development of AIDS include:

- African American and Hispanic populations
- Homosexual and bisexual men who do not practice safe sex
- Individuals with multiple sexual partners
- Adolescents who do not practice safe sex
- Heterosexual intravenous drug users
- Homosexual and bisexual men who also use intravenous drugs
- Heterosexual men and women who have had sex with a person from one of the previously mentioned groups
- Persons with hemophilia and others who have received blood transfusions
- Infants born to mothers carrying the AIDS virus
- Persons who are occupationally exposed (Centers for Disease Control [CDC], 2001; Davidson, 2004)

AIDS in Adolescents

In some developing countries, as many as 50% of young adults between the ages of 25 and 35 years are infected with the AIDS virus. In the United States, new HIV infections among young people between the ages of 15 and 24 years has been estimated to be 40,000 per year for the last few years. Given the fact that the average time of onset from infection to the development of AIDS is approximately 10 years, these young adults were probably infected as teenagers (CDC, 2000; Weiss, 2001).

Several factors have contributed to the rise of HIV infection in adolescents. Teens who engage in sexual exploration, including bisexual experimentation, generally have a sense of infallibility, or believe that HIV can be cured. "Russian roulette group sex" is an example of experimentation in which members of the group engage in sex knowing that one person in the group has HIV. The excitement is in the risk of becoming HIV-infected. Furthermore, lack of adequate protection by young teens places girls at high risk because immature cervixes are more likely to submit to infection (Ivantic-Doucette & Haglund, 2004).

Making decisions about disclosure is difficult for teens, who may lack social experiences and skills. Their fear of the loss of friends, family, and other supports, or lack of knowledge about the phenomena of the illness, often delays them from seeking help (Ferri, 1995; Weiss, 2001).

AIDS in the Older Adult

The number of elderly persons with HIV/AIDS continues to rise. According to the CDC (2000), 11% of all new AIDS cases in the United States occur in people age 50 years and older. In the past, little attention had been given to this group in the areas of prevention, education, psychosocial support or treatment because older people and their health care providers did not consider older adults to be at risk for contracting the AIDS virus. Individuals may live for many years with HIV infection but be asymptomatic. With aging, the immune system weakens, possibly leading to subtle signs of HIV. However, these signs may be attributed to normal physiologic changes during the aging process. Additionally, HIV testing may not be requested because of the belief that HIV infection affects young people or those who abuse substances. Older adults also may be too embarrassed to ask about the possibility of an infection. Consequently, as a result of a delay in the diagnosis of HIV, older adults often present with a more advanced disease process (CDC, 2000; Willard & Dean, 2000; Fox-Seaman, 2005; Norman, 2006).

Clinical Picture Associated With AIDS

The AIDS virus attacks an individual's immune system and emerges in the form of one or more of 12 **secondary infectious diseases** or **opportunistic infectious diseases** (an infection that occurs as a result of the individual's weak or compromised immune system resulting from AIDS, cancer, or immunosuppressive

drugs such as chemotherapy). Although the average time of the development of AIDS is about 10 years, HIV can occur between 6 months and 5 years after exposure to the virus. However, some people may carry the virus without showing symptoms of the disease for an indefinite period.

Secondary or Opportunistic Infectious Diseases

The two most common secondary or opportunistic infectious diseases found in AIDS clients are *Pneumocystis carinii* pneumonia and Kaposi's sarcoma, a rare form of skin cancer. *Pneumocystis carinii* pneumonia is characterized by a chronic, nonproductive cough and dyspnea that may be severe enough to result in hypoxemia and cognitive impairment. Kaposi's sarcoma presents with a blue-purple–tinted skin lesion.

Other most common infections are *Toxoplasma gondii,* caused by protozoa; *Cryptococcus neoformans* and *Candida albicans,* caused by fungi; *Mycobacterium avium-intracellulare,* caused by bacteria; and viruses such as the herpes simplex virus and cytomegalovirus.

All of these infectious diseases associated with AIDS have extremely painful, debilitating, and devastating physical and psychosocial effects (Figure 34-2). The physical symptoms may include:

- Nausea and vomiting
- Constant fever
- Chronic headaches
- Diarrhea
- Painful mouth infections
- Hypotension
- Liver and kidney failure
- Severe respiratory distress
- Incontinence
- Central nervous system dysfunction with psychomotor retardation

Early Symptomatic HIV Infection

Early symptomatic HIV infection (also known as **AIDS-related complex [ARC]**) is the stage of viral infection caused by HIV in which symptoms have begun to manifest, but before the development of AIDS (North Arundel Hospital, 2003). It is characterized by chronically swollen lymph nodes and persistent fever, cough, weight loss, debilitating fatigue, diarrhea, night sweats,

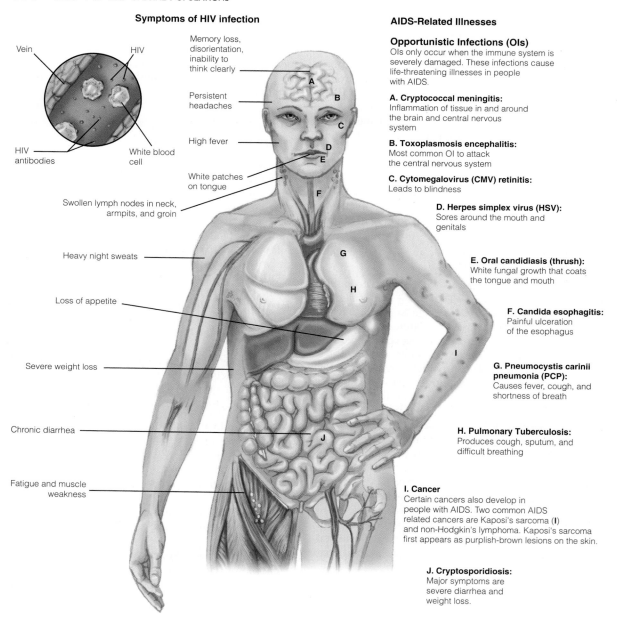

Symptoms of HIV infection

Vein

HIV

HIV antibodies

White blood cell

Memory loss, disorientation, inability to think clearly

Persistent headaches

High fever

White patches on tongue

Swollen lymph nodes in neck, armpits, and groin

Heavy night sweats

Loss of appetite

Severe weight loss

Chronic diarrhea

Fatigue and muscle weakness

AIDS-Related Illnesses

Opportunistic Infections (OIs)
OIs only occur when the immune system is severely damaged. These infections cause life-threatening illnesses in people with AIDS.

A. Cryptococcal meningitis:
Inflammation of tissue in and around the brain and central nervous system

B. Toxoplasmosis encephalitis:
Most common OI to attack the central nervous system

C. Cytomegalovirus (CMV) retinitis:
Leads to blindness

D. Herpes simplex virus (HSV):
Sores around the mouth and genitals

E. Oral candidiasis (thrush):
White fungal growth that coats the tongue and mouth

F. Candida esophagitis:
Painful ulceration of the esophagus

G. Pneumocystis carinii pneumonia (PCP):
Causes fever, cough, and shortness of breath

H. Pulmonary Tuberculosis:
Produces cough, sputum, and difficult breathing

I. Cancer
Certain cancers also develop in people with AIDS. Two common AIDS related cancers are Kaposi's sarcoma (**I**) and non-Hodgkin's lymphoma. Kaposi's sarcoma first appears as purplish-brown lesions on the skin.

J. Cryptosporidiosis:
Major symptoms are severe diarrhea and weight loss.

FIGURE 34.2 Symptoms of HIV infection and AIDS-related illness.

and pain. One third to one half of these individuals will go on to develop AIDS, whereas the others will show no progression of the disease. Additional information pertaining to the medical aspect of AIDS and its impact on health care providers can be obtained in medical–surgical nursing textbooks. Extensive data is also available online (see Internet Resources on the Student Resource CD-ROM).

HIV Infection and Neuropsychiatric Syndromes

Clients infected with the AIDS virus may develop an extensive array of **neuropsychiatric syndromes** (neurologic symptoms occurring as the result of organic disturbances of the central nervous system that constitute a recognizable psychiatric condition) such as HIV-associated dementia and HIV encephalopathy (Shahrokh & Hales, 2003). HIV-associated dementia is found in a large portion of clients infected with HIV; however, other causes of dementia (eg, vascular dementia or dementia secondary to substance abuse) also must be considered. HIV encephalopathy, a less severe form of neurologic dysfunction, is characterized by impaired cognitive functioning and reduced mental activity that interferes with activities of daily living, work, and social functioning. Delirium in HIV-infected clients is underdiagnosed. The etiology of dementia in HIV-infected clients can also cause clinical symptoms of delirium (Sadock & Sadock, 2003). (See Chapter 27 for additional information about clinical symptoms of dementia, delirium, and other cognitive disorders.) Box 34-1 lists the neurologic manifestations associated with HIV/AIDS.

BOX 34.1 NEUROLOGIC MANIFESTATIONS ASSOCIATED WITH HIV/AIDS

Cognitive impairment (eg, ARC or dementia)

Delirium secondary to opportunistic infections, neoplasms, cerebrovascular changes, metabolic abnormalities, or medication used in the management of HIV/AIDS

Personality change

Mood disorder secondary to organic changes

Delusional disorder secondary to organic changes

Psychosis secondary to AIDS–dementia complex

Drug–drug interactions between psychotropics and antiretrovirals

Extrapyramidal symptoms secondary to the use of antipsychotic agents

Myelopathy

Demyelinating neuropathies

Psychosocial Impact of AIDS

AIDS is frequently described as a tragic and complex phenomenon that provokes a shattering emotional and psychosocial impact on all who are involved with the illness. Indeed, AIDS connects medicine and psychiatry to a greater degree than any other major illness. Certain population groups have been identified as at risk for the psychosocial impact of AIDS, including:

- Clients in various stages of the illness
- Sexual partners and family of individuals with AIDS
- Individuals at particular risk for contracting the disease based on epidemiologic data
- Individuals with a mental disorder (eg, substance abuse) who fear exposure but refuse to be tested

The most serious psychosocial problems occur for those clients who actually have the disease. Most people with AIDS are relatively young, were previously healthy, and had not experienced a major medical illness. The confirmation of this diagnosis can be catastrophic for the client, eliciting a series of emotional and social reactions. These reactions include:

- A loss of self-esteem
- Fear of the loss of physical attractiveness and rapid changes in body image
- Feelings of isolation and stigmatization
- An overwhelming sense of hopelessness and helplessness
- A loss of control over their lives

In addition, emotional crises may result from the client's increasing isolation as he or she attempts to cope with the nearly universal stigma faced on a daily basis. AIDS clients experience rejection from all parts of society, including significant others, families, friends, social agencies, landlords, and health care workers. For many, this constant rejection causes a re-living of the "coming-out process," with a heightening of the associated anxiety, guilt, and internalized self-hatred. The fear of spreading AIDS to others can lead to further isolation and abandonment, commonly at a time when there is an ever-greater need for physical and emotional support. Clients with AIDS may respond with intense anger and hostility as their conditions deteriorate and they confront the everyday realities of this illness: loss of job and home, forced changes in lifestyle, the perceived lack of response by the medical community, and the often crippling expense associated with the illness.

HIV Infection and Psychiatric Disorders

Several comorbid psychiatric disorders have been observed in clients with HIV infection or AIDS. They include, but are not limited to, substance abuse, anxiety disorders, depressive disorders, adjustment disorders, and psychotic disorders.

The frequency of suicidal ideation and suicide attempts may increase in clients who are informed of the presence of HIV infection or AIDS, especially if they have inadequate social or financial support, experience relapses, or face difficult social issues relating to their sexual identity or sexual preferences (Sadock & Sadock, 2003). Box 34-2 describes the behavioral manifestations associated with HIV infection and AIDS. (See specific chapters for information regarding symptoms of and nursing interventions for substance abuse, anxiety, depression, adjustment reaction, and psychosis.)

The Worried Well

Individuals in high-risk groups who, although they test negative for the AIDS virus, have anxiety about contracting the virus are referred to as the *worried well*.

BOX 34.2 BEHAVIORAL MANIFESTATIONS ASSOCIATED WITH HIV/AIDS

Confrontation (eg, anger, aggressiveness, hostility, or impulsivity)

Impaired social functioning

Impaired occupational functioning

Overwhelming stress and anxiety due to preoccupation with clinical phenomena of HIV/AIDS

Sleep disturbances unrelated to stress, mood, or psychosocial problems but rather due to neuroendocrine dysfunctions, systemic inflammation, or obstructive sleep apnea

Lack of sexual function or interest due to fear of transmission of HIV, rejection by a partner, or hypogonadism

Suicide due to partial remission with an uncertain survival time after preparing oneself to die

---

Clinical symptoms of generalized anxiety disorder, panic disorder, obsessive–compulsive disorder, or hypochondriasis may develop if they do not receive reassurance that they are free of the AIDS virus (Sadock & Sadock, 2003). (See specific chapters for information regarding symptoms of and nursing interventions for anxiety and anxiety-related disorders).

Grief Reaction to HIV/AIDS

A four-stage grief reaction by clients diagnosed with AIDS has been described (Nichols, 1983). The reaction is similar to the pattern designated by Kübler-Ross in dying patients (Kübler-Ross, 1969; Nichols, 1983).

First Stage

The initial stage consists of shock, numbness, and disbelief. The severity of the reaction may depend on existing support systems for the individual. During this period, clients report sleep problems and an experience of depersonalization and derealization. For some, the acknowledgment of the AIDS diagnosis causes severe emotional paralysis or regression.

Second Stage

The second stage is denial, in which the person may attempt to ignore the diagnosis of AIDS. Although it may serve a necessary psychic function, this denial can cause the client to engage in behaviors that are both self-destructive and potentially dangerous to others. Some clients begin to plunge into complete isolation, avoiding human contact as much as possible.

Third Stage

In the third stage, the individual begins to question why he or she contracted AIDS. Expressions of guilt and anger are frequent as the client seeks to understand the reason for his or her illness. Homosexual or bisexual men may experience feelings of **homophobia** (ie, the unreasonable fear or hatred of homosexuals or homosexuality) and believe that God is punishing them for their homosexual preference.

Fourth or Final Stage

The fourth or final stage, that of resolution and acceptance, depends on the individual's personality and ego integration. This stage may be signified by the acceptance of the illness and its limitations, a sense of peace and dignity, and a preparation for dying. As the debilitating symptoms progress, however, other clients may become increasingly despondent and depressed, stop eating, express suicidal ideation, and develop almost-psychotic fixations and obsessions with their illness. A significant and growing number of AIDS clients make successful suicide attempts.

Effects of AIDS on Family Dynamics

The family of an AIDS client experiences severe psychological stress and trauma. The issue of the individual's sexuality and lifestyle, of which the family often was not aware, may create an additional crisis when they are confronted with the knowledge that their son, daughter, or sibling has a terminal illness. The pressure on the family system causes members to respond with quiet anger, confusion, and possible rejection of the AIDS client and his or her entire lifestyle. Families may blame the client's partner for the condition, but simultaneously find themselves forced to include the partner in their grief and in their attempts to cope with the illness.

Coleman (1988) describes the diagnosis of AIDS as creating a further challenge to the fragile balance of roles in the family system. An adult child who has been functioning independently for many years must now rely again on parental support to meet daily self-care needs. Parents are confronted with a change in their new retired lifestyle as the dying child comes home. Families also are forced to assume financial responsibility, which can further magnify their anger, guilt, and frustration. Some families are able to achieve resolution of their own painful psychological conflicts and provide the necessary physical and emotional support to the AIDS client. A significant number of families, however, become fixed in their rejection, grief, and anger and are never able to resolve the distance and estrangement from the family member with AIDS.

In response to this familial abandonment, the individual with AIDS often develops an alternate family that assumes the support and caretaker role. This new family may include a gay partner and close gay and straight friends who significantly alter their lifestyles to care for the client. These friends experience the same sense of loss, isolation, and bereavement as the more traditional family, but are denied the customary social support systems and public recognition for their role. Clinical Example 34-1 depicts the effects of AIDS on family dynamics.

THE NURSING PROCESS

ASSESSMENT

Assessment is a clearly defined activity, but may be difficult to initiate due to the sensitive nature of the topic of AIDS. The psychiatric–mental health nurse may find it difficult to ask clients about any history of drug use, their sexual activity, or the presence of alternative sexual lifestyles. It is important that personal issues and attitudes of the nursing staff do not interfere with the assessment and application of the nursing process. Early recognition of psychiatric disorders associated with HIV/AIDS is important to enhance one's understanding of clients' behavior.

The psychiatric–mental health nurse's understanding of the clinical phenomena of HIV/AIDS plays a critical role during assessment. Nurses consistently have underestimated the frequency and intensity of HIV signs and symptoms (Holzemer, 2002). For example, AIDS in the older adult raises unique assessment and treatment concerns. AIDS-dementia complex may be confused with other dementias that occur in the elderly, and cognitive impairment may be attributed to the aging process. Failure to assess or diagnose HIV infection denies the client proper treatment and care (Whipple & Scura, 1996; Willard & Dean, 2000).

Phases of Assessment

Clients may enter the health care system at different phases of their illness depending on their biopsychosocial and spiritual needs. Ripich (1997) discusses three phases of the HIV continuum (ie, from the time the client tests positive with HIV infection to the development of AIDS, including the progression of the disease). Following is a discussion of the psychiatric–mental

THE EFFECTS OF AIDS DIAGNOSIS ON FAMILY DYNAMICS

MP, a 41-year old male, left home to attend college in California at the age of 18 years. Following graduation, at the age of 22 years, MP chose to remain in California and work as an electronic engineer at a major corporation. He became sexually involved with another male employee, GW, who was 3 years his senior. MP's parents were not aware of his sexual relationship with GW. At the age of 39 years, MP was diagnosed as HIV-positive. Approximately 1 year later, he began to exhibit clinical symptoms of AIDS.

Although MP was unable to continue to work, GW continued to stay with him and was quite supportive in all aspects of his life. MP became quite ill and was hospitalized with a diagnosis of *Pneumocystis carinii* pneumonia. GW notified MP's parents of his hospitalization. When MP's parents arrived at the hospital, MP told them about his lifestyle and illness. Both parents reacted with disbelief but remained in California until MP was released from the hospital.

Approximately 9 months later, MP called his parents and asked them if he could return home because he was no longer able to perform his activities of daily living independently and did not want to remain a burden to GW. His parents, who were now retired, agreed to let him return home. When MP arrived home, his parents were shocked by his physical appearance because MP had lost a significant amount of weight since they had last seen him. He looked quite pale and appeared to tire easily. They also noted that MP had difficulty concentrating and was unable to remember details of previous conversations.

Although MP no longer had medical benefits, his parents agreed to provide financial support as he entered the terminal phase of AIDS and received palliative medical and nursing care through hospice. Both of MP's parents were quite active in the church, and, with MP's permission, asked the parish priest to provide spiritual support for the entire family. MP died a few months later, following his 48th birthday.

health nurse's role in the assessment of each of the phases. (Note: The focus of discussion here is on assessment and treatment of the psychosocial impact of HIV/AIDS. The reader is referred to medical–surgical texts for a complete discussion of the complex medical assessment and treatment.)

Early-Phase Assessment. Clients who first learn that they are HIV-positive are considered to be in the early phase of the HIV continuum. The major thrust of the assessment at this time is to obtain data that will enable the nurse to (1) formulate a plan of care to improve or stabilize the client's emotional and physical well-being and (2) empower the client to maintain a sense of control over as many aspects of his or her life as possible.

As noted in Box 34-3, the client in the early phase of HIV/AIDS may exhibit various clinical phenomena when told that he or she is HIV-positive. The client is faced with many difficult decisions because life goals may not be achievable, and living day to day becomes the ultimate goal (Ripich, 1997).

The initial assessment of the client suspected of having HIV infection or AIDS generally occurs in the primary care setting unless the client has been admitted to an acute care hospital or an inpatient psychiatric setting, or requests testing while receiving psychiatric–mental health care as an outpatient. The initial assessment usually includes a comprehensive history and physical evaluation including a review of the client's present complaints, baseline laboratory testing, nutritional assessment, psychosocial assessment, and determination of the client's knowledge of the disease

---

BOX 34.3 CLINICAL PHENOMENA OF EARLY-PHASE HIV/AIDS

- Denial
- Shock, anger, panic
- Fear of incapacitation
- Fear of physical and mental deterioration
- Fear of deformity and pain
- Shame
- Disappointment
- Depression
- Suicidal ideation
- Sudden awareness that death is possible

process (Burnett, 2001). Formal neurologic and psychological testing is often conducted to determine the extent of the disease process. Clients are generally referred to the psychiatric–mental health nurse or other mental health professionals to rule out the presence of a comorbid neuropsychiatric syndrome or psychiatric disorder (Kongable, 1998).

The psychiatric–mental health nurse assesses the client for:

- Clinical symptoms of anxiety and depression (eg, fatigue, insomnia)
- Clinical symptoms of impaired memory or cognitive impairment
- Suicidal ideation
- Substance abuse or chemical dependency
- Domestic-violence issues
- Legal issues
- Effective coping skills
- Any fears or myths about the disease
- Adequate support systems (eg, family or significant others, spiritual, financial, legal)
- The initial stage of the grief process (eg, denial)
- Medical support system to evaluate physical concerns or complaints (Burnett, 2001)

Middle-Phase Assessment. During the middle phase, the HIV-infected client begins to experience symptoms that will ultimately result in a decline in health. Clinical phenomena, listed in Box 34-4, challenge coping mechanisms such as denial, as the client realizes he or she is losing control due to uncertainty about the future. The nurse assesses the client's:

- Knowledge of the progression of the disease process
- Knowledge of and consent to treatment options
- Coping skills as the disease process progresses
- Self-esteem
- Perception of body image
- Desires regarding the use of life-support systems, emergency measures, and hospice care

Concerns verbalized by family members or significant others are identified.

Late-Phase Assessment. By the late phase, the client ideally has reached a realistic level of acceptance of his or her health status and uncertain future and may elect to begin a *life-review process* (ie, reflecting on one's life and finding peace with it) and make final preparations for death (Ripich, 1997). During the late phase of the HIV continuum, the nurse assesses the client for:

- Changes in mental status (eg, clinical symptoms of dementia, delirium, acute psychosis, severe anxiety, personality change, depression, or suicidal ideation)
- An ability to maintain independence and control of his or her environment
- Physical or cognitive changes that interfere with activities of daily living
- Any concerns about changes in medical status

Box 34-5 lists the clinical phenomena related to late-phase HIV/AIDS.

BOX 34.4 CLINICAL PHENOMENA OF MIDDLE-PHASE HIV/AIDS

- Sense of isolation and alienation from partner, family, or friends
- Anger and acting-out behavior
- Low self-esteem
- Feelings of guilt, helplessness, vulnerability, and loss of control
- Fear of violence secondary to homophobia or social stigma
- Changes in physical appearance
- Passivity
- Paranoia or ideas of reference
- Depression

BOX 34.5 CLINICAL PHENOMENA OF LATE-PHASE HIV/AIDS

- Ambivalence about dying alone or with loved ones present
- Attempt to disengage or emotionally detach oneself from others
- Ambivalence regarding the ability to control the dying process
- Desire to complete a life review process with or without friends and family present
- Desire to have spiritual needs addressed before death
- Resolution regarding death in the form of acceptance or passive resignation

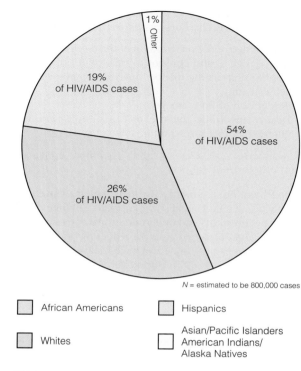

N = estimated to be 800,000 cases

☐ African Americans   ☐ Hispanics

☐ Whites   ☐ Asian/Pacific Islanders
American Indians/
Alaska Natives

FIGURE 34.3 Frequency of HIV/AIDS cases reported in various cultures according to 2000 Centers For Disease Control and Prevention report.

Transcultural Considerations

A significant aspect of assessment is the need to be aware of the prevalence of the HIV virus in different cultures. Boyle (2003) discusses the HIV/AIDS pandemic and the fact that the HIV virus disproportionately affects selected groups, especially African Americans and Hispanics. Of equal concern, minority women are particularly at risk, especially in rural areas (Boyle, 2003). Figure 34-3 depicts, by culture, the frequency of HIV/AIDS in the United States (CDC, 2000). Table 34-1 compares the epidemiology of HIV/AIDS among men and women of different cultures (CDC, 2000).

Cultural Beliefs and Myths. During the assessment, the psychiatric–mental health nurse needs to be aware of cultural beliefs and myths that may be expressed by the client in an attempt to justify HIV infection or AIDS. Although research has identified the etiology of AIDS, several cultural myths explain the cause inaccurately

TABLE 34.1 Epidemiology of HIV/AIDS Among Men and Women of Different Cultures

CULTURE	WOMEN	MEN
African American	64%	50%
Hispanic	18%	20%
White	18%	30%
Heterosexual	75%	15%
MSM*	n/a	42%
IDU**	25%	25%

*Men having sex with men.
**Infected by drug use.

SOURCE: Centers for Disease Control and Prevention. (2000). *Epidemiology of AIDS*. Retrieved from http://www.cdc.gov/

(Ripich, 1997; Trzcianowska & Mortensen, 2001). For example, some cultural myths state that AIDS:

- Is a form of punishment for wrongdoing
- Has occurred as a message to teach people to get along with each other
- Is the result of a sick world
- Is the result of a government germ-warfare experiment

Another myth is that the cause of AIDS has been fabricated to allow pharmaceutical companies and the health care system to profit financially from the sale of expensive drugs and use of specific treatment protocols.

It is important to recognize that such myths exist. Be sure to assess the client for beliefs in such myths. The psychiatric–mental health nurse must be prepared to discuss them if the client or a family member introduces the subject.

Ethnic Issues of Homophobia and Stigmatization. Not only is it imperative that the nurse be aware of cultural beliefs and myths about AIDS, but the ethnic issues of homophobia and **stigmatization** (ie, to set a mark of disgrace or shame upon an individual) may also need to be addressed during the initial assessment.

Norman (1996) discusses the problems of homophobia and stigmatization of men having sex with men in ethnic communities of color as well as in the society at large. Social and emotional isolation, disapproval, prejudice, judgments of shame and immorality, and even violence may occur. Attitudes of various ethnic communities may be influenced by organized religion, conceptualizations of men having sex with men, and the value placed on civil liberties. Dual standards for men and women extend to cultural attitudes toward monogamy, expression of sexuality, talking about sexuality, condom use, who may initiate sexual intercourse, and reproduction. A client may be reluctant to seek treatment unless he or she knows that the health care providers will respect his or her individuality and alternative lifestyle. (See Chapter 26 regarding transcultural considerations when conducting a sexual history.)

Assessment for Immune Recovery Syndrome

Since the emergence and widespread use of highly active antiretroviral therapy (HAART) in the treatment of AIDS, clients and health care providers have seen significant decreases in AIDS-related diseases and death (Grodesky, 2002). Although it is beyond the scope of this text to discuss the complex medical treatment of HIV/AIDS, it is important to mention that the psychiatric–mental health nurse must be able to distinguish among significant adverse effects of psychoactive drugs, HAART therapy, and symptoms resulting from the immune recovery process. Additional information regarding the immune recovery syndrome may be obtained online (see Internet Resources on the Student Resource CD-ROM).

Assessment As a Secondary Prevention

Secondary prevention of HIV during mental health care visits for clients who are at risk is as critical with HIV as it is for breast, cervical, or prostate cancer (Konkle-Parker, 1998). The psychiatric–mental heath nurse should tell the client that he or she is not being singled out, but rather is being given an opportunity to discuss sensitive issues that could place him or her at risk for HIV infection. A nonjudgmental approach is essential while obtaining a history of blood transfusions, drug use, and unprotected sex. The importance of HIV testing for those clients at risk should also be discussed.

NURSING DIAGNOSES

Formulating nursing diagnoses for the client with HIV/AIDS can be challenging, given the complexity of the illness, the client's psychosocial needs, and neurologic changes that occur as the client progresses through the different stages. See the accompanying Examples of North American Nursing Diagnosis Association (NANDA) Nursing Diagnoses for the client with HIV/AIDS.

OUTCOME IDENTIFICATION

The psychiatric–mental health nurse collects data to formulate a plan of care and works collaboratively with the medical health care provider to establish outcomes that:

- Address psychosocial issues such as living with a chronic illness and dying
- Empower the client to maintain a sense of control over his or her life during the progression of the disease
- Educate the client about HIV disease, infection control, available treatments, and medications

---

EXAMPLES OF NANDA NURSING DIAGNOSES/ HIV/AIDS

- Ineffective Health Maintenance related to lack of motivation to seek treatment for HIV/AIDS
- Disturbed Thought Processes related to neurologic changes as evidenced by a decline in cognition
- Anticipatory Grieving related to knowledge that HIV/AIDS is a terminal illness
- Death Anxiety as evidenced by statement, "I'm afraid to die," during individual therapy
- Hopelessness related to deterioration of physical condition secondary to HIV/AIDS
- Impaired Social Interaction related to alienation from others secondary to low self-concept
- Ineffective Coping related to altered appearance (significant weight loss) due to HIV/AIDS disease process
- Deficient Knowledge regarding illness and safe use of medication
- Situational Low Self-Esteem related to loss of independence and autonomy secondary to debilitating illness
- Spiritual Distress related to challenges to belief system secondary to terminal illness

- Monitor health status and manage symptoms
- Promote adequate nutrition and other health-maintenance goals
- Provide palliative care (Schultz & Videbeck, 2005)

PLANNING INTERVENTIONS AND IMPLEMENTATION

Major clinical advances that began in 1996 have dramatically changed the treatment and course of HIV/AIDS. These significant gains have come from a clearer understanding of the pathogenesis of HIV infection, the development of stronger and more effective therapeutic agents, the development of combination therapies, and the use of carefully selected complementary therapies. A holistic, multidisciplinary approach that augments the available treatment and management options for clients is used to improve palliative outcomes and enhance overall well-being.

Early-Phase Planning and Implementation

Nursing interventions for clients with HIV/AIDS vary according to the feelings and clinical phenomena exhibited. During the early phase, the nurse encourages the client to express thoughts and feelings, assists the client in accepting the diagnosis, and reassures the client that professional help is available. Crisis intervention, counseling, client education, and referral to support groups are examples of interventions used during this stage as personal values and internal conflicts are explored. If the client verbalizes thoughts about death or suicide, interventions are planned to help the person explore such thoughts and feelings. If a suicide plan is revealed, its lethality is determined and appropriate interventions are used (see Chapter 31).

Middle-Phase Planning and Implementation

Clinical phenomena of the middle phase may last for years. They include changes in physical appearance such as weight loss, somatic preoccupation in anticipation of changes in physical status, and an actual decline in physical condition as the illness progresses. Medical problems may include infections such as toxoplasmosis, herpesvirus, cryptococcal meningitis, lymphomas, and toxic effects of treatment. Central nervous system

pathology may contribute to deficits in intellectual, cognitive, and sensorimotor function and disturbances in personality or behavior. Interventions for clinical symptoms related to dementia, delirium, depression, anxiety, and personality disorders are discussed in previous chapters. Because symptoms progress differently for each client, individualizing the plan of care is important to address deficits in the client's ability to meet basic needs, as well as to meet the client's psychosocial needs.

Assistance With Meeting Basic Needs. After the client's clinical symptoms have been identified and the client's preferences and resources regarding the best possible approach to care are known, interventions are provided by the psychiatric–mental health nurse personally or in collaboration with members of the treatment team if a multidisciplinary treatment team approach is used.

Interventions usually focus on the progression of intellectual and cognitive dysfunction, impaired sensorimotor function, and the presence of personality or behavioral disturbances (Ripich, 1997). They include:

- Assisting the client with activities of daily living if the client has impaired sensorimotor function or intellectual and cognitive dysfunction
- Providing adequate nutrition
- Providing an environment that includes safety measures and support to prevent injury secondary to impaired sensorimotor function or confusion
- Monitoring vital signs and laboratory results during HAART therapy to minimize adverse effects
- Providing relief of symptoms such as pain, cough, and diarrhea as the clinical symptoms of HIV/AIDS progress
- Providing opportunities for the client to socialize with friends and family

Medication Management. The nurse must be fully aware of the pharmacokinetic and pharmacodynamic properties of the prescribed psychotropic agents and antiretroviral drugs used to treat HIV/AIDS. Because of the potential for medication interactions, appropriate dosages for psychotropic agents (eg, antidepressants, antianxiety agents, neuroleptic agents) are calculated based on the guidelines used for older adult populations. A medication typically starts with a low dose, builds up slowly, and achieves a significantly lower peak than that targeted in seronegative individuals. It is recommended that medication be prescribed by an expert in the treatment of mental illness and HIV/AIDS or by a member of a consultation team that contains experts in the various subfields. All clients need to be monitored closely for early signs of adverse effects or drug–drug interactions, as well as medication compliance, because adverse effects are both more prevalent and more severe in clients with HIV/AIDS disease (Whitaker, 1999).

Caution must be exercised when prescribing psychotropic drugs to clients taking protease inhibitors. Because both classifications of drugs are similarly metabolized, the serum levels of psychotropic drugs are generally increased. Antidepressant and antipsychotic agents are prescribed at 25% of the usual recommended dosage. Benzodiazepines should be avoided because they compromise cognitive function (Sadock & Sadock, 2003).

Assistance With Emotional Needs. The nurse also provides interventions for special concerns verbalized by the client and his or her partner, family, and friends (see Supporting Evidence for Practice 34-1). For example, sexuality and safe-sex education are discussed with the client and partner if desired, healthy lifestyles are explored, and family therapy is provided to discuss rejection or reconciliation issues.

Interactive therapies are provided to assist the client in:

- Verbalizing feelings and fears related to disfigurement and loss of control
- Finding new meaning in life while adapting to limitations of his or her illness
- Coping with possible condemnation and rejection from society, family, friends, and health care workers
- Maintaining continuing communication among all involved social and medical agencies and providers
- Resolving multiple and complex financial and legal concerns
- Reconciling with estranged family members or significant others
- Facing and discussing death and dying issues while maintaining respect and dignity
- Discussing and exploring ethical and moral beliefs about rational suicide

Late-Phase Planning and Implementation

In the late phase, death is relatively near. The nurse provides palliative care interventions. Because fewer invasive procedures and examinations are performed

---

SUPPORTING EVIDENCE FOR PRACTICE 34.1

Understanding the Various Factors that Promote the Progression of AIDS

PROBLEM UNDER INVESTIGATION / How do serum cortisol levels, coping strategies, stressful events, social support, and depression affect the disease progression of AIDS?

SUMMARY OF RESEARCH / A sample of 82 homosexual men with HIV type-1 infection were evaluated every 6 months for all measurements except social support, which was assessed yearly for 7.5 years. Subjects were given a battery of scales and questionnaires to assess stressful life events, depressive symptoms, and coping skills. Four serum cortisol levels were drawn initially at 20-minute intervals, along with a CD4 count. These counts were drawn periodically to measure disease progression. Adjustment was made for race, baseline CD4 count, viral load, and cumulative average antiretroviral drugs.

Results indicated that subjects with higher average serum cortisol levels, higher cumulative average stressful life events, lower cumulative satisfaction with social support, and those who used denial as a coping mechanism had a faster progression of AIDS.

SUPPORT FOR PRACTICE / The results of this study, along with other studies by the same researchers, provide strong evidence that psychosocial interventions such as the presence of adequate social support and positive coping skills and the stabilization of clinical symptoms of depression may slow the progression of AIDS.

SOURCE: Leserman, J., Petitto, J. M., Golden, R. N., Gaynes, B. N., Gu, H., Perkins, D. O., et al. (2000). Impact of stressful life events, depression, social support, coping, and cortisol on progression of AIDS. The American Journal of Psychiatry, 157(8), 1221–1228.

in the late phase of AIDS, most interventions focus on symptom management, such as for cognitive dysfunction due to HIV-associated dementia and for HIV encephalopathy. The wishes of the client set forth in a living will or relegated by durable power of attorney to a family member or significant other are respected and implemented at this time. In some instances, a health care surrogate may be designated to make decisions (Coyne, Lyne, & Watson, 2002).

The nurse remains available and assists the client in expressing his or her feelings regarding this final stage of life. Clients often want to review happier times or talk about regrets during a life-review process. The nurse encourages the client to express feelings and may ask if there are friends or relatives to call or messages to send.

The needs of family members and significant others are also considered; the nurse assists them in understanding and experiencing their own grief. This may be done without the physical presence of the client (Lego, 1996; Ripich, 1997).

Client and Family Education

HIV/AIDS education generally begins when the client is first diagnosed as being HIV-positive. Ideally, members of the family or a significant other would be involved during this process. The nurse considers the cognitive and intellectual abilities of the client and family members or significant other to avoid any misunderstanding about the disease process and treatment, including alternative therapies.

Most communities have established full-service agencies to educate clients and family members about HIV/AIDS. These agencies are often composed of volunteers from the community and health professionals who work together to provide education to individuals with HIV/AIDS and their families. The comprehensive services provided include, for example, 24-hour telephone hotlines, community AIDS clinics, educational groups, financial counseling, and hospice services.

Community Support Groups. Support groups have become the key element in providing treatment. These groups, established by community and gay-oriented organizations to respond to this health crisis and to lessen the isolation of people with AIDS, involve a variety of concerned volunteers. Through use of the buddy system, and with the assistance of trained professionals, these specialized groups provide emotional and physical support, assistance with daily chores, legal and financial planning, and advocacy with the appropriate social and government agencies. Lawyers can minimize some of the emotional trauma by helping the individual make crucial decisions regarding hospital visitation rights, treatment options, power of attorney, and disposition of property. Hirsch and Enlow (1985) describe the benefit of helping the person with AIDS retain legal and personal control over his or her life for as long as possible.

Continuum of Care

Many hospitals and long-term care units have responded to the demand for continuum of care by providing a special care unit for clients with AIDS, specifically designed to address the particular medical and psychological needs of the AIDS client. They are staffed by health care professionals and gay volunteer counselors who have been trained in working with the terminally ill client. Chapter 8 provides additional information about the concept of continuum of care.

EVALUATION

Traditional evaluation strategies are effective when stated outcomes reflect realistic, attainable expectations. In other words, outcomes should reflect the uncertainty of the client's life. Failure to develop such outcomes often results in client frustration (Ripich, 1997).

During the evaluation process, the nurse may identify the need to make several adjustments because of the progression of the disease process and development or existence of a comorbid mental illness. Continuum of care is evaluated to determine whether all possible support systems are in place as the client deals with the final stage of life. Chapter 7 addresses loss, grief, and end-of-life care. See Nursing Plan of Care 34-1: The Client With AIDS.

NURSING PLAN OF CARE 34.1

THE CLIENT WITH AIDS

Gary, age 38, a single white man, has been seeing a nurse therapist weekly for 8 months with complaints of anxiety, sleep disturbances, and angry outbursts. Gary is a banker with a master's degree in business administration. He is a member of the Jaycees, an active member of his church, and the captain of his bank's softball team. He grew up in the Midwest and remains close to his parents and younger brothers, although they reside in another state. A gourmet cook, Gary had planned to retire early and travel around the world with his significant other. He is homosexual and was diagnosed with AIDS 5 months prior to beginning individual therapy. Although he tested seropositive, he is asymptomatic at present.

DSM-IV-TR DIAGNOSIS: Adjustment disorder with anxiety

ASSESSMENT: Personal strengths: Asymptomatic; college education; actively involved in sports, church, and the community; financially solvent; supportive family and significant other; motivated for treatment.

Weaknesses: Ineffective coping skills

NURSING DIAGNOSIS: Ineffective Coping related to diagnosis of AIDS as evidenced by outbursts of anger

OUTCOME: The client will identify personal coping patterns to reduce anger.

Planning/Implementation	Rationale
Assess the client's present coping status.	The client may not recognize positive coping skills.
Encourage verbalization of cause of anger.	Verbalizing anger about his illness is an initial step toward dealing constructively with his personal feelings.
Validate the client's anger regarding his illness.	Validating the client's thoughts, especially negative thoughts, may relieve some of the client's anger and enable him to cope effectively with his feelings.

NURSING DIAGNOSIS: Anxiety related to confirmation of AIDS diagnosis and threat to biologic integrity as evidenced by client's verbalization of anxiety.

OUTCOME: The client will verbalize an increase in psychological and physiologic comfort.

Planning/Implementation	Rationale
Make observations to the client about his anxious behavior.	The client may not be aware of the relationship between his anger about his illness and his anxious behavior.
Encourage the client to express feelings about his illness.	The more specific the client can be about his feelings, the better equipped he will be to deal with his illness.
Provide information about HIV/AIDS.	Providing the client with information about AIDS gives him an opportunity to ask questions and may reduce his anger and anxiety.

(Continued on following page)

NURSING DIAGNOSIS: Disturbed Sleep Pattern related to anxiety response secondary to the diagnosis of AIDS

OUTCOME: The client will identify techniques to induce sleep.

Planning/Implementation	Rationale
Assess the client's usual bedtime routine.	The client may identify external stimuli or verbalize habits that interfere with relaxation.
Educate the client about sleep hygiene practices such as the avoidance of caffeine, alcohol, or exercise prior to bedtime.	The client may never have had a need to purposefully relax before retiring.

EVALUATION: Gary's ability to control his anger, his level of physiologic and psychological comfort, and his sleep pattern are evaluated. The progression of Gary's illness and the need for medical intervention are also evaluated during each visit.

KEY CONCEPTS

◆ Although acquired immunodeficiency syndrome (AIDS) emerged in 1981 and human immunodeficiency virus (HIV) was identified in 1986, at this time there is neither a cure for the disease nor a preventive vaccine.

◆ Global statistics, representative of HIV/AIDS cases in Africa, Asia, Europe, and North America have remained fairly constant during the years 2001 through 2005, with an estimated 39.4 million cases. In the United States, at the beginning of 2004, approximately 1,039,000 to 1,185,000 individuals were infected with HIV, and an estimated 405,925 individuals were living with AIDS.

◆ The AIDS virus attacks an individual's immune system and emerges in the form of one or more of 12 secondary infectious diseases or malignant cancer. All of the AIDS-related diseases have painful, debilitating, and devastating physical and psychological effects.

◆ Neuropsychiatric syndromes caused by the AIDS virus include AIDS-related complex (ARC), HIV-associated dementia, and HIV encephalopathy.

◆ The confirmation of AIDS can be catastrophic for the client, eliciting a series of emotional and social reactions. Clients may experience a comorbid psychiatric disorder such as anxiety, depression, or psychosis or exhibit clinical symptoms of a grief reaction to AIDS.

◆ Individuals who test negative for the AIDS virus but exhibit anxiety about contracting the virus are referred to as the *worried well*.

◆ The family of a client with HIV/AIDS often experiences severe psychological stress and trauma that challenges the fragile balance of roles in the family system.

◆ Assessment is difficult to initiate because of the sensitive nature of the topic. The psychiatric–mental health nurse may find it difficult to ask clients about any history of drug use, sexual activity, or the presence of alternative sexual lifestyles.

◆ Clients may enter the health care system at different phases of their illness depending on their biopsychosocial and spiritual needs. The major thrust of assessment is to obtain data that will enable the nurse to formulate a plan of care to improve or stabilize the emotional and physical well-being of clients and to empower clients to maintain a sense of control over as many aspects of their lives as possible

◆ Assessment is ongoing as clients experience the clinical phenomena of the different phases of the disease process.

◆ Major clinical advances have dramatically changed the treatment and management of HIV/AIDS due to a clearer understanding of the pathogenesis of HIV infection, the development of stronger and more effective therapeutic agents, the development of combination therapies, and the use of carefully selected complementary therapies.

◆ Most communities have established full-service agencies to provide continuum of care for HIV/AIDS clients and their families.

◆ During the evaluation process, the nurse may identify the need to make several adjustments to the plan of care because of the progression of the disease and development or existence of a comorbid mental illness. Continuum of care is also evaluated to determine whether all possible support systems are in place as the client experiences the final stage of life.

For additional study materials, please refer to the Student Resource CD-ROM located in the back of this textbook.

 ## CHAPTER WORKSHEET

CRITICAL THINKING QUESTIONS

1. Review nursing history to learn about other epidemics to which nurses have responded. How are the social, economic, and political conditions surrounding those epidemics similar to conditions surrounding the AIDS epidemic? How are the conditions different?
2. Considering developmental, social, and psychological issues, what would you tell a group of sexually active teenagers about AIDS?
3. Nurses on the forefront of providing care for clients with AIDS in the home and hospice environments are seldom recognized by the media. What strategies would you use to create media interest in this remarkable work?

REFLECTION

According to the chapter opening quote by Sadock and Sadock, clients with HIV infection may develop neuropsychiatric phenomena. Prepare an educational tool to inform HIV-infected clients and their families or significant others about the neuropsychiatric syndromes and psychiatric disorders associated with AIDS. What approach would you use? Explain the rationale for your approach. Would you provide the clients and other attendees an opportunity to interact with you and others during the discussion?

NCLEX-STYLE QUESTIONS

1. A 32-year-old homosexual male has recently been diagnosed with *Pneumocystis carinii* pneumonia as a result of AIDS. He is hospitalized and receiving treatment on a medical–surgical unit. He tells the nurse, "I did everything the doctor told me when I was diagnosed as having HIV and it didn't matter. I still got sick." The nursing diagnosis most appropriate for this client is
   a. Disturbed Thought Processes related to neurologic changes
   b. Ineffective Coping related to altered appearance
   c. Hopelessness related to deterioration of physical condition
   d. Deficient Knowledge regarding handling the illness

2. The nurse understands that which of the following is the most important factor affecting the client's ability to cope with the diagnosis of AIDS?
   a. Existing support systems
   b. Knowledge of the disease
   c. Attitude of the physician
   d. Complexity of treatment regimen

3. The nurse assesses the client recently diagnosed with AIDS for which of the following expected psychological responses?
   a. Anxiety and depression
   b. Cognitive impairment
   c. Delusions and hallucinations
   d. Somatic symptoms

4. The plan of care for a client in the late phase of HIV/AIDS includes which of the following?
   a. Ensuring adequate financial support
   b. Encouraging a life review
   c. Monitoring for depression
   d. Recognizing fear of deformity

5. Which intervention would the nurse implement to ensure the continuum of care for a client with HIV/AIDS?
   a. Assisting family to discuss feelings about client's diagnosis

b. Encouraging client to learn about the disease process
c. Helping client identify fears related to dying
d. Referring client to community AIDS support groups

6. A client diagnosed with AIDS is in the third stage of a grief reaction. Which of the following would the nurse expect to find? Select all that apply.
a. Derealization
b. Denial
c. Questioning why
d. Anger
e. Shock
f. Belief that God is punishing him or her

Selected References

Aegis.com. (2006). A brief history of AIDS/HIV. Retrieved May 15, 2006, from http://www.aegis.com/topics/timeline

Associated Press. (2000, June 10). AIDS' origin traced back to early '30's. *Orlando Sentinel.*

Avert.org. (2006). History of AIDS. Retrieved May 15, 2006, from http://www.avert.org/historyi.htm

Boyle, J. S. (2003). Transcultural perspectives in the nursing care of adults. In M. M. Andrews & J. S. Boyle (Eds.), *Transcultural concepts in nursing care* (3rd ed., pp. 181–208). Philadelphia: Lippincott Williams & Wilkins.

Burnett, D. W. (2001). First steps: Initial assessment of HIV patients. *ADVANCE for Nurse Practitioners, 9*(5), 59–60, 63–64.

Centers for Disease Control and Prevention. (2000). Epidemiology of AIDS. Retrieved March 4, 2004, from http://www.cdc.gov

Centers for Disease Control and Prevention. (2001). HIV/AIDS: General information. Retrieved March 3, 2004, from http://www.cdc.gov

Coleman, D. (1988). Nursing care of the AIDS patient. *In AIDS: A health management response.* Rockwell, MD: Aspen.

Coyne, P. J., Lyne, M. E., & Watson, A. C. (2002). Symptom management in people with AIDS. *American Journal of Nursing, 102*(9), 48–55.

Davidson, M. R. (2004). Sexually transmitted infections: Screening and counseling. *Clinician Reviews, 14*(6), 56–62.

Ferri, R. S. (1995). HIV and adolescents: A primary care perspective. *ADVANCE for Nurse Practitioners, 3*(7).

Fohn.net. (2006). The history of AIDS. Retrieved May 15, 2006, from http://fohn.net/history-of-aids/

Fox-Seaman, G. A. (2005). HIV and other STDs in older adults. *ADVANCE for Nurse Practitioners, 13*(2), 61–64.

Grodesky, M. J. (2002). Immune recovery syndrome with HAART therapy: A clinical perspective. *ADVANCE for Nurse Practitioners, 10*(3), 87–88.

Hirsch, D., & Enlow, R. (1985). *The effects of the acquired immune deficiency syndrome on gay lifestyle and the gay individual.* New York: New York Academy of Science.

Holzemer, W. L. (2002). HIV and AIDS: The symptom experience. *American Journal of Nursing, 102*(4), 48–52.

Ivantic-Doucette, K., & Haglund, K. (2004). Adolescents and HIV: The coming storm. *ADVANCE for Nurse Practitioners, 4*(12), 79–82.

Kongable, G. L. (1998). Psychosocial aspects of medically compromised persons. In M. A. Boyd & M. A. Nihart (Eds.), *Psychiatric nursing: Contemporary practice* (pp. 972–996). Philadelphia: Lippincott Williams & Wilkins.

Konkle-Parker, D. (1998). Early HIV detection and treatment. *ADVANCE for Nurse Practitioners, 6*(9), 63–66.

Kübler-Ross, E. (1969). *On death and dying.* London: Macmillan.

Lego, S. (1996). The client with HIV infection. In S. Lego (Ed.), *Psychiatric nursing: A comprehensive reference* (2nd ed., pp. 338–344). Philadelphia: Lippincott-Raven.

Leserman, J., Petitto, J. M., Golden, R. N., Gaynes, B. N., Gu, H., Perkins, D. O., et al. (2000). Impact of stressful life events, depression, social support, coping, and cortisol on progression of AIDS. *The American Journal of Psychiatry, 157*(8), 1221–1228.

MacNeil, J. S. (2006). Psych disorders common in kids with HIV. *Clinical Psychiatry News, 34*(2), 2.

Nichols, S. (1983). Psychiatric aspects of AIDS. *Psychosomatics, 24.*

Norman, J. C. (1996). *Essentials of nursing management: HIV-AIDS.* Irvine, CA: Continuing Medical Education, Inc.

Norman, J. C. (2006). HIV/AIDS: Epidemic update for Florida. *CME resource: Continuing education for Florida nurses, 131*(2), 27–68.

North Arundel Hospital. (2003). Early symptomatic HIV infection. Retrieved September 16, 2003, from http://www.northarundel.com/ency/article/000603.htm

Ripich, S. (1997). The client on the human immunodeficiency virus spectrum. In B. S. Johnson (Ed.), *Psychiatric-mental health nursing: Adaptation and growth* (4th ed., pp. 953–967). Philadelphia: Lippincott-Raven.

Sadock, B. J., & Sadock, V. A. (2003). *Kaplan and Sadock's synopsis of psychiatry: Behavioral sciences/clinical psychiatry* (9th ed.). Philadelphia: Lippincott Williams & Wilkins.

Schultz, J. M., & Videbeck, S. L. (2005). *Lippincott's manual of psychiatric nursing care plans* (7th ed.). Philadelphia: Lippincott Williams & Wilkins.

Seattle Biomedical Research Institute. (2003). HIV/AIDS. Retrieved December 15, 2003, from http://www.sbri.org/diseases/hiv_aids.asp

Shahrokh, N., & Hales, R. E. (Eds.). (2003.) *American psychiatric glossary* (8th ed.). Washington, DC: American Psychiatric Press.

Trzcianowska, H., & Mortensen, E. (2001). HIV and AIDS: Separating fact from fiction. *American Journal of Nursing, 101*(6), 53–59.

Tucker, M. E. (2006). HIV/AIDS incidence falls among African Americans. *Clinical Psychiatry News, 34*(4), 19.

United Nations. (2006). A global overview of the AIDS epidemic. Retrieved April 5, 2006, from http://www.unaids.org/bangkok2004/GAR2004_htmo/GAR2004_03_en.htm

Weiss, B. (2001). HIV in adolescents: Prevention and identification are pivotal. *ADVANCE for Nurse Practitioners, 9,* 44–50.

Whipple, B., & Scura, K. W. (1996). The overlooked epidemic: HIV in older adults. *American Journal of Nursing, 96*(2).

Whitaker, R. (1999). Psychopharmacological treatment issues in HIV disease. *Psychiatric Times, 16*(8), 24–30.

Willard, S., & Dean, L. M. (2000). AIDS in the older adult: Aging raises unique treatment concerns. *ADVANCE for Nurses, 1*(12), 12–15.

Suggested Readings

American Journal of Nursing. (2000). News: The third decade of the HIV epidemic. *American Journal of Nursing, 100*(10), 36–37.

American Psychiatric Association. (2000). *Diagnostic and statistical manual of mental disorders* (4th ed., text revision). Washington, DC: Author.

Baldwin, J. (2001). AIDS may escape diagnosis in older people. *Geriatric Times, 2*(1), 6–8.

Barroso, J. (2002). HIV-related fatigue. *American Journal of Nursing, 102*(5), 83–86.

Boschert, S. (2004). Extent of New York's HIV epidemic emerging. *Clinical Psychiatry News, 32*(6), 75.

Boschert, S. (2004). HIV drugs change cognitive impairment risk. *Clinical Psychiatry News, 32*(5), 42.

Carpenito-Moyet, L. M. (2006). *Handbook of nursing diagnosis* (11th ed.). Philadelphia: Lippincott Williams & Wilkins.

DeSantis, J. P., & Patsdaughter, C. A. (2005). A changing course: HIV takes toll on ethnic and sexual minorities. *ADVANCE for Nurse Practitioners, 13*(4), 47–48, 50.

Doerfler, E. (2002). Sweetening the toxic cocktail: Managing side effects of HIV medications. *ADVANCE for Nurse Practitioners,* 52–58.

Easter, S., & Farrell, M. (2004). HIV and the elderly. *Vital Signs, 14*(6), 15–18.

Ferri, R. S. (2000). The new AIDS paradigm: Living with metabolic complications. *ADVANCE for Nurse Practitioners, 8*(9), 69–70.

Goldrick, B. (2004). HIV advances. *American Journal of Nursing, 104*(5), 37–38.

Johnson, D. L. (2002). Metabolic complications in HIV infection: In search of underlying mechanisms. *ADVANCE for Nurse Practitioners, 10*(7), 45–49.

Quinn, T. C. (1998). Epidemiology of HIV infections: International and U.S. perspectives. *Hopkins HIV Report, 10*(3), 11–12.

Whitaker, R. (1999). Significance of community psychiatry to HIV disease. *Psychiatric Times, 16*(1), 58–64.

Yeargen, P., & Johnson, C. (2001). Home care for patients with AIDS. *ADVANCE for Nurse Practitioners, 9*(1), 61, 63–64.

CHAPTER 35 / SERIOUSLY AND PERSISTENTLY MENTALLY ILL, HOMELESS, OR INCARCERATED CLIENTS

*Hundreds of thousands of vulnerable Americans are eking out a pitiful existence
on city streets, under ground in subway tunnels, or in jails and prisons due to the
misguided efforts of civil rights advocates to keep the severely mentally ill out
of hospitals and out of treatment.   —TORREY & ZDANDOWICZ, 1999*

*It is estimated that there are approximately 9 million people incarcerated in prisons worldwide,
with 2 million in the United States. An exhaustive research of 62 psychiatric surveys of 22,790
prisoners found that psychiatric disorders are much more prevalent in the prison population
than in the general population.   —DANESH, 2002*

LEARNING OBJECTIVES

AFTER STUDYING THIS CHAPTER, YOU SHOULD BE ABLE TO:

1. Articulate the effect of a serious and persistent mental illness on the life of a client so affected.
2. Discuss the relationship between serious and persistent mental illness and the problems of homelessness and incarceration.
3. Explain how deinstitutionalization, transinstitutionalization, and lack of community services have contributed to the current problems of those with serious and persistent mental illness.
4. Describe the groups of individuals comprising the homeless population.
5. Identify those clients with serious and persistent mental illness who are at risk for incarceration.
6. Compare and contrast mental health and social service treatments for nursing-home residents, the homeless, and the incarcerated who are experiencing serious and persistent mental illness.
7. Articulate the impact of managed care on the mental health treatment and continuum of care of those with serious and persistent mental illness.
8. Discuss the effect of a member of the family having serious and persistent mental illness.
9. Summarize important nursing assessments for the client with serious and persistent mental illness.
10. Determine nursing implementations that are important for a client with serious and persistent mental illness.
11. Construct a nursing plan of care for a client with serious and persistent mental illness.

KEY TERMS

Assertive Community Treatment (ACT) model
Clubhouse program
Deinstitutionalization
Empowerment Model of Recovery
Hate crime
Impulse control disorders
Integrated Model Program (IMPACT)
Mercy bookings
Respite care for the homeless
Serious and persistent mental illness (SPMI)
Transinstitutionalization
Welcome Home Ministries

Serious and persistent mental illness **(SPMI),** also referred to as *severe and persistent mental illness,* is the current accepted term denoting a variety of psychiatric–mental health problems that lead to tremendous disability. Although commonly associated with illnesses such as schizophrenia, the term *SPMI* includes people with wide-ranging psychiatric diagnoses (eg, bipolar disorder, severe major depression, substance-related disorders, and personality disorders) persisting over long periods (ie, years) and causing disabling symptoms that significantly impair functioning.

The symptoms of SPMI can be ongoing throughout the lives of some individuals, whereas others may experience periods of remission. Every aspect of living can be affected by the illness, including family and social relationships, physical health status, the ability to obtain employment and housing, and even the ability to accomplish routine activities of daily living. Persons with SPMI are often shunned by society and isolated from the community. Their behavior is often bizarre, including such actions as responding to hallucinations by shouting in public or talking or gesturing to themselves. Their appearance may be disheveled because hygiene and other self-care activities are neglected due to the severity of the symptoms. Often, these persons are unable to live independently and need assisted-living situations. Such clients go through the revolving doors of acute psychiatric care. They may be sent to group homes, to one of the few remaining state institutions, or to jails, or they may become homeless. Understanding this population and their special problems and needs is important for the psychiatric–mental health nurse.

This chapter focuses on the role of the psychiatric–mental health nurse and the application of the nursing process related to the current needs of individuals with SPMI. These clients often have coexisting problems such as homelessness, a dual diagnosis, or involvement with the judicial system.

Scope of Serious and Persistent Mental Illness

According to the World Health Organization, major depression, bipolar disorder, schizophrenia, and substance-related disorders account for four of the ten leading causes of disability globally. Each year, approximately 23% of American adults are diagnosed with a psychiatric–mental health disorder, and 5.4% of these adults are said to be seriously and persistently mentally ill (Medscape Resource Center, 2004). The association of SPMI with poverty and poor health care creates a need for comprehensive psychiatric–mental health care and the use of social services to address issues related to independent living. Factors such as substandard housing, unemployment or underemployment, poor nutrition, lack of preventive care, and limited access to medical care create severe stressors for individuals affected with mental illness (United States Department of Health and Human Services, 1999). Figure 35-1 shows the states that provide some form of insurance benefits for mental illness as of June 2003. At the time of publication, four states had no laws addressing mental health insurance coverage: Idaho, Wyoming, Iowa, and Alaska.

The physical health of individuals with SPMI is worse than the physical health of those without SPMI. Poor living conditions related to the failure to provide for basic needs in a stable environment contribute to this poor physical health status. In fact, people with SPMI die an average of 10 to 15 years earlier than the general population. Unhealthy lifestyle habits, excessive smoking, lack of physical exercise, and poor nutrition contribute to the increased health risk. Fifty percent of people with SPMI are estimated to have a known comorbid medical disorder (Farnam, Zipple, Tyrell, & Chittinanda, 1999).

Factors Related to the Current Problems of the Seriously and Persistently Mentally Ill

Three factors have contributed to the current problems associated with SPMI. These factors, complex and related to the history of psychiatric–mental health treatment over the last several decades, include deinstitutionalization, transinstitutionalization, and the lack of community services to provide for the multiple needs of the seriously and persistently mentally ill.

Deinstitutionalization

Deinstitutionalization, the process by which large numbers of psychiatric–mental health clients were discharged from public psychiatric facilities during the last 40 years, created an influx of seriously and persis-

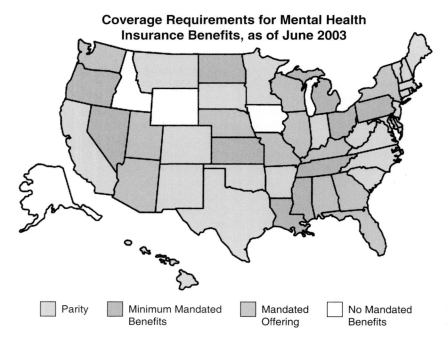

Coverage Requirements for Mental Health Insurance Benefits, as of June 2003

Parity | Minimum Mandated Benefits | Mandated Offering | No Mandated Benefits

FIGURE 35.1 States that provide some form of insurance benefits for mental illness as of June 2003.

tently mentally ill clients sent back into the community to receive outpatient care. Deinstitutionalization is a major factor in the current problems of the mentally ill. Since 1960, more than 90% of state psychiatric hospital beds have been eliminated. This process began in 1955, and accelerated with the Civil Rights legislation of the 1960s as well as the withdrawal of federal-government financing for state-hospital clients in the 1970s (see Chapter 8). See Clinical Example 35-1 for an example.

Transinstitutionalization

Transinstitutionalization is the process of transferring state-hospital clients to other facilities. Nursing-home placement and incarceration remain a significant component of transinstitutionalization. According to Andrew Sperling, director of policy for the National Alliance for the Mentally Ill (NAMI), it appears that there are still a large number of people with SPMI being placed in nursing homes (MacNeil, 2001). Furthermore, America's jails and prisons are now surrogate psychiatric hospitals for thousands of individuals with the most severe brain diseases (Treatment Advocacy Center [TAC], 2003).

Inappropriate Use and Lack of Community Services

The initial plans for deinstitutionalization involved federal funding for community mental health centers with the goal of providing early diagnosis and timely treatment in a community setting, rather than in large state hospitals removed from the community. The belief was that these mental health centers would eliminate the need for state hospitals. However, cost shifting by the federal government to state governments for these mental health centers led to inadequate and insufficient money for treatment. In addition, issues of insufficiently trained personnel and funding mechanisms were not addressed (Smoyak, 2000). Large numbers of clients who were deinstitu-

CLINICAL EXAMPLE 35.1

A CLIENT AFTER DEINSTITUTIONALIZATION

EM was among the large population of clients released from state hospitals from 1960 to 1980. Hospitalized since adolescence, she was in her thirties when released and was unable to function in society. Without family support and lacking fundamental resources or employment skills, she became permanently dependent on social services. EM was admitted to the hospital after police were called by her landlord and neighbors, who complained that she was knocking on doors in the middle of the night and threatening people with harm. Her apartment contained large amounts of trash and was infested with cockroaches. The landlord began eviction proceedings soon after she was hospitalized. This was her 16th hospital admission for mental illness.

tionalized were actually transferred to nursing homes and other similar institutions. Those who did not qualify for nursing-home care were released to hastily established group homes, boarding homes, personal-care facilities, or the streets. Today, funding for after-care community services continues to decline (Sadock & Sadock, 2003).

Categories of Seriously and Persistently Mentally Ill Clients

The categories of seriously and persistently mentally ill clients who provide challenges to the psychiatric-mental health nurse include nursing-home residents, the homeless, and the incarcerated. Each group is discussed below.

Nursing-Home Residents

An act of Congress and a Supreme Court decision to perform pre-admission screening and resident reviews (PASRRs) prior to admission have not stopped the inappropriate placement of mentally ill adults into nursing homes that do not provide psychiatric services (see Chapter 8). According to the Inspector General's office, there are people in nursing homes who are seriously and persistently mentally ill (eg, schizophrenia, bipolar disorder, and personality disorder) and in need of more than casual mental health services. For example, 3.8% of clients with chronic schizophrenia reside in nursing homes (Begley, 2002). Researchers in San Diego found that although older people with schizophrenia did not have more physical illnesses than non–mentally ill people in the same age range, their illnesses were often more severe (Cohen, 2001). Of the top primary diagnoses at the time of admission for nursing-home residents, mental disorders ranked second (17%) only to diseases of the circulatory system (27%) (Clinical Psychiatry News, 2001).

Federal agencies have accepted state recommendations to improve nursing-home admission criteria for clients with mental illness and to provide appropriate mental health services. However, the individual states must agree to initiate programs (eg, availability of on-site mental health services and reimbursement for services) and remove certain barriers for reform to occur (MacNeil, 2001).

The Homeless

Homeless individuals and families are those who are sleeping in places not meant for human habitation (eg, cars, parks, sidewalks, or abandoned buildings) or who sleep in emergency shelters as a primary nighttime residence. Other individuals may be considered homeless if they:

- Live in transitional or supportive housing
- Ordinarily sleep in transitional or supportive housing but are spending 30 or fewer consecutive days in a hospital or other institution
- Are being evicted within a week from a private dwelling and without resources to obtain access to alternative housing
- Are being discharged from an institution in which they resided for more than 30 consecutive days and without resources to obtain access to alternative housing (United States Department of Housing and Urban Development, 2002)

Although several national estimates are available about homelessness, many are dated or are based on dated information. By its very nature, homelessness is impossible to measure with 100% accuracy. Researchers use different methods to measure homelessness. One method, *point-in-time counts,* attempts to count all the people who are literally homeless on a given day or during a given week. A second method, *period prevalence counts,* attempts to count the number of people who are homeless over a given period of time. The high turnover in the homeless population documented in various studies suggests that many people experience homelessness but do not remain homeless. For example, over time some people will find housing and escape homelessness, whereas new people will lose housing and become homeless (National Coalition for the Homeless [NCH], 2005a).

Recent studies suggest that the United States generates homelessness at a much higher rate than had been previously thought. The best approximation of homelessness is from an Urban Institute study in the year 2000, which states that about 3.5 million people—1.35 million of them children—are likely to experience homelessness in a given year (NCH, 2005a).

Clients deinstitutionalized from 1970 through the 1990s often ended up homeless due to lack of adequate psychiatric–mental health and social services. Statistics released by the Treatment Advocacy Center in 1999 indicate that 200,000 individuals with schizophrenia or bipolar disorder are homeless. In addition, the loss of state hospital beds caused a significant portion of the population with SPMI, who would have been in state hospitals, to become homeless. Homelessness among those with SPMI usually occurs as a result of several factors, including lack of family involvement, inability to pay rent, bizarre behaviors, and commitment to a psychiatric institution. A new wave of deinstitutionalization, and the denial of services or premature and unplanned discharge brought about by managed care arrangements, also may be contributing to the continued presence of the homeless population (NCH, 2005b).

Risk Factors for Homelessness. Several risk factors have been described for homelessness among persons with SPMI (Caton & Shront, 1994). These include:

- Presence of positive symptoms of schizophrenia
- Concurrent drug or alcohol abuse
- Presence of a personality disorder
- High rate of disorganized family functioning from birth to age 18
- Lack of current family support

See Clinical Example 35-2 for an example.

Although mental illness can precipitate homelessness, the crisis of being homeless can also compound the problem of mental illness. That is, the stressors of not being able to meet basic needs, and of being

---

CLINICAL EXAMPLE 35.2

THE HOMELESS CLIENT WITH SPMI

DN was removed from her parents' home at the age of 8 after physical and sexual abuse. She lived in five different foster homes until the age of 15, when she was placed in a group home. At age 17, she ran away from the group home and lived on the streets or in shelters in between the times she was hospitalized. DN's situation includes risk factors for homelessness, including the presence of positive symptoms of schizophrenia (hallucinations and delusions), a personality disorder, and a chaotic family experience until age 18.

---

exposed to the elements and other risks to safety such as violence, can all increase the severity and persistence of mental illness.

Special Populations of the Homeless. Health care providers today are confronted with the changing face of the homeless. Following is a list of the groups that comprise the homeless (NCH, 2005c):

- 39% of children under the age of 18 years; 42% of these children were under the age of 5 years
- 25% ages 25 to 34 years
- 6% were ages 55 to 60 years
- 41% were single men and 14% were single women
- 49% were African American; 35% Caucasian, 13% Hispanic, 2% Native American, and 1% Asian
- Veterans (approximately 40% of the homeless population)
- HIV/AIDS victims (approximately 3%–20% of the homeless population)
- Domestic-violence victims (approximately 50% of all women and children experiencing homelessness are fleeing domestic violence.)
- Substance abusers (unable to estimate due to refusal to admit to illegal use of substances)
- 23% of individuals who are diagnosed as SPMI

The rates of both chronic and acute health problems are extremely high among the homeless, who are far more likely to suffer from every category of chronic health problem. In addition, the problems associated with homelessness, although affecting every aspect of living, can have specific consequences depending on the age and gender of the individual affected.

Children, Adolescents, and Young Adults. Numerous psychiatric–mental health problems that manifest in adolescence and young adulthood have their roots in early childhood. Studies have also shown that an important risk factor for infants and children is the occurrence of psychopathology in the primary caregivers (Office of Disease Prevention and Health Promotion [ODPHP], 1998). For example, preschool and school-age children of women who are homeless and mentally ill are at high risk for physical and emotional illnesses, as well as developmental delays. Poor nutrition, chronic stress of the caregiver who is homeless, and lack of access to preventive health care are contributing factors. The adolescent population is at high risk for being physically and sexually abused. They are also at high risk for using drugs and alcohol to cope with homelessness.

Women. Women who are homeless have often experienced domestic violence. When mental illness is present, the combination of the illness and lack of adequate resources is a causative factor in homelessness. A history of unwanted pregnancies and sexually transmitted diseases, and the risk for rape and violence, also are common in homeless women.

The Elderly. The elderly, although constituting a small percentage of the homeless population, generally have problems related to dementia often caused by chronic use of substances. A study of elderly homeless men identified that this population was poorer, in poorer health, and more likely to have alcohol-use disorders than their younger counterparts (DeMallie, North, & Smith, 1997).

Hate Crimes Against the Homeless. **Hate crime** is defined by the U.S. Congress as a crime in which the defendant intentionally selects a victim (or in the case of a property crime, the property that is the object of the crime) because of the victim's race, color, or national origin.

The federal law to combat hate crimes (Title 18 U.S.C. §245) was passed in 1968. It mandated that the government must prove both that the crime occurred because of a victim's membership in a designated group and because the victim was engaged in certain specified federally protected activities (eg, serving on a jury, voting, attending public school). Federal bias crime laws such as the Hate Crimes Statistics Act of 1990 and the Hate Crimes Sentencing Enhancement Act of 1994 further clarified the definition of hate crime by stating that the crime occurs because of "actual or perceived race, color, national origin, ethnicity, gender, disability, or sexual orientation of any person"(NCH, 2006).

During the last several years, advocates and homeless-shelter workers have received news reports of homeless individuals, including children, being harassed, kicked, set on fire, beaten to death, and even decapitated. During the year 2005, a total of 86 hate crimes were committed in 22 states plus Puerto Rico. Of the 86 acts, 13 resulted in death. Ages of the victims ranged from 22 to 70 years. The age range of the perpetrators of the hate crimes ranged from 13 to 75 years. A majority of the victims (62) were male (NCH, 2006).

Most hate violence is committed by individual citizens who harbor a strong resentment toward a certain group of people; who violently act out their resentment toward the perceived growing economic power of a particular racial or ethnic group; or who take advantage of vulnerable and disadvantaged persons to satisfy their own pleasure. Teens who are "thrill seekers" are the most common perpetrators of violence against the homeless (NCH, 2006). See Chapter 33 for additional information regarding hate crimes.

The Incarcerated

The process of deinstitutionalization has also resulted in a significant population of clients with SPMI being maintained in jails and prisons. Since the 1970s, when state mental institutions were closed, correctional facilities now house more individuals with SPMI than ever before (Yurkovich, Smyer, & Dean, 2000). According to a study by the Human Rights Watch, jails and prisons have become the nation's default mental health system. Approximately 400,000 Americans in jail and prison (compared with 300,000 in 1999) have SPMI—more than four times the number in state mental institutions. The percentage of female inmates who are mentally ill is considerably higher than that of male inmates (Butterfield, 2003). Moreover, according to one estimate, more than 40% of persons with a mental illness have been arrested at least once. Additional statistics comparing the seriously and persistently mentally ill incarcerated population with the general prison population were reported by the Bureau of Justice Statistics (2001):

• One of eight state prisoners received mental health counseling or therapy by mid-2000.

- Offenders between the ages of 45 and 54 years were most likely to be identified as seriously and persistently mentally ill.
- Mentally ill state prison inmates were twice as likely as general population inmates to have lived in a shelter within the last year.
- 50% of mentally ill offenders reported having three or more prior sentences.
- 33% of mentally ill federal inmates were convicted of a violent offense, compared with 13% of general population inmates.
- 53% of mentally ill state inmates were convicted of a violent offense, compared with 46% of general population inmates.
- 10% of state prisoners received psychotropic medication.
- 50% of state prison facilities provided mental health services.
- 66% of hospitalized state prisoners who were released obtained mental health services.

Factors Related to Incarceration. Those with psychiatric–mental illness are often incarcerated because community-based programs are non-existent, are filled to capacity, or are inconveniently located. Other factors include the failure to address clients' mental health problems and obstacles to commitment to psychiatric care by the legal structure. Persons with a mental illness are incarcerated for overt, aggressive behavior caused by psychotic symptoms such as hallucinations or delusions; vagrancy; trespassing; disorderly conduct; alcohol-related charges; or failure to pay for a meal. Generally, the offense leading to incarceration occurs as a result of either the effect of the mental illness itself or the problem of mental illness coexisting with a substance-abuse disorder. See Clinical Example 35-3.

Mercy bookings, defined as arrests made by police to protect individuals with SPMI, are surprisingly common. This is especially true for women, who are easily victimized, even raped, on the streets (TAC, 2003).

The jails and prisons lack necessary services for effective treatment of the mentally ill, and thus have become warehouses for those with nowhere else to go. In a National Institute of Justice survey, prison administrators described their mental health programs as grossly understaffed and in urgent need of program development and intervention by mental health organizations (McEwen, 1995). Often, persons with mental illness remain incarcerated for longer periods of time than do persons without mental illness who are in prison for the same charges. Unfortunately, jails and prisons usually exacerbate the clinical symptoms of mental illness, either because individuals are not given the necessary medication to control their symptoms, or because they are placed in solitary confinement (TAC, 2003).

Clients at Risk for Incarceration. Most crimes for which the seriously and persistently mentally ill are arrested are minor. However, some mentally ill offenders require incarceration to protect society. These offenders often include individuals with impulse control disorders, sexual disorders, substance-abuse disorders, bipolar disorders, personality disorders, and, as noted earlier, psychotic disorders.

The Client With an Impulse Control Disorder. Many psychological problems are characterized by a loss of control or a lack of control in specific situations. Usually this lack of control is part of a pattern of behavior that also involves other maladaptive thoughts and actions, such as substance abuse (Psychology Information Online, 2003).

Impulse control disorders are characterized by a person's failure to resist an impulse despite negative consequences, thus not preventing oneself from performing an act that will be harmful to self or others. This includes the failure to stop gambling and the impulse to engage in violent behavior (eg, road rage), sexual behavior, fire starting, stealing, and self-abusive behavior. Researchers believe that impulse control problems may be related to functions in specific parts of the brain, and may be caused by a hormonal imbalance or the abnormal transmission of nerve impulses. Although the specific etiology is unknown, a person

---

CLINICAL EXAMPLE 35.3

THE CLIENT WITH SPMI WHO IS INCARCERATED

FR was never able to secure employment due to his SPMI and has depended on welfare and group-home living. He had a substance-abuse problem and when drinking would frequently destroy property or become involved in fights. Thus, he has a history of being incarcerated. FR also has a history of obesity and diabetes mellitus, has had one myocardial infarction, and continues to smoke and not manage his diabetes well.

TABLE 35.1 Examples of Impulse Control Disorders

TYPE OF DISORDER	DESCRIPTION OF DISORDER
Intermittent explosive	The client exhibits episodes of aggressive behavioral outbursts in either the destruction of property or physical assaults on others. The degree of aggressive behavior is in proportion to a precipitating factor. Legal problems usually occur as a result of destruction of property, assault, or domestic violence.
Kleptomania	The client feels tension, experiences a compulsive need to steal items, and then experiences a sense of pleasure at the time of the theft. The items are not stolen for their monetary value nor are they stolen to express vengeance. Clients are often charged with shoplifting.
Pathological gambling	The client experiences persistent maladaptive gambling that creates serious problems interfering with his or her personal life and work. Financial problems often occur and the client may engage in criminal activity to cover financial losses.
Pyromania	The client experiences an increasing sense of tension or affective arousal and deliberately and purposefully sets a fire, resulting in a sense of intense pleasure or relief. Firesetting, also referred to as *arson*, generally results in the destruction of property and may destroy life—resulting in legal problems for the client.

SOURCES: Psychology Information Online. (2003). *Impulse control disorders*. Retrieved December 16, 2003, from http://www.psychologyinfo.com/problems/impulse_control.html; Sadock, B. J., & Sadock, V. A. (2003). *Kaplan & Sadock's synopsis of psychiatry: Behavioral sciences/clinical psychiatry* (9th ed.). Philadelphia: Lippincott Williams & Wilkins.

who has had a head injury or the diagnosis of temporal lobe epilepsy is at higher risk for developing an impulse control disorder. Diagnosis is only made after all other medical and psychiatric disorders that might account for the symptoms have been ruled out (Psychology Information Online, 2003). Examples of impulse control disorders that often lead to incarceration are listed in Table 35-1.

The Client With a Sexual Disorder. Individuals with the diagnosis of a sexual disorder may be incarcerated due to exhibitionism, voyeurism, rape, or pedophilic behavior. Alexander (1999) examined 79 studies covering 10,988 offenders who received outpatient treatment. Findings indicated that:

- Treated offenders reoffended at a rate of 11% when compared with 17.6% of offenders who were not treated.
- True incest offenders have lower reoffense rates when compared with other types of child molesters.
- Men treated with more traditional methods during incarceration before 1980 reoffended at a rate of 12.8%, whereas men treated after 1980 by present-day methods including behavioral therapy reoffended at a rate of 7.4% of probationary sentences.

The Client With a Substance-Related Disorder. More than 90% of inmates with SPMI who are incarcerated have life-long drug or alcohol disorders. Their reported rates of current substance-use problems, including the abuse of alcohol, range from 62% to 72%. More than half of incarcerated mentally ill clients report having used drugs or alcohol while committing their current offense (Watson, Hanrahan, Luchins, & Lurigio, 2001). Clients with a dual diagnosis are more likely to become homeless, to be hospitalized, to have greater difficulty sustaining employment, and to be noncompliant with treatment. Figure 35-2 depicts the co-occurrence of SPMI and substance use disorders in adults age 18 years or older.

The Client With Bipolar Disorder. The prevalence of bipolar disorder in the prison population is approximately 6%, compared with 1% in the community at large. Prominent bipolar symptoms such as agitation, impulsivity, poor judgment, and psychosis increase the risk of criminal behavior. Comorbidity with a substance-use disorder is greater than with any other Axis I disorder. Offenses for which clients with bipolar disorder are usually incarcerated cover a broad spectrum, but violent crimes are twice as common as property or drug-use

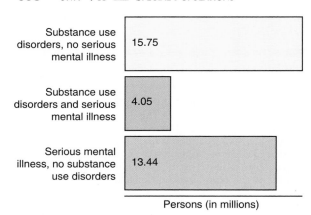

Substance use disorders, no serious mental illness — 15.75

Substance use disorders and serious mental illness — 4.05

Serious mental illness, no substance use disorders — 13.44

Persons (in millions)

Note: Based on 68,126 face-to-face interviews with a representative sample conducted from January to December 2002.
Source: Substance Abuse and Mental Health Services Administration

FIGURE 35.2 Co-occurrence of serious and persistent mental illness and substance use disorders in adults age 18 years or older, 2002.

crimes. Crimes of noncompliance (ie, failure to heed the police) are also frequently committed (Sherman, 2001).

The Client With a Personality Disorder. Individuals with a personality disorder make up a large proportion of the violent mentally ill; antagonistic and hostile traits are noted in eight of the different personality disorders (Kravitz & Silberberg, 2001). Antisocial, borderline, and schizotypal personality disorders are the most common types noted in clients who are incarcerated.

Clients with antisocial personality disorder fail to conform to social norms with respect to lawful behaviors. They violate the rights of others and repeatedly perform acts that are grounds for arrest. Clinical features also include deceitfulness, impulsivity, irritability and aggressiveness, recklessness, irresponsibility, lack of remorse, and the presence of a conduct disorder before the age of 15 years.

Clients with borderline personality disorder exhibit impulsivity that is potentially self-damaging. They have difficulty controlling anger, thereby posing a threat to the safety of others, and they exhibit transient stress-related paranoid behavior. Clients with the diagnosis of schizotypal personality disorder exhibit suspiciousness or paranoid thoughts; odd or peculiar behavior; excessive social anxiety; and odd beliefs or magical thinking that influence behavior inconsistent with

social norms. These clients are all at risk for incarceration because of their propensity or natural inclination to commit unlawful acts (American Psychiatric Association, 2000; Sadock & Sadock, 2003).

Risk for Suicide Among Incarcerated Clients. Related to the problem of the lack of treatment for mental illness in jails and prisons is the problem of suicide. Suicide is the leading cause of death in jails, and most jail suicides occur in the mentally ill population (eg, clients with schizophrenia or bipolar disorder); (TAC, 2003).

The characteristics of individuals who commit suicide during incarceration include the presence of a significant mental illness, a history of suicide attempts, older age, a lengthy sentence, and segregated or isolated housing (Hayes, 1995). Incarcerated individuals with SPMI often have a difficult time integrating into the prison population because of the illness's effect on their behavior. In addition, they have difficulty communicating and relating to others. Bizarre behavior is disquieting to other non-ill inmates, who frequently react with violence against those with cognitive or behavioral disorders, thereby making life in jail a brutal experience for them. Consequently, many of the mentally ill, who are isolated or segregated from the population at large and receive little or no treatment for their illness, are at risk for self-destructive behavior. For each successful suicide in jail, there are many others that are unsuccessful (TAC, 2003).

THE NURSING PROCESS

ASSESSMENT

The assessment of clients with SPMI, including the homeless or incarcerated, can be challenging. For example, homeless clients with SPMI often view the mental health system with suspicion and apprehension. Furthermore, about 50% to 75% of the incarcerated youth nationwide suffer from SPMI and are legally entitled to mental health services; however, access to care is limited because of confusion about consent and confidentiality, and lack of continuity of care across placement changes. The nurse may need to work closely with a social worker, case manager, or other support persons to obtain sufficient data to develop a plan of care that addresses the individual needs of these clients (Christensen, 2005; Mahoney, 2004).

Wendling (2006) discusses the possibility of inadequate assessment and misdiagnosis of clients with SPMI who are frequently hospitalized. For example, less than 50% of clients with the diagnosis of bipolar disorder received the same diagnosis upon readmission to the same facility within 30 days, and 90% of the clients with schizoaffective disorder were later diagnosed with bipolar disorder, major depression, or schizophrenia. Client factors that may impede the assessment process include poor reporting or deliberate misrepresentation of clinical symptoms, refusal to participate in interviews, and over-identification with a diagnosis because benefits or services are tied to a specific diagnosis. Therefore, assessment of a client with SPMI must be comprehensive, focusing on physical health status, current clinical symptoms, self-care abilities, living situation, coping skills and available support systems, compliance with medications, and the presence of substance abuse. Information regarding previous treatment, including hospitalization, should be obtained if available. Assessment may occur in a variety of settings including the hospital, long-term care facility (eg, nursing home or assisted-living facility), jail or prison, homeless shelter, or clinic.

Physical Health Status

A general physical assessment is performed using either a head-to-toe approach or a review-of-systems approach. Admission assessment forms from the specific health care facility guide this assessment. Problems related to lack of attention to physical health, often an issue with the SPMI client, are noted. Poor nutrition, chronic smoking, and sedentary lifestyle are risk factors for chronic health problems such as heart and lung disease, obesity, and diabetes mellitus.

Current Clinical Symptoms

Usually the client's psychiatric diagnosis is one of the major psychotic disorders, such as schizophrenia or bipolar disorder. However, the client may exhibit clinical symptoms related to personality disorder, lack of impulse control, substance abuse, or inappropriate sexual behavior. (Refer to Chapters 21, 22, 24, 25, and 26 respectively, for specific assessment information related to these disorders.) Assessment for hallucinations or delusions, associative looseness, changes in affect, loss of reality contact, impaired judgment, and excessive anxiety or agitation is important. The client

also is questioned about thoughts of self-harm or the desire to harm others. If the nurse encounters the client in an acute psychiatric facility or an institutional setting, he or she assesses the reason for the admission as well as the presence of stressors leading up to admission. Clear, direct communication in a calm, quiet environment is key. Sufficient time must be allowed for the client to respond to assessment questions.

Self-Care Abilities

Assess the client's self-care abilities and the ability to provide for basic physical needs (eg, grooming, bathing, feeding, toileting). Many clients with SPMI experience frequent decompensation (ie, return of psychotic symptoms) and find that negotiating activities of daily living can become overwhelming whether they reside in an institutional setting or are homeless (Delaney, 1998).

Current Living Situation

Because homelessness is a common problem for clients with SPMI, ask about the client's current living situation. If homelessness is a problem, establish the circumstances, including how long the client has been homeless and whether the client uses available shelters. Often, the client may live in an assisted-living situation, such as a group home or boarding home. Living situations of clients who reside in a nursing home or who are incarcerated are also assessed. Question clients to describe how they get along with the other clients and staff in these situations.

Coping Skills and Support Systems

Because the nursing plan of care builds on the client's strengths, assess for evidence of the client's coping skills and areas of functioning that are satisfactory.

Questions about the client's available support systems are important in determining resources available for assistance. If family members maintain involvement with the non-institutionalized client, the nurse determines the level of daily assistance, monitoring, and crisis intervention provided (Saunders, 1997). If a family member accompanies the client, ask the family member about the impact of the client's problems on family functioning. Saunders (1997) suggests asking additional assessment questions about the effect of the SPMI on the family, including what specific situations are especially difficult for the family to handle. The family member also is asked how the client's illness has affected relationships with family and friends. This information helps to determine the level of isolation that exists in the family as a result of the client's illness (Saunders, 1997). When family involvement is limited or absent, ask about other people with whom the client interacts on a regular basis. Case managers and mental health personnel working with the client may be the primary support systems.

Compliance With Medication

Because noncompliance with prescribed psychotropic medications is a major reason for the reoccurrence of symptoms, ask about the use of medications. Clients who are seriously and persistently mentally ill are generally placed on psychotropic medication to treat psychosis, depression, anxiety, or substance-use disorder. Determine whether the client takes prescribed medications on a daily basis and evaluate for any adverse effects that the client finds distressing. Adverse effects are often present and may be one of the reasons for noncompliance. The nurse uses a screening tool, such as the Abnormal Involuntary Movement Scale (AIMS) (discussed in Chapter 16), to assess for extrapyramidal adverse effects if the client is taking antipsychotic or neuroleptic medication.

Substance-Abuse Problems

Because substance abuse is often a problem for the client with SPMI and often contributes to arrest and incarceration, assessment is key. A screening tool, such as the CAGE questionnaire for alcoholism discussed in Chapter 25, is useful in determining the coexistence of a substance-abuse problem. Questions focus on the specific substances and the amount, frequency, and length of time used. The client also is asked whether he or she has received any treatment for substance abuse. Inadequate treatment often leads to continued substance abuse and repeated incarceration (Watson et al., 2001).

NURSING DIAGNOSES

Many nursing diagnoses can apply to the client with SPMI. Priorities are established on the basis of the client's physical health status, potential for harm to self or others, current symptomatic behaviors, self-care abilities, coping skills, and available support systems.

EXAMPLES OF NANDA NURSING DIAGNOSES / CLIENT WITH SERIOUS AND PERSISTENT MENTAL ILLNESS

- Interrupted Family Processes related to presence of persistent mental illness in a member
- Ineffective Health Maintenance related to inability to access services for health care
- Imbalanced Nutrition: More Than Body Requirements related to high-fat, high-carbohydrate diet
- Ineffecive Role Performance related to presence of persistent mental illness
- Disturbed Thought Processes related to presence of delusions and/or associative looseness
- Chronic Low Self-Esteem related to multiple psychiatric hospitalizations and failure to establish independent lifestyle
- Hopelessness related to lack of resources necessary to establish and maintain a home
- Impaired Social Interaction related to lack of, or inability to use, social and communication skills
- Ineffective Coping related to inability to handle problems of daily living
- Noncompliance (failure to take prescribed psychotropic medications or participate in long-term psychiatric treatment) related to uncomfortable side effects of medications and/or denial of mental illness
- Risk for Violence: Self-Directed or Other-Directed related to presence of command hallucinations, impairment in reality contact, or increased agitation
- Disturbed Sensory Perception (Visual and/ or Auditory) related to presence of hallucinations
- Social Isolation related to failure to establish and maintain interactions with others

---

See the accompanying Examples of North American Nursing Diagnosis Association (NANDA) Nursing Diagnoses box.

OUTCOME IDENTIFICATION

The concept of SPMI describes a population of mentally ill people, not a *Diagnostic and Statistical Manual of Mental Disorders, 4th Edition, Text Revision (DSM-IV-*

TR) diagnosis, living in a variety of environments (eg, at home or in a nursing home, homeless shelter, or prison), who are recipients of interventions by a multidisciplinary team that focuses on a biosocial rather than a purely medical approach. Functional outcomes, especially social and occupational, are generally more important than symptomatic outcomes (Spollen, 2003).

Outcomes for clients who are living alone, homeless, reside in long-term care facilities, or are incarcerated may vary. However, outcomes generally focus on maintaining client safety; establishing and maintaining client self-care; establishing client trust and facilitating interaction with staff and peers; and decreasing the presence of delusional thinking and hallucinatory experiences. Other outcomes include increased positive self-statements, having the client agree to take prescribed psychotropic medications, and the provision of family support when available. Long-term goals, which depend upon the client's specific diagnosis, focus on the client's ability to remain symptom-free; establish and maintain an independent living situation or adjust to an alternative living situation; increase social interaction; and participate in ongoing treatment programs. Provisions for continuum of care include coordination of the multiple social services necessary for the client to live in the community. See the accompanying Examples of Stated Outcomes box.

PLANNING INTERVENTIONS

The nurse encounters clients with SPMI in various settings, including the home, inpatient unit, hospital emergency room, mental health clinic, long-term care facility, homeless shelter, or corrections facility. Planning nursing interventions is dependent on the nurse's ability to assess the client and to establish and maintain a therapeutic relationship. The nurse uses listening skills to provide client support. Delaney, Rogers-Pitula, and Perraud (2000) state that the client will feel supported by the nurse when the nurse listens and communicates recognition and understanding. The client with a history of SPMI has usually experienced rejection by others, and the nurse's communication of care and concern is important.

IMPLEMENTATION

Since deinstitutionalization, the psychiatric–mental health nurse in the public sector may encounter the client in community clinics; community, academic, and

state hospitals; long-term care facilities; and correctional settings. Furthermore, mandatory outpatient psychiatric–mental health treatment may occur through the avenues of civil commitment, pretrial diversion, or probation, or because a client is declared unfit to stand trial. Table 35-2 lists types of outpatient treatment that may be mandated for mentally ill clients (Silberberg, Vital, & Brakel, 2001).

Various approaches have been used when providing interventions for clients who are seriously and persistently mentally ill. They include:

- Providing a safe environment
- Promoting physical health
- Providing medication management and education

EXAMPLES OF STATED OUTCOMES/ CLIENT WITH SERIOUS AND PERSISTENT MENTAL ILLNESS

- The family will verbalize knowledge of coping measures useful when dealing with a persistently mentally ill family member.
- The client will utilize referrals for services necessary to maintain health.
- The client will maintain healthy diet consisting of low-fat, adequate protein and carbohydrate intake.
- The client will accept necessary assistance to function in expected roles.
- The client will demonstrate reality-based thoughts without presence of delusional thinking.
- The client will identify positive aspects of self-functioning in several areas of life.
- The client will use resources necessary to establish and maintain a home.
- The client will use social and communication skills in establishing successful interactions with others.
- The client will establish coping measures to handle activities of daily living.
- The client will take prescribed psychotropic medications and participate in long-term psychiatric treatment.
- The client will maintain safety of self and others.
- The client will verbalize decrease or absence of hallucinatory experiences.
- The client will identify and interact with people who are supportive and helpful.

TABLE 35.2 Types of Mandated Outpatient Treatment for Mentally Ill Offenders

Outpatient civil commitment	As specified by each state's mental health code, the detainee appears in a civil court rather than a criminal court. The criminal event is offered as evidence that civil dangerousness exists and the detainee is mandated to receive outpatient mental health treatment.
Pretrial diversion	The defendant negotiates a pretrial diversion by agreeing to undergo outpatient treatment in return for the elimination or reduction of charges, pretrial jail time, or both.
Probation	Also referred to as *court-supervised release,* the defendant, after entering a plea of guilt or being convicted on criminal charges, is given a court-supervised release in lieu of incarceration. A series of conditions include: • No further criminal violations • Reporting requirements to a designated agency or official • No firearms or other dangerous weapons • No out-of-state travel without court approval • Home visits by the probation officer
Fitness to stand trial	If a defendant is declared unfit to stand trial, outpatient treatment is imposed by the criminal court as a less restrictive alternative to hospitalization. The defendant will return to court for trial when psychiatry determines that the defendant's clinical symptoms have resolved and the defendant is able to stand trial.

SOURCE: Silberberg, J. M., Vital, T. L., & Brakel, S. J. (2001). Breaking down barriers to mandated outpatient treatment for mentally ill offenders. *Psychiatric Annals, 31*(7), 433–440.

- Using cognitive–behavioral therapy to orient the client to reality, promote self-care, enhance self-esteem, and provide support
- Employing psychosocial rehabilitation to teach the client various skills
- Using the Assertive Community Treatment (ACT) model to provide comprehensive care
- Providing continuum of care

The combination of medication management with the cognitive-behavioral approach or with psychosocial rehabilitation has proven to be effective in the treatment of clients with SPMI (Delaney, 1998).

Providing a Safe Environment

If the client is hospitalized, institutionalized, or incarcerated, the nurse establishes and maintains an environment that promotes and protects client safety. It is vitally important for the nurse to identify clients at risk for suicide. Suicide precautions, safety rounds, and consistent rules and expectations for client behavior on the unit are important in the promotion of safety (Yurkovich et al., 2000). If the client demonstrates agita-

tion, de-escalation techniques are used, such as reducing environmental stimuli, talking to the client in a calm and controlled manner, and encouraging him or her to talk about feelings and issues. The nurse protects the client from the consequences of acting-out behaviors by offering the client medication to decrease agitation or the use of a quiet room to promote calm.

Promoting Physical Health

The nurse uses a wellness-education approach to improve the health status of the client. The client is encouraged to stop smoking, improve nutrition, and increase physical activity and exercise. Regular routine screenings such as Pap tests, mammograms, and prostate screenings are also encouraged.

Providing Medication Management and Education

Medication management usually consists of neuroleptics or atypical antipsychotics to decrease the positive and negative symptoms of schizophrenia or to stabilize the mood of clients with bipolar disorder; antidepressants for clients who primarily exhibit clinical symptoms of depression; and anxiolytics for clients who exhibit clinical symptoms of anxiety (see Chapter 16 for specific medications). Differences in the environmental settings such as shelters or correctional facilities can affect prescribing decisions and add a level of complexity to pharmacologic management. For example, if medication is prescribed three times a day to a client in a correctional facility, the possibility exists that the client will get only one or two dosages because of security emergencies or unexpected detainee movement in the system. Depot medications may be prescribed. However, clients are at risk for developing adverse reactions that may not be detected in a timely fashion (Kravitz & Silberberg, 2001).

Client education focuses on the illness and the prescribed psychotropic medications. Finnell (2005) suggests utilizing the Stages of Change Model (See Chapter 25) during medication management to determine the client's commitment to adherence. Once the client agrees to take the medication as directed, encourage the client to keep a record of times the medication is taken and any changes in symptoms. Christensen (2005) suggests providing psychotropic samples to outpatient clients to ensure medication compliance. Clients may not have insurance coverage, access to a pharmacy, or the financial means to pay for prescribed medication. Symptom control is emphasized as the goal.

Using Cognitive-Behavioral Therapy

The cognitive-behavioral therapy approach for clients with SPMI involves improving their ability to test reality; promoting self-care; enhancing self-esteem; and providing support. During therapy, the nurse establishes concrete goals with the client and focuses on the development of coping skills and problem-solving techniques. Nursing interventions are used to remotivate the client, increase his or her sense of control, and increase socialization skills (see Chapter 14) (Blair, 1996).

Orienting to Reality. Clients with SPMI often have difficulty recognizing or accepting reality. During cognitive-behavioral therapy, the nurse employs various techniques to help clients improve their ability to test reality and regain control of their environment. The nurse may reinforce reality through the use of a calendar and large poster boards that include the date, weather, names of staff, and schedule of activities for

the unit or clinic if the client is seen on an outpatient basis. When the client experiences hallucinations or delusions, the nurse intervenes by accepting that the hallucinatory voice or delusional thought is real to the client. Explaining to the client that the nurse neither believes what the client believes, nor hears what the client hears, reinforces reality. Malhotra (2006) suggests telling the client that it is important to remember that hallucinations and delusions are created in one's mind. Explain to the client that a video camera or tape recorder cannot capture hallucinations or delusions. Suggest that the client ask a trusted family member or friend to verify what is heard. A helpful technique includes directing the client to tell the voices that they hear to go away. This technique helps the client learn to push the voices aside rather than pay attention to what they are saying.

Focusing on something concrete in the immediate environment also helps the client by distracting him or her from the voices or the delusional thought. Simple physical activities, such as writing, drawing, or using an exercise bike, can redirect energy to acceptable activities and help distract the client.

When a client demonstrates loose associations, the nurse clarifies the meaning of the client's communication and focuses the client on "here-and-now" issues. Telling the client that the nurse does not understand what the client is trying to say is important feedback to the client's communication. Encouraging the client to explain in another way communicates the nurse's interest in understanding the client's experience.

Promoting Self-Care. Clients with SPMI often neglect personal hygiene. They may not have access to supplies or may lack motivation to attend to personal hygiene. During cognitive-behavioral therapy, the nurse encourages the client to maintain personal hygiene, and uses techniques such as positive reinforcement to improve the client's efforts. Telling the client in a matter-of-fact manner that it is time to take a shower, and then providing the materials needed for showering, provides necessary cues. If the client is completely unable to perform self-care, the nurse provides care in an accepting, nonjudgmental manner. The nurse continues to encourage the client in self-care measures, however. A regular routine for hygiene activities helps to structure the client's day and reinforces these activities on a daily basis.

Enhancing Self-Esteem. The client with SPMI often has great difficulty feeling positive about him- or herself because of repeated failures in multiple areas of living. During cognitive-behavioral therapy, the nurse communicates respect for the client and identifies those areas in which the client has been able to function. Encouraging the client to identify positive self-statements and provide examples of positive functioning promotes self-esteem. Other nursing interventions may include:

- Identifying positive coping skills
- Helping the client use problem-solving for identified problems
- Teaching assertiveness skills
- Encouraging participation in support groups in which others are experiencing similar problems

Providing Support. During cognitive-behavioral therapy, the nurse provides support to the client by listening with empathy to the client's story. Most likely, the client with SPMI has been subjected to multiple instances of rejection on the basis of appearance and behaviors. The nurse enhances the client's feelings of being understood through the use of active listening skills. Remember that the client's perspective is important because it determines what the client views as problems, as well as how the client will respond to perceived problems. For example, the nurse may believe that the client's major problem is the experience of hallucinations, while the client may be focusing on his or her current living situation as the primary problem. Schofield (1998) suggests using an empowerment education approach that shifts focus from the client's illness to health, and from the nurse's perspective to the client's perspective. The **Empowerment Model of Recovery** describes mental illness as a combination of severe emotional distress and an interruption of a person's place in the community and social role. The model emphasizes that emotional distress is a temporary disruption in life (White, 2005). Utilizing this approach, the nurse focuses on the client's priorities and goals to promote empowerment.

National Empowerment Center. The National Empowerment Center, Inc. (NEC), is a consumer/survivor/ex-patient–run organization that communicates a message of recovery, empowerment, hope, and healing to people who have been labeled with mental illness. Members of the organization believe that recovery and empowerment are not the privilege of a few, but rather are possible for each person diagnosed with a mental illness whether on the back ward of a state mental institution or working as an executive in a corporation. NEC has a toll-free information and referral line (800-769-3728) to provide information to mental

health consumers. The organization keeps updated lists of consumer-run organizations and advocacy groups (eg, independent living centers, disability rights groups) in all 50 states (NEC, 2005).

Employing the Psychosocial Rehabilitation Approach

The psychosocial rehabilitation approach is appropriate for settings such as the mental health center, partial hospitalization unit, and outpatient programs. One of the most hopeful aspects of a psychosocial rehabilitation approach is the use of the Clubhouse program to provide continued social support and meaningful pre-vocational training.

The **Clubhouse program** is a voluntary, participatory group of clients who work together to secure and sustain employment, locate and maintain appropriate housing, and participate in recreational and social activities. The nurse uses elements of this approach by teaching the client social skills, such as how to introduce oneself to another, how to ask for assistance in a store, and how to talk to someone in a social setting. The nurse also teaches the client the skills necessary for independent living, such as housekeeping, shopping, and cooking. Basic employment-skills training is another part of psychosocial rehabilitation appropriate for the client who desires a job (Delaney, 1998).

Using the Assertive Community Treatment (ACT) Model

The **Assertive Community Treatment (ACT) model** is a team treatment approach designed to provide comprehensive, community-based psychiatric treatment, rehabilitation, and support to persons with SPMI who often have coexisting problems (eg, homelessness or substance abuse) or are involved with the judicial system (see Chapter 8). It is an evidence-based practice that evolved in the late 1960s and has been implemented in more than 30 U.S. cities as well as in other countries including Australia, Sweden, Canada, England, and the United Kingdom. The Department of Veterans Affairs has also implemented ACT. Services, which include initial and ongoing assessments and psychiatric–mental health care, are available 24 hours a day, 365 days a year (Assertive Community Treatment Association, 2003). Box 35–1 describes the basic principles of ACT. Despite the efficacy of ACT, the demand for such services far outpaces the supply. The National Institute of Mental Health estimates that on any given day in any given year, 40% of the 2.3 million American adults with bipolar disorder and 2.2 million with schizophrenia do not get treatment for their conditions (Mahoney, 2005).

Providing Continuum of Care

The psychiatric–mental health nurse works as a team member in planning continued treatment for the client with SPMI. Coordination of services, including the social services necessary for community living and continued psychotherapeutic support, is important. Team treatment meetings and communication with assigned case managers enhances client support on an ongoing basis. Clients are urged to remain in the Clubhouse program because it emphasizes wellness and health and can reduce recidivism in clients with SPMI.

A pilot program by Unity Health System in Rochester, NY, provides continuum of care for homeless clients. The **Integrated Model Program (IMPACT)**, based on Assertive Community Treatment, is funded by a 3-year, $1.6 million grant from the Substance Abuse and Mental Health Services Administration (SAMHSA). It allows clients to have access to whatever level of treatment they need (eg, day treatment, partial hospitalization, outpatient care). The goal of the program is to reduce clients' hospital admissions and criminal involvement, improve their quality of life, and prepare them to become employed (Frieden, 2004).

Respite care for the homeless is another form of continuum of care that is currently available for clients with SPMI. The homeless medical respite unit is a unique form of care offering recuperative services for clients who are too sick to be on the street or in shelters, but who are not sick enough to need acute inpatient beds. A 90-bed respite center in Boston tends to the medical and psychosocial needs of homeless clients. It provides nursing, dental, and psychiatric care; physical rehabilitation; assistance in applying for benefits; and referrals to other services. There are currently 30 respite care centers within the United States (Walsh, 2004).

Not all programs that provide continuum of care are government funded. For example, **Welcome Home Ministries** (WHM) is a voluntary organization started by a nurse who received her master's degree in theology and became an ordained minister. The program is briefly described in the next section.

Welcome Home Ministries (WHM). Recognizing that the transition from life in correctional facilities to life on the outside can be difficult for a woman, WHM, a faith-based community program in California, supports women who have recently been released from prison (see Chapter 8). Most of the clients are white women older than 30 years who have less than a high school education, have been addicted to drugs for more than 10 years, and are estranged from their families. Clients are supported as they maintain drug recovery, find a safe place to stay, complete probation, complete their education, find a job, and resume relationships with their families (Parsons & Warner-Robbins, 2002). Not all clients who are recipients of

---

BOX 35.1 BASIC PRINCIPLES OF THE ASSERTIVE COMMUNITY TREATMENT (ACT) MODEL

- The ACT multidisciplinary team, which includes a psychiatrist and mental health nurse, serves as the client's primary care provider.
- Services are provided in a variety of community settings such as the client's home, parks, local restaurants, or nearby stores.
- Treatment plans, which are modified as needed, are developed with input by the client and are based on individualized needs and strengths, hopes and desires.
- Team members utilize a proactive approach, assisting clients to participate in and continue treatment so that they may live independently and recover from disability.
- Services are long-term (ie, many years), due to impairments associated with serious and persistent mental illness.
- Clients are encouraged to participate in community employment and vocational rehabilitation.
- Substance-abuse services are provided by the team as needed.
- Psychoeducational services are provided to teach clients about mental illness and the skills needed to improve their illnesses and lives.
- Family support and education are provided with active involvement by the client.
- The team promotes client participation in community activities and membership in organizations of the client's choice.
- Accessibility to health care services and health education is provided.

SOURCE: Assertive Community Treatment Association. (2003). *Act model.* Retrieved December 16, 2003, from http://www.actassociation.org/actModel/

continuum of care in programs such as ACT or WHM have success stories.

Concerns About Continuum of Care for Homeless Clients.
Virtually every homeless person with SPMI has had prior experience with the mental health service delivery system. The complex problems of this population also illustrate the importance of providing additional services to augment psychiatric–mental health treatment. These services include targeting and improving physical health status, locating housing, and providing appropriate services so that individuals with mental illness can maintain their housing (ODPHP, 1998). Providing these services is costly and often results in fragmentation. Goldman (2000) describes fragmentation in the community-support movement for clients with SPMI. Studies on issues such as employment, income support, transportation, and housing, which have been included with treatment, have revealed fragmentation of the system of services needed. A lack of adequate resources that are comprehensive and coordinated continues to be a major issue in the treatment of clients with SPMI.

Concerns About Continuum of Care for Incarcerated Clients.
Discharge planning and follow-up (ie, continuum of care) are the key components of correctional-facility psychiatric–mental health programs, although they are the weakest elements of programs nationwide. Released offenders have a variety of service needs that must be addressed. Case management that begins in the correctional facility and continues into the community can provide continuing contact between community-treatment staff and criminal-justice staff. Linkage should be made to the following programs if continuum of care is to occur:

- Entitlement to Supplemental Security Income (SSI) and Medicaid
- Money management and representative payee programs
- Mental health treatment, including that for dual diagnosis if present
- Psychosocial rehabilitation
- Housing
- Medical care (Watson et al., 2001)

Concerns About Managed Care.
The managed-care system was founded in the 1990s, with the primary motive of reducing expenditures by withholding services that are considered unnecessary and substituting less expensive services (Parron, 1999). Managed care requires using less costly alternative treatments whenever possible. Therefore, brief sessions of psychotherapy have replaced the former, lengthy model of psychotherapeutic sessions. Psychotropic drugs are ordered as a first choice.

The shorter length of stays in acute care facilities and the reliance on medication as the first, and sometimes only, treatment can be problematic. Hospitalization provides a stopgap-type approach to the problem of SPMI. The client is admitted during an acute psychotic episode and, in many cases, the episode is related to the fact that the client has not used prescribed medication or followed the prescription for continued treatment given at the previous inpatient admission. For many clients with SPMI, acceptance of the illness and of the need to take medication is difficult; therefore, noncompliance is common. For other clients, the unpleasant adverse effects of neuroleptic or atypical antipsychotic medications contribute to refusal to continue taking them. One study suggests that noncompliance with neuroleptic or atypical antipsychotic medications accounts for at least 40% of all rehospitalizations and at least 33% of all acute care inpatient costs for people with SPMI (Friedrich, Lively, & Buckwalter, 1999).

Educating the Family

The nurse provides assistance to families coping with a member having SPMI by using a psychoeducational approach. After assessing the family's areas of concern, the nurse teaches them about the illness, symptom management, use of medications, and measures to enhance the client's medication compliance. The nurse also encourages the family members to use support groups such as NAMI. The family members are encouraged to maintain normal daily activities and to participate in social and recreational activities that are pleasurable.

EVALUATION

The nurse evaluates the outcomes of client care and the degree to which established goals have been met. For clients with SPMI, care is ongoing and includes the provision of support necessary for community living. Recurrence of symptoms is common. When services are coordinated and comprehensive, the client may receive support to avoid hospitalization and maintain community housing and support systems. See Nursing Plan of Care 35-1: The Client With Serious and Persistent Mental Illness.

THE CLIENT WITH SERIOUS AND PERSISTENT MENTAL ILLNESS

DM is a 24-year-old unemployed single female who was readmitted to the psychiatric inpatient unit following a suicide attempt in which she had taken an overdose of prescribed psychotropic medications along with alcohol. Shortly after taking the pills and alcohol, she called 911 and asked for help. She spent 2 days in the medical–surgical unit and was transferred to the psychiatric unit when medically stable.

Upon her admission, the nurse notes a flat affect, drooping eyelids, uncombed and greasy hair, and a general disheveled appearance with poorly fitting, unkempt clothing. DM's voice is a monotone and she answers questions in a brief manner.

According to chart data, DM lives in a rent-subsidized apartment by herself. She had been homeless for the first 3 months of this current year. This was her 19th psychiatric admission, with the first admission occurring when she was 9 years old. Past history reveals that her father and older brothers physically and sexually abused her and that she lived in a series of foster homes and group homes from the ages of 10 to 18. She also has a history of drinking alcohol and smoking pot, beginning at age 9. During adolescence, she abused cocaine and heroin and resorted to prostitution to obtain money for drugs. She has been noncompliant with past treatment recommendations, including outpatient treatment and psychotropic medications.

DSM–IV–TR DIAGNOSIS: Schizoaffective disorder, depressive type: Posttraumatic stress disorder; Alcohol abuse; Cannabis abuse

ASSESSMENT: Personal strengths: Has some insight as evidenced by verbalizing, "I know I need to stay on the medications and continue in counseling in order to get better." Recognizes factors leading to readmission: stopping medications, experiencing flashbacks related to abuse history, and isolating herself in her apartment. Has a GED and has taken several college courses. Likes to write in a journal and also writes poetry. Has a good singing voice and has been in a church choir in the past

Weaknesses: Expresses self-hatred stating, "I know I'm worthless and no good. I can't stay out of the hospital or live on my own." Lacks a support system, identifying only a case manager as her primary support person. Verbalizes little motivation to stop using alcohol and drugs and has been unable to obtain and keep a job

---

NURSING DIAGNOSIS: Risk for Self-Directed Violence related to persistence of suicidal thoughts

OUTCOME: The client will remain safe in the hospital environment, verbalizing an absence of suicidal thoughts.

Planning/Implementation	Rationale
Implement suicidal precautions, establishing one-to-one supervision.	DM needs constant supervision and limitation of opportunities to harm herself.
Encourage DM to sign a "no self-harm" contract.	Signing a contract may lower DM's risk of suicide and enable her to attend activities.
Encourage DM to write thoughts and feelings in a journal sharing this with the nurse–therapist and doctor.	Writing thoughts and feelings enables DM to externalize her feelings.

(Continued on following page)

NURSING DIAGNOSIS: Chronic Low Self-Esteem related to past history of abuse and feelings of shame and guilt about her inability to stay out of the hospital

OUTCOME: DM will verbalize at least three personal strengths within the next 3 days.

Planning/Implementation	Rationale
Use active listening skills in assisting DM to talk about issues of concern related to past history.	Discussing her feelings can help DM to identify, accept, and work through her feelings even if they are painful or otherwise uncomfortable.
Help DM identify positive aspects about herself.	DM's feeling of low-self esteem are real to her. Positive feedback presents a different viewpoint that DM can begin to integrate into her thoughts.

NURSING DIAGNOSIS: Ineffective Coping related to reliance on abusive substances when feeling overwhelmed by problems

OUTCOME: DM will select the location and times for attending AA meetings upon discharge.

Planning/Implementation	Rationale
Help DM identify reasons to stop use of alcohol and drugs.	DM may recognize the relatedness of ineffective coping and problematic behavior.
Provide DM with literature about AA.	DM may not understand the dynamics of AA.
Encourage DM to verbally commit to attending an AA meeting the same day she is discharged.	Problems for clients who have dual diagnosis are often complicated and require ongoing community support.

NURSING DIAGNOSIS: Social Isolation related to withdrawal from others when feeling depressed.

OUTCOME: The client will actively participate in group therapies and community meetings during hospitalization.

Planning/Implementation	Rationale
Teach DM social skills.	DM may have little or no knowledge of social interaction skills.
Discuss with the client the benefits of interacting with others.	Interacting with DM and providing feedback provides a concrete example of the benefits of interacting for DM.

NURSING DIAGNOSIS: Risk for Noncompliance with outpatient treatment/medication recommendations related to past history.

OUTCOME: DM will sign a behavioral agreement to follow recommendations for outpatient treatment and prescribed psychotropic medications.

Planning/Implementation	Rationale
Discuss with DM past history of noncompliance, identifying factors related to noncompliance.	DM may have inadequate or incomplete information about appropriate treatment for her diagnosis.
Review DM's knowledge of prescribed psychotropic medication.	DM may be more likely to conform if she feels fully informed about the reason for medication.
Identify any adverse effects experienced by DM when taking medication.	DM may be noncompliant because of adverse effects of prescribed medication.
Help DM write a specific behavioral contract identifying outpatient treatment recommendations.	Writing a specific behavioral contact is an effective method of minimizing treatment noncompliance.

EVALUATION: Evaluation focuses on the achievement of the specified outcomes. The nurse provides specific data, indicating that the client has achieved the outcomes and identifying the effect of the nursing implementations. In this case the client remained safe in the hospital environment and reported an absence of thoughts of suicide. The client identified three positive areas of strength, including the use of a journal to identify feelings, willingness to participate in the treatment plans, and concern for other clients on the psychiatric unit. During inpatient treatment, the client attended an AA meeting and was able to commit to attending a meeting in her community on the day of discharge. The client participated in all group therapies on the unit and wrote a specific behavioral contract agreeing to participate in an outpatient treatment program.

Data for this care plan were adapted from an unpublished paper (Fall, 2000) by Patricia Catalogna, Student Nurse from Luzerne County Community College.

KEY CONCEPTS

◆ Statistics indicate that four of the ten leading causes of disability globally are major depression, bipolar disorder, schizophrenia, and substance-related disorders. Each year, approximately 23% of American adults are diagnosed with a mental disorder, and 5.4% of these adults are said to be seriously and persistently mentally ill.

◆ People with serious and persistent mental illness (SPMI) have disabling symptoms that significantly impair functioning over their lifetime.

◆ Deinstitutionalization, transinstitutionalization, and lack of community services contribute to the current problems and issues of the seriously and persistently mentally ill.

◆ Categories of seriously and persistently mentally ill clients who provide challenges to the psychiatric–mental health nurse include nursing-home residents, the homeless, and the incarcerated.

◆ Factors contributing to homelessness of the SPMI population include the presence of positive symptoms of schizophrenia, concurrent drug or alcohol abuse, the presence of a personality disorder, and lack of family support. In addition, the problems associated with homelessness can have special consequences in regard to the age and gender of the individual affected, such as children, women, and the elderly.

◆ Clients with the diagnosis of impulse control disorder, sexual disorder, substance-related disorder, bipolar disorder, and personality disorder are at risk for incarceration.

◆ Suicide is the leading cause of death in correctional facilities. Most suicides in correctional facilities occur in the mentally ill population.

◆ Settings in which the nurse may assess clients with SPMI include the hospital, long-term care facility, jail or prison, homeless shelter, or clinic.

◆ Assessment of the client with SPMI focuses on current clinical symptoms, self-care abilities, current living situation, coping skills and support systems, medication compliance, and the presence of substance abuse.

◆ Nursing diagnoses are multiple, and priorities are established on the basis of the client's physical health status, potential for harm to self or others, current symptomatic behaviors, self-care abilities, coping skills, and available support systems.

◆ Outcomes focus on maintaining client safety, establishing and maintaining self-care, establishing trust and interaction with staff and others, decreasing symptomatic behaviors, increasing self-esteem, and maintaining medication compliance.

◆ Implementation focuses on providing a safe environment, promoting physical health, providing medication management and education, using cognitive–behavioral therapy including orienting to reality, promoting self-care, enhancing self-esteem, and providing support by using approaches such as the psychosocial rehabilitation approach or the ACT model, providing continuum of care, and educating the family.

◆ Coordination of services, team treatment meetings, and communication with assigned case managers enhance client support during continuum of care. Clients are urged to continue in programs that emphasize wellness and health to reduce recidivism.

◆ The nurse uses a psychoeducational approach to assist families coping with a member having SPMI.

◆ Lack of adequate resources that are comprehensive and coordinated continues to be a major issue in the treatment of homeless clients. Discharge planning and continuum of care are the weakest elements of correctional-facility mental health programs.

◆ The impact of managed care on the continuum of care includes brief treatments, shortened hospital stays, and reliance on medications to control symptoms.

For additional study materials, please refer to the Student Resource CD-ROM located in the back of this textbook.

CHAPTER WORKSHEET

CRITICAL THINKING QUESTIONS

1. Interview several clients with multiple rehospitalizations in psychiatric–mental health inpatient care and ask about factors related to readmission. Identify common factors that clients discuss. How could you use these data in preventing readmission of these clients?

2. What topics would you include in an educational program for families of clients experiencing SPMI?
3. What services are available in your community for clients with SPMI?
4. Construct a nursing plan of care for a client with a diagnosis of schizophrenia, undifferentiated type, who has persistent hallucinations and is currently homeless. What are the priority nursing diagnoses and realistic outcomes for this client? How could the nurse establish a therapeutic relationship with this client?

REFLECTION

The chapter opening quotes include statistics that indicate the need for psychiatric–mental health nurses to provide care for the seriously and persistently mentally ill, homeless, or incarcerated clients. Reflect on your psychiatric nursing curriculum. Most curriculums address the issues of chronic mental illness, but may not address psychosocial needs of the homeless or incarcerated client. Are the psychosocial needs of these clients included in the curriculum? If not, determine why. If they are addressed, are the nursing interventions realistic? Explain your answers.

NCLEX-STYLE QUESTIONS

1. The nurse identifies which factor as being most related to an increased risk of homelessness in a client with a history of serious and persistent mental illness?
   a. Lack of family involvement
   b. History of physical illness
   c. Poor hygiene
   d. Lack of education

2. The nurse uses which of the following interventions to establish rapport and provide support for the client with serious and persistent mental illness?
   a. Teaching social skills
   b. Providing cognitive restructuring
   c. Listening to client's story
   d. Establishing reality contact

3. A client tells the nurse about hearing voices for many years, telling him that he is worthless.

Which action by the nurse would be most effective?

a. Directing the client to tell the voices he hears to go away

b. Listening carefully to the message of the voices

c. Telling the client that the voices are only his imagination

d. Exploring with the client the origin of the voices

4. Which assessment finding would be most important for a client with a severe and persistent mental illness who is incarcerated?

a. Physical illness

b. Hallucinations and delusions

c. Suicidal thoughts

d. Aggressive tendencies

5. The nurse assists the client with a serious and persistent mental illness to take a shower and change clothes on the basis of which rationale?

a. It is easier for the nurse to provide care rather than wait for the client to initiate it.

b. The nurse's assistance positively reinforces the client to maintain personal hygiene.

c. The client will feel better if hygiene needs are met.

d. The client will be offensive to peers if not clean.

6. Which of the following would the nurse identify as an impulse control disorder? Select all that apply.

a. Kleptomania

b. Antisocial personality

c. Pathological gambling

d. Pyromania

e. Intermittent explosive disorder

f. Bipolar disorder

Selected References

Alexander, M. (1999). An analysis of sex offender studies: Sexual abuse. *Journal of Research and Treatment, 11*(2).

American Psychiatric Association. (2000). *Diagnostic and statistical manual of mental disorders* (4th ed., text revision). Washington, DC: Author.

Assertive Community Treatment Association. (2003). ACT model. Retrieved December 16, 2003, from http://www.actassociation.org/actModel/

Begley, S. (2002, March). The schizophrenic mind. *Newsweek,* 44–51.

Blair, D.T. (1996). Integration and synthesis: Cognitive–behavioral therapies within the biological paradigm. *Journal of Psychosocial Nursing and Mental Health Services, 34*(12), 26–30.

Bureau of Justice Statistics. (2001). Mental health treatment in state prisons, 2000. Retrieved December 16, 2003, from http://www.ojp.usdoj.gov/bjs/pub/pdf/mhtsp00.pdf

Butterfield, F. (2003, October). Study finds hundreds of thousands of inmates mentally ill. Retrieved April 9, 2006, from http://www.nytimes.com

Caton, C. M., & Shront, P. E. (1994). Risk factors for homelessness among schizophrenic men: A case-control study. *American Journal of Public Health, 84,* 265–270.

Christensen, R. (2005). Homeless, not hopeless: 4 strategies for successful interventions. *Current Psychiatry, 4*(6), 94.

Clinical Psychiatry News. (2001). Data watch: Top primary diagnoses at admission for nursing home residents. *Clinical Psychiatry News, 29*(4), 45.

Cohen, C. (2001). Schizophrenia and the aging population. *Psychiatric Times, 18*(12), 37–40.

Danesh, F. S. (2002). Serious mental disorder in 23,000 prisoners: A systematic review of 62 surveys. *Lancet, 359*(9306), 545–550.

Delaney, C. (1998). Reducing recidivism: Medication versus psychosocial rehabilitation. *Journal of Psychosocial Nursing and Mental Health Services, 36*(11), 28–32.

Delaney, K. R., Rogers-Pitula, C., & Perraud, S. (2000). Psychiatric hospitalization and process description: What will nursing add? *Journal of Psychosocial Nursing and Mental Health Services, 38*(3), 7–13.

DeMallie, D.A., North, M. D., & Smith, E. M. (1997). Psychiatric disorders among the homeless: A comparison of older and younger groups. *The Gerontologist, 37*(1), 61–66.

Farnam, C. R., Zipple, A. M., Tyrell, W., & Chittinanda, D. (1999). Health status risk factors of people with severe and persistent mental illness. *Journal of Psychosocial Nursing and Mental Health Services, 37*(6), 16–21.

Finnell, D. S. (2005). Promote medication adherence, one stage at a time. *Current Psychiatry, 4*(8), 88.

Frieden, J. (2004). Hospital program targets homeless. *Clinical Psychiatry News, 32*(6), 1, 57.

Friedrich, R. M., Lively, S., & Buckwalter, K. C. (1999). Well siblings: Living with schizophrenia: Impact of associated behaviors. *Journal of Psychosocial Nursing and Mental Health Services, 37*(8), 11–19.

Goldman, H. (2000, February/March). The program on chronic mental illness. *Perspectives: A Mental Health Magazine.* Retrieved May 10, 2001, from http://www.mentalhelp.net/poc/view_index.php

Hayes, L. M. (1995). *Prison suicide: An overview and guide to prevention.* Washington, DC: U.S. Justice Department, National Institute of Corrections.

Kravitz, H. M., & Silberberg, J. M. (2001). Correctional psychiatry: Effective and safe linkage of mentally ill offenders. *Psychiatric Annals, 31*(7), 405–406.

MacNeil, J. S. (2001). Mentally ill still dumped into nursing homes. *CNS News, 3*(4), 1, 14.

Mahoney, D. (2004). Addressing the needs of juvenile offenders. *Clinical Psychiatry News, 32*(10), 53.

Mahoney, D. (2005). Assertive community treatment. *Clinical Psychiatry News, 33*(7), 46.

Malhotra, H. K. (2006). Tips to cope with hallucinations. *NeuroPsychiatry Reviews, 7*(20), 10.

McEwen, T. (1995). *National assessment program: 1994 survey results* (NIJ Publication No. 150856, pp. 67-68). Washington, DC: National Institute of Justice.

Medscape Resource Center. (2004). Management of serious mental illness. Retrieved April 2, 2004, from http://www.medscape.com/pages/editorial/resourcecenters

National Coalition for the Homeless. (2005a, June). How many people experience homelessness? NCH fact sheet #2. Retrieved April 3, 2006, from http://www.nationalhomeless.org/numbers.html

National Coalition for the Homeless. (2005b, July). Mental illness and homelessness. NCH fact sheet #5. Retrieved April 3, 2006, from http://nationalhomeless.org/factmentalillnessandhomelessness.html

National Coalition for the Homeless. (2005c, June). Who is homeless? NCH fact sheet #3. Retrieved April 3, 2006, from http://nationalhomeless.org/factwhoishomeless.html

National Empowerment Center, Inc. (2005). Programs and services. Retrieved January 31, 2005, from http://www.power2u.org/what.html

National Coalition for the Homeless. (2006, January). Hate crimes and violence against people experiencing homelessness: NCH fact sheet #21. Retrieved April 3, 2006, from http://www.nationalhomeless.org/facthatecrimes.html

Office of Disease Prevention and Health Promotion. (1998). Healthy People 2010 objectives: Draft for public comment. Mental health and mental disorders. Retrieved October 23, 2000, from http://www.health.gov/hpcomments/2010Draft/pdf/mental.pdf

Parron, C. (1999). Caring under managed care: The effect of case management on state psychiatric clients. *Journal of Psychosocial Nursing and Mental Health Services, 37*(10), 16-21.

Parsons, M. L., & Warner-Robbins, C. (2002). Holistic nursing on the front lines. *American Journal of Nursing, 102*(6), 73-77.

Psychology Information Online. (2003). *Impulse control disorders.* Retrieved December 16, 2003, from http://www.psychologyinfo.com/problems/impulse_control.html

Sadock, B. J., & Sadock, V. A. (2003). *Kaplan & Sadock's synopsis of psychiatry: Behavioral sciences/clinical psychiatry* (9th ed.). Philadelphia: Lippincott Williams & Wilkins.

Saunders, J. (1997). Walking a mile in their shoes: Symbolic interactionism for families living with severe mental illness. *Journal of Psychosocial Nursing and Mental Health Services, 35*(6), 8-13.

Schofield, R. (1998). Empowerment education for individuals with serious mental illness. *Journal of Psychosocial Nursing and Mental Health Services, 36*(11), 35-40.

Sherman, C. (2001). Inpatient today, inmate tomorrow. *Clinical Psychiatry News, 29*(12), 1-2.

Silberberg, J. M., Vital, T. L., & Brakel, S. J. (2001). Breaking down barriers to mandated outpatient treatment for mentally ill offenders. *Psychiatric Annals, 31*(7), 433-440.

Smoyak, S. (2000). The history, economics, and financing of mental health care. Part 3: The present. *Journal of Psychosocial Nursing and Mental Health Services, 38*(11), 32-38.

Spollen, J. M. (2003). Perspectives in serious mental illness. *Medscape Psychiatry & Mental Health, 8*(1). Retrieved August 16, 2003, from http://www.medscape.com/viewarticle/455499_print

Torrey, E. F., & Zdandowicz, M. T. (1999, July). Deinstitutionalization hasn't worked. *Washington Post.*

Treatment Advocacy Center. (2003). Fact sheet: Criminalization of Americans with severe mental illnesses. Retrieved December 16, 2003, from http://www.psychlaws.org/GeneralResources/Fact3.htm

United States Department of Health and Human Services. (1999). *Mental health: A report of the Surgeon General.* Washington, DC: DHHS, Substance Abuse and Mental Health Services Administration, Center for Mental Health Services, NIH, NIMH.

United States Department of Housing and Urban Development. (2002). Homeless assistance. Retrieved December 16, 2003, from http://www.hud.gov/offices/cpd/homeless/index.cfm

Walsh, N. (2004). Homeless respite care may cut risk of hospital readmission. *Clinical Psychiatry News, 32*(4), 112.

Watson, A., Hanrahan, P., Luchins, D., & Lurigio, A. (2001). Paths to jail among mentally ill persons: Service needs and service characteristics. *Psychiatric Annals, 31*(7), 421-429.

Wendling, P. (2006). Misdiagnosis common at readmission. *Clinical Psychiatry News, 34*(5), 2.

White, R. (2005). An empowerment model of recovery from severe mental illness: An expert interview with Daniel B. Fisher, MD, PhD. Retrieved January 31, 2005, from http://www.medscape.com/viewarticle/496394

Yurkovich, E., Smyer, T., & Dean, L. (2000). Health maintenance behaviors of individuals with severe and persistent mental illness in a state prison. *Journal of Psychosocial Nursing and Mental Health Services, 38*(6), 21-31.

Suggested Readings

Frankenburg, F. R. (2006). It's not easy being emperor. *Current Psychiatry, 5*(5), 73-76, 79-80.

Evans, J. (2004). For women, gambling turns pathological faster. *Clinical Psychiatry News, 32*(8), 47.

Keefe, S. (2006). Understanding human behavior. Emphasis on recovery and patient empowerment has forever changed the psychiatric nursing landscape. *ADVANCE for Nurses, 7*(5), 29–30, 38.

Leard-Hansson, J., & Guttmacher, L. (2005). Substance abuse and SPMI patients. *Clinical Psychiatry News, 33*(1), 31.

McQuistion, H. L., Goisman, R. M., & Tennison, C. R. (2000). Psychosocial rehabilitation: Issues and answers for psychiatry. Retrieved October 23, 2000, from http://www.comm. psych.pitt.edu/finds/psychosocial.html

Mahoney, D. (2006). Addressing homelessness and substance abuse. *Clinical Psychiatry News, 34*(3), 56.

Mullin, K. A., & Ambrosia, T. (2005). Role of the nurse practitioner in providing health care for the homeless. *American Journal for Nurse Practitioners, 9*(9), 37–40, 43–44.

Roche, T. (2000, July 10). The chief and his ward: When the mentally ill have no place to go, they go to jail. *Time, 156*(19), 82–84.

Splete, H. (2004). Serious mental disorders not getting treated. *Clinical Psychiatry News, 32*(7), 82.

Note: Page numbers followed by the letter *b* refer to boxed material. Page numbers followed by the letter *f* refer to figures; those followed by the letter *t* refer to tables.